Atlas *of* NEURORANATOMY

Atlas *of* NEUROANATOMY

With Systems Organization and Case Correlations

Joseph J. Warner, M.D.

Assistant Professor of Neuroscience, Department of Neuroscience and University of Florida Brain Institute; University of Florida College of Medicine, Gainesville; Consulting Neurologist, Lake City Medical Center, Lake City, Florida; Private Practice, Neurological Sciences Center, Lake City, Florida

Foreword by

Martin A. Samuels, M.D.

Professor of Neurology, Harvard Medical School, Boston; Neurologist-in-Chief, Brigham and Women's Hospital, Boston

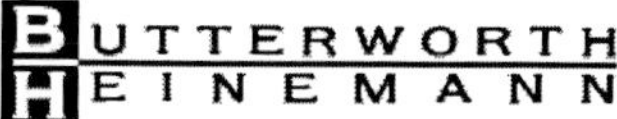

Boston • Oxford • Auckland • Johannesburg • Melbourne • New Delhi

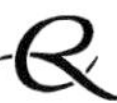 member of the Reed Elsevier group

Every effort has been made to ensure that the drug dosage schedules within this text are accurate and conform to standards accepted at time of publication. However, as treatment recommendations vary in the light of continuing research and clinical experience, the reader is advised to verify drug dosage schedules herein with information found on product information sheets. This is especially true in cases of new or infrequently used drugs.

 Recognizing the importance of preserving what has been written, Butterworth–Heinemann prints its books on acid-free paper whenever possible.

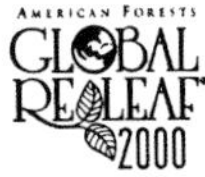

Butterworth–Heinemann supports the efforts of American Forests and the Global ReLeaf program in its campaign for the betterment of trees, forests, and our environment.

Library of Congress Cataloging-in-Publication Data

Warner, Joseph J.
Atlas of neuroanatomy : with systems organization and case correlations / Joseph J. Warner ; foreword by Martin A. Samuels.
p. ; cm.
Includes index.
ISBN 0-7506-7250-1 (alk. paper)
1. Neuroanatomy—Atlases. I. Title.
[DNLM: 1. Central Nervous System—anatomy & histology—Atlases. 2. Central Nervous System Diseases—physiopathology—Atlases. WL 17 W282a 2000]
QM451 .W35 2000
611'.8'0222—dc21 00-023285

British Library Cataloguing-in-Publication Data
A catalogue record for this book is available from the British Library.

The publisher offers special discounts on bulk orders of this book.
For information, please contact:
Manager of Special Sales
Butterworth–Heinemann
225 Wildwood Avenue
Woburn, MA 01801-2041
Tel: 781-904-2500
Fax: 781-904-2620

For information on all Butterworth–Heinemann publications available, contact our World Wide Web home page at: http://www.bh.com

10 9 8 7 6 5 4 3 2 1

Printed in the United States of America

This book is dedicated to Lieutenant Commander Terry G. Briggs, U.S. Navy (Retired). His contribution to this work has included the illumination of an important perspective of the study of neuroanatomy and pathophysiology.

As "state-of-the-art" basic science and clinical research in the neurological sciences has advanced into the twenty-first century, new applications in terms of diagnostic and therapeutic intervention have revolutionized patient care. A wide spectrum of research, from molecular biology through higher neural function, has resulted in the elucidation of many aspects of neuroanatomy, neurophysiology, and neuropathology with a major impact on neurology, neurosurgery, psychiatry, and related clinical disciplines. Given the rapid pace of these developments, it is imperative that we not lose sight of the primary objective for these endeavors, the individual patient.

Professionals who embark upon scientific and clinical studies must understand the significance of this dedication.

My own background in neurology has included studies of the nervous system from basic science and clinical perspectives, ranging from feline research paradigms combining stereotactic neurosurgery, electrophysiology, and cytoarchitectonic analysis, to studies of behavioral neurology, human neuroanatomy, histopathology, and systems organization. As a neurologist, I have emphasized neuroanatomic and pathophysiologic correlations in case analysis, reflective of a vertically integrated approach to the study of the human nervous system.

No length of experience in research or patient care fully prepares a professional for the occurrence of a neurologically devastating illness in an individual as close as a family member. Approximately nine months prior to the completion of this book, the apparently indiscriminate nature by which serious neurologic illness could strike declared itself. No longer was the illness simply a "diagnostic entity" nor was Terry Briggs a "case" with applicable statistics for survival over time. This was a human being with a unique personality, an individual with a strength of character in the face of severe adversity who served as an inspiration to those around him. I vividly recall a statement he had made to me after he knew of his diagnosis. With a serious demeanor, he calmly stated, "my future is history." Despite knowledge of the available statistics for his survival over time, he maintained his faith, determination, and his sense of humor, providing strength for himself and for those around him. During a discussion we had with reference to his latest MRI, he wryly commented, "I guess the tumor is stable, but I'm not so sure about the character who's got it."

Terry Briggs has consented for the inclusion of his case in this book so that others may benefit from its study. I believe that his contribution is far greater than that of providing his own case for analysis. We, as professionals, must remember that every "case" is unique. Patients should not be considered as diagnostic entities or as statistics. The diagnostic and therapeutic approach should be individualized for each patient. The philosophy of Dr. Norman Geschwind would well be remembered in this context: that each patient should be studied thoroughly, each patient provides a unique opportunity for the advancement of our professional knowledge, and each patient should be considered as a human being, deserving of compassion and the best care we can provide.

CONTENTS

FOREWORD

Clinical neurology differs from other medical fields in that it depends to an enormous extent on the localization of disease processes. Classic history taking, the traditional neurological examination, and modern imaging techniques all depend for their validity on the clinician's ability to understand structural and functional neuroanatomy.

Joseph Warner's *Atlas of Neuroanatomy* is the most important contribution to the teaching of relevant neuroanatomy in recent memory. Dr. Warner, a neurologist, has spent his entire career fastidiously collecting and personally preparing pathologic specimens that are aimed at elucidating the whole panoply of normal and pathological anatomy. The dissections are magnificent, photographed beautifully and labeled with precision and clarity. Major areas, such as the motor system, eye movement control pathways, and vestibular anatomy contain drawings of the functional connections, richly illustrated with beautifully analyzed case histories, imaging studies, and relevant neurochemical pathways, such as those for norepinephrine, dopamine, and serotonin.

Dr. Warner's training and practice as a neurologist are reflected in the authentic nature of the clinical problems, the solutions to which only yield to a detailed understanding of the neuroanatomy. Above and beyond the academic usefulness of the Atlas, the beauty of the diagrams and photographs—all created by Dr. Warner himself—is truly a tour de force, reflecting his lifelong love affair with the nervous system.

Dr. Warner's *Atlas of Neuroanatomy* will be the new gold standard against which future works will be judged. It will become a classic that will be found on the bookshelves of all serious neurologists, neurosurgeons, psychiatrists, neuroscientists, neuroradiologists, neuropathologists, and students of neuroanatomy. All of us who value the art and science of neurological medicine welcome this remarkable one-man work as a main contribution to our field.

Martin A. Samuels, M.D.

PREFACE

The selection of clinical, pathologic, and neuroimaging cases for teaching and research purposes began during my residency and clinical fellowship in Neurology at Harvard Medical School. With the encouragement and cooperation of Dr. Win Schoene and Dr. James Morris of the Division of Neuropathology at the Brigham and Women's Hospital, Harvard Medical School, I completed several neuropathologic case analyses. I personally executed all phases of this process for each case, from the resection of neural tissues at autopsy through dissection, photography, and neurohistologic slide preparation and photomicroscopy. Clinical records along with any available neuroradiologic studies were obtained for correlation. This work provided the opportunity for the study and documentation of normal as well as neuropathologic cases in conjunction with detailed clinical data. Thorough neurologic evaluation in the context of a major emphasis on principles of neuroanatomy and pathophysiology was also encouraged throughout my residency by several of the Harvard neurology faculty, including Drs. Martin A. Samuels, David Dawson, Michael Ronthal, and Norman Geschwind. Through numerous discussions, conferences, and other interactions with Dr. Geschwind, my special clinical interest in behavioral neurology continued to grow in conjunction with detailed neuroanatomic and physiologic study.

Upon completion of my residency and clinical fellowship in Neurology at Harvard Medical School, I joined the faculty of the University of Florida College of Medicine with a joint appointment in the Departments of Neurology and Neuroscience. My work with neuroanatomy, systems physiology, and neuropathology (in conjunction with basic science research and clinical case investigations) has continued for the past eighteen years. A major factor that stimulated the development of the *Atlas of Neuroanatomy* was my teaching of graduate students, medical students, and residents in neuroscience and neurology. Medical Neuroscience, given by the Department of Neuroscience at the University of Florida College of Medicine, is an intensive five-week, full-time laboratory and lecture-based course. This course integrates basic human neuroanatomy, neurohistology, neuroimaging, neurophysiology, and neurochemistry with the study of basic systems organization and illustrative clinical correlations. I have been an active member of the course faculty for over sixteen years. My extensive involvement in the teaching of medical neuroscience has been a major determinant of the format of the *Atlas of Neuroanatomy*. Even during its evolution, earlier versions of this book had been designated by the faculty of the University of Florida College of Medicine as a mandatory text for the Medical Neuroscience course. This resource was used by graduate and medical students, residents in neurology and neurosurgery, and neuroscience faculty. The resulting evaluations, comments, and reviews were invaluable in further development and refinement of the content and format of the text. Each year, additions and revisions were made in response to the identification of areas of specific conceptual difficulty encountered by students and teaching staff. Furthermore, modifications were based upon discussions with my colleagues, addressing specific limitations in currently available texts and references in the neurological sciences.

The scope of this work includes gross external, sectional, and special dissection neuroanatomy, neurohistology, detailed stained sectional anatomy of the spinal cord, brainstem and diencephalon, cerebrovascular anatomy, correlative neuroimaging, and principles of systems organization. An extensive section featuring illustrative clinical and neuropathologic case presentations is included for contrast and comparison with normal neuroanatomy and to emphasize functional correlations and principles of systems organization. A major objective of this approach has been the development of a reference for medical students, graduate students, residents, post-doctoral fellows, and faculty that is consistent with the increasing movement toward vertical curricular integration in medical schools throughout the United States and internationally.

Materials used for the book are based on my collection, including over 35,000 slide images derived from the anatomic and histologic study of over 400 brains and numerous spinal cord dissections; along with a large collection of clinical neuroimaging studies, including angiography, computerized tomography, and magnetic resonance imaging. Procedures that I developed for the special studies of normal and pathologic specimens have been included as well. These include (1) postmortem combined angiography and ventriculography (presented at the 1999 Society for Neuroscience Annual Meeting), (2) modified staining procedures, and (3) specific post-fixation techniques in conjunction with infrared specimen imaging (selected for presentation at the 2000 Society for Neuroscience Annual Meeting). Included in this edition are images and diagrams that have been particularly useful in the teaching of medical neuroscience and for study in conjunction with case analysis for residents and faculty in the neurological sciences.

Joseph J. Warner, M.D.

ACKNOWLEDGMENTS

I consider this section of the book one of the most important, albeit susceptible to errors of omission. There are, without question, individuals not specifically listed who have made a contribution through their assistance, support, and enthusiasm. I extend my gratitude to all those who have contributed in some way to the development of this book, including my patients, both past and present.

First, I would like to thank Terry Briggs and his family, whose cooperation, encouragement, and understanding certainly added a new dimension to the clinicopathologic case analyses in Part VIII of this book. Their contribution is more completely explained in the Dedication.

Several of my colleagues have been instrumental in providing collaborative and academic support necessary for the integration of neuroanatomy, systems organization, and pathophysiology with case correlations. Floyd Thompson, Ph.D., of the Department of Neuroscience at the University of Florida College of Medicine, was instrumental in the development of my research interest in neurophysiology. Our collaboration over many years on research projects involving the physiology of cortical and subcortical motor systems has undoubtedly influenced my approach to the section that includes schematic diagrams of neural connectivity and systems organization. The contributions of William Schoene, M.D., James Morris, M.D., Martin A. Samuels, M.D., and Norman Geschwind, M.D., are discussed in the preface. These and other members of the faculty of Harvard Medical School have made a lasting impression on my approach to clinical and pathologic case analysis and the necessity for the integration of clinical neurology, neuroradiology, neuroanatomy, and pathophysiology for teaching, research, and patient care. I also appreciate the encouragement and support shown by my fellow residents in the Harvard Neurology Program.

As discussed in the Preface, the teaching of medical neuroscience has served both as an impetus as well as a guide for the development and refinement of this book. Specific University of Florida faculty are deserving of special mention in this regard for their encouragement, advice, and assistance. Dr. William Luttge, Director of the University of Florida Brain Institute, facilitated the establishment of my neuroanatomy and histopathology laboratory in the Department of Neuroscience, and has provided necessary support and collaboration for my teaching endeavors in the medical neuroscience course. Dr. Luttge has encouraged the publication of this book since its inception several years ago. Dr. W. J. Streit and Dr. Tanya McGraw Ferguson have provided invaluable assistance and collaboration with respect to the coordination of our teaching efforts and the integration of materials from the *Atlas of Neuroanatomy* into the medical neuroscience course. Dr. Lynn Romrell, Associate Dean of Medical Education, has also been supportive of various aspects of the laboratory and teaching activities that have been major factors in the development of this book.

I must recognize the efforts of Susan Pioli and Cheri Dellelo of Butterworth–Heinemann. Through her enthusiasm for this project, her expertise in medical publishing, and her energetic approach, Susan was instrumental in realizing the completion of this book. Cheri's efforts in the coordination of various aspects of this project are certainly appreciated as well. Their patience and encouragement through some difficult times has been indispensable.

Acknowledgments would not be complete without including individuals whose contribution, although perhaps indirectly related to this edition, has nevertheless been invaluable on a long-term basis. Those deserving special mention include Carol and James Strouse, Joseph John Warner, Maria Eugenia Barbier, and Helen Caldwell.

Atlas *of* NEUROANATOMY

PART I: MAJOR DIVISIONS OF THE CENTRAL NERVOUS SYSTEM: INTRODUCTION AND OVERVIEW

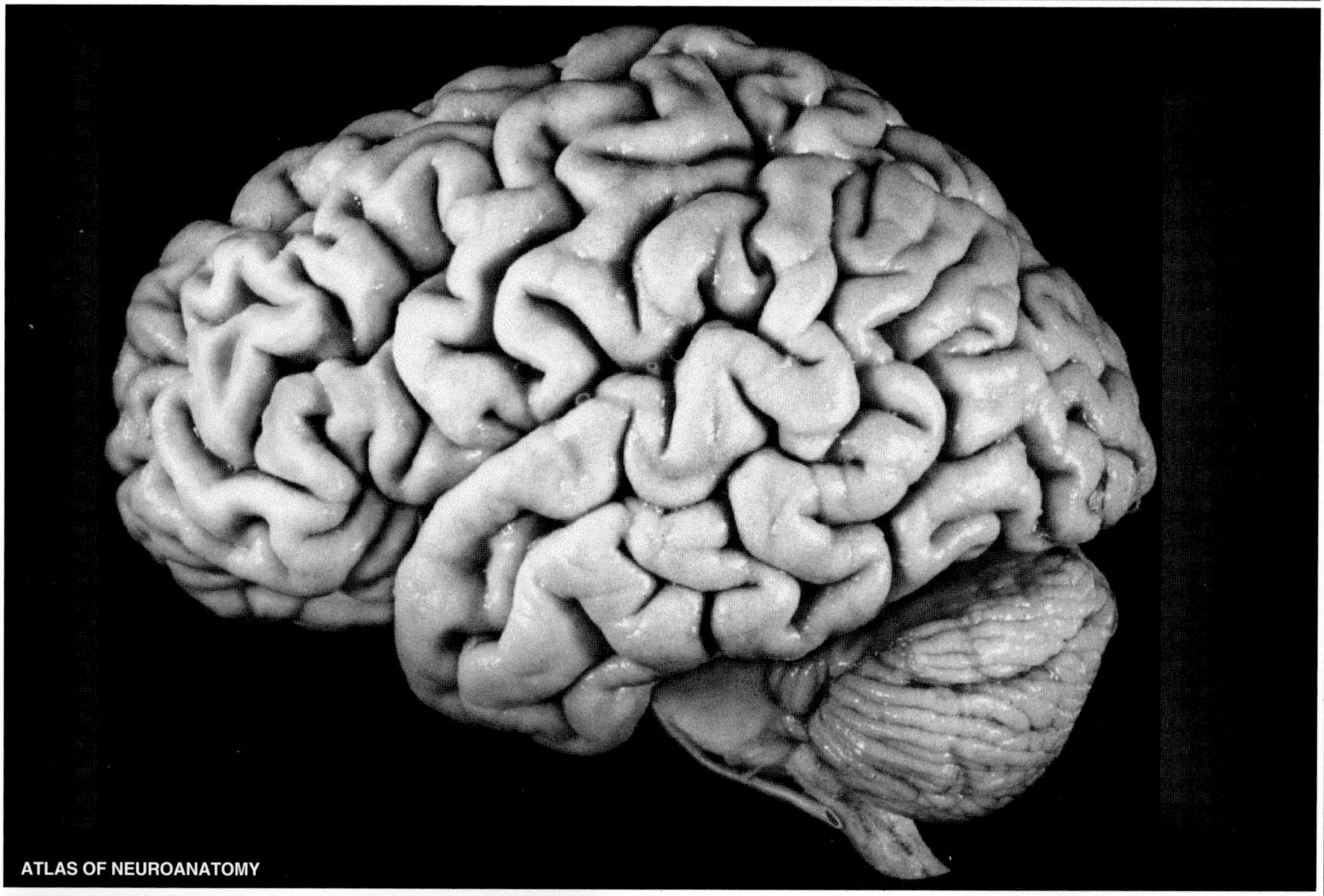

ATLAS OF NEUROANATOMY

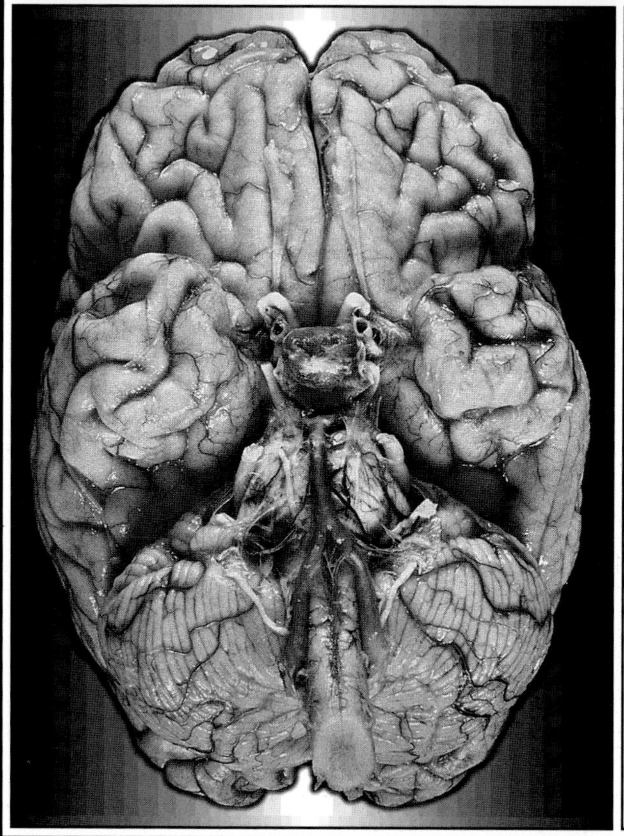

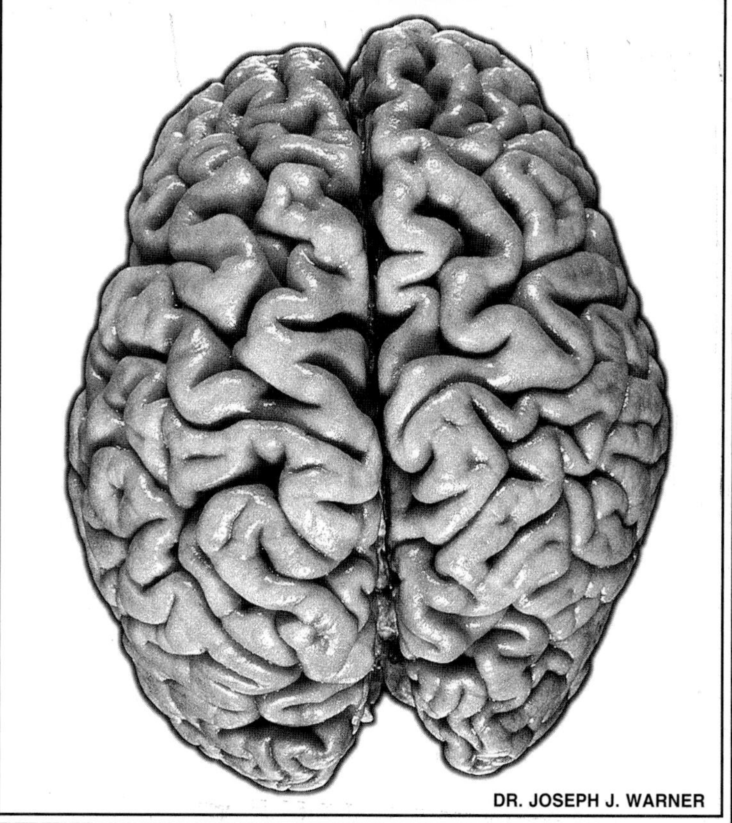

CRANIAL DISSECTION: BASE OF THE SKULL AND DURA INTACT, WITH RESECTION OF THE DURA OVERLYING THE RIGHT DORSOLATERAL FRONTAL LOBE AND EXPOSURE OF THE ARACHNOID MEMBRANE

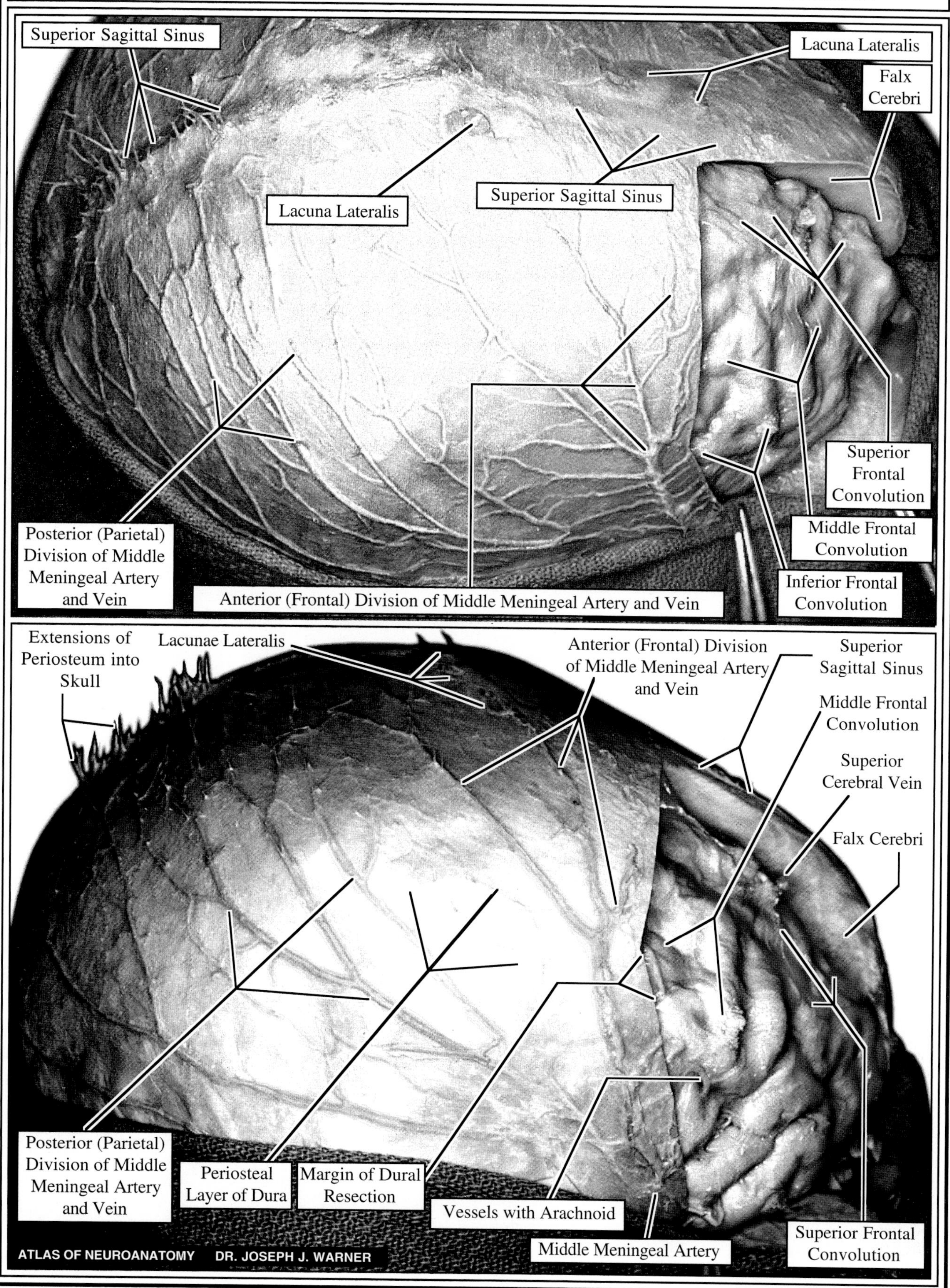

CRANIAL DISSECTION: DURA RESECTED OVER THE RIGHT FRONTAL LOBE DEMONSTRATING THE SUBJACENT ARACHNOID MEMBRANE

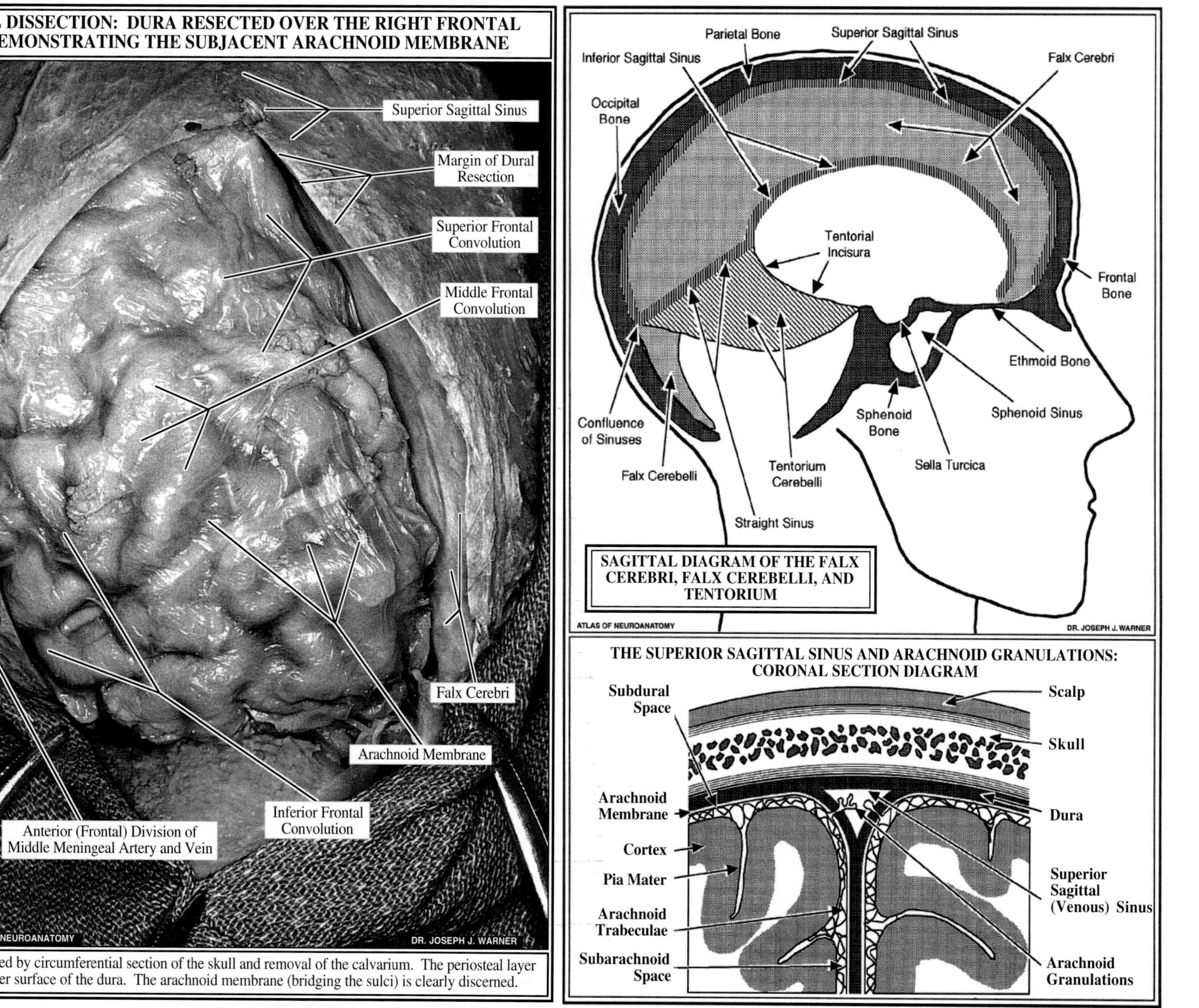

The dura is exposed by circumferential section of the skull and removal of the calvarium. The periosteal layer comprises the outer surface of the dura. The arachnoid membrane (bridging the sulci) is clearly discerned.

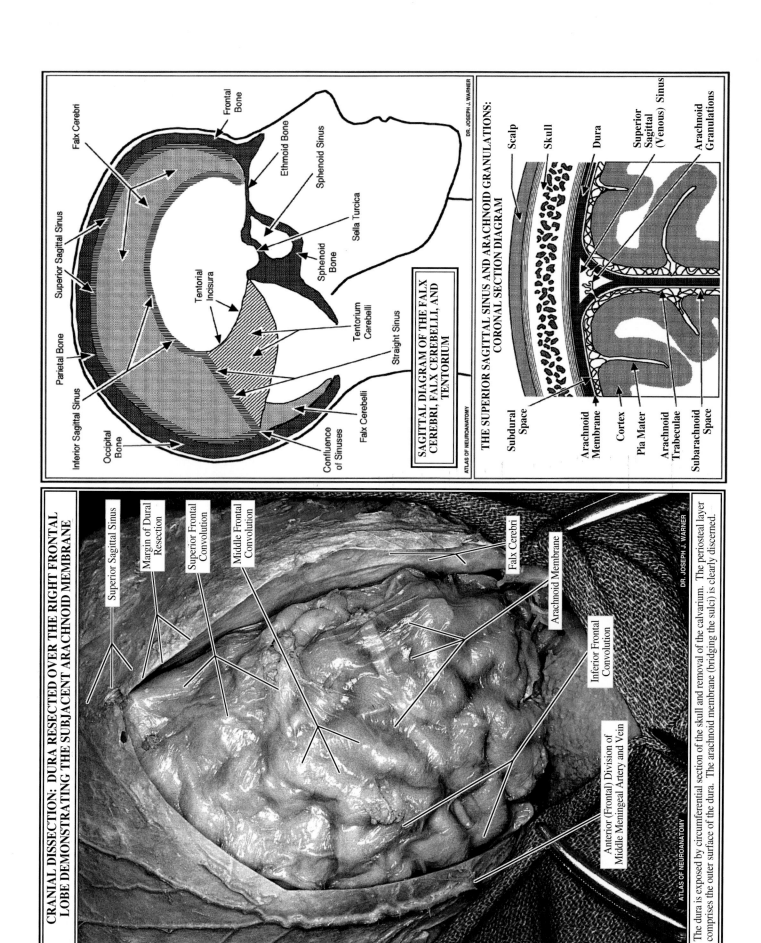

THE DURA, ARACHNOID MEMBRANE AND SURFACE VASCULATURE OF THE DORSAL ASPECT OF THE BRAIN: (A) DURA INTACT, AND (B) DURA REFLECTED FROM THE LEFT CEREBRAL HEMISPHERE

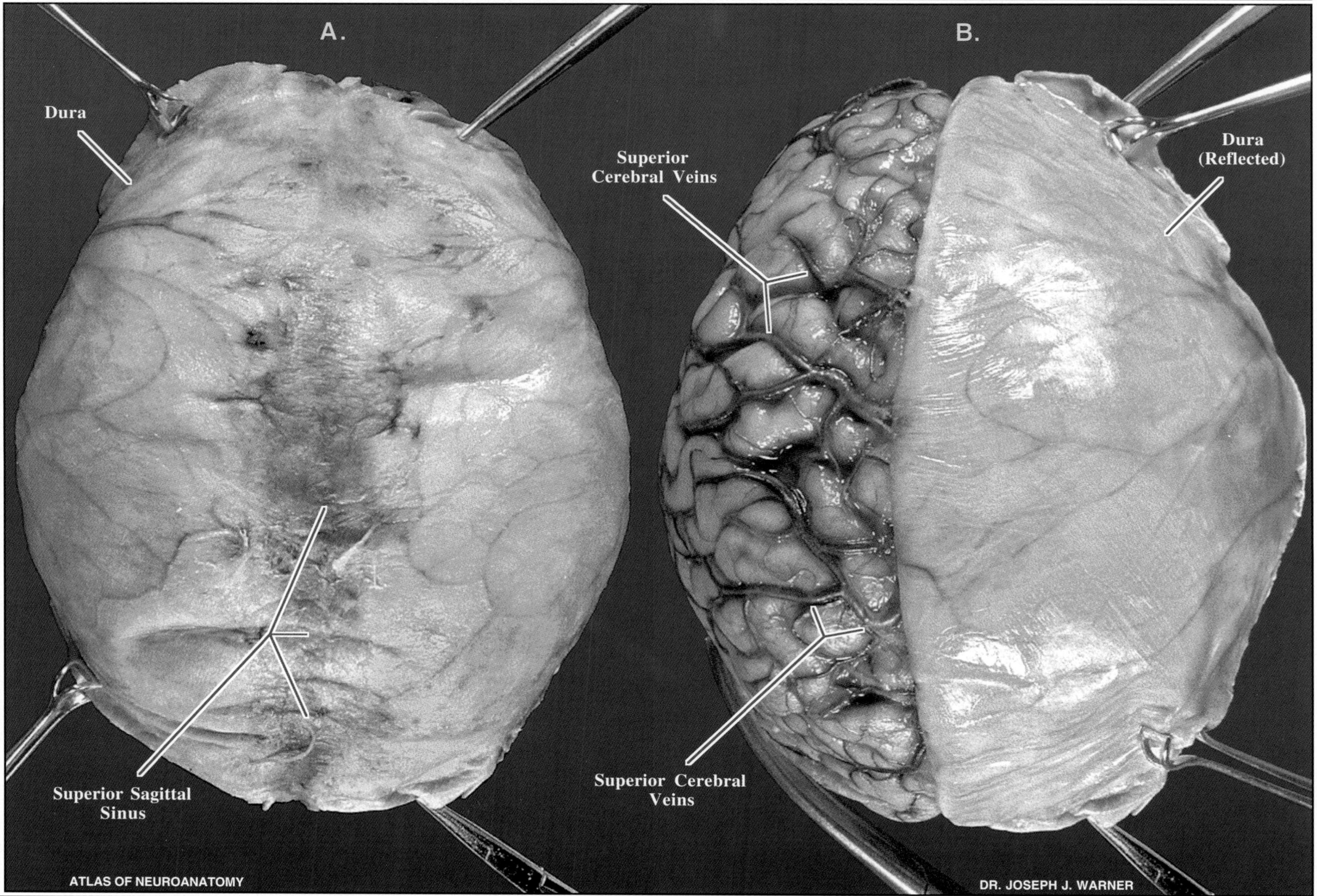

A.

Dura

Superior Sagittal Sinus

B.

Superior Cerebral Veins

Dura (Reflected)

Superior Cerebral Veins

ATLAS OF NEUROANATOMY

DR. JOSEPH J. WARNER

DORSOLATERAL ASPECT OF THE BRAIN: DURA REFLECTED FROM THE LEFT HEMISPHERE DEMONSTRATING THE ARACHNOID MEMBRANE, SURFACE VASCULATURE, AND GYRAL MORPHOLOGY

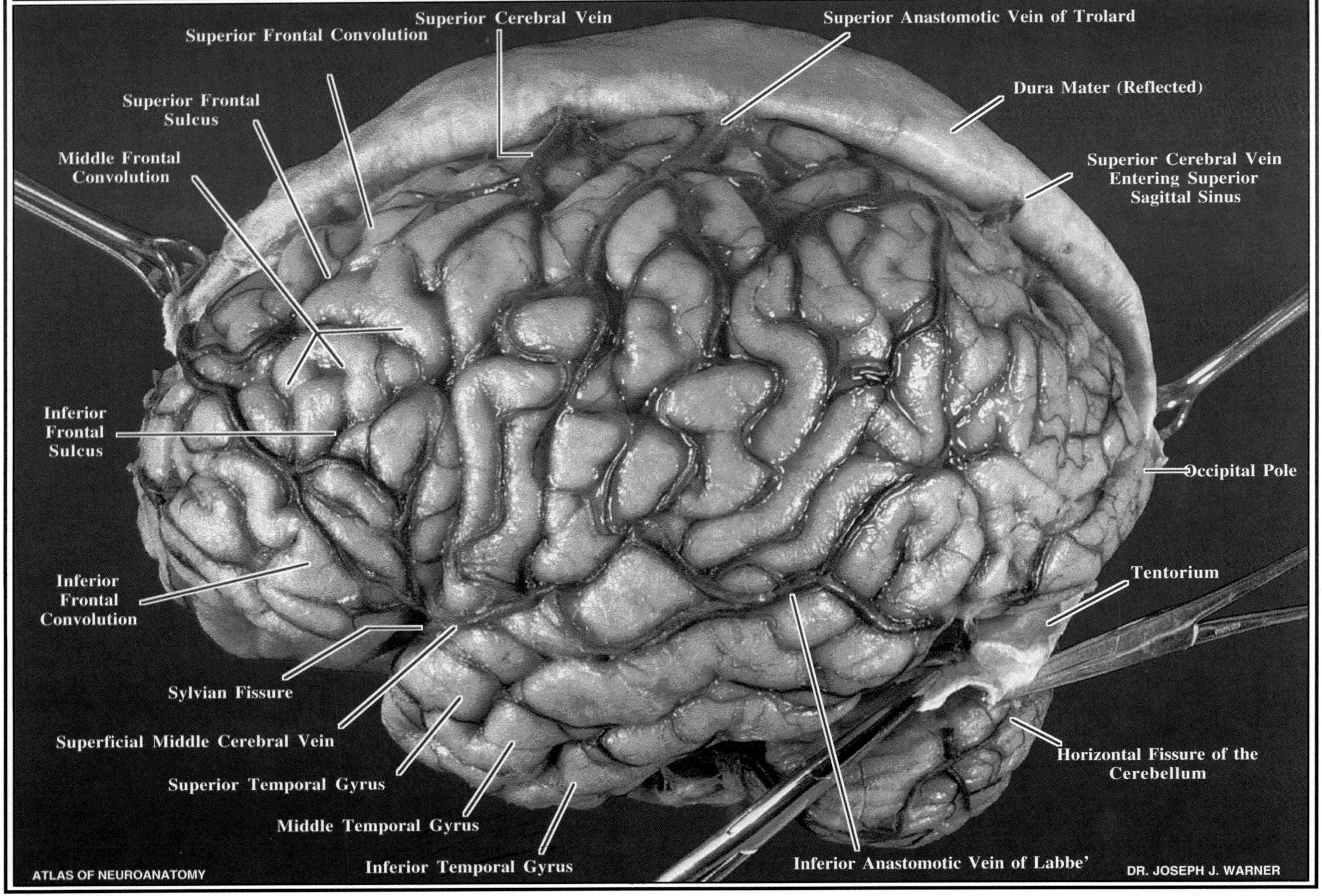

ATLAS OF NEUROANATOMY

DR. JOSEPH J. WARNER

CRANIOCERVICAL SAGITTAL SECTION: DURAL STRUCTURES

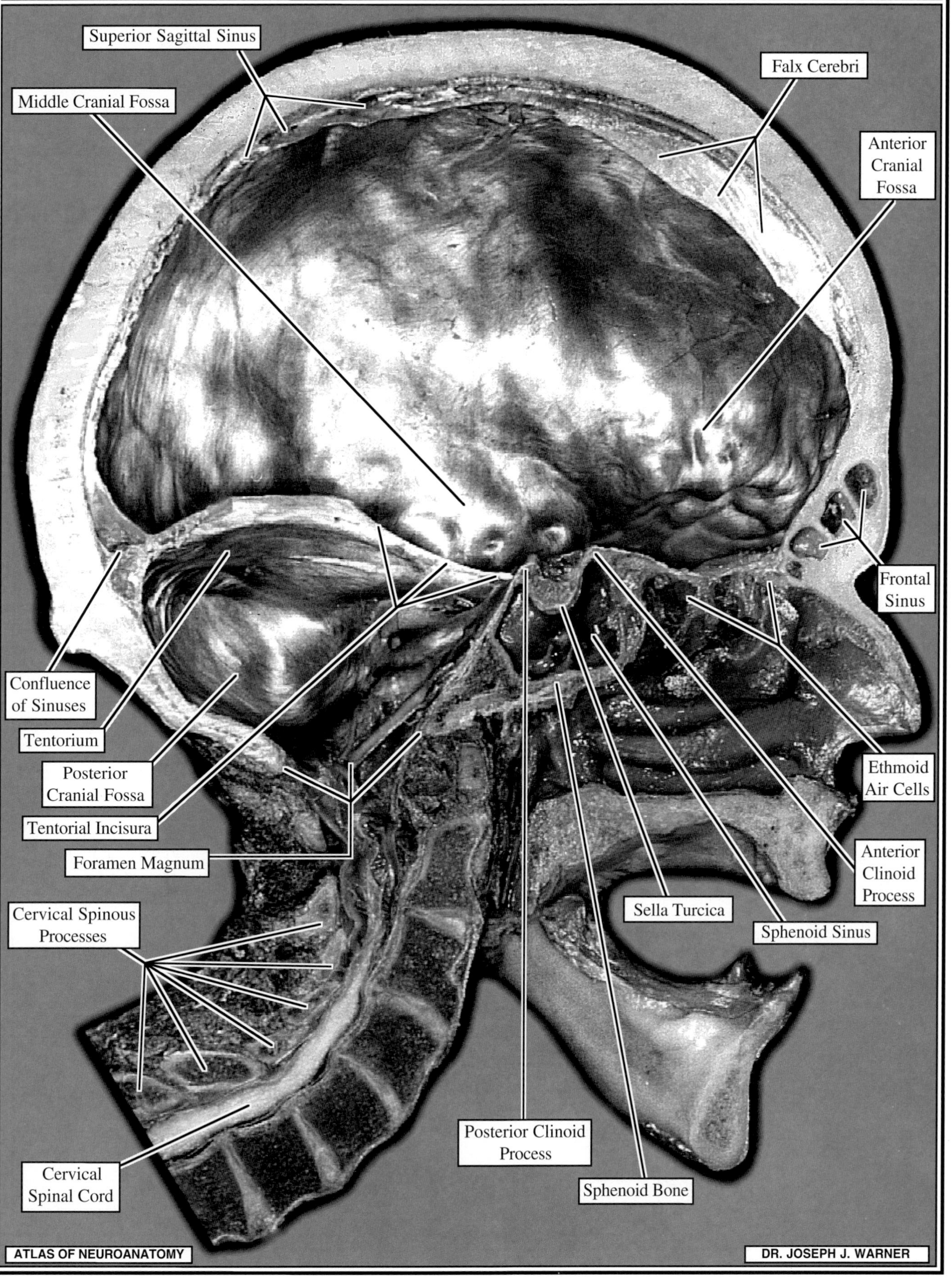

Superior Sagittal Sinus
Middle Cranial Fossa
Falx Cerebri
Anterior Cranial Fossa
Frontal Sinus
Confluence of Sinuses
Tentorium
Posterior Cranial Fossa
Tentorial Incisura
Foramen Magnum
Ethmoid Air Cells
Anterior Clinoid Process
Sella Turcica
Sphenoid Sinus
Cervical Spinous Processes
Cervical Spinal Cord
Posterior Clinoid Process
Sphenoid Bone

ATLAS OF NEUROANATOMY

DR. JOSEPH J. WARNER

CRANIOCERVICAL HEMISECTION: INTERNAL CRANIAL ANATOMY, DURA INTACT

CRANIAL HEMISECTION: MEDIAL TO LATERAL PERSPECTIVE (Figure at right)

INTERNAL VIEW OF THE VENTRAL AND LATERAL CRANIUM, DURA INTACT (Figure below)

The complex surface contour of the floor of the anterior and middle cranial fossae is a contributory factor in the specific susceptibility of certain brain regions to structural damage from closed-head trauma. Such areas include the anterior temporal lobes and orbitofrontal cortex.

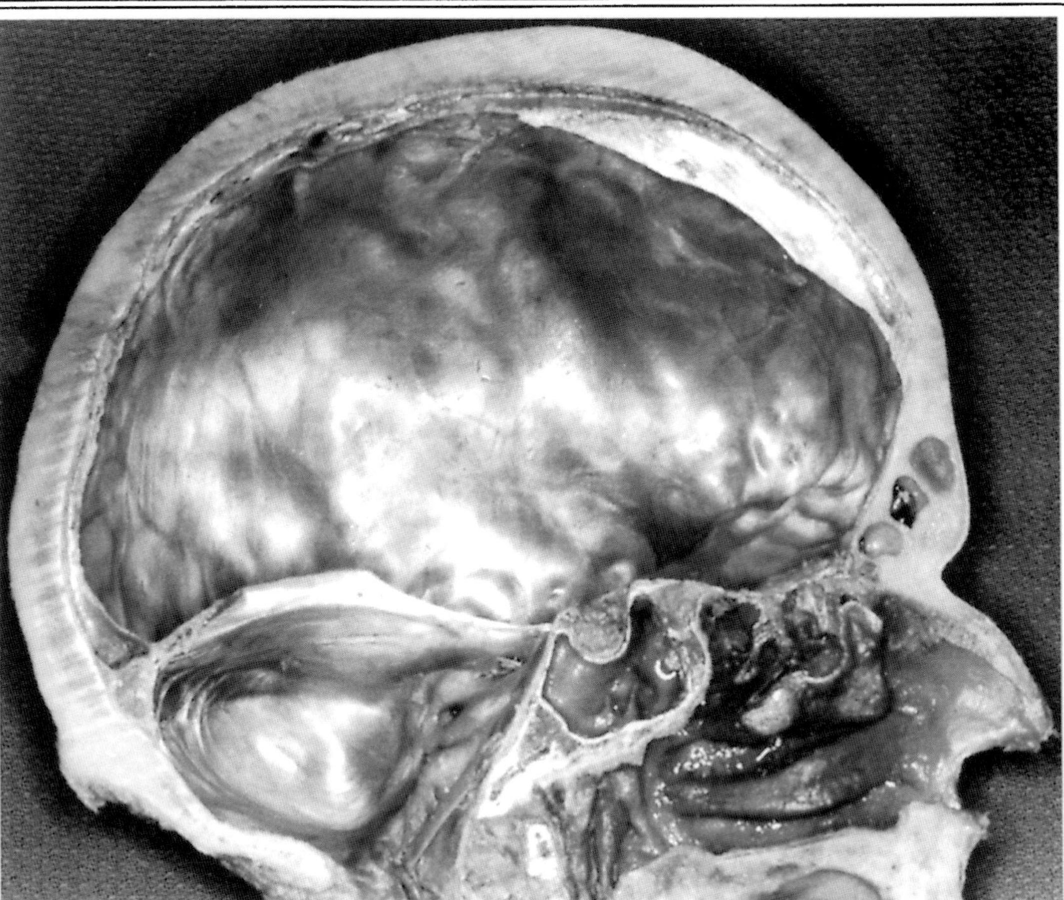

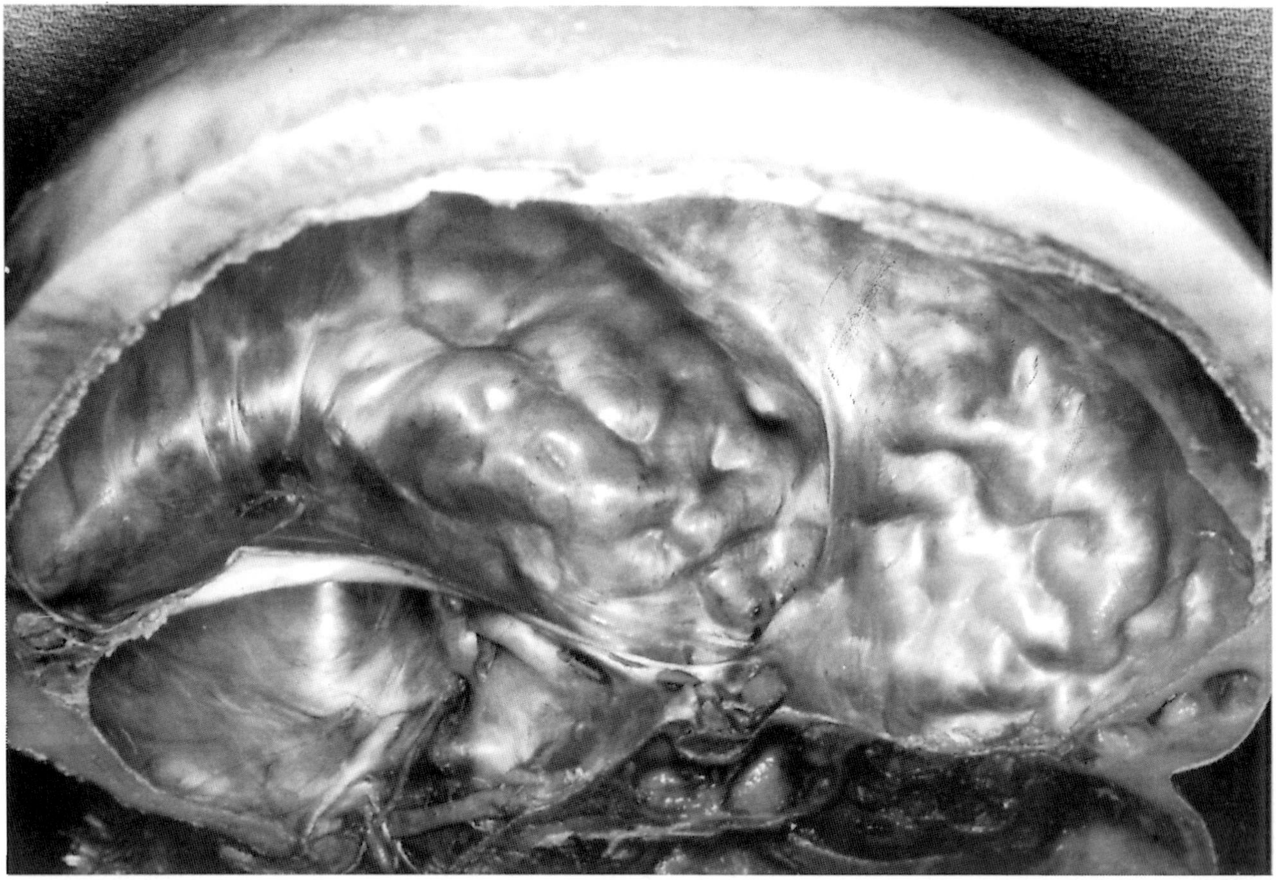

DORSAL ASPECT OF THE BRAIN, VASCULATURE AND ARACHNOID MEMBRANE INTACT, DEMONSTRATING THE ARACHNOID GRANULATIONS

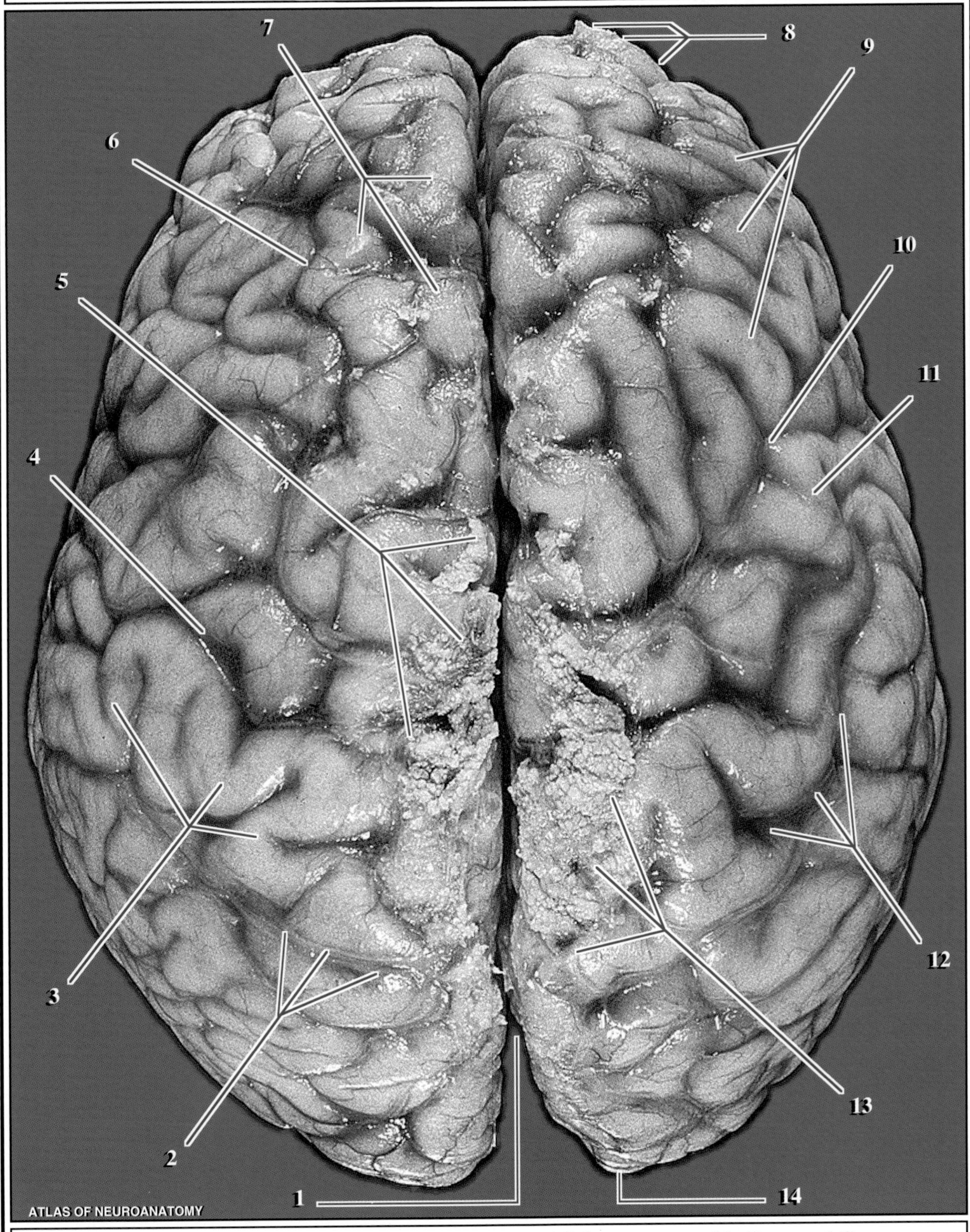

1. Interhemispheric Fissure
2. Superior Cerebral Vein
3. Postcentral Gyrus
4. Rolandic Fissure (Central Sulcus)
5. Arachnoid Granulations
6. Superior Frontal Sulcus
7. Superior Frontal Convolution
8. Frontal Pole
9. Middle Frontal Convolution
10. Precentral Sulcus
11. Precentral Gyrus
12. Postcentral Sulcus
13. Arachnoid Granulations
14. Occipital Pole

DR. JOSEPH J. WARNER

DORSAL ASPECT OF THE BRAIN: ARACHNOID MEMBRANE AND VASCULATURE INTACT, WITH MAGNIFIED VIEW OF THE ARACHNOID GRANULATIONS

MAP OF THE MAGNIFIED AREA OF THE DORSAL VIEW OF THE BRAIN

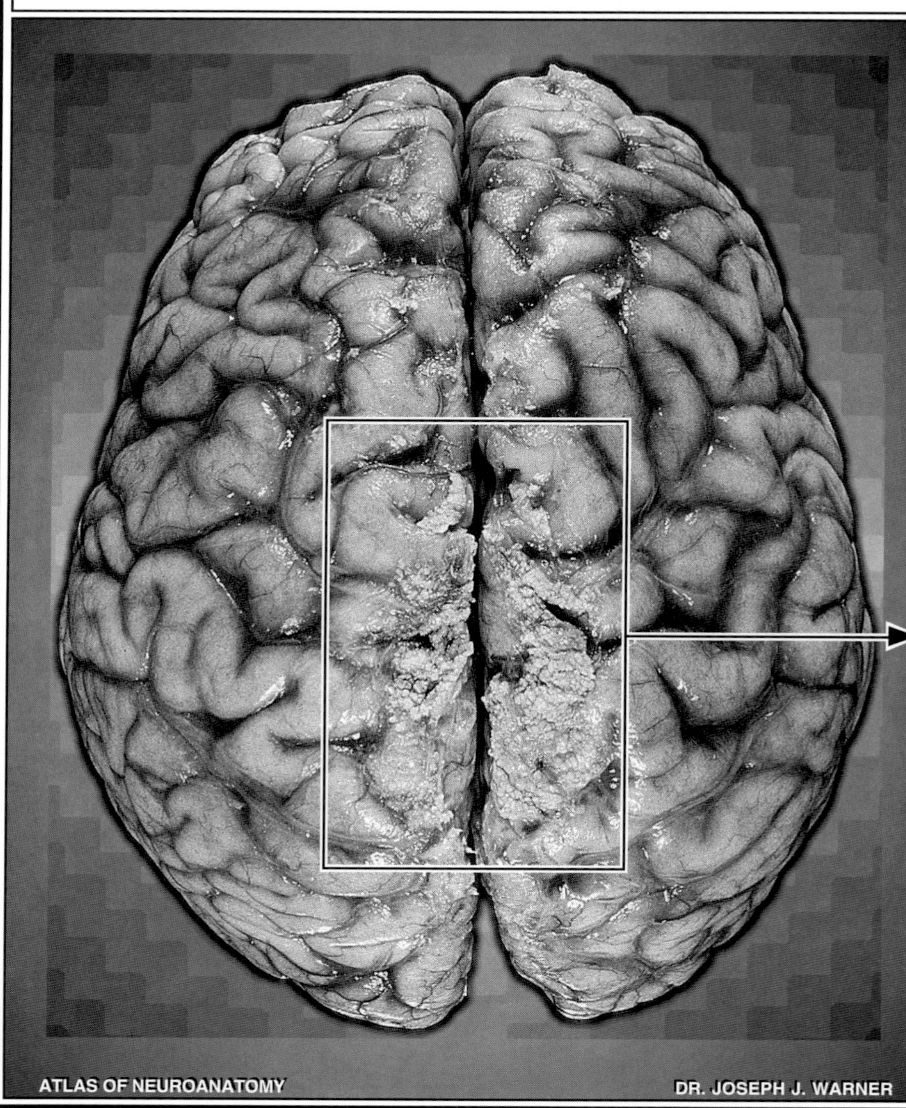

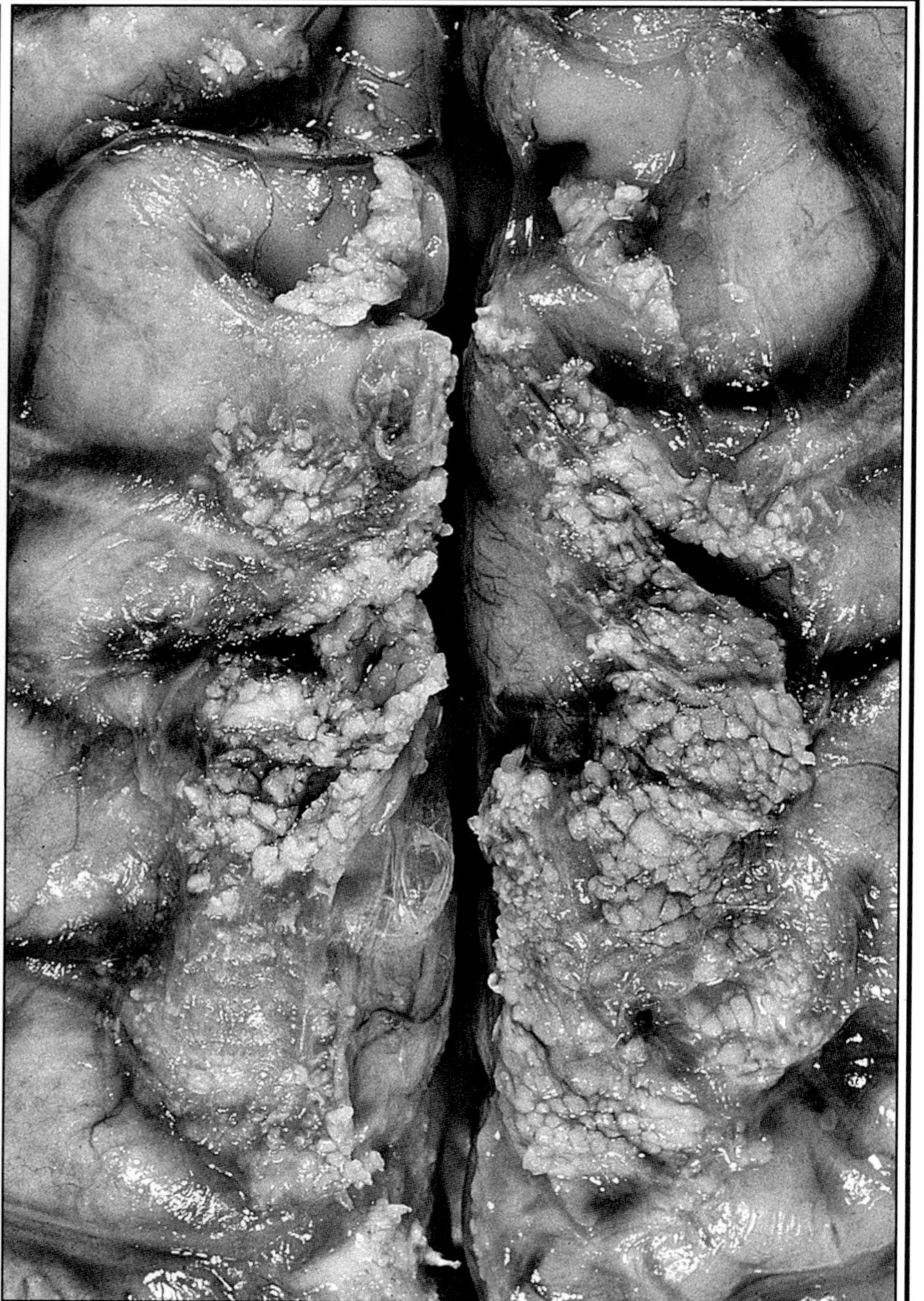

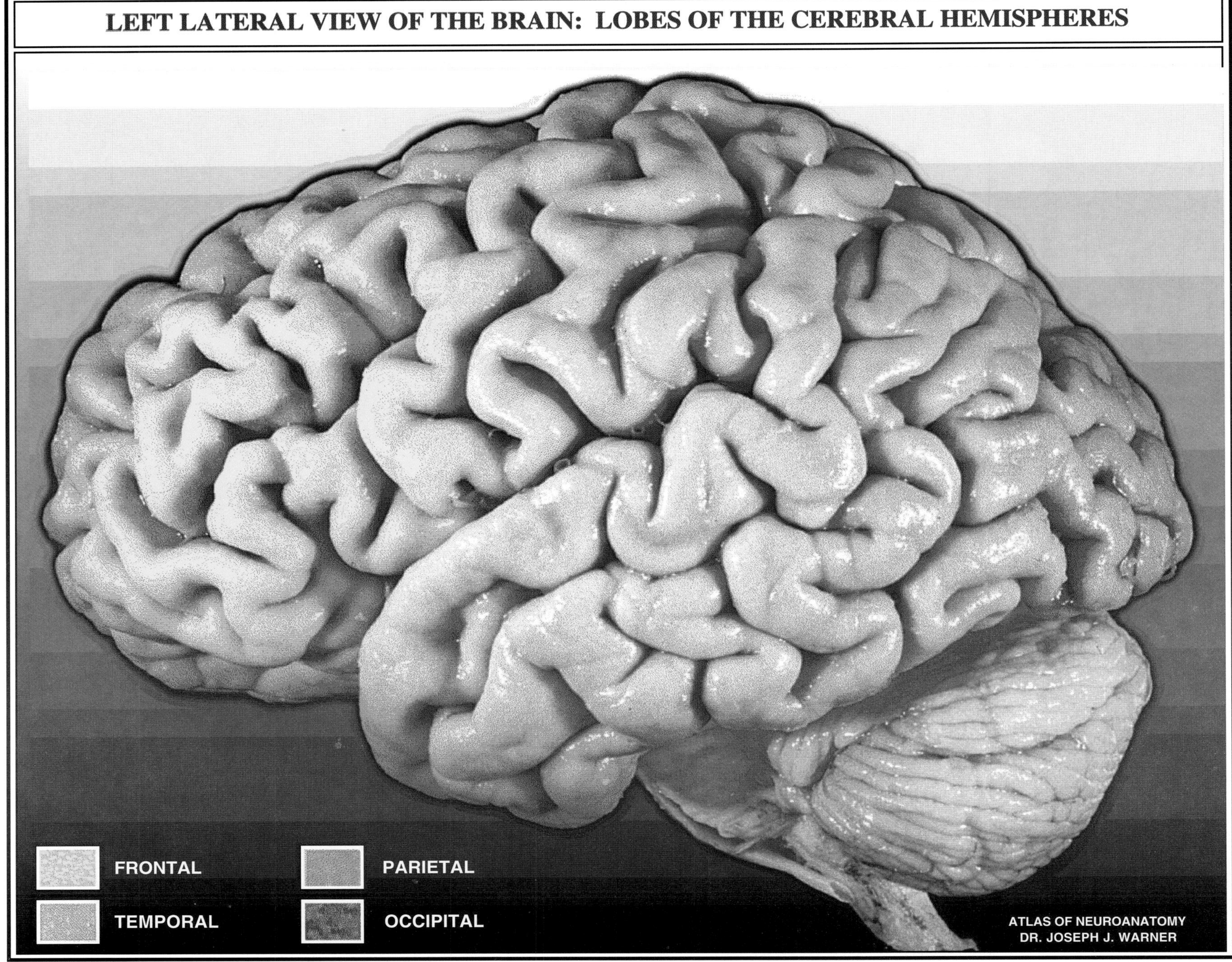
LEFT LATERAL VIEW OF THE BRAIN: LOBES OF THE CEREBRAL HEMISPHERES
FRONTAL
PARIETAL
TEMPORAL
OCCIPITAL
ATLAS OF NEUROANATOMY
DR. JOSEPH J. WARNER

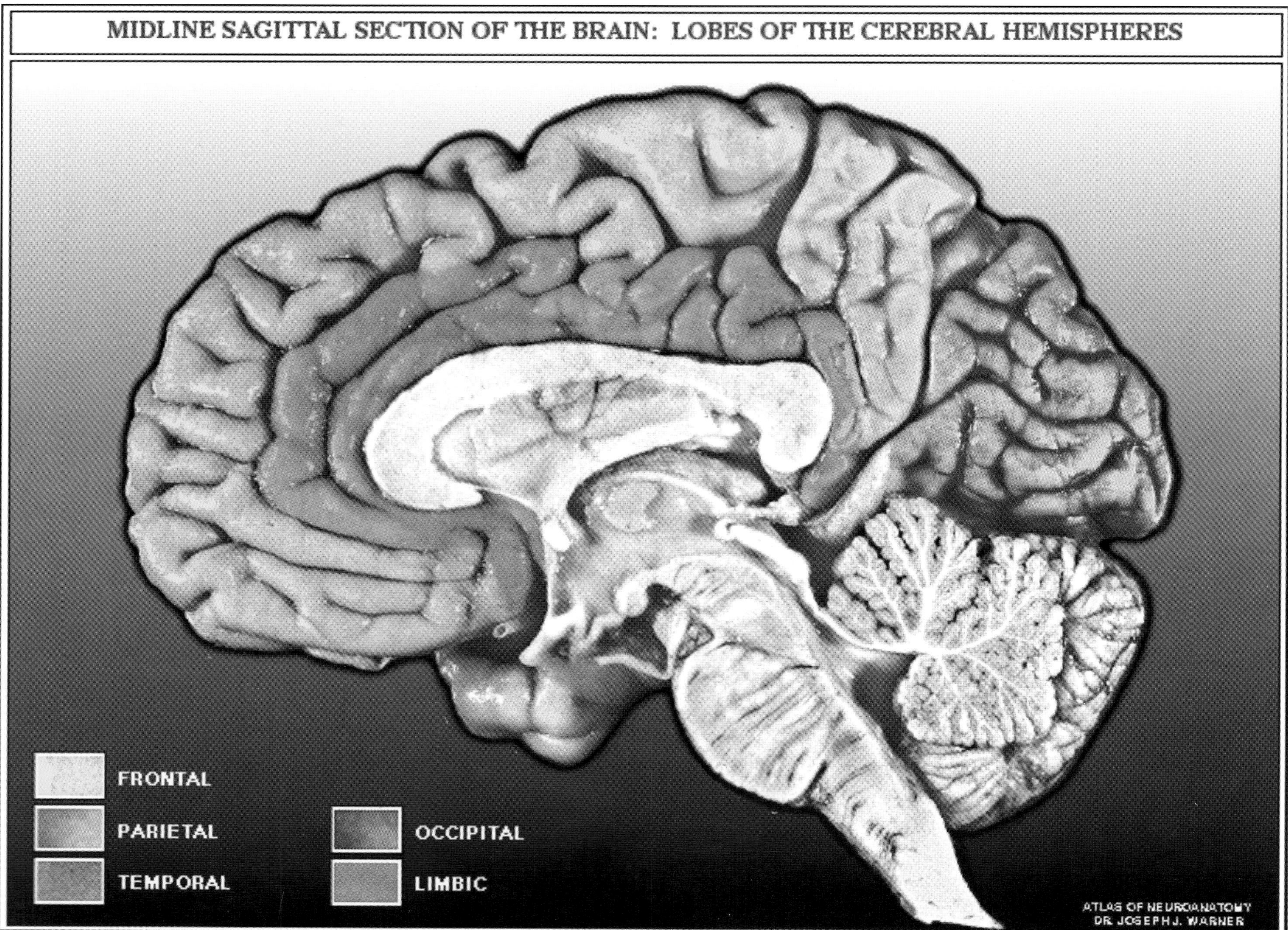
MIDLINE SAGITTAL SECTION OF THE BRAIN: LOBES OF THE CEREBRAL HEMISPHERES
FRONTAL
PARIETAL
TEMPORAL
OCCIPITAL
LIMBIC
ATLAS OF NEUROANATOMY
DR. JOSEPH J. WARNER

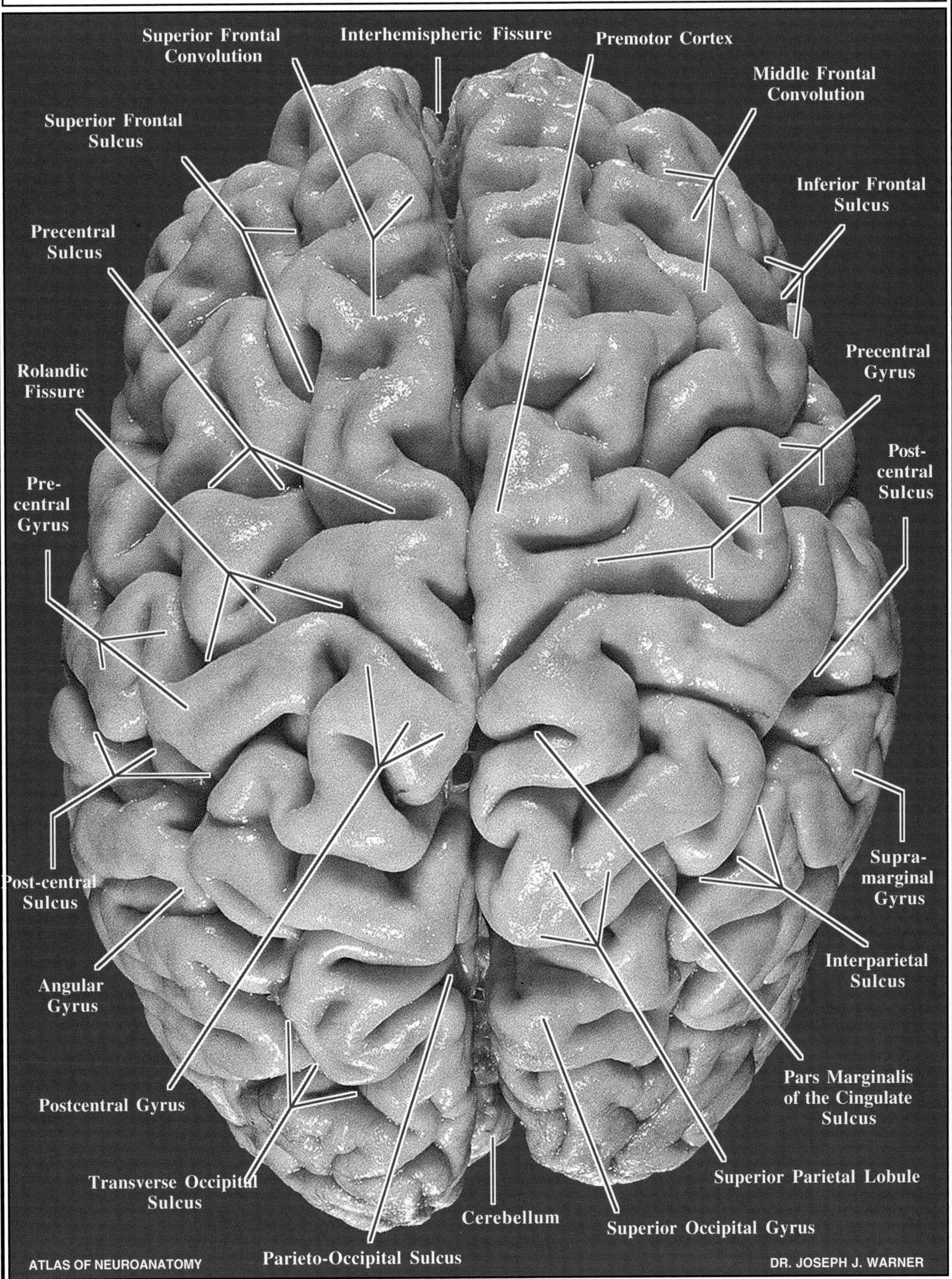
DORSAL ASPECT OF THE BRAIN, ARACHNOID MEMBRANE RESECTED
Superior Frontal Convolution
Interhemispheric Fissure
Premotor Cortex
Middle Frontal Convolution
Superior Frontal Sulcus
Inferior Frontal Sulcus
Precentral Sulcus
Precentral Gyrus
Rolandic Fissure
Post-central Sulcus
Pre-central Gyrus
Post-central Sulcus
Supra-marginal Gyrus
Interparietal Sulcus
Angular Gyrus
Pars Marginalis of the Cingulate Sulcus
Postcentral Gyrus
Superior Parietal Lobule
Transverse Occipital Sulcus
Cerebellum
Superior Occipital Gyrus
Parieto-Occipital Sulcus
ATLAS OF NEUROANATOMY
DR. JOSEPH J. WARNER

DORSAL VIEW OF THE BRAIN: ARACHNOID MEMBRANE RESECTED

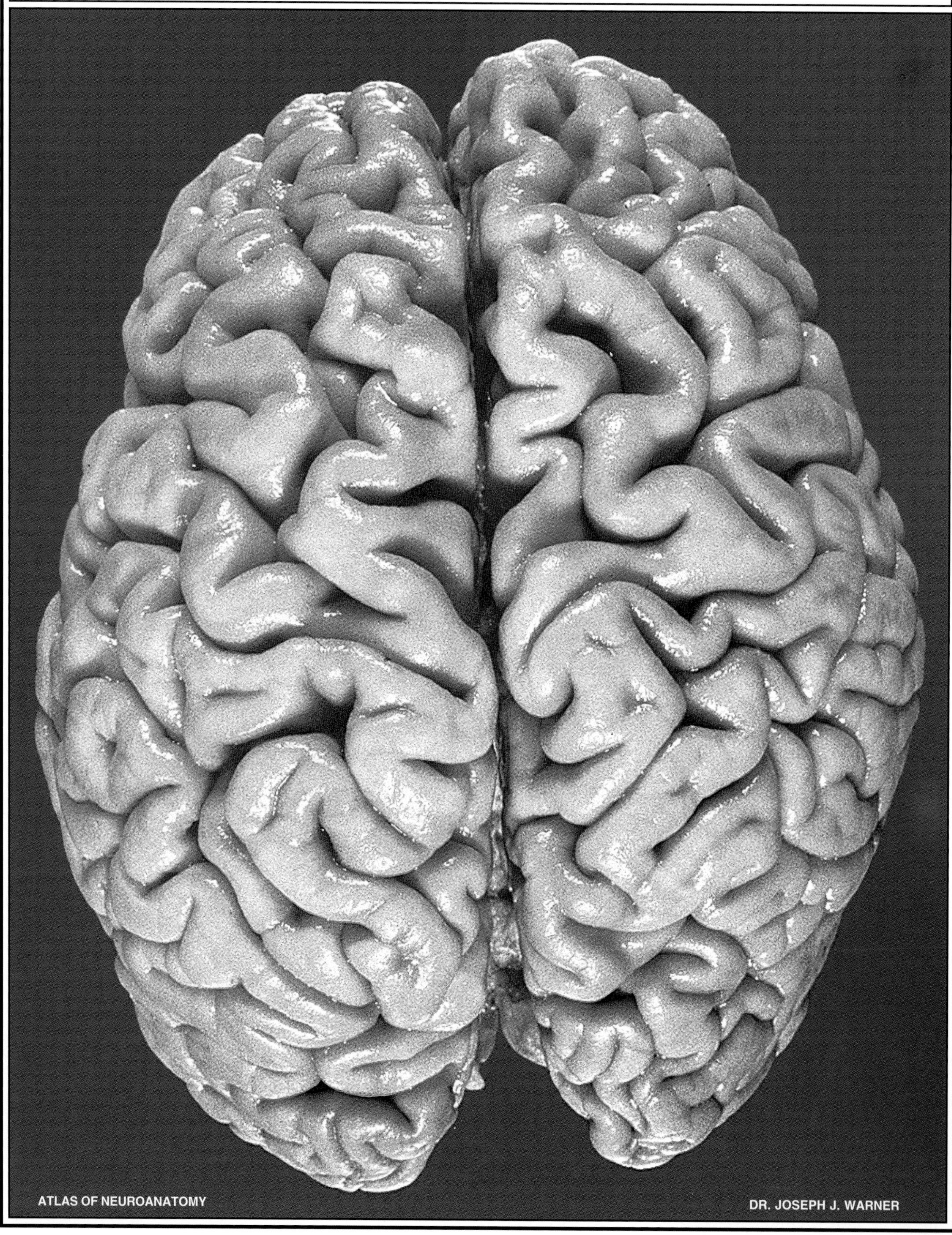

ATLAS OF NEUROANATOMY

DR. JOSEPH J. WARNER

DORSAL VIEW OF THE BRAIN: ARACHNOID MEMBRANE RESECTED

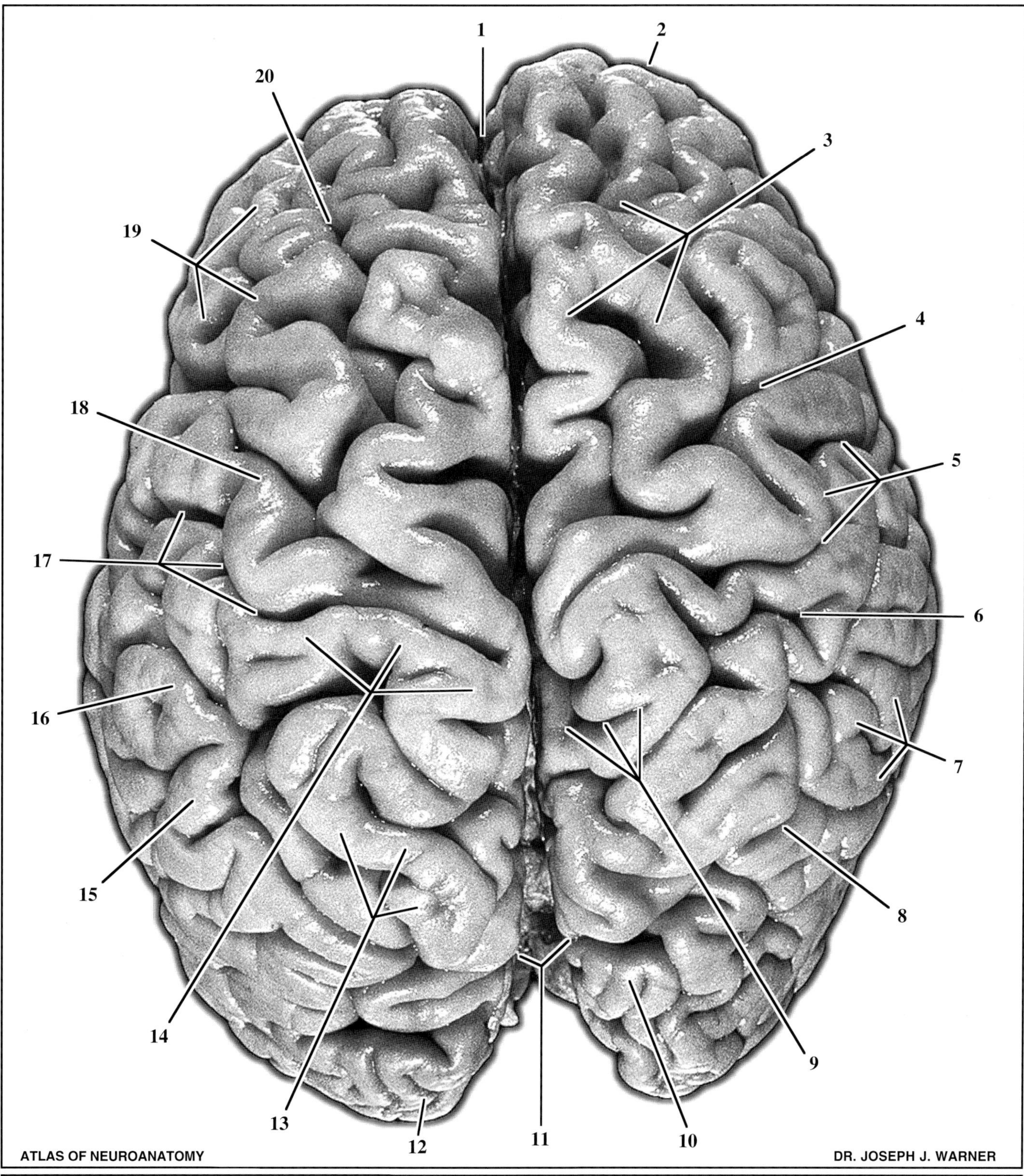

ATLAS OF NEUROANATOMY

DR. JOSEPH J. WARNER

1. Interhemispheric Fissure
2. Frontal Pole
3. Superior Frontal Convolution
4. Precentral Sulcus
5. Rolandic Fissure (Central Sulcus)
6. Postcentral Sulcus
7. Inferior Parietal Lobule
8. Interparietal Sulcus
9. Pars Marginalis of the Cingulate Sulcus
10. Superior Occipital Gyrus
11. Parieto-Occipital Sulcus
12. Occipital Pole
13. Superior Parietal Lobule
14. Postcentral Gyrus
15. Angular Gyrus
16. Supramarginal Gyrus
17. Rolandic Fissure (Central Sulcus)
18. Precentral Gyrus
19. Middle Frontal Convolution
20. Superior Frontal Sulcus

LEFT LATERAL VIEW OF THE BRAIN, ARACHNOID RESECTED: GYRAL MORPHOLOGY

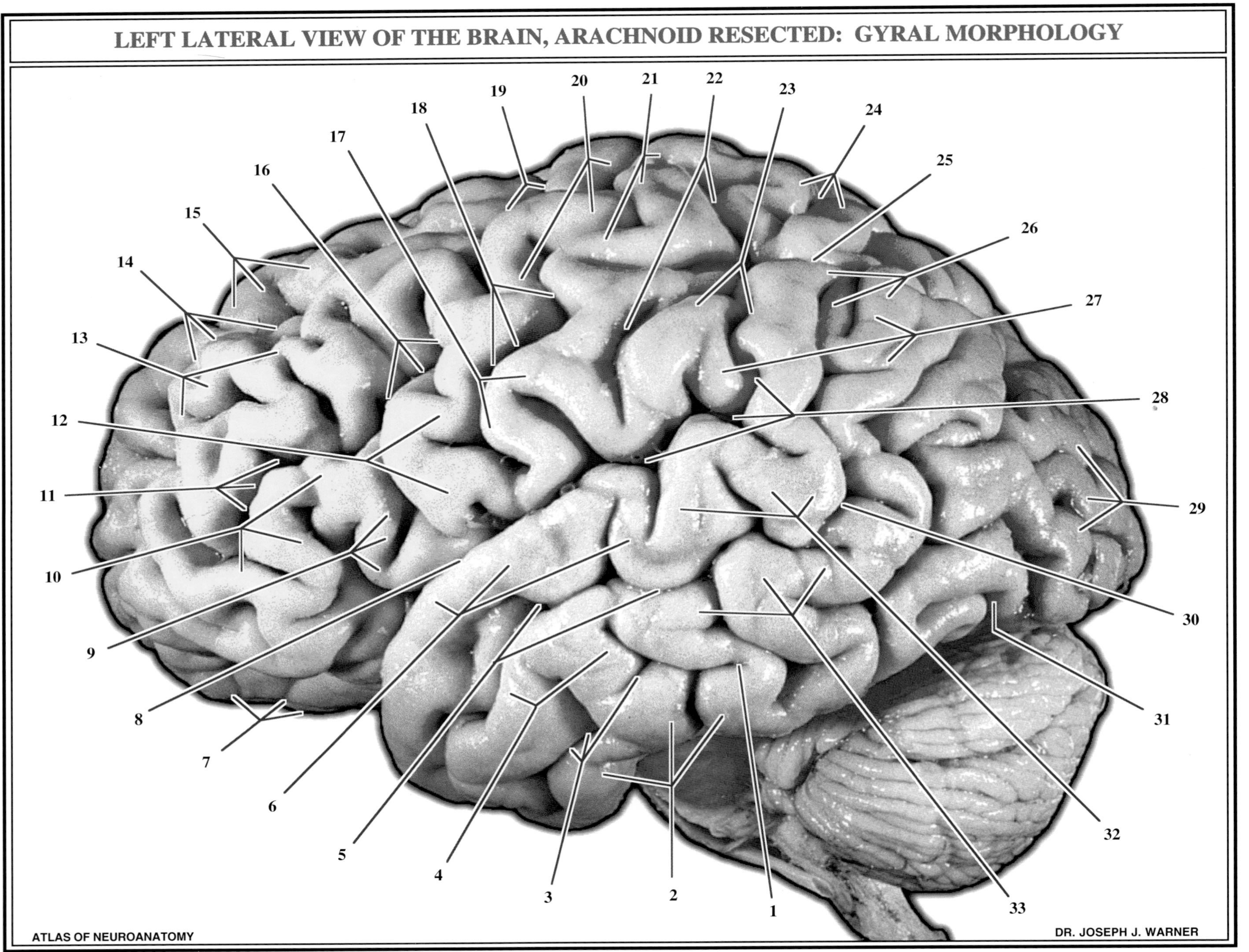

LEFT LATERAL VIEW OF THE BRAIN (ARACHNOID RESECTED); GYRAL MORPHOLOGY: KEY TO NUMBERED STRUCTURES

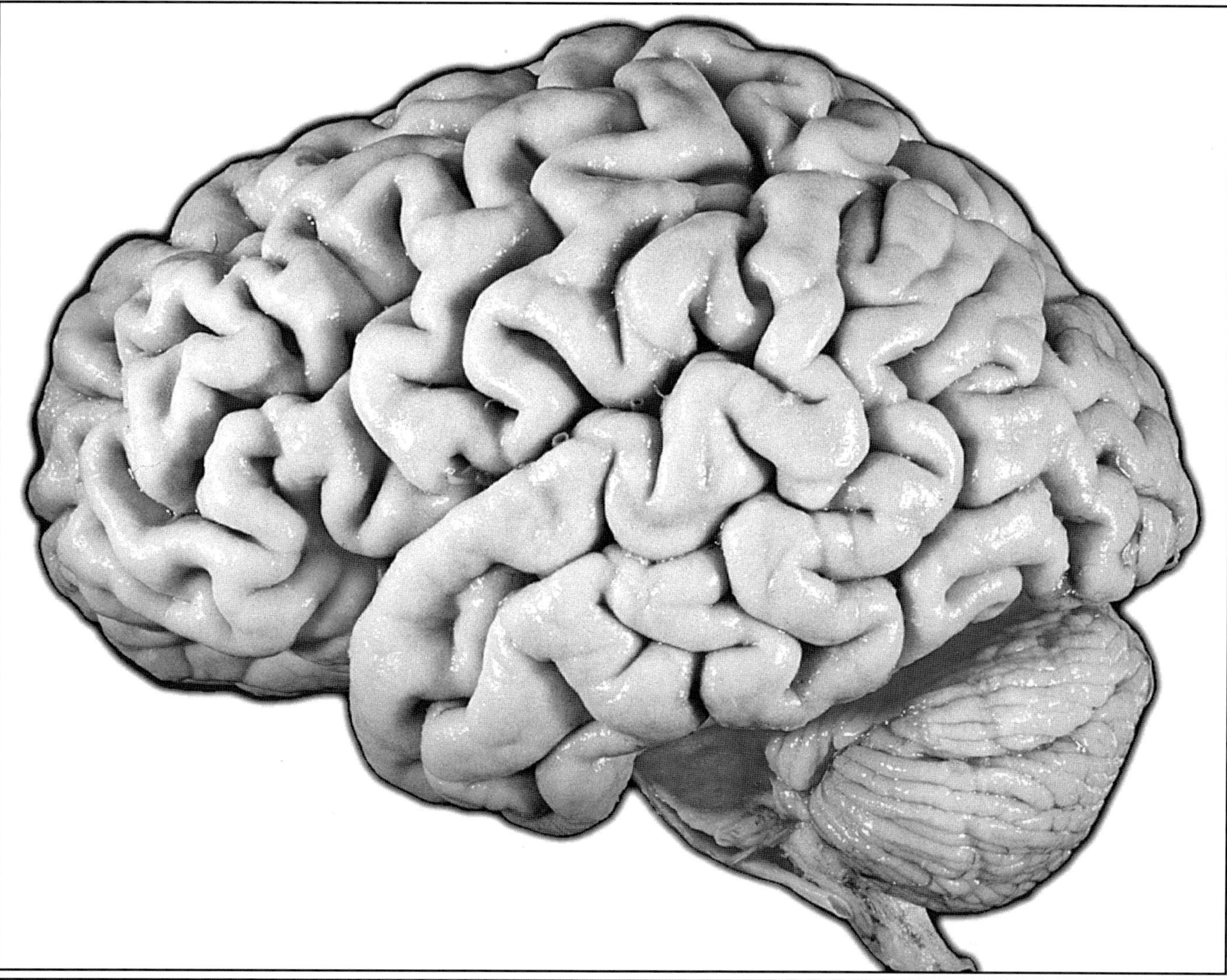

1. Middle Temporal Sulcus
2. Inferior Temporal Gyrus
3. Middle Temporal Sulcus
4. Middle Temporal Gyrus
5. Superior Temporal Sulcus
6. Superior Temporal Gyrus
7. Orbitofrontal Gyri
8. Sylvian Fissure
9. Frontal Opercular Region
10. Inferior Frontal Convolution
11. Inferior Frontal Sulcus
12. Precentral Gyrus
13. Middle Frontal Convolution
14. Superior Frontal Sulcus
15. Superior Frontal Convolution
16. Precentral Sulcus
17. Postcentral Gyrus
18. Rolandic Fissure (Central Sulcus)
19. Precentral Sulcus
20. Precentral Gyrus
21. Postcentral Gyrus
22. Postcentral Sulcus
23. Supramarginal Gyrus
24. Superior Parietal Lobule
25. Interparietal Sulcus
26. Angular Gyrus
27. Inferior Parietal Lobule
28. Sylvian Fissure
29. Lateral Occipital Gyri
30. Superior Temporal Sulcus
31. Preoccipital Notch
32. Superior Temporal Gyrus
33. Middle Temporal Gyrus

Surface anatomy of the cerebral hemispheres is quite variable. However, basic similarities are clearly discernible with respect to the major divisions. The primary sensory and motor areas are characterized by surface morphologic features that are quite comparable between brains. Other areas, such as the prefrontal cortex, demonstrate greater variability. Thus, areas such as the precentral and postcentral gyri are readily identifiable on the basis of surface morphology, in contrast to the superior, middle, and inferior frontal convolutions, which are often discontinuous or incompletely demarcated by the superior and inferior frontal sulci. The gyri and sulci of the lateral aspect of the temporal lobe are also characterized by variations in relative size and continuity. The study of gyral morphology must therefore include the direct comparison of several specimens.

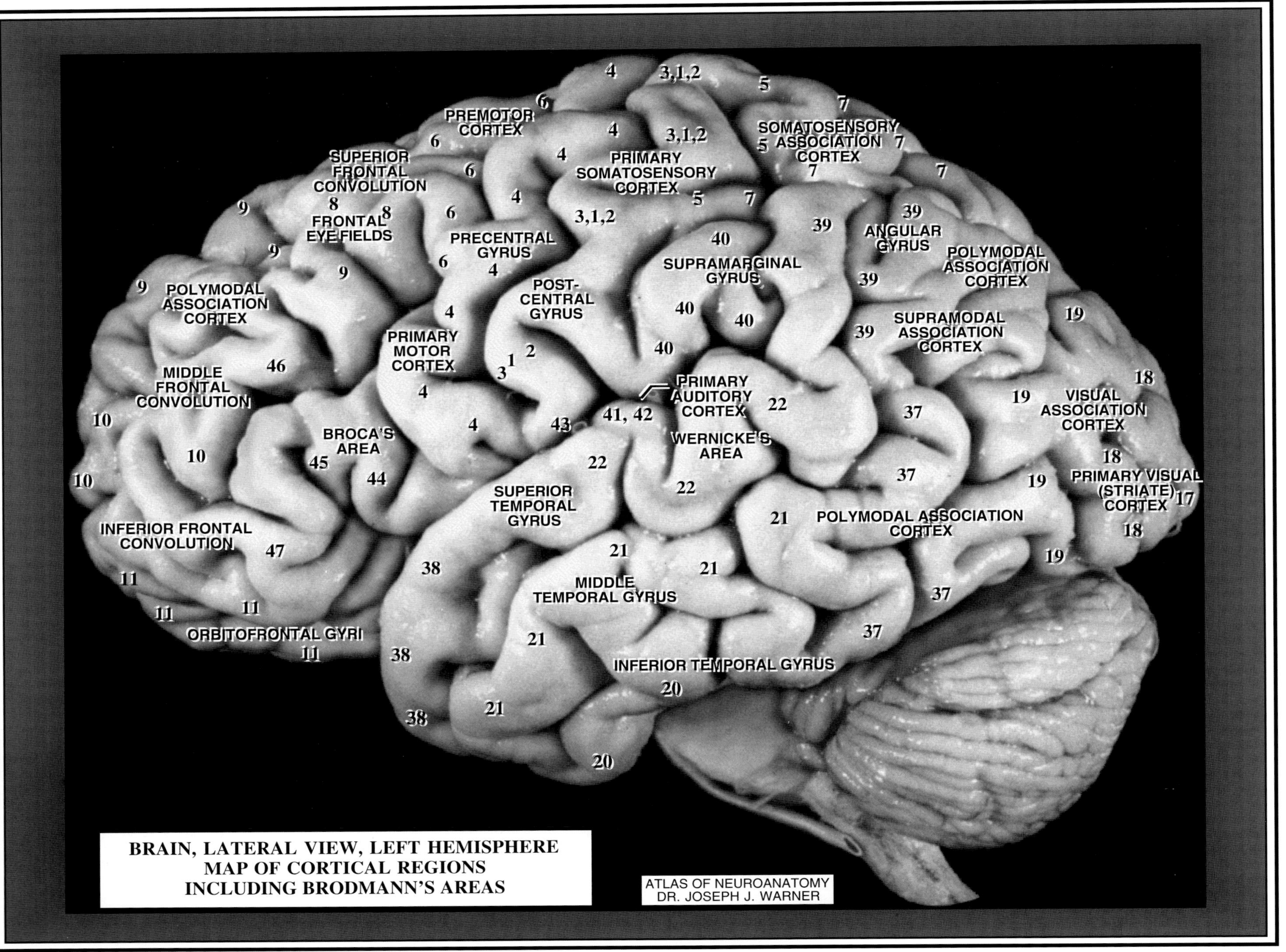

BRAIN, LATERAL VIEW, LEFT HEMISPHERE
MAP OF CORTICAL REGIONS
INCLUDING BRODMANN'S AREAS

CORONAL (FRONTAL) VIEW OF THE CEREBRAL HEMISPHERES: ARACHNOID MEMBRANE INTACT

This external rostral to caudal perspective of the cerebral hemispheres demonstrates the concave ventral contour of the frontal lobes. Their anatomic configuration is reflective of the contour of the anterior cranial fossa, the floor of which includes the roofs of the orbits. The ventral position of the medial aspect of the orbitofrontal surface (relative to the lateral aspect) conforms to the olfactory groove in the anterior cranial fossa.

The anterior aspect of the temporal pole is visible just ventral to the caudal aspect of the left frontal lobe. Given the normal anatomic asymmetry of the cerebral hemispheres, the unilateral appearance of the temporal pole is a frequent characteristic of this view of the brain.

The arachnoid membrane is intact in this specimen. Bridging the sulci, this membrane is transparent or translucent. This allows visualization of the surface vasculature over the brain.

The prominent vessels shown include the superior cerebral veins, a major component of the surface venous drainage of the cerebral hemispheres. The arachnoid granulations are clearly discernible on either side of the interhemispheric fissure.

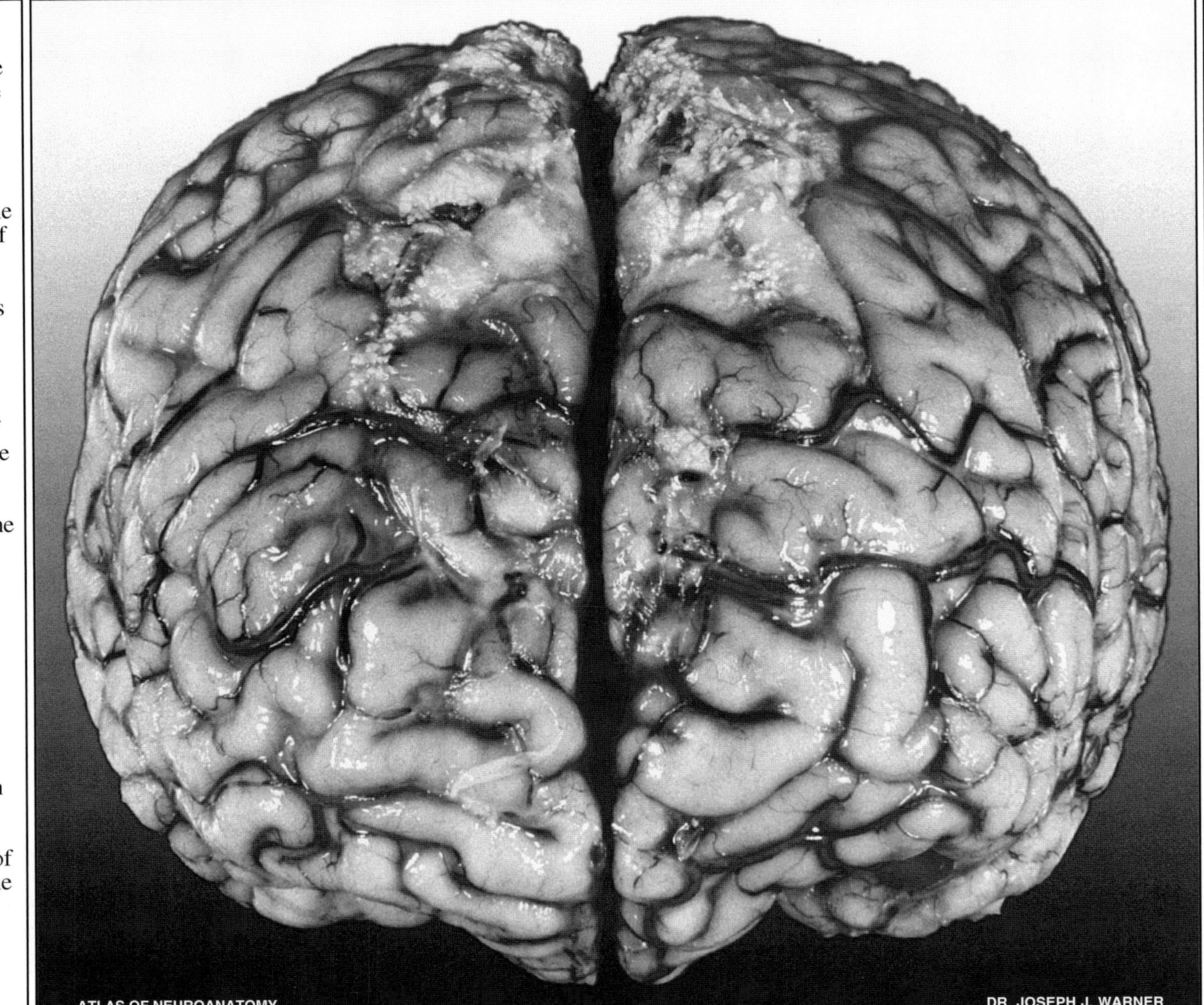

CEREBRAL HEMISPHERES, ROSTRAL ASPECT: VIEW ALIGNED WITH THE LONGITUDINAL AXIS OF THE BRAINSTEM

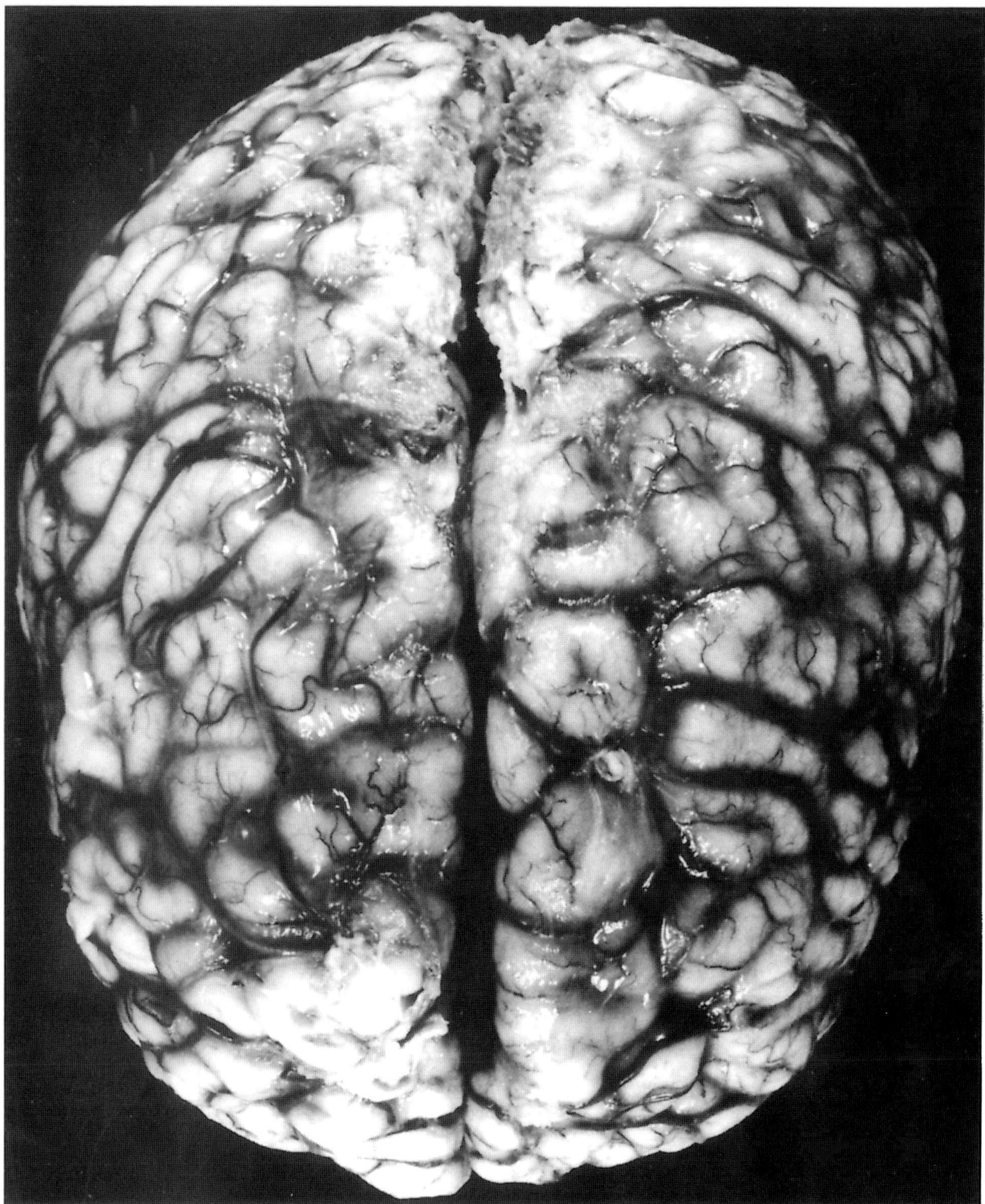

In this view, the brain has been rotated from a coronal perspective (along the rostrocaudal axis of the cerebral hemispheres). The axis of rotation is a line perpendicular to the sagittal plane. The rostral aspect of the brain has been rotated ventrally, thus demonstrating the dorsal surface of the frontal lobes in a view along the longitudinal axis of the brainstem. The arachnoid granulations are longitudinally distributed along each side of the interhemispheric fissure. Coursing subjacent to the arachnoid layer, distal branches of the anterior and middle cerebral arteries as well as superior cerebral veins are visible.

CAUDAL ASPECT OF THE BRAIN DEMONSTRATING THE CEREBRAL HEMISPHERES, CEREBELLUM, AND ROSTRAL CERVICAL SPINAL CORD

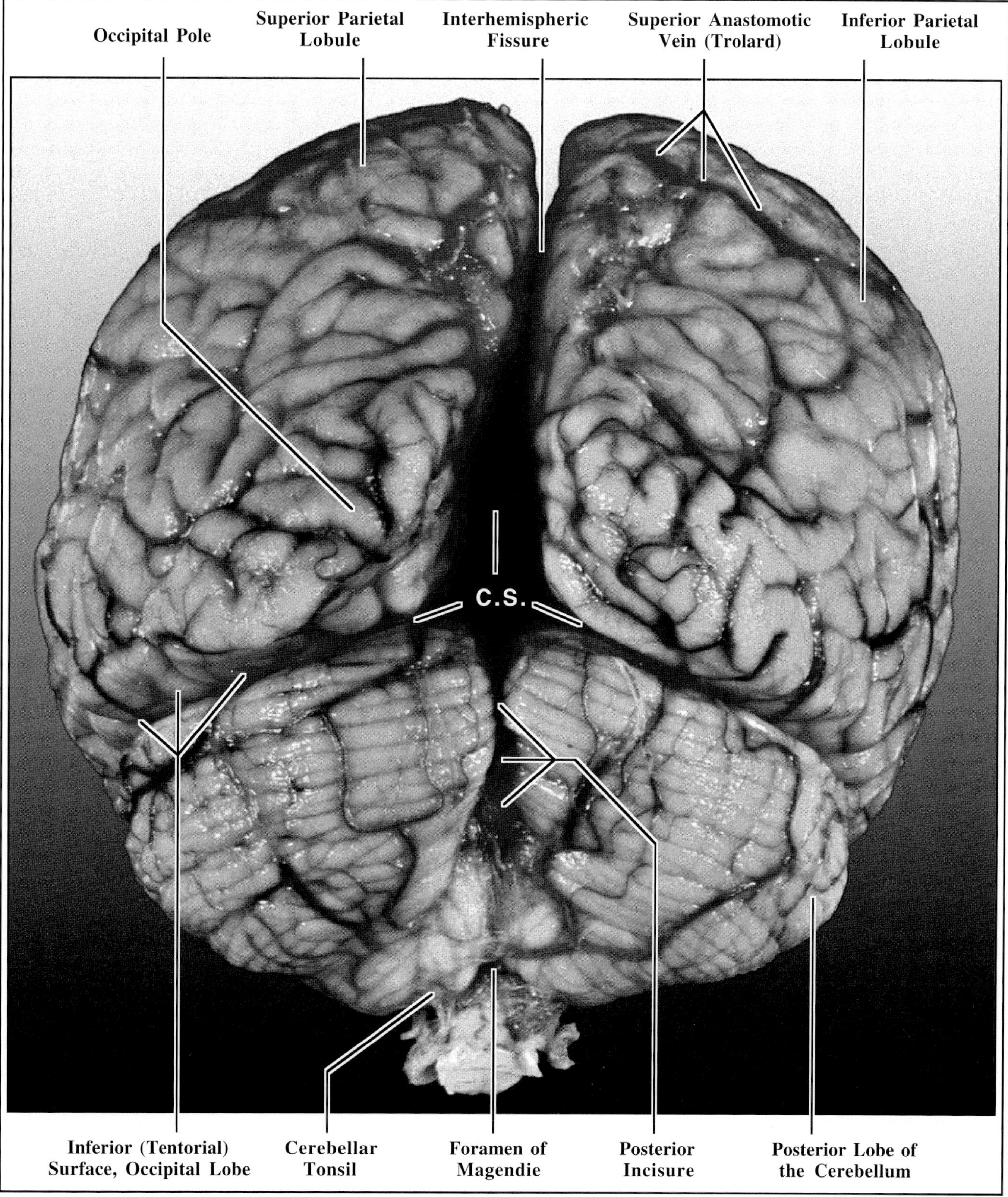

Located in the interhemispheric fissure, the falx cerebri extends between the superior sagittal, inferior sagittal, and straight sinuses. The falx cerebelli is located in the posterior incisure between the cerebellar hemispheres. The confluence of sinuses (C.S. in the figure) marks the junction between the superior sagittal, straight, and transverse sinuses. Each transverse sinus courses circumferentially around the tentorium cerebelli, then begins an inferior curve at the transition to the sigmoid sinus.

VENTRAL VIEW OF THE BRAIN, SPECIMEN RESECTED FROM THE CRANIUM WITH THE PITUITARY IN SITU: ARACHNOID MEMBRANE, VASCULATURE, AND DORSAL ASPECT OF THE DURA INTACT

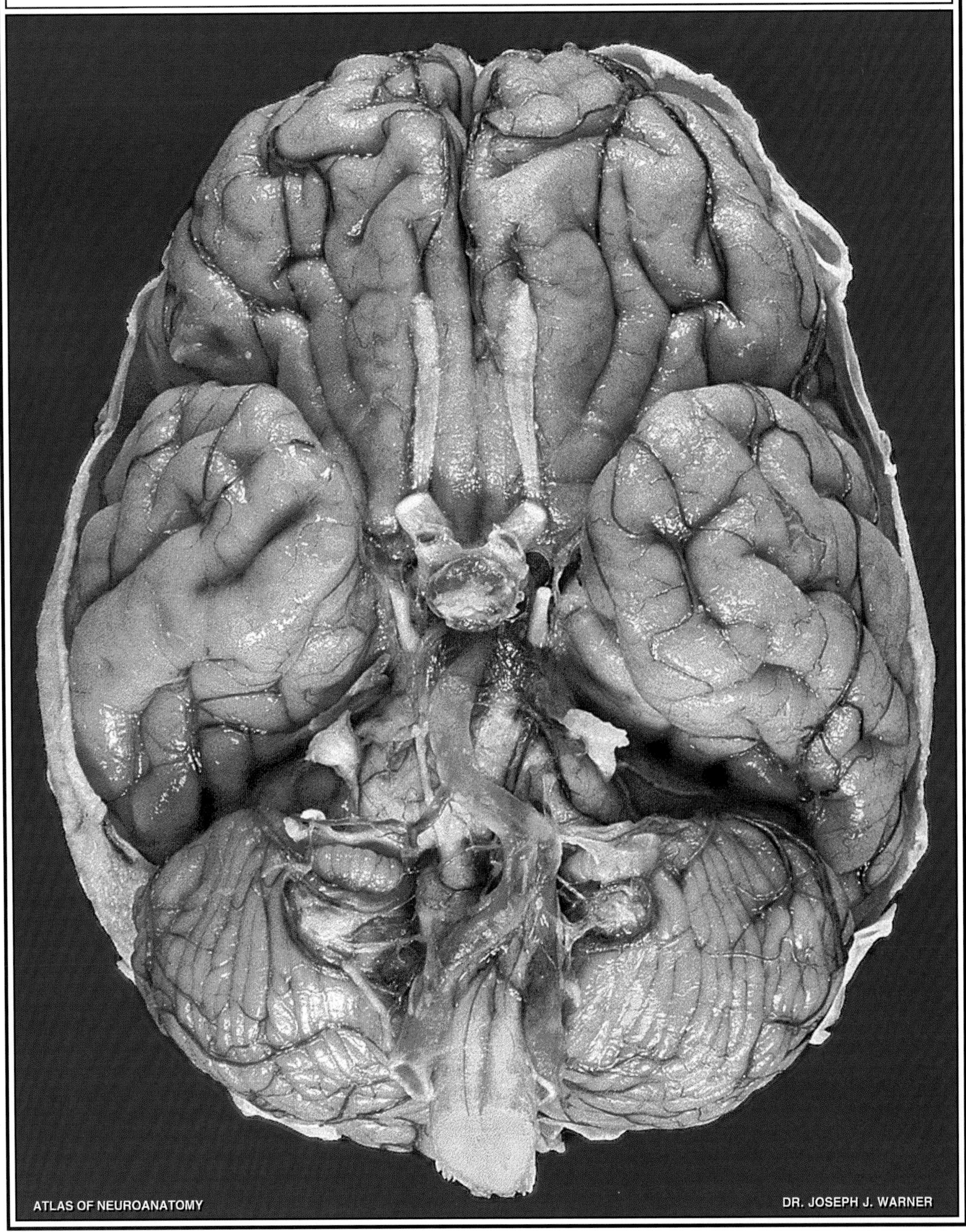

VENTRAL VIEW OF THE BRAIN, SPECIMEN RESECTED FROM THE CRANIUM WITH THE PITUITARY IN SITU: ARACHNOID MEMBRANE, VASCULATURE, AND DORSAL ASPECT OF THE DURA INTACT

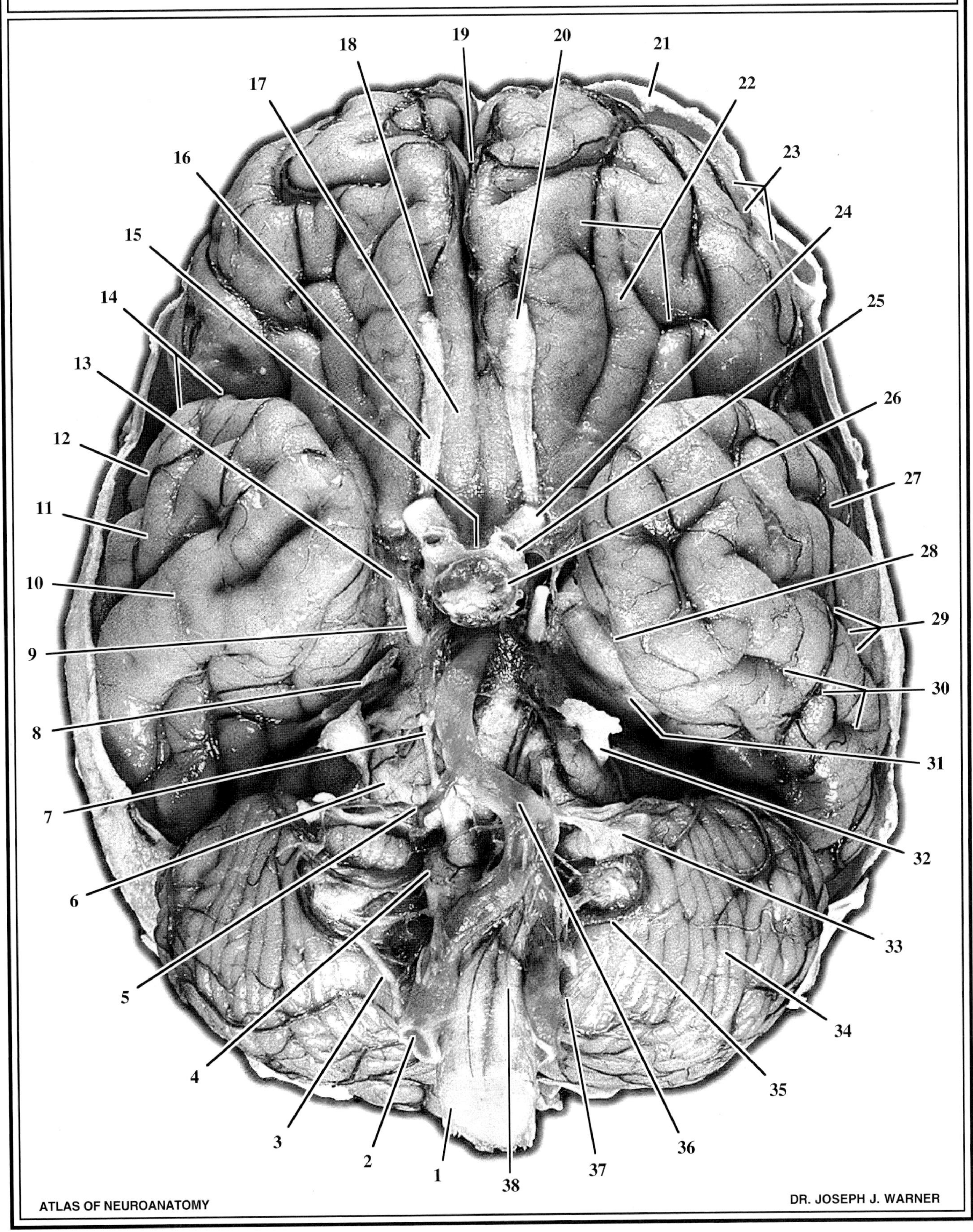

ATLAS OF NEUROANATOMY

DR. JOSEPH J. WARNER

VENTRAL VIEW OF THE BRAIN, SPECIMEN RESECTED FROM THE CRANIUM WITH THE PITUITARY IN SITU; ARACHNOID MEMBRANE, VASCULATURE, AND DORSAL ASPECT OF THE DURA INTACT: KEY TO NUMBERED STRUCTURES

KEY TO NUMBERED STRUCTURES

1. Rostral Cervical Spinal Cord
2. Vertebral Artery
3. Spinal Accessory (XI) Nerve
4. Inferior Olive
5. Anterior Inferior Cerebellar Artery
6. Middle Cerebellar Peduncle
7. Abducens (VI) Nerve
8. Resection Margin of Tentorium
9. Oculomotor (III) Nerve
10. Inferior Temporal Gyrus
11. Middle Temporal Gyrus
12. Superior Temporal Gyrus
13. Uncus
14. Anterior Temporal Pole (ventral to Sylvian Fissure)
15. Optic Chiasm
16. Olfactory Tract
17. Gyrus Rectus
18. Olfactory Sulcus
19. Interhemispheric Fissure
20. Olfactory Bulb
21. Dura
22. Orbitofrontal Gyri
23. Inferior Frontal Convolution
24. Optic (II) Nerve
25. Internal Carotid Artery
26. Pituitary Gland
27. Superior Temporal Sulcus
28. Collateral Sulcus
29. Middle Temporal Sulcus
30. Inferior Temporal Sulcus
31. Parahippocampal Gyrus
32. Trigeminal (V) Nerve
33. Flocculus
34. Posterior Lobe of the Cerebellum
35. Posterior Inferior Cerebellar Artery
36. Basilar Artery
37. Cerebellar Tonsil
38. Medullary Pyramid

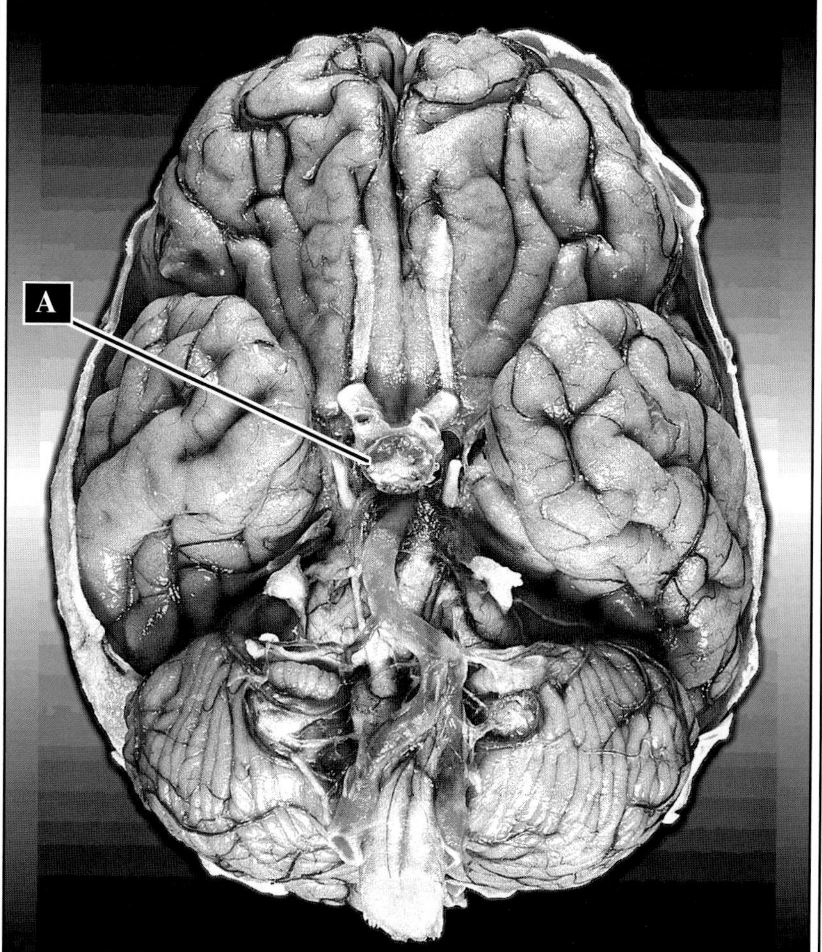

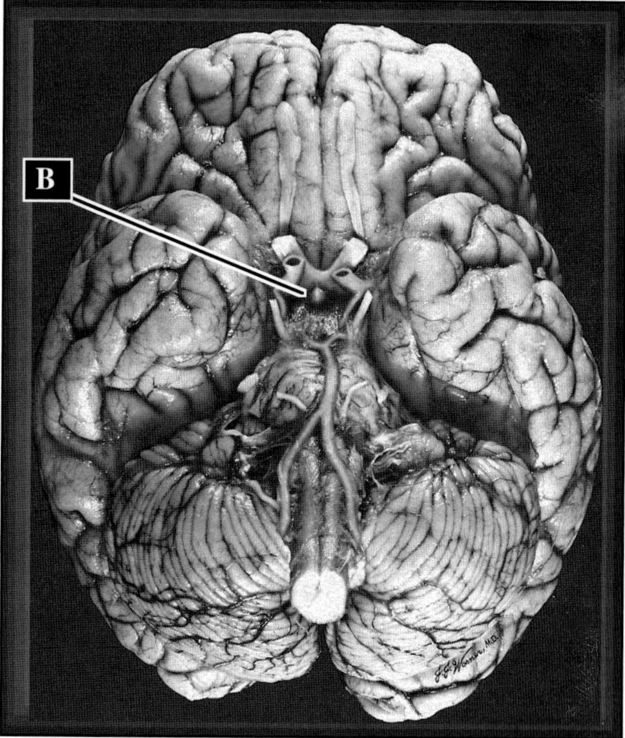

The anatomic variability between brains is readily appreciated upon examination of several specimens. This variability applies to the cerebrovasculature, gyral morphology, and major aspects of hemispheric configuration. Ventral and lateral temporal gyri demonstrate significant variations between brains, and their study should include comparative identification. (Several autopsy brains have been included in the coverage of major divisions and external morphology.) Compare the specimen with the pituitary in situ (A) with the ventral view in which the pituitary is removed (B). The position of the pituitary is such that tumors of the gland may compress the optic chiasm, resulting in a bitemporal hemianopsia or similar visual field deficit.

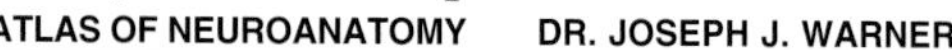

VENTRAL VIEW OF THE BRAIN, SPECIMEN RESECTED FROM THE CRANIUM WITH THE PITUITARY IN SITU: ARACHNOID MEMBRANE AND VASCULATURE INTACT

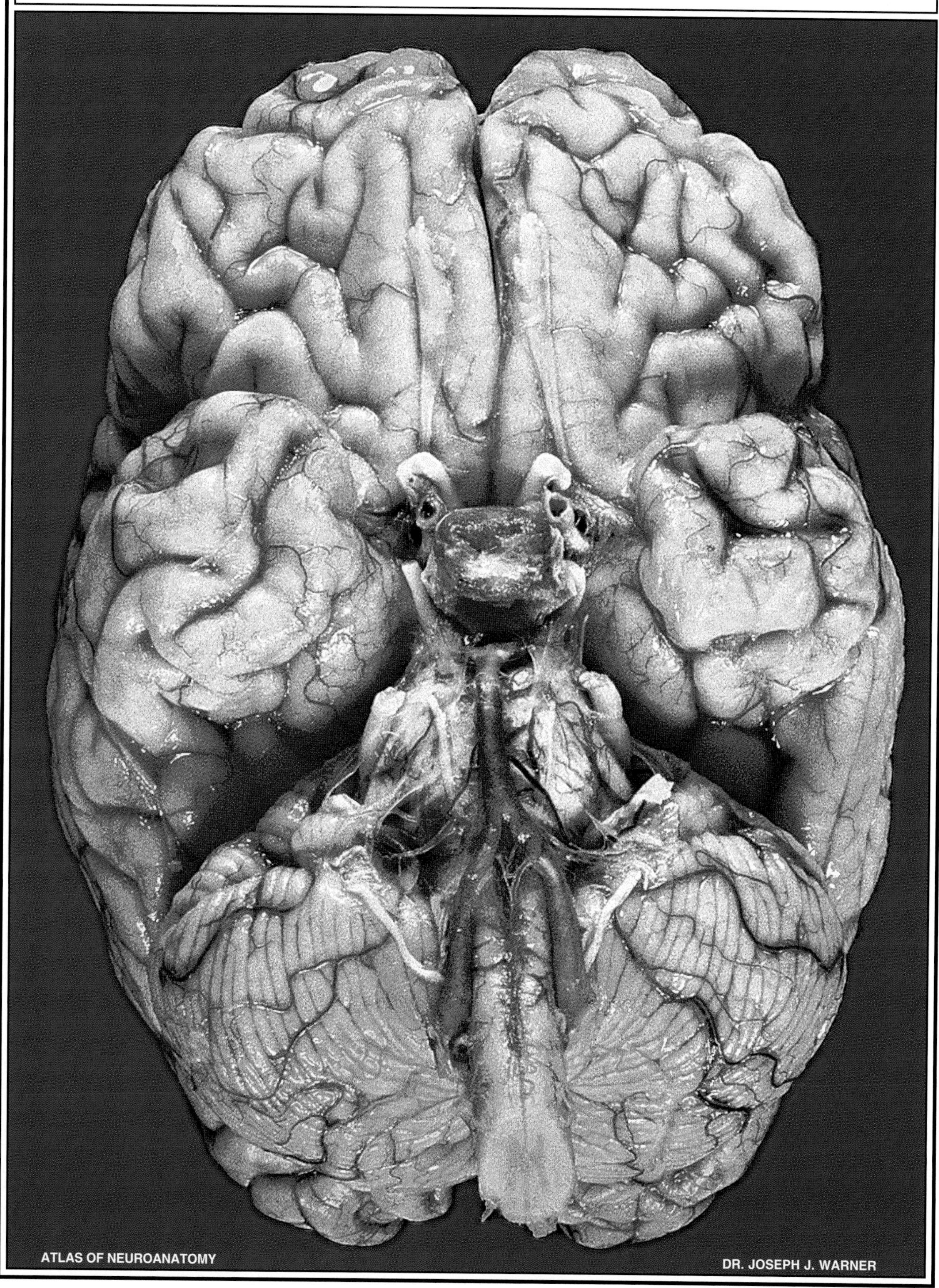

VENTRAL VIEW OF THE BRAIN, SPECIMEN RESECTED FROM THE CRANIUM WITH THE PITUITARY IN SITU: ARACHNOID MEMBRANE AND VASCULATURE INTACT

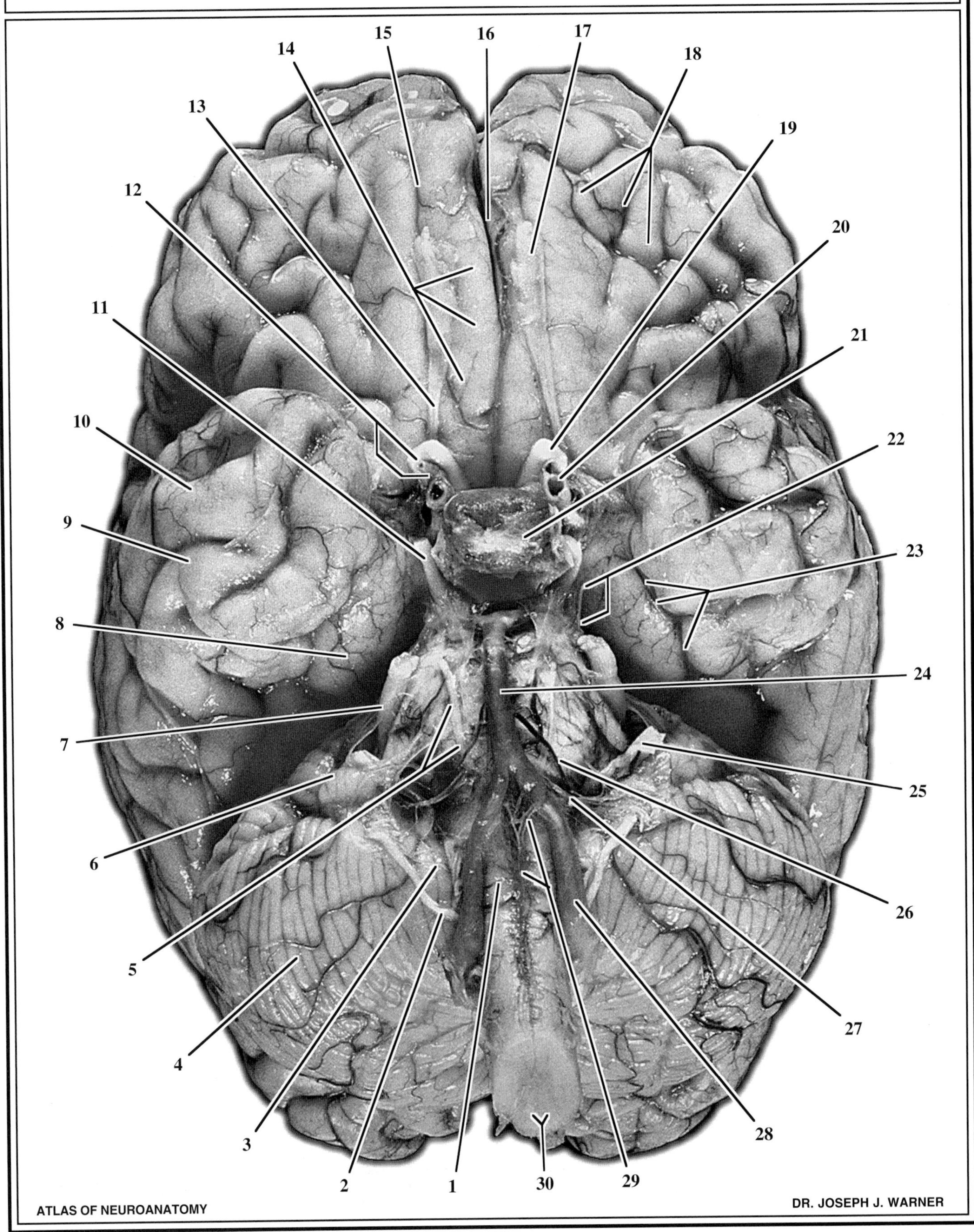

VENTRAL VIEW OF THE BRAIN, SPECIMEN RESECTED FROM THE CRANIUM WITH THE PITUITARY IN SITU; ARACHNOID MEMBRANE AND VASCULATURE INTACT: KEY TO NUMBERED STRUCTURES

KEY TO NUMBERED STRUCTURES

1. Medullary Pyramid
2. Spinal Accessory (XI) Nerve
3. Cerebellar Tonsil
4. Posterior Lobe of the Cerebellum
5. Abducens (VI) Nerve
6. Flocculus
7. Trigeminal (V) Nerve
8. Parahippocampal Gyrus
9. Inferior Temporal Gyrus
10. Middle Temporal Gyrus
11. Oculomotor (III) Nerve
12. Ophthalmic Artery**
13. Olfactory Tract
14. Gyrus Rectus
15. Olfactory Sulcus
16. Interhemispheric Fissure
17. Olfactory Bulb
18. Orbitofrontal Gyri
19. Optic Nerve
20. Internal Carotid Artery
21. Pituitary Gland
22. Trochlear (IV) Nerve
23. Collateral Sulcus
24. Basilar Artery
25. Facial (VII) Nerve
26. Anterior Inferior Cerebellar Artery
27. Posterior Inferior Cerebellar Artery
28. Vertebral Artery
29. Anterior Spinal Artery*
30. Fasciculus Gracilis and Cuneatus

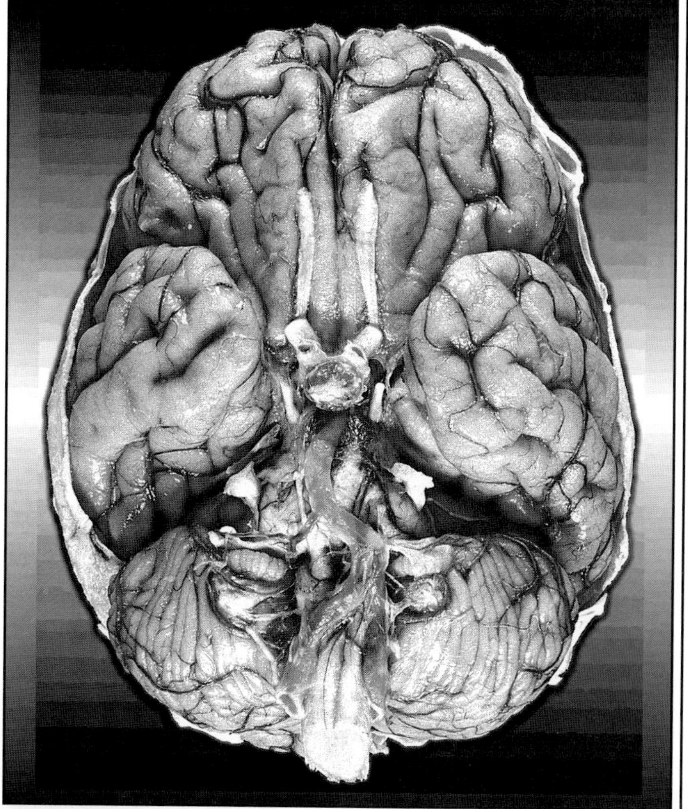

A comparison of these two specimens (ventral views, pituitary intact) demonstrates the marked variability characteristic of the vertebrobasilar arterial system. In the specimen with the dorsal aspect of the dura intact, the basilar artery is mildly tortuous, in contrast to the second specimen in which the basilar artery is relatively straight, following the midline ventral to the pons. The posterior inferior cerebellar arteries form prominent tonsillar loops in the first specimen, whereas in the second, these vessels are hypoplastic (although identifiable). *The anterior spinal artery is well visualized in the second specimen. Each vertebral artery gives rise to a vessel which joins its contralateral homologue. The confluence of these two vessels forms the single anterior spinal artery along the ventral median sulcus of the medulla. **Note the clear visualization of the right ophthalmic artery arising from the internal carotid ventral to the optic nerve. By dissection of the cavernous sinus (and sella turcica), the ophthalmic artery was preserved.

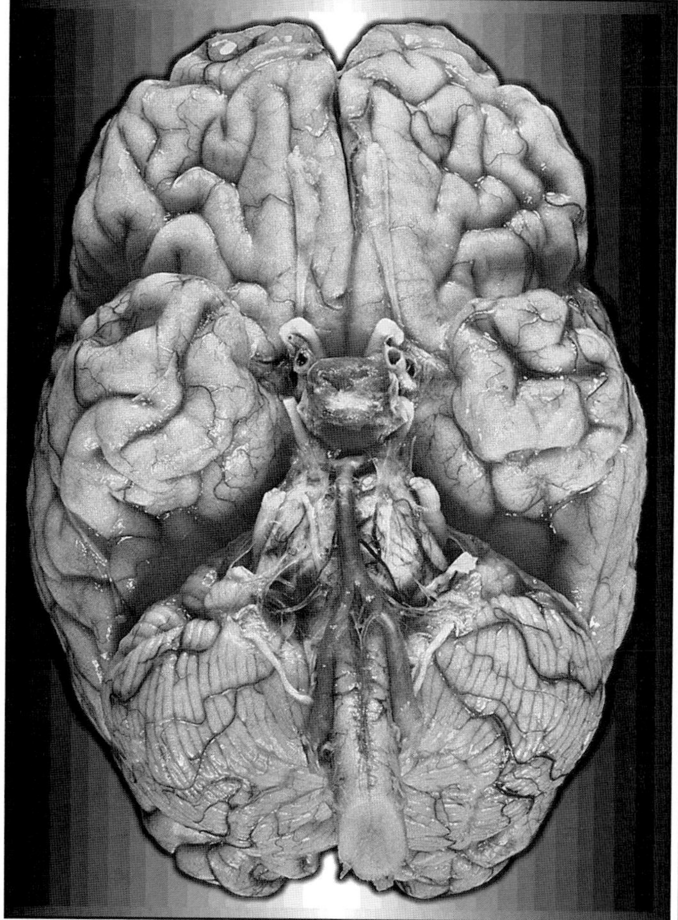

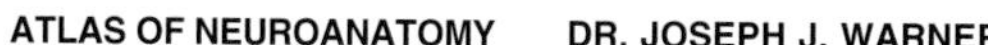

VENTRAL ASPECT OF THE BRAIN: VASCULATURE AND ARACHNOID MEMBRANE INTACT

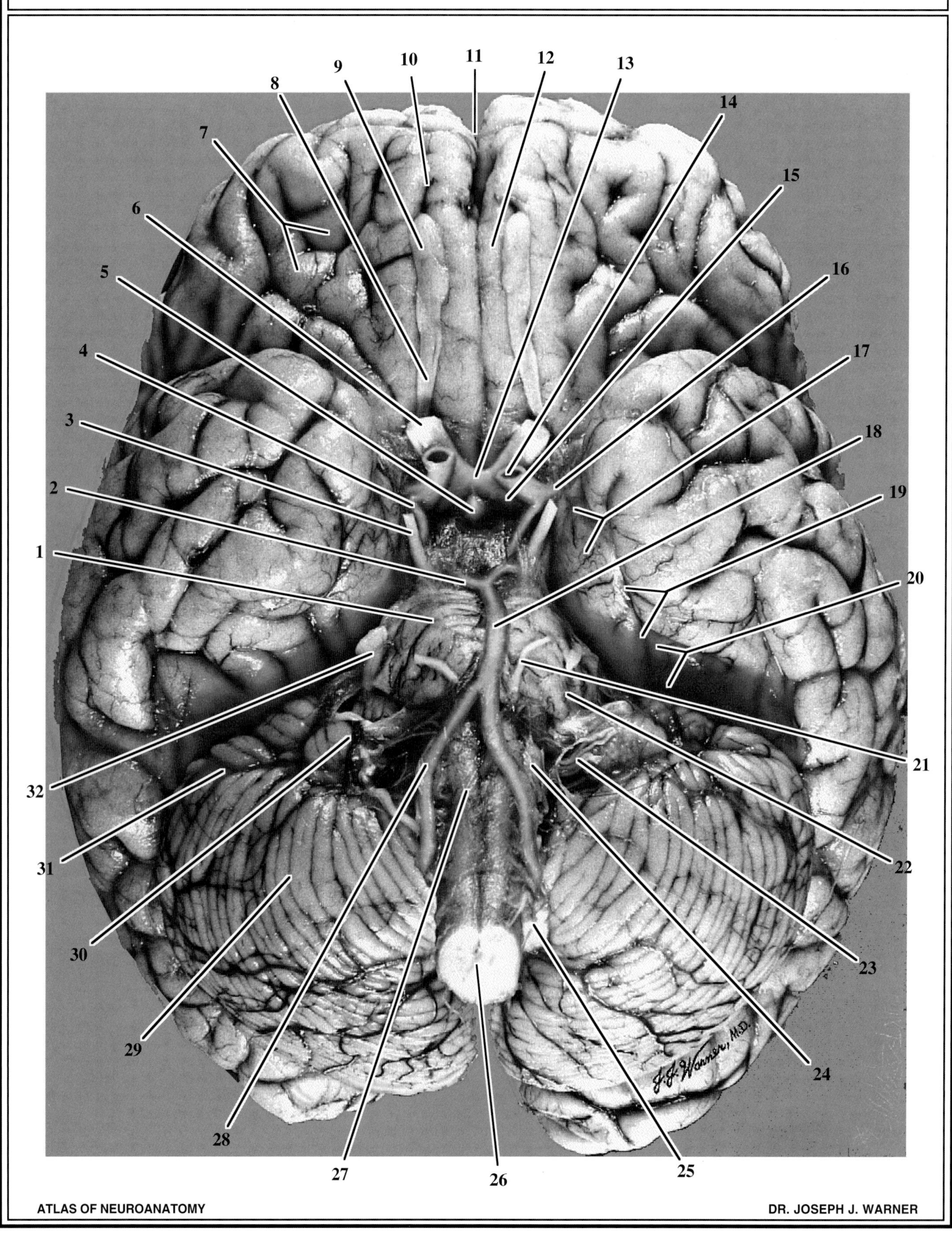

CEREBRAL HEMISPHERES, VENTRAL ASPECT: BRAINSTEM RESECTED (HORIZONTAL TRANSECTION THROUGH LEVEL OF THE DECUSSATION OF THE SUPERIOR CEREBELLAR PEDUNCLES)

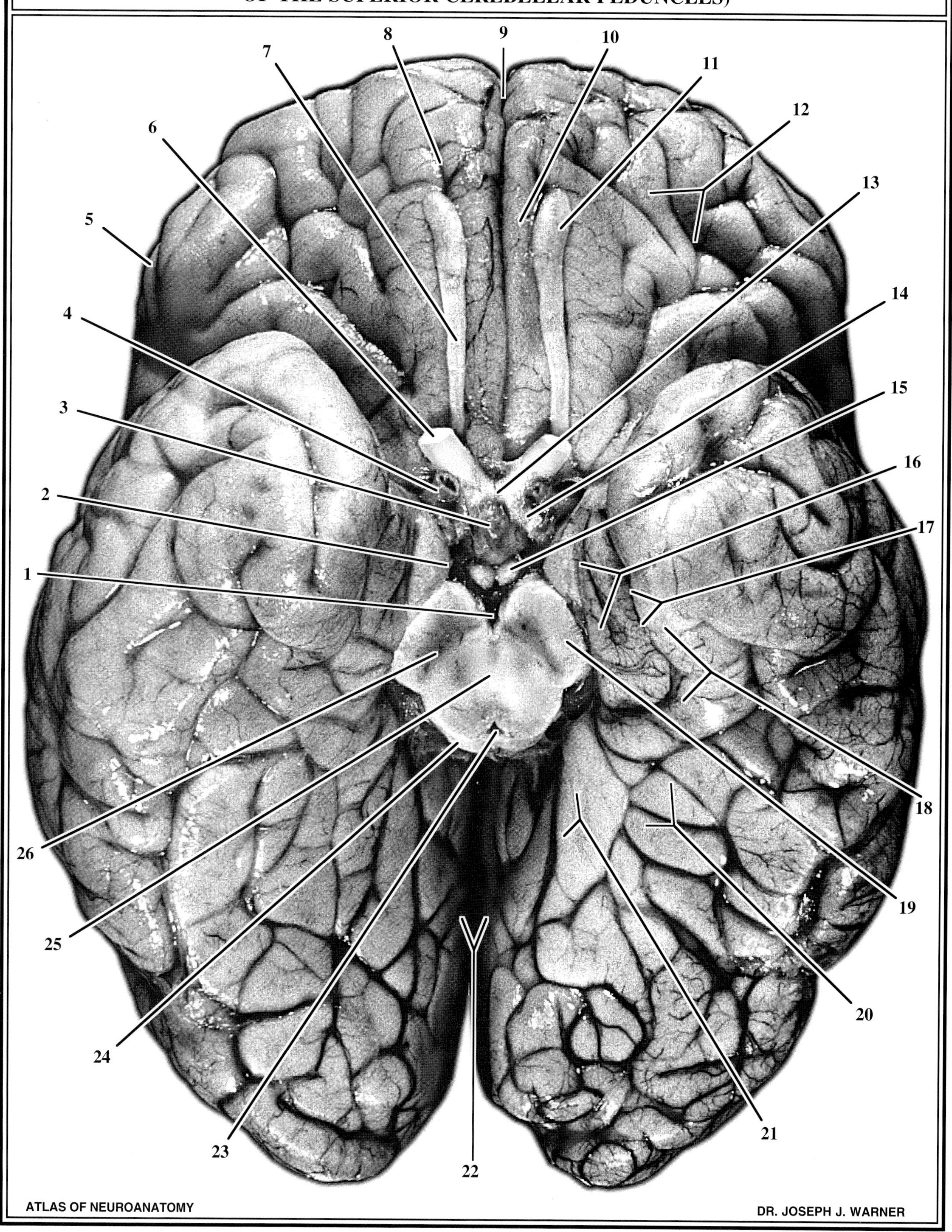

VENTRAL ASPECT OF THE BRAIN, VASCULATURE AND ARACHNOID INTACT: KEY TO NUMBERED STRUCTURES

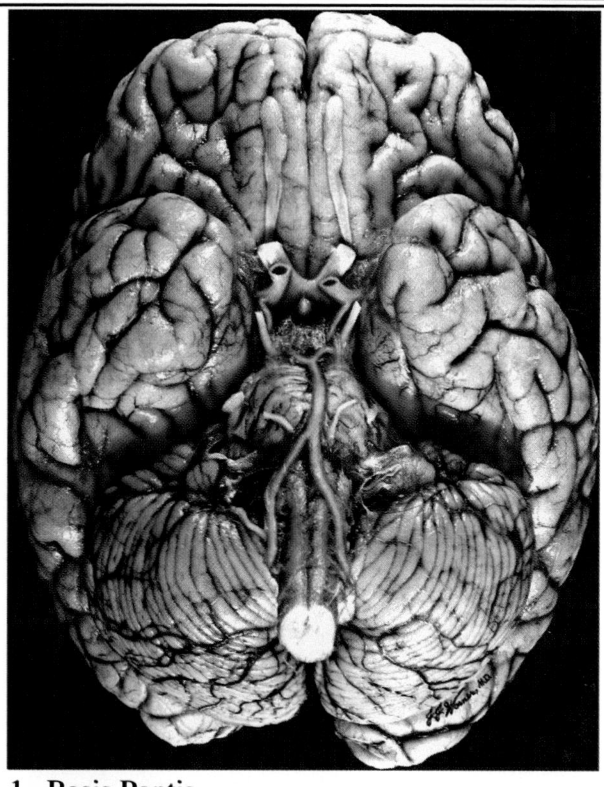

1. Basis Pontis
2. Superior Cerebellar Artery*
3. Oculomotor Nerve
4. Posterior Communicating Artery
5. Infundibulum
6. Optic Nerve
7. Orbitofrontal Gyri
8. Olfactory Tract
9. Olfactory Bulb
10. Olfactory Sulcus
11. Interhemispheric Fissure
12. Gyrus Rectus
13. Optic Chiasm
14. Internal Carotid Artery
15. Optic Tract
16. Internal Carotid Artery**
17. Parahippocampal Gyrus
18. Basilar Artery
19. Collateral Sulcus
20. Fusiform Gyrus
21. Abducens (VI) Nerve
22. Middle Cerebellar Peduncle
23. Vagus (X) Nerve
24. Inferior Olive
25. Cerebellar Tonsil
26. Pyramidal Decussation
27. Medullary Pyramid
28. Vertebral Artery
29. Posterior Lobe of Cerebellum
30. Flocculus (Dorsal to VII and VIII Nerves)
31. Posterolateral Fissure of the Cerebellum
32. Trigeminal (V) Nerve

* The posterior cerebral artery is covered by arachnoid membrane in this view.

** Proximal to the trifurcation into branches of the middle cerebral artery.

CEREBRAL HEMISPHERES, VENTRAL ASPECT, BRAINSTEM RESECTED (HORIZONTAL TRANSECTION THROUGH LEVEL OF THE DECUSSATION OF THE SUPERIOR CEREBELLAR PEDUNCLES): KEY TO NUMBERED STRUCTURES

1. Interpeduncular Fossa
2. Uncus
3. Infundibulum
4. Internal Carotid Artery
5. Inferior Frontal Convolution
6. Optic Nerve
7. Olfactory Tract
8. Olfactory Sulcus
9. Interhemispheric Fissure
10. Gyrus Rectus
11. Olfactory Bulb
12. Orbitofrontal Gyri
13. Optic Chiasm
14. Optic Tract
15. Mammillary Body
16. Parahippocampal Gyrus
17. Collateral Sulcus
18. Fusiform Gyrus
19. Cerebral Peduncle
20. Fusiform Gyrus
21. Lingular Gyrus
22. Area 17 Calcarine Cortex (banks of the Calcarine Fissure)
23. Aqueduct of Sylvius
24. Inferior Colliculus
25. Decussation of the Superior Cerebellar Peduncles
26. Substantia Nigra

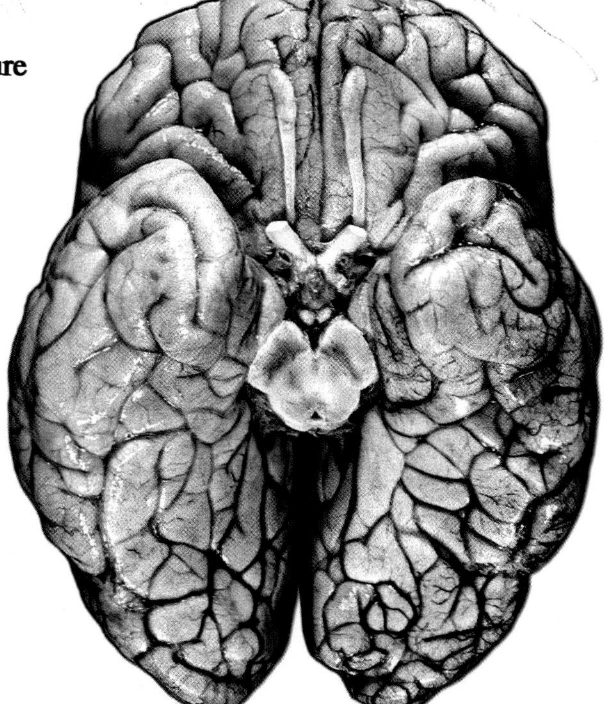

VENTRAL ASPECT OF THE BRAIN: ARACHNOID MEMBRANE RESECTED, DEMONSTRATING THE CIRCLE OF WILLIS

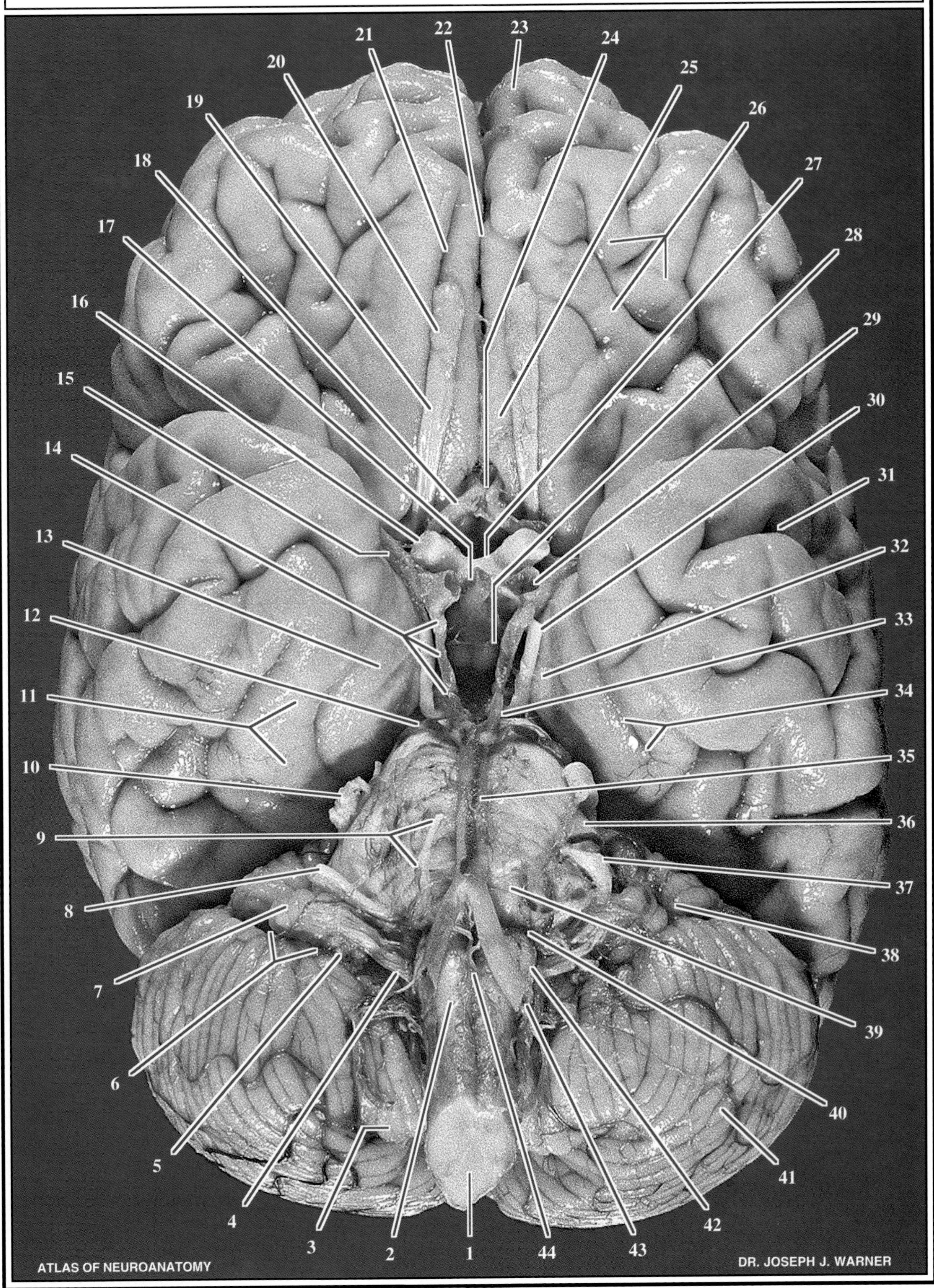

VENTRAL ASPECT OF THE BRAIN: ARACHNOID RESECTED, DEMONSTRATING THE CIRCLE OF WILLIS

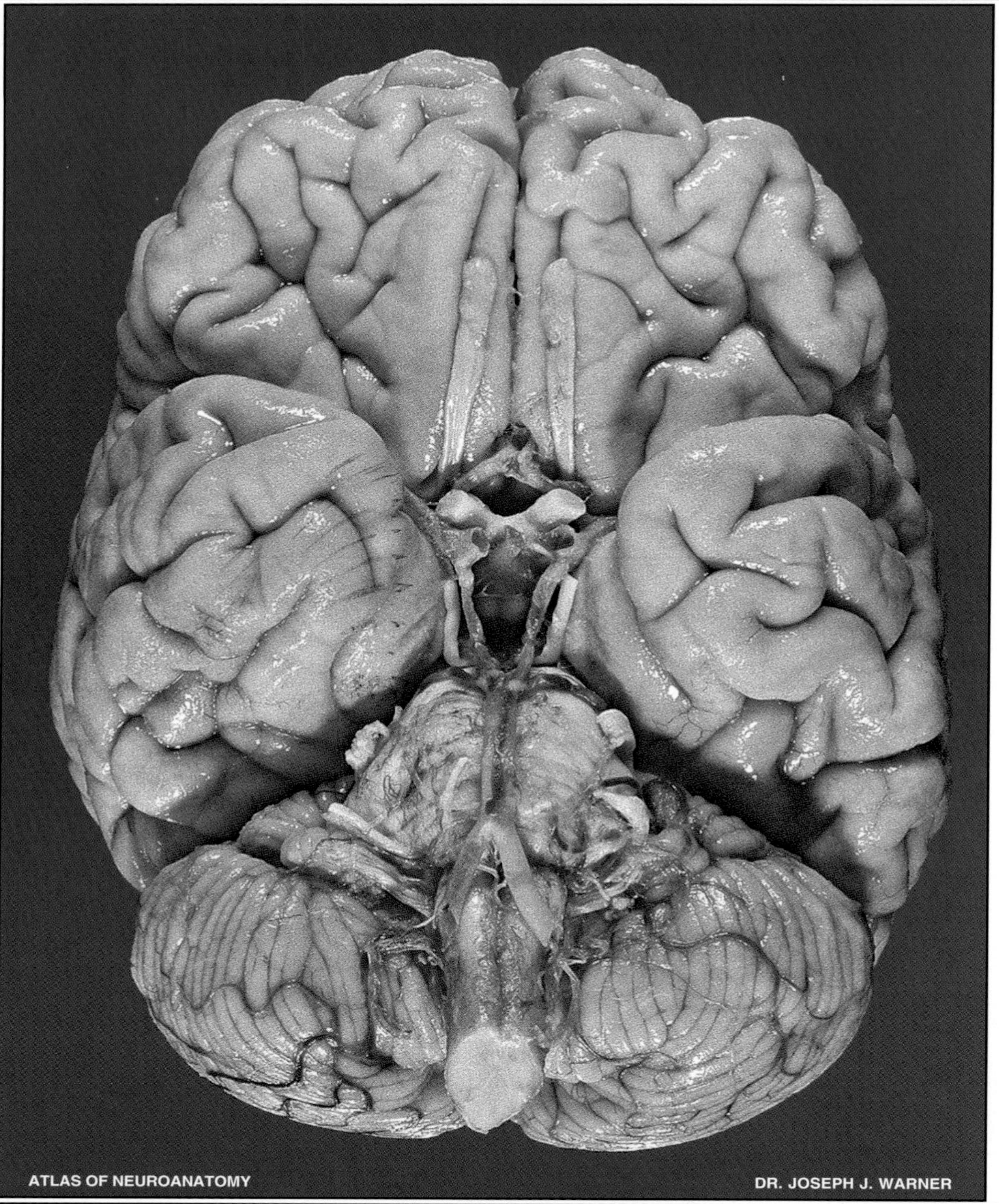

ATLAS OF NEUROANATOMY

DR. JOSEPH J. WARNER

KEY TO NUMBERED STRUCTURES

1. Rostral Cervical Spinal Cord
2. Medullary Pyramid
3. Cerebellar Tonsil
4. Vagus (X) Nerve
5. Choroid Plexus adjacent to the Foramen of Luschka
6. Posterolateral Fissure
7. Flocculus
8. Facial (VII) Nerve
9. Abducens (VI) Nerve
10. Trigeminal (V) Nerve
11. Fusiform Gyrus
12. Superior Cerebellar Artery
13. Parahippocampal Gyrus
14. Posterior Communicating Artery
15. Middle Cerebral Artery
16. Optic (II) Nerve
17. Pituitary Stalk
18. Anterior Cerebral Artery
19. Olfactory Tract
20. Olfactory Bulb
21. Olfactory Sulcus
22. Interhemispheric Fissure
23. Frontal Pole
24. Anterior Communicating Artery
25. Gyrus Rectus
26. Orbitofrontal Gyri
27. Optic Chiasm
28. Mammillary Body
29. Internal Carotid Artery
30. Oculomotor (III) Nerve
31. Superior Temporal Sulcus
32. Uncus
33. Junction of the Posterior Cerebral and Posterior Communicating Arteries
34. Collateral Sulcus
35. Basilar Artery
36. Middle Cerebellar Peduncle
37. Vestibulocochlear (VIII) Nerve
38. Anterior Lobe of the Cerebellum
39. Basis Pontis
40. Pontomedullary Sulcus
41. Posterior Lobe of the Cerebellum
42. Inferior Olive
43. Vertebral Artery
44. Anterior Spinal Artery

VENTROANTERIOR ASPECT OF THE BRAIN: VIEW ALONG AN AXIS PARALLEL TO THE PLANE OF THE SYLVIAN FISSURE

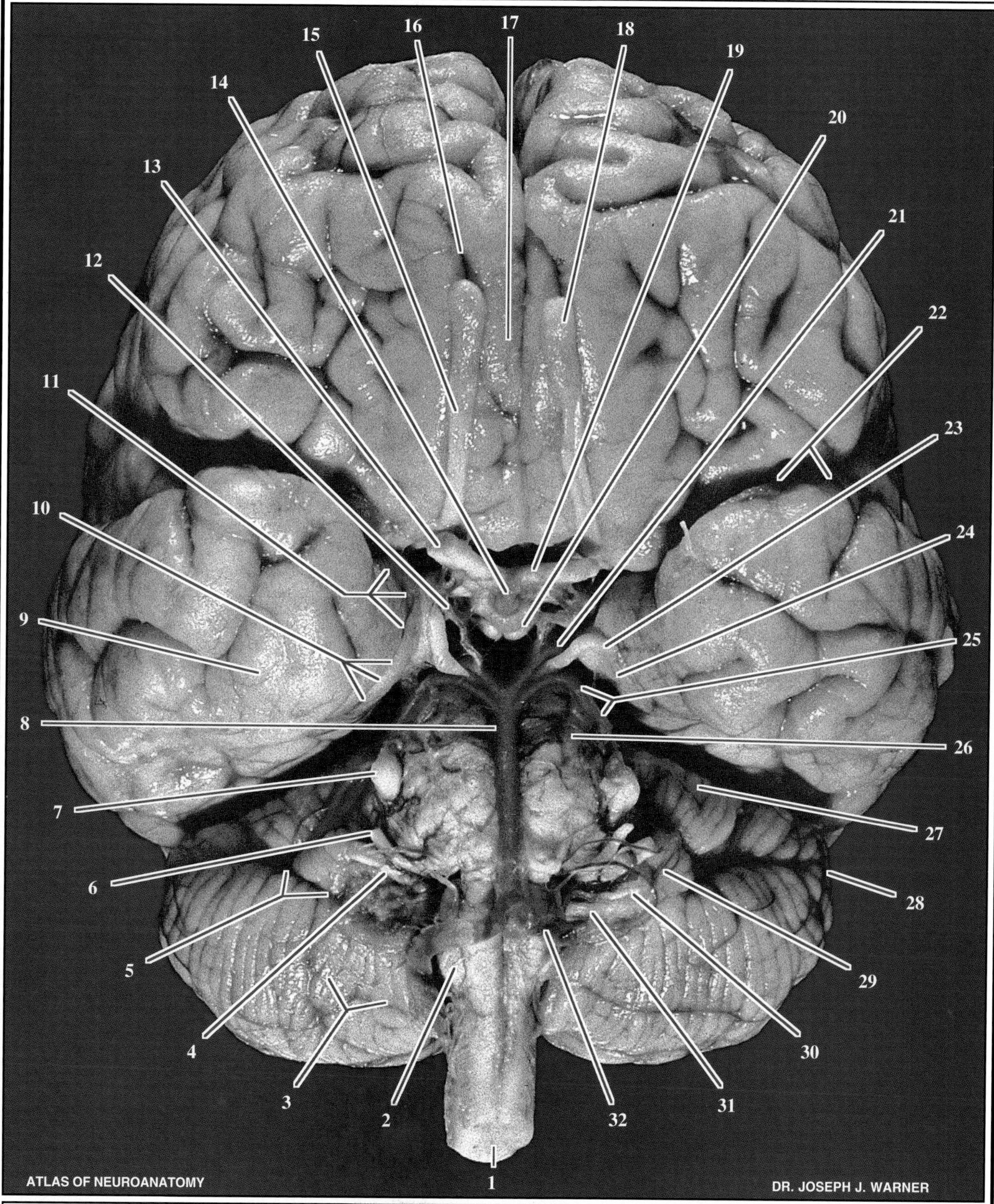

This perspective of the ventral aspect of the brainstem provides a view of the oculomotor (III) nerves as they course between the superior cerebellar and posterior cerebral arteries. The posterolateral fissure is clearly demonstrated in relation to the flocculus and the anterior and posterior lobes of the cerebellum.

VENTROANTERIOR ASPECT OF THE BRAIN; VIEW ALONG AN AXIS PARALLEL TO THE PLANE OF THE SYLVIAN FISSURE: KEY TO STRUCTURES AND ORIENTATION

KEY TO NUMBERED STRUCTURES

1. Rostral Cervical Spinal Cord
2. Inferior Olive
3. Posterior Lobe of the Cerebellum
4. Vestibulocochlear (VIII) Nerve
5. Posterolateral Fissure
6. Facial (VII) Nerve
7. Trigeminal (V) Nerve
8. Basilar Artery
9. Inferior Temporal Gyrus
10. Collateral Sulcus
11. Rhinal Fissure
12. Posterior Communicating Artery
13. Optic (II) Nerve
14. Pituitary Stalk
15. Olfactory Tract
16. Olfactory Sulcus
17. Gyrus Rectus
18. Olfactory Bulb
19. Optic Chiasm
20. Mammillary Body
21. Posterior Cerebral Artery
22. Sylvian Fissure
23. Oculomotor (III) Nerve
24. Parahippocampal Gyrus
25. Superior Cerebellar Artery
26. Basis Pontis
27. Anterior Lobe of the Cerebellum
28. Horizontal Fissure of the Cerebellum
29. Flocculus
30. Glossopharyngeal (IX) Nerve
31. Vagus (X) Nerve
32. Vertebral Artery

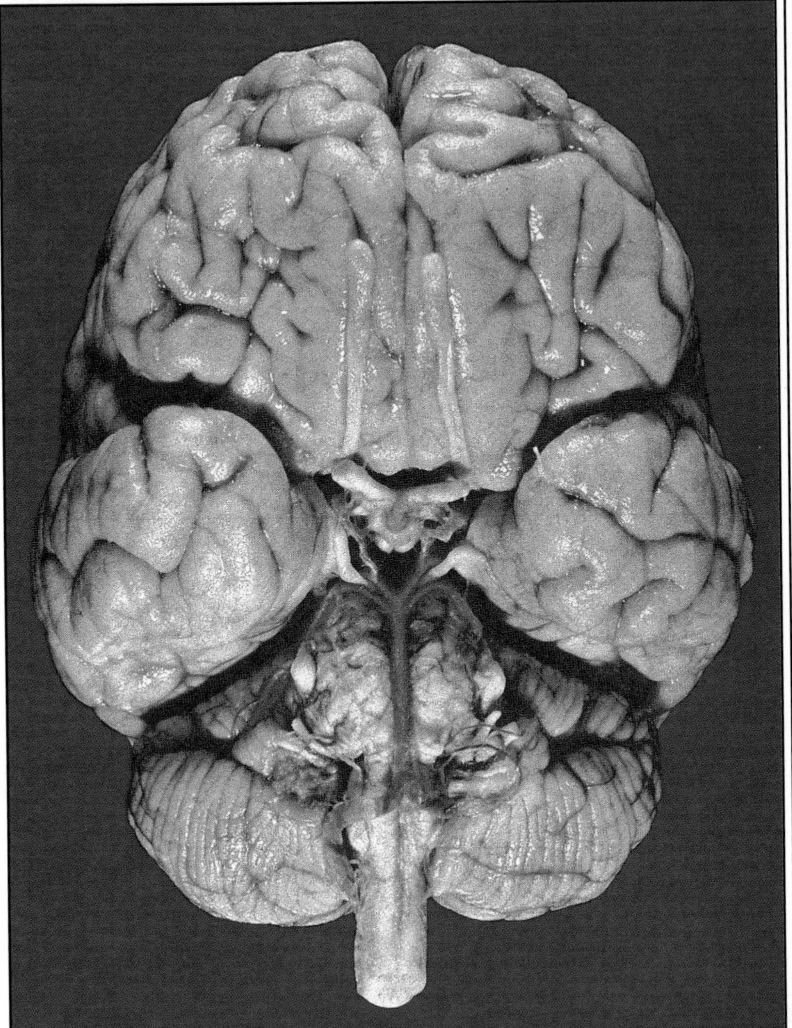

The collateral sulcus is located between the parahippocampal and fusiform gyri. This sulcus extends rostrally and is contiguous with the rhinal fissure, which curves laterally around the temporal pole to approach the Sylvian fissure. The rhinal fissure is generally not visualized from the ventral perspective. Orientation of the specimen such that it is viewed along an axis parallel to the Sylvian fissure (as mapped on the lateral view of the brain) allows the collateral sulcus to be followed rostrally to the rhinal fissure. Examination of the ventromedial aspect of the temporal lobe also demonstrates this anatomic relationship.

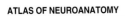

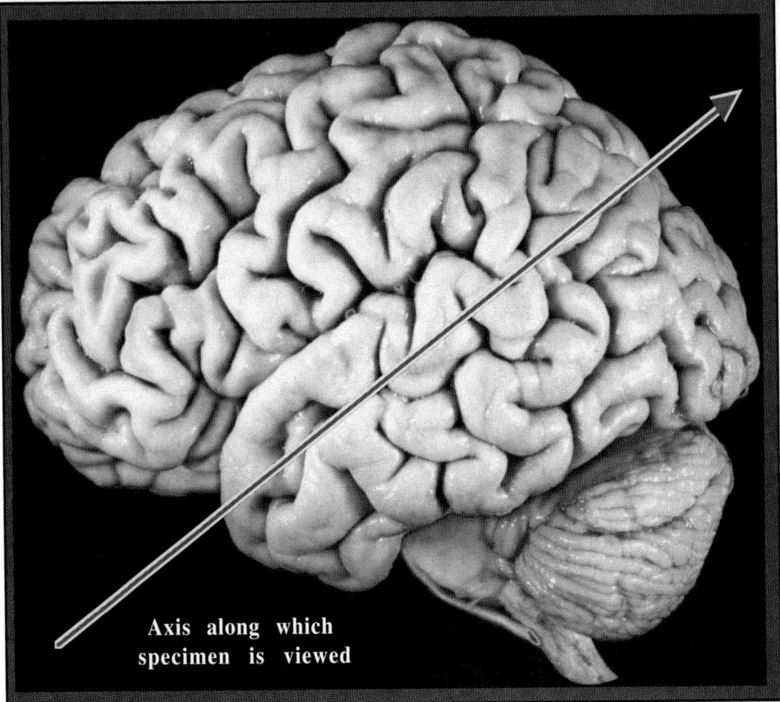

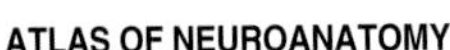

RIGHT VENTROLATERAL VIEW OF THE BRAIN: ARACHNOID AND VASCULATURE INTACT

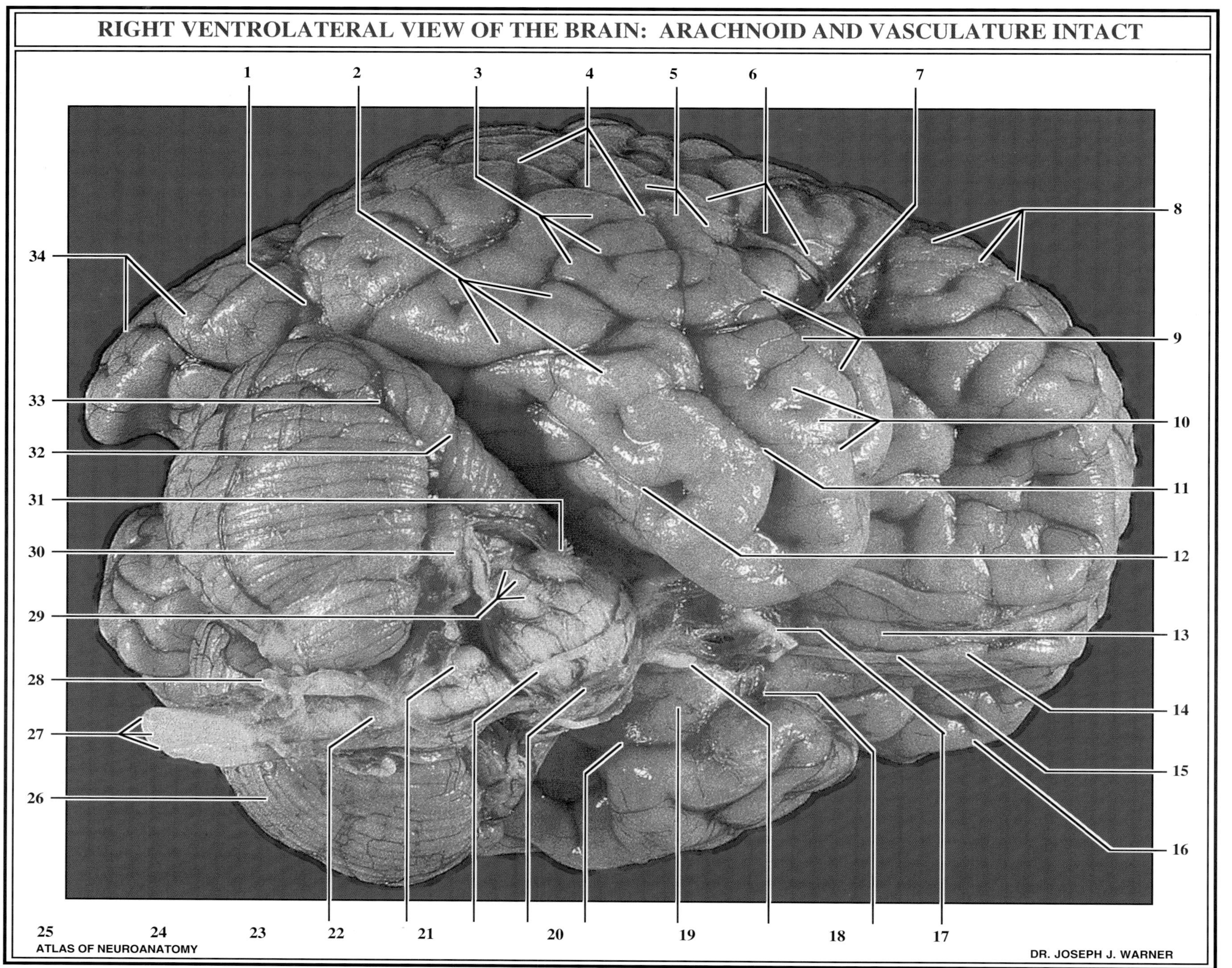

DR. JOSEPH J. WARNER

RIGHT VENTROLATERAL VIEW OF THE BRAIN; ARACHNOID AND VASCULATURE INTACT: KEY TO NUMBERED STRUCTURES

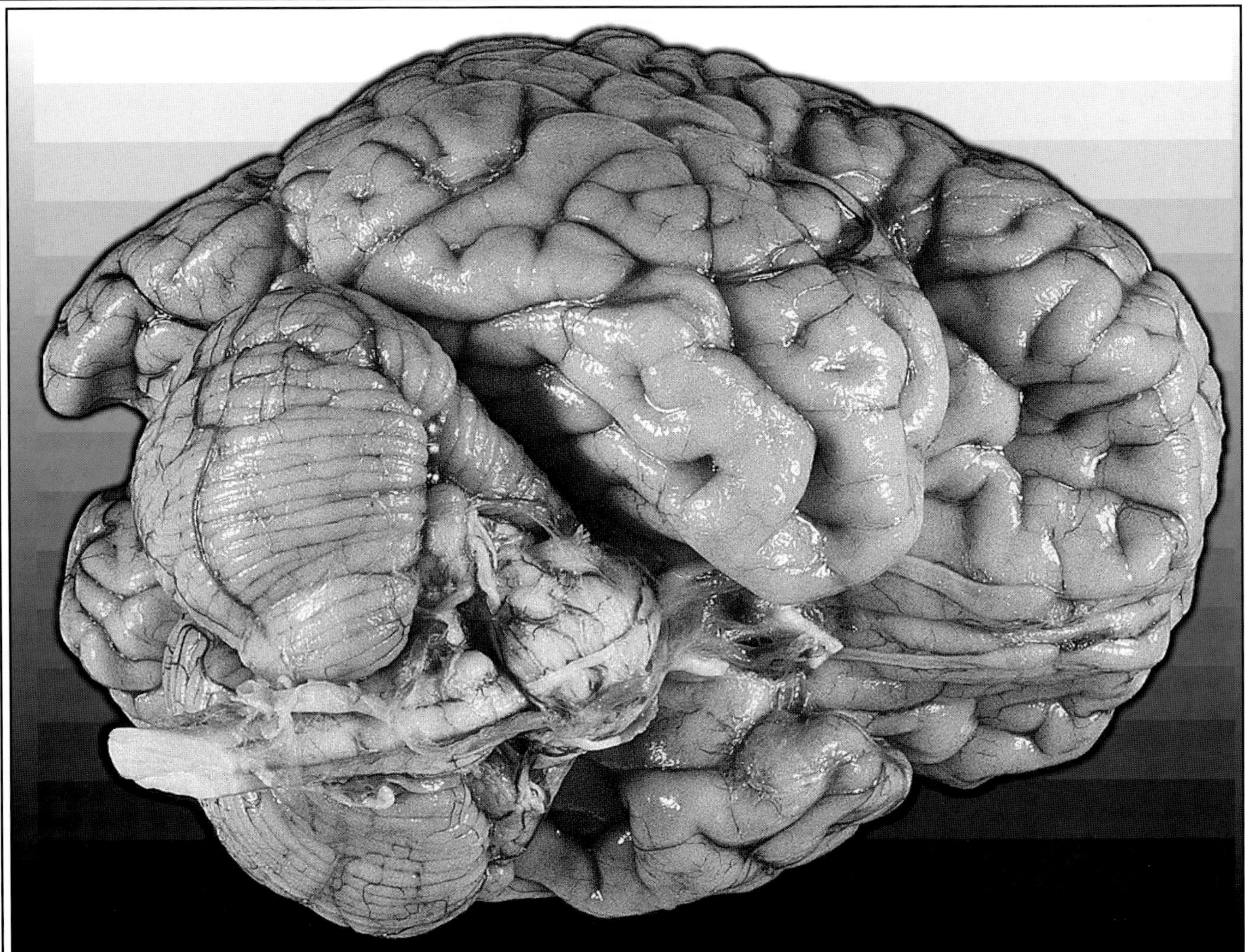

KEY TO NUMBERED STRUCTURES

1. Preoccipital Notch
2. Inferior Temporal Gyrus
3. Middle Temporal Gyrus
4. Superior Temporal Sulcus
5. Superior Temporal Gyrus
6. Sylvian Fissure
7. Superior Temporal Gyrus
8. Inferior Frontal Convolution
9. Superior Temporal Sulcus
10. Middle Temporal Gyrus
11. Middle Temporal Sulcus
12. Inferior Temporal Sulcus
13. Gyrus Rectus
14. Olfactory Bulb
15. Olfactory Tract
16. Orbitofrontal Gyri
17. Optic (II) Nerve
18. Rhinal Fissure
19. Oculomotor (III) Nerve
20. Parahippocampal Gyrus
21. Collateral Sulcus
22. Basilar Artery
23. Abducens (VI) Nerve
24. Inferior Olive
25. Medullary Pyramid
26. Posterior Lobe of the Cerebellum
27. Dorsal Columns (Fasciculus Gracilis and Cuneatus) of the Rostral Cervical Spinal Cord
28. Vertebral Artery
29. Middle Cerebellar Peduncle
30. Flocculus
31. Trigeminal (V) Nerve
32. Primary Fissure of the Cerebellum
33. Horizontal Fissure of the Cerebellum
34. Occipital Lobe

MIDLINE SAGITTAL SECTION OF THE BRAIN, COMPLETE: ARACHNOID AND CEREBROVASCULATURE INTACT

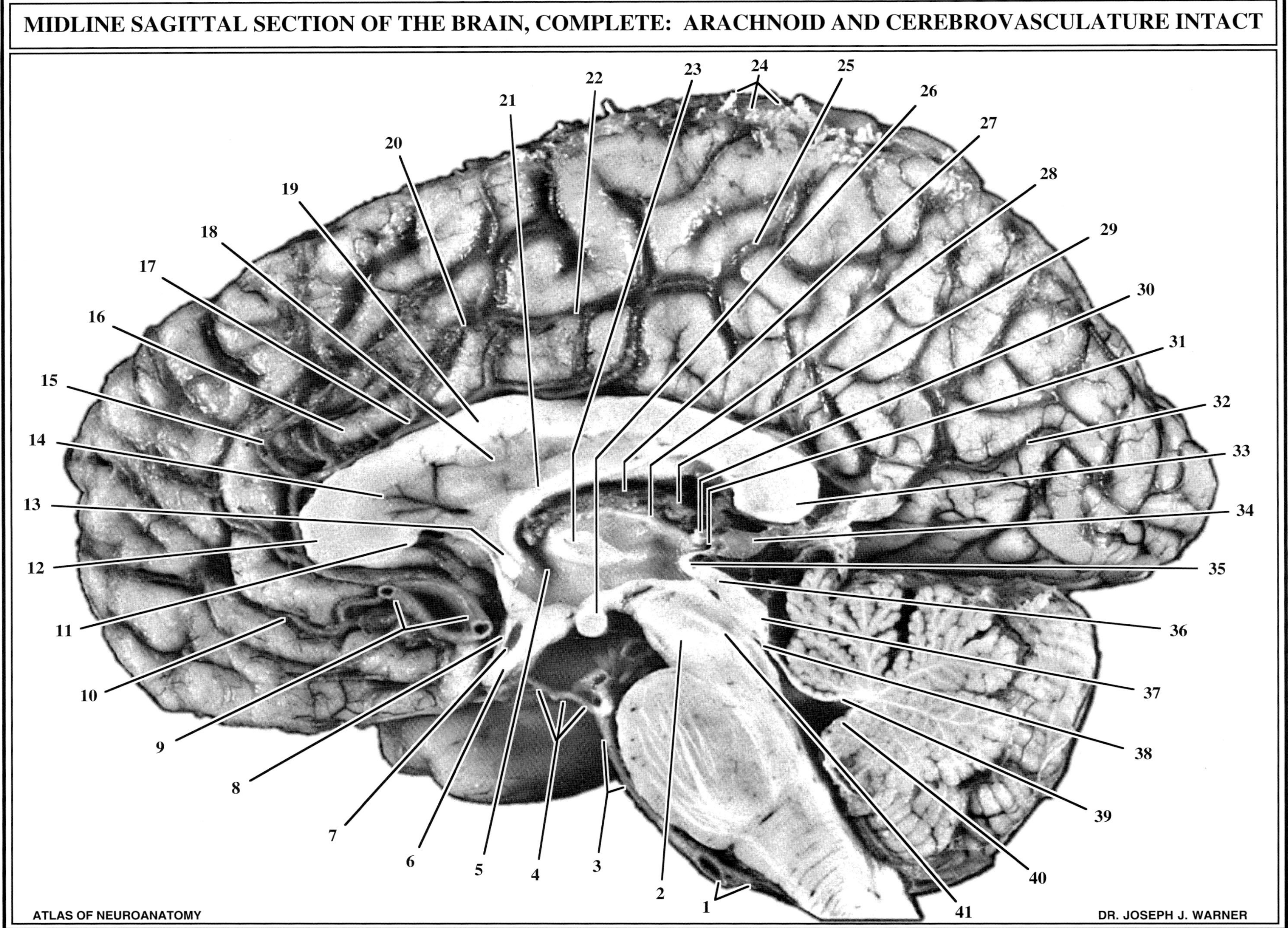

DR. JOSEPH J. WARNER

MIDLINE SAGITTAL SECTION OF THE BRAIN, COMPLETE; ARACHNOID AND CEREBROVASCULATURE INTACT: KEY TO NUMBERED STRUCTURES

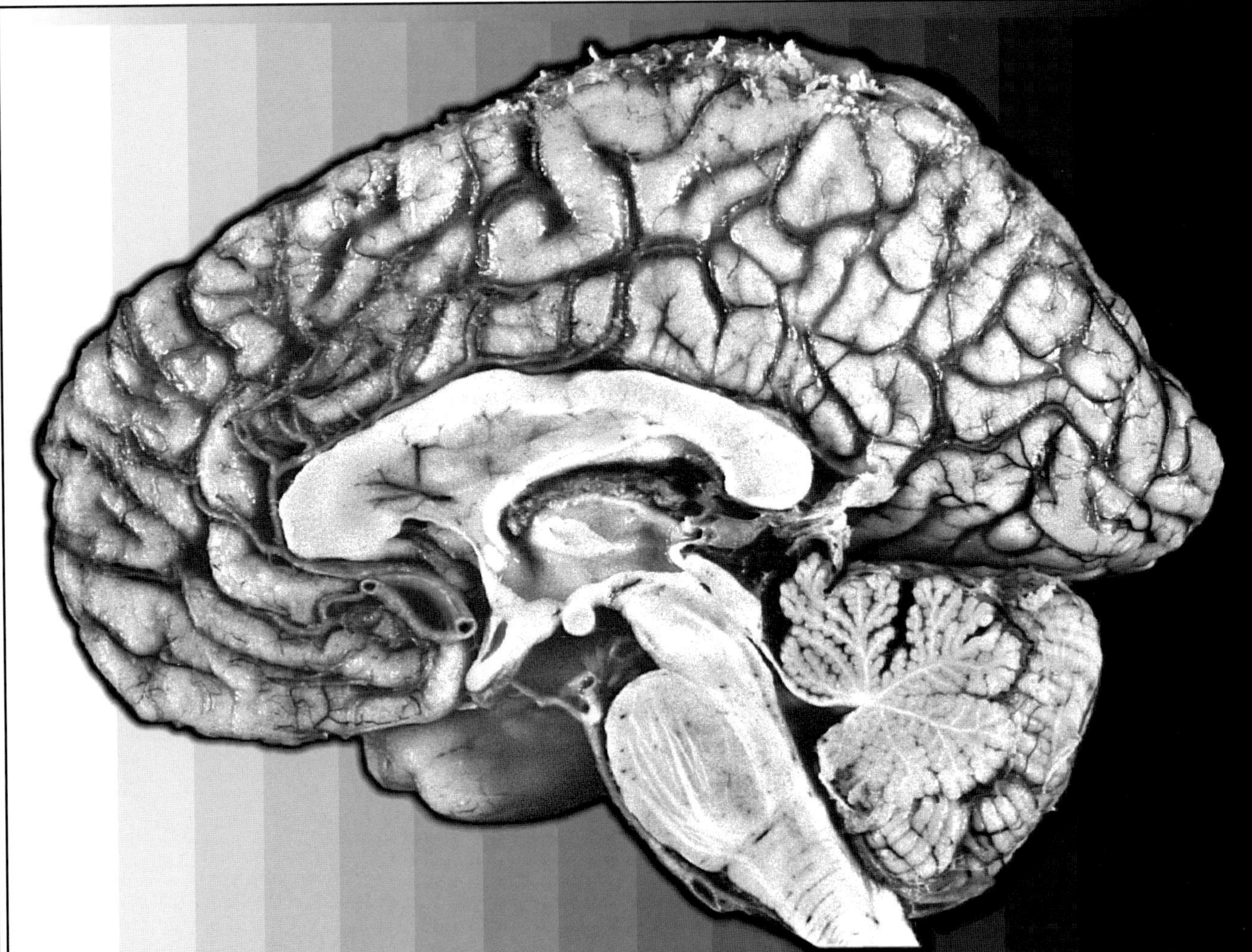

1. Vertebral Arteries
2. Decussation of the Superior Cerebellar Peduncles
3. Basilar Artery
4. Posterior Communicating Artery
5. Foramen of Monro
6. Optic Chiasm
7. Supraoptic Recess of the Third Ventricle
8. Lamina Terminalis
9. Anterior Cerebral Artery
10. Frontopolar Artery
11. Rostrum of the Corpus Callosum
12. Genu of the Corpus Callosum
13. Anterior Commissure
14. Septal Vein
15. Callosomarginal Branch, Anterior Cerebral Artery
16. Cingulate Gyrus
17. Pericallosal Branch, Anterior Cerebral Artery
18. Septum Pellucidum
19. Body of the Corpus Callosum
20. Callosomarginal Branch, Anterior Cerebral Artery
21. Fornix
22. Cingulate Sulcus
23. Massa Intermedia
24. Arachnoid Granulations
25. Pars Marginalis (extension of the Cingulate Sulcus)
26. Mammillary Body
27. Internal Cerebral Vein
28. Stria Medullaris
29. Choroid Plexus
30. Habenula
31. Pineal Recess of the Third Ventricle
32. Calcarine Fissure
33. Splenium of the Corpus Callosum
34. Pineal Body
35. Posterior Commissure
36. Superior Colliculus
37. Inferior Colliculus
38. Aqueduct of Sylvius
39. Superior Medullary Velum
40. Inferior Medullary Velum
41. Medial Longitudinal Fasciculus

MIDLINE SAGITTAL SECTION OF THE BRAIN, COMPLETE: ARACHNOID RESECTED

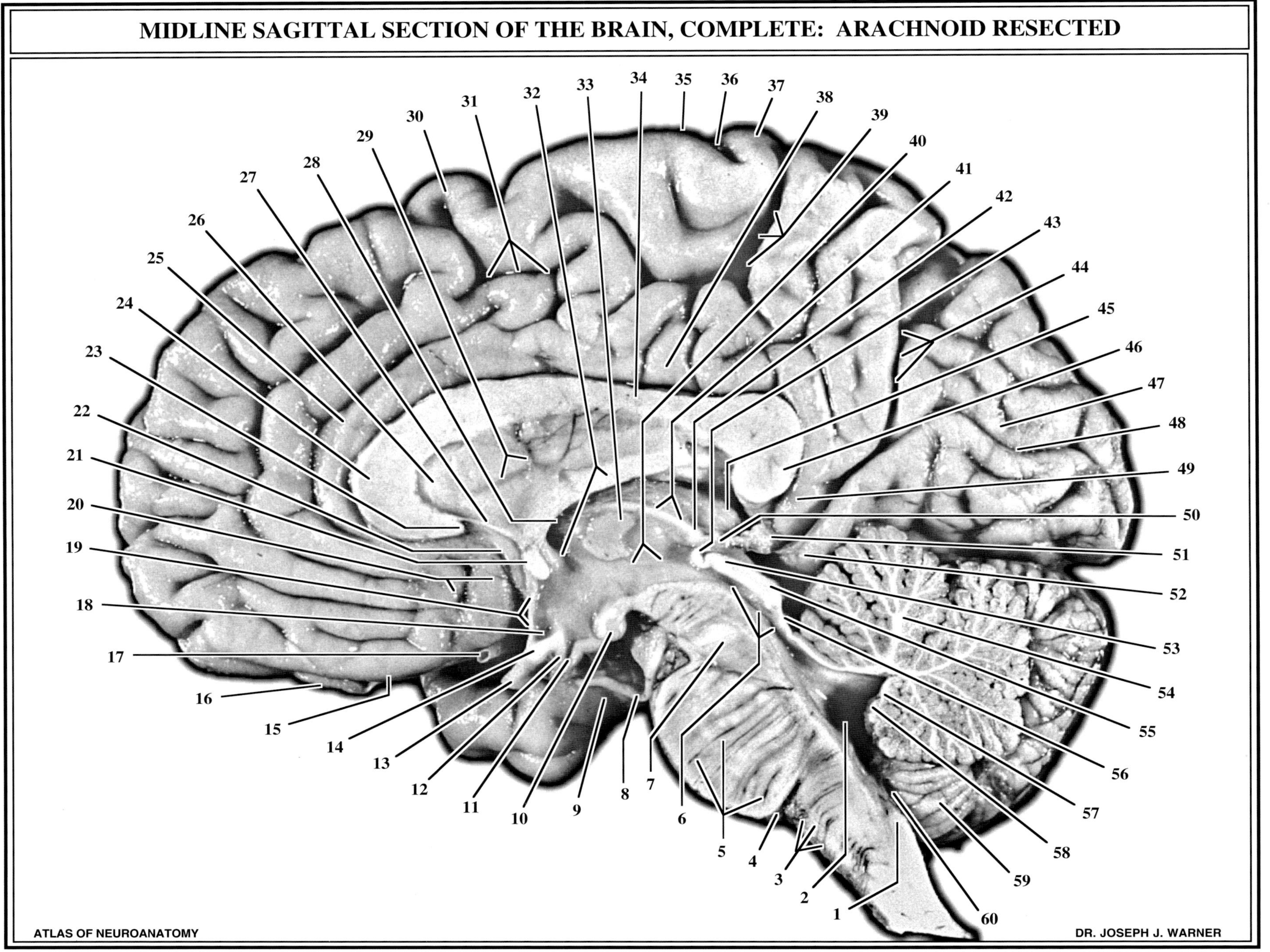

ATLAS OF NEUROANATOMY

DR. JOSEPH J. WARNER

MIDLINE SAGITTAL SECTION OF THE BRAIN, COMPLETE; ARACHNOID RESECTED: KEY TO NUMBERED STRUCTURES

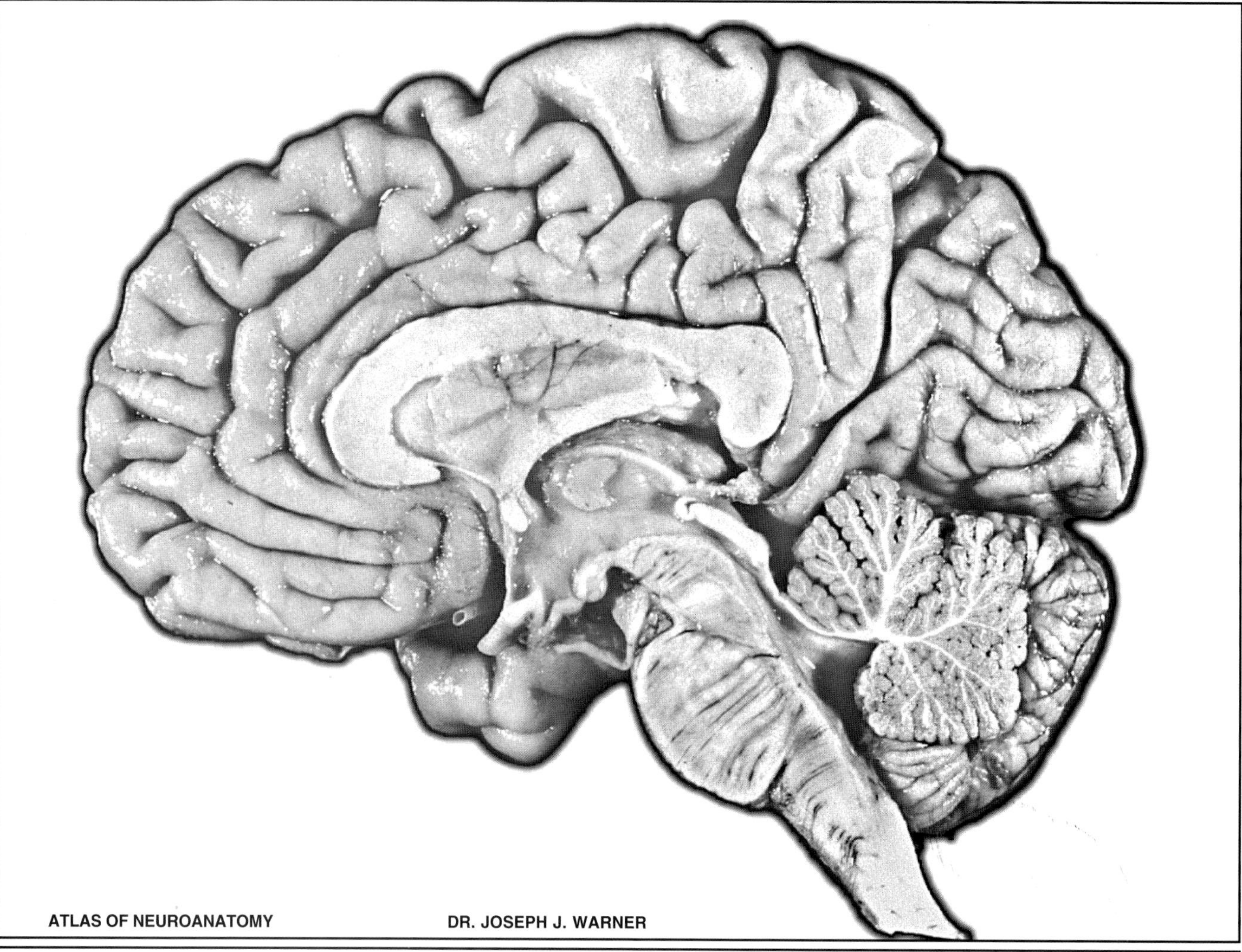

1. Gracile Tubercle
2. Fourth Ventricle
3. Paramedian Medullary Arteries
4. Pontomedullary Sulcus
5. Paramedian Pontine Arteries
6. Aqueduct of Sylvius
7. Decussation of the Superior Cerebellar Peduncle
8. Oculomotor (III) Nerve
9. Parahippocampal Gyrus
10. Mammillary Body
11. Infundibular Recess of the Third Ventricle
12. Infundibulum
13. Optic (II) Nerve
14. Optic Chiasm
15. Gyrus Rectus
16. Olfactory Bulb
17. Anterior Cerebral Artery
18. Supraoptic Recess of the Third Ventricle
19. Lamina Terminalis
20. Paraolfactory Gyri
21. Anterior Commissure
22. Paraterminal Gyrus
23. Rostrum of the Corpus Callosum
24. Genu of the Corpus Callosum
25. Cingulate Gyrus
26. Septum Pellucidum
27. Lamina Terminalis
28. Foramen of Monro
29. Septal Veins
30. Superior Frontal Convolution
31. Cingulate Sulcus
32. Fornix
33. Massa Intermedia
34. Body of the Corpus Callosum
35. Precentral Gyrus
36. Rolandic Fissure (Central Sulcus)
37. Postcentral Gyrus
38. Cingulate Gyrus
39. Pars Marginalis of the Cingulate Sulcus
40. Hypothalamic Sulcus
41. Stria Medullaris
42. Habenula
43. Posterior Commissure
44. Parieto-Occipital Sulcus
45. Pulvinar Nucleus of the Thalamus
46. Splenium of the Corpus Callosum
47. Calcarine (Striate) Cortex
48. Calcarine Fissure
49. Isthmus of the Gyrus Fornicatus
50. Pineal Recess, Third Ventricle
51. Pineal Body
52. Lingular Gyrus
53. Superior Colliculus
54. Superior Cerebellar Vermis
55. Inferior Colliculus
56. Superior Medullary Velum
57. Inferior Medullary Velum
58. Nodulus
59. Cerebellar Tonsil
60. Foramen of Magendie

MIDLINE SAGITTAL SECTION OF THE FELINE BRAIN AND ROSTRAL SPINAL CORD

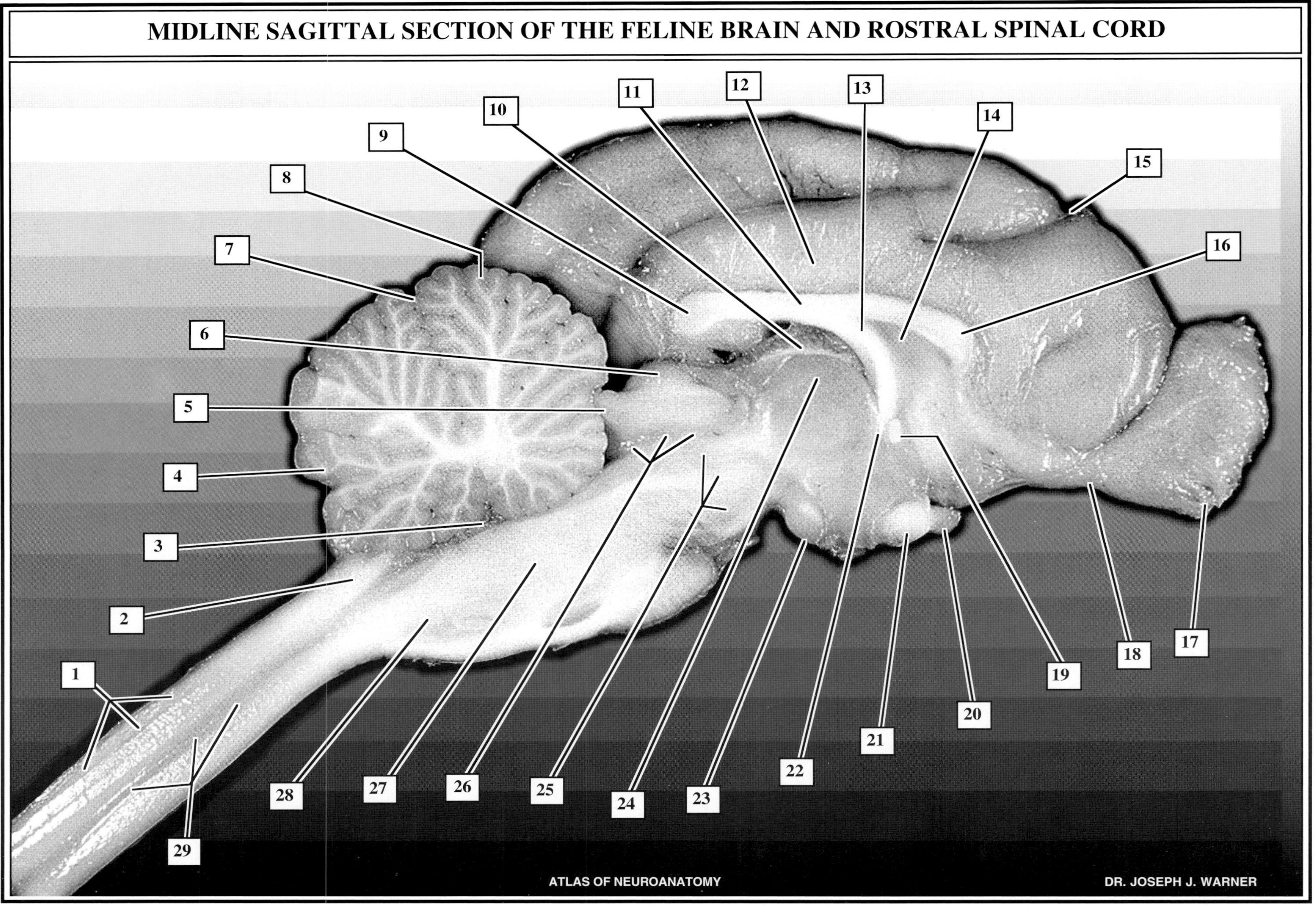

MAJOR DIVISIONS OF THE CENTRAL NERVOUS SYSTEM: ORIENTATION OF THE NEURAXIS AND COMPARATIVE SAGITTAL MORPHOLOGY

KEY TO NUMBERED STRUCTURES ON THE FELINE BRAIN

1. Fasciculus Gracilis
2. Gracile Tubercle
3. Fourth Ventricle
4. Caudal Lobe of the Cerebellum
5. Caudal Colliculus
6. Rostral Colliculus
7. Primary Fissure of the Cerebellum
8. Rostral Lobe of the Cerebellum
9. Splenium of the Corpus Callosum
10. Stria Medullaris
11. Body of the Corpus Callosum
12. Cingulate Gyrus
13. Fornix
14. Septum Pellucidum
15. Cruciate Sulcus
16. Genu of the Corpus Callosum
17. Olfactory Bulb
18. Olfactory Tract
19. Rostral Commissure
20. Optic Nerve
21. Optic Chiasm
22. Fornix
23. Mammillary Body
24. Thalamus
25. Mesencephalon
26. Mesencephalic Aqueduct
27. Pons
28. Medulla
29. Central Canal

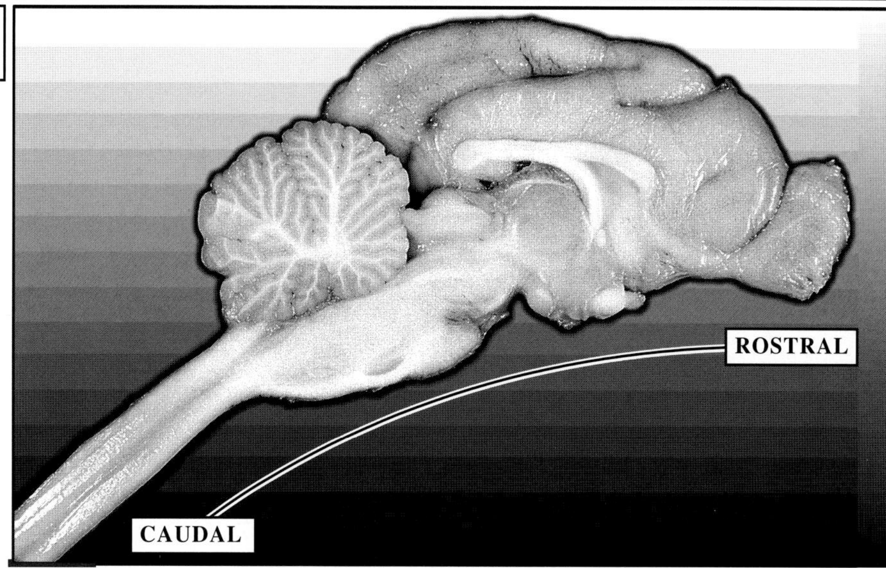

The feline central nervous system is exemplary of a *curvilinear neuraxis,* which is horizontally oriented. The axis of the brainstem and spinal cord is approximately parallel to that of the cerebral hemispheres. Therefore, the feline brain has a rostral and a caudal commissure, corresponding to the human anterior and posterior commissures, respectively. However, the angle between the axis of the human cerebrum (A) and the brainstem and spinal cord (B) is accompanied by the application of distinct anatomic terminology. Thus, the feline *rostral* and *caudal* colliculi correspond to the human *superior* and *inferior* colliculi.

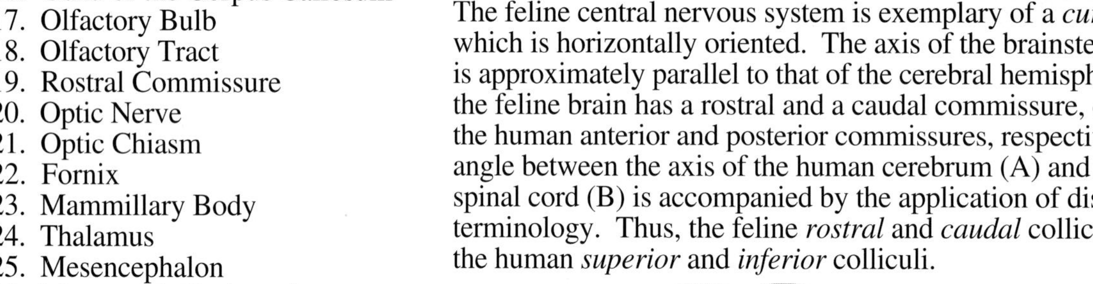

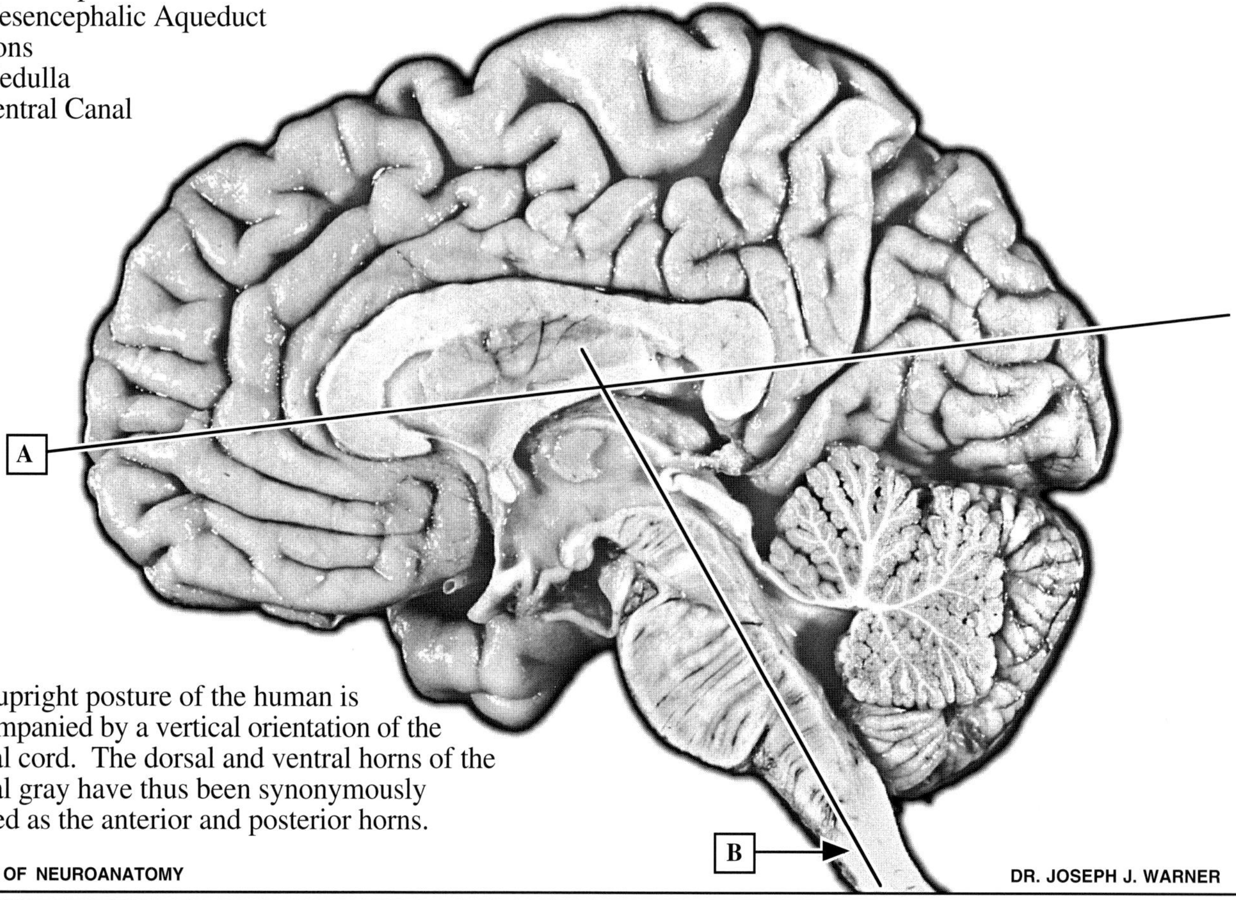

A

B

The upright posture of the human is accompanied by a vertical orientation of the spinal cord. The dorsal and ventral horns of the spinal gray have thus been synonymously named as the anterior and posterior horns.

MIDLINE SAGITTAL SECTION OF THE BRAIN, COMPLETE: BRODMANN'S AREAS

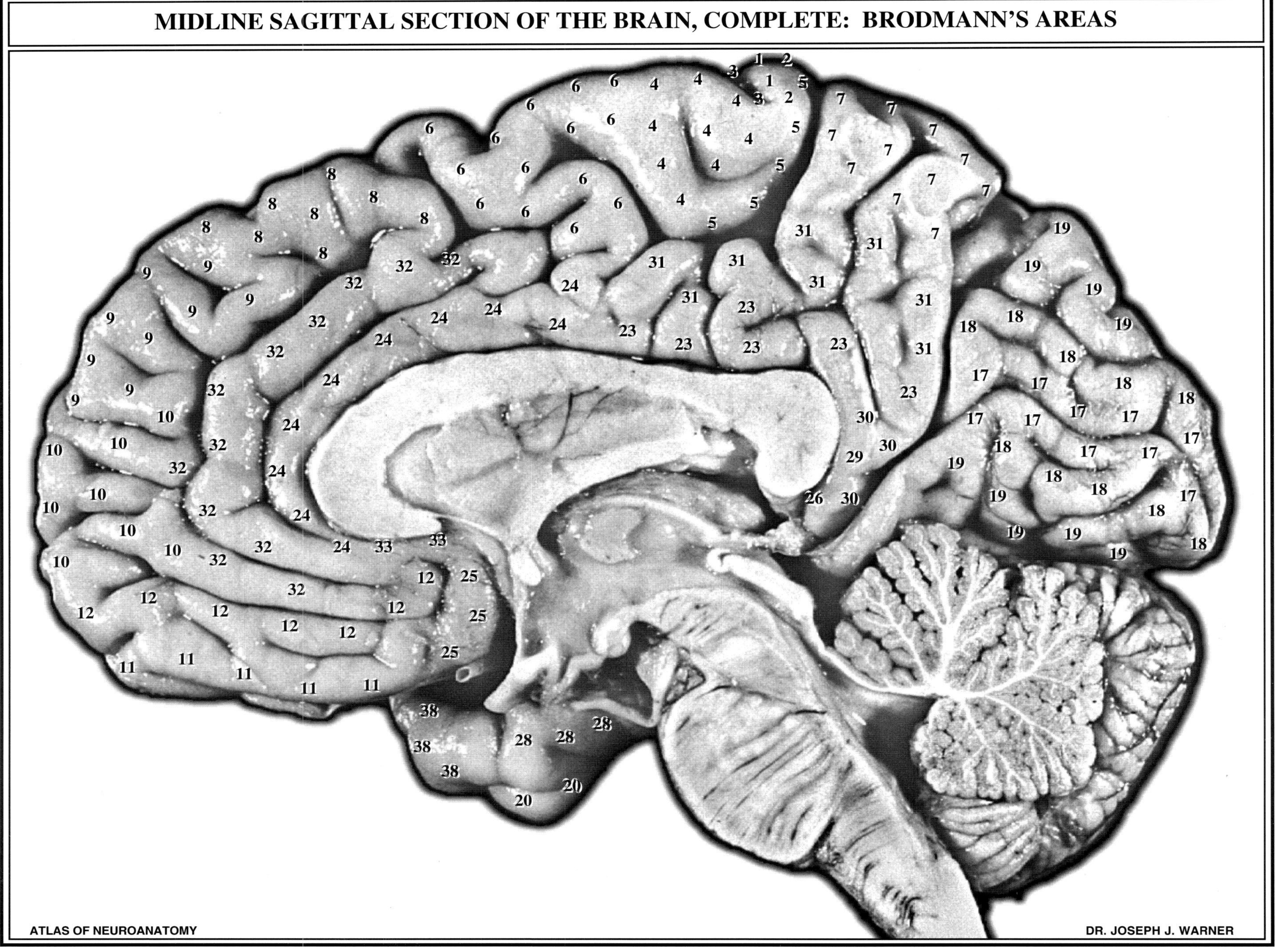

DR. JOSEPH J. WARNER

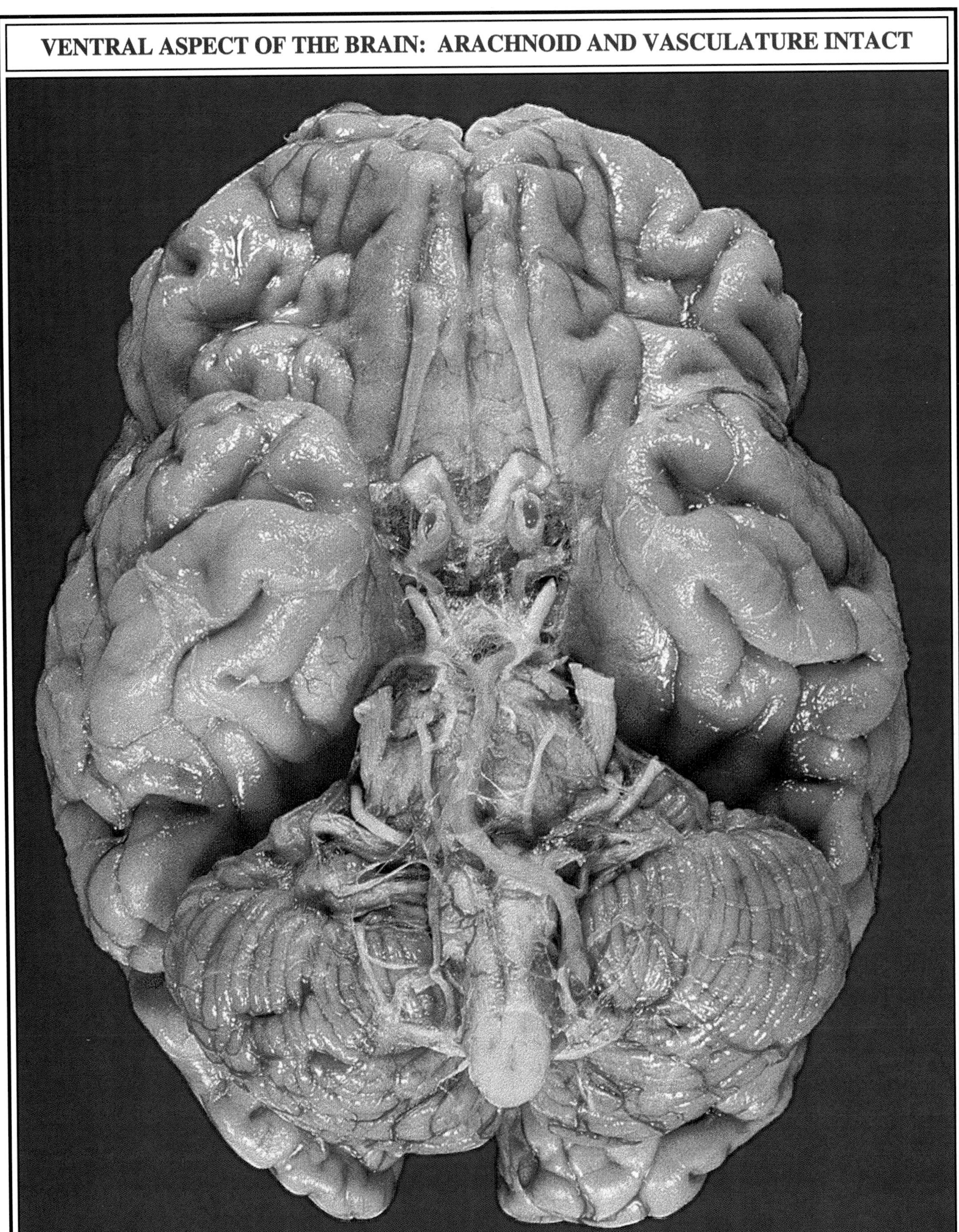
VENTRAL ASPECT OF THE BRAIN: ARACHNOID AND VASCULATURE INTACT
ATLAS OF NEUROANATOMY
DR. JOSEPH J. WARNER

VENTRAL ASPECT OF THE BRAIN: ARACHNOID AND VASCULATURE RESECTED FROM THE VENTRAL BRAINSTEM AND DIENCEPHALON

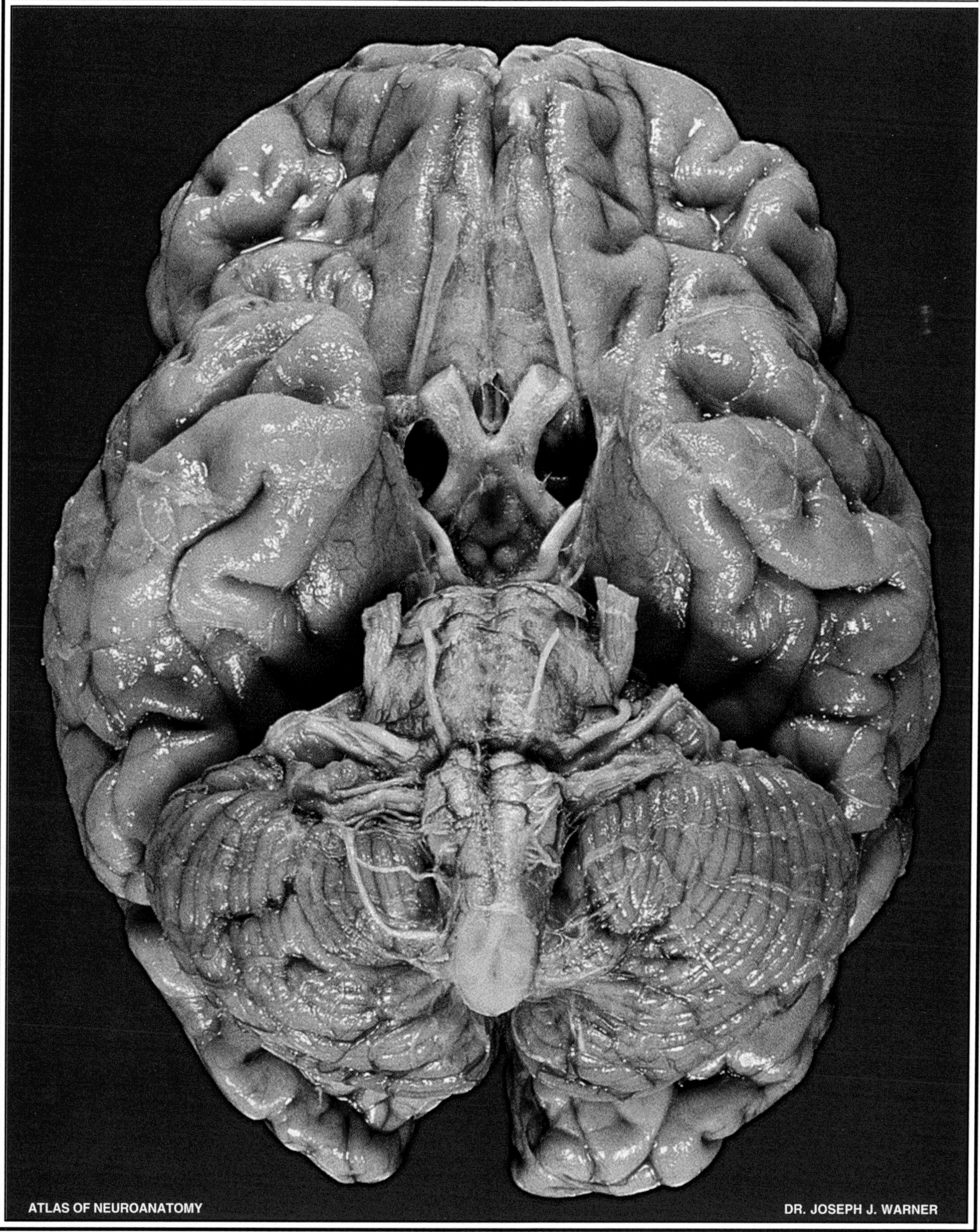

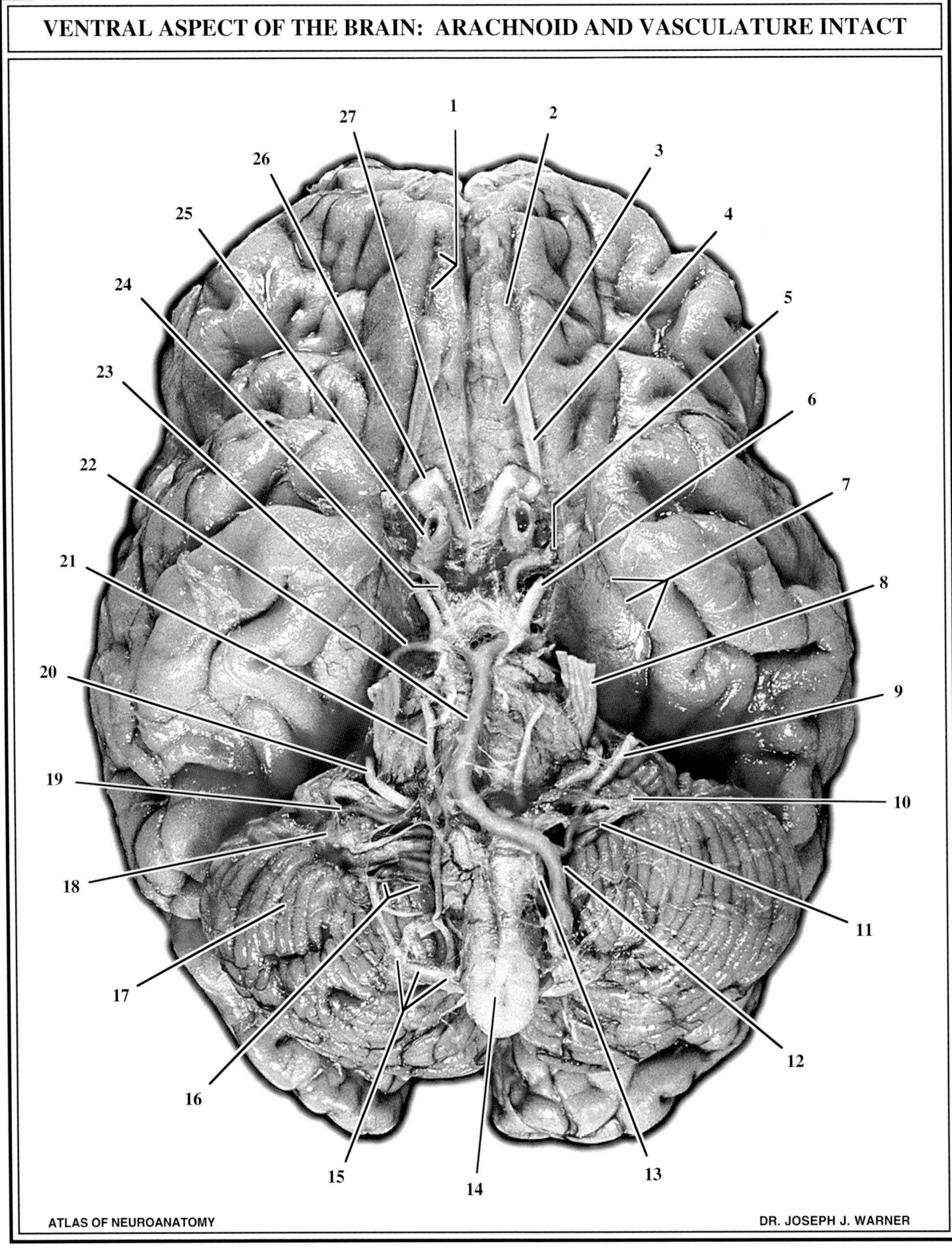
VENTRAL ASPECT OF THE BRAIN: ARACHNOID AND VASCULATURE INTACT
1
2
3
4
5
6
7
8
9
10
11
12
13
14
15
16
17
18
19
20
21
22
23
24
25
26
27
ATLAS OF NEUROANATOMY
DR. JOSEPH J. WARNER

VENTRAL ASPECT OF THE BRAIN: ARACHNOID AND VASCULATURE RESECTED FROM THE VENTRAL BRAINSTEM AND DIENCEPHALON

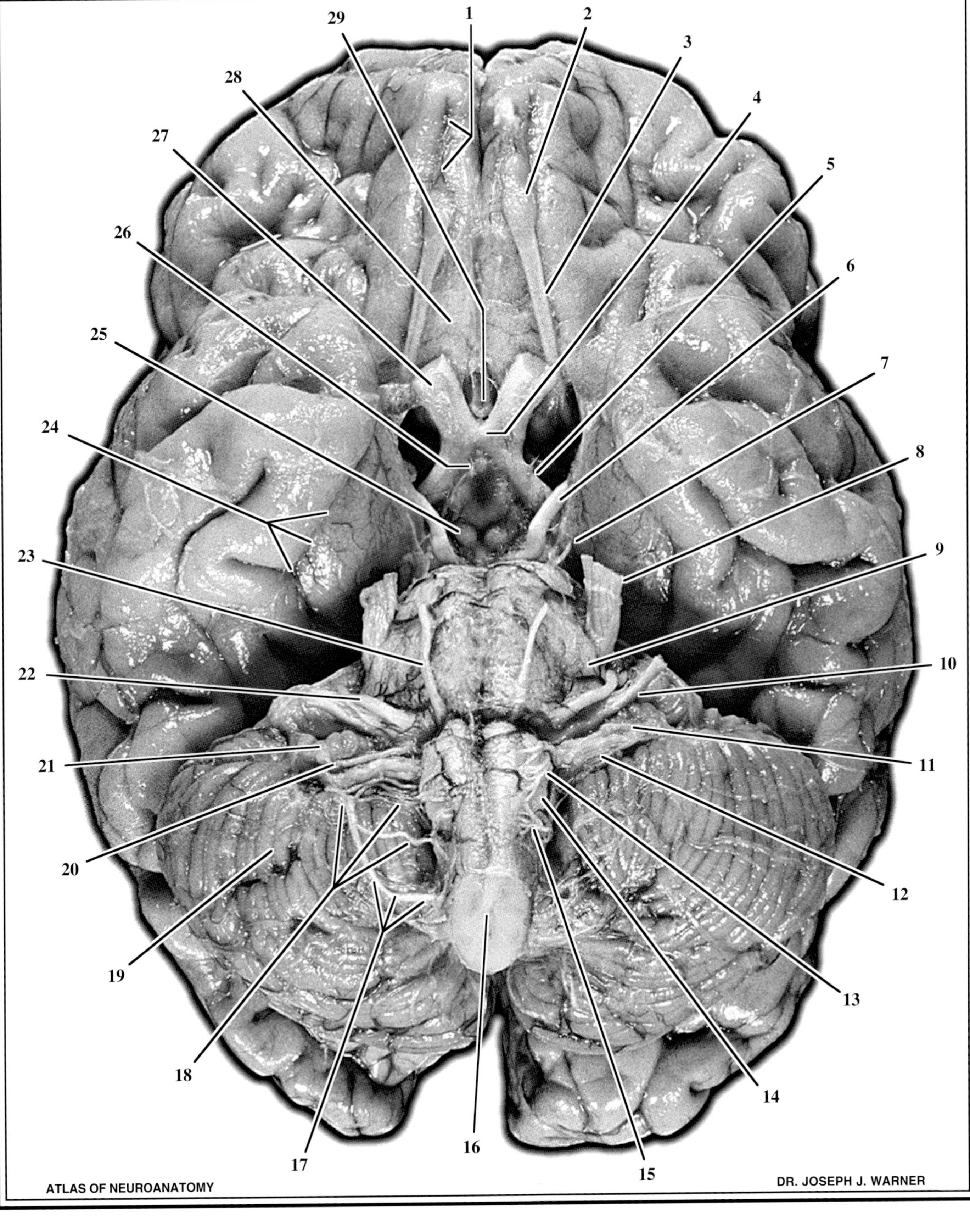

29 1 2 3 28 4 27 5 26 6 25 7 24 8 23 9 22 10 21 11 20 12 19 13 18 14 17 16 15

VENTRAL ASPECT OF THE BRAIN; DISSECTION OF THE ARACHNOID, VASCULATURE, AND CRANIAL NERVES: KEY TO NUMBERED STRUCTURES

ARACHNOID AND VASCULATURE INTACT: KEY

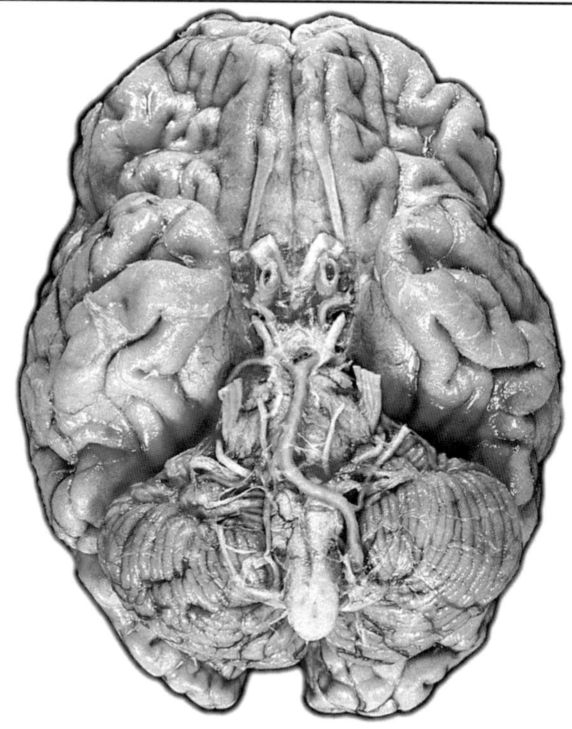

1. Olfactory Sulcus
2. Olfactory Bulb
3. Gyrus Rectus
4. Olfactory Tract
5. Middle Cerebral Artery
6. Oculomotor (III) Nerve
7. Collateral Sulcus
8. Trigeminal (V) Nerve
9. Vestibulocochlear (VIII) Nerve
10. Glossopharyngeal (IX) Nerve
11. Vagus (X) Nerve
12. Vertebral Artery
13. Inferior Olive
14. Pyramidal Decussation
15. Spinal Accessory (XI) Nerve
16. Bulbar Root of the Accessory (XI) Nerve
17. Posterior Lobe of the Cerebellum
18. Flocculus
19. Anterior Inferior Cerebellar Artery
20. Facial (VII) Nerve
21. Abducens (VI) Nerve
22. Basilar Artery
23. Superior Cerebellar Artery
24. Posterior Communicating Artery
25. Internal Carotid Artery
26. Optic (II) Nerve
27. Optic Chiasm

ARACHNOID AND VASCULATURE RESECTED: KEY

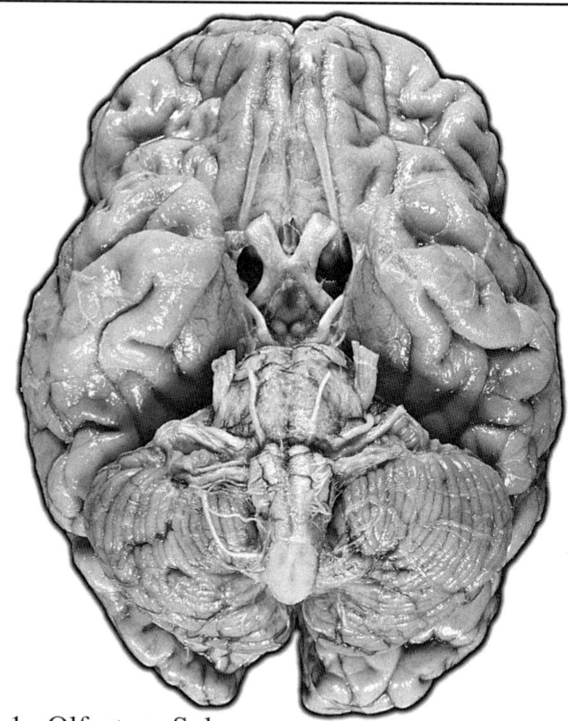

1. Olfactory Sulcus
2. Olfactory Bulb
3. Olfactory Tract
4. Optic Chiasm
5. Optic Tract
6. Oculomotor (III) Nerve
7. Trochlear (IV) Nerve
8. Trigeminal (V) Nerve
9. Middle Cerebellar Peduncle
10. Vestibulocochlear (VIII) Nerve
11. Glossopharyngeal (IX) Nerve
12. Vagus (X) Nerve
13. Fascicles of the Hypoglossal (XII) Nerve
14. Inferior Olive
15. Fascicles of the Hypoglossal (XII) Nerve
16. Pyramidal Decussation
17. Spinal Accessory (XI) Nerve
18. Spinal Accessory (XI) Nerve (Bulbar Roots)
19. Posterior Lobe of the Cerebellum
20. Glossopharyngeal (IX) Nerve
21. Flocculus
22. Facial (VII) Nerve
23. Abducens (VI) Nerve
24. Collateral Sulcus
25. Mammillary Body
26. Pituitary Stalk
27. Optic (II) Nerve
28. Gyrus Rectus
29. Anterior Communicating Artery

VENTRAL ASPECT OF THE BRAIN

THE GUIDEWIRES DEMONSTRATE THE TROCHLEAR (IV) NERVES, WHICH COURSE ANTERIORLY FROM THE DORSAL MESENCEPHALON TOWARD THE CAVERNOUS SINUS

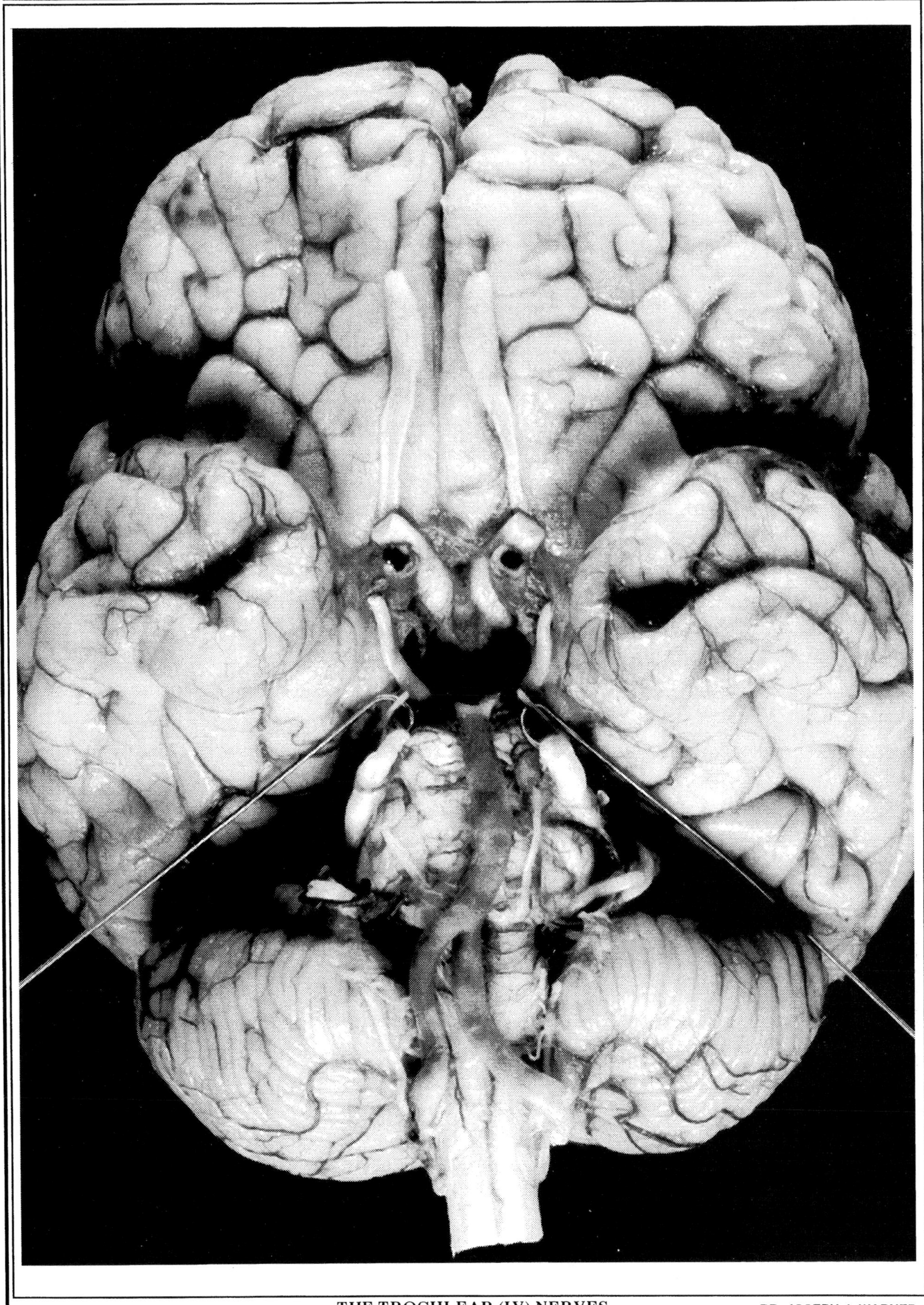

THE TROCHLEAR (IV) NERVES

THE TROCHLEAR (IV) NERVES	THE GUIDEWIRES DEMONSTRATE THE TROCHLEAR (IV) NERVES. THE CELL BODIES OF ORIGIN OF EACH NERVE ARE LOCATED IN THE CONTRALATERAL IV NERVE NUCLEUS.

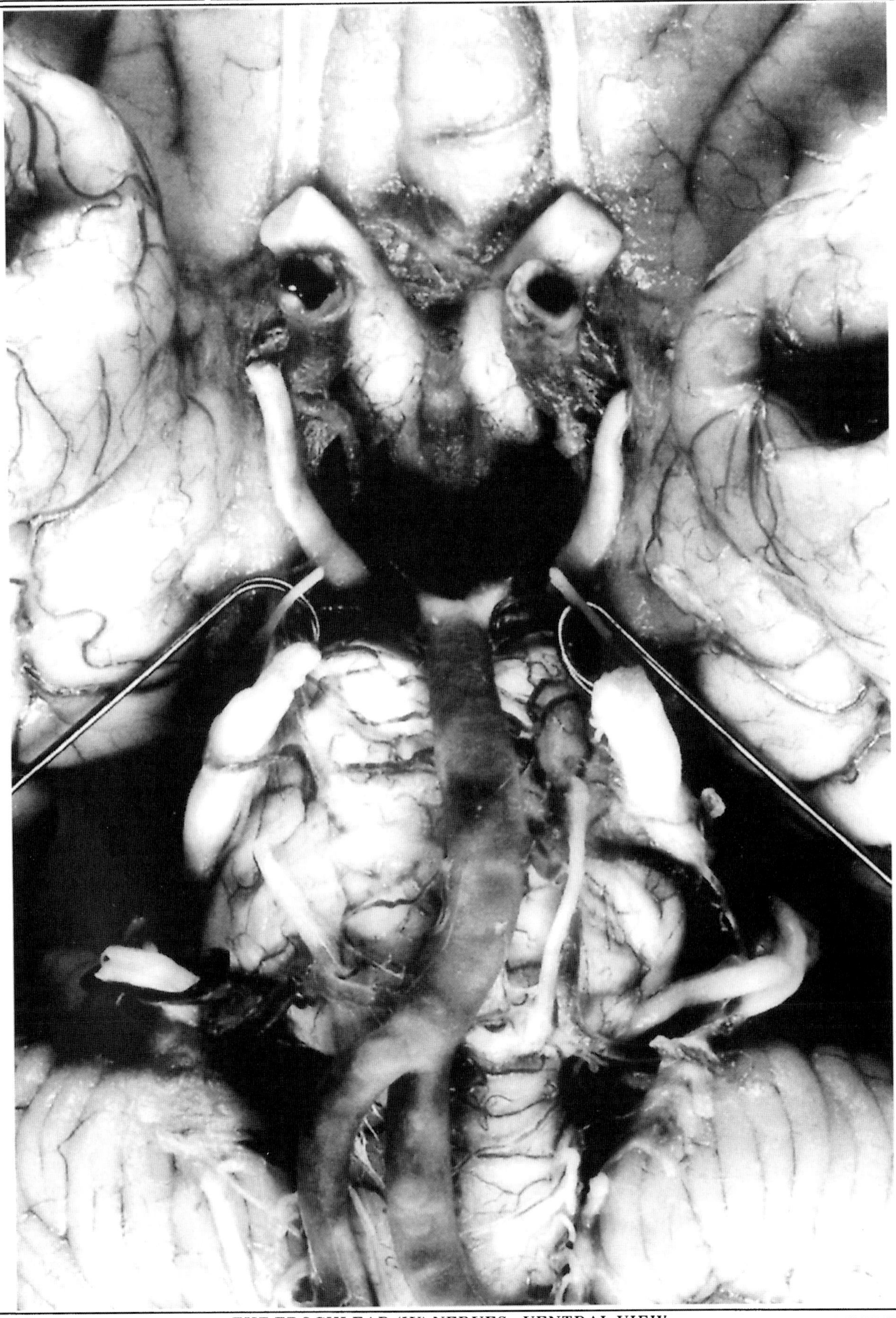

THE TROCHLEAR (IV) NERVES: VENTRAL VIEW

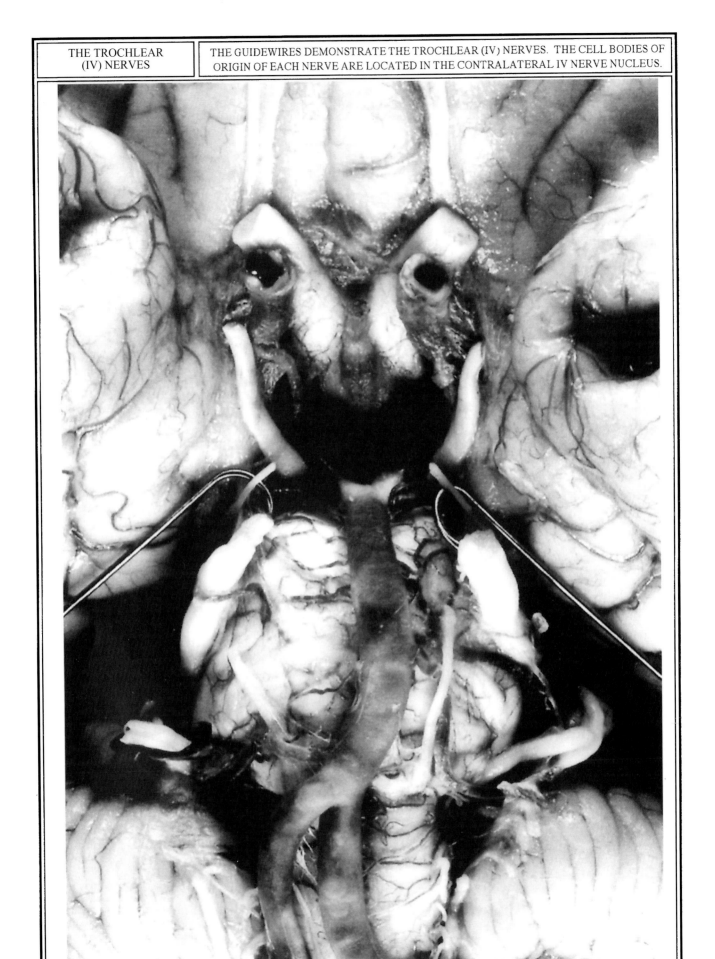

COURSE OF THE TROCHLEAR (IV) NERVE: VENTROLATERAL ASPECT OF THE BRAIN

The cerebellum has been retracted ventrally, exposing the lateral aspect of the mesencephalon. The guidewire to the right surrounds the Trigeminal Nerve. The left guidewire is medial to the Trochlear Nerve.

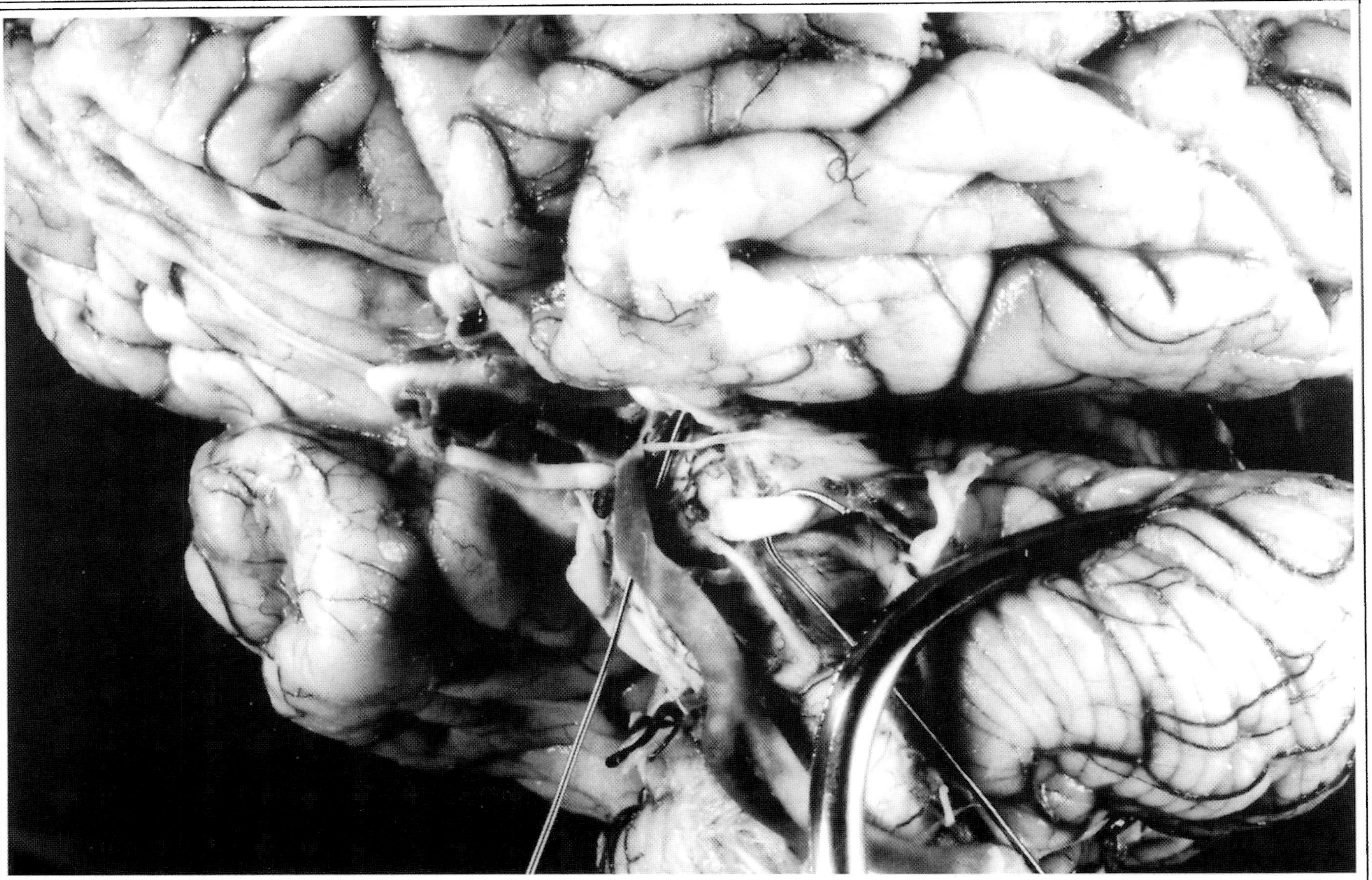

THE GLASS ROD DEMONSTRATES FASCICLES OF THE HYPOGLOSSAL (XII) NERVE. SPINAL AND BULBAR COMPONENTS OF THE ACCESSORY (XI) NERVE ARE DISCERNIBLE.

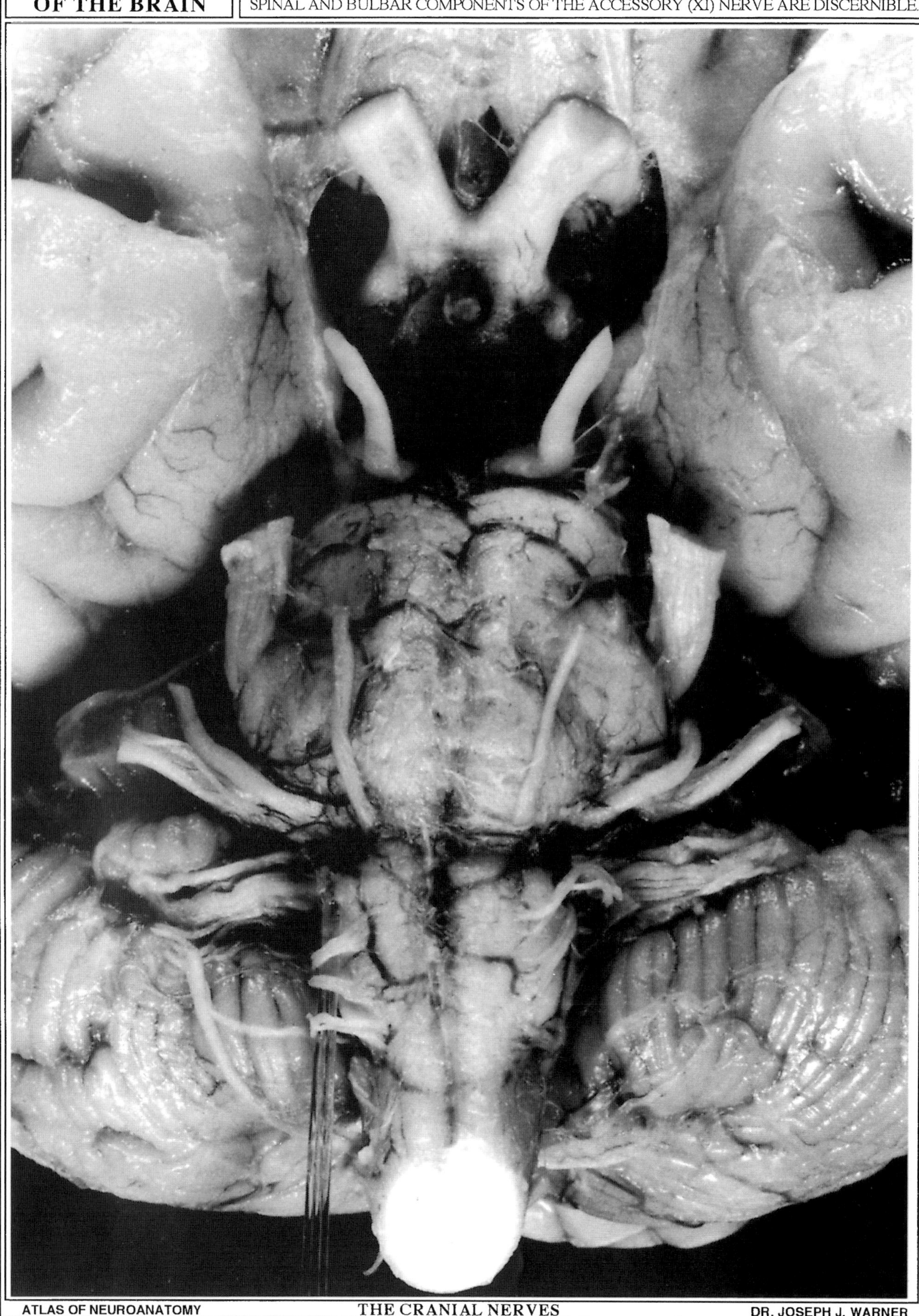

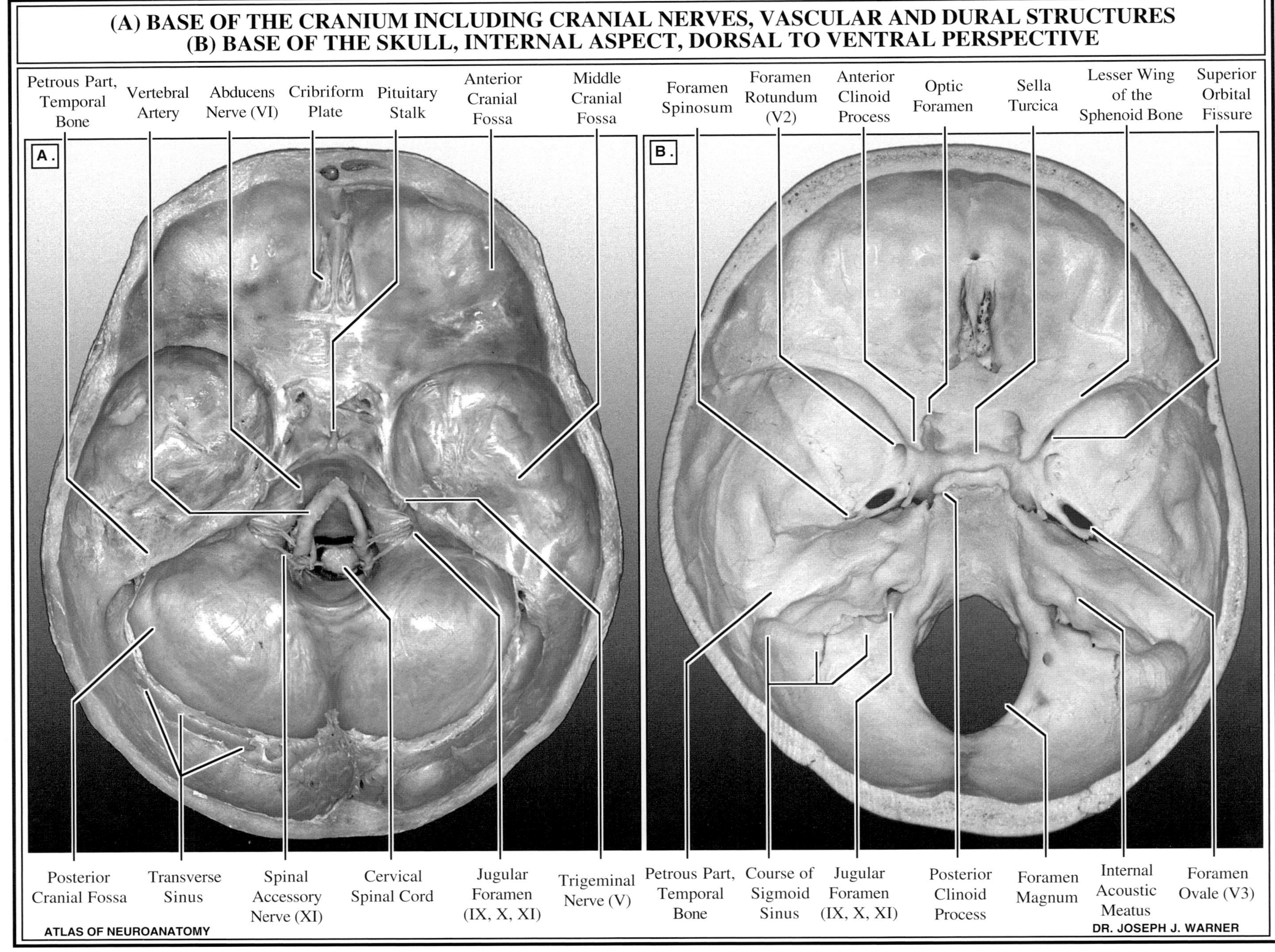
(A) BASE OF THE CRANIUM INCLUDING CRANIAL NERVES, VASCULAR AND DURAL STRUCTURES
(B) BASE OF THE SKULL, INTERNAL ASPECT, DORSAL TO VENTRAL PERSPECTIVE
A.
Petrous Part, Temporal Bone
Vertebral Artery
Abducens Nerve (VI)
Cribriform Plate
Pituitary Stalk
Anterior Cranial Fossa
Middle Cranial Fossa
Posterior Cranial Fossa
Transverse Sinus
Spinal Accessory Nerve (XI)
Cervical Spinal Cord
Jugular Foramen (IX, X, XI)
Trigeminal Nerve (V)
B.
Foramen Spinosum
Foramen Rotundum (V2)
Anterior Clinoid Process
Optic Foramen
Sella Turcica
Lesser Wing of the Sphenoid Bone
Superior Orbital Fissure
Petrous Part, Temporal Bone
Course of Sigmoid Sinus
Jugular Foramen (IX, X, XI)
Posterior Clinoid Process
Foramen Magnum
Internal Acoustic Meatus
Foramen Ovale (V3)
ATLAS OF NEUROANATOMY
DR. JOSEPH J. WARNER

BASE OF THE SKULL INCLUDING THE DURA, CRANIAL NERVES, AND PROXIMAL VASCULATURE: MAGNIFIED VIEW PERPENDICULAR TO THE CLIVUS

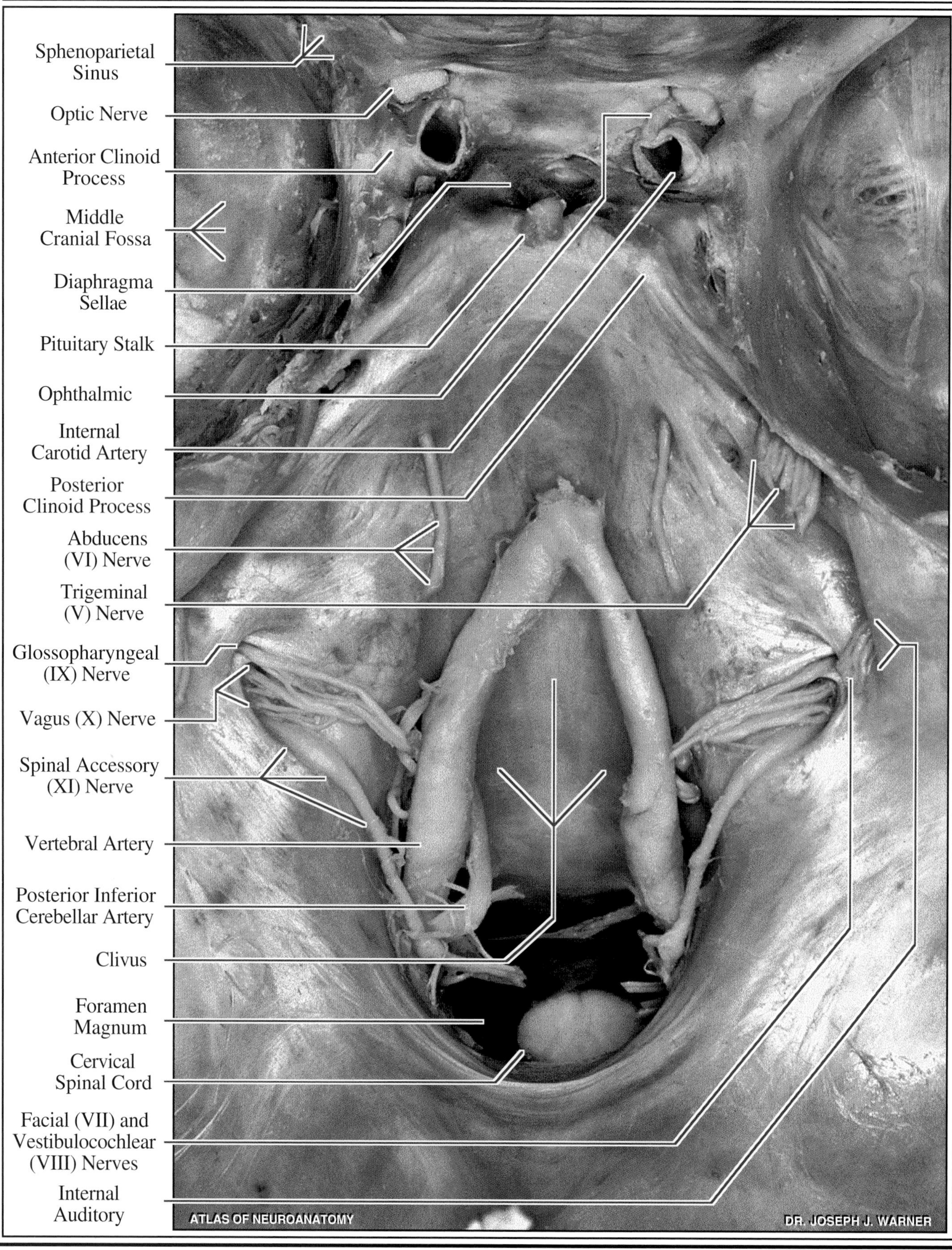

ANTEROLATERAL VIEW OF THE SKULL, INCLUDING REFERENCES TO CRANIAL NERVES AND OTHER NEURAL STRUCTURES

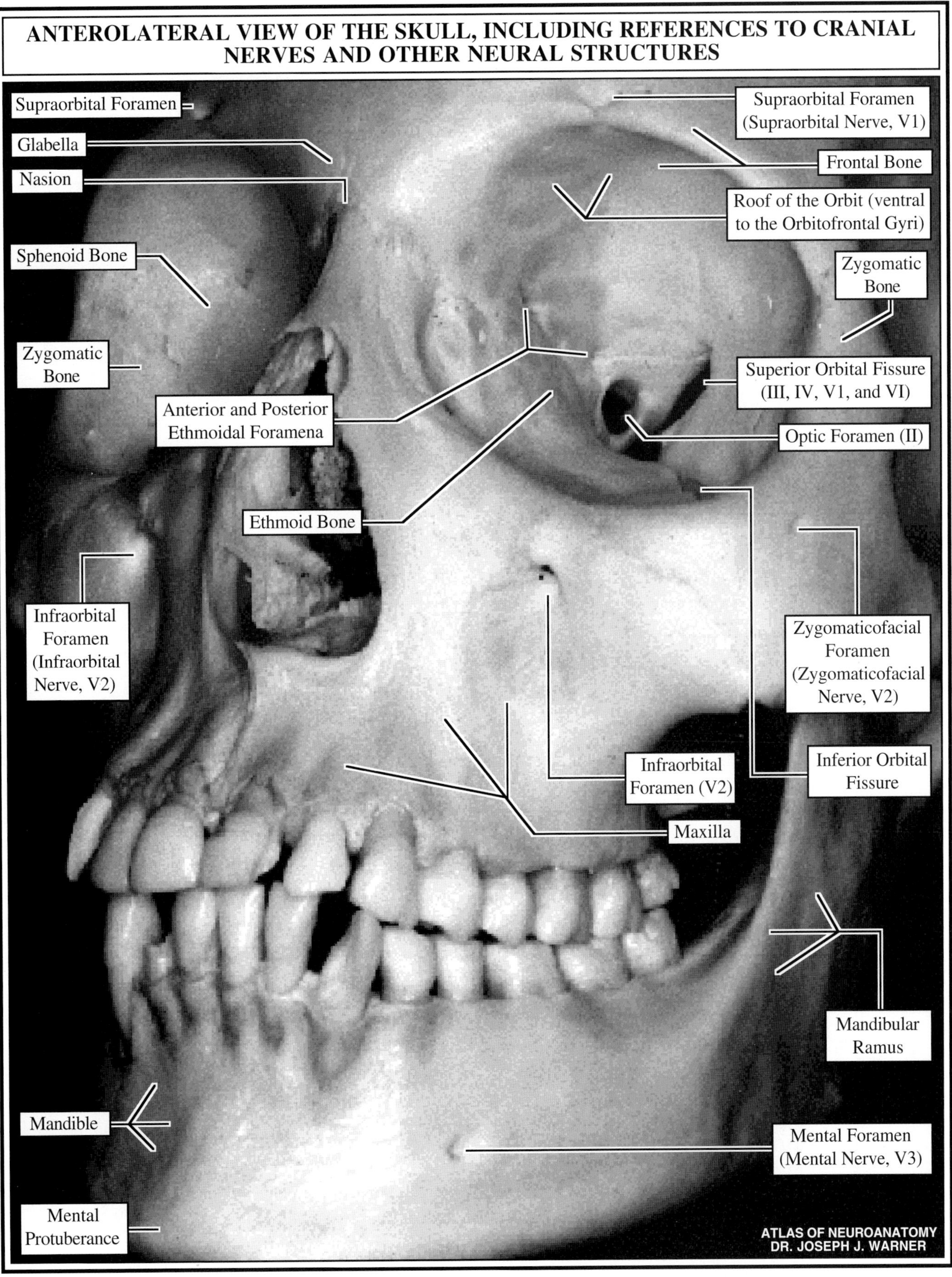

CAUDAL ASPECT OF THE CEREBELLUM: ARACHNOID AND VASCULATURE INTACT

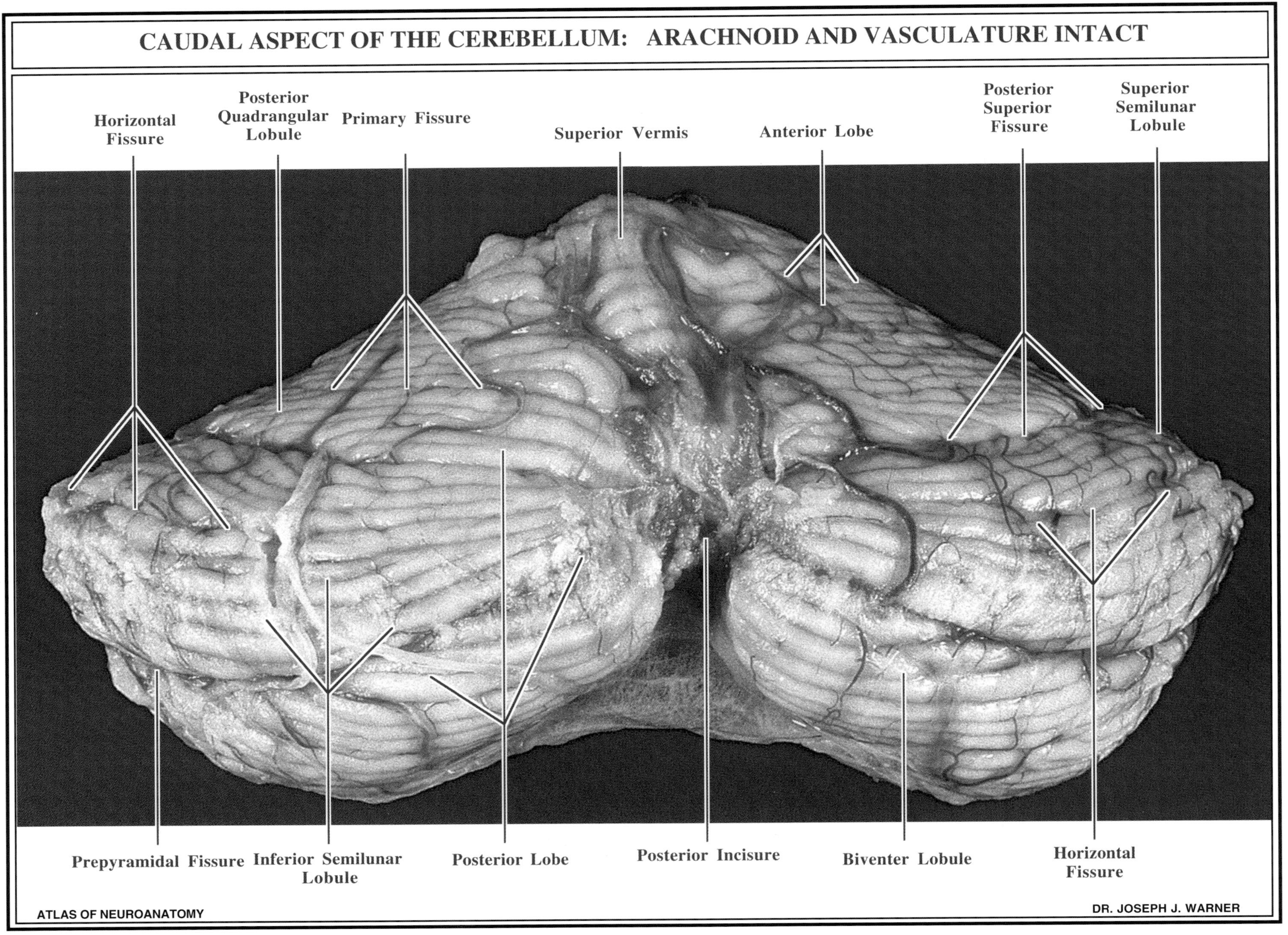

DIAGRAM OF THE CEREBELLUM: ANATOMIC AND FUNCTIONAL DIVISIONS

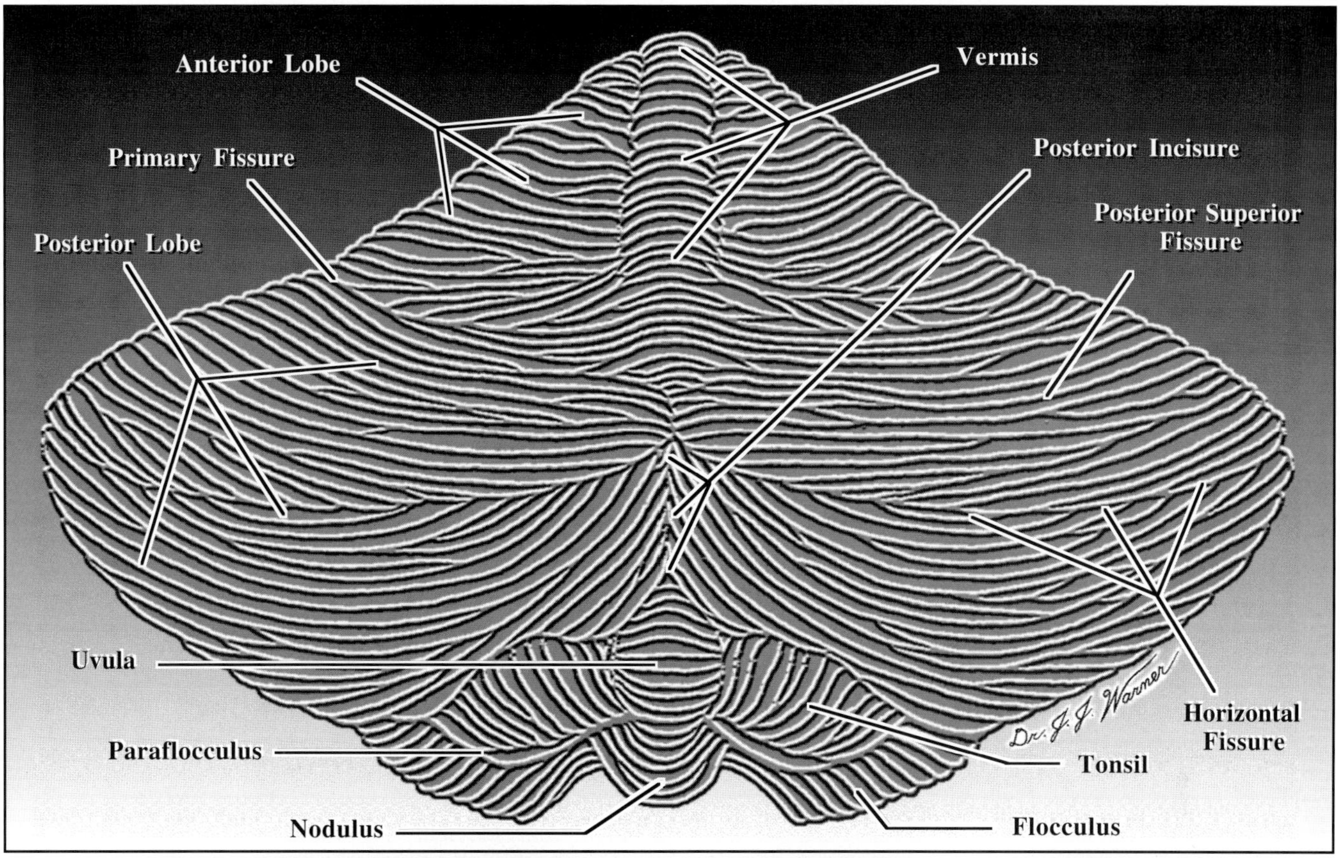

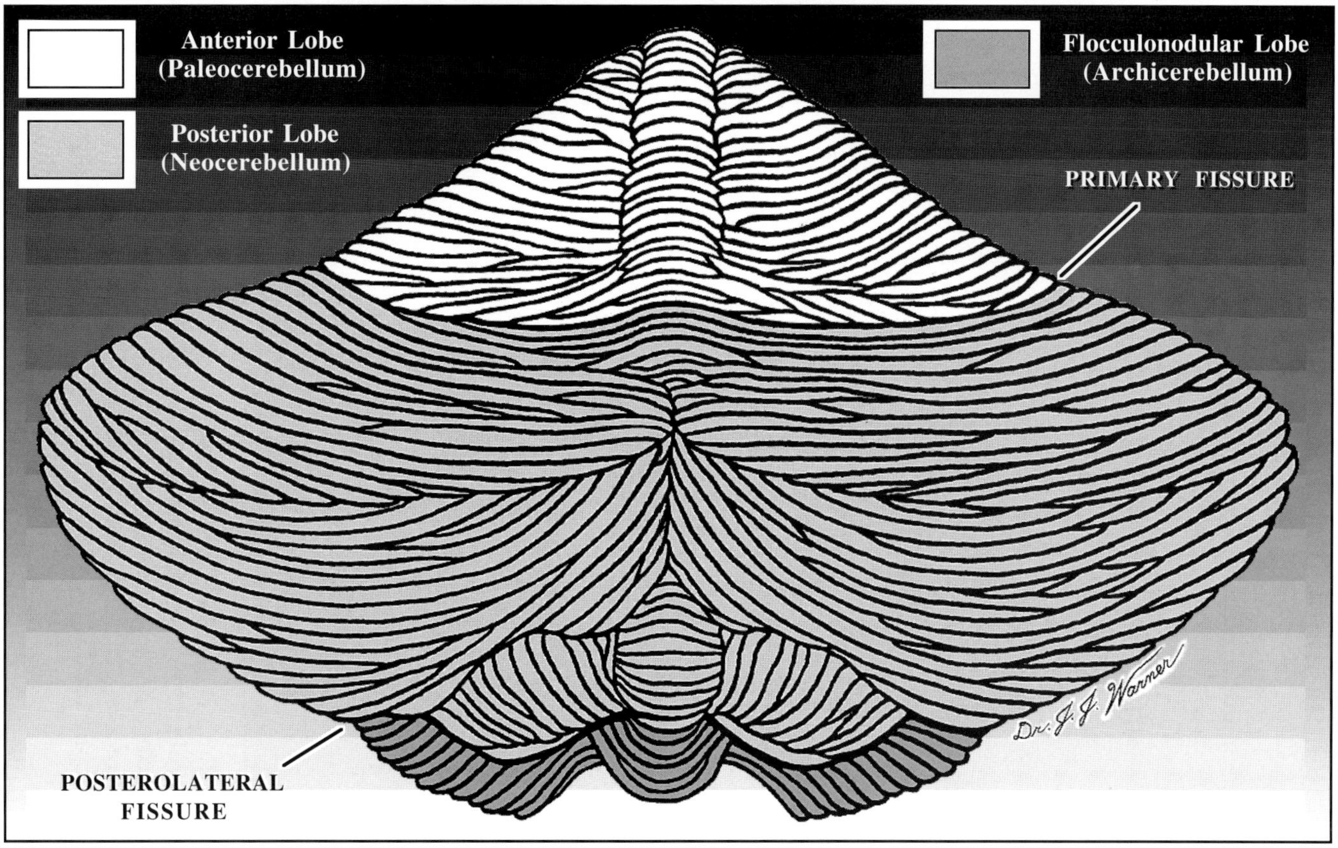

In this representation of the cerebellum, the anterior inferior regions have been retracted ventrally and dorsally. Thus, the flocculonodular lobe, normally not visible in this projection, is demonstrated diagrammatically.

CEREBELLUM, ANTERIOR ASPECT: RESECTED FROM THE BRAINSTEM BY TRANSECTION OF THE SUPERIOR, MIDDLE, AND INFERIOR CEREBELLAR PEDUNCLES

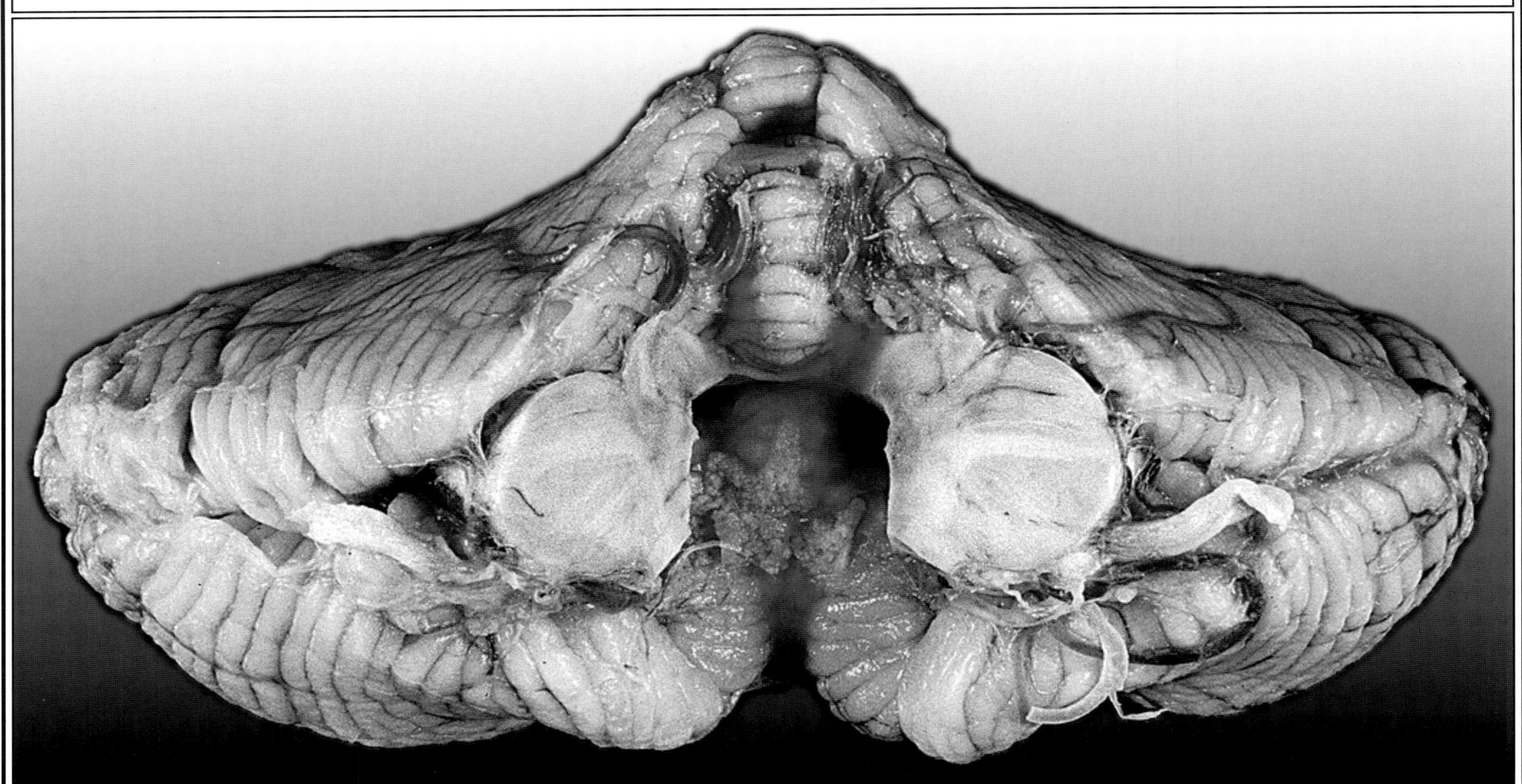

The cerebellum is demonstrated in the anatomically horizontal position, viewed from the anterior to posterior direction. The superior surface of the cerebellum is normally juxtaposed to the inferior surface of the tentorium. In this view, the superior biconcave contour of the cerebellum is clearly evident and conforms to the contour of the inferior surface of the occipital lobes.

Note the position of the superior cerebellar vermis in relation to the intermediate and lateral zones of the cerebellum. In contrast to the configuration of the superior surface, the posterolateral and inferior surfaces of the cerebellum are biconvex, reflecting the contour of the posterior cranial fossa. Just superior to the foramen magnum, the cerebellar tonsils extend ventrally, caudal to the pontomedullary sulcus.

CEREBELLUM, ANTERIOR ASPECT: RESECTED FROM THE BRAINSTEM BY TRANSECTION OF THE SUPERIOR, MIDDLE, AND INFERIOR CEREBELLAR PEDUNCLES

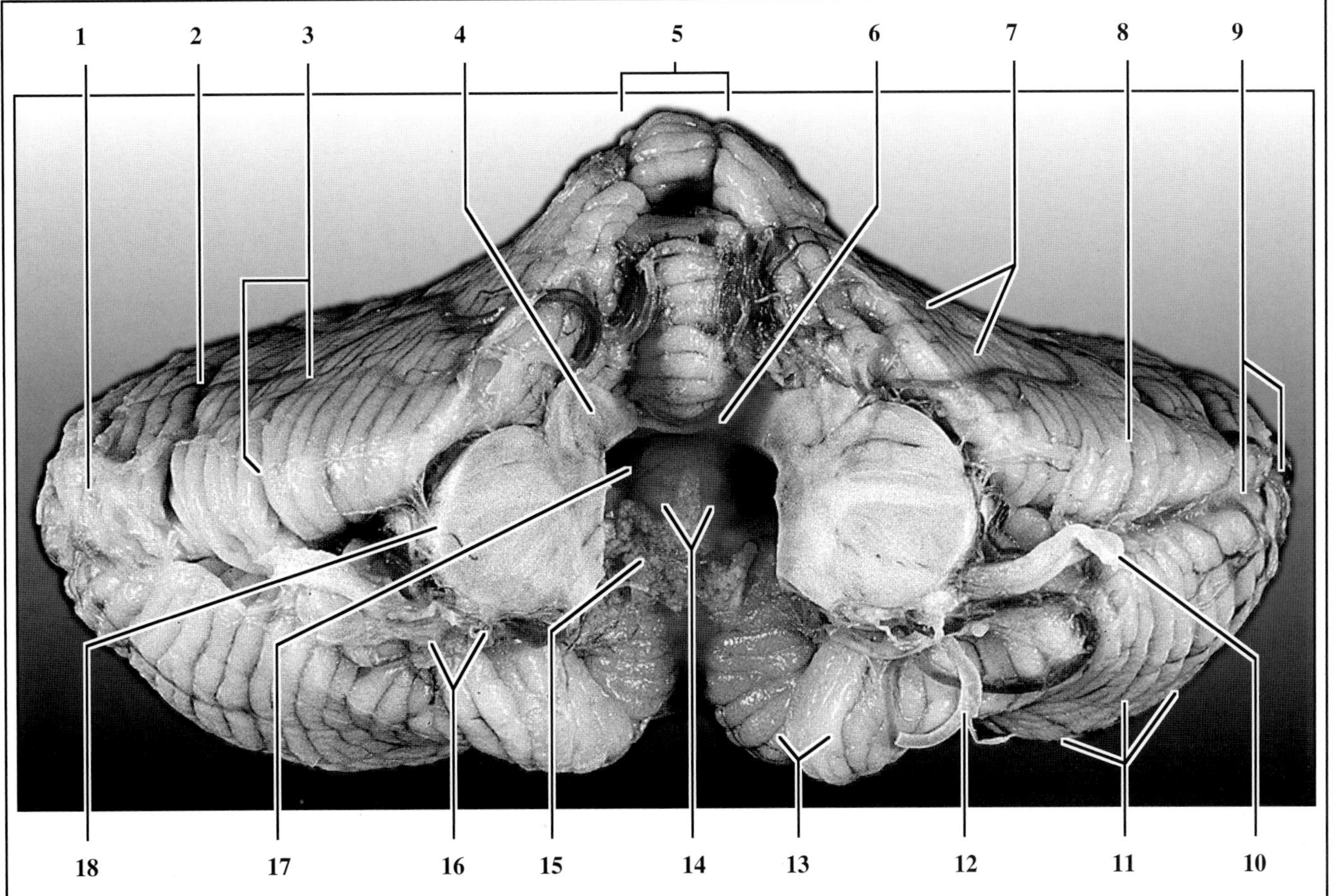

The primary fissure of the cerebellum is the deepest of all cerebellar sulci, and demarcates the division between the anterior and posterior lobes. The horizontal fissure passes circumferentially around each cerebellar hemisphere, extending from either side of the vermis to the anterolateral surface of the posterior lobe. This fissure is continuous with the posterolateral fissure, which passes anteromedially between the flocculus and paraflocculus, and between the nodulus and uvula (a division of the inferior cerebellar vermis). In examining the ventral surface of a complete brain, the flocculus is exposed by medial retraction of the emerging facial (VII), vestibulocochlear (VIII), and glossopharnygeal (IX) nerves. The posterolateral fissure may thus be followed toward the midline. The flocculus (covered by other structures in this dissection) is adjacent to the inferolateral aspect of the middle cerebellar peduncle on the anterior aspect of the cerebellum. The superior cerebellar vermis is clearly separated from the nodulus by the anterior medullary velum. This demarcation is demonstrated in the dissection above. The roof of the fourth ventricle includes the anterior medullary velum, the anterior surface of the nodulus covered by the posterior (inferior) medullary velum. Choroid plexus is visible over the latter structures.

KEY TO NUMBERED STRUCTURES

1. Lateral Zone, Posterior Lobe of the Cerebellum
2. Posterior Superior Fissure
3. Primary Fissure
4. Superior Cerebellar Peduncle
5. Cerebellar Vermis
6. Anterior Medullary Velum
7. Anterior Lobe of the Cerebellum
8. Primary Fissure
9. Horizontal Fissure
10. Vestibulocochlear (VIII) Nerve
11. Posterior Lobe (inferior surface)
12. Posterior Inferior Cerebellar Artery
13. Cerebellar Tonsil
14. Nodulus
15. Choroid Plexus
16. Posterolateral Fissure
17. Fourth Ventricle
18. Middle Cerebellar Peduncle

CEREBELLUM, ANTERIOR ASPECT; RESECTED FROM THE BRAINSTEM BY TRANSECTION OF THE SUPERIOR, MIDDLE, AND INFERIOR CEREBELLAR PEDUNCLES: MAGNIFIED VIEW

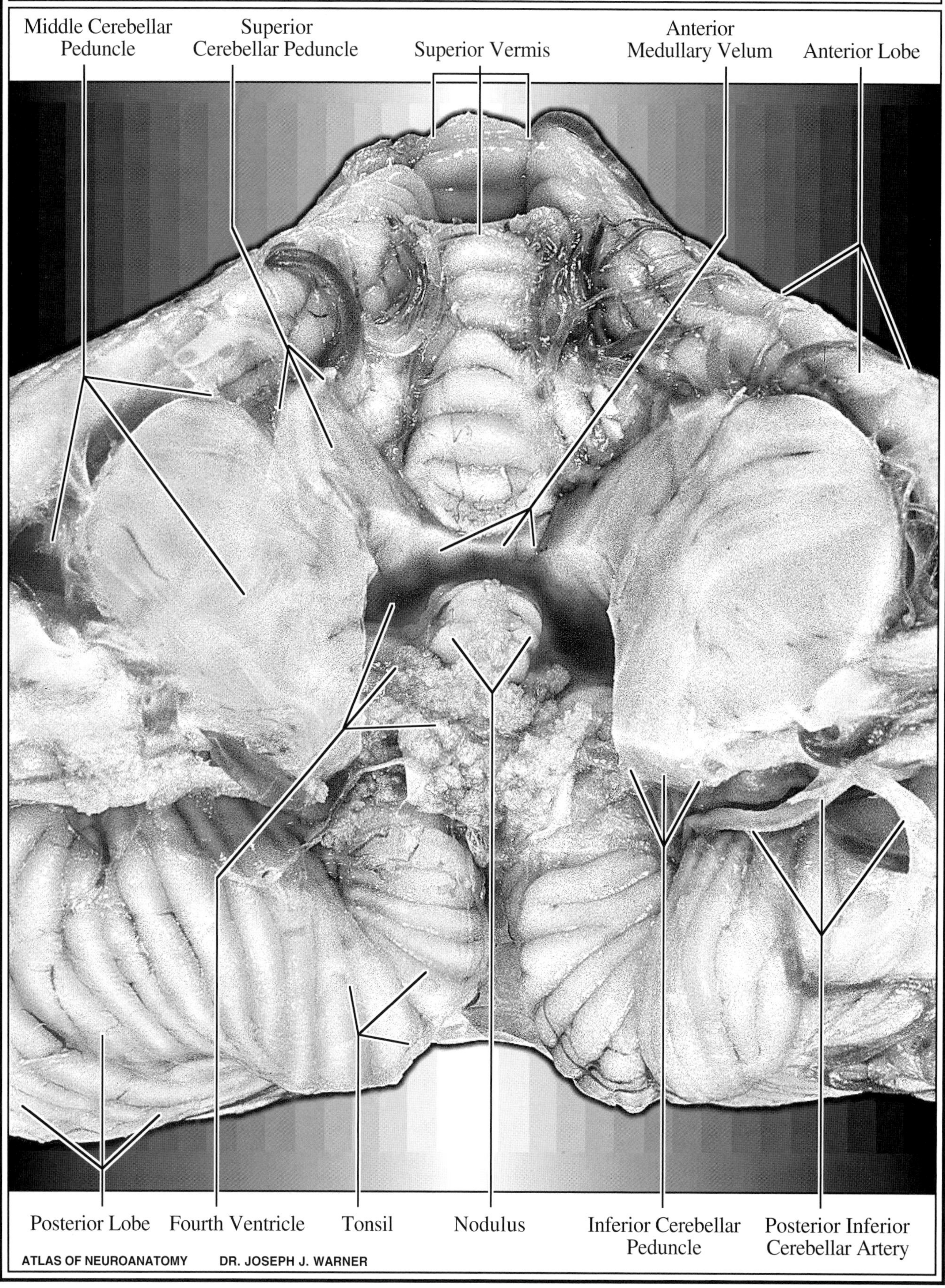

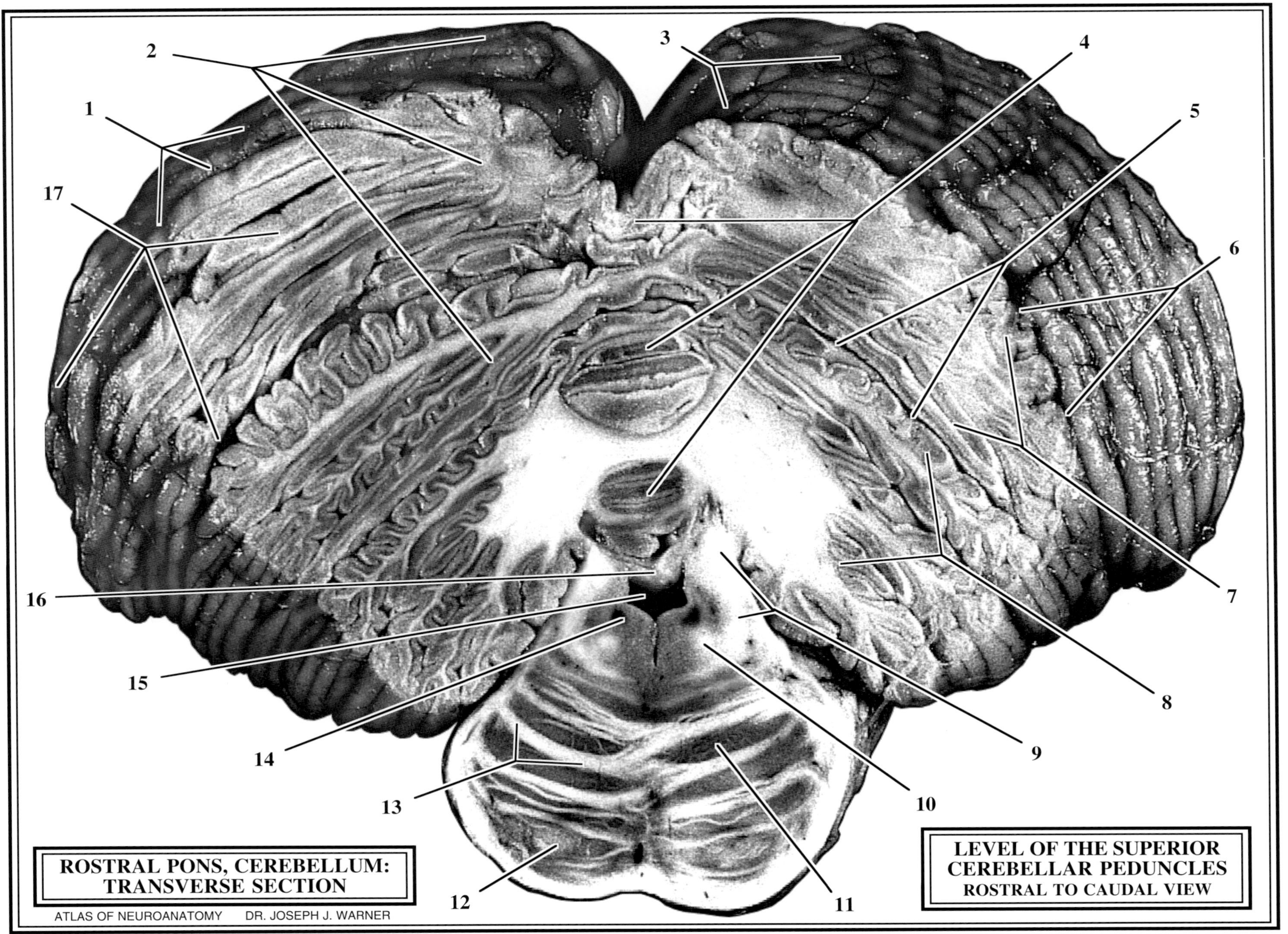
2
3
4
1
5
17
6
16
7
15
8
14
9
13
10
12
11
ROSTRAL PONS, CEREBELLUM:
TRANSVERSE SECTION
ATLAS OF NEUROANATOMY
DR. JOSEPH J. WARNER
LEVEL OF THE SUPERIOR
CEREBELLAR PEDUNCLES
ROSTRAL TO CAUDAL VIEW

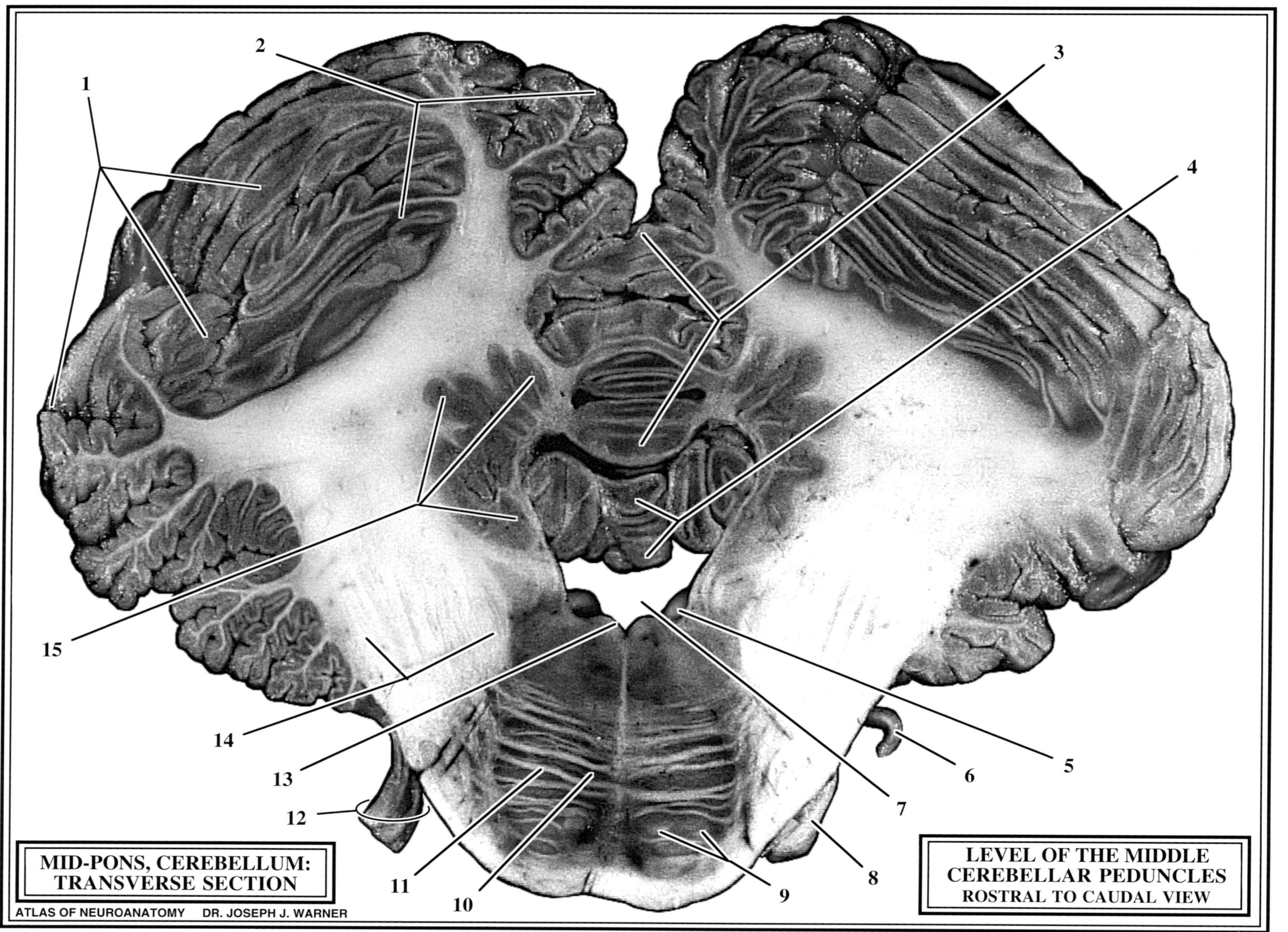
1
2
3
4
15
14
13
12
11
10
9
8
7
6
5
MID-PONS, CEREBELLUM:
TRANSVERSE SECTION
ATLAS OF NEUROANATOMY DR. JOSEPH J. WARNER
LEVEL OF THE MIDDLE
CEREBELLAR PEDUNCLES
ROSTRAL TO CAUDAL VIEW

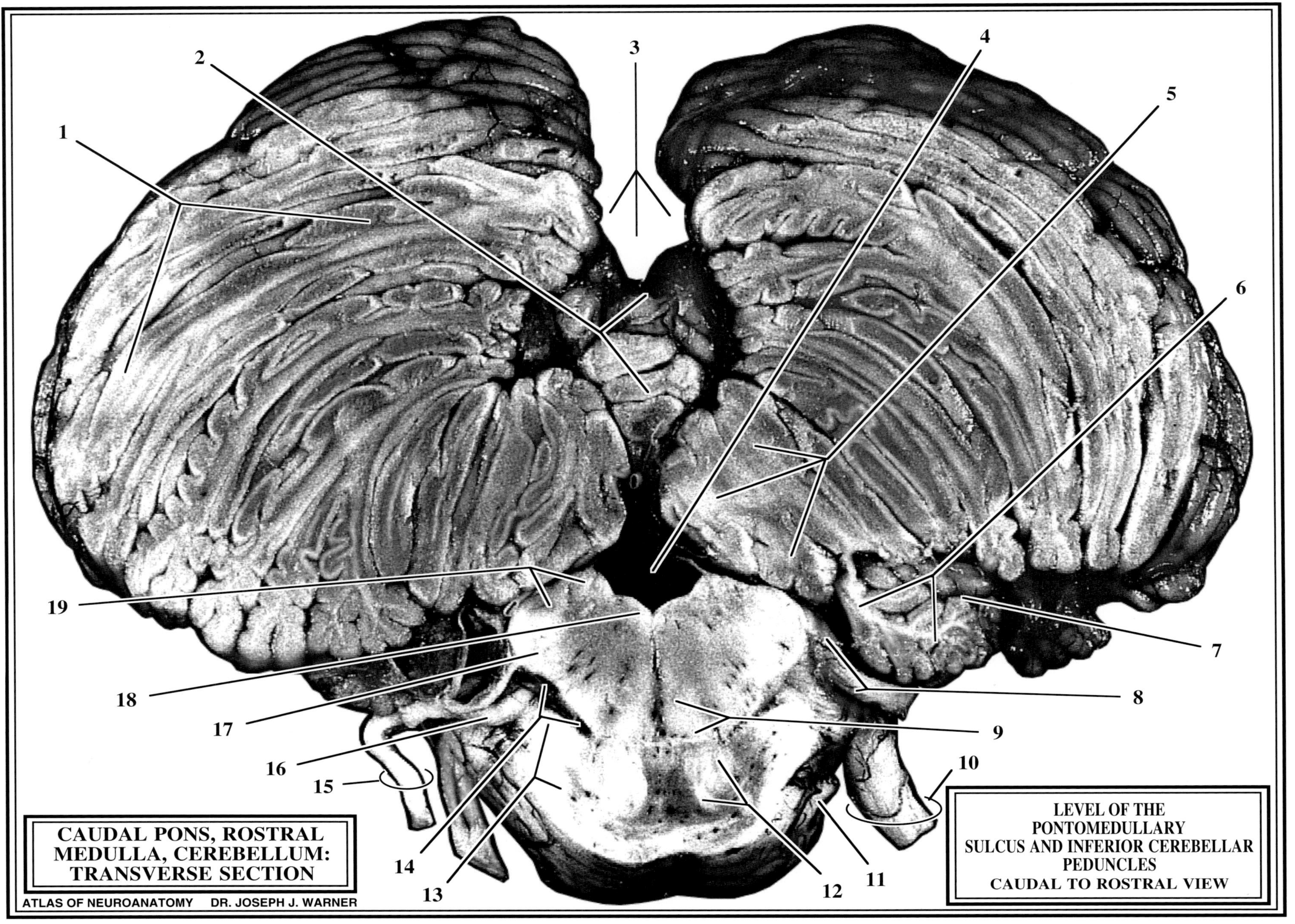
1
2
3
4
5
6
7
8
9
10
11
12
13
14
15
16
17
18
19
CAUDAL PONS, ROSTRAL MEDULLA, CEREBELLUM: TRANSVERSE SECTION
ATLAS OF NEUROANATOMY DR. JOSEPH J. WARNER
LEVEL OF THE PONTOMEDULLARY SULCUS AND INFERIOR CEREBELLAR PEDUNCLES
CAUDAL TO ROSTRAL VIEW

PONS, CEREBELLUM, AND PONTOMEDULLARY JUNCTION: MAP OF SECTION ORIENTATIONS AND KEY TO STRUCTURES

REFERENCED TO PARASAGITTAL SECTION, 15μ, KLUVER-BARRERA TECHNIQUE

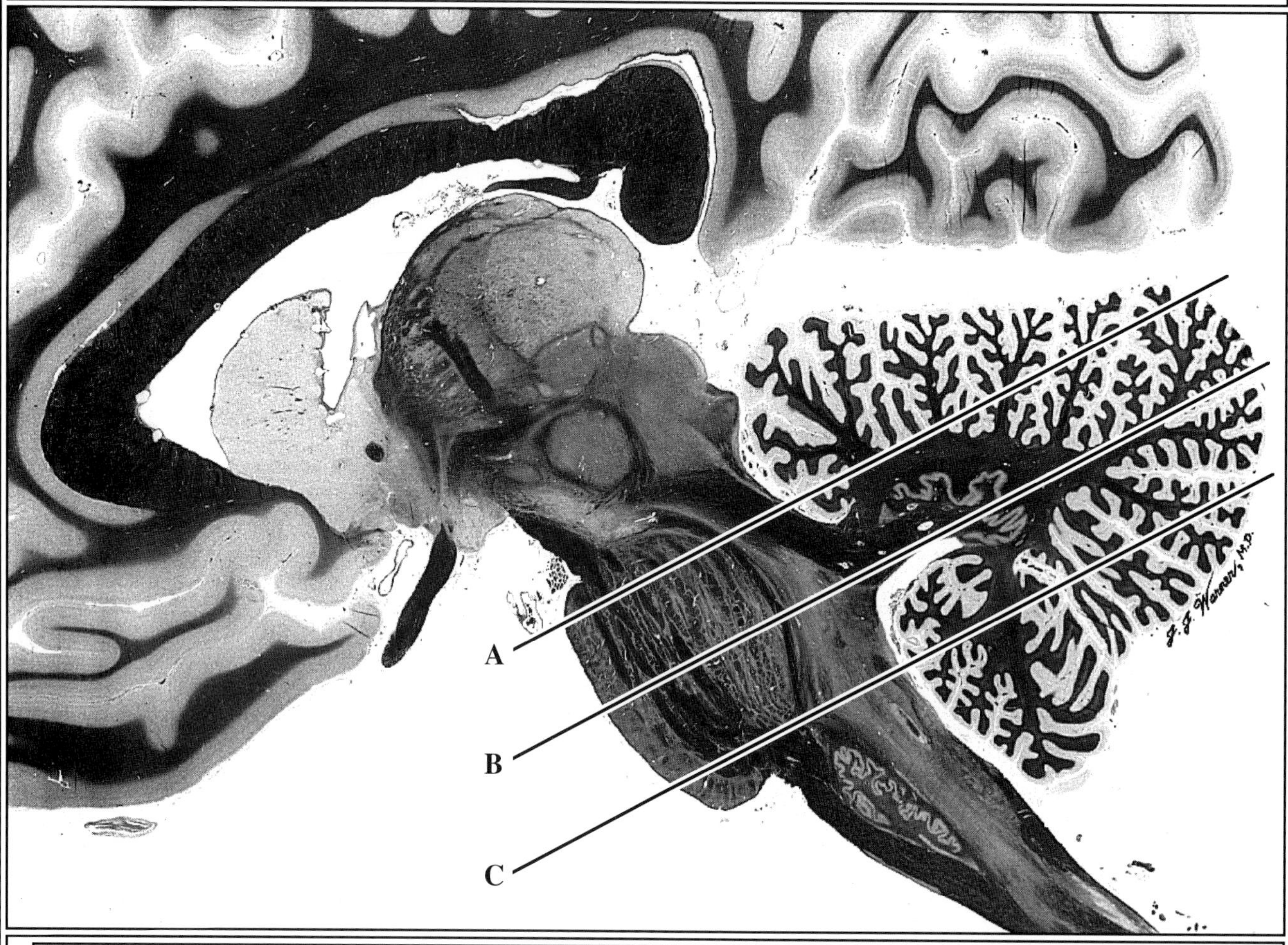

KEY TO NUMBERED STRUCTURES FOR EACH LEVEL (REFER TO ORIENTATION MAPS)

A. ROSTRAL PONS AND CEREBELLUM: LEVEL OF THE SUPERIOR CEREBELLAR PEDUNCLES

1. Superior Semilunar Lobule
2. Intermediate Zone
3. Horizontal Fissure
4. Vermis of Cerebellum
5. Primary Fissure
6. Posterior Superior Fissure
7. Posterior Quadrangular Lobule
8. Anterior Lobe of Cerebellum
9. Superior Cerebellar Peduncle
10. Central Tegmental Tract
11. Pontine Nuclei (Pontine Gray)
12. Corticobulbar, Corticospinal Tracts
13. Transverse Pontocerebellar Fibers
14. Locus Coeruleus
15. Fourth Ventricle (rostral aspect)
16. Anterior Medullary Velum
17. Posterior Lobe of Cerebellum

B. MID-PONS AND CEREBELLUM: LEVEL OF THE MIDDLE CEREBELLAR PEDUNCLES

1. Lateral Zone (Cerebrocerebellum)
2. Intermediate Zone
3. Vermis (Midline Cerebellum)
4. Nodulus
5. Contour of Vestibular and Vagal Nuclei
6. Facial (VII) Nerve
7. Fourth Ventricle
8. Trigeminal (V) Nerve
9. Corticobulbar, Corticospinal Tracts
10. Pontine Nuclei (Gray)
11. Transverse Pontocerebellar Fibers
12. Trigeminal (V) Nerve
13. Facial Colliculus
14. Middle Cerebellar Peduncle
15. Dentate Nucleus of the Cerebellum

C. CAUDAL PONS, ROSTRAL MEDULLA, AND CEREBELLUM: LEVEL OF THE PONTOMEDULLARY SULCUS AND THE INFERIOR CEREBELLAR PEDUNCLES

1. Inferior Semilunar Lobule
2. Cerebellar Vermis
3. Posterior Incisure
4. Fourth Ventricle
5. Cerebellar Tonsil
6. Flocculus
7. Posterolateral Fissure
8. Vestibulocochlear (VIII) Nerve
9. Medial Lemniscus
10. Trigeminal (V) Nerve
11. Abducens (VI) Nerve
12. Corticobulbar, Corticospinal Tracts
13. Middle Cerebellar Peduncle
14. Pontomedullary Sulcus
15. Facial (VII) Nerve
16. Glossopharyngeal (IX) Nerve
17. Inferior Cerebellar Peduncle
18. Hypoglossal Trigone
19. Vestibular Nuclear Complex

MAJOR DIVISIONS OF THE CENTRAL NERVOUS SYSTEM: HORIZONTAL SECTION REFERENCE DIAGRAM

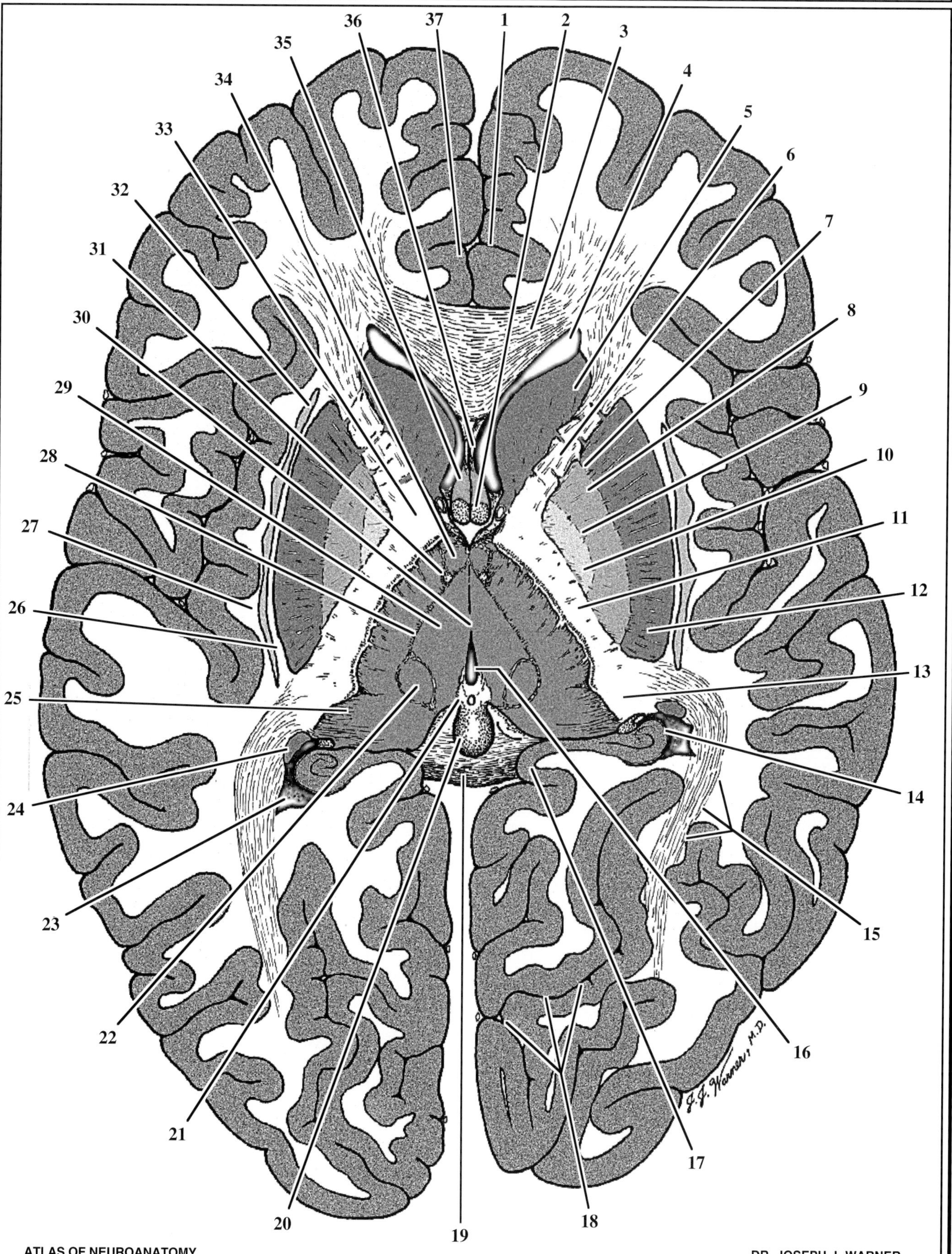

MAJOR DIVISIONS OF THE CENTRAL NERVOUS SYSTEM; HORIZONTAL SECTION REFERENCE DIAGRAM: ANATOMIC RELATIONSHIPS BETWEEN THE THALAMUS, THE CORPUS STRIATUM, AND THE INTERNAL CAPSULE

The presentation of major divisions of the central nervous system must, by necessity, include an examination of the major diencephalic and telencephalic structures on sectioned specimens, even prior to the systematic detailed study of sectional neuroanatomy. In this volume, certain sections are presented as major *reference levels*, as they demonstrate essential points of the spatial organization of subcortical structures and components of the ventricular system. One of these reference planes is that which includes the caudate nucleus, thalamus, lenticular nucleus, and internal capsule in horizontal section.

The internal capsule consists of a massive arrangement of ascending and descending fiber tracts, which include thalamocortical and corticofugal projections. This white matter structure has a geometric configuration that is fundamentally characterized by (1) *divergence in a ventral to dorsal direction,* and (2) an anterior limb, genu, and posterior limb that form *an obtuse angle medial to the lenticular nucleus*. Of course, this is an oversimplification that does not apply to the retrolenticular or sublenticular components of the internal capsule. However, this model is quite useful in understanding the appearance of the structure in various planes of section. Two additional points are to be emphasized. *(1) With the exception of nucleus accumbens ventral to the anterior limb, the internal capsule and corona radiata separate the caudate nucleus from the lenticular nucleus. (2) The posterior limb of the internal capsule separates the thalamus from the lenticular nucleus.*

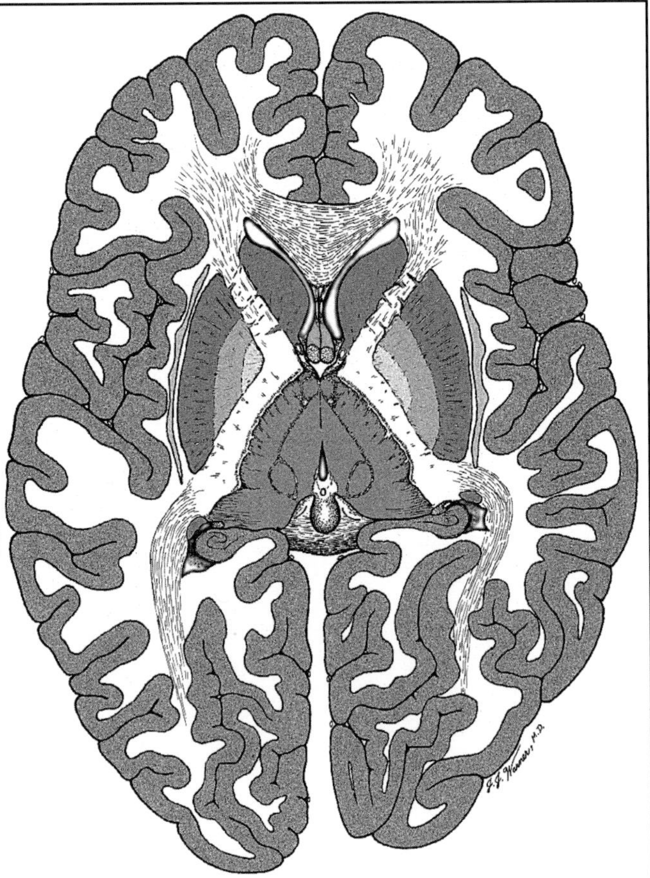

These principles, which apply to horizontal, coronal, and sagittal planes, are essential to the three-dimensional conceptualization of subcortical neuroanatomy.

KEY TO NUMBERED STRUCTURES

1. Cingulate Sulcus
2. Fornix
3. Genu of the Corpus Callosum
4. Anterior Horn of the Lateral Ventricle
5. Head of the Caudate Nucleus
6. Anterior Limb of the Internal Capsule
7. External Medullary Lamina
8. Globus Pallidus II
9. Internal Medullary Lamina
10. Globus Pallidus I
11. Posterior Limb of the Internal Capsule
12. Putamen
13. Retrolenticular Component of the Internal Capsule
14. Hippocampal Formation
15. Optic (Geniculocalcarine) Radiations
16. Third Ventricle
17. Isthmus of the Gyrus Fornicatus
18. Calcarine Fissure
19. Splenium of the Corpus Callosum
20. Pineal Body
21. Habenula
22. Centromedian Nucleus of the Thalamus
23. Temporal Horn of the Lateral Ventricle
24. Tail of the Caudate Nucleus
25. Putamen
26. External Capsule
27. Extreme Capsule
28. Internal Medullary Lamina of the Thalamus
29. Dorsomedial Nucleus of the Thalamus
30. Massa Intermedia
31. Mammillothalamic Tract
32. Claustrum
33. Genu of the Internal Capsule
34. Anterior Nucleus of the Thalamus
35. Septal Nuclei
36. Septum Pellucidum
37. Cingulate Cortex

MAJOR DIVISIONS: HORIZONTAL SECTION REFERENCE DIAGRAM

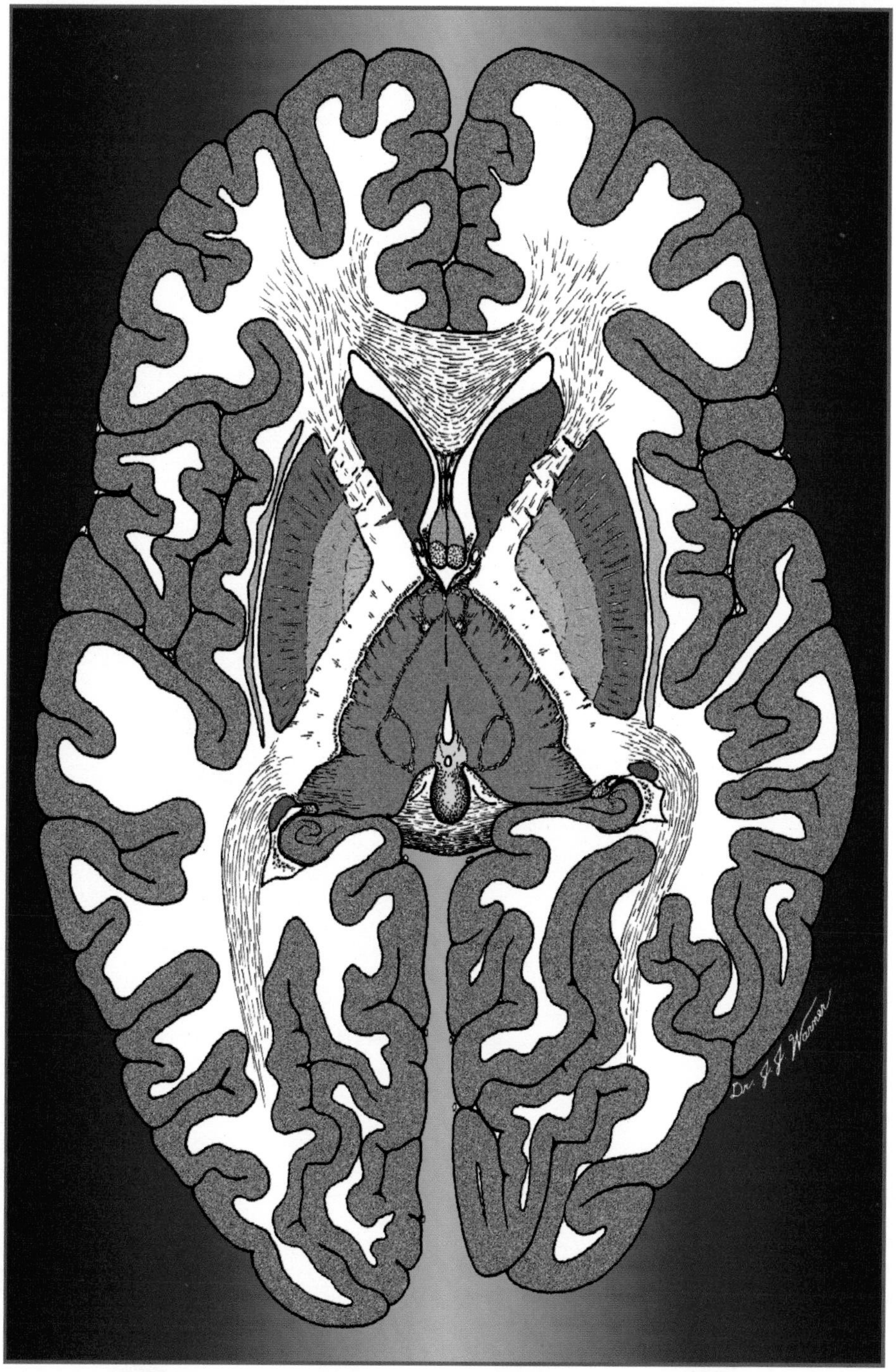

DIENCEPHALON
Thalamus
Metathalamus
Hypothalamus
Subthalamus
Epithalamus

SUBTHALAMUS
Zona Incerta
Fields of Forel
Prerubral Fields
Subthalamic Nucleus

EPITHALAMUS
Pineal Body
Habenula
Habenular Commissure
Stria Medullaris
Epithelial Roof of the Third Ventricle

METATHALAMUS
Medial Geniculate Nucleus
Lateral Geniculate Nucleus

KEY TO STRUCTURES

A. Caudate Nucleus
B. Putamen
C. Globus Pallidus II
D. Globus Pallidus I
E. Claustrum
F. Thalamus
G. Septal Nuclei
H. Epithalamus

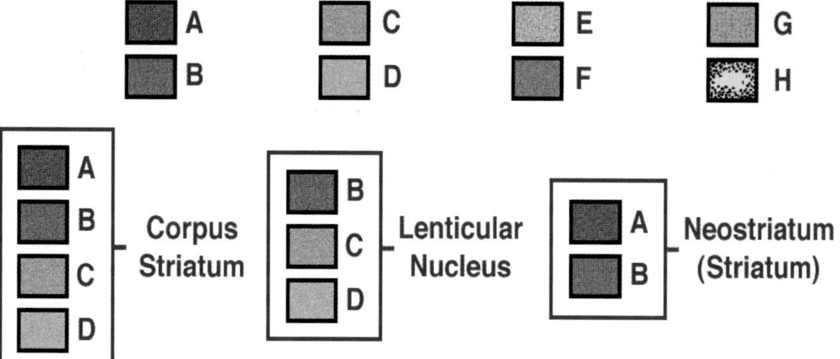

BASAL GANGLIA (TELENCEPHALIC)

Globus Pallidus I & II
Putamen
Caudate Nucleus
Amygdaloid Nuclear Complex

MAJOR DIVISIONS OF THE CENTRAL NERVOUS SYSTEM; REFERENCE CORONAL SECTION: LEVEL OF THE MAMMILLARY BODIES AND THE ANTERIOR NUCLEUS OF THE THALAMUS

STRUCTURAL KEY

A

B

C

D

E

F

G

H

I

A. Caudate Nucleus
B. Putamen
C. Globus Pallidus II
D. Globus Pallidus I
E. Amygdala
F. Subthalamus
G. Hypothalamus
H. Thalamus
I. Epithalamus

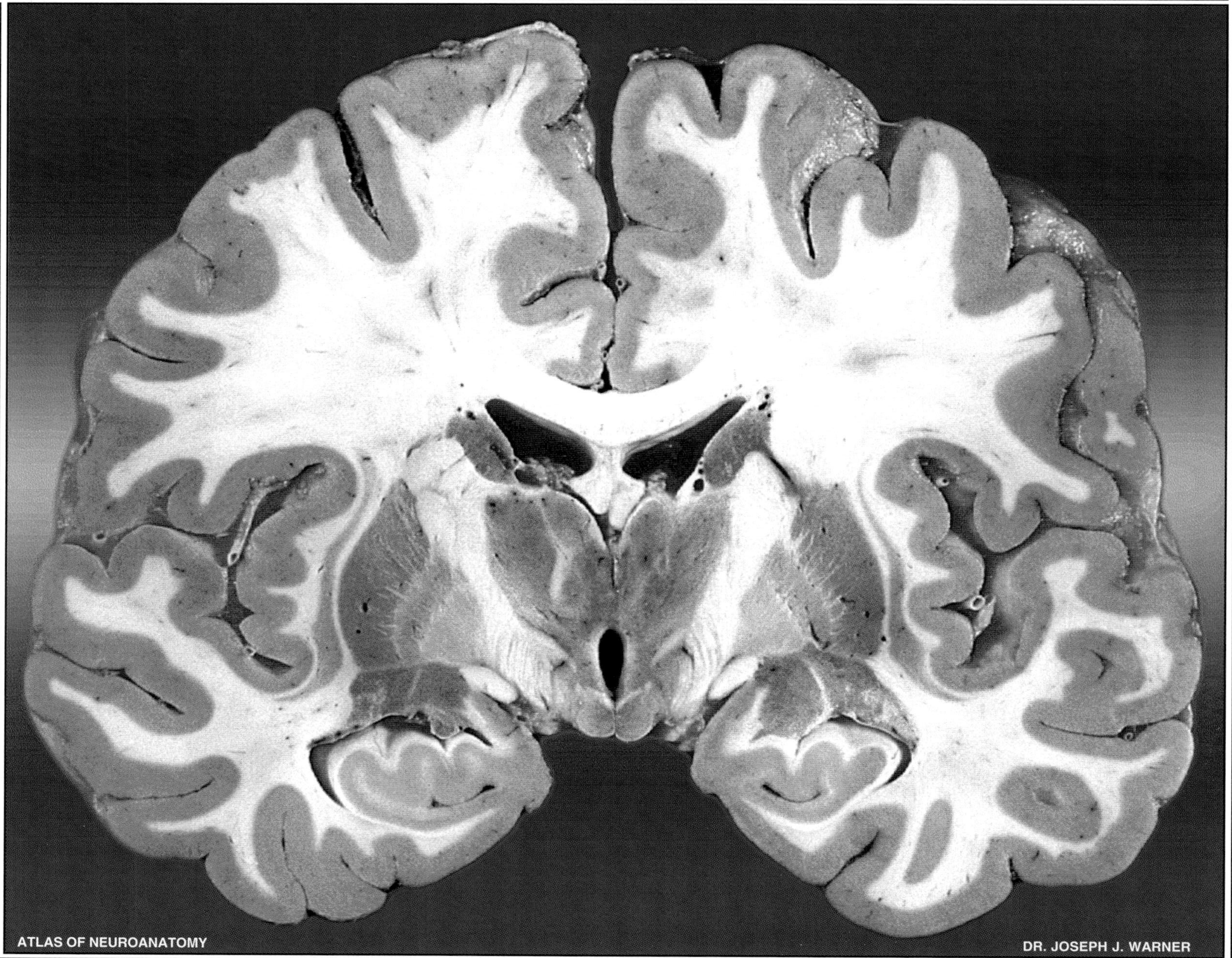

ATLAS OF NEUROANATOMY

DR. JOSEPH J. WARNER

THE INTERNAL CAPSULE: THREE-DIMENSIONAL CHARACTERISTICS

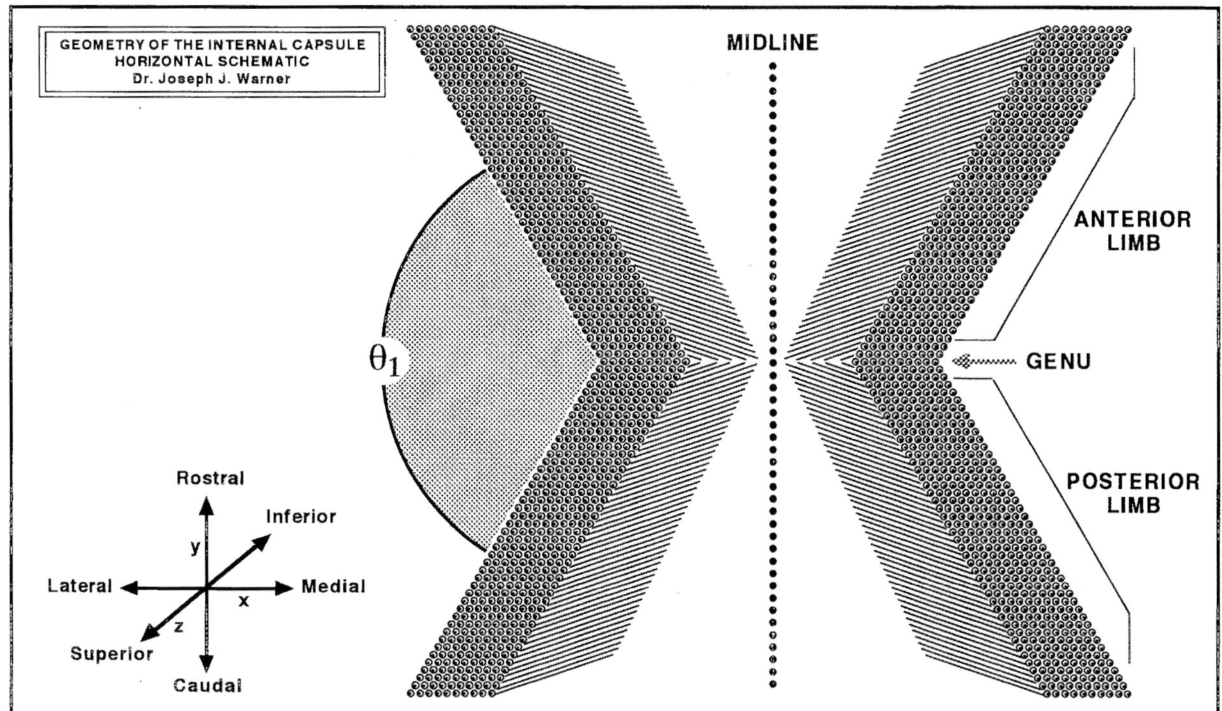

Consideration of the geometric configuration of the internal capsule is useful in analyzing the orientation of sections which include this structure. The characteristic appearance of the internal capsule in horizontal, sagittal, and coronal sections is determined by its three-dimensional configuration. Two components of the internal capsule of each hemisphere, the anterior and posterior limb, form an obtuse angle (**θ_1**, referring to figure). The vertex of this angle (located at the genu) points toward the midline. Furthermore, each internal capsule diverges from the midline (angle **θ_2**, referring to figure) in a ventral to dorsal direction.

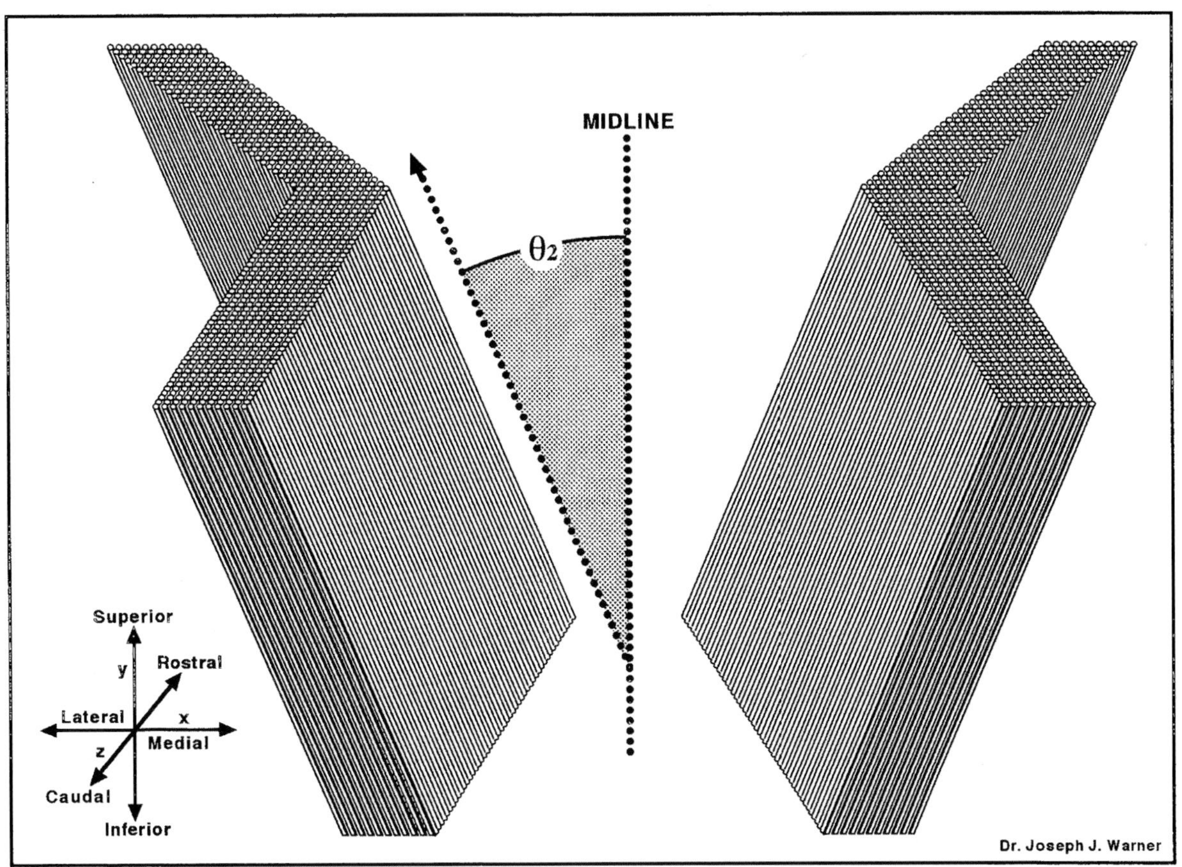

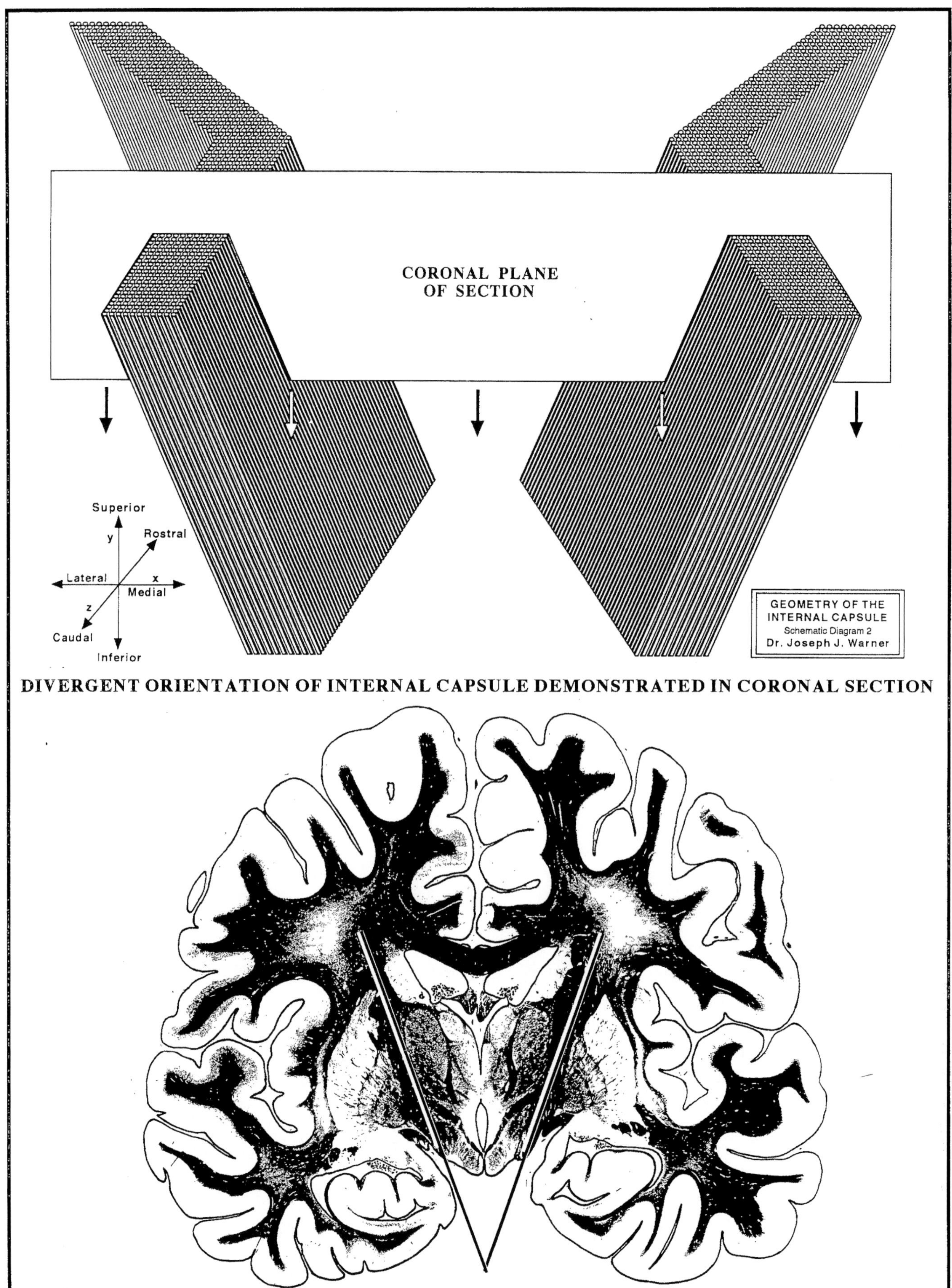
CORONAL PLANE
OF SECTION
Superior
y
Rostral
Lateral
x
Medial
z
Caudal
Inferior
GEOMETRY OF THE
INTERNAL CAPSULE
Schematic Diagram 2
Dr. Joseph J. Warner
DIVERGENT ORIENTATION OF INTERNAL CAPSULE DEMONSTRATED IN CORONAL SECTION

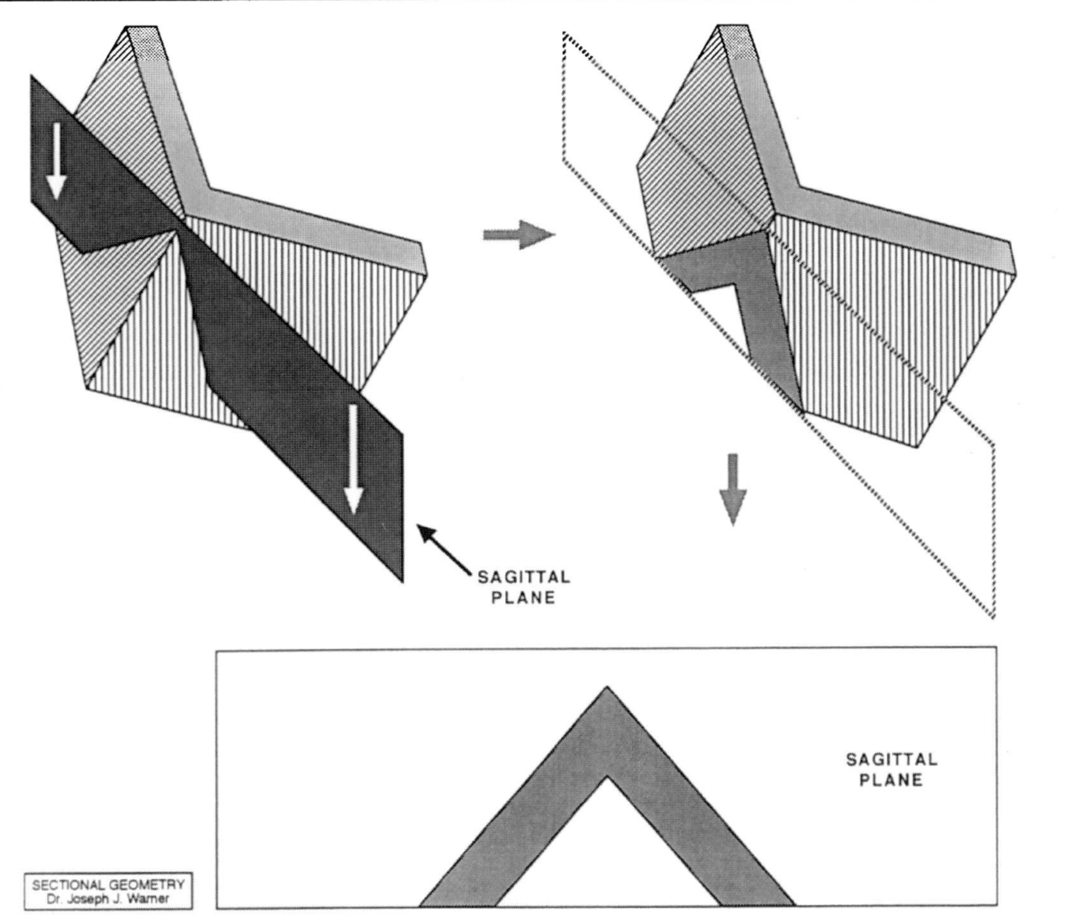

GEOMETRY OF INTERNAL CAPSULE DEMONSTRATED IN SAGITTAL SECTION

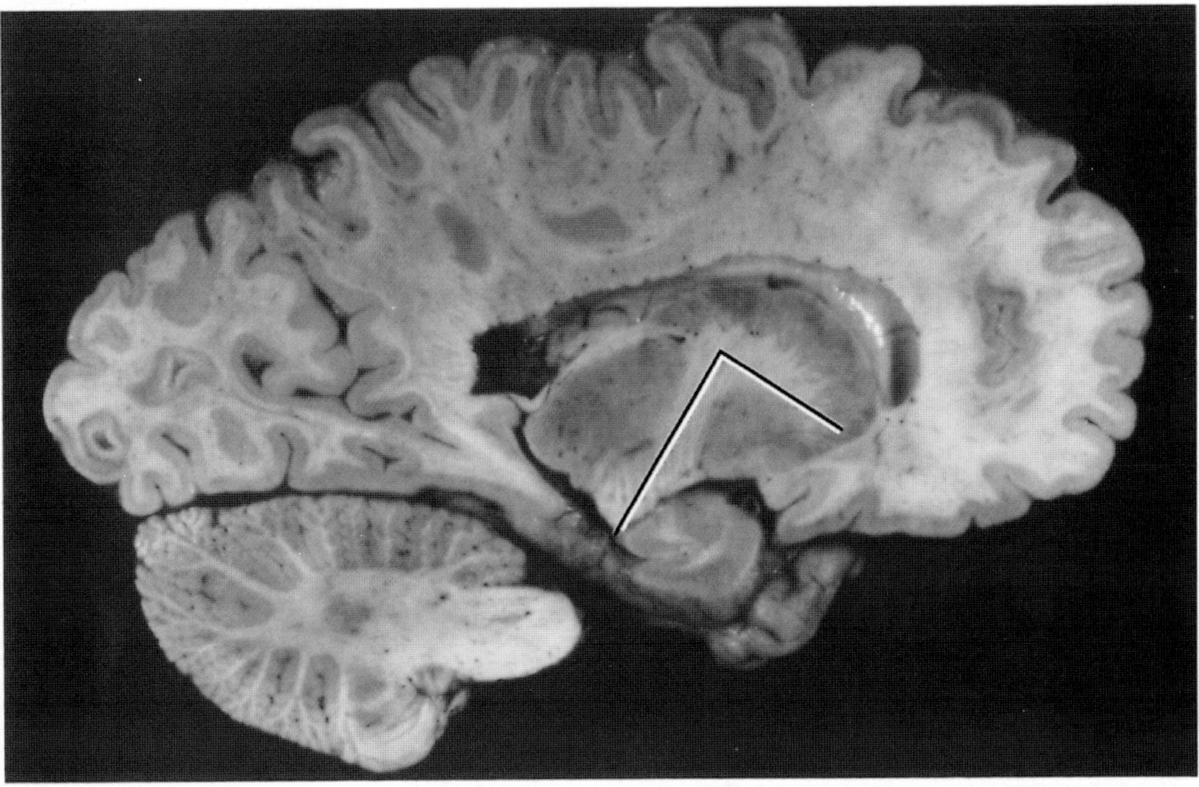

The genu of the internal capsule is at the vertex of the angle formed by the anterior and posterior limbs. Thus, a sagittal section plane passes through the genu at a level more dorsal than either the anterior or posterior limb.

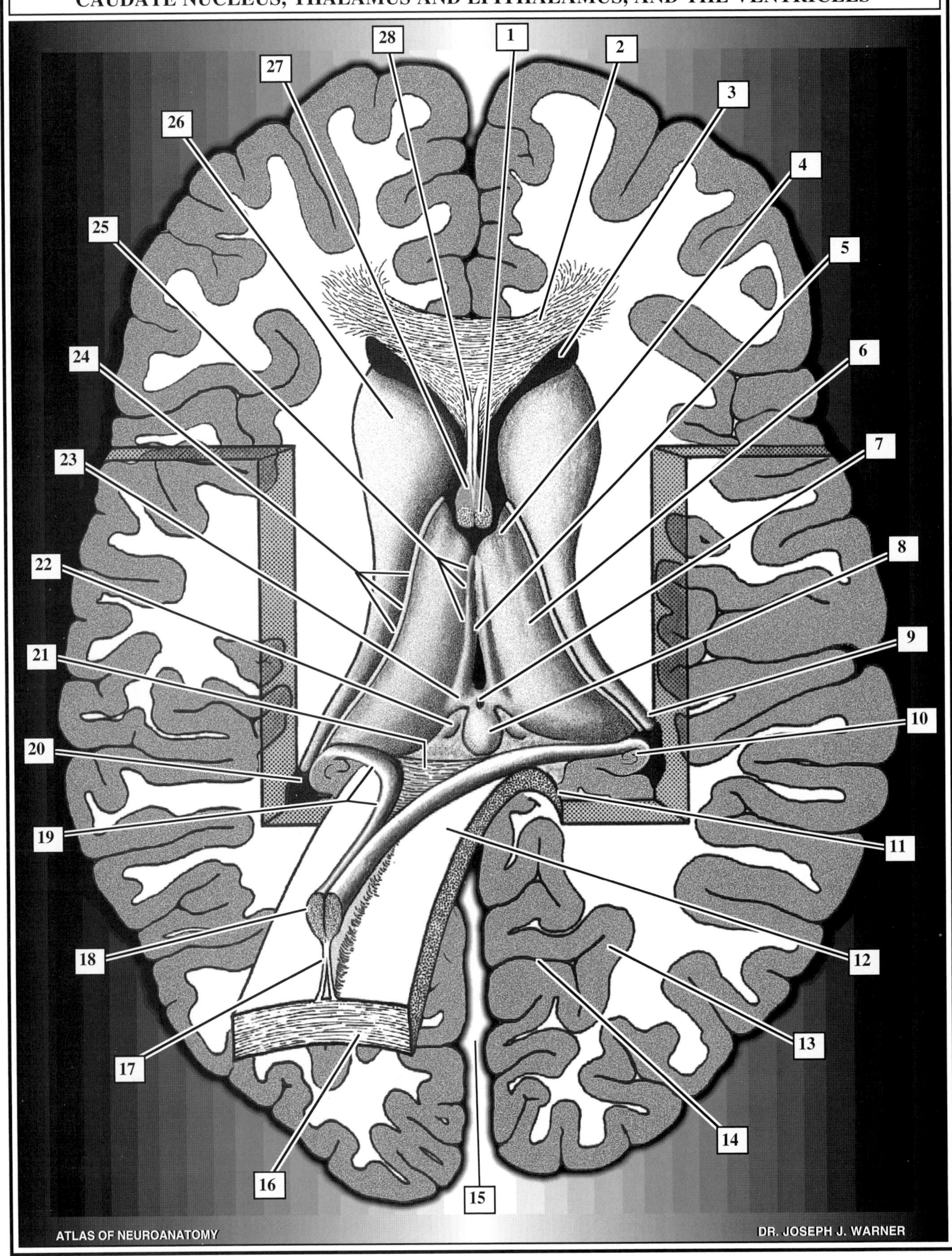
DIAGRAM OF A DISSECTION OF THE CEREBRAL HEMISPHERES: SECTION AND RETRACTION OF THE CORPUS CALLOSUM AND FORNIX TO DEMONSTRATE THE CAUDATE NUCLEUS, THALAMUS AND EPITHALAMUS, AND THE VENTRICLES
1
2
3
4
5
6
7
8
9
10
11
12
13
14
15
16
17
18
19
20
21
22
23
24
25
26
27
28
ATLAS OF NEUROANATOMY
DR. JOSEPH J. WARNER

DIAGRAM OF A DISSECTION OF THE CEREBRAL HEMISPHERES: SECTION AND RETRACTION OF THE CORPUS CALLOSUM AND FORNIX TO DEMONSTRATE THE CAUDATE NUCLEUS, THALAMUS AND EPITHALAMUS, AND THE VENTRICLES

Diagram (A) represents the dissection of the basal ganglia, thalamus, and epithalamus through initial horizontal section dorsal to the corpus callosum, followed by longitudinal section of the corpus callosum bilaterally. A more ventral horizontal section is utilized to section the genu of the corpus callosum, rostral aspect of the fornix, septal nuclei, and septum pellucidum. Dorsal retraction of these structures with separation of the fornix from the dorsal thalamus exposes the lateral and ventral aspects of the body of each lateral ventricle, as well as the roof of the third ventricle. Deeper horizontal section through the white matter (sparing the caudate nucleus) transects fibers of the corona radiata. [The conventional horizontal section through the extreme dorsal thalamus (B) demonstrates the normal anatomic relationship of the fornix to the caudate nucleus, thalamus, and lateral ventricles.] Note that these structures are encountered in more dorsal planes than horizontal sections which include the lenticular nucleus. A variation of this dissection (which includes bilateral circumferential section of the corona radiata and complete resection of the corpus callosum) demonstrates the dorsal brainstem and diencephalon (Refer to figure of special dissection).

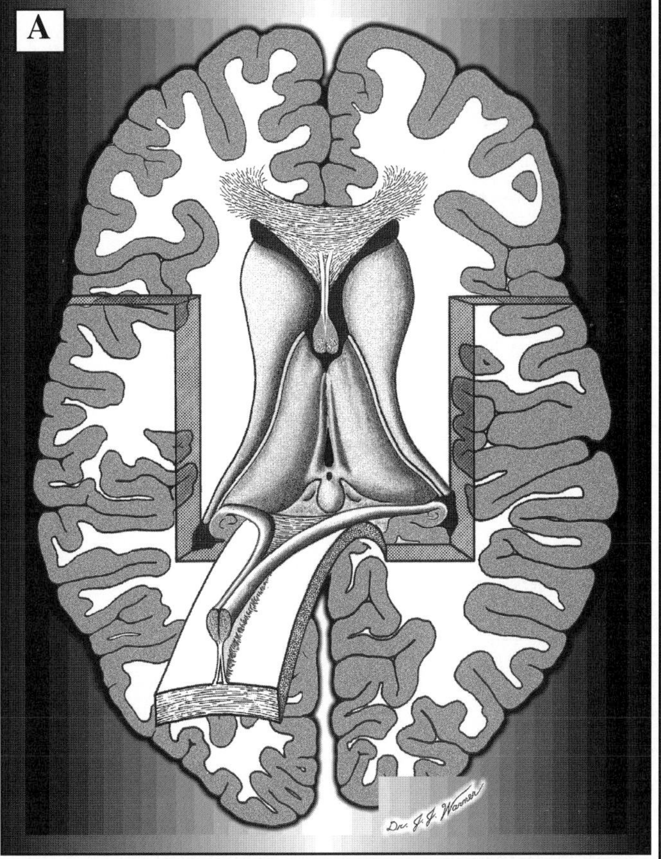

KEY TO NUMBERED STRUCTURES

1. Fornix
2. Genu of the Corpus Callosum
3. Anterior Horn of the Lateral Ventricle
4. Anterior Tubercle of the Thalamus
5. Massa Intermedia ventral to Taenia Thalami
6. Lamina Affixa of the Thalamus
7. Pineal Recess of the Third Ventricle
8. Pineal Body
9. Tail of the Caudate Nucleus
10. Hippocampal Formation
11. Splenium of the Corpus Callosum
12. Body of the Corpus Callosum (forms the roof of the bodies of the Lateral Ventricles)
13. Area 17 Striate Cortex
14. Calcarine Fissure
15. Interhemispheric Fissure
16. Retracted surface of the Corpus Callosum
17. Septum Pellucidum
18. Fornix
19. Crus of the Fornix
20. Atrium/Temporal Horn of the Lateral Ventricle
21. Hippocampal Commissure
22. Superior Colliculus
23. Habenula
24. Stria Terminalis and Thalamostriate Vein
25. Stria Medullaris
26. Head of the Caudate Nucleus
27. Septal Nuclei
28. Septum Pellucidum

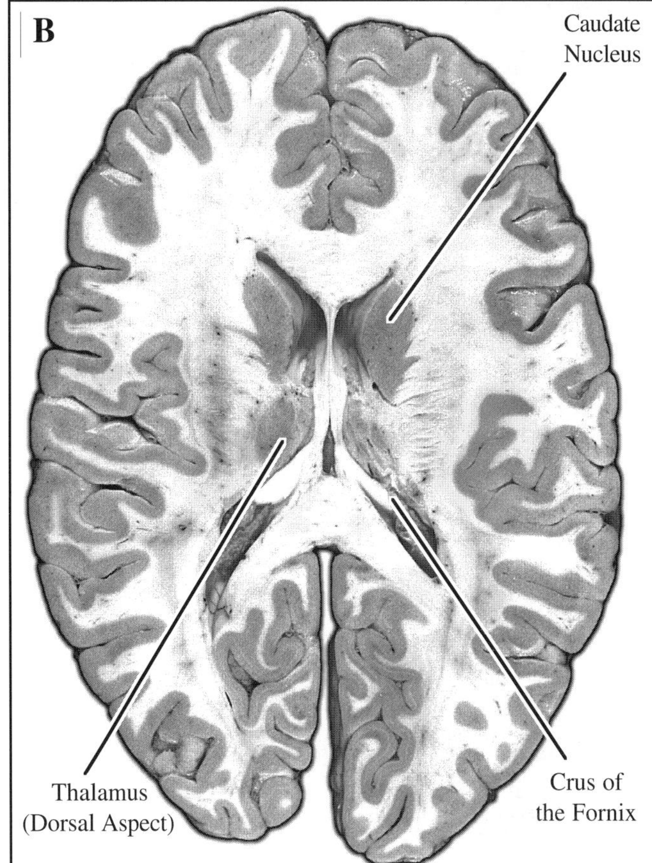

DORSAL ASPECT OF THE MESENCEPHALON, DIENCEPHALON, AND CEREBELLUM

(1) RESECTION OF THE CORPUS CALLOSUM, FORNIX, AND CHOROID PLEXUS * (2) CIRCUMFERENTIAL SECTION OF THE CORONA RADIATA

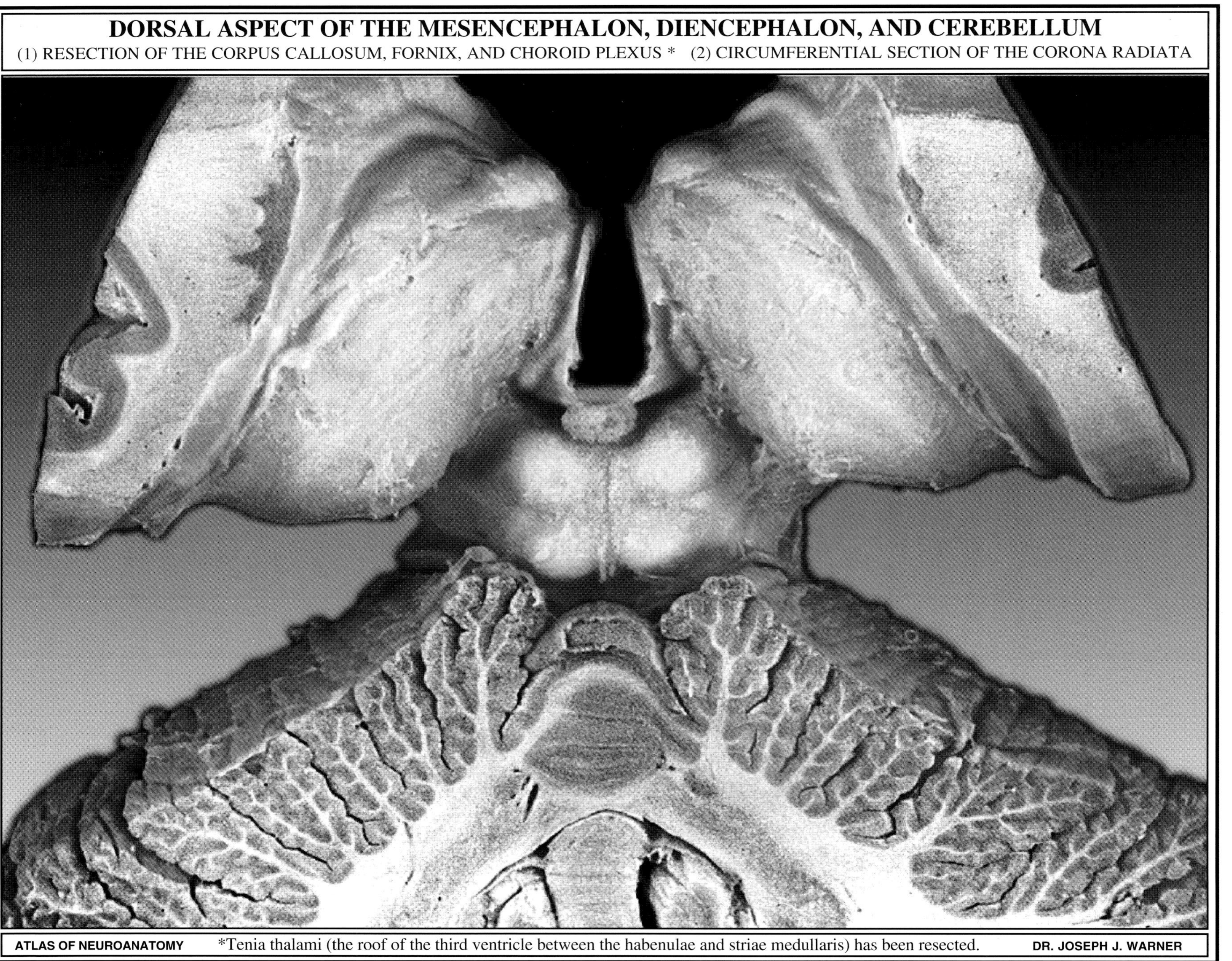

*Tenia thalami (the roof of the third ventricle between the habenulae and striae medullaris) has been resected.

DORSAL ASPECT OF THE MESENCEPHALON, DIENCEPHALON, AND CEREBELLUM

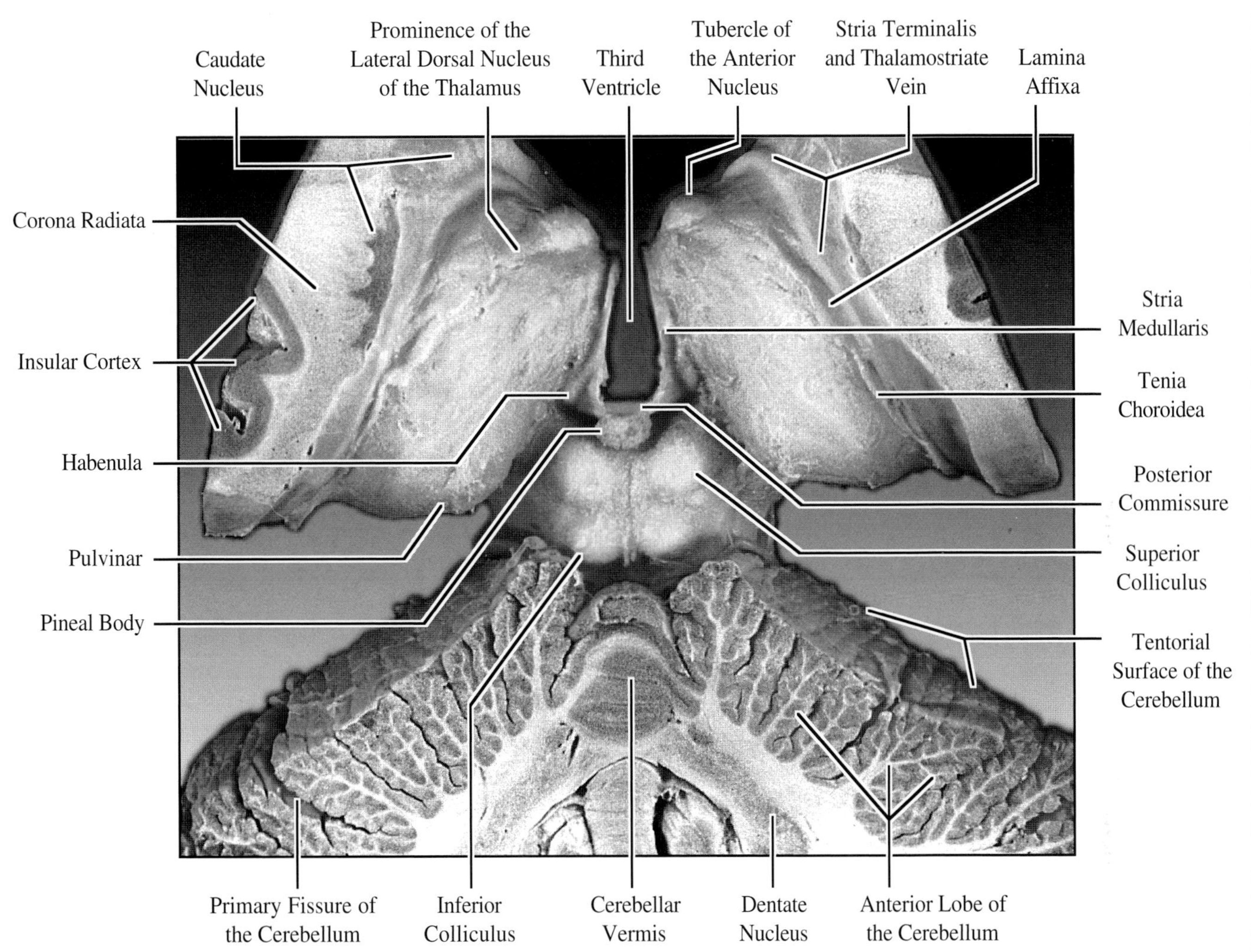

The methodology of this dissection is a key to understanding the important neuroanatomic relationships between the diencephalon and telencephalic structures. Telencephalic structures dorsal and caudal to the corpus callosum are resected. The lateral ventricles are exposed by resection of the corpus callosum from the genu through the splenium and circumferential sectioning of the corona radiata. Choroid plexus is dissected from each lateral ventricle. The rostral aspect of the septum pellucidum and fornices are sectioned adjacent to the anterior commissure, then retracted dorsally and caudally, with separation of the fornix from the lamina affixa (on the dorsal surface of the thalamus) bilaterally. This exposes the dorsal surface of the thalamus. Caudally, the fornices are transected (as they course from the temporal lobes) and removed. Removal of the fornices and choroid plexus also involves longitudinal separation from the tenia choroidea bilaterally. The third ventricle is exposed by resection of the tenia thalami (roof of the third ventricle between each stria medullaris and habenula). The tenia choroidea, tenia thalami, and tela choroidea are best examined on stained coronal sections. These bridging structures form the distinct cerebrospinal fluid compartments of the ventricular system. (Magnified examination of gross specimens is optimal to visualize the demarcation of the lateral ventricles, the third ventricle, and the subarachnoid space). The Aqueduct of Sylvius passes ventral to the posterior commissure, continues caudally, roofed by the corpora quadrigemina (superior and inferior colliculi), and opens into the fourth ventricle. The caudate nucleus is demonstrated in the lateral wall of the lateral ventricle, demarcated from the thalamus by the stria terminalis and thalamostriate vein. Deep insular cortex is visible (lateral to the corona radiata) bilaterally.

DORSAL ASPECT OF THE MESENCEPHALON, DIENCEPHALON, AND CEREBELLUM: VIEW OF THE EPITHALAMUS AND THE THIRD VENTRICLE

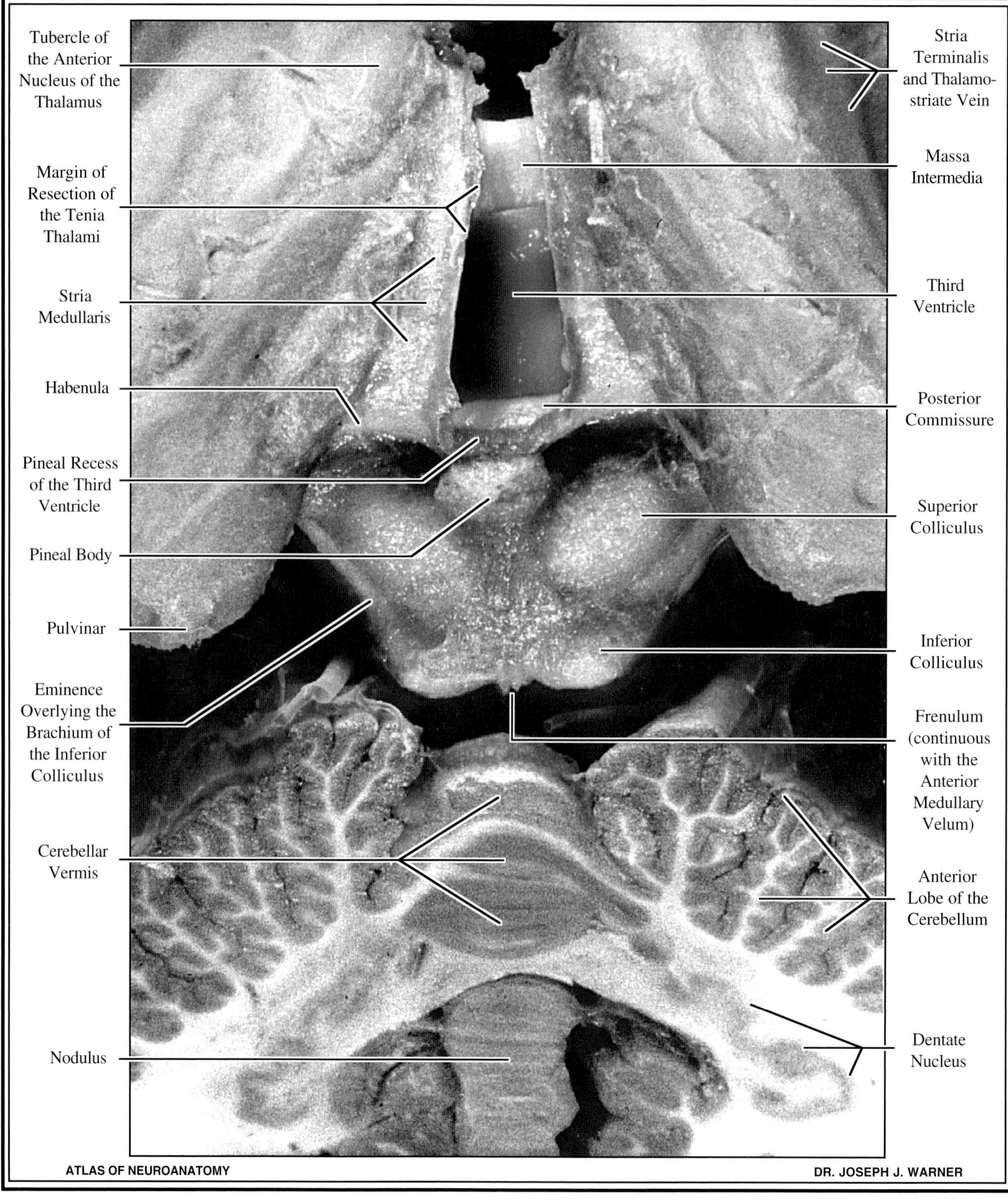

DORSAL ASPECT OF THE MESENCEPHALON AND DIENCEPHALON: ROOF OF THE THIRD VENTRICLE AND ROSTRAL CHOROID PLEXUS INTACT

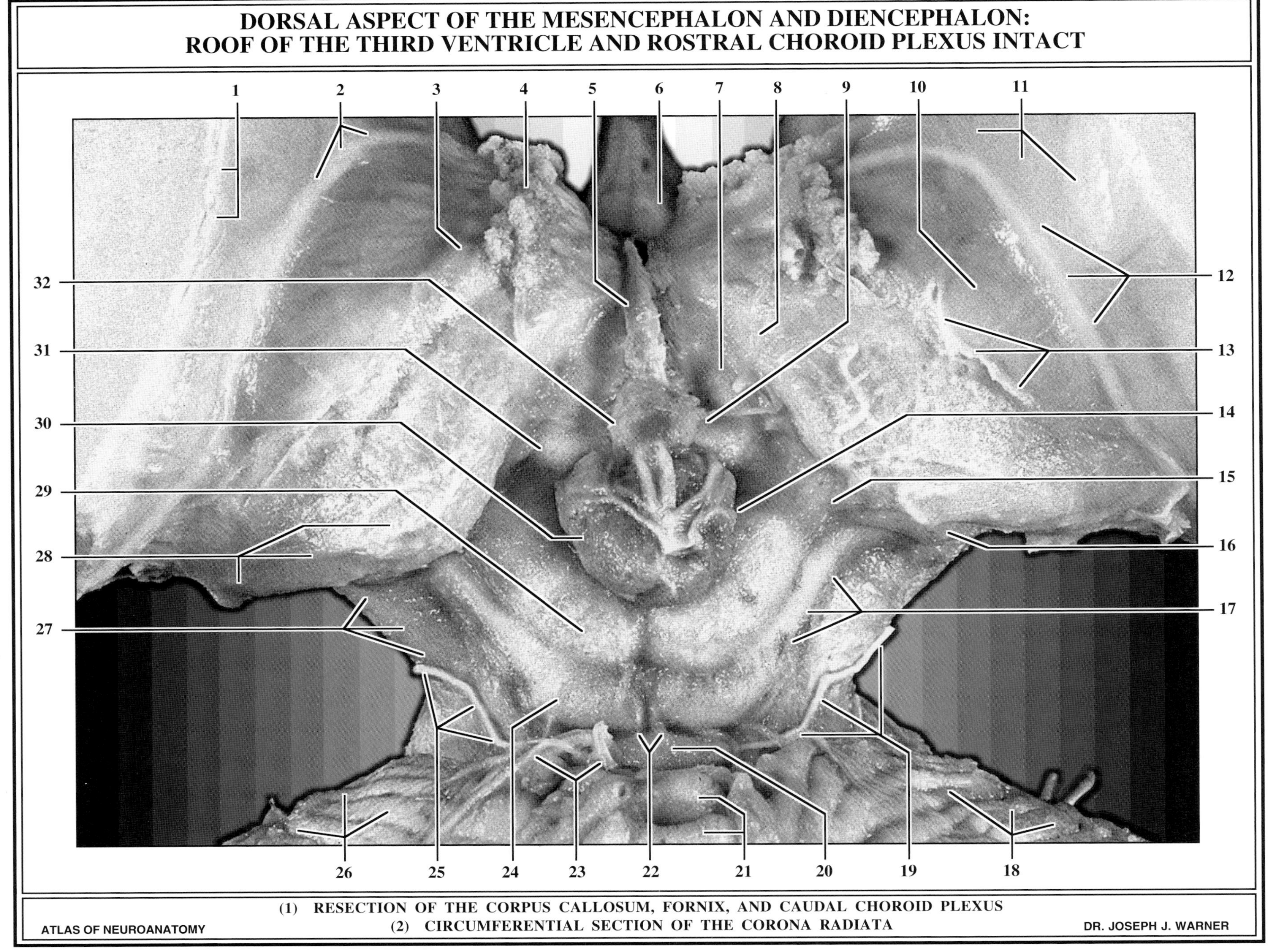

(1) RESECTION OF THE CORPUS CALLOSUM, FORNIX, AND CAUDAL CHOROID PLEXUS
(2) CIRCUMFERENTIAL SECTION OF THE CORONA RADIATA

DR. JOSEPH J. WARNER

DORSAL ASPECT OF THE MESENCEPHALON AND DIENCEPHALON: ROOF OF THE THIRD VENTRICLE AND ROSTRAL CHOROID PLEXUS INTACT

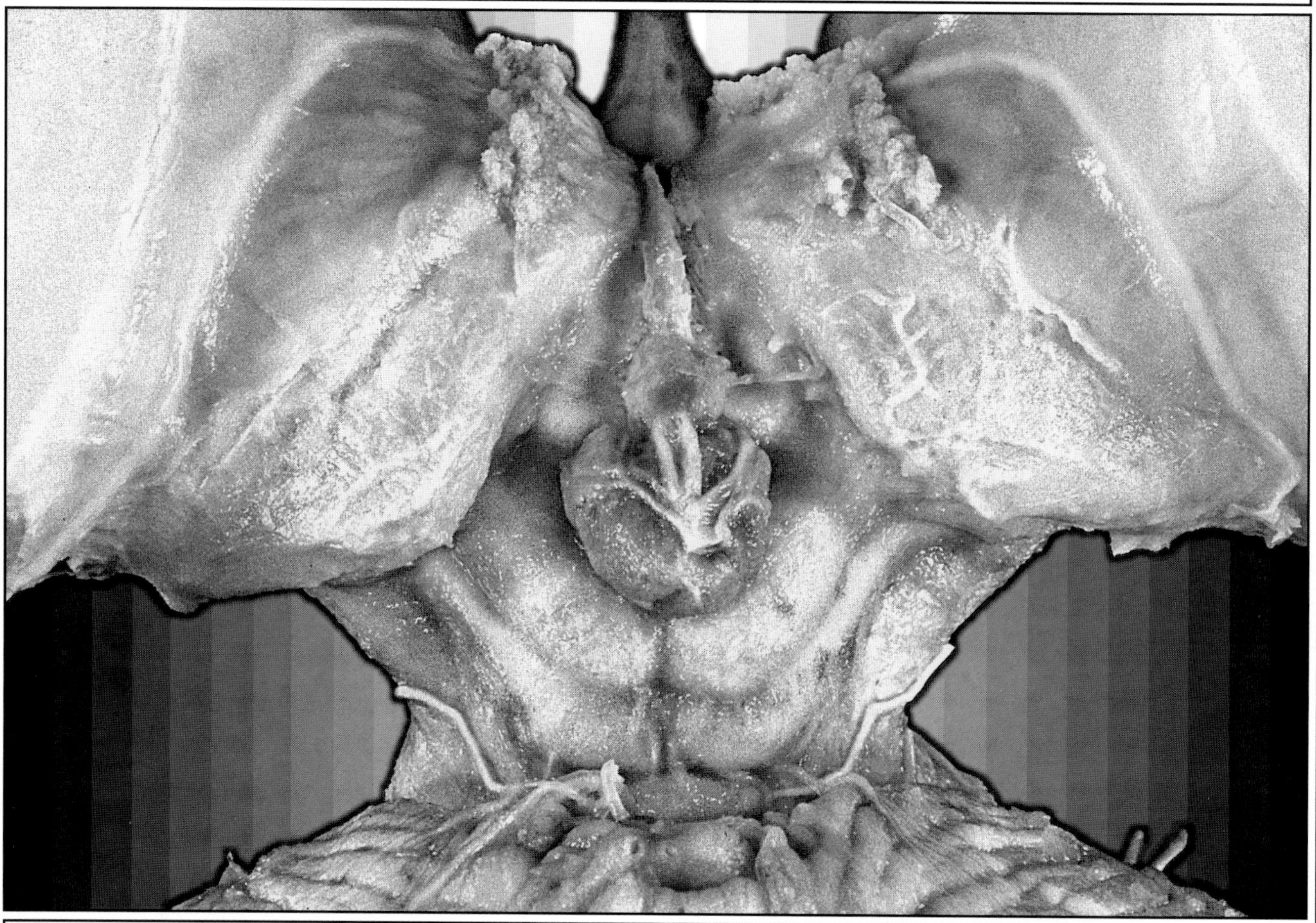

KEY TO NUMBERED STRUCTURES

1. Intersection of the lateral wall of the lateral ventricle with the resection surface of the corona radiata
2. Stria Terminalis and Thalamostriate Vein
3. Dorsal contour of the Lateral Dorsal Nucleus of the Thalamus
4. Choroid Plexus overlying the Anterior Nucleus of the Thalamus
5. Velum Interpositum, Taenia Thalami
6. Fornix (transected)
7. Stria Medullaris
8. Surface of the Thalamus exposed by resection of the Fornix (the Dorsomedial Nucleus is subjacent to this region)
9. Habenular Commissure
10. Dorsal surface of the Lateral Posterior Nucleus of the Thalamus
11. Caudate Nucleus
12. Stria Medullaris and Thalamostriate Vein
13. Taenia Choroidea
14. Tectal Vein (courses dorsal to the Pineal Body to join the Great Vein of Galen)*
15. Brachium of the Superior Colliculus
16. Medial Geniculate Nucleus
17. Brachium of the Inferior Colliculus
18. Anterior Lobe of the Cerebellum
19. Trochlear (IV) Nerve
20. Rostral aspect of the Anterior Medullary Velum
21. Central Lobule of the Cerebellum (dorsal to the Lingula)
22. Frenulum
23. Precentral Cerebellar Veins (transected dorsal to the Inferior Colliculus)
24. Inferior Colliculus
25. Trochlear (IV) Nerve
26. Quadrangular Lobule of the Cerebellum
27. Cerebral Peduncle (dorsolateral surface)
28. Pulvinar Nucleus of the Thalamus
29. Superior Colliculus
30. Pineal Body*
31. Habenula
32. Transition between Velum Interpositum and arachnoid layers of the Quadrigeminal

*Note: This dissection requires transection of the arachnoid adhesions and accompanying vasculature between the dorsal aspect of the Pineal Body and the Great Vein of Galen, which is resected.

VENTRAL ASPECT OF THE PONS AND MESENCEPHALIC - DIENCEPHALIC JUNCTION: EXTERNAL MORPHOLOGY OF THE CEREBRAL PEDUNCLES AND SURROUNDING STRUCTURES

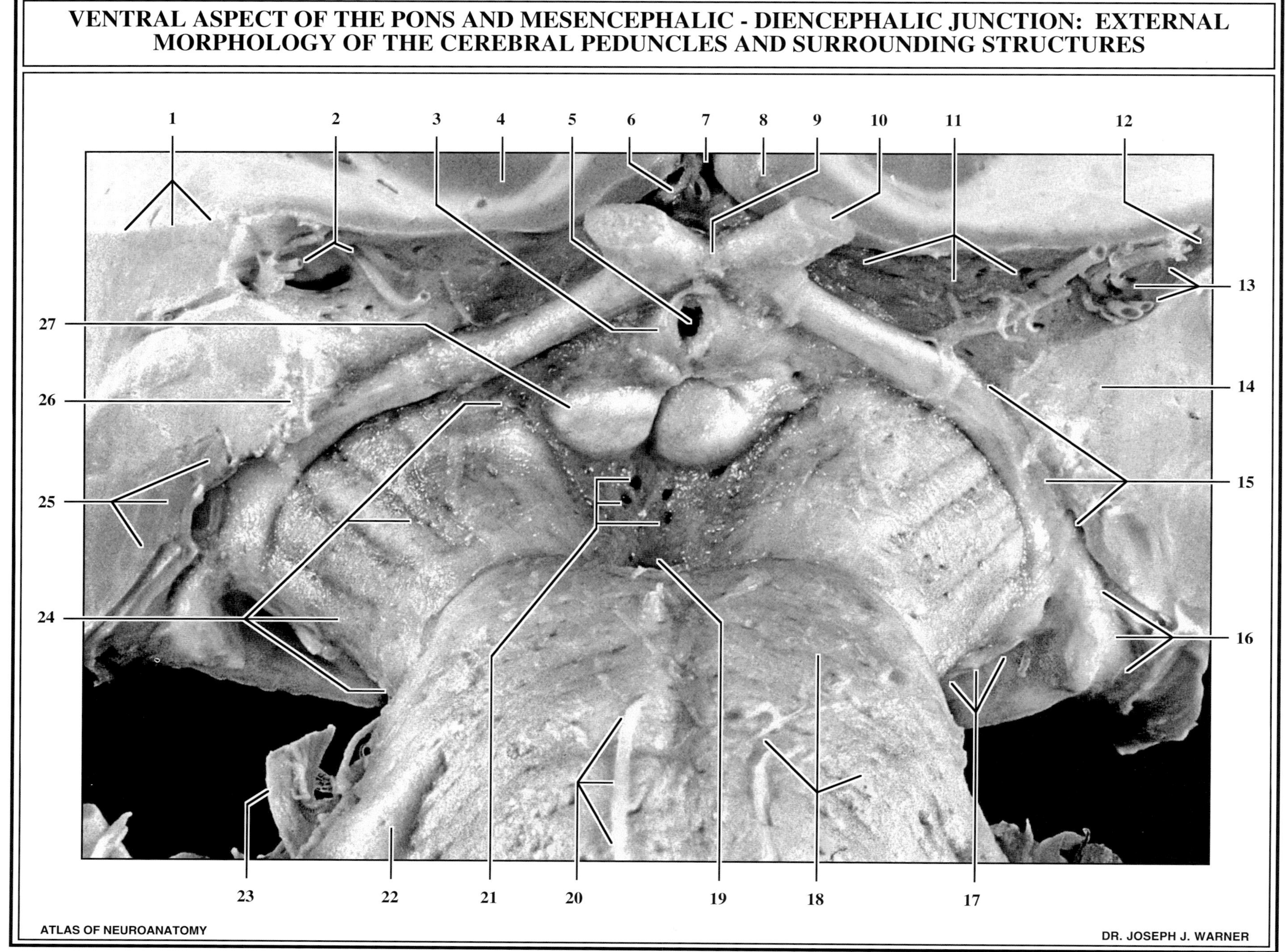

DR. JOSEPH J. WARNER

VENTRAL ASPECT OF THE PONS AND MESENCEPHALIC - DIENCEPHALIC JUNCTION: EXTERNAL MORPHOLOGY OF THE CEREBRAL PEDUNCLES AND SURROUNDING STRUCTURES

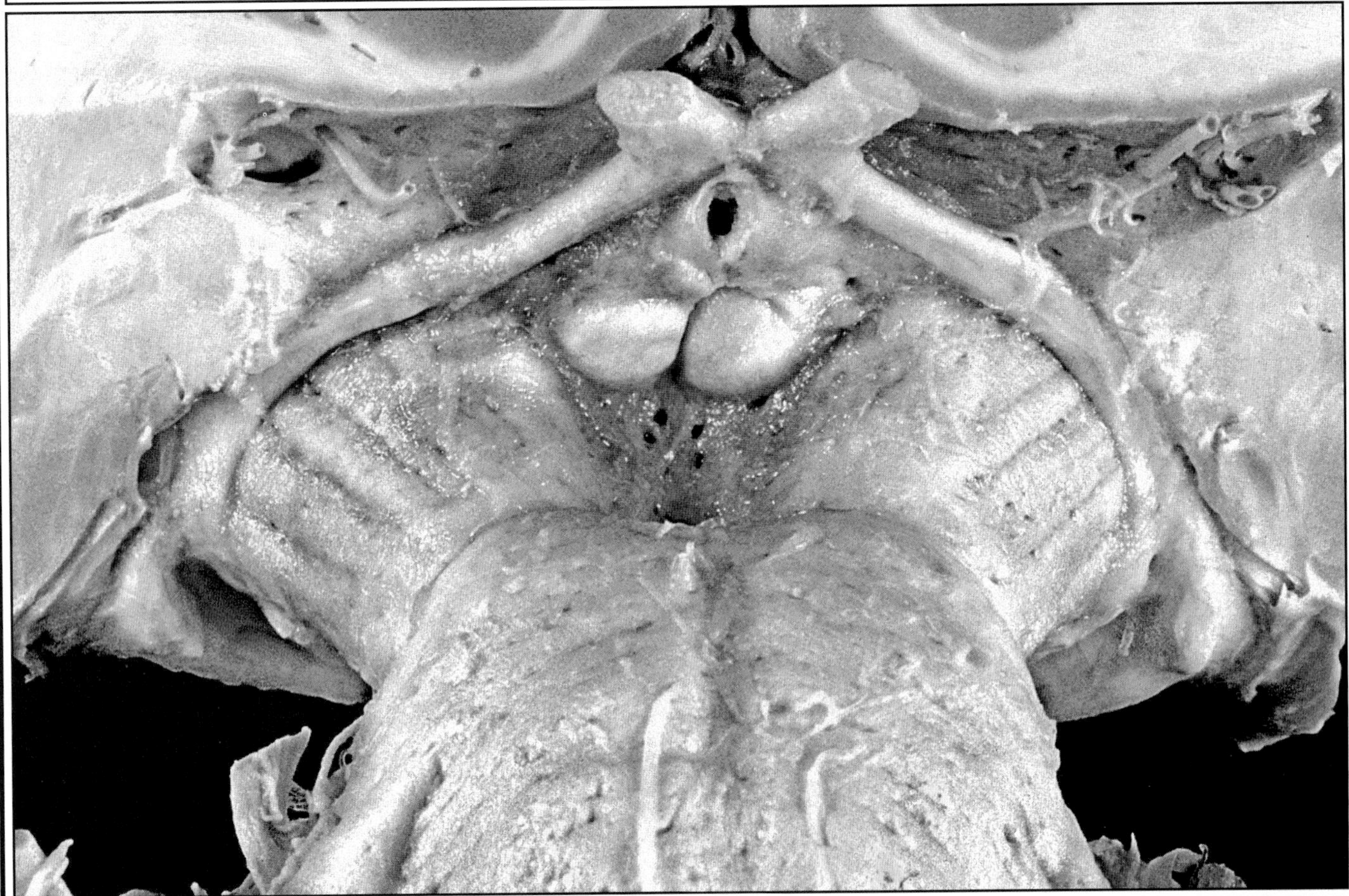

KEY TO NUMBERED STRUCTURES

1. Intersection of Coronal and Horizontal Planes of Telencephalic Resection*
2. Lateral Striate Arteries
3. Infundibulum
4. Nucleus Accumbens
5. Infundibular Recess of the Third Ventricle
6. Anterior Cerebral Artery
7. Interhemispheric Fissure
8. Paraterminal Gyrus
9. Optic Chiasm
10. Optic Nerve
11. Anterior Perforated Substance
12. Sylvian Fissure
13. Lateral Striate Branches of the Middle Cerebral Artery
14. Amygdala
15. Optic Tract
16. Lateral Geniculate Nucleus
17. Brachium of the Superior Colliculus
18. Basis Pontis
19. Interpeduncular Fossa
20. Abducens (VI) Nerve
21. Perivascular Spaces of the Posteromedial Arterial Group (including the Thalamo-perforating Arteries)
22. Middle Cerebellar Peduncle
23. Trigeminal (V) Nerve
24. Cerebral Peduncle
25. Medial Temporal Lobe (ventrolateral to the Optic Tract)
26. Uncus
27. Mammillary Body

*Following resection of the arachnoid membrane and major vessels, the cerebral hemispheres were coronally sectioned dorsal to the optic chiasm, sparing the latter. Ventral telencephalic structures caudal to that coronal plane were circumferentially resected to expose the optic tract and lateral geniculate nucleus bilaterally. The oculomotor nerves were resected to visualize the medial aspect of the cerebral peduncles and the interpeduncular fossa. The anterior perforated substance is clearly demonstrated dorsal and lateral to the optic chiasm. The optic tract courses circumferentially around the cerebral peduncles to terminate in the lateral geniculate nucleus. The brachium of the superior colliculus is discernible as a medial group of fibers which continues dorsomedially from the lateral geniculate nucleus to the tectal region.

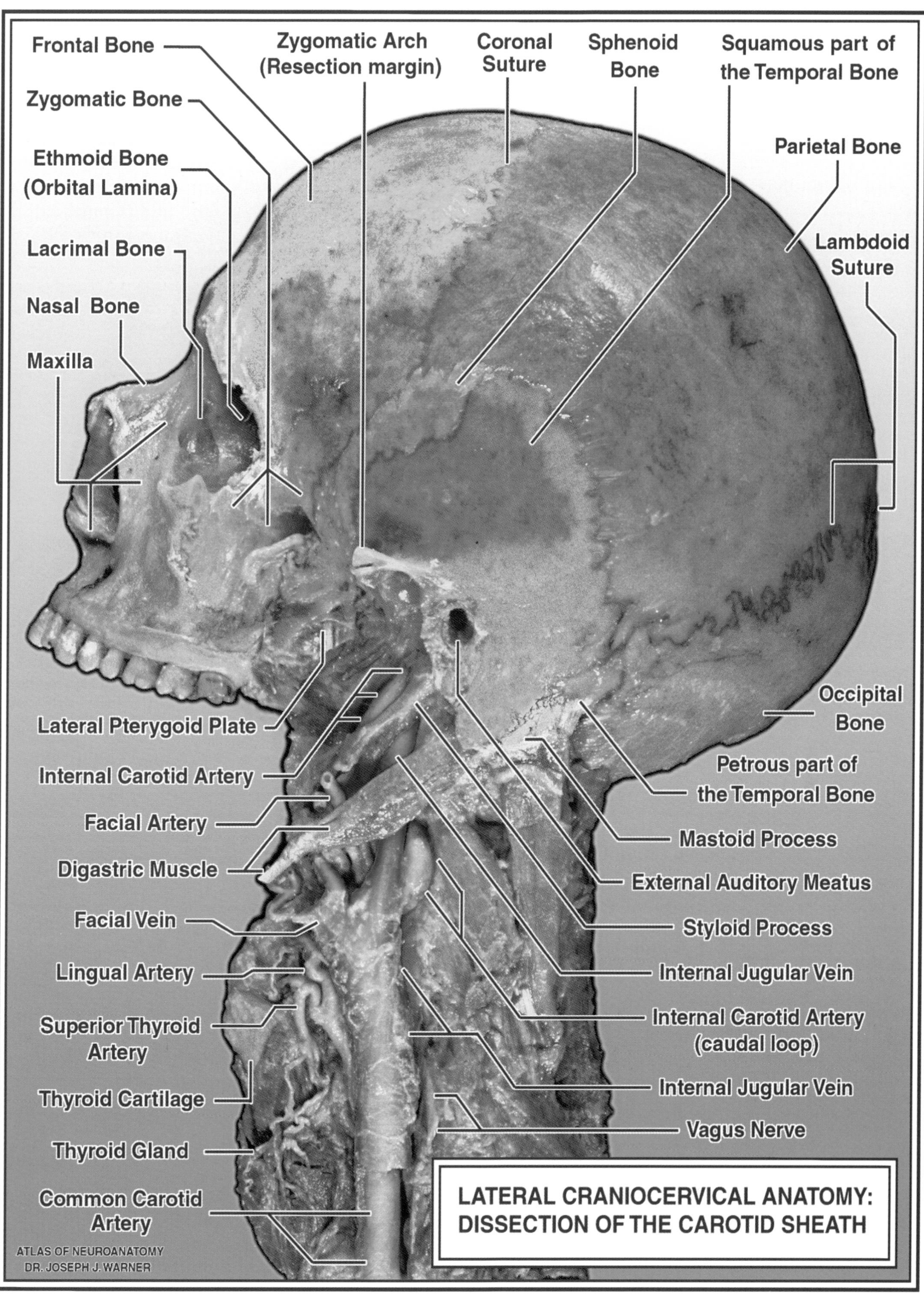
Frontal Bone
Zygomatic Arch
(Resection margin)
Coronal
Suture
Sphenoid
Bone
Squamous part of
the Temporal Bone
Zygomatic Bone
Ethmoid Bone
(Orbital Lamina)
Parietal Bone
Lacrimal Bone
Lambdoid
Suture
Nasal Bone
Maxilla
Occipital
Bone
Lateral Pterygoid Plate
Petrous part of
the Temporal Bone
Internal Carotid Artery
Facial Artery
Mastoid Process
Digastric Muscle
External Auditory Meatus
Facial Vein
Styloid Process
Lingual Artery
Internal Jugular Vein
Superior Thyroid
Artery
Internal Carotid Artery
(caudal loop)
Internal Jugular Vein
Thyroid Cartilage
Vagus Nerve
Thyroid Gland
Common Carotid
Artery
LATERAL CRANIOCERVICAL ANATOMY:
DISSECTION OF THE CAROTID SHEATH
ATLAS OF NEUROANATOMY
DR. JOSEPH J. WARNER

SAGITTAL CRANIOCERVICAL DISSECTION: RADIOGRAPH, LATERAL PROJECTION

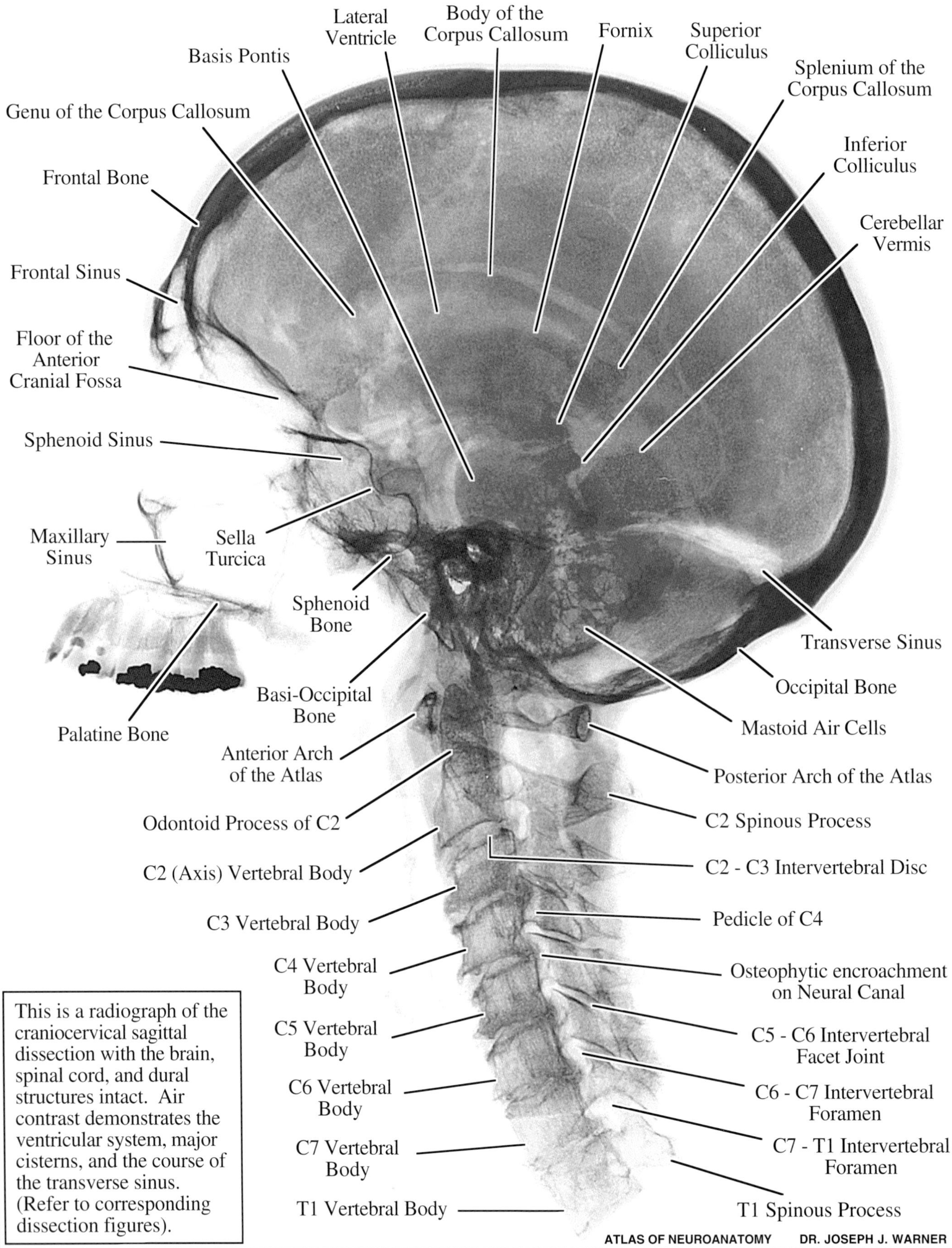

Lateral Ventricle
Body of the Corpus Callosum
Fornix
Superior Colliculus
Basis Pontis
Splenium of the Corpus Callosum
Genu of the Corpus Callosum
Inferior Colliculus
Frontal Bone
Cerebellar Vermis
Frontal Sinus
Floor of the Anterior Cranial Fossa
Sphenoid Sinus
Maxillary Sinus
Sella Turcica
Sphenoid Bone
Transverse Sinus
Occipital Bone
Basi-Occipital Bone
Mastoid Air Cells
Palatine Bone
Anterior Arch of the Atlas
Posterior Arch of the Atlas
C2 Spinous Process
Odontoid Process of C2
C2 - C3 Intervertebral Disc
C2 (Axis) Vertebral Body
C3 Vertebral Body
Pedicle of C4
C4 Vertebral Body
Osteophytic encroachment on Neural Canal
C5 Vertebral Body
C5 - C6 Intervertebral Facet Joint
C6 Vertebral Body
C6 - C7 Intervertebral Foramen
C7 Vertebral Body
C7 - T1 Intervertebral Foramen
T1 Vertebral Body
T1 Spinous Process

This is a radiograph of the craniocervical sagittal dissection with the brain, spinal cord, and dural structures intact. Air contrast demonstrates the ventricular system, major cisterns, and the course of the transverse sinus. (Refer to corresponding dissection figures).

MIDLINE SAGITTAL CRANIOCERVICAL SECTION: DEMONSTRATION OF THE FALX CEREBRI, MIDLINE VENOUS SINUSES, BRAIN AND SPINAL CORD

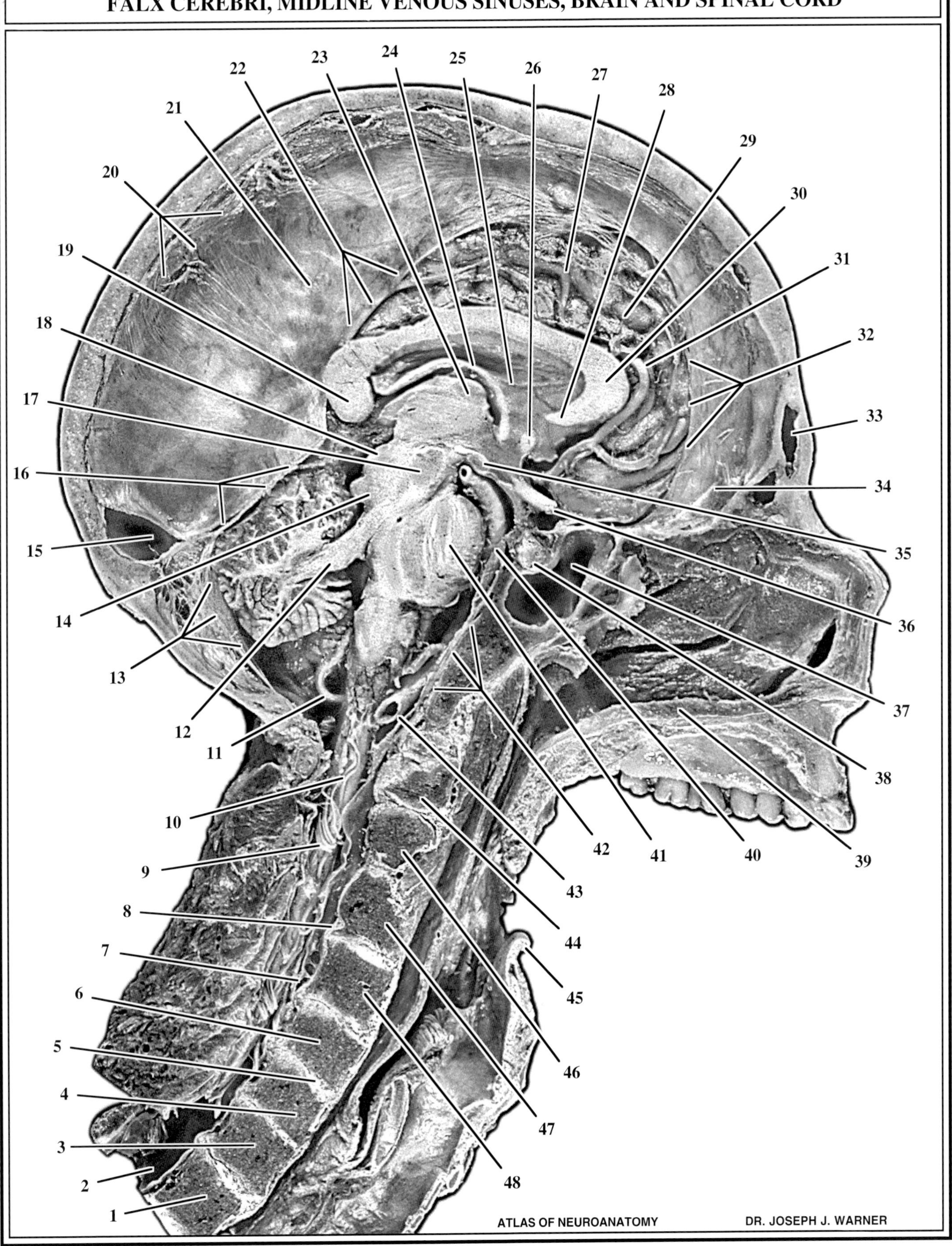

ATLAS OF NEUROANATOMY DR. JOSEPH J. WARNER

MIDLINE SAGITTAL CRANIOCERVICAL SECTION: DEMONSTRATION OF THE FALX CEREBRI, MIDLINE VENOUS SINUSES, BRAIN, AND SPINAL CORD

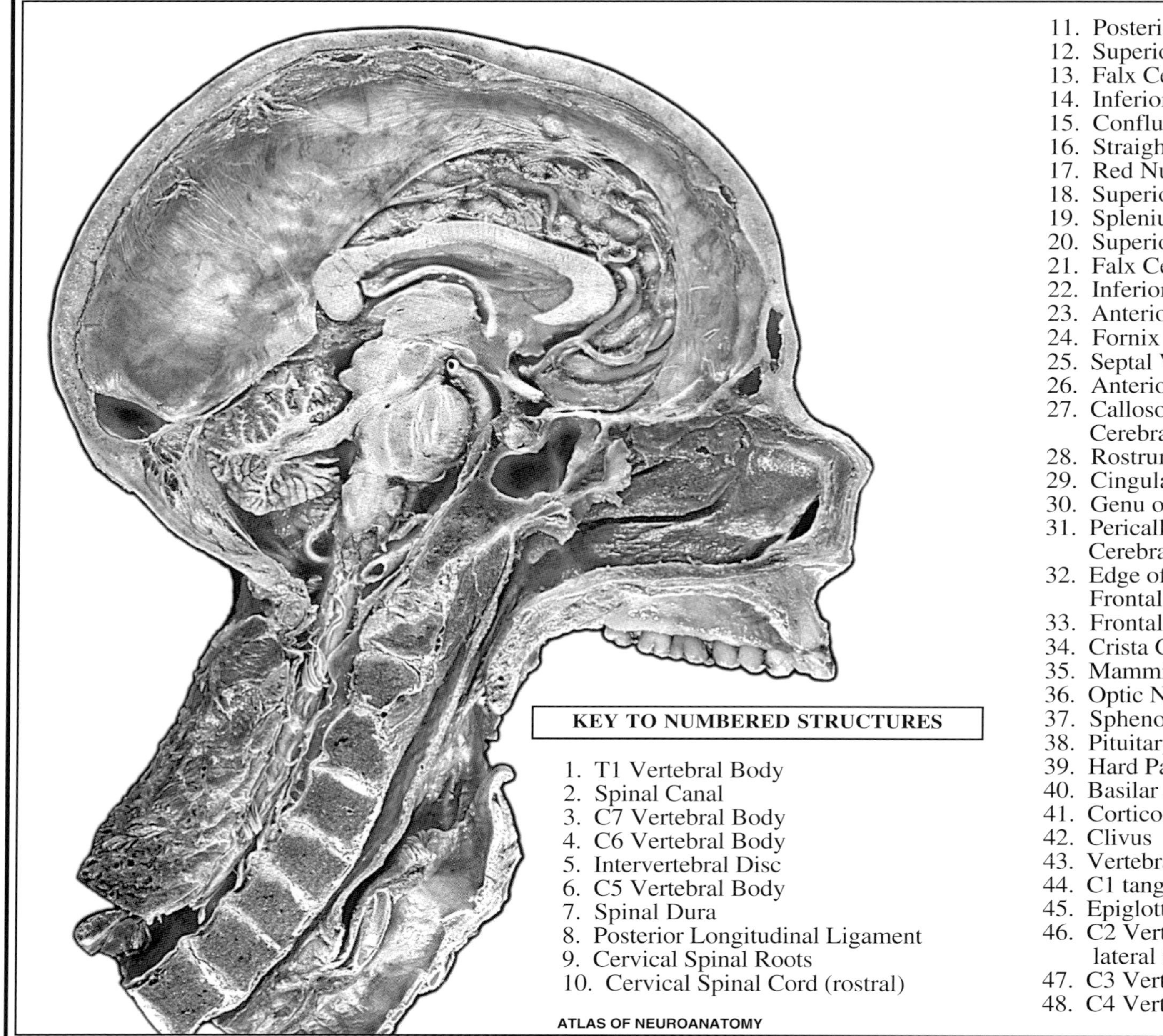

KEY TO NUMBERED STRUCTURES

1. T1 Vertebral Body
2. Spinal Canal
3. C7 Vertebral Body
4. C6 Vertebral Body
5. Intervertebral Disc
6. C5 Vertebral Body
7. Spinal Dura
8. Posterior Longitudinal Ligament
9. Cervical Spinal Roots
10. Cervical Spinal Cord (rostral)
11. Posterior Inferior Cerebellar Artery
12. Superior Cerebellar Peduncle
13. Falx Cerebelli
14. Inferior Colliculus
15. Confluence of Sinuses
16. Straight Sinus
17. Red Nucleus
18. Superior Colliculus
19. Splenium of the Corpus Callosum
20. Superior Sagittal Sinus
21. Falx Cerebri
22. Inferior Sagittal Sinus
23. Anterior Nucleus of the Thalamus
24. Fornix
25. Septal Vein
26. Anterior Commissure
27. Callosomarginal Branch of the Anterior Cerebral Artery
28. Rostrum of the Corpus Callosum
29. Cingulate Gyrus
30. Genu of the Corpus Callosum
31. Pericallosal Branch of the Anterior Cerebral Artery
32. Edge of the Falx Cerebri between the Frontal Poles
33. Frontal Sinus
34. Crista Galli
35. Mammillary Body
36. Optic Nerve
37. Sphenoid Sinus
38. Pituitary Gland
39. Hard Palate
40. Basilar Artery
41. Corticospinal, Corticobulbar Fibers
42. Clivus
43. Vertebral Artery
44. C1 tangentially sectioned lateral to Dens
45. Epiglottis
46. C2 Vertebral Body (Axis) slightly lateral to the Odontoid Process (Dens)
47. C3 Vertebral Body
48. C4 Vertebral Body

DR. JOSEPH J. WARNER

SAGITTAL CRANIOCERVICAL DISSECTION: RADIOCONTRAST VENTRICULOGRAPHY, LATERAL PROJECTION

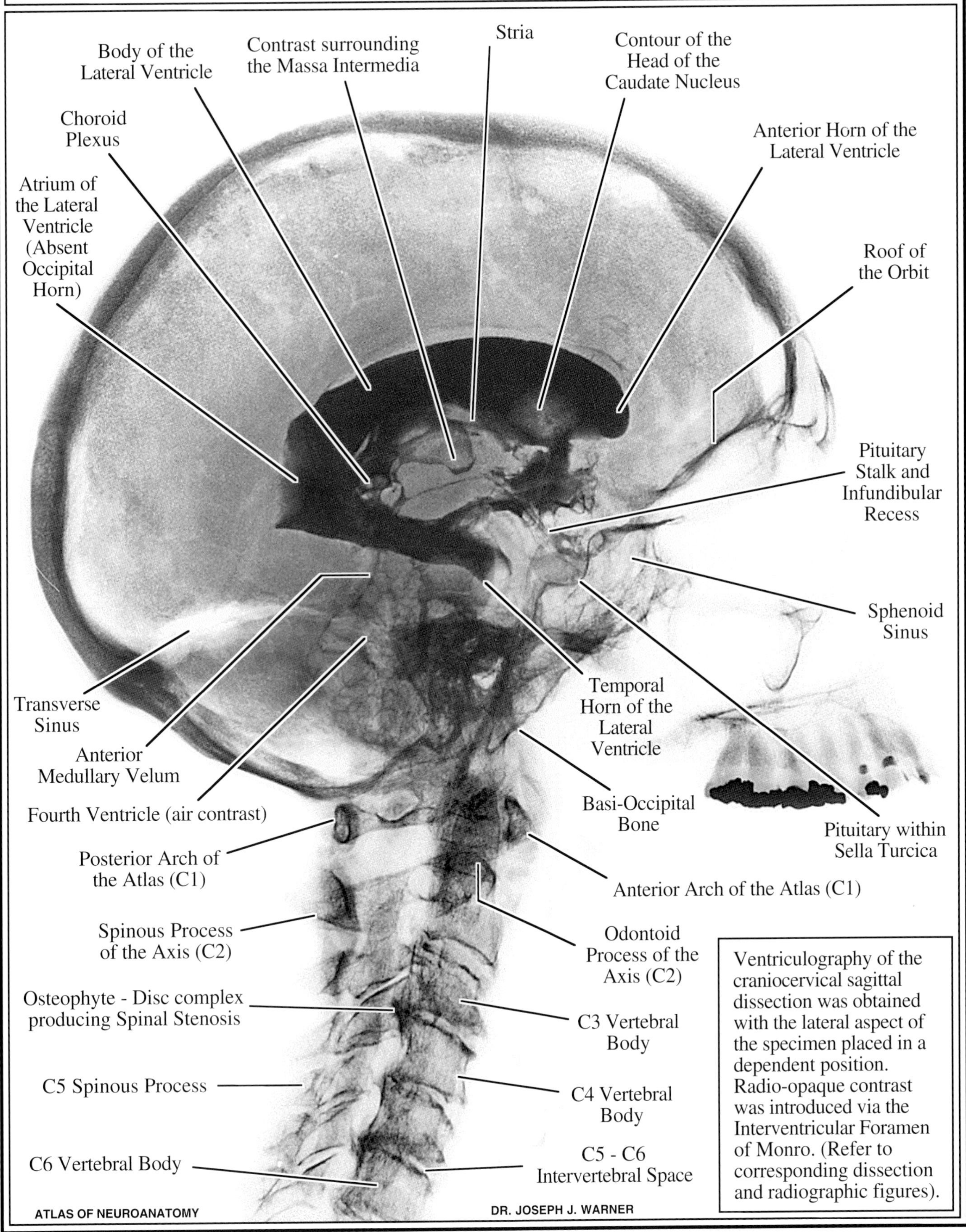

Ventriculography of the craniocervical sagittal dissection was obtained with the lateral aspect of the specimen placed in a dependent position. Radio-opaque contrast was introduced via the Interventricular Foramen of Monro. (Refer to corresponding dissection and radiographic figures).

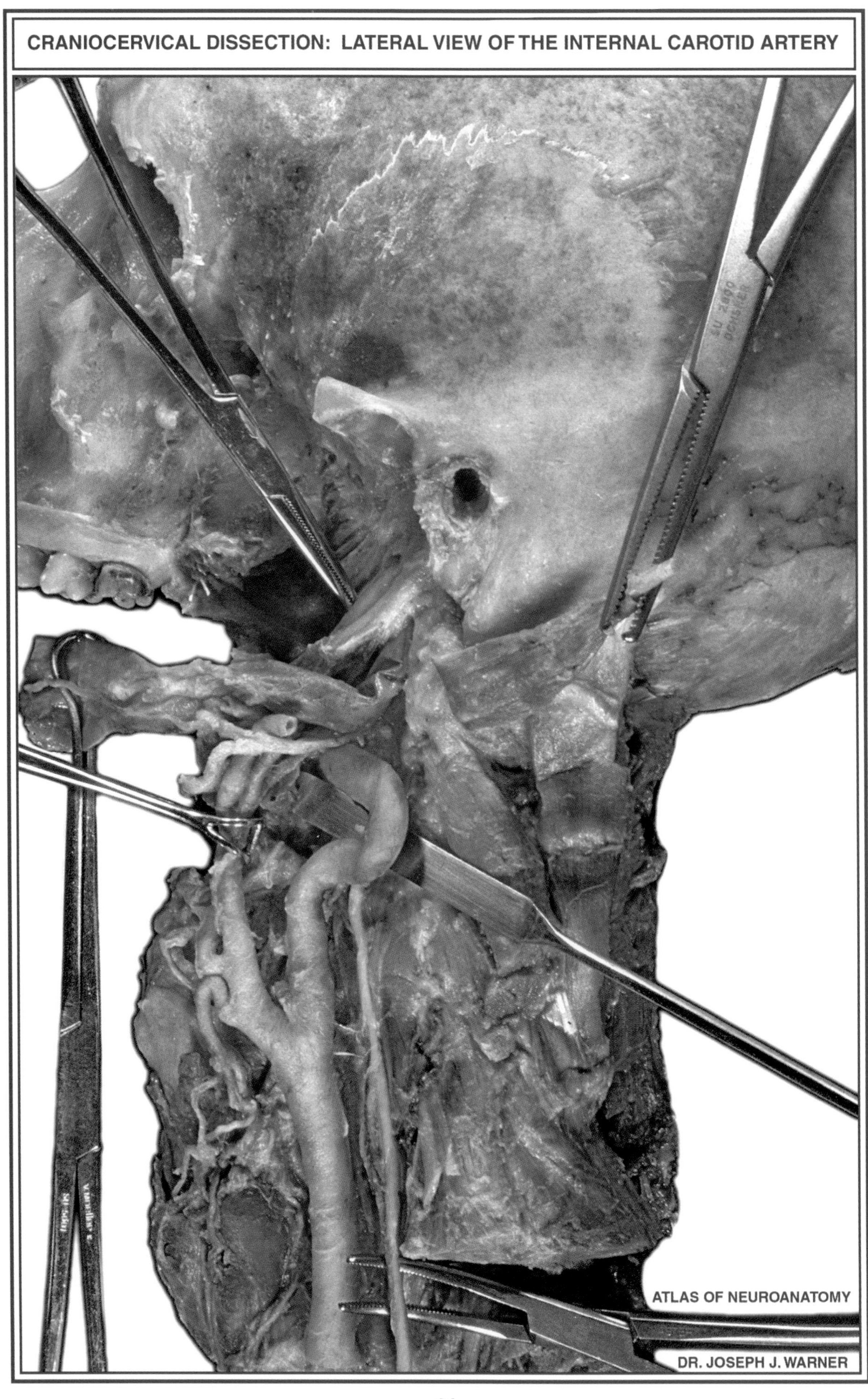

CRANIOCERVICAL DISSECTION: LATERAL VIEW OF THE INTERNAL CAROTID ARTERY

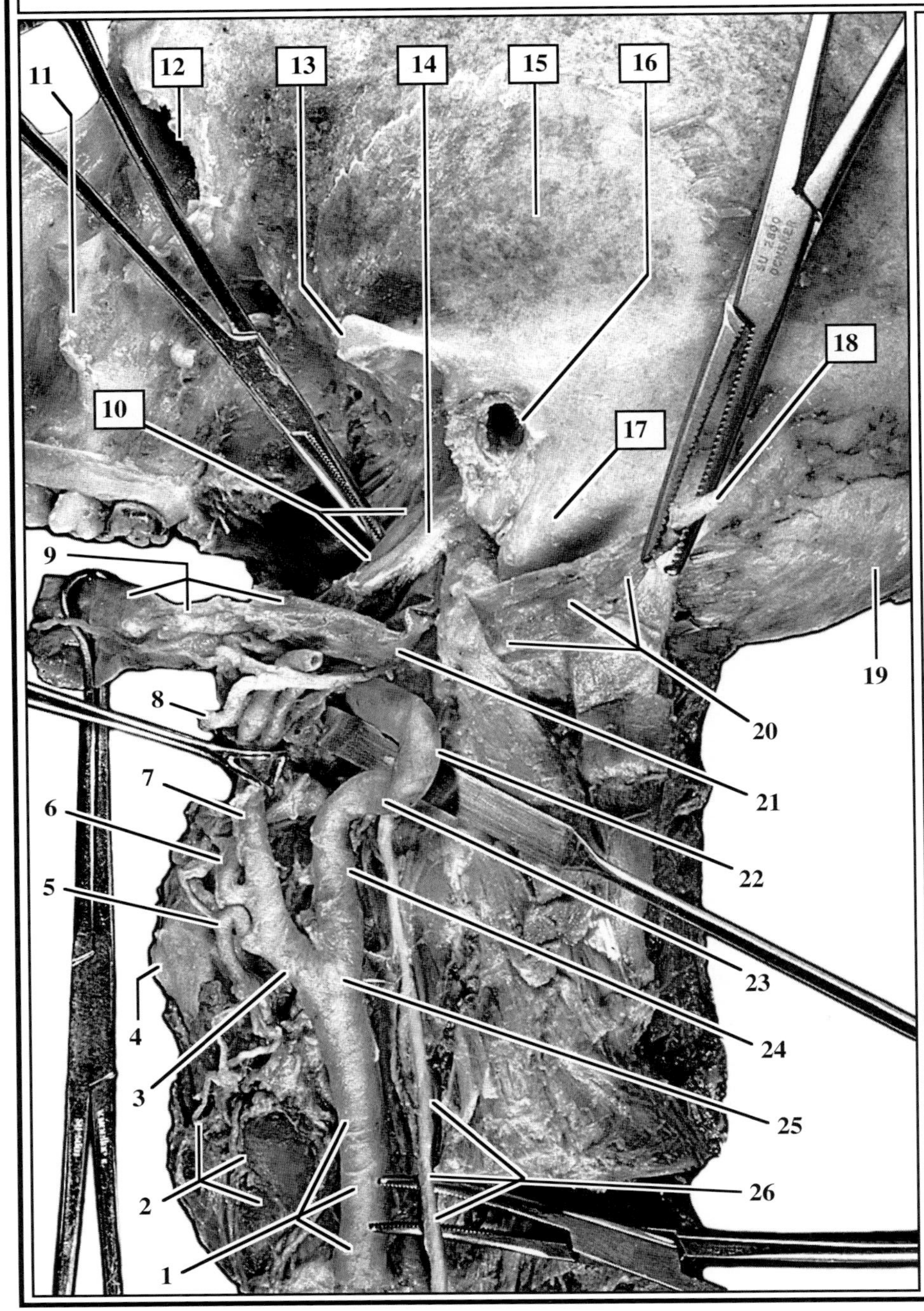

In this craniocervical dissection, the zygomatic arch, lateral wall of the orbit, and the entire mandible were resected. The posterior portion of the digastric muscle was retracted posteriorly. Following dissection of the carotid sheath, the internal jugular vein was reflected laterally and rostrally. The resulting exposure revealed the common carotid artery, the carotid bifurcation, and the course of the internal carotid artery into the base of the skull medial to the styloid process. The vagus nerve is demonstrated along the internal and common carotid arteries. The hypoglossal nerve has been reflected rostrally, along with the internal jugular vein. The external carotid artery, distal to the superior thyroid artery, is retracted slightly in an anterior direction. The internal carotid artery in this specimen is characterized by a a tortuous course as it approaches the styloid process. An impression, left by the internal jugular vein, is visible along the posteriorly convex loop of the internal carotid artery.

KEY TO NUMBERED STRUCTURES

1. Internal Carotid Artery
2. Thyroid Gland
3. Proximal Segment, External Carotid Artery
4. Thyroid Cartilage
5. Superior Thyroid Artery
6. Lingual Artery
7. External Carotid Artery
8. Hypoglossal Nerve
9. Internal Jugular Vein (reflected laterally and rostrally)
10. Internal Carotid Artery (course medial to the Styloid Process)
11. Maxilla
12. Lateral Rim of the Orbit (Frontal Bone)
13. Resected Margin of the Zygomatic Arch
14. Styloid Process
15. Squamous Part of the Temporal Bone
16. External Auditory Meatus
17. Mastoid Process
18. Tendon of the Digastric Muscle
19. Occipital Bone
20. Digastric Muscle (reflected laterally and caudally)
21. Internal Jugular Vein
22. Caudal Loop of the Internal Carotid Artery
23. Impression of the Internal Jugular Vein
24. Internal Carotid Artery
25. Bifurcation of the Common Carotid Artery
26. Vagus Nerve

SAGITTAL CRANIOCERVICAL DISSECTION: CAROTID ANGIOGRAPHY FOLLOWING RADIOCONTRAST VENTRICULOGRAPHY, LATERAL PROJECTION

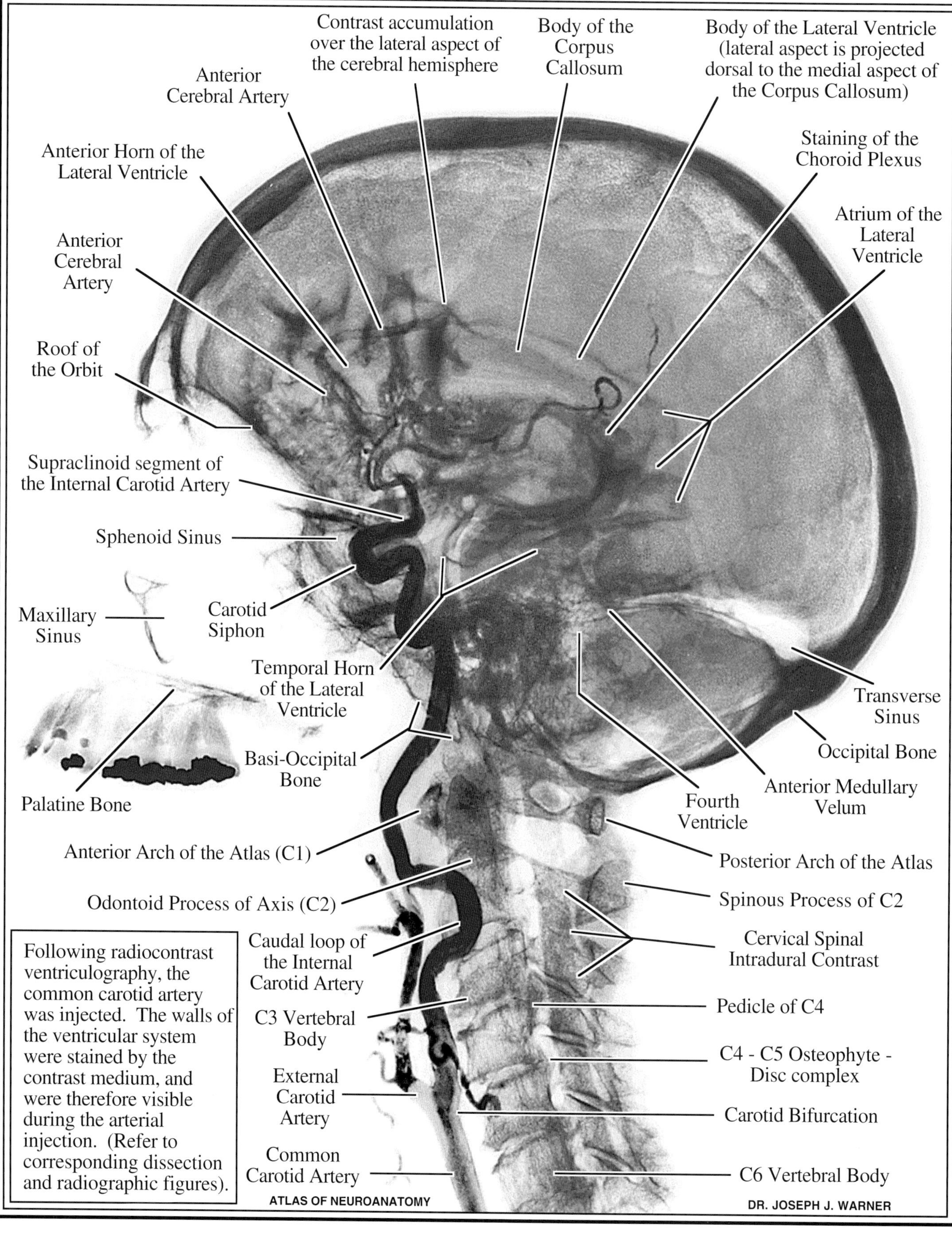

Following radiocontrast ventriculography, the common carotid artery was injected. The walls of the ventricular system were stained by the contrast medium, and were therefore visible during the arterial injection. (Refer to corresponding dissection and radiographic figures).

MIDLINE CRANIOCERVICAL SAGITTAL DISSECTION: RESECTION OF ROSTRAL CEREBRUM WITH ILLUSTRATION OF DURA, CRANIUM, AND CERVICAL SPINE

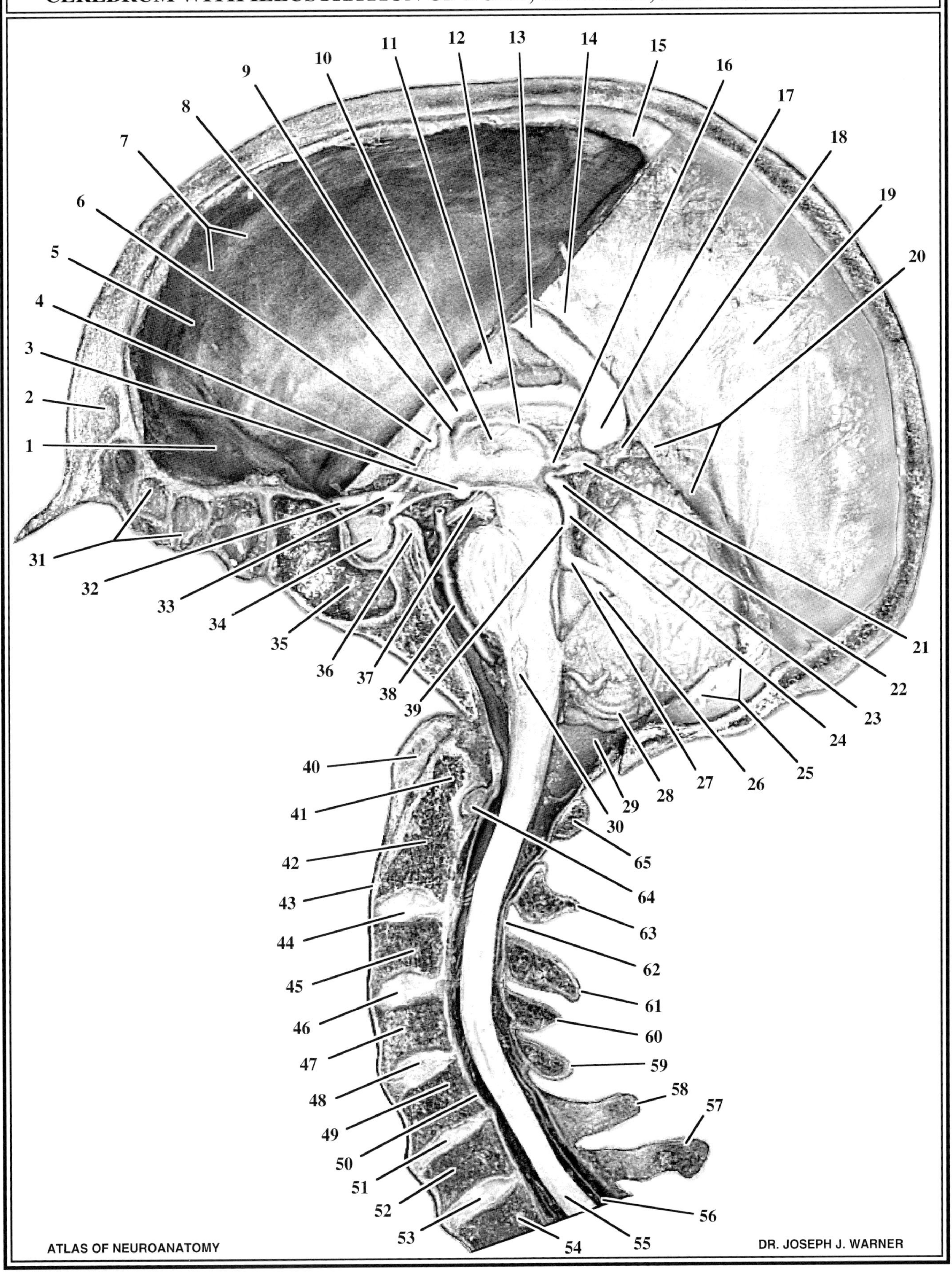

MIDLINE CRANIOCERVICAL SAGITTAL DISSECTION: RESECTION OF ROSTRAL CEREBRUM WITH ILLUSTRATION OF DURA, CRANIUM, AND CERVICAL SPINE

The dissection procedure included sagittal section of the head and neck, followed by oblique coronal section of the right cerebral hemisphere and falx cerebri. The entire right cerebral hemisphere and falx cerebri rostral to the plane of section (S) were then removed, sparing the right wall of the superior sagittal sinus This exposed the inner surface of the dura in the anterior cranial fossa and overlying the right frontoparietal region.

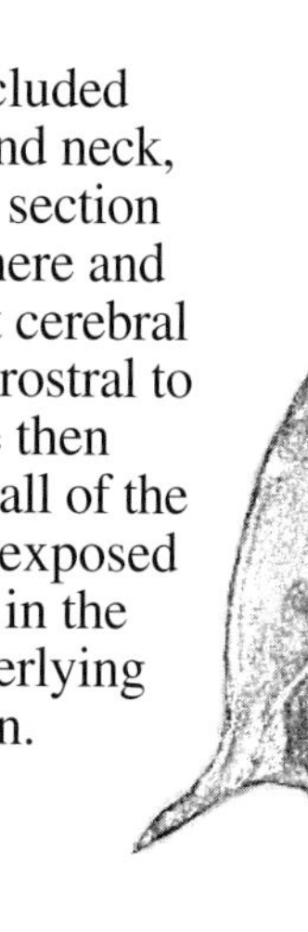

KEY TO NUMBERED STRUCTURES

1. Floor of Anterior Cranial Fossa (Roof of the Orbit)
2. Frontal Sinus
3. Mammillary Body
4. Lamina Terminalis
5. Anterior Cranial Fossa
6. Anterior Commissure
7. Dura, layer facing arachnoid
8. Foramen of Monro
9. Fornix
10. Massa Intermedia
11. Septum Pellucidum
12. Stria Medullaris
13. Corpus Callosum
14. Inferior Sagittal Sinus
15. Right Wall of the Superior Sagittal Sinus
16. Habenula
17. Splenium of Corpus Callosum
18. Great Vein of Galen
19. Falx Cerebri
20. Straight Sinus
21. Pineal
22. Superior Cerebellar Vermis
23. Superior Colliculus
24. Inferior Colliculus
25. Falx Cerebelli
26. Fourth Ventricle
27. Superior Cerebellar Peduncle
28. Cerebellar Tonsil
29. Cisterna Magna, level of Foramen Magnum
30. Inferior Olivary Nucleus
31. Ethmoid Air Cells
32. Optic Nerve
33. Optic Chiasm
34. Pituitary Gland
35. Sphenoid Sinus
36. Posterior Clinoid Process
37. Oculomotor Nerve
38. Basilar Artery
39. Aqueduct of Sylvius
40. Anterior Arch of Atlas (C1)
41. Odontoid Process of Axis
42. Axis (C2)
43. Anterior Longitudinal Ligament
44. C2 - C3 Intervertebral Disc
45. Vertebral Body of C3
46. C3 - C4 Intervertebral Disc
47. Vertebral Body of C4
48. C4 - C5 Intervertebral Disc
49. Vertebral Body of C5
50. Posterior Longitudinal Ligament
51. C5 - C6 Intervertebral Disc
52. Vertebral Body of C6
53. C6 - C7 Intervertebral Disc
54. Vertebral Body of C7
55. Cervical Spinal Cord
56. Dura
57. C7 Spinous Process
58. C6 Spinous Process
59. C5 Spinous Process
60. C4 Spinous Process
61. C3 Spinous Process
62. Ligamentum Flavum
63. C2 Spinous Process
64. Transverse Ligament of Atlas
65. Posterior Arch of Atlas (C1)

CRANIOCERVICAL DISSECTION WITH EXPOSURE OF POSTERIOR AND INFERIOR CEREBELLUM, DORSAL MEDULLA, CERVICAL SPINAL CORD, AND VERTEBRAE

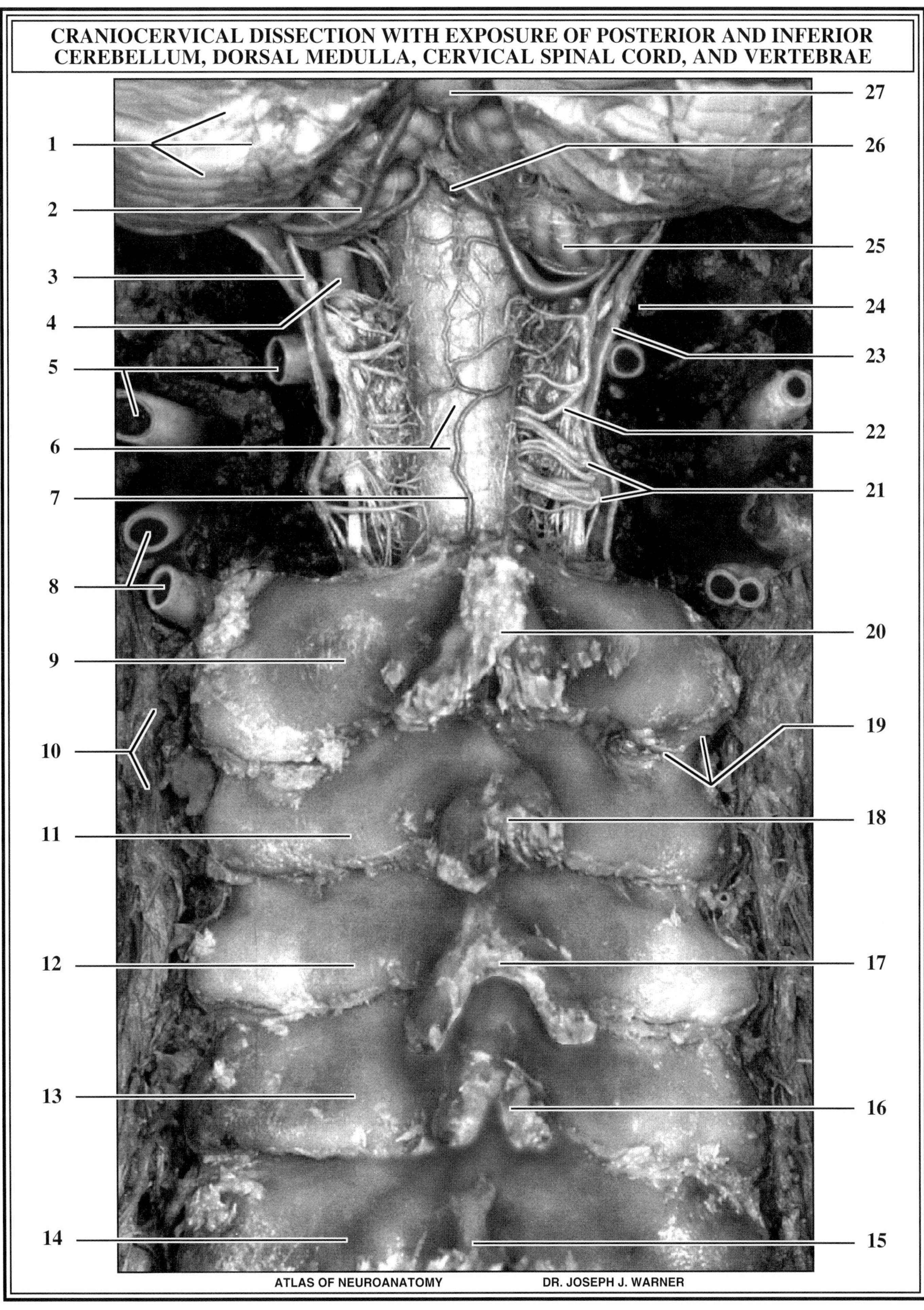

ATLAS OF NEUROANATOMY DR. JOSEPH J. WARNER

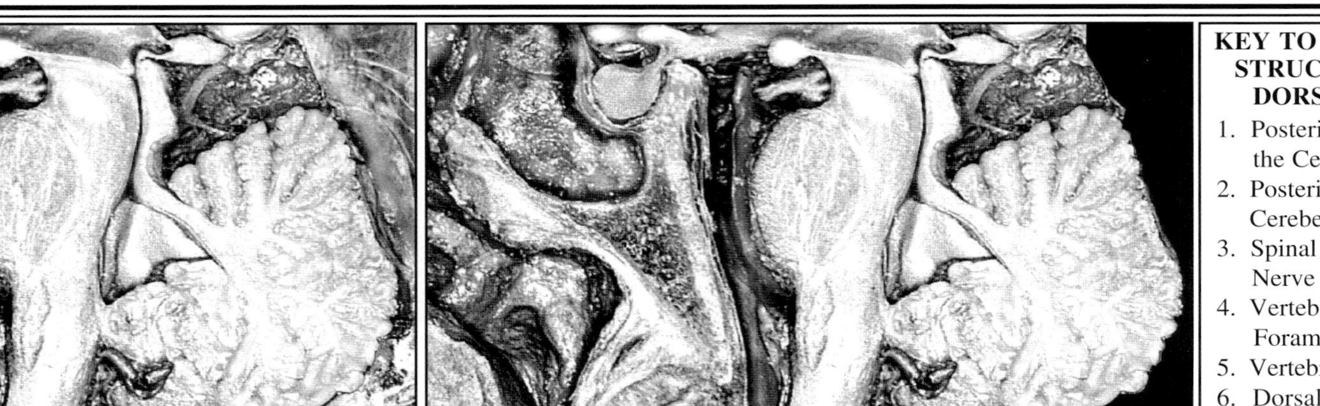

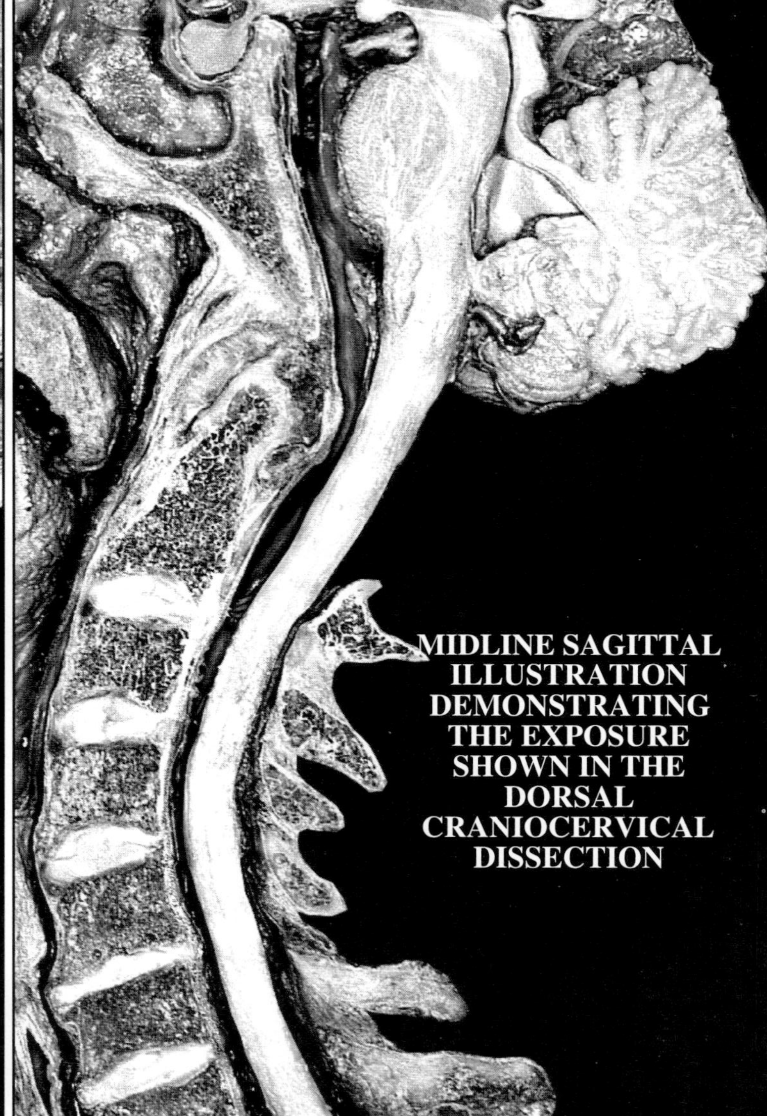

MIDLINE SAGITTAL ILLUSTRATION DEMONSTRATING THE EXPOSURE SHOWN IN THE DORSAL CRANIOCERVICAL DISSECTION

KEY TO NUMBERED STRUCTURES ON DORSAL VIEW

1. Posterior Lobe of the Cerebellum
2. Posterior Inferior Cerebellar Artery
3. Spinal Accessory Nerve
4. Vertebral Artery at Foramen Magnum
5. Vertebral Artery
6. Dorsal Columns, Cervical Spinal Cord
7. Dorsal Venous Plexus, Spinal Cord
8. Vertebral Artery
9. C2 Lamina
10. Paraspinous Musculature
11. C3 Lamina
12. C4 Lamina
13. C5 Lamina
14. C6 Lamina
15. C6 Spinous Process
16. C5 Spinous Process
17. C4 Spinous Process
18. C3 Spinous Process
19. Margin of Intervertebral Articular Facet
20. C2 Spinous Process
21. Cervical Spinal Roots
22. Spinal Root, Spinal Accessory Nerve
23. Dura
24. Level of Foramen Magnum
25. Cerebellar Tonsil
26. Obex, Dorsal Medulla
27. Cerebellar Nodulus

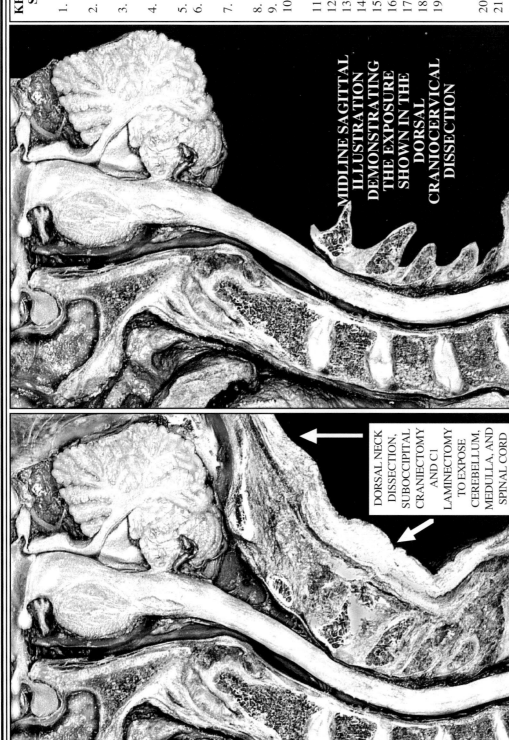

CRANIOCERVICAL DISSECTION WITH EXPOSURE OF THE POSTERIOR AND INFERIOR ASPECT OF THE CEREBELLUM, THE DORSAL MEDULLA, CERVICAL SPINAL CORD, AND VERTEBRAE

The diagrams above demonstrate the exposure shown in the dorsal craniocervical dissection,with exposure of the posterior and inferior aspect of the cerebellum, the medulla, rostral cervical spinal cord, vertebrae (C2 and below), and paraspinous musculature. The vertebral artery is sectioned where its course crosses the plane of dissection, thus demonstrating the lumen at multiple points (refer to A-P and lateral projection vertebral angiograms to examine the course of this vessel).

CRANIOCERVICAL DISSECTION: ARTERIAL AND VENOUS INJECTION WITH EXPOSURE OF THE DORSAL CEREBELLUM, CAUDAL MEDULLA, AND ROSTRAL CERVICAL SPINAL CORD

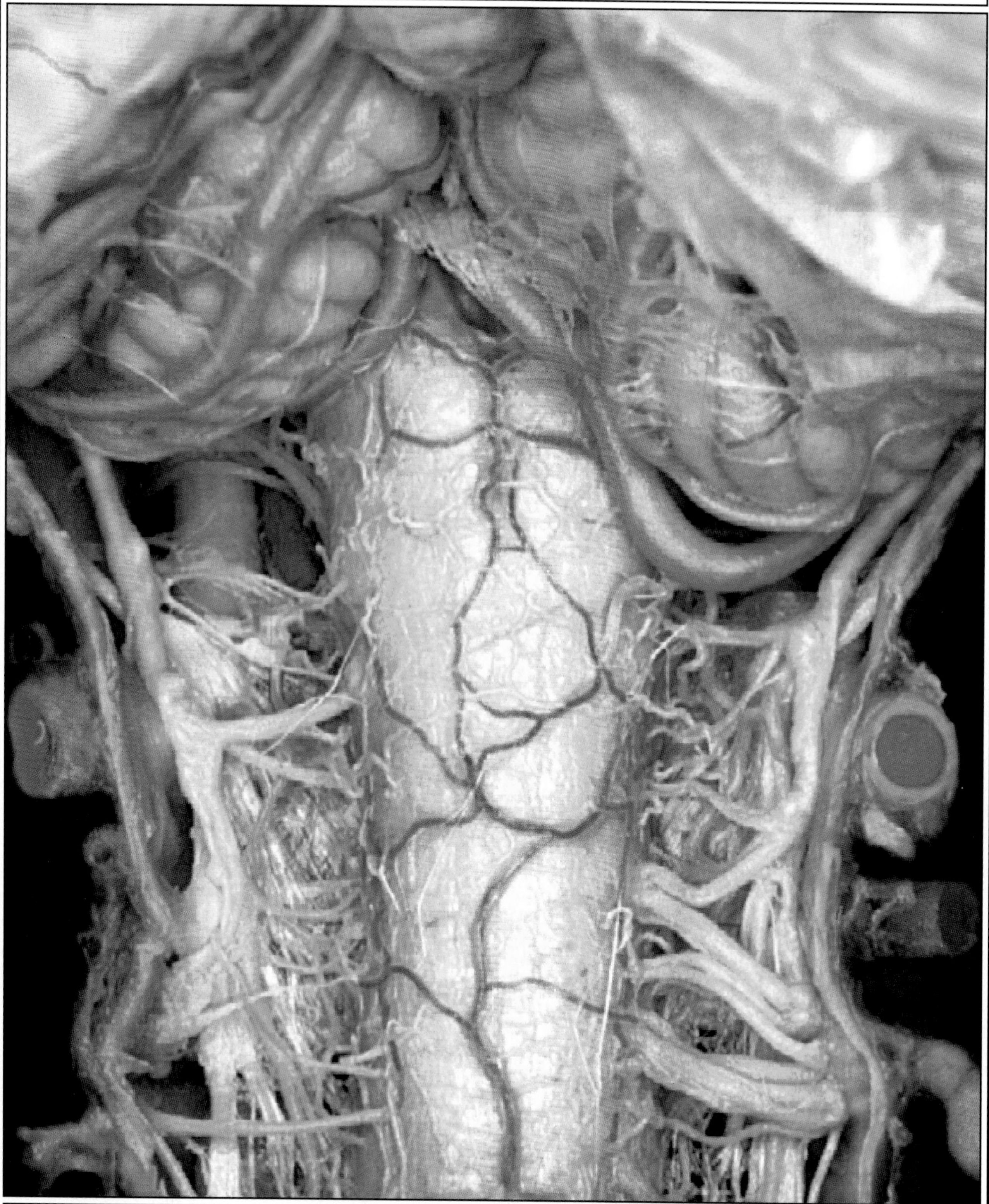

Arterial (red) and venous (blue) injections were performed. Occipital craniectomy and C1 - C2 laminectomy with resection of the dorsal aspect of the dura demonstrates the neural and vascular structures. The venous plexus overlying the dorsal cervical spinal cord is well visualized. Fibers of the spinal component of the accessory nerve (XI) course rostrally, in contrast to the lateral orientation of the dorsal roots of C1 and C2.

CERVICOTHORACIC AND CRANIAL DISSECTION DEMONSTRATING THE COURSE OF EACH VERTEBRAL ARTERY INTO THE TRANSVERSE FORAMEN OF THE CERVICAL SPINE

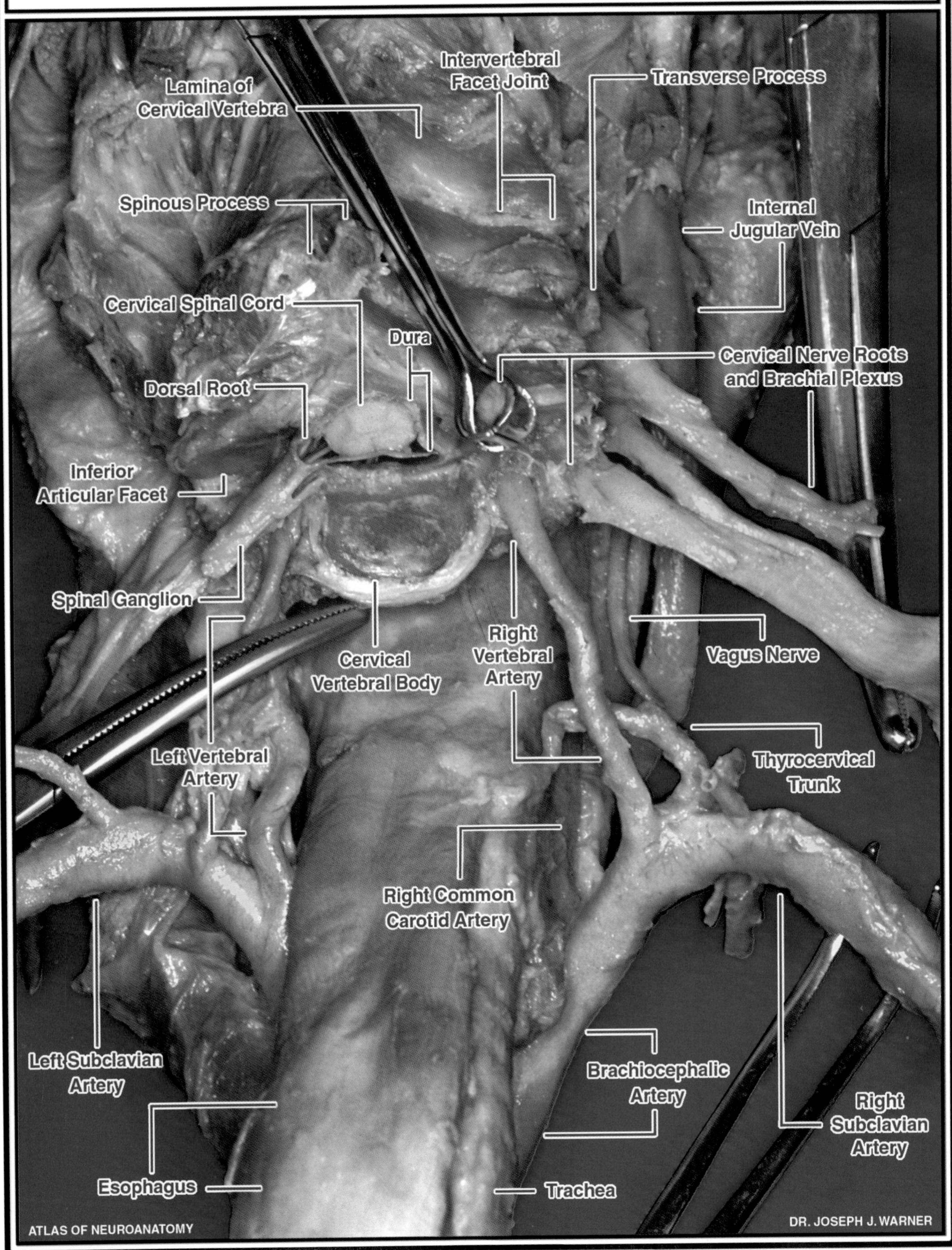

CRANIOSPINAL DISSECTION DEMONSTRATING THE PROXIMAL COURSE OF THE VERTEBRAL ARTERY, THE CERVICAL VERTEBRAE, AND THE CERVICAL SPINAL CORD

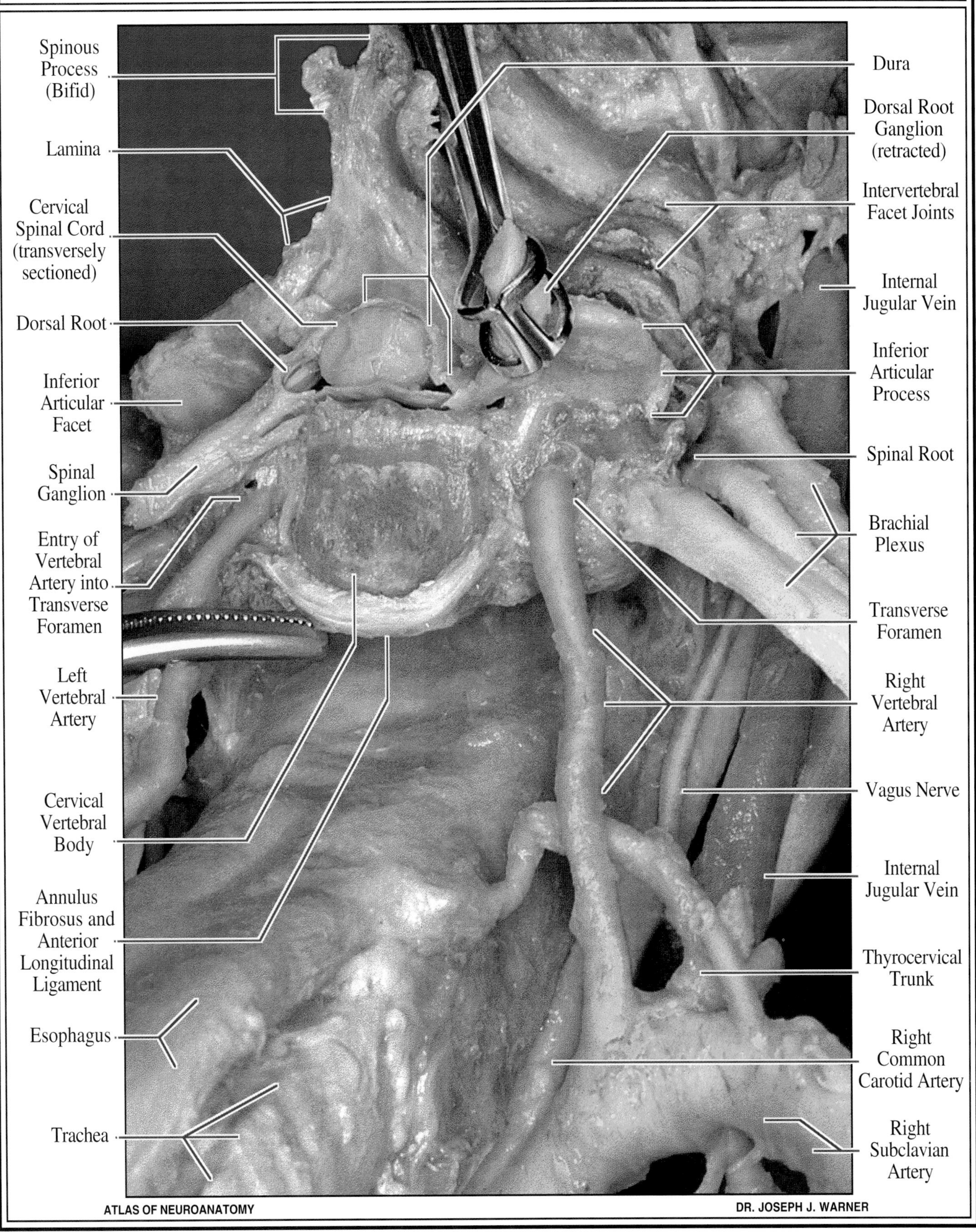

VENTRAL ASPECT OF THE THORACOLUMBAR SPINAL CORD, INCLUDING THE SPINAL ROOTS AND VASCULATURE: DURA REFLECTED LATERALLY

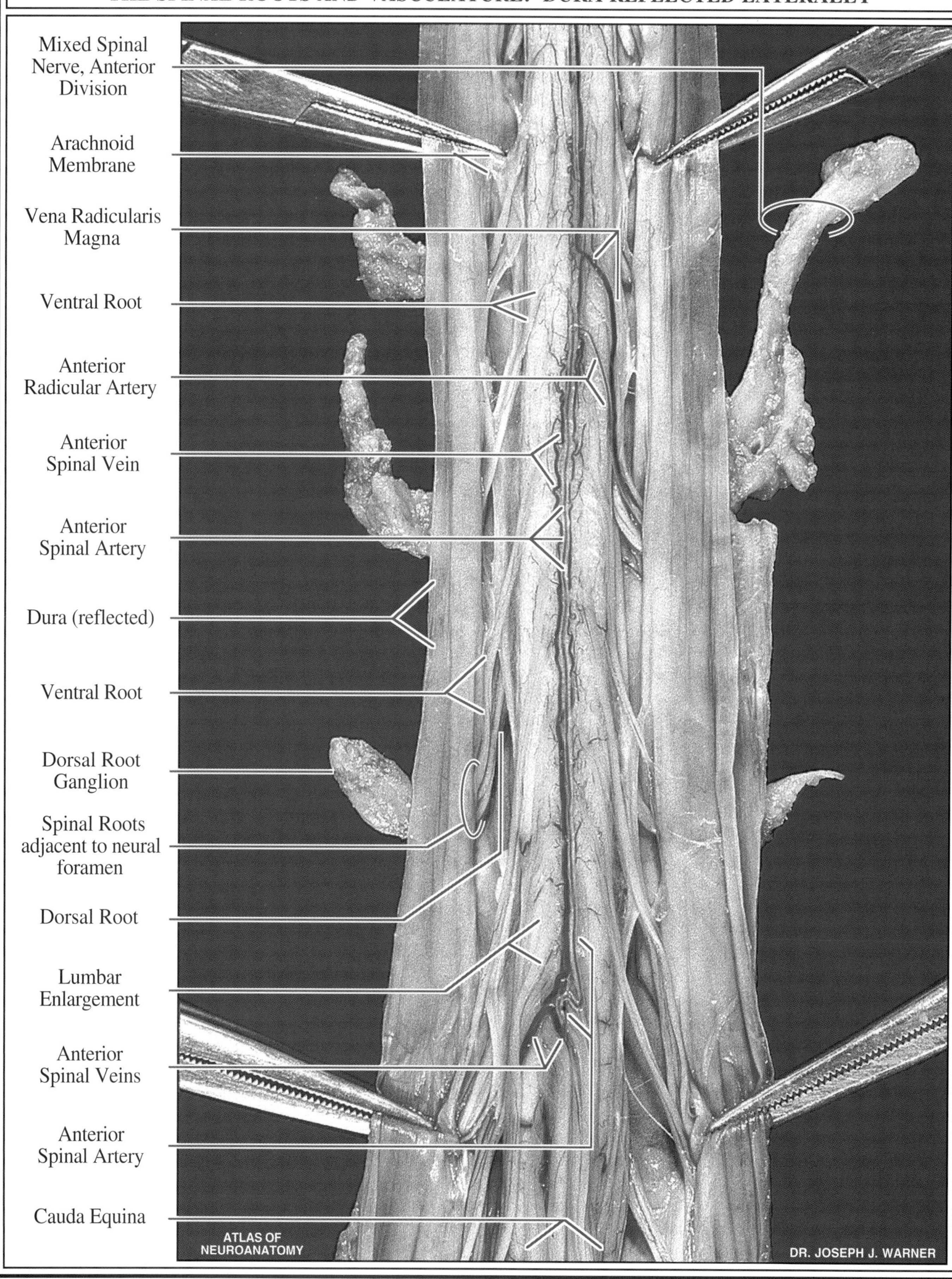

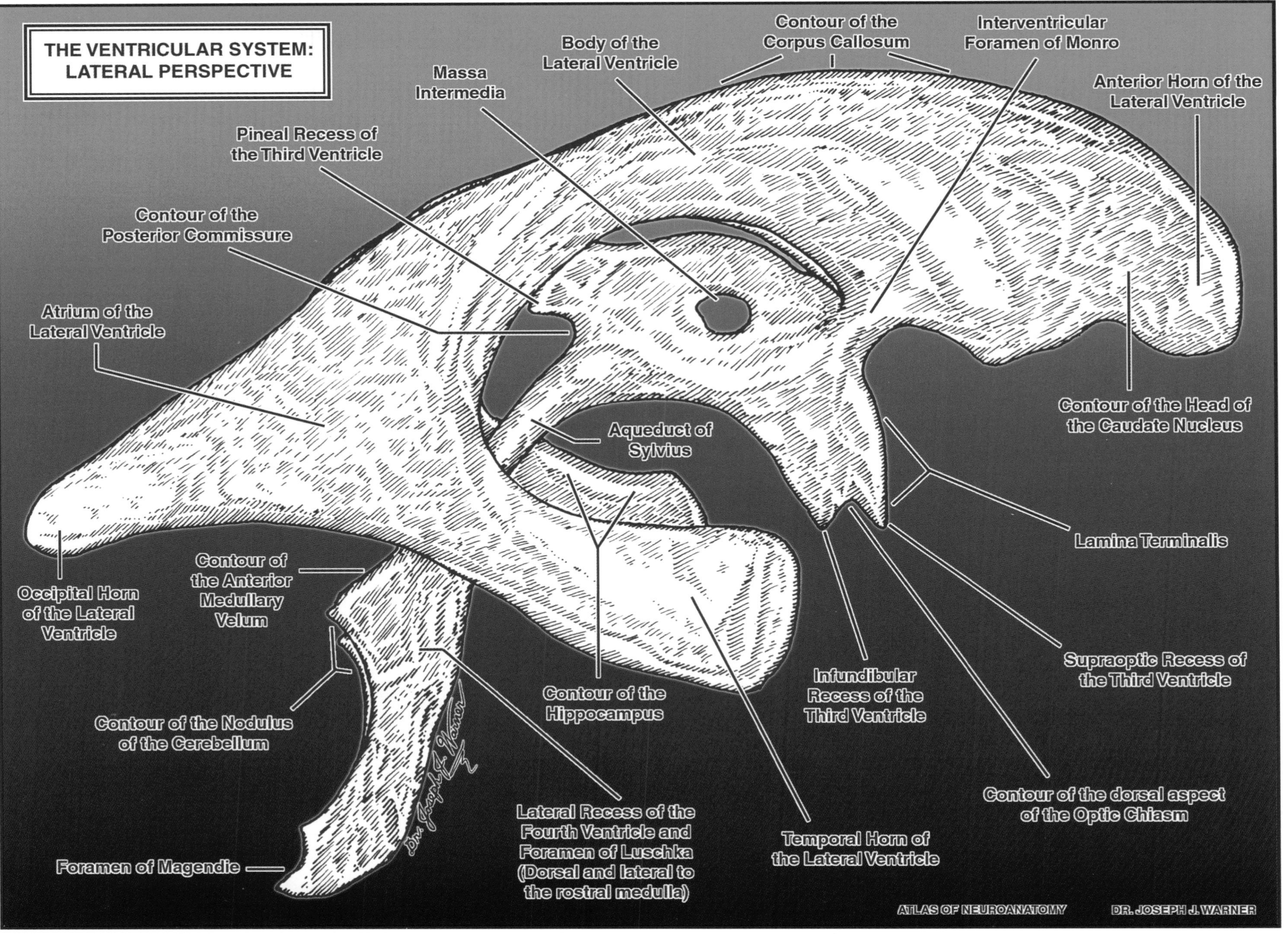
THE VENTRICULAR SYSTEM: LATERAL PERSPECTIVE
Contour of the Corpus Callosum
Interventricular Foramen of Monro
Body of the Lateral Ventricle
Massa Intermedia
Anterior Horn of the Lateral Ventricle
Pineal Recess of the Third Ventricle
Contour of the Posterior Commissure
Atrium of the Lateral Ventricle
Aqueduct of Sylvius
Contour of the Head of the Caudate Nucleus
Lamina Terminalis
Occipital Horn of the Lateral Ventricle
Contour of the Anterior Medullary Velum
Supraoptic Recess of the Third Ventricle
Contour of the Hippocampus
Infundibular Recess of the Third Ventricle
Contour of the Nodulus of the Cerebellum
Contour of the dorsal aspect of the Optic Chiasm
Lateral Recess of the Fourth Ventricle and Foramen of Luschka (Dorsal and lateral to the rostral medulla)
Temporal Horn of the Lateral Ventricle
Foramen of Magendie
ATLAS OF NEUROANATOMY
DR. JOSEPH J. WARNER

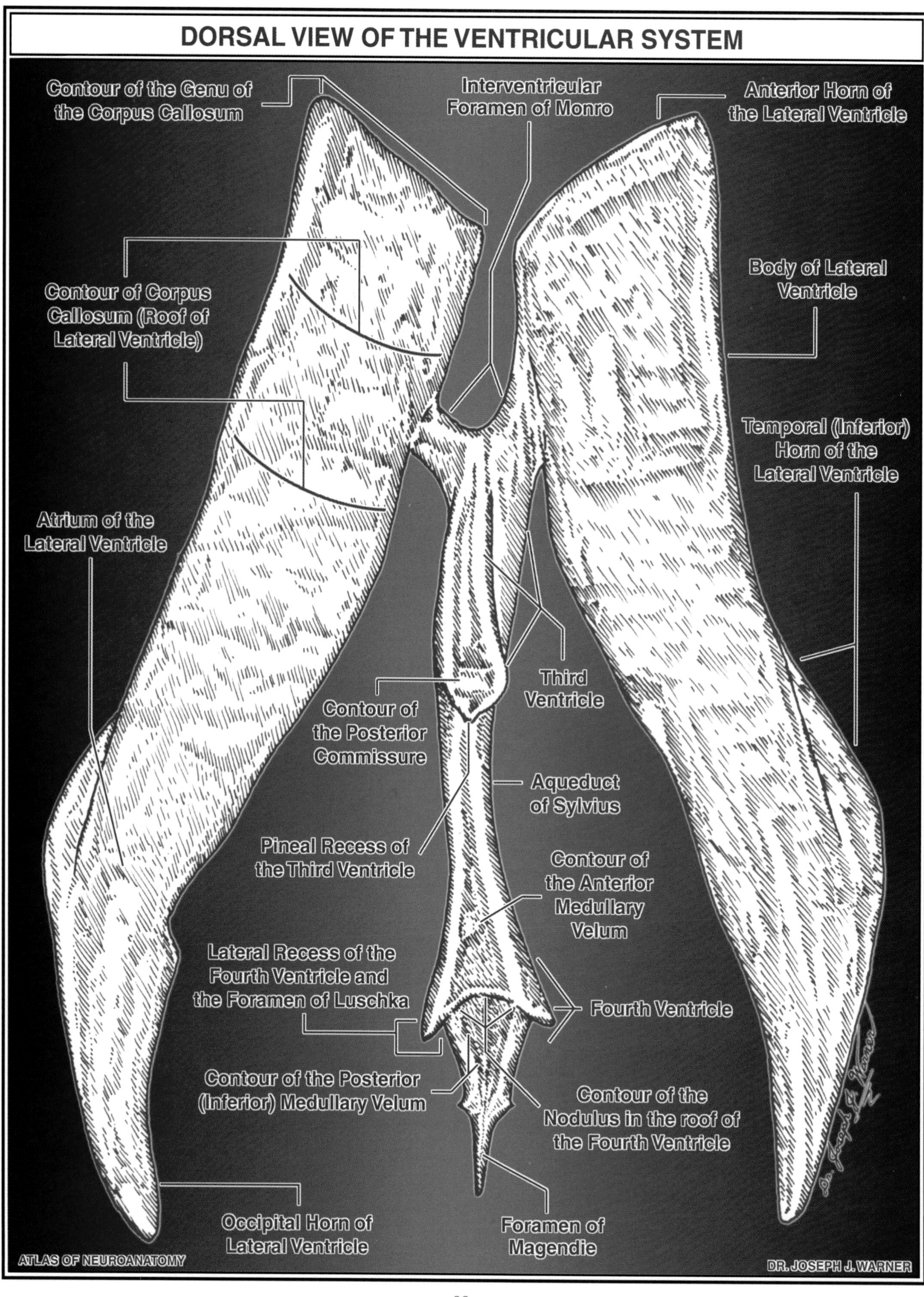
DORSAL VIEW OF THE VENTRICULAR SYSTEM
Contour of the Genu of the Corpus Callosum
Interventricular Foramen of Monro
Anterior Horn of the Lateral Ventricle
Contour of Corpus Callosum (Roof of Lateral Ventricle)
Body of Lateral Ventricle
Temporal (Inferior) Horn of the Lateral Ventricle
Atrium of the Lateral Ventricle
Third Ventricle
Contour of the Posterior Commissure
Aqueduct of Sylvius
Pineal Recess of the Third Ventricle
Contour of the Anterior Medullary Velum
Lateral Recess of the Fourth Ventricle and the Foramen of Luschka
Fourth Ventricle
Contour of the Posterior (Inferior) Medullary Velum
Contour of the Nodulus in the roof of the Fourth Ventricle
Occipital Horn of Lateral Ventricle
Foramen of Magendie
ATLAS OF NEUROANATOMY
DR. JOSEPH J. WARNER

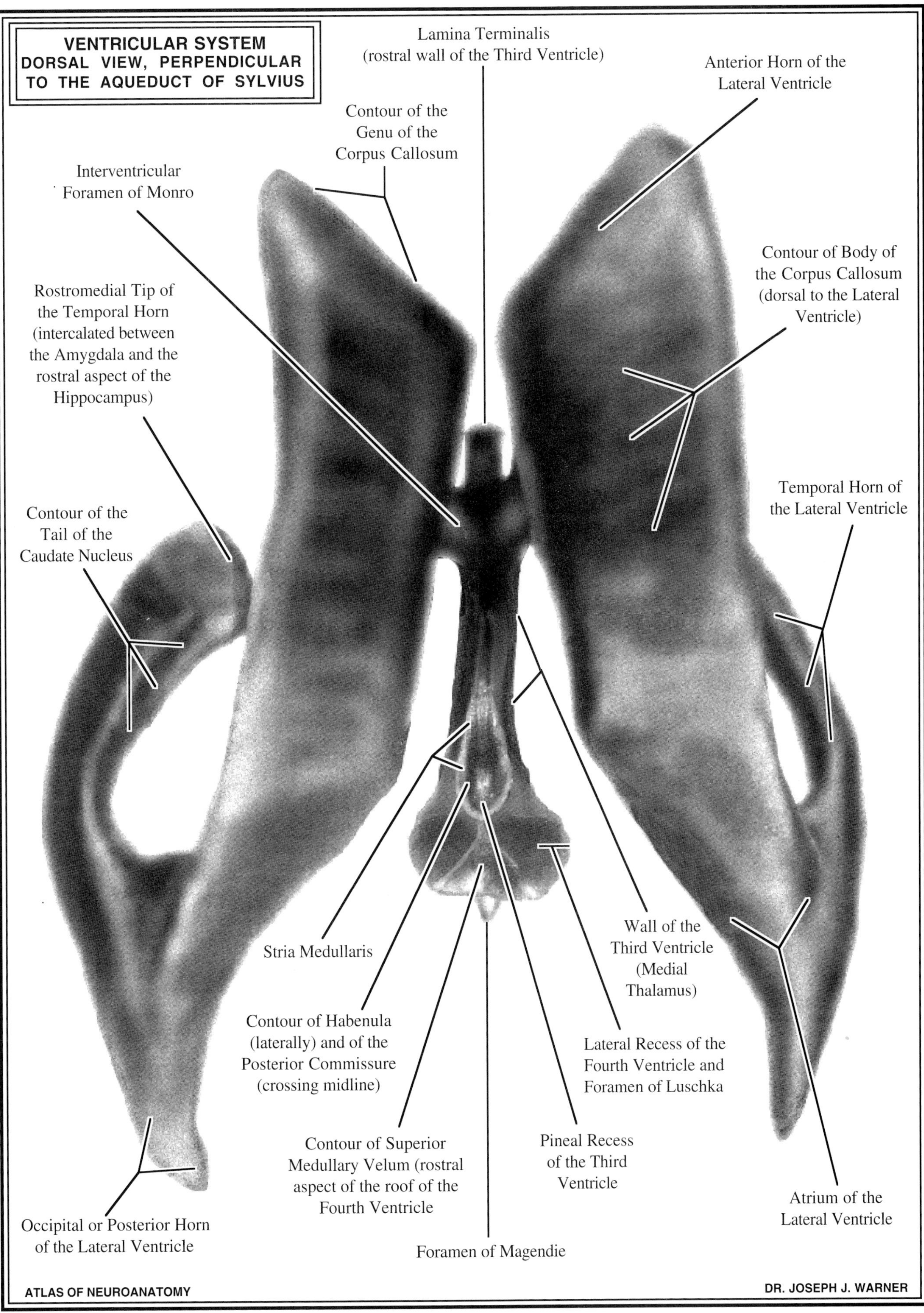
VENTRICULAR SYSTEM
DORSAL VIEW, PERPENDICULAR TO THE AQUEDUCT OF SYLVIUS
Lamina Terminalis (rostral wall of the Third Ventricle)
Anterior Horn of the Lateral Ventricle
Contour of the Genu of the Corpus Callosum
Interventricular Foramen of Monro
Contour of Body of the Corpus Callosum (dorsal to the Lateral Ventricle)
Rostromedial Tip of the Temporal Horn (intercalated between the Amygdala and the rostral aspect of the Hippocampus)
Temporal Horn of the Lateral Ventricle
Contour of the Tail of the Caudate Nucleus
Stria Medullaris
Wall of the Third Ventricle (Medial Thalamus)
Contour of Habenula (laterally) and of the Posterior Commissure (crossing midline)
Lateral Recess of the Fourth Ventricle and Foramen of Luschka
Contour of Superior Medullary Velum (rostral aspect of the roof of the Fourth Ventricle)
Pineal Recess of the Third Ventricle
Atrium of the Lateral Ventricle
Occipital or Posterior Horn of the Lateral Ventricle
Foramen of Magendie

SECTION OF THE BRAIN PARALLEL TO THE LONGITUDINAL AXIS OF THE BRAINSTEM: RESECTION DEMONSTRATING THE CAUDAL ASPECT OF THE LATERAL VENTRICLES, THE DORSAL THALAMUS, FORNIX, CHOROID PLEXUS, STRIA TERMINALIS AND THALAMOSTRIATE VEIN, AND THE CAUDATE NUCLEUS

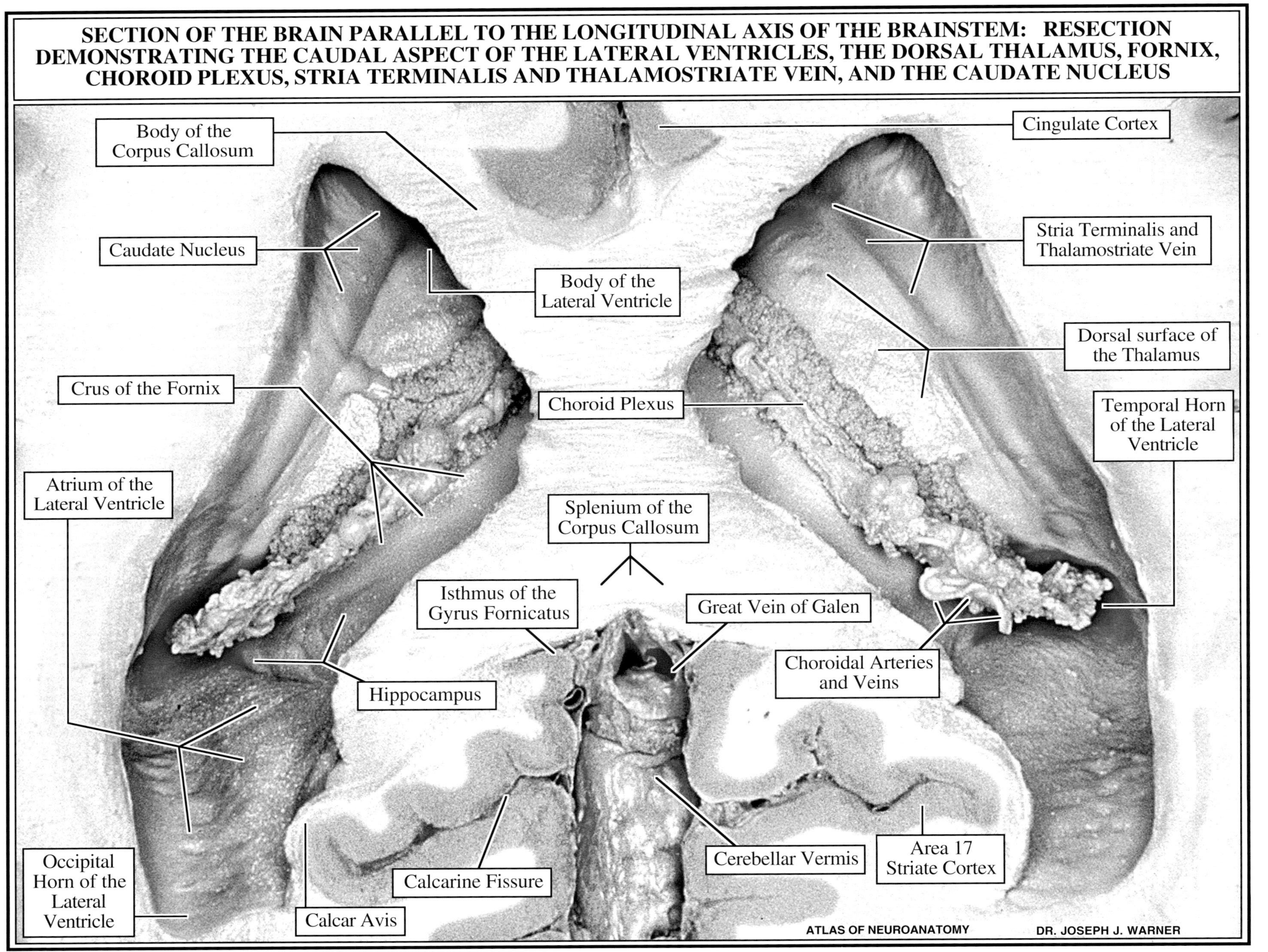

HORIZONTAL SECTION (MAGNIFIED DORSAL TO VENTRAL VIEW); LEVEL OF THE FORAMEN OF MONRO, MASSA INTERMEDIA, AND THE PINEAL RECESS OF THE THIRD VENTRICLE: SECTION MAP WITH REFERENCE TO THE VENTRICULAR SYSTEM

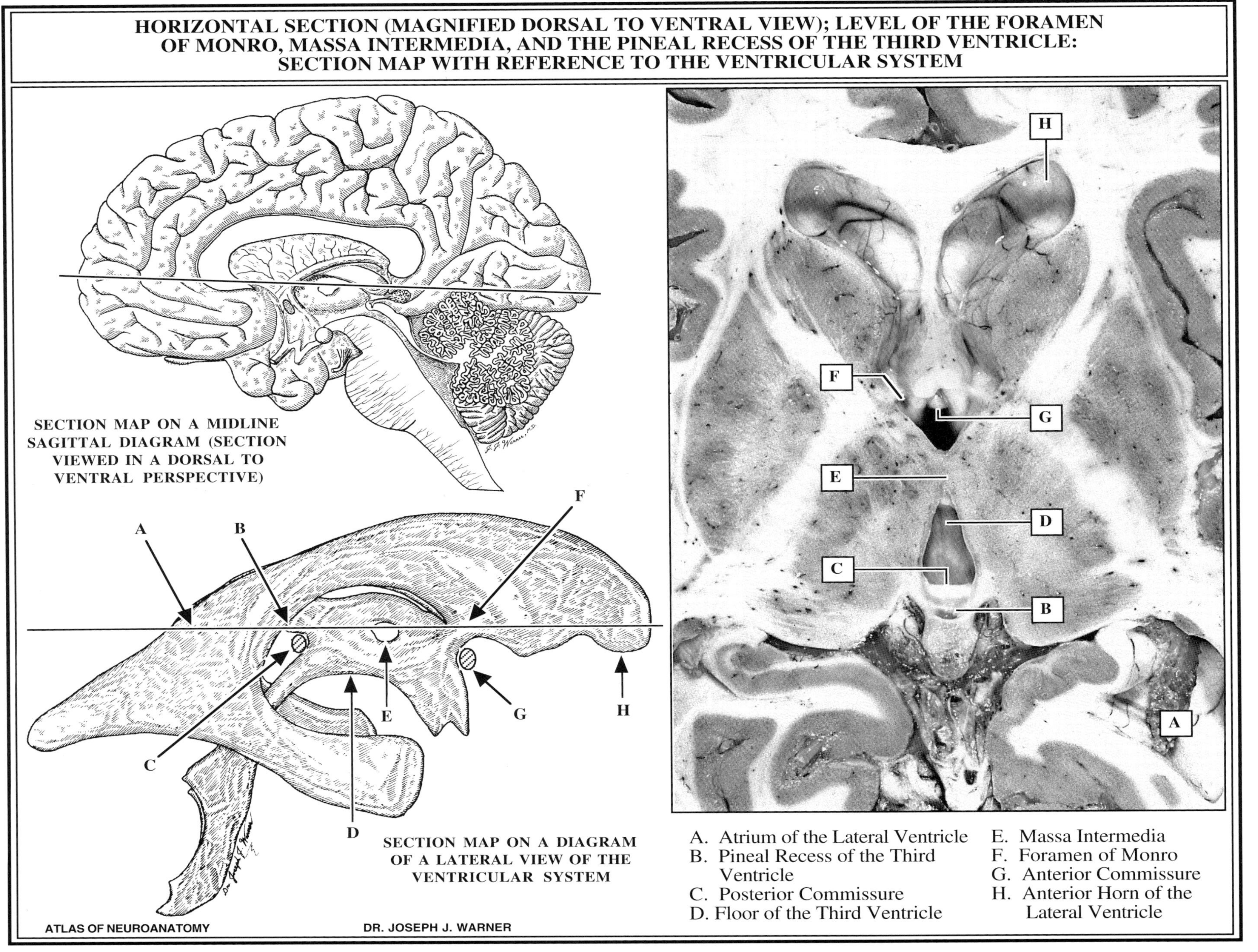

SECTION MAP ON A MIDLINE SAGITTAL DIAGRAM (SECTION VIEWED IN A DORSAL TO VENTRAL PERSPECTIVE)

SECTION MAP ON A DIAGRAM OF A LATERAL VIEW OF THE VENTRICULAR SYSTEM

A. Atrium of the Lateral Ventricle
B. Pineal Recess of the Third Ventricle
C. Posterior Commissure
D. Floor of the Third Ventricle
E. Massa Intermedia
F. Foramen of Monro
G. Anterior Commissure
H. Anterior Horn of the Lateral Ventricle

OBLIQUE SECTION OF THE CEREBRAL HEMISPHERES DEMONSTRATING THE LEFT LATERAL VENTRICLE: DORSAL TO VENTRAL PERSPECTIVE

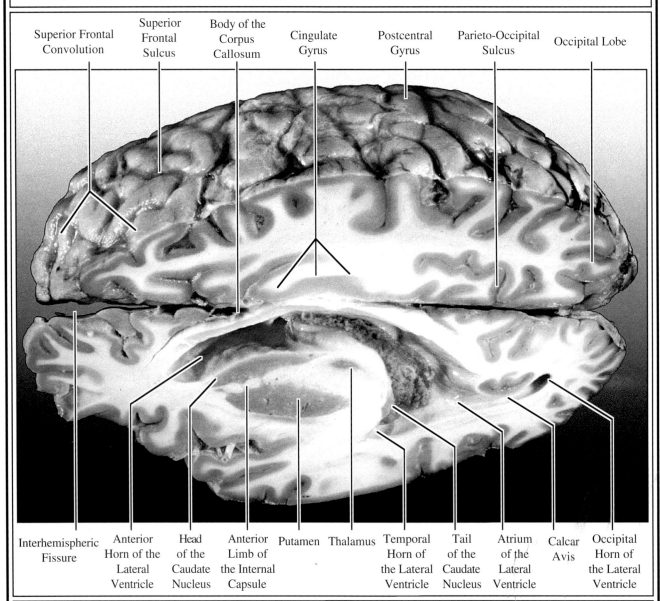

Superior Frontal Convolution
Superior Frontal Sulcus
Body of the Corpus Callosum
Cingulate Gyrus
Postcentral Gyrus
Parieto-Occipital Sulcus
Occipital Lobe

Interhemispheric Fissure
Anterior Horn of the Lateral Ventricle
Head of the Caudate Nucleus
Anterior Limb of the Internal Capsule
Putamen
Thalamus
Temporal Horn of the Lateral Ventricle
Tail of the Caudate Nucleus
Atrium of the Lateral Ventricle
Calcar Avis
Occipital Horn of the Lateral Ventricle

SECTION ORIENTATION (A) AND DIRECTION IN WHICH THE SPECIMEN IS VIEWED (B).

The cerebral hemispheres have been sectioned in an oblique plane (A) perpendicular to the coronal plane. The plane of section passes through the superior parasagittal region of the right hemisphere, crossing the interhemispheric fissure immediately dorsal to the corpus callosum. The dorsolateral aspect of the left hemisphere has been resected to expose the anterior horn, body, atrium, occipital horn, and temporal horns of the left lateral ventricle. This view provides a direct dorsal to ventral perspective (B), demonstrating the relative position of the various regions of the lateral ventricle with respect to the midline (interhemispheric fissure). The lateral position of the temporal horn relative to the remainder of the lateral ventricle is well delineated by this dissection.

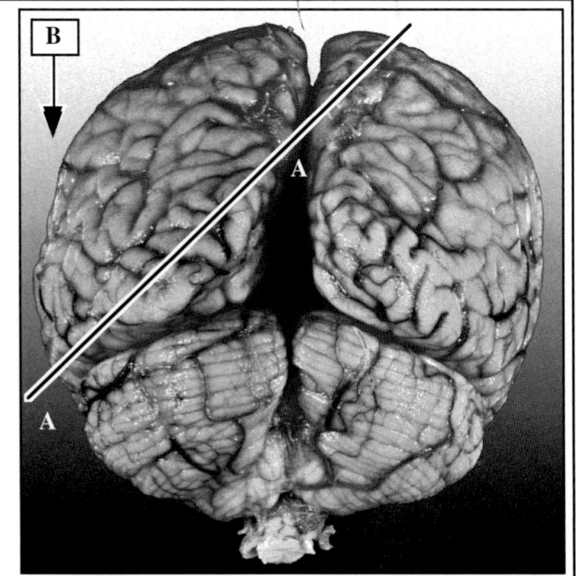

OBLIQUE SECTION OF THE CEREBRAL HEMISPHERES DEMONSTRATING THE LEFT LATERAL VENTRICLE: DIRECTION OF VIEW PERPENDICULAR TO THE PLANE OF SECTION

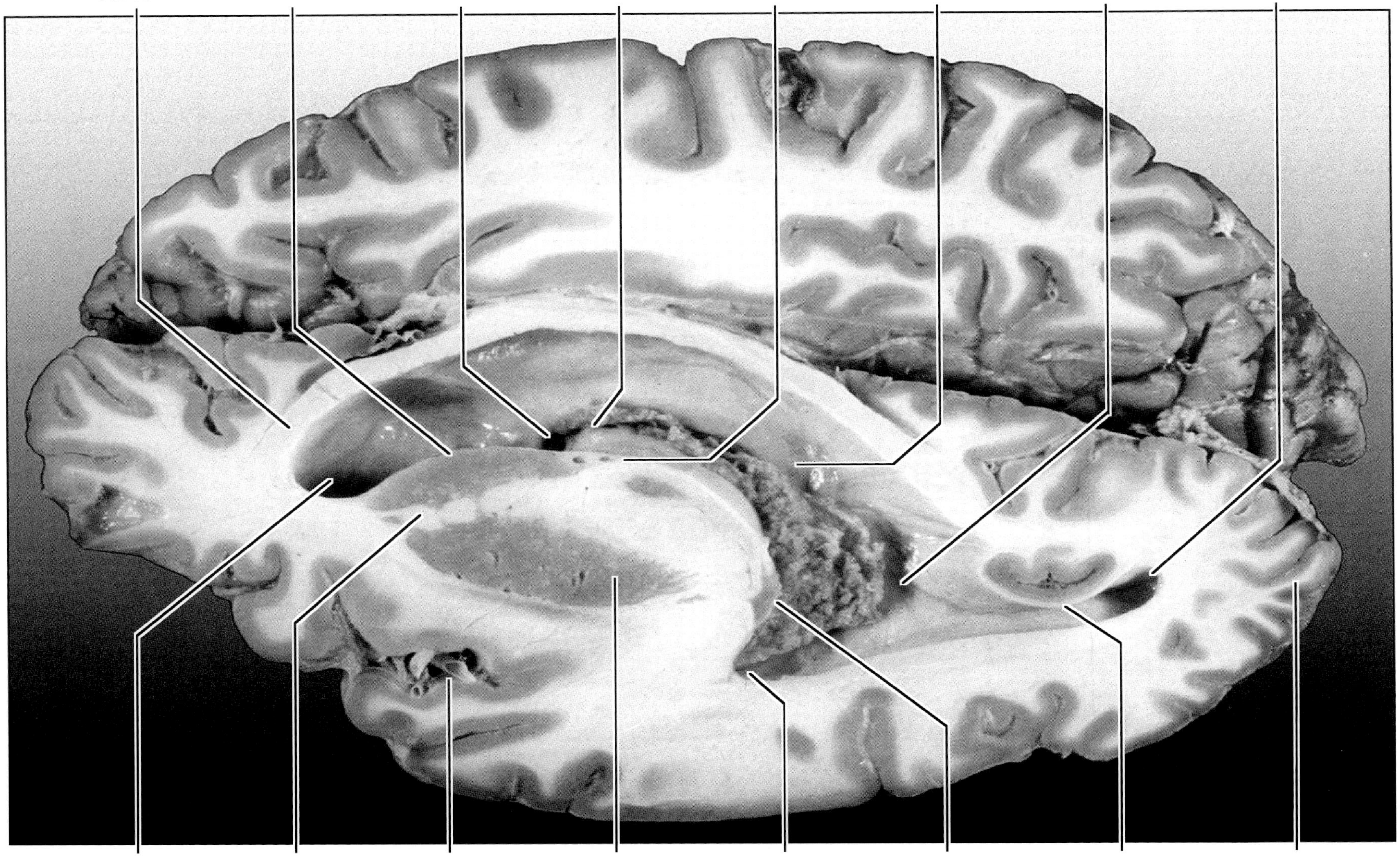

Genu of the Corpus Callosum

Head of the Caudate Nucleus

Interventricular Foramen of Monro

Anterior Tubercle of the Thalamus

Stria Terminalis and Thalamostriate Vein

Fornix

Atrium of the Lateral Ventricle

Occipital Horn of the Lateral Ventricle

Anterior Horn of the Lateral Ventricle

Anterior Limb of the Internal Capsule

Sylvian Fissure

Putamen

Temporal Horn of the Lateral Ventricle

Tail of the Caudate Nucleus

Calcar Avis

Occipital Pole

FLUOROSCOPIC VENTRICULOGRAPHY OF AN AUTOPSY SPECIMEN: LATERAL PROJECTION

Radiocontrast was injected into the ventricular system via cannulation of the foramen of Magendie, with the brain inverted 180 degrees from anatomic position. (Radiocontrast, due to its density, flows according to the position of the brain relative to gravity). The contrast flowed through the fourth ventricle and the aqueduct of Sylvius into the third ventricle. To fill each lateral ventricle, the brain was rotated (during injection) to direct the contrast material through each interventricular foramen of Monro. Subsequently, the brain was rotated about an axis perpendicular to the sagittal plane, sequentially placing (1) the occipital lobes and (2) the temporal lobes in a dependent position. This resulted in contrast flow into the temporal horns of each lateral ventricle. The brain was then inverted, accompanied by air entry into the third and fourth ventricles. Thus, they appear radiolucent as compared to the radiodense lateral ventricles.

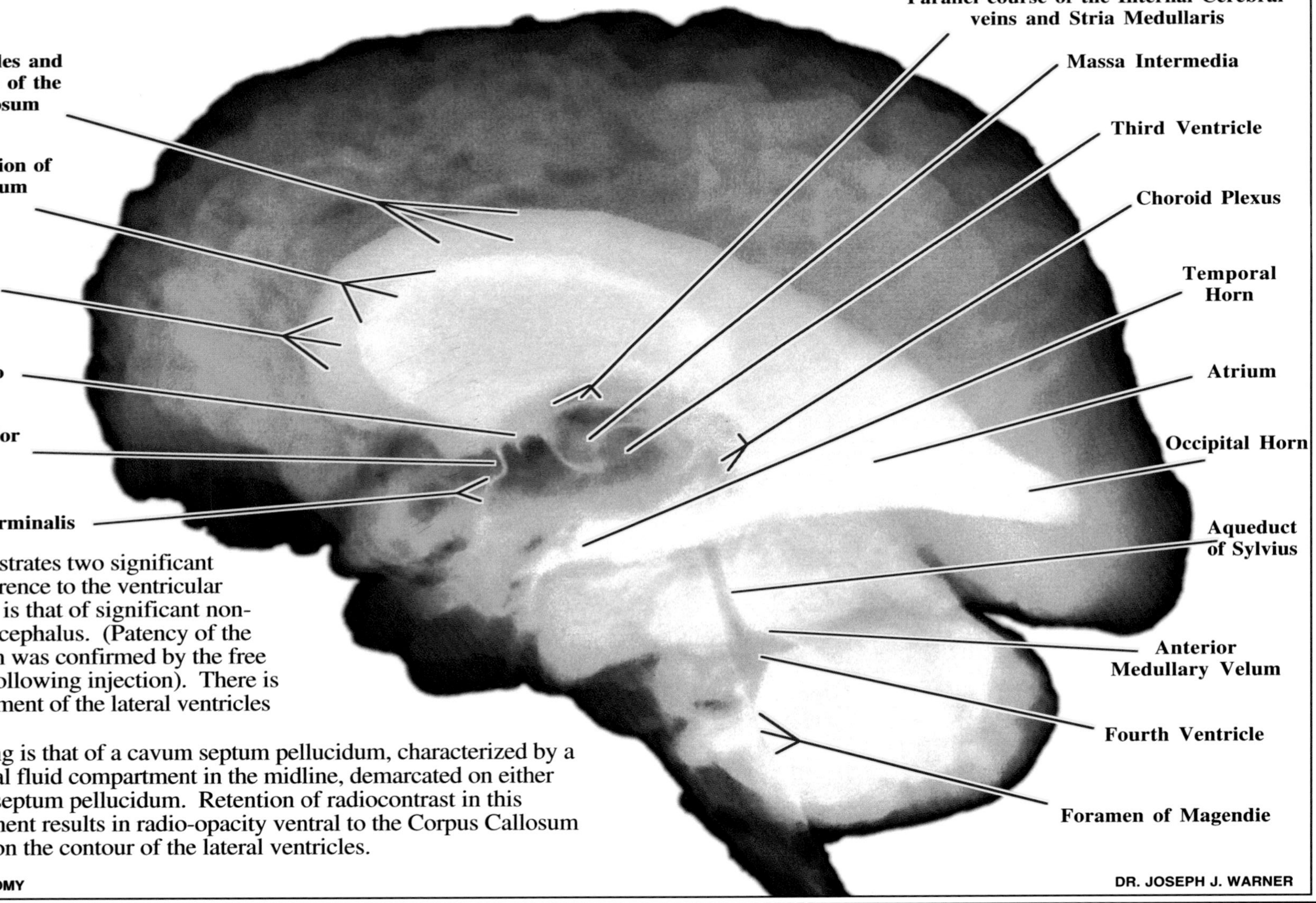

This brain demonstrates two significant findings with reference to the ventricular system. The first is that of significant non-obstructive hydrocephalus. (Patency of the ventricular system was confirmed by the free flow of contrast following injection). There is particular enlargement of the lateral ventricles in this case.

The second finding is that of a cavum septum pellucidum, characterized by a large cerebrospinal fluid compartment in the midline, demarcated on either side by a double septum pellucidum. Retention of radiocontrast in this midline compartment results in radio-opacity ventral to the Corpus Callosum superimposed upon the contour of the lateral ventricles.

FLUOROSCOPIC VENTRICULOGRAPHY OF AN AUTOPSY SPECIMEN DEMONSTRATING HYDROCEPHALUS AND CAVUM SEPTUM PELLUCIDUM:
DORSAL TO VENTRAL PROJECTION (BRAIN HORIZONTALLY ORIENTED)

Under fluoroscopic monitoring, the brain was rotated to vertically orient the plane of the interhemispheric fissure. The specimen was placed with the ventral aspect downward, with the projection axis perpendicular to the horizontal plane. Contrast injection 45 minutes prior to fluoroscopy allowed for the radio-opaque staining of the choroid plexus and ventricular walls. Repeat injection was performed during fluorososcopy.

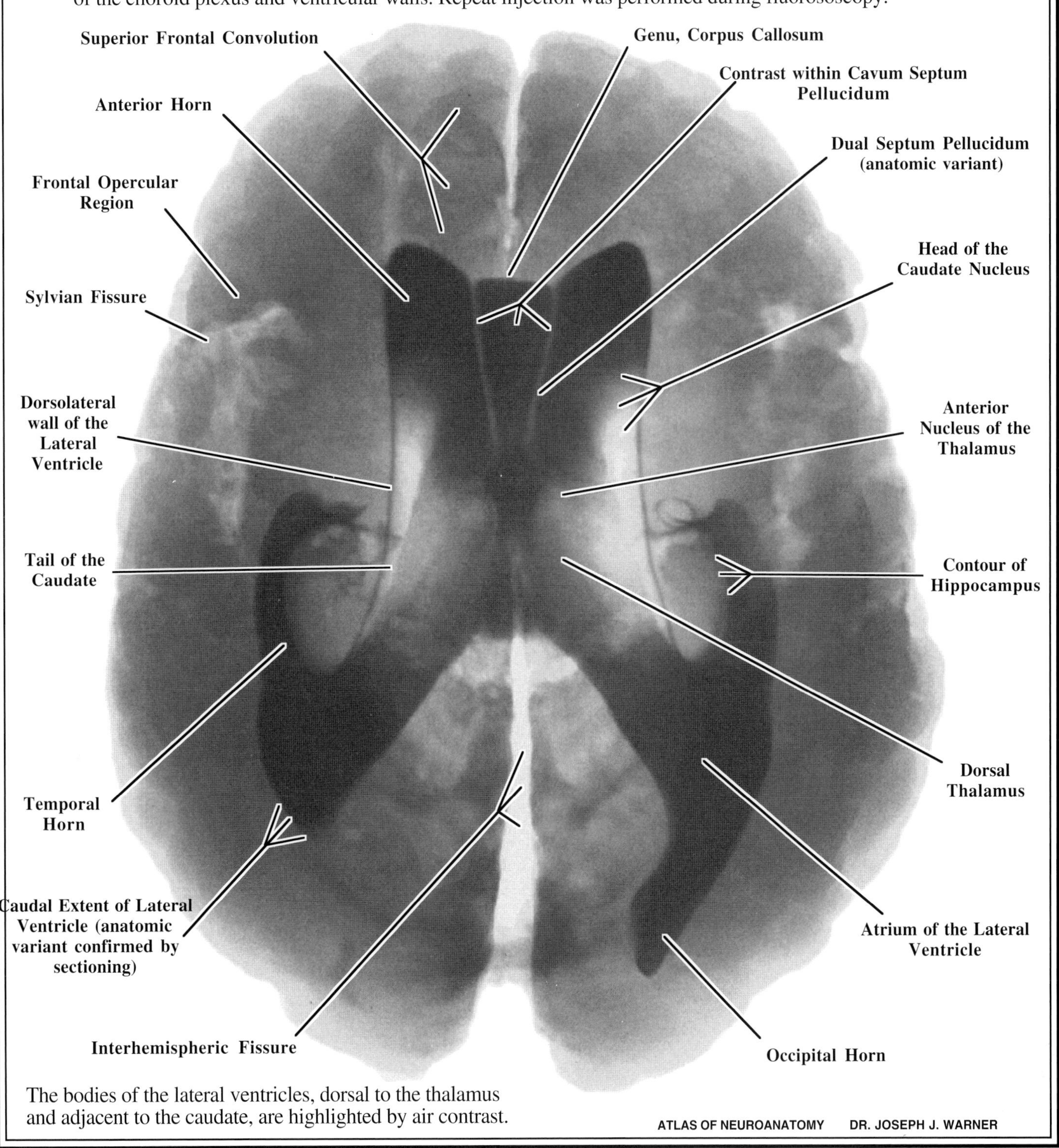

The bodies of the lateral ventricles, dorsal to the thalamus and adjacent to the caudate, are highlighted by air contrast.

FLUOROSCOPIC VENTRICULOGRAPHY OF AN AUTOPSY SPECIMEN DEMONSTRATING HYDROCEPHALUS AND CAVUM SEPTUM PELLUCIDUM:

VENTRAL TO DORSAL PROJECTION (COLOR ENHANCED STUDY)

Under fluoroscopic monitoring, the brain was rotated to vertically orient the plane of the Interhemispheric Fissure. The specimen was placed with the dorsal aspect downward, with the projection axis perpendicular to the horizontal plane. Contrast injection 45 minutes prior to fluoroscopy allowed for the radio-opaque staining of the choroid plexus and ventricular walls. Repeat injection was performed during fluorososcopy.

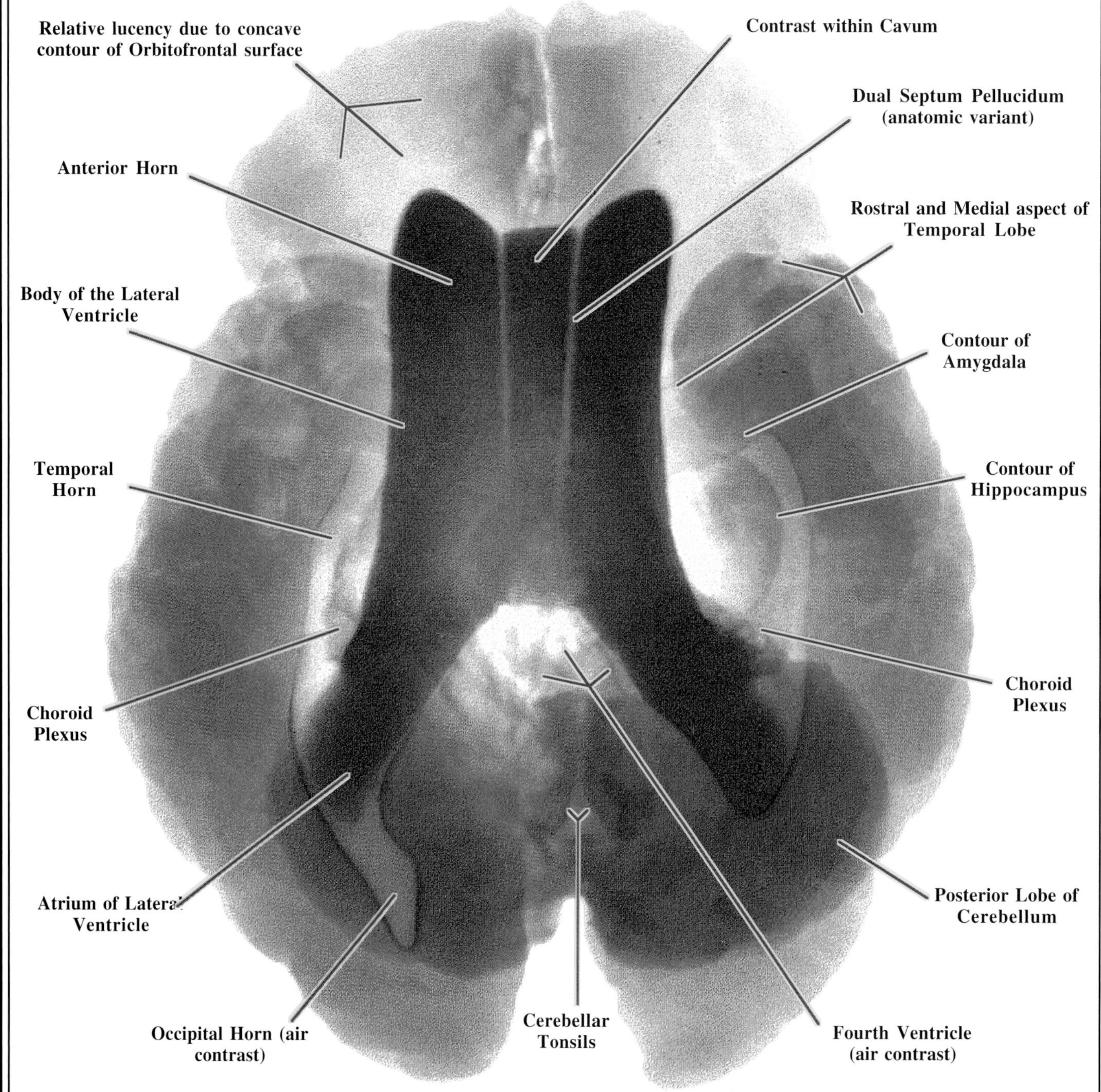

This orientation results in flow of contrast from the temporal horns into the bodies of the lateral ventricles. The atria and dorsal ventricular structures are radio-opaque, whereas the temporal horns demonstrate air contrast radiolucency.

FLUOROSCOPIC VENTRICULOGRAPHY OF AN AUTOPSY SPECIMEN DEMONSTRATING HYDROCEPHALUS AND CAVUM SEPTUM PELLUCIDUM: PROJECTION ALONG THE CAUDAL TO ROSTRAL AXIS

Under fluoroscopic monitoring, the brain was rotated such that the rostrocaudal axis was perpendicular to the horizontal plane. The contrast had been placed in the ventricles approximately 45 minutes prior to this filming. This time interval allowed for the diffusion of iodinated radiocontrast through the ependymal lining of the ventricles (with retention in the ventricular walls) as well as radio-opaque staining of the choroid plexus.

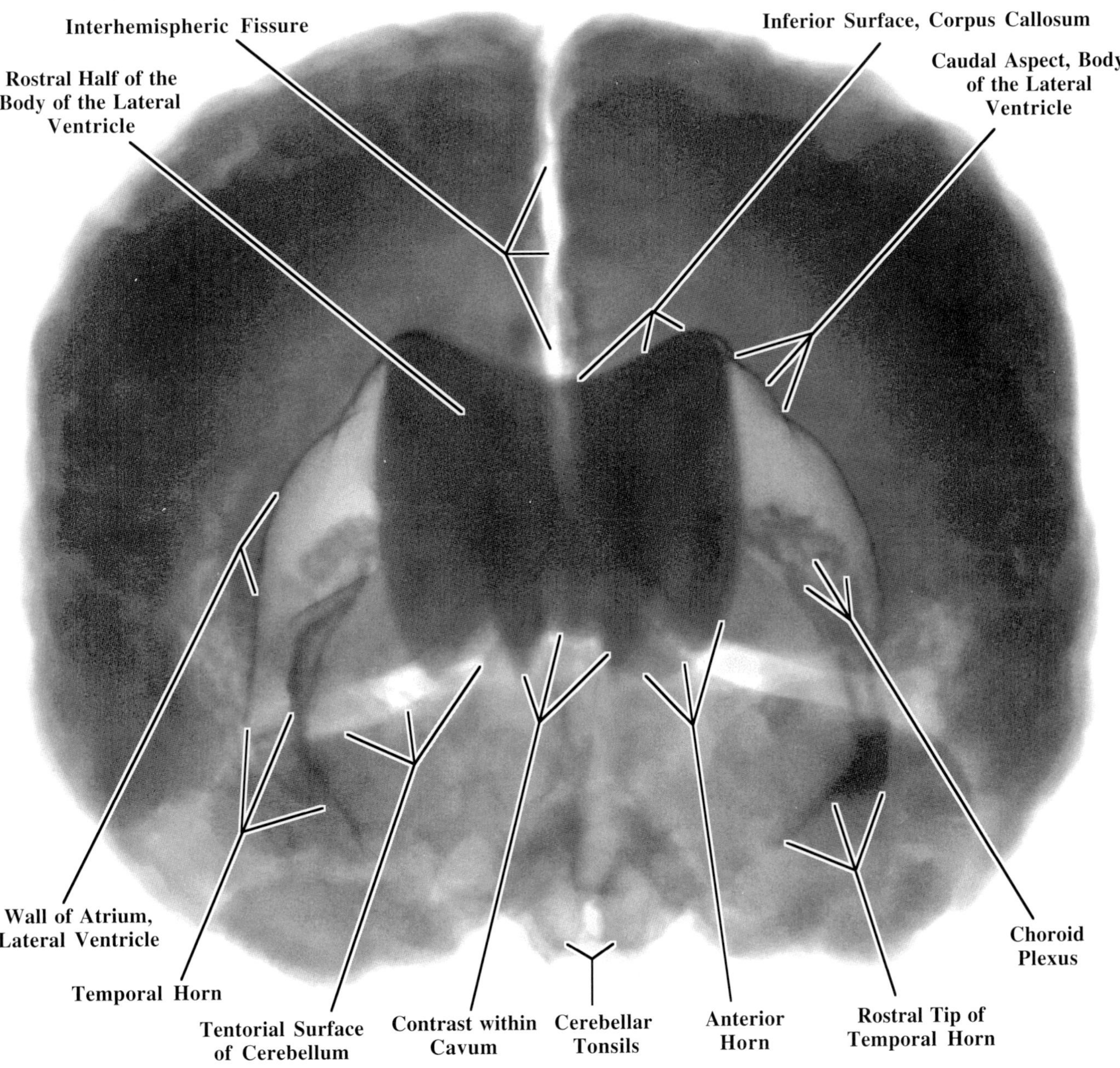

Orientation of this specimen (rostral aspect downward) has thus resulted in flow of contrast into the anterior horns and bodies of the lateral ventricles. The rostral tips of the temporal horns demonstrate contrast radio-opacity as well. Radiolucency within the caudal aspect of the ventricular system appears in marked contrast to the radio-opaque ventricular walls and choroid plexus.

Landmarks to the orientation of this specimen include visualization of the tentorial surface of the cerebellum, the cerebellar tonsils, and the interhemispheric fissure. The relative X-ray lucency of brain parenchyma results in an apparent juxtaposition of these landmarks and the ventricular system (e.g. superimposition of the temporal horns over the cerebellum in this projection).

FLUOROSCOPIC VENTRICULOGRAPHY OF AN AUTOPSY SPECIMEN DEMONSTRATING HYDROCEPHALUS AND CAVUM SEPTUM PELLUCIDUM:
ROSTRAL - CAUDAL PROJECTION, AXIS PARALLEL TO THE SYLVIAN FISSURE

Under fluoroscopic monitoring, the brain was rotated to vertically orient the planes of the Sylvian and Interhemispheric Fissures. Contrast injection 45 minutes prior to fluoroscopy allowed for the radio-opaque staining of the choroid plexus and ventricular walls. Repeat injection was performed during fluorososcopy to increase contrast of the ventricles in comparison to the density of the brain along this axis.

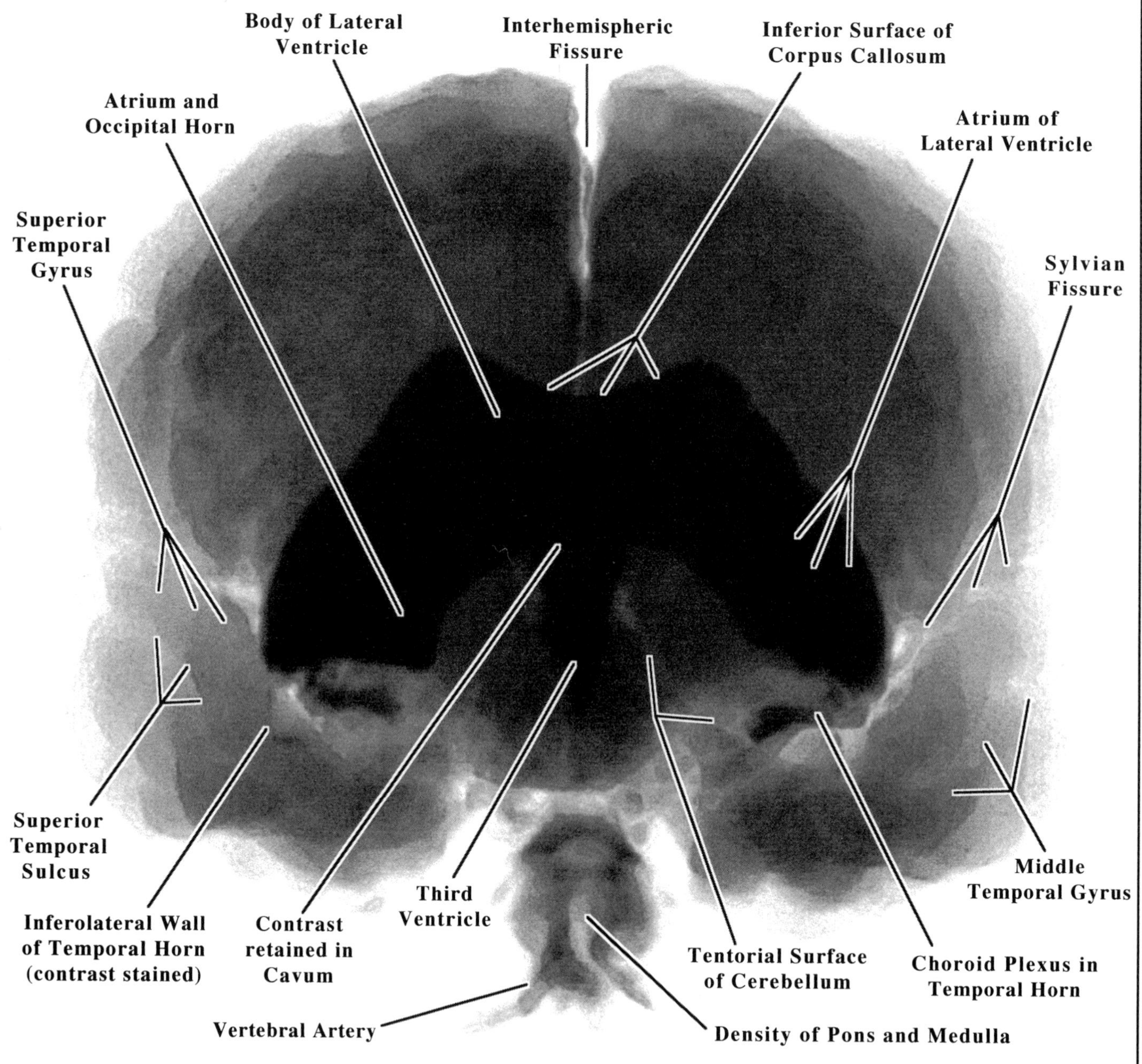

Orientation of this specimen (occipital lobes downward) has resulted in flow of contrast into the atria and caudal aspects of the bodies and temporal horns of the lateral ventricles. Radio-opacity thus delineates the caudal aspect of the ventricular system within the cerebral hemispheres. The choroid plexus is visualized (due to contrast staining) more rostrally within the temporal horns of the lateral ventricles. Important orientation landmarks include the Interhemispheric and Sylvian Fissures, the temporal lobes, brainstem and vertebral arteries.

HORIZONTAL SECTION OF A BRAIN WITH CAVUM SEPTUM PELLUCIDUM AND HYDROCEPHALUS, MAGNIFIED DORSAL TO VENTRAL VIEW: DISSECTION FOLLOWING TOLUIDINE BLUE MARKED RADIOCONTRAST VENTRICULOGRAPHY AND ANGIOGRAPHY

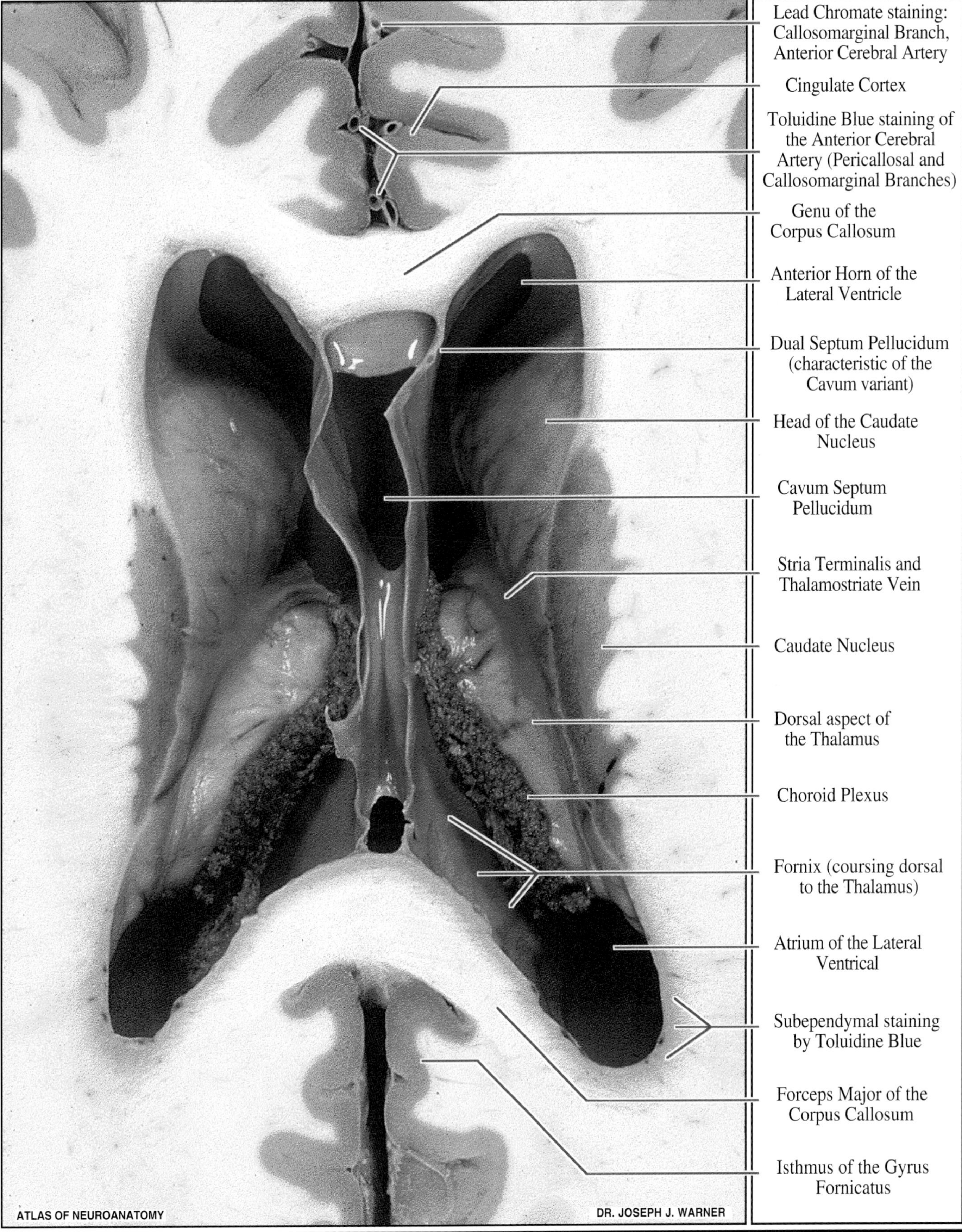

Lead Chromate staining: Callosomarginal Branch, Anterior Cerebral Artery

Cingulate Cortex

Toluidine Blue staining of the Anterior Cerebral Artery (Pericallosal and Callosomarginal Branches)

Genu of the Corpus Callosum

Anterior Horn of the Lateral Ventricle

Dual Septum Pellucidum (characteristic of the Cavum variant)

Head of the Caudate Nucleus

Cavum Septum Pellucidum

Stria Terminalis and Thalamostriate Vein

Caudate Nucleus

Dorsal aspect of the Thalamus

Choroid Plexus

Fornix (coursing dorsal to the Thalamus)

Atrium of the Lateral Ventrical

Subependymal staining by Toluidine Blue

Forceps Major of the Corpus Callosum

Isthmus of the Gyrus Fornicatus

HORIZONTAL SECTION OF A BRAIN WITH CAVUM SEPTUM PELLUCIDUM AND HYDROCEPHALUS, LEVEL OF THE ANTERIOR COMMISSURE AND SUPERIOR COLLICULUS (VENTRAL TO DORSAL PERSPECTIVE): DISSECTION FOLLOWING TOLUIDINE BLUE MARKED RADIOCONTRAST VENTRICULOGRAPHY AND ANGIOGRAPHY

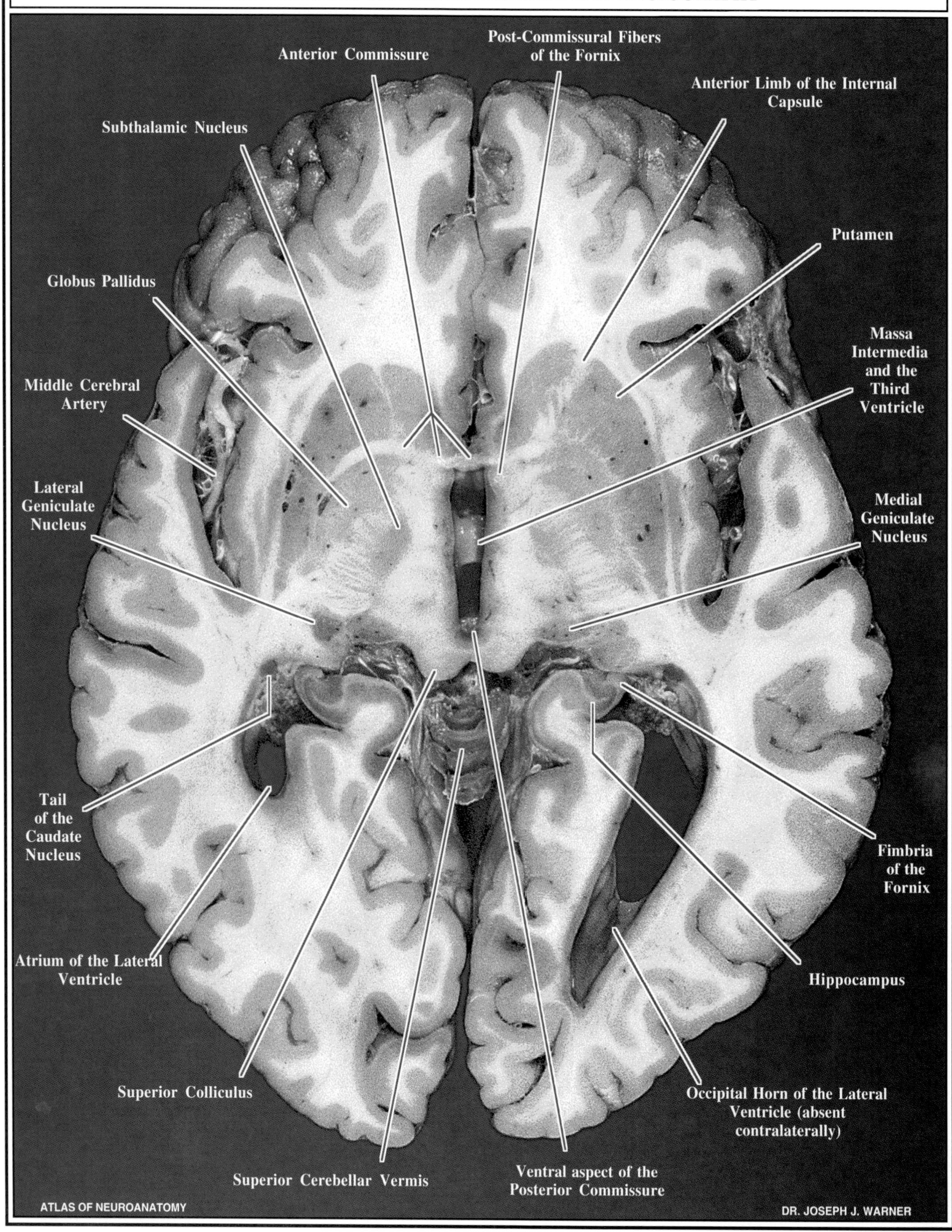

SIMULTANEOUS FLUOROSCOPIC VENTRICULOGRAPHY AND CEREBRAL ANGIOGRAPHY: PROJECTION ALONG THE DORSAL-VENTRAL AXIS

Under fluoroscopic monitoring, the brain was rotated to vertically orient the plane of the interhemispheric fissure. Via cannulation of the foramen of Magendie, radio-opaque contrast was injected into the ventricular system. The brain (fixed previously) was then suspended in deionized water. Radiolucent vascular clamps were placed on both supraclinoid carotid arteries and one vertebral artery. A catheter was sutured in place in the remaining vertebral artery. An aqueous suspension of $BaSO_4$ and $PbCrO_4$ was then injected, demonstrating the carotid and vertebrobasilar systems.

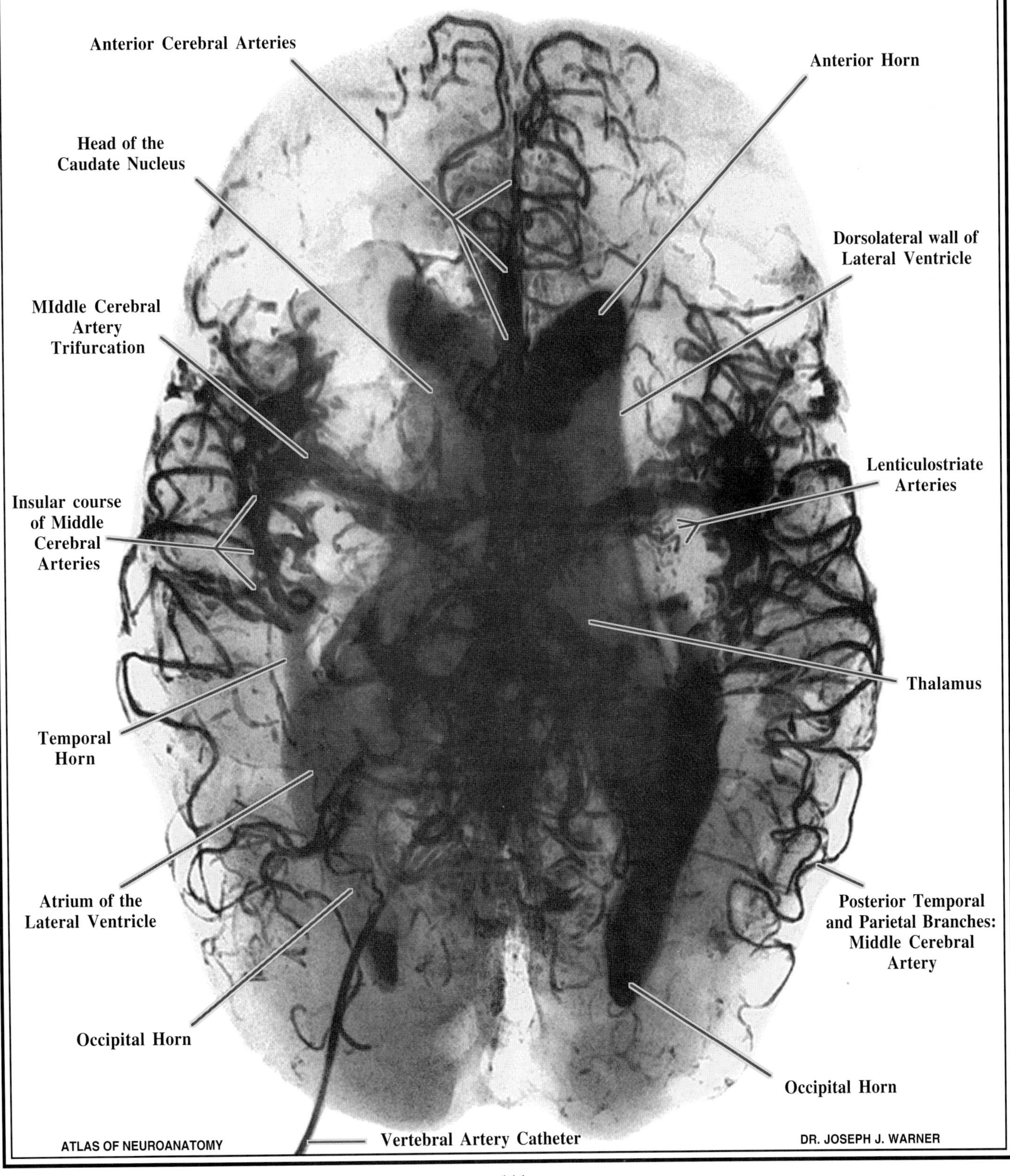

SIMULTANEOUS FLUOROSCOPIC VENTRICULOGRAPHY AND CEREBRAL ANGIOGRAPHY: LATERAL PROJECTION

Radiocontrast was injected into the ventricular system via cannulation of the foramen of Magendie, with the brain inverted 180 degrees from anatomic position. The contrast flowed through the fourth ventricle and the aqueduct of Sylvius into the third ventricle. To fill each lateral ventricle, the brain was rotated (during injection) to direct the contrast material through each interventricular foramen of Monro.

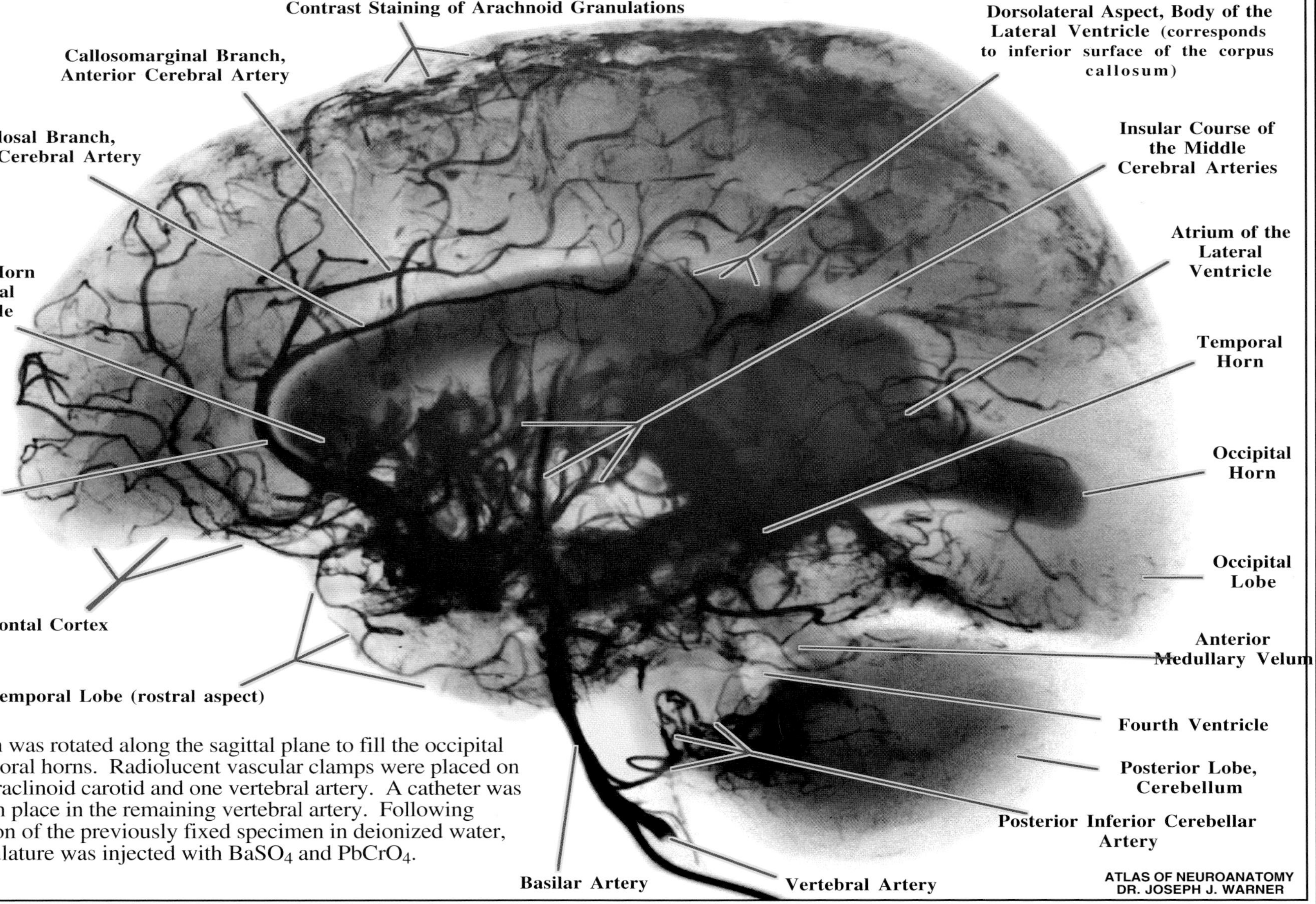

The brain was rotated along the sagittal plane to fill the occipital and temporal horns. Radiolucent vascular clamps were placed on each supraclinoid carotid and one vertebral artery. A catheter was sutured in place in the remaining vertebral artery. Following suspension of the previously fixed specimen in deionized water, the vasculature was injected with $BaSO_4$ and $PbCrO_4$.

DIAGRAM OF THE CERVICOCRANIAL ARTERIAL SYSTEM AND THE CIRCLE OF WILLIS

KEY TO NUMBERED STRUCTURES

1. Arch of the Aorta
2. Brachiocephalic Artery
3. Left Common Carotid Artery
4. Left Subclavian Artery
5. Right Common Carotid Artery

6, 7. Vertebral Artery (right, left)

8. Right Subclavian Artery

9, 10. Bifurcation of the Common Carotid Artery (right, left)

11, 12. External Carotid Artery (right, left)

13, 14. Carotid Sinus (right, left)

15, 16. Internal Carotid Artery (left, right)

17, 18. Carotid Siphon (right, left)

19, 20. Ophthalmic Artery (right, left)

21, 22. Internal Carotid Artery, Supraclinoid Segment (right, left)

23, 24. Anterior Cerebral Artery (right, left)

25. Anterior Communicating Artery

26, 27. Middle Cerebral Artery (right, left)

28, 29. Lenticulostriate Arteries (right, left)

30, 31. Middle Cerebral Arteries (in Sylvian Fissure) (right, left)

32, 33. Posterior Communicating Artery (right, left)

34, 35. Posterior Cerebral Artery (right, left)

36, 37. Superior Cerebellar Artery (right, left)

38, 39. Pontine Arteries (right, left)

40, 41. Anterior Inferior Cerebellar Artery (right, left)

42, 43. Posterior Inferior Cerebellar Artery (right, left)

44. Anterior Spinal Artery
45. Basilar Artery

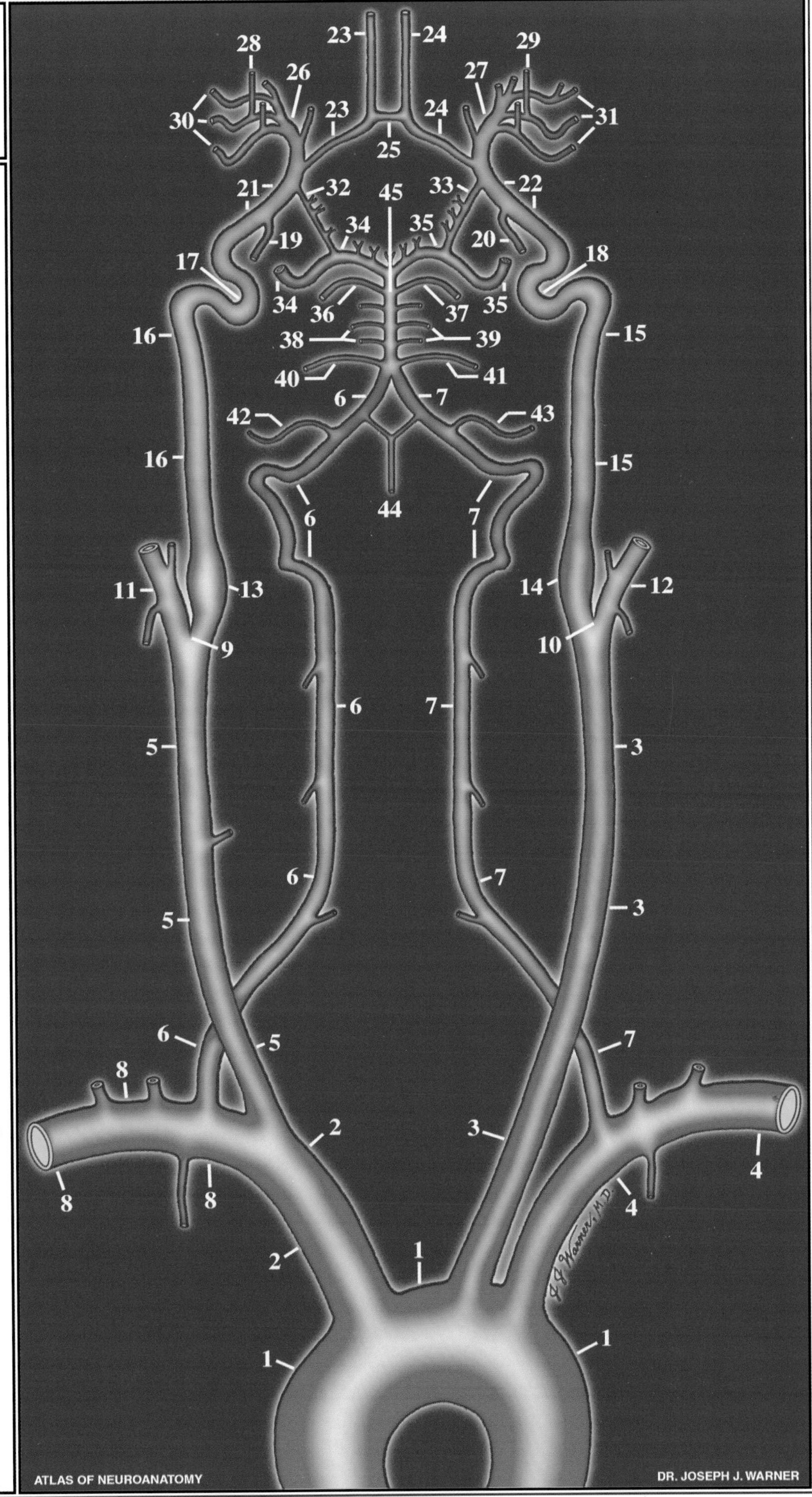

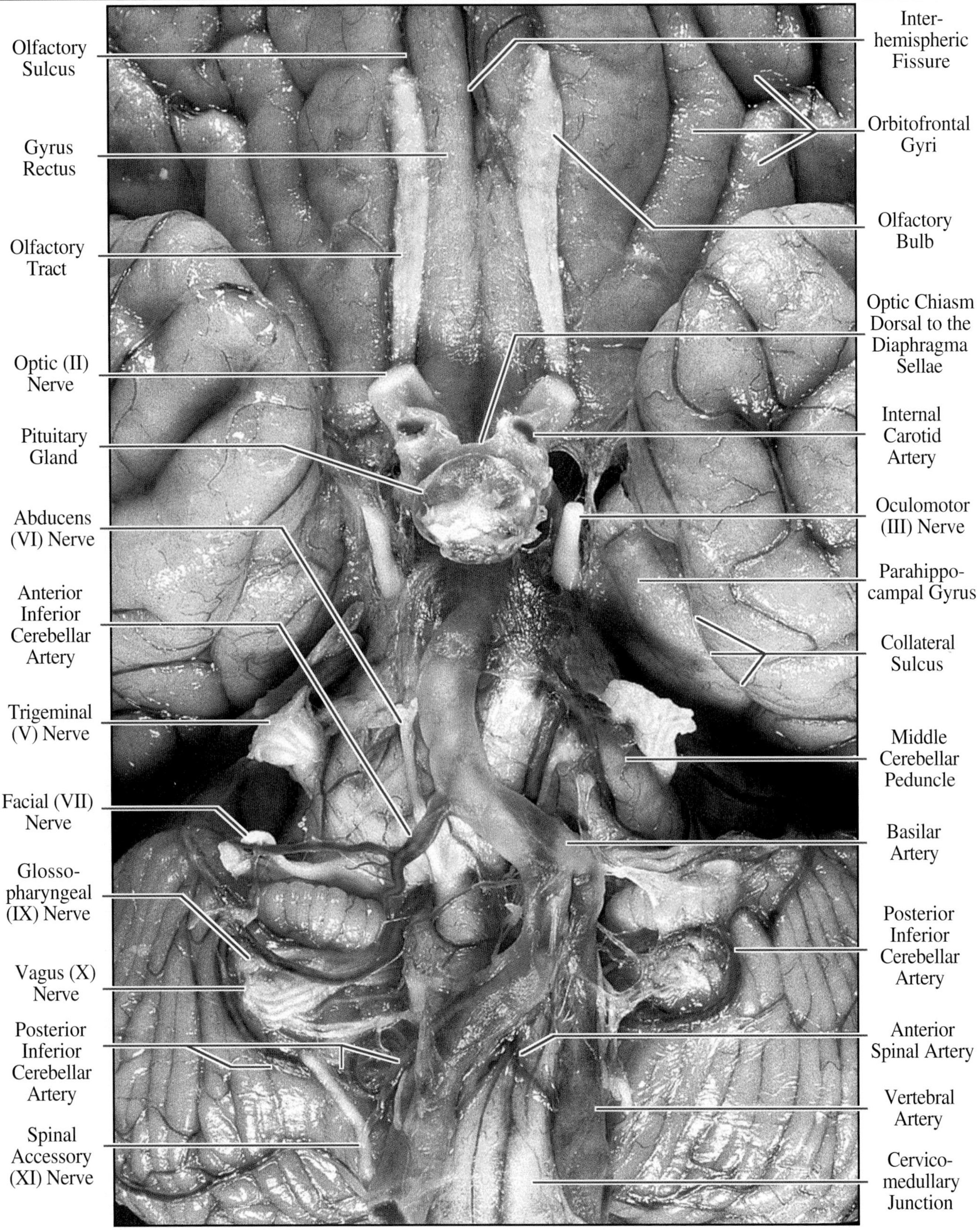

CEREBROVASCULATURE: VENTRAL ASPECT OF THE BRAIN, PITUITARY INTACT

Olfactory Sulcus
Gyrus Rectus
Olfactory Tract
Optic (II) Nerve
Pituitary Gland
Abducens (VI) Nerve
Anterior Inferior Cerebellar Artery
Trigeminal (V) Nerve
Facial (VII) Nerve
Glosso-pharyngeal (IX) Nerve
Vagus (X) Nerve
Posterior Inferior Cerebellar Artery
Spinal Accessory (XI) Nerve
Inter-hemispheric Fissure
Orbitofrontal Gyri
Olfactory Bulb
Optic Chiasm Dorsal to the Diaphragma Sellae
Internal Carotid Artery
Oculomotor (III) Nerve
Parahippo-campal Gyrus
Collateral Sulcus
Middle Cerebellar Peduncle
Basilar Artery
Posterior Inferior Cerebellar Artery
Anterior Spinal Artery
Vertebral Artery
Cervico-medullary Junction

CEREBROVASCULATURE: VENTRAL ASPECT OF THE BRAIN, ARACHNOID RESECTED

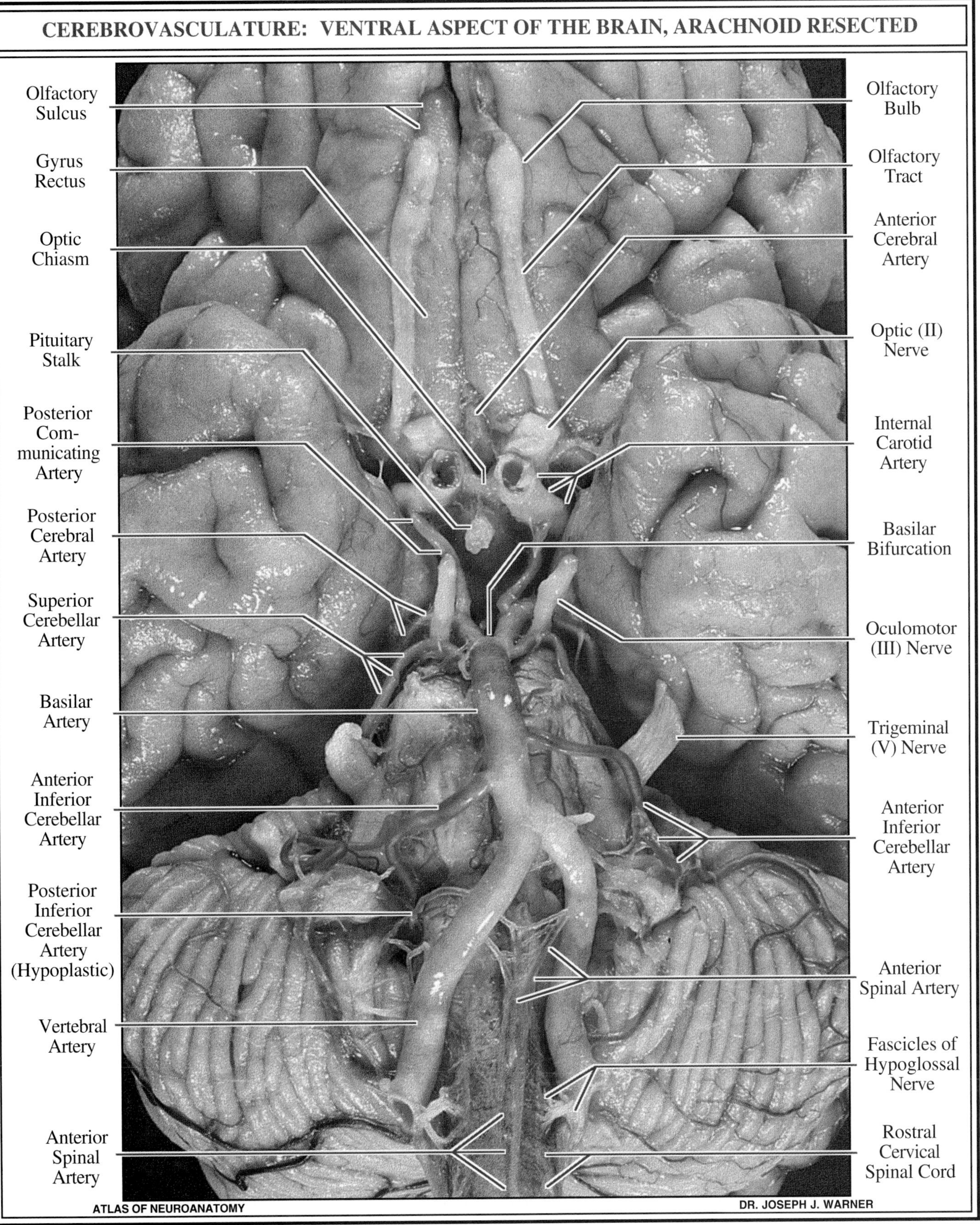

DISSECTION OF THE ARTERIAL CEREBROVASCULATURE

The illustrations which follow demonstrate the dissected intracranial arterial system, including the vascular supply to the brainstem, cerebellum, and cerebral hemispheres. At the center of this system is the Circle of Willis, which serves as the major collateral system between the vertebrobasilar and internal carotid arterial cerebrovascular supplies. This is the point of initiation of the vascular dissections used in the following illustrations. Vessels were prepared by dissection from autopsy brain specimens. This technique involves extensive resection of the arachnoid membrane to expose and mobilize the cerebrovascular system, with each vessel traced distally from the Circle of Willis. Once isolated from the brain, the arterial tree is arranged such that the ventral aspect of the Circle of Willis is oriented toward the observer. The distal vasculature is then allowed to follow this orientation by flotation in a shallow fluid-filled chamber over a submerged glass plate. Long vessels, such as the anterior cerebral arteries, are arranged radially from the Circle of Willis. Posterior fossa vasculature is similarly arranged from the vertebrobasilar axis. The fluid is slowly drained while maintaining appropriate vascular orientation, and the specimens are subsequently photographed. Vessels are fixed in 10% neutral buffered formalin (phosphate).

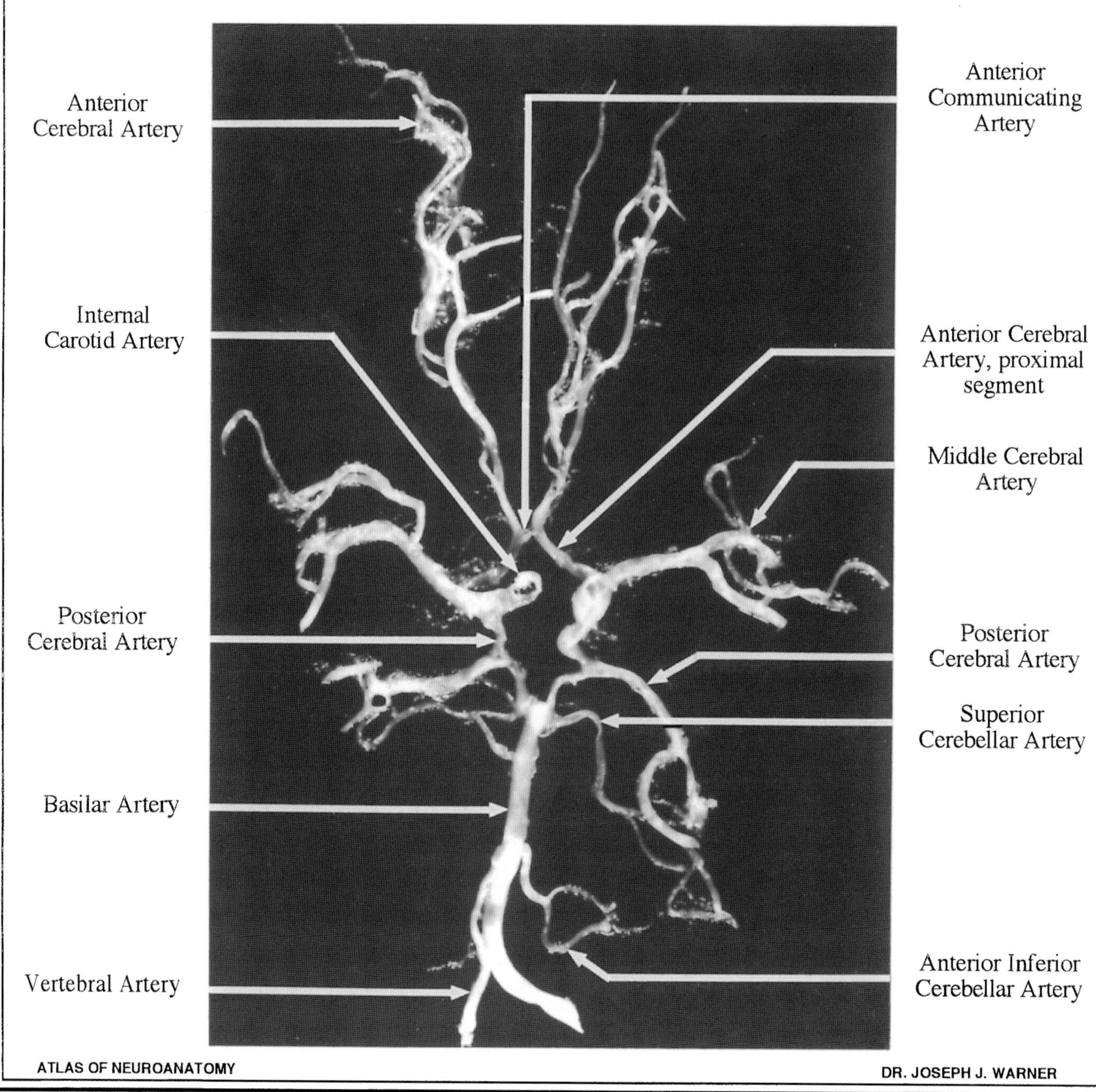

DISSECTION OF THE ARTERIAL CEREBROVASCULATURE

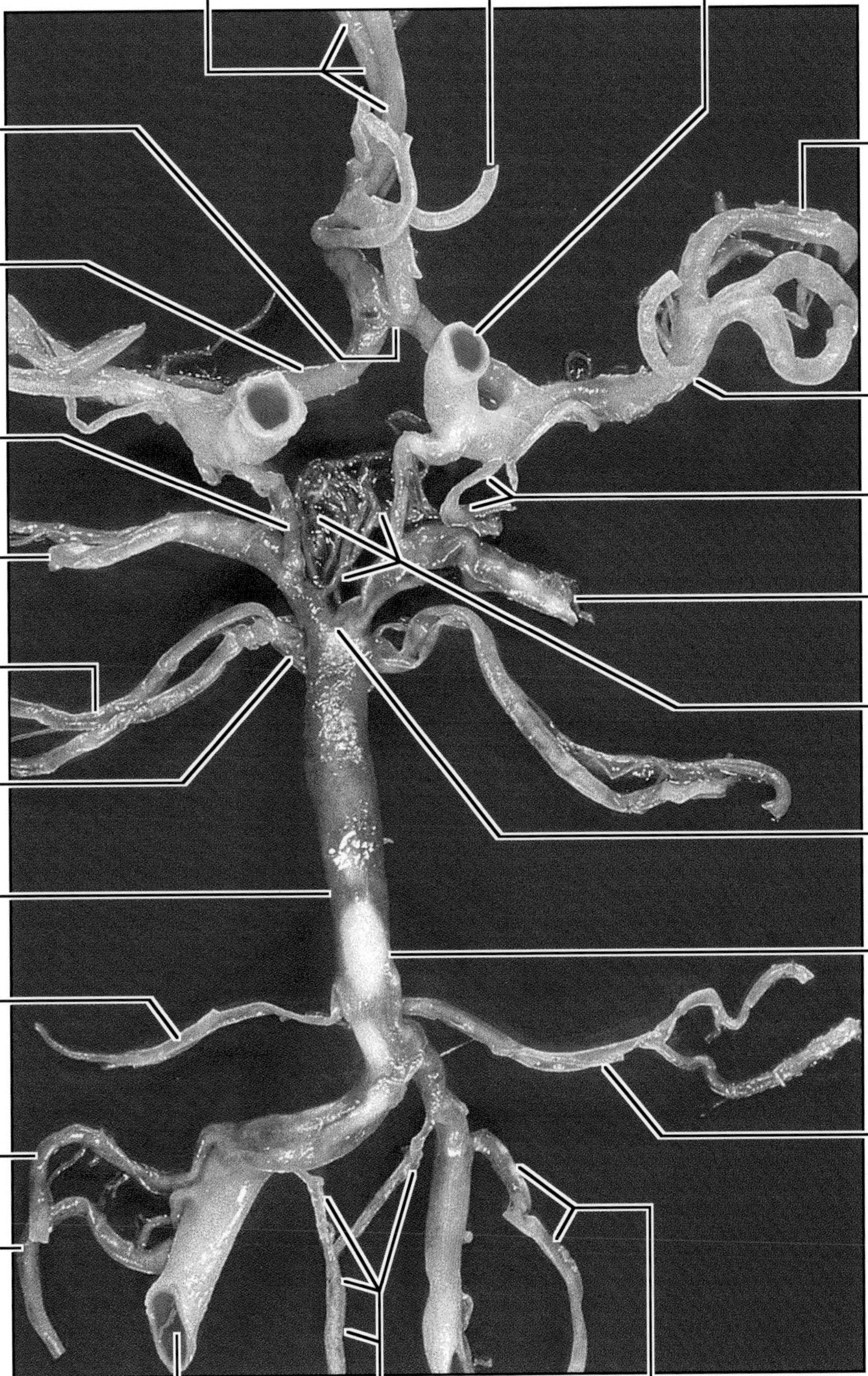

Anterior Cerebral Arteries, Pericallosal Branches

Anterior Cerebral Artery, Callosomarginal Branch

Internal Carotid Artery

Anterior Communicating Artery

Middle Cerebral Arteries, Sylvian Course

Anterior Cerebral Artery (proximal segment, dorsal to optic chiasm)

Trifurcation of Middle Cerebral Artery

Posterior Communicating Artery

Anterior Choroidal Artery

Posterior Cerebral Artery

Posterior Cerebral Artery

Superior Cerebellar Arteries (paired)

Thalamopeduncular Penetrating Arteries

Common Trunk of Paired Superior Cerebellar Arteries

Bifurcation of the Basilar Artery

Basilar Artery

Atherosclerotic Plaque

Anterior Inferior Cerebellar Artery

Anterior Inferior Cerebellar Artery

Posterior Inferior Cerebellar Arteries (paired, anatomic variant)

Vertebral Artery

Anterior Spinal Artery (note the confluence of vessels arising from each vertebral artery)

Posterior Inferior Cerebellar Artery

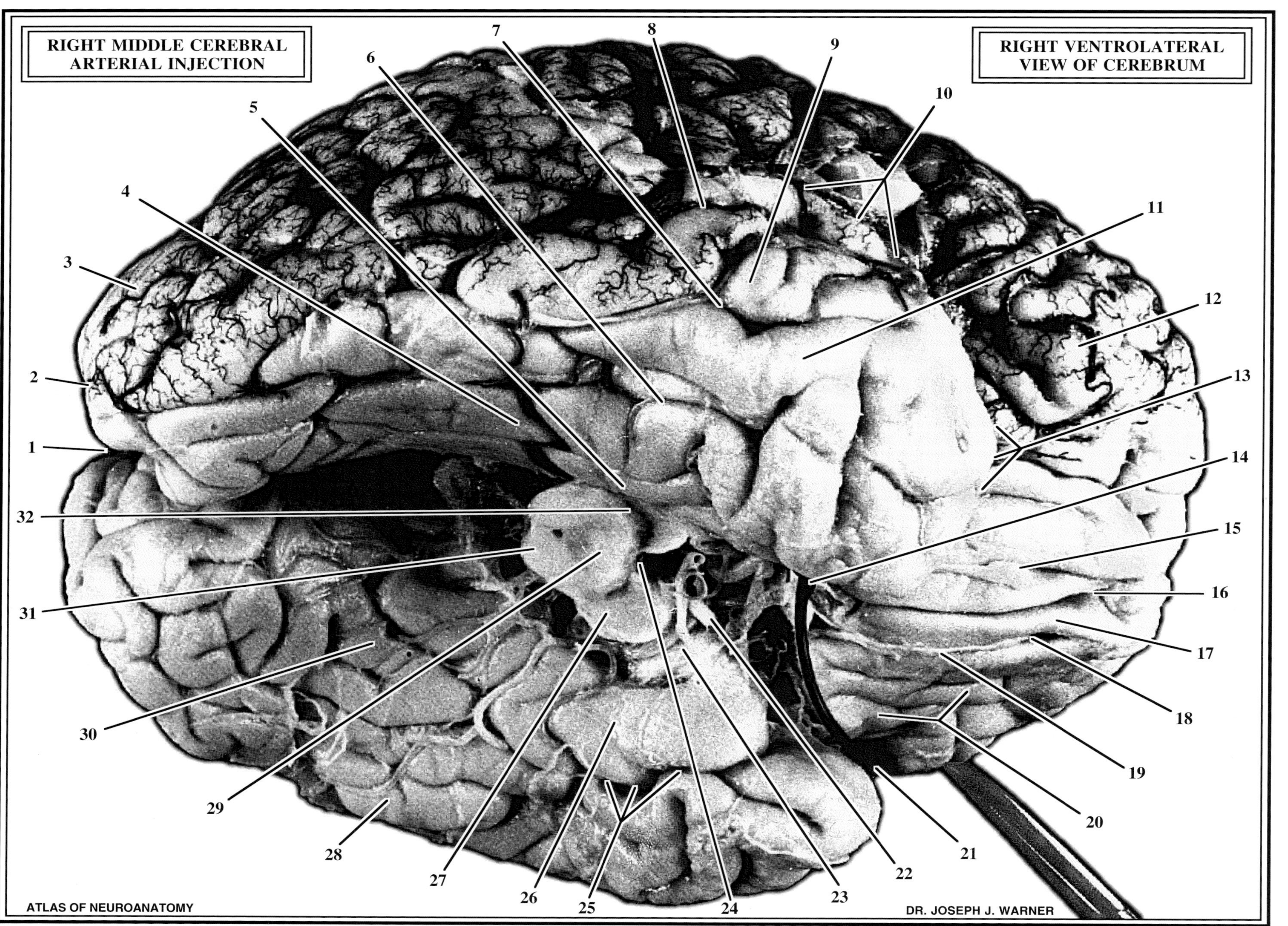
RIGHT MIDDLE CEREBRAL ARTERIAL INJECTION
RIGHT VENTROLATERAL VIEW OF CEREBRUM
1
2
3
4
5
6
7
8
9
10
11
12
13
14
15
16
17
18
19
20
21
22
23
24
25
26
27
28
29
30
31
32
ATLAS OF NEUROANATOMY
DR. JOSEPH J. WARNER

RIGHT MIDDLE CEREBRAL ARTERIAL INJECTION
RIGHT VENTROLATERAL VIEW OF CEREBRUM
KEY TO NUMBERED STRUCTURES AND MAP OF MAGNIFIED VIEW

1. Interhemispheric Fissure
2. Right Occipital Pole
3. Caudal extent of perfusion by MCA injection (this area is generally in the watershed between the posterior and middle cerebral arterial distributions)
4. Fusiform Gyrus
5. Parahippocampal Gyrus
6. Inferior Temporal Sulcus
7. Middle Temporal Sulcus
8. Superior Temporal Sulcus
9. Middle Temporal Gyrus
10. Superior Temporal Gyrus
11. Inferior Temporal Gyrus
12. Inferior Frontal Convolution
13. Rostral aspect of temporal lobe
14. Injection cannula near entry into right Middle Cerebral Artery
15. Olfactory Bulb
16. Interhemispheric Fissure
17. Gyrus Rectus
18. Olfactory Sulcus
19. Olfactory Tract
20. Orbitofrontal Gyri
21. Injection Cannula
22. Oculomotor Nerve
23. Uncus
24. Interpeduncular Fossa
25. Collateral Sulcus
26. Parahippocampal Gyrus
27. Cerebral Peduncle
28. Inferior Temporal Gyrus of the Left Hemisphere
29. Decussation of Superior Cerebellar Peduncle
30. Fusiform Gyrus (left)
31. Inferior Colliculus
32. Substantia Nigra

The injection of the right middle cerebral artery was accomplished through passage of a cannula through the supraclinoid segment of the right internal carotid artery. The cannula was advanced distal to the posterior communicating, anterior choroidal, and anterior cerebral arteries. The tip of the cannula was proximal to the origin of the individual divisions of the middle cerebral artery. To eliminate significant backfill and perfusion of proximal vessels with pressure injection, the terminal aspect of the carotid artery was ligated around the cannula, followed by ligation of the anterior cerebral and posterior communicating arteries. (With selective injection, flow through distal collaterals may result in limited perfusion beyond the normal territory of the middle cerebral artery under physiologic conditions.)

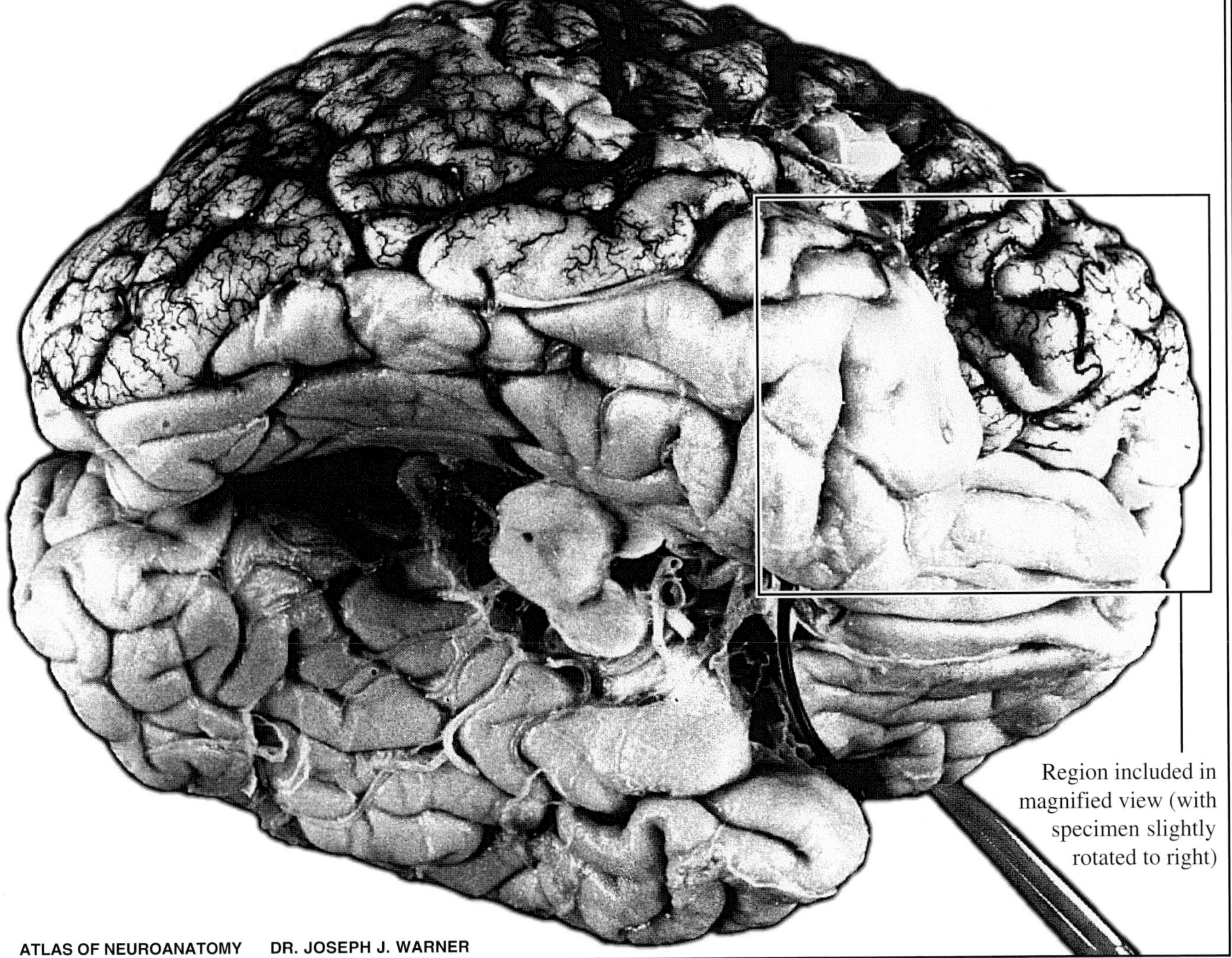

Region included in magnified view (with specimen slightly rotated to right)

RIGHT MIDDLE CEREBRAL ARTERY INJECTION: VENTROLATERAL ASPECT OF THE FRONTAL AND ANTERIOR TEMPORAL LOBES

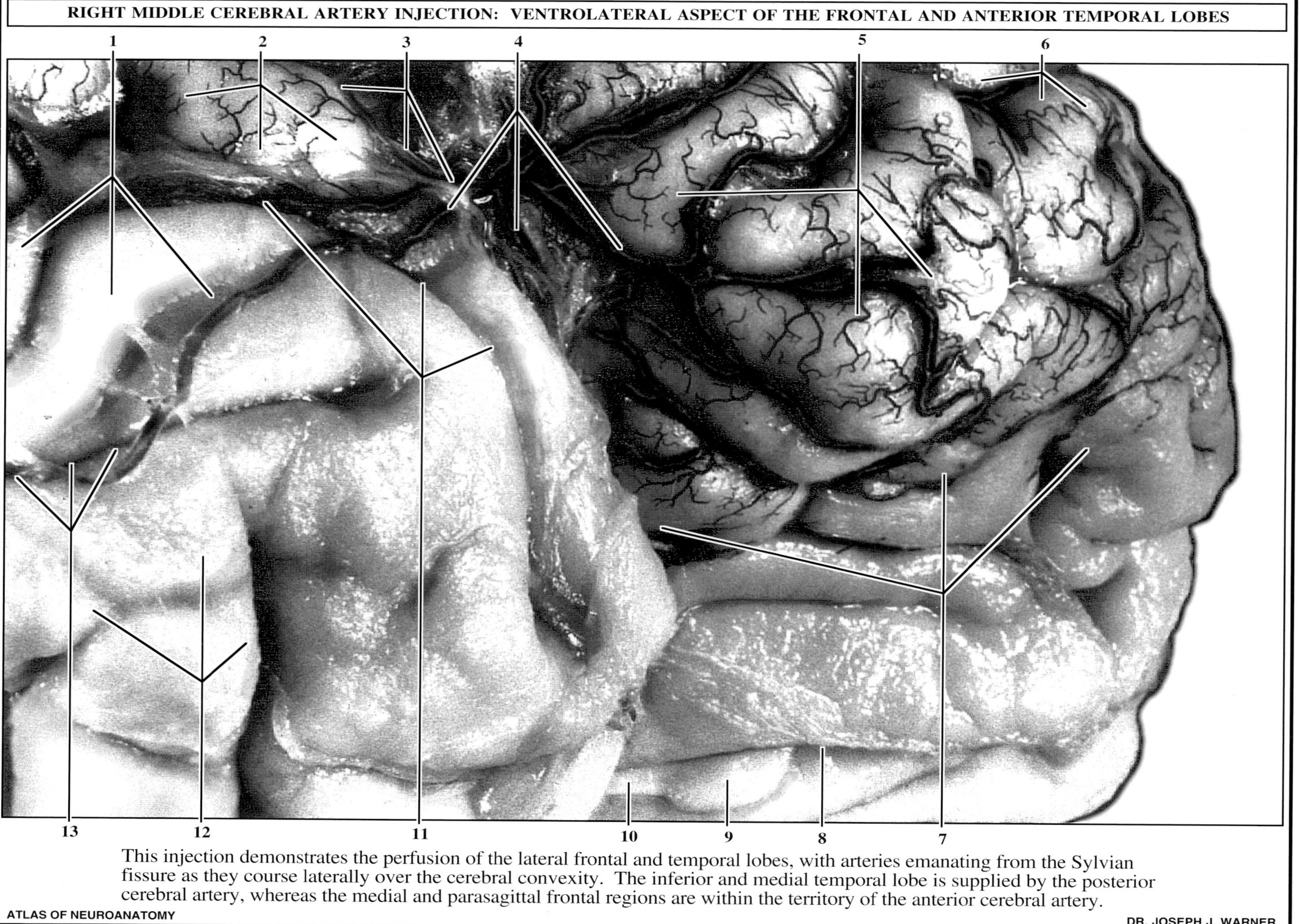

This injection demonstrates the perfusion of the lateral frontal and temporal lobes, with arteries emanating from the Sylvian fissure as they course laterally over the cerebral convexity. The inferior and medial temporal lobe is supplied by the posterior cerebral artery, whereas the medial and parasagittal frontal regions are within the territory of the anterior cerebral artery.

RIGHT MIDDLE CEREBRAL ARTERY INJECTION: MAGNIFIED VIEW OF THE VENTROLATERAL ASPECT OF THE FRONTAL AND TEMPORAL LOBES

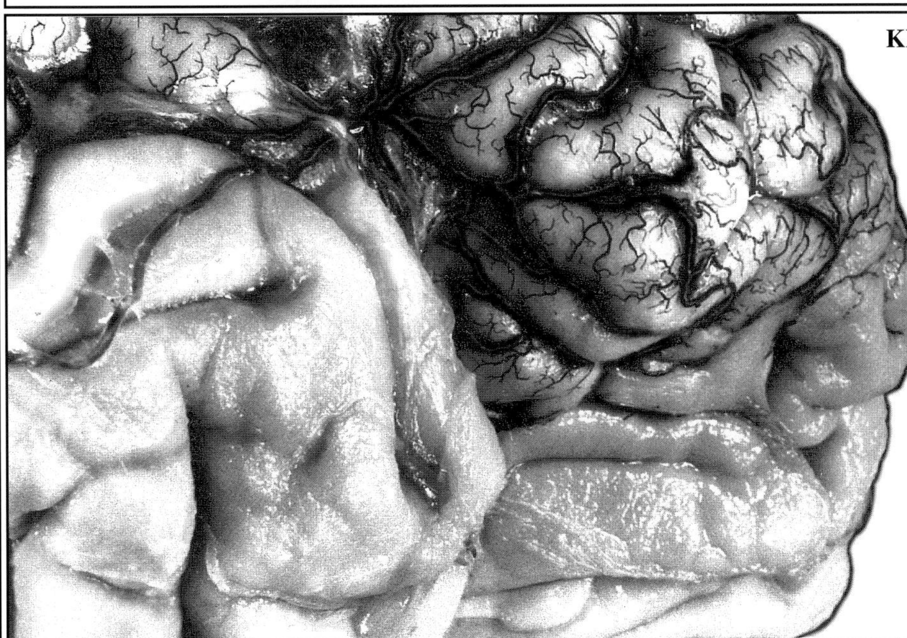

KEY TO NUMBERED STRUCTURES

1. Middle Temporal Gyrus
2. Superior Temporal Gyrus
3. Sylvian Fissure
4. Middle Cerebral Artery (branches emerging from the Sylvian Fissure)
5. Inferior Frontal Convolution
6. Middle Frontal Convolution
7. Orbitofrontal Gyri
8. Olfactory Sulcus
9. Olfactory Bulb
10. Olfactory Tract
11. Superior Temporal Sulcus
12. Inferior Temporal Gyrus
13. Inferior Temporal Sulcus

RIGHT MIDDLE CEREBRAL ARTERY INJECTION: MAGNIFIED VIEW OF THE LATERAL PARIETO-OCCIPITAL SURFACE

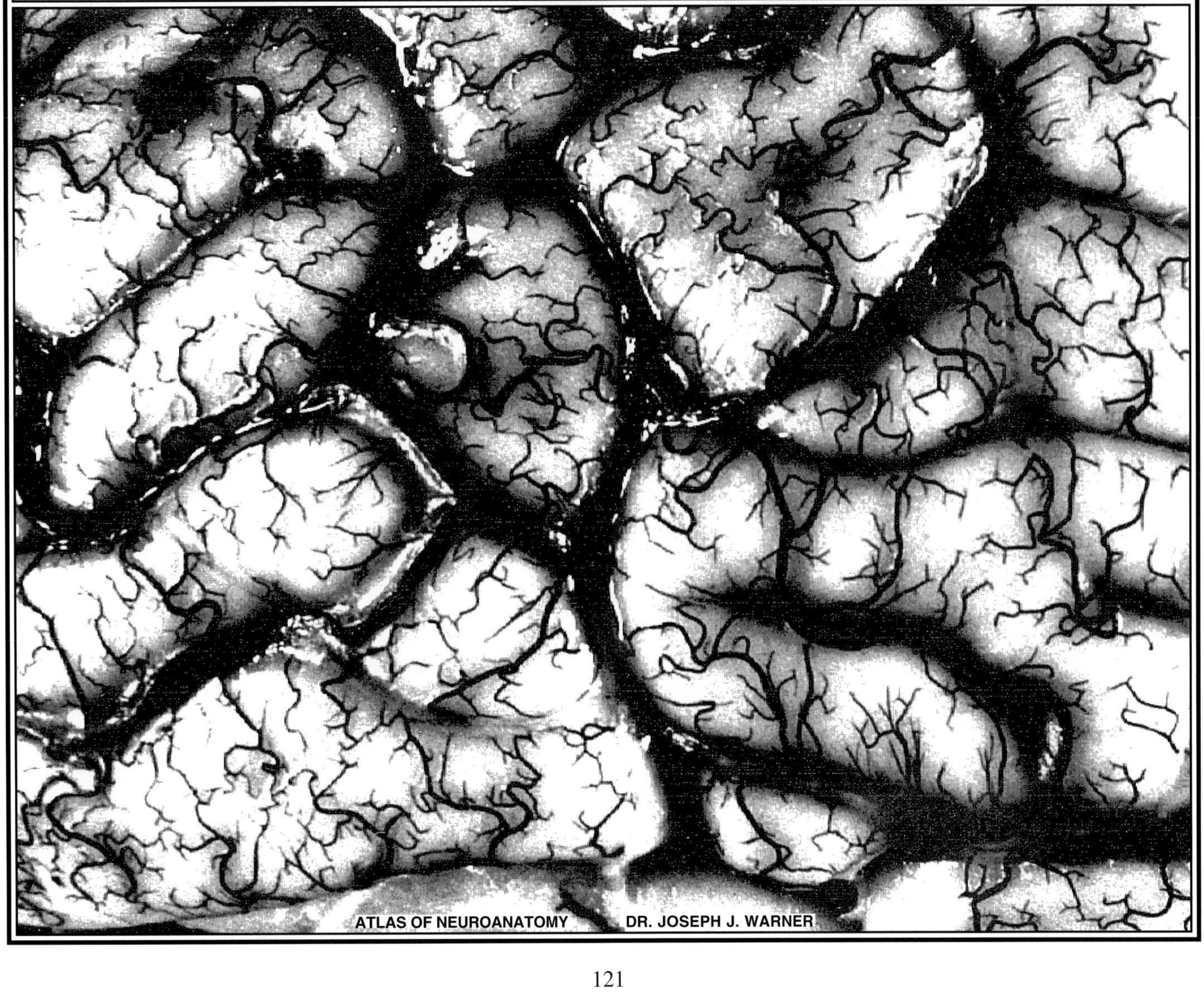

RIGHT MIDDLE CEREBRAL ARTERY INJECTION: LATERAL ASPECT OF THE PARIETO-OCCIPITAL REGION

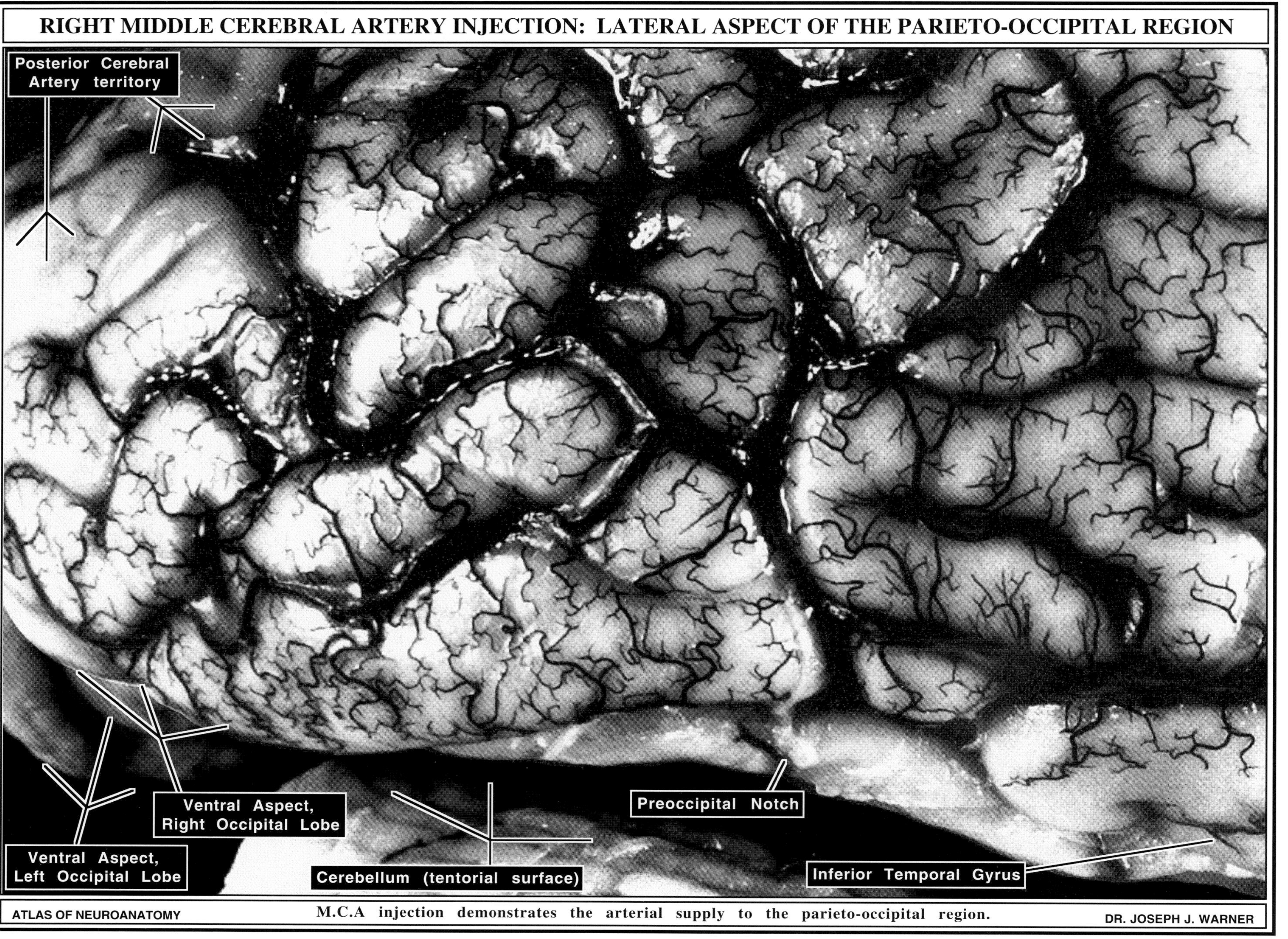

M.C.A injection demonstrates the arterial supply to the parieto-occipital region.

MIDLINE SAGITTAL SECTION OF THE BRAIN: ARACHNOID AND VASCULATURE INTACT

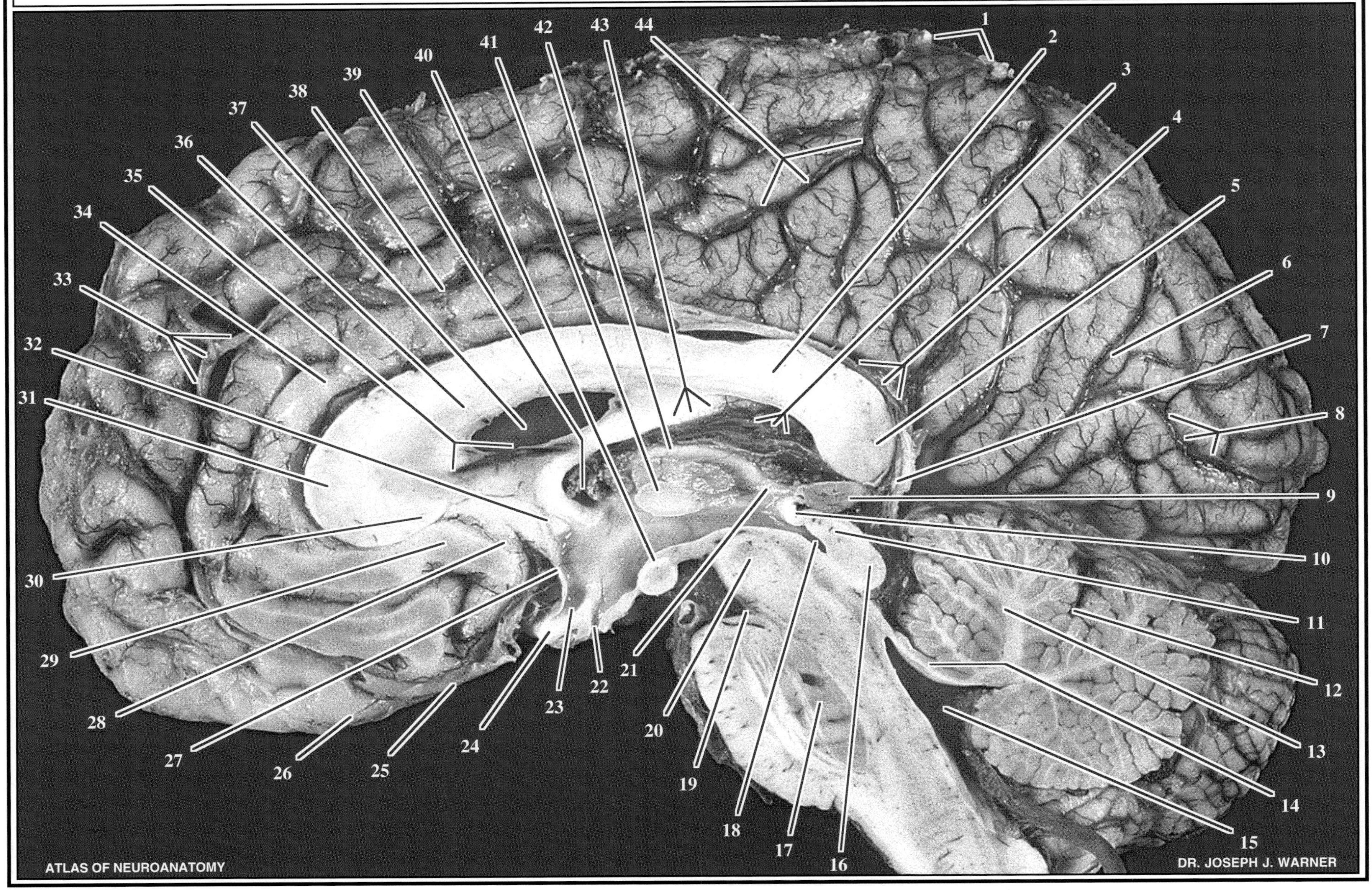

MIDLINE SAGITTAL SECTION OF THE BRAIN; ARACHNOID INTACT, DEMONSTRATING MEDIAL CORTICAL SURFACE VASCULATURE AND THE PARAMEDIAN VENOUS SYSTEM: KEY TO NUMBERED STRUCTURES

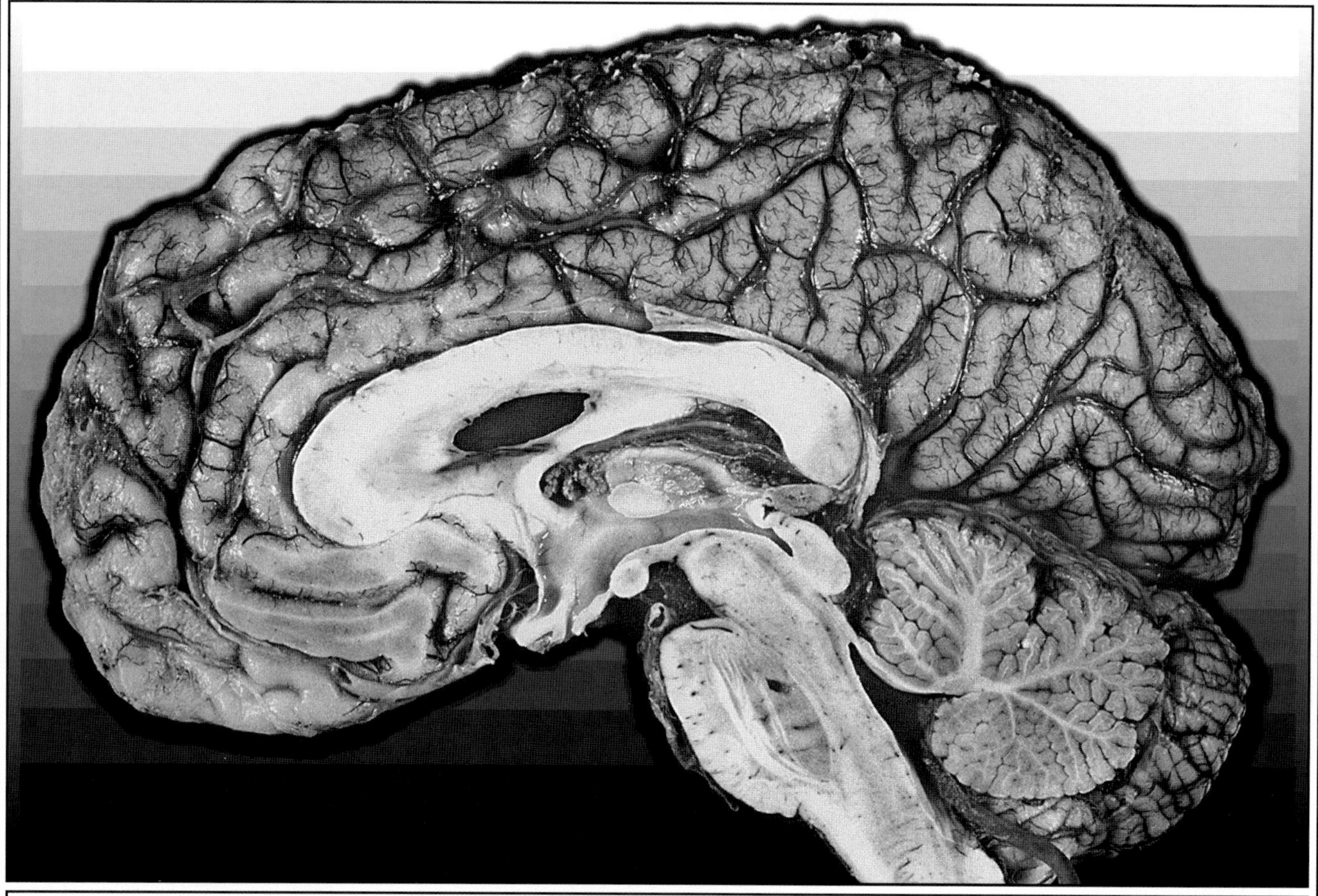

KEY TO NUMBERED STRUCTURES

1. Arachnoid Granulations
2. Body of the Corpus Callosum
3. Internal Cerebral Vein
4. Inferior Sagittal Sinus
5. Splenium of the Corpus Callosum
6. Parieto-Occipital Sulcus
7. Great Vein of Galen
8. Calcarine Fissure
9. Pineal Body
10. Posterior Commissure
11. Superior Colliculus
12. Primary Fissure of the Cerebellum
13. Superior Vermis of the Cerebellum
14. Superior Medullary Velum
15. Fourth Ventricle
16. Inferior Colliculus
17. Pontine Nuclei
18. Aqueduct of Sylvius
19. Interpeduncular Fossa
20. Red Nucleus
21. Habenula
22. Infundibular Recess of the Third Ventricle
23. Supraoptic Recess of the Third Ventricle
24. Optic Chiasm
25. Anterior Cerebral Artery
26. Gyrus Rectus
27. Lamina Terminalis
28. Paraterminal Gyrus
29. Subcallosal Gyrus
30. Rostrum of the Corpus Callosum
31. Genu of the Corpus Callosum
32. Anterior Commissure
33. Callosomarginal Branch, Anterior Cerebral Artery
34. Cingulate Gyrus
35. Septal Vein
36. Septum Pellucidum
37. Caudate Nucleus (lateral wall of the Lateral Ventricle)
38. Cingulate Sulcus
39. Foramen of Monro
40. Mammillary Body
41. Massa Intermedia
42. Stria Medullaris
43. Fornix
44. Pars Marginalis (extension of the Cingulate Sulcus)

INTRAOPERATIVE PHOTOGRAPH OF CEREBRAL CORTICAL VASCULATURE

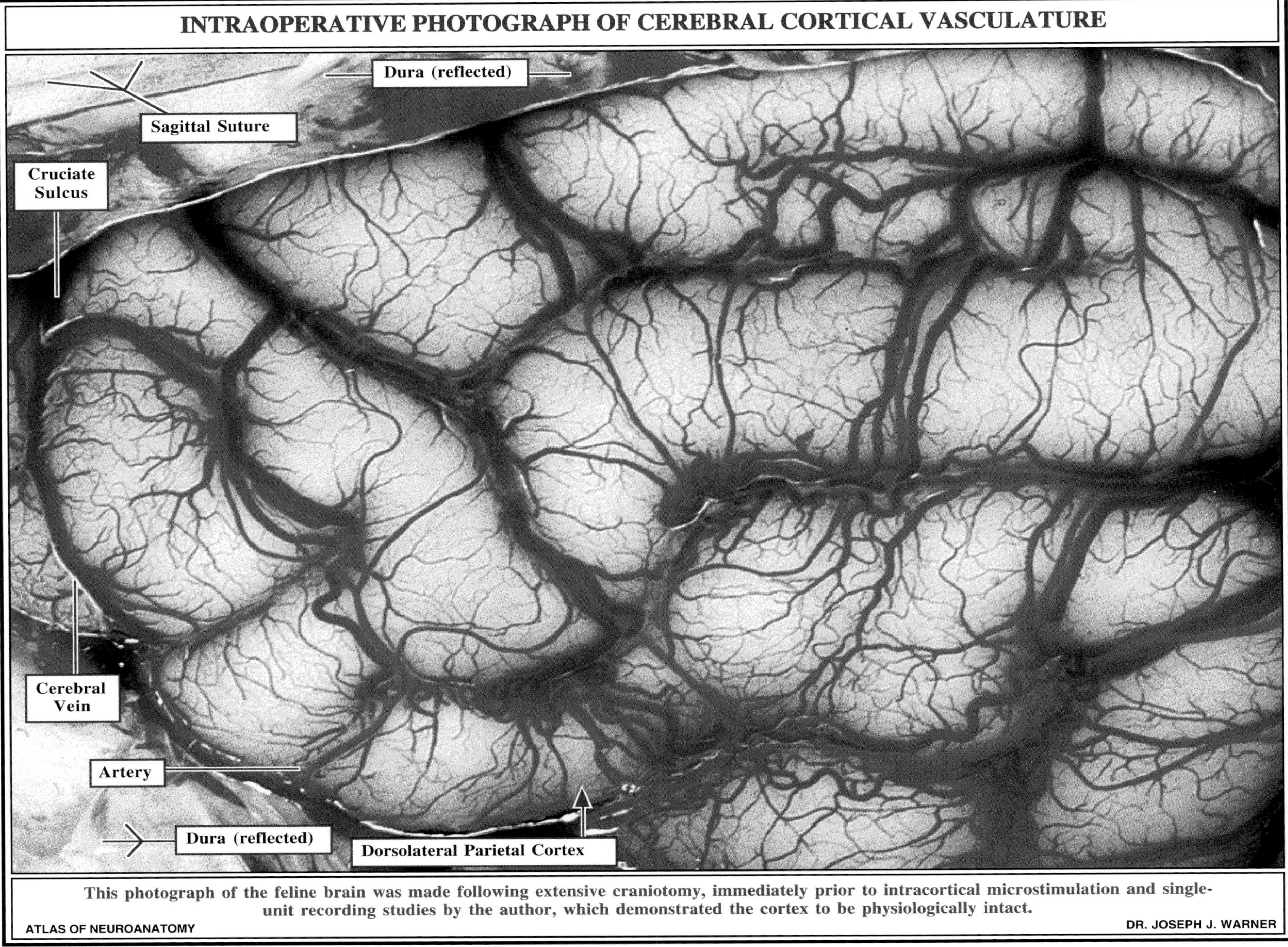

This photograph of the feline brain was made following extensive craniotomy, immediately prior to intracortical microstimulation and single-unit recording studies by the author, which demonstrated the cortex to be physiologically intact.

CAROTID ANGIOGRAM, LATERAL PROJECTION, ARTERIAL PHASE

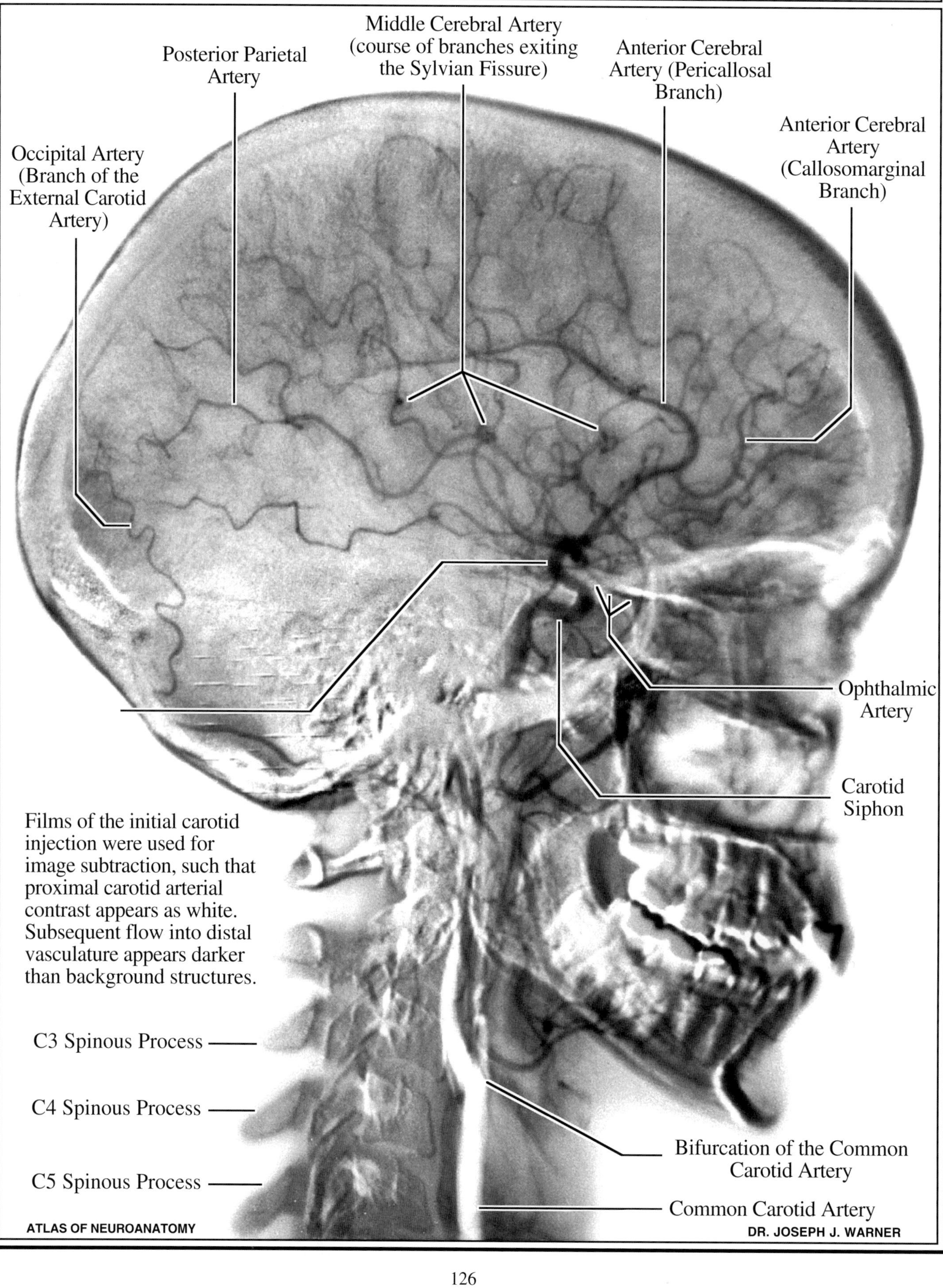

Middle Cerebral Artery (course of branches exiting the Sylvian Fissure)

Posterior Parietal Artery

Anterior Cerebral Artery (Pericallosal Branch)

Anterior Cerebral Artery (Callosomarginal Branch)

Occipital Artery (Branch of the External Carotid Artery)

Ophthalmic Artery

Carotid Siphon

Films of the initial carotid injection were used for image subtraction, such that proximal carotid arterial contrast appears as white. Subsequent flow into distal vasculature appears darker than background structures.

C3 Spinous Process

C4 Spinous Process

C5 Spinous Process

Bifurcation of the Common Carotid Artery

Common Carotid Artery

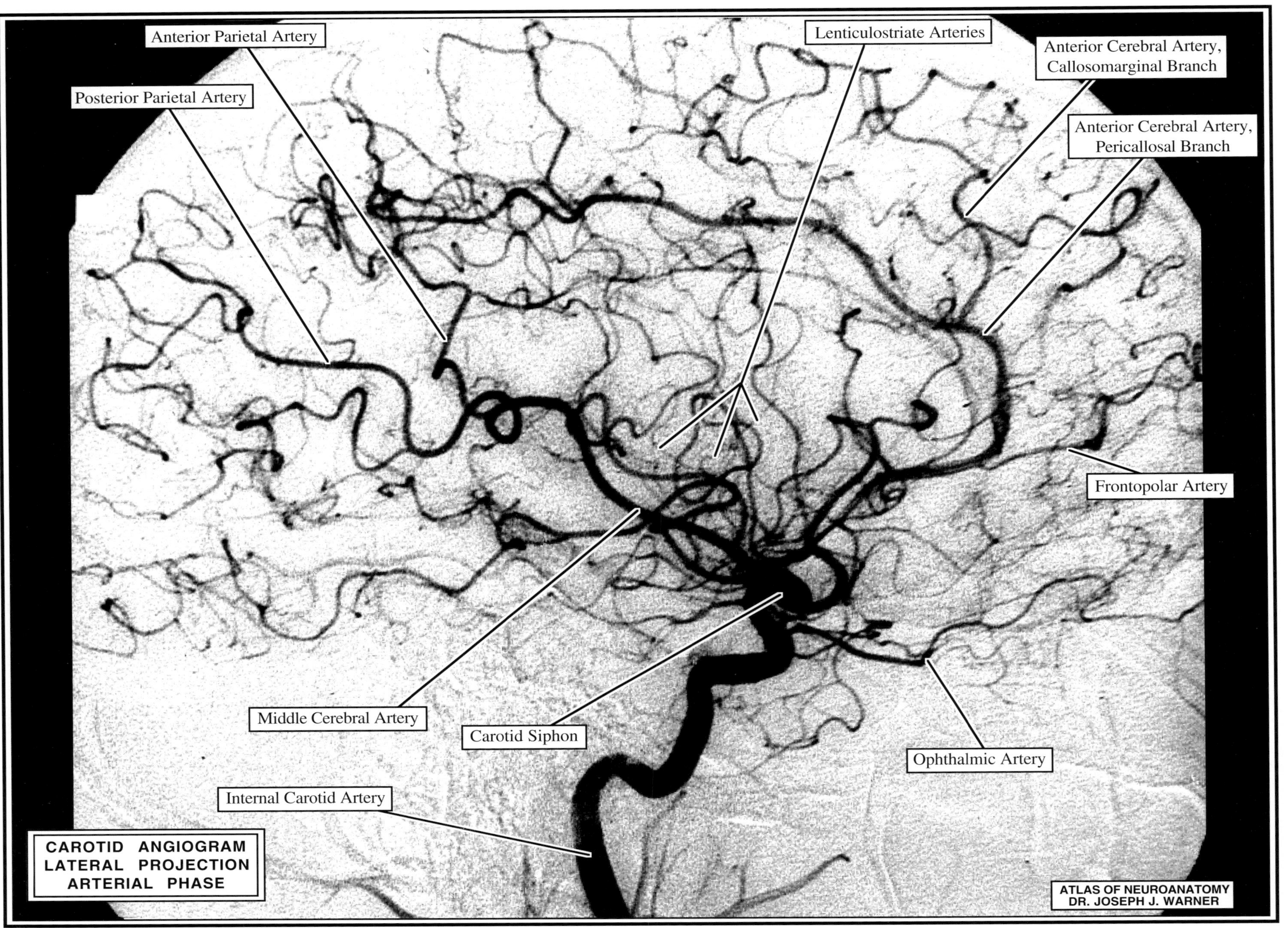
Anterior Parietal Artery
Posterior Parietal Artery
Lenticulostriate Arteries
Anterior Cerebral Artery, Callosomarginal Branch
Anterior Cerebral Artery, Pericallosal Branch
Frontopolar Artery
Middle Cerebral Artery
Carotid Siphon
Ophthalmic Artery
Internal Carotid Artery
CAROTID ANGIOGRAM
LATERAL PROJECTION
ARTERIAL PHASE
ATLAS OF NEUROANATOMY
DR. JOSEPH J. WARNER

RIGHT CAROTID ANGIOGRAM, ARTERIAL PHASE, TOWNE PROJECTION; DEMONSTRATING FLOW INTO THE CONTRALATERAL ANTERIOR AND MIDDLE CEREBRAL ARTERIES VIA THE ANTERIOR COMMUNICATING ARTERY

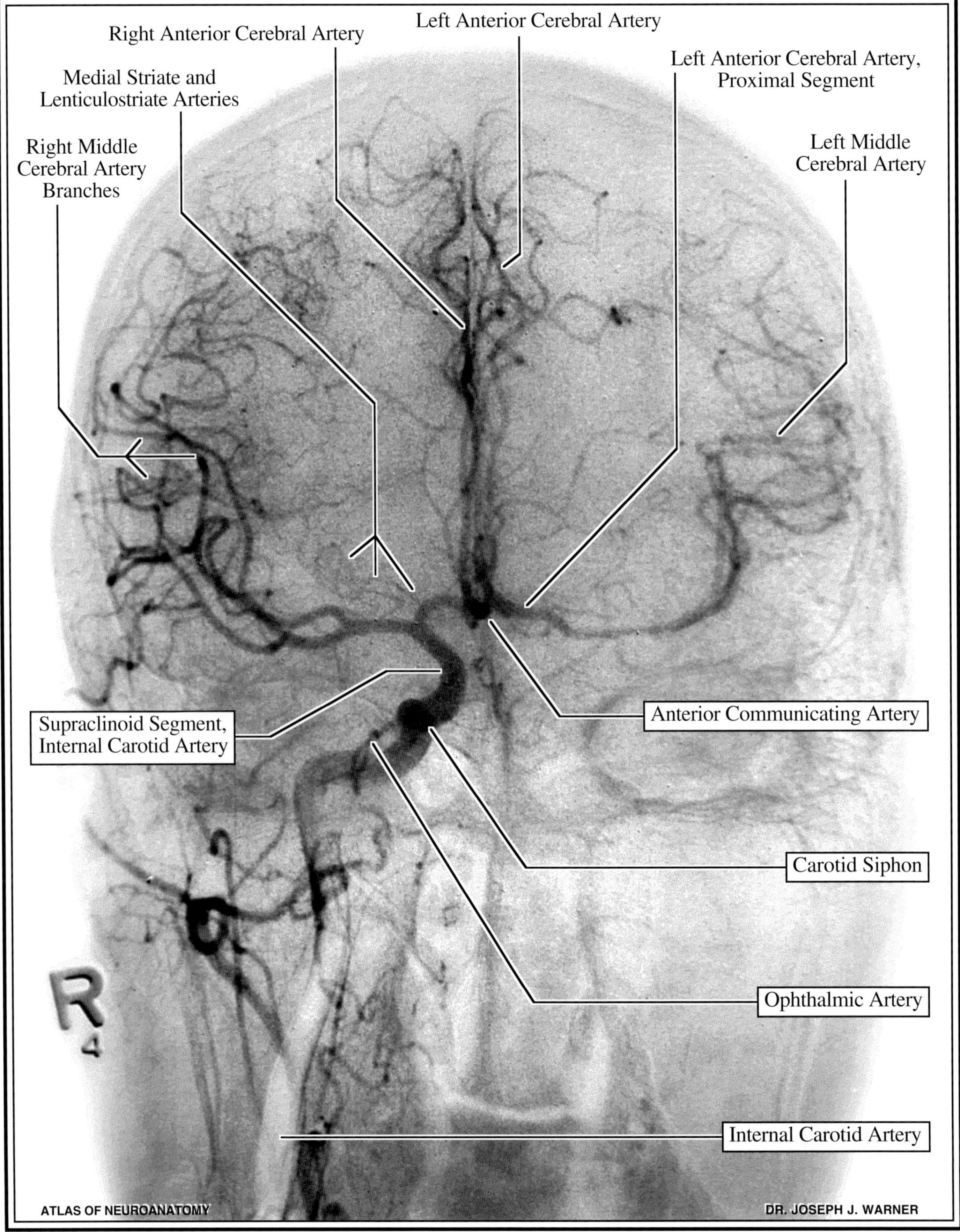

RIGHT AND LEFT CAROTID ARTERIOGRAMS IN A PATIENT WITH BILATERAL PERSISTENCE OF THE FETAL ORIGIN OF THE POSTERIOR CEREBRAL ARTERIES: LATERAL PROJECTION

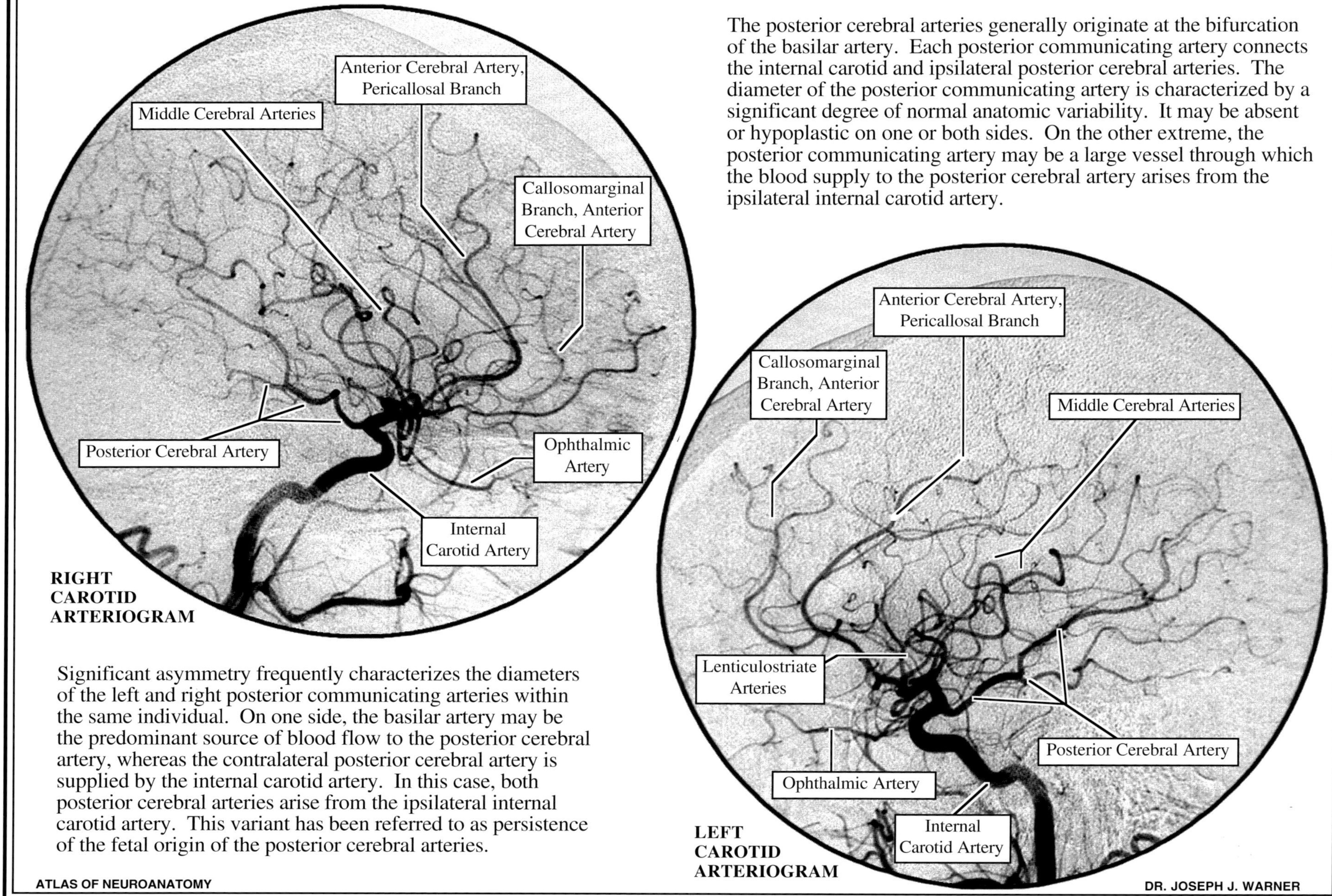

The posterior cerebral arteries generally originate at the bifurcation of the basilar artery. Each posterior communicating artery connects the internal carotid and ipsilateral posterior cerebral arteries. The diameter of the posterior communicating artery is characterized by a significant degree of normal anatomic variability. It may be absent or hypoplastic on one or both sides. On the other extreme, the posterior communicating artery may be a large vessel through which the blood supply to the posterior cerebral artery arises from the ipsilateral internal carotid artery.

Significant asymmetry frequently characterizes the diameters of the left and right posterior communicating arteries within the same individual. On one side, the basilar artery may be the predominant source of blood flow to the posterior cerebral artery, whereas the contralateral posterior cerebral artery is supplied by the internal carotid artery. In this case, both posterior cerebral arteries arise from the ipsilateral internal carotid artery. This variant has been referred to as persistence of the fetal origin of the posterior cerebral arteries.

RIGHT AND LEFT CAROTID ARTERIOGRAMS IN A PATIENT WITH BILATERAL PERSISTENCE OF THE FETAL ORIGIN OF THE POSTERIOR CEREBRAL ARTERIES: TOWNE VARIANT OF THE A-P PROJECTION

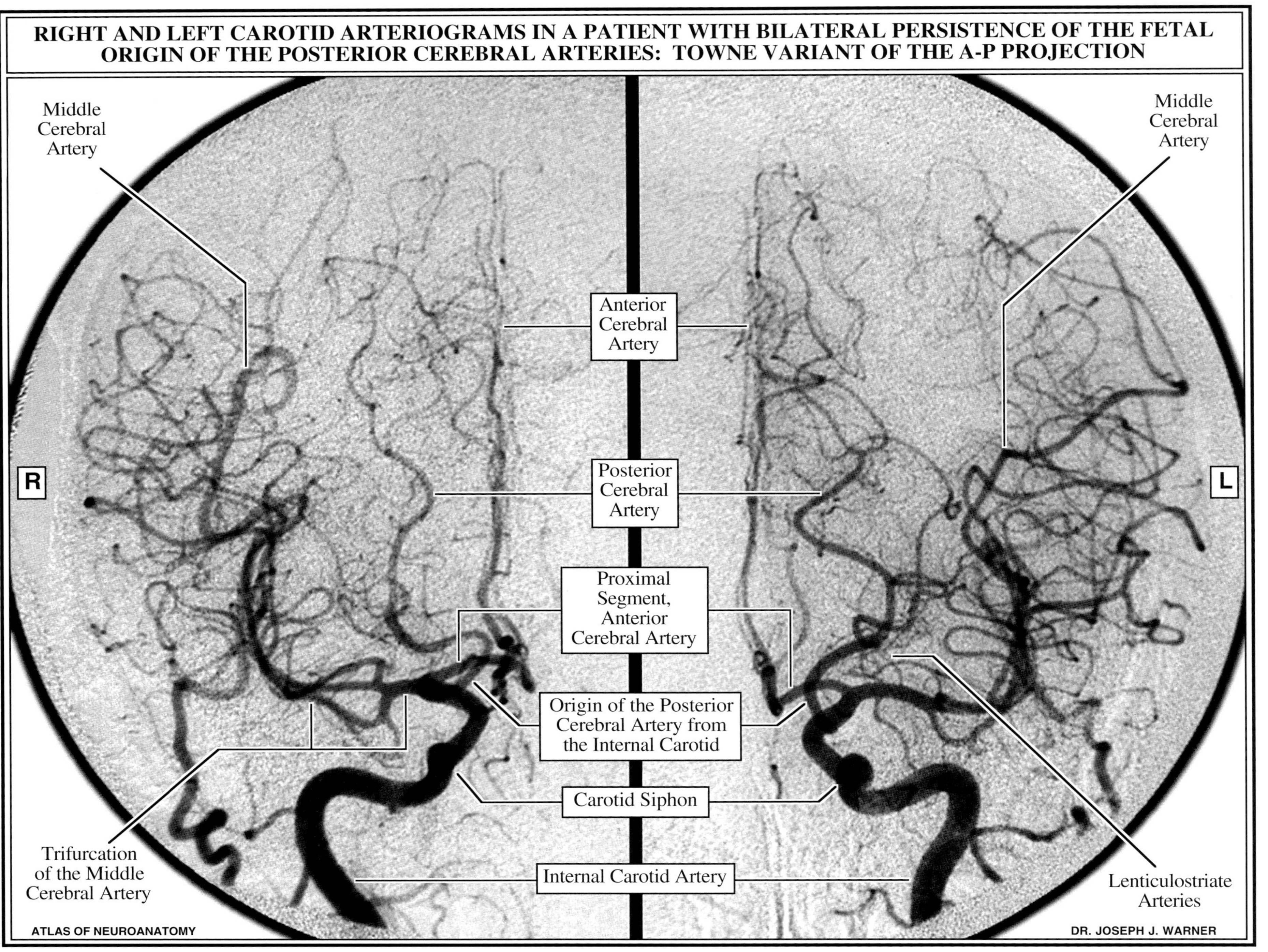

VERTEBRAL ANGIOGRAM, LATERAL PROJECTION, ARTERIAL PHASE

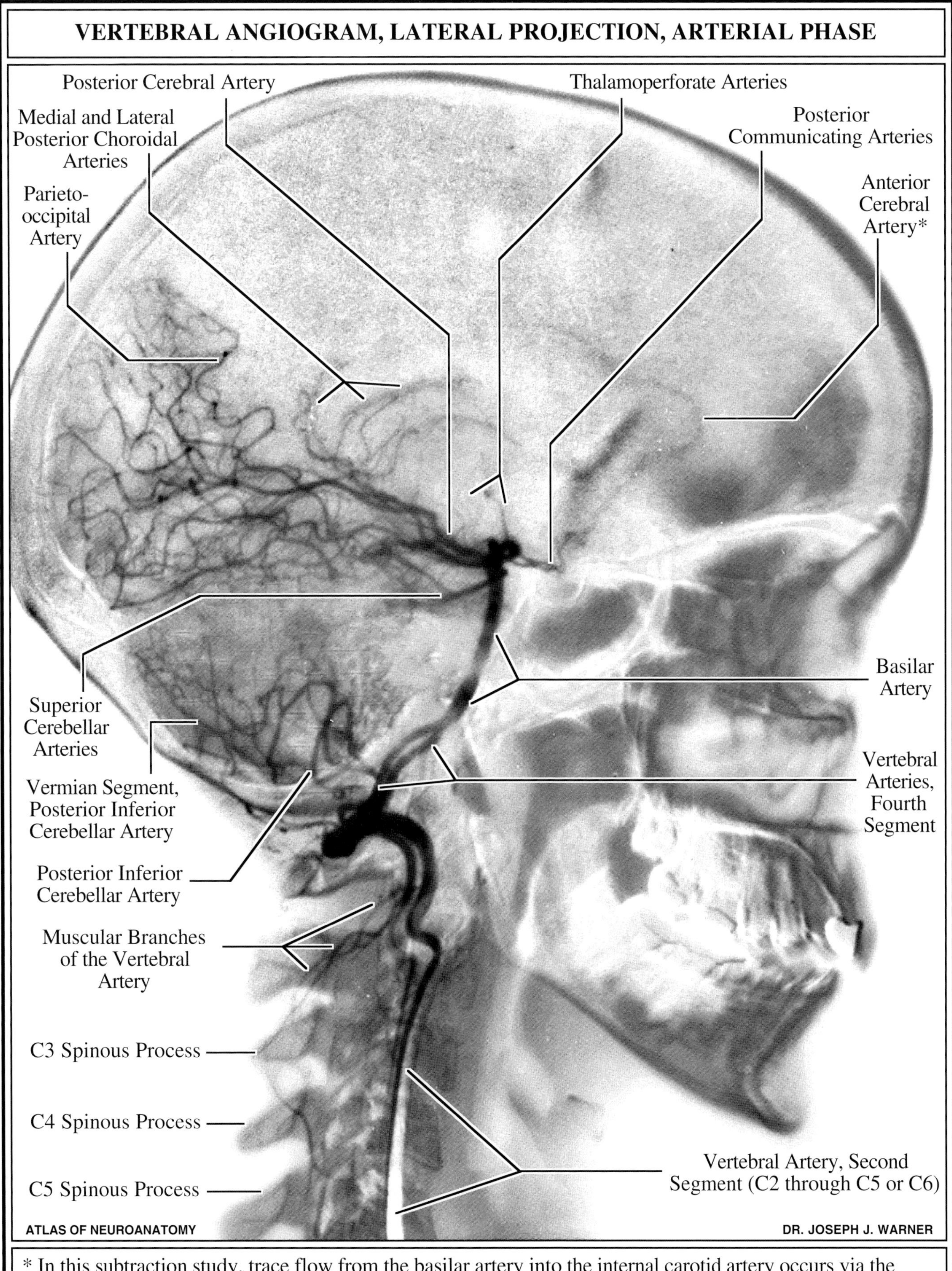

DR. JOSEPH J. WARNER

* In this subtraction study, trace flow from the basilar artery into the internal carotid artery occurs via the posterior communicating arteries. Anterograde contrast flow is thus discernible in the anterior cerebral artery.

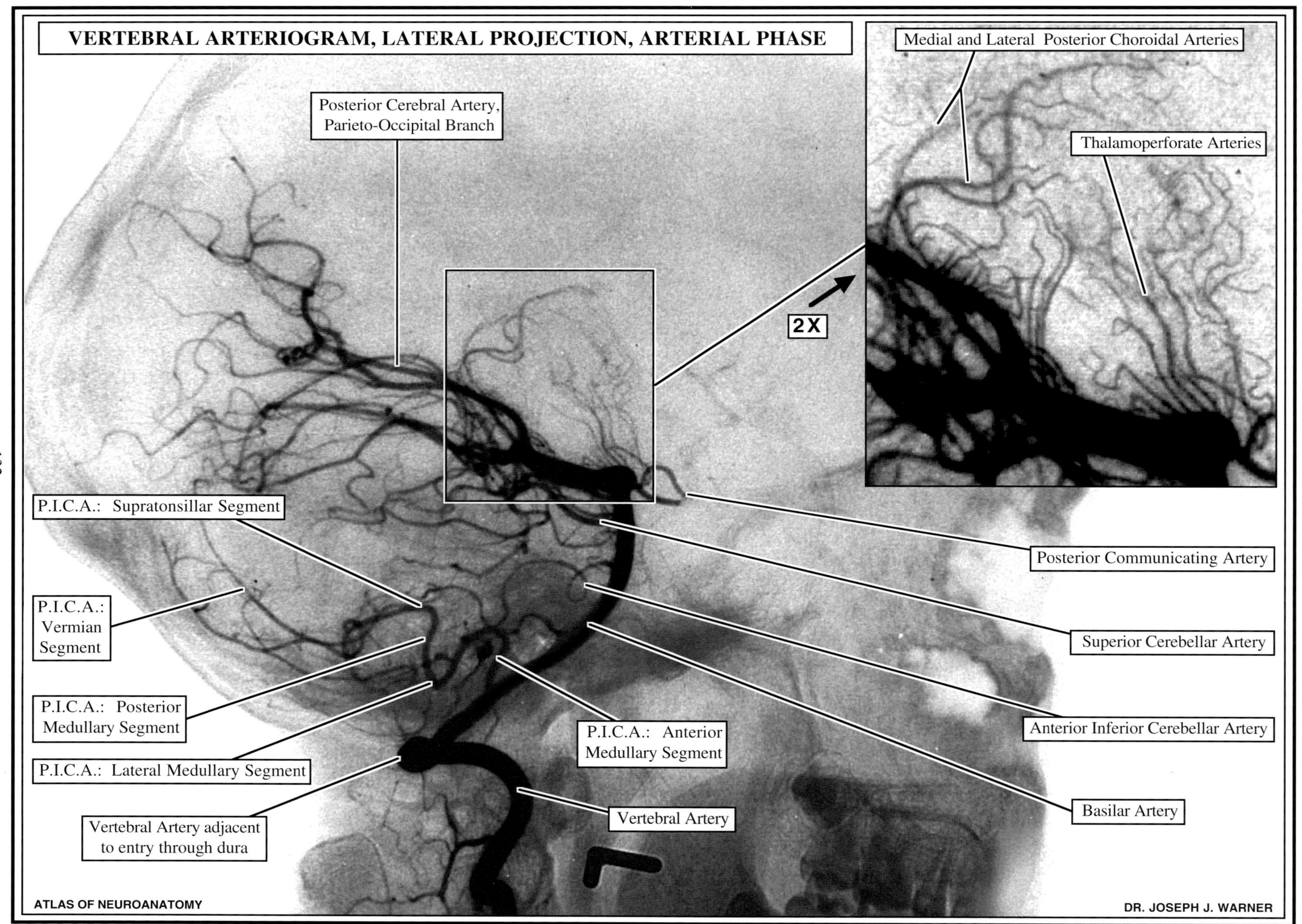
VERTEBRAL ARTERIOGRAM, LATERAL PROJECTION, ARTERIAL PHASE
Posterior Cerebral Artery, Parieto-Occipital Branch
Medial and Lateral Posterior Choroidal Arteries
Thalamoperforate Arteries
2X
P.I.C.A.: Supratonsillar Segment
P.I.C.A.: Vermian Segment
P.I.C.A.: Posterior Medullary Segment
P.I.C.A.: Lateral Medullary Segment
Vertebral Artery adjacent to entry through dura
P.I.C.A.: Anterior Medullary Segment
Vertebral Artery
Posterior Communicating Artery
Superior Cerebellar Artery
Anterior Inferior Cerebellar Artery
Basilar Artery
ATLAS OF NEUROANATOMY
DR. JOSEPH J. WARNER

VERTEBRAL ANGIOGRAM (TOWNE VARIATION OF THE ANTEROPOSTERIOR PROJECTION, ARTERIAL PHASE): DURING RIGHT VERTEBRAL INJECTION, RETROGRADE FLOW TOWARD THE FIRST SEGMENT OF THE LEFT VERTEBRAL ARTERY DEMONSTRATES THE VERTEBROBASILAR SYSTEM BILATERALLY

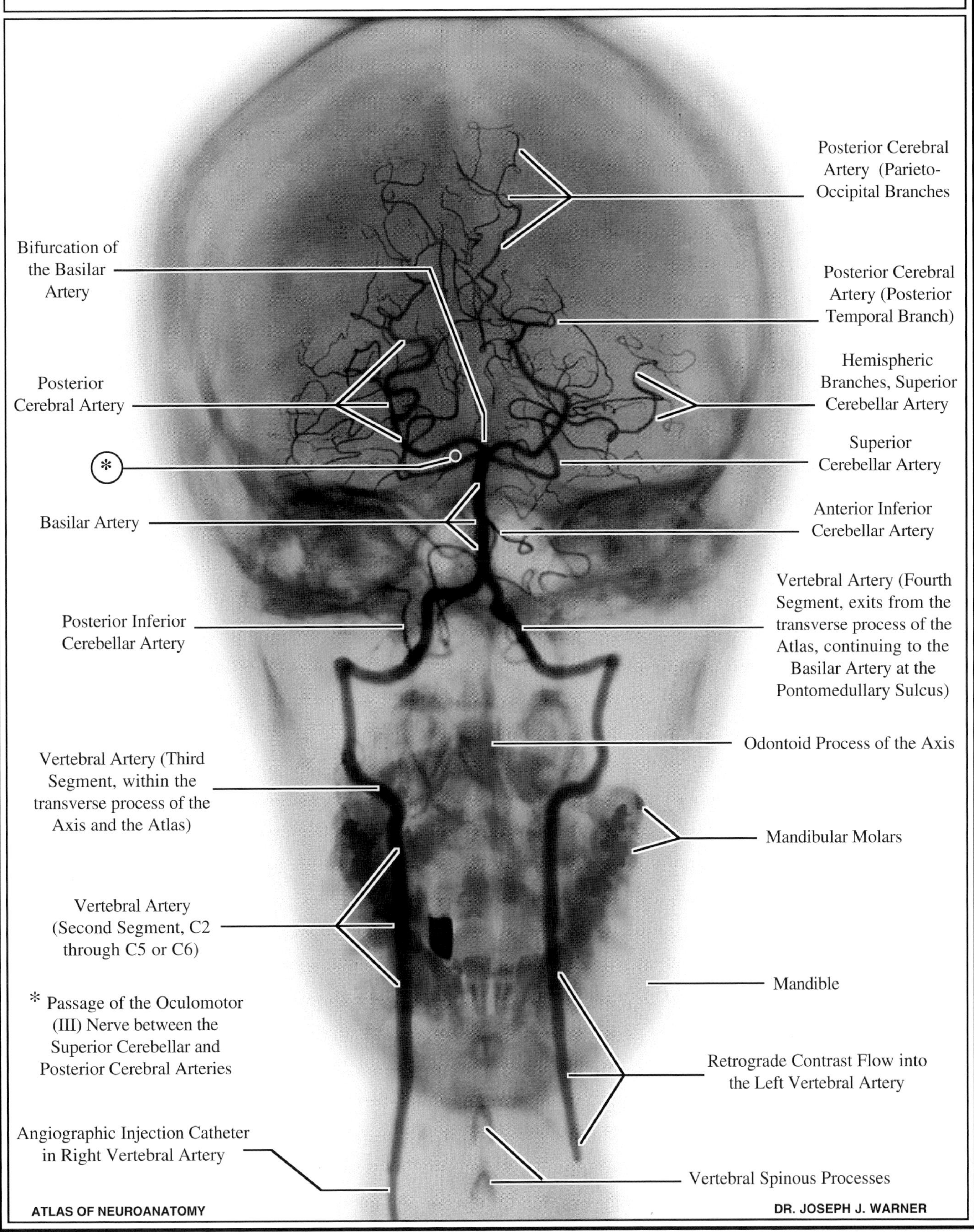

SELECTIVE VERTEBRAL ARTERIOGRAM, OBLIQUE PROJECTION DEMONSTRATING THE CERVICOCRANIAL COURSE OF THE VERTEBRAL AND BASILAR ARTERIES

The vertebral artery originates from the subclavian artery, which on the left arises from the aortic arch distal to the left common carotid artery. On the right, the brachiocephalic artery arises from the aorta and subsequently bifurcates into the right common carotid artery and the right subclavian artery. The right vertebral artery originates from the subclavian artery distal to this bifurcation. Both vertebral arteries course rostrally from the thorax through the cervical region. At the level of the sixth cervical vertebra, each vertebral artery passes through the transverse foramen. As the vertebral arteries course rostrally, they pass through the transverse foramina of the cervical vertebrae through the level of C3. At the level of C2, each vertebral artery courses laterally, then turns rostrally to pass through the atlas (C1). Each artery subsequently curves medially, then rostrally to enter the foramen magnum.

KEY TO LABELED STRUCTURES ON ARTERIOGRAM AND DIAGRAM OF THE CEREBROVASCULATURE

R
B
P
Internal Carotid Artery
C3
C6
Common Carotid Artery
Vertebral Arteries
Subclavian Artery
Brachiocephalic Artery
Ascending Aorta

A. Contrast within arterial catheter

B. Basilar Artery

C. Transverse Foramen of the Sixth Cervical Vertebra

F. Vertebral Artery passing through the Transverse Foramina from C6 rostrally

I. Intervertebral disc space (T1-T2)

P. Posterior Inferior Cerebellar Artery

R. Basilar bifurcation to Posterior Cerebral Artery

T. Thoracic Vertebral Bodies (T2-T4)

V. Contrast reflux into the contralateral Vertebral Artery

Cervical and thoracic vertebrae are labeled adjacent to the course of the vertebral artery and arterial catheter.

ATLAS OF NEUROANATOMY

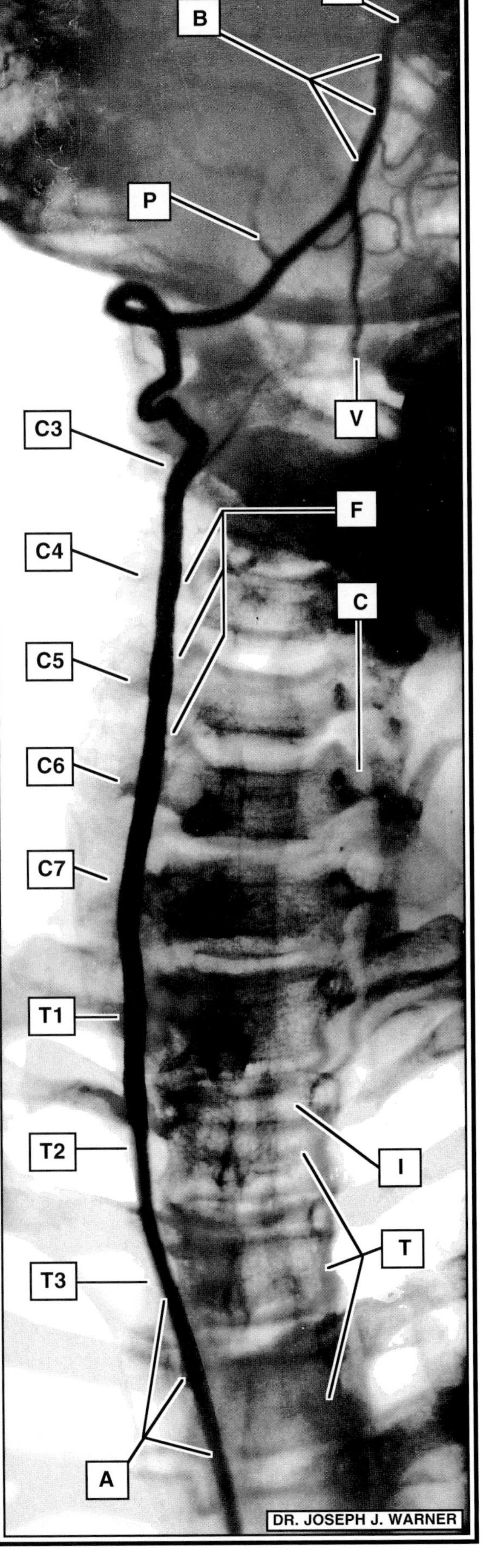

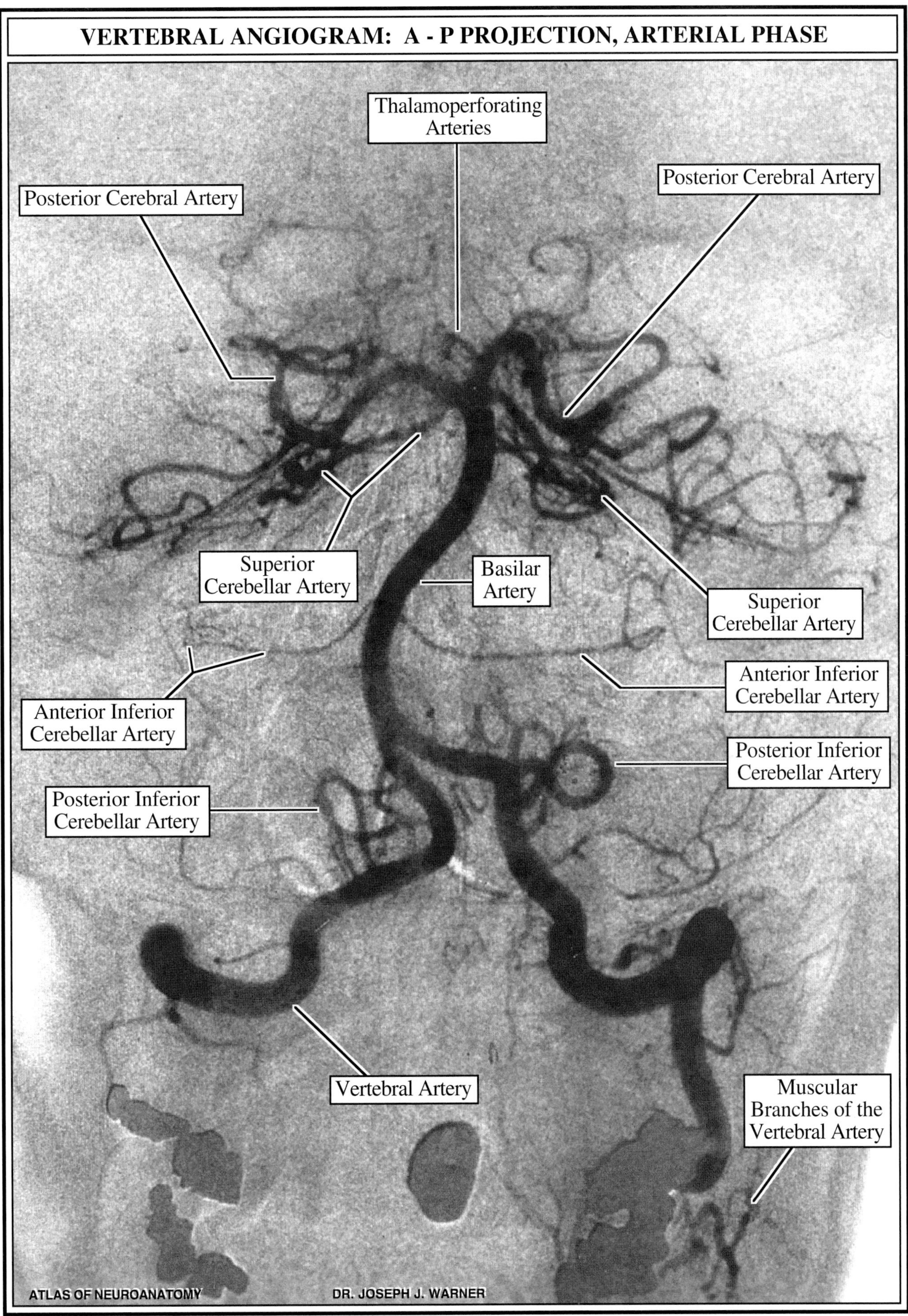
VERTEBRAL ANGIOGRAM: A - P PROJECTION, ARTERIAL PHASE
Thalamoperforating Arteries
Posterior Cerebral Artery
Posterior Cerebral Artery
Superior Cerebellar Artery
Basilar Artery
Superior Cerebellar Artery
Anterior Inferior Cerebellar Artery
Anterior Inferior Cerebellar Artery
Posterior Inferior Cerebellar Artery
Posterior Inferior Cerebellar Artery
Vertebral Artery
Muscular Branches of the Vertebral Artery
ATLAS OF NEUROANATOMY
DR. JOSEPH J. WARNER

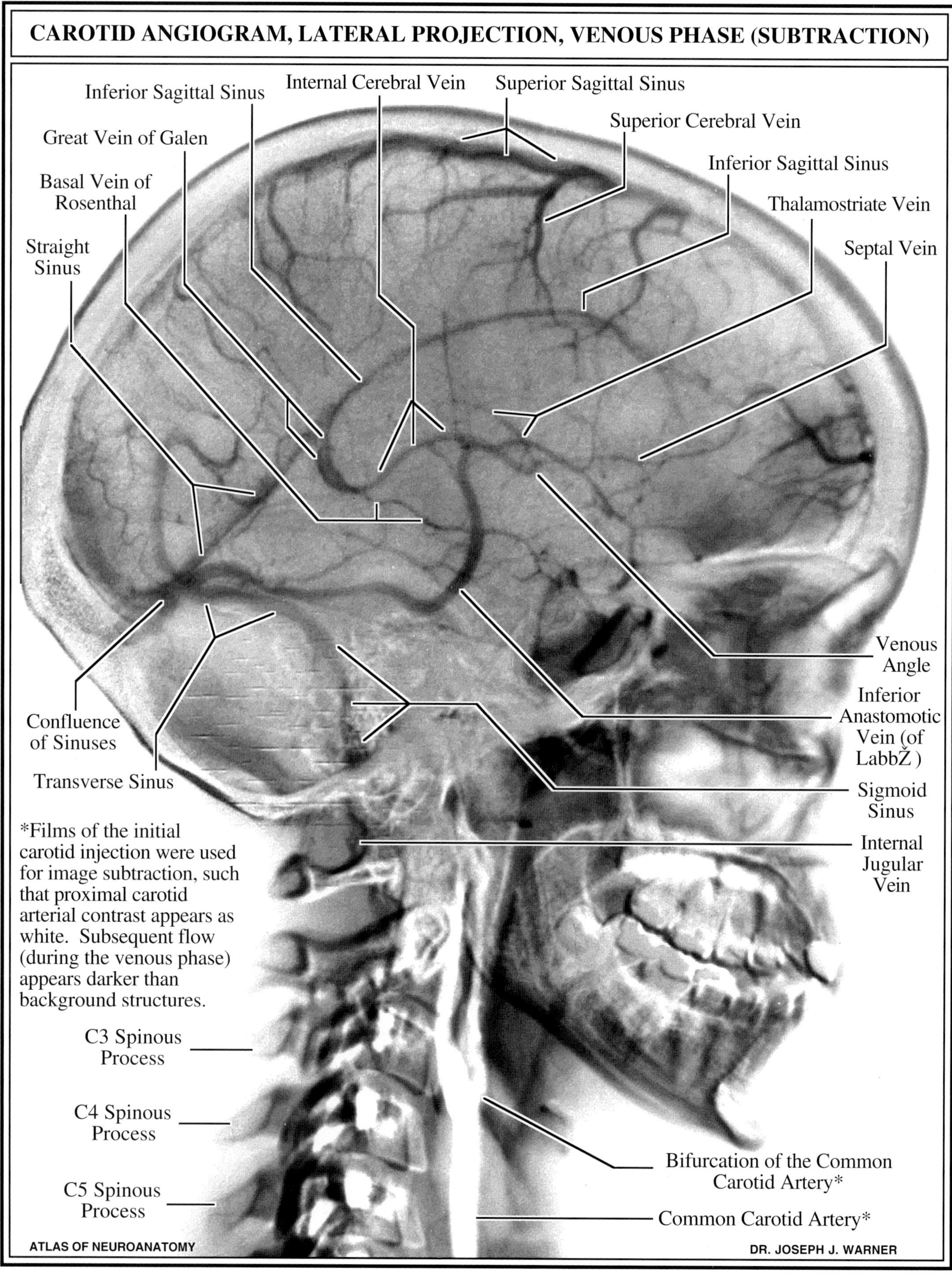
CAROTID ANGIOGRAM, LATERAL PROJECTION, VENOUS PHASE (SUBTRACTION)
Inferior Sagittal Sinus
Internal Cerebral Vein
Superior Sagittal Sinus
Superior Cerebral Vein
Great Vein of Galen
Inferior Sagittal Sinus
Basal Vein of Rosenthal
Thalamostriate Vein
Straight Sinus
Septal Vein
Venous Angle
Inferior Anastomotic Vein (of LabbŽ)
Confluence of Sinuses
Sigmoid Sinus
Transverse Sinus
Internal Jugular Vein
*Films of the initial carotid injection were used for image subtraction, such that proximal carotid arterial contrast appears as white. Subsequent flow (during the venous phase) appears darker than background structures.
C3 Spinous Process
C4 Spinous Process
C5 Spinous Process
Bifurcation of the Common Carotid Artery*
Common Carotid Artery*
ATLAS OF NEUROANATOMY
DR. JOSEPH J. WARNER

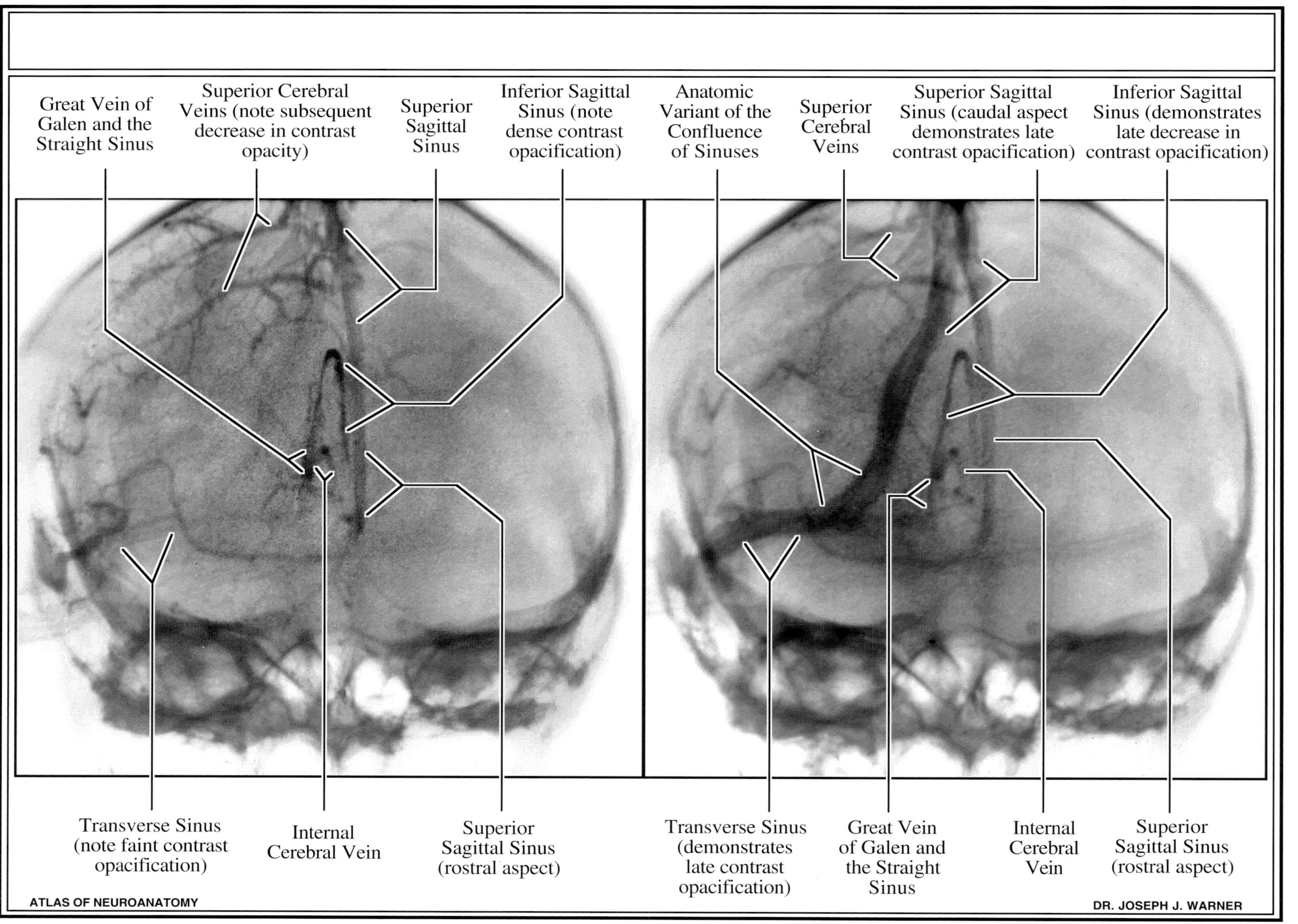
Great Vein of Galen and the Straight Sinus
Superior Cerebral Veins (note subsequent decrease in contrast opacity)
Superior Sagittal Sinus
Inferior Sagittal Sinus (note dense contrast opacification)
Anatomic Variant of the Confluence of Sinuses
Superior Cerebral Veins
Superior Sagittal Sinus (caudal aspect demonstrates late contrast opacification)
Inferior Sagittal Sinus (demonstrates late decrease in contrast opacification)
Transverse Sinus (note faint contrast opacification)
Internal Cerebral Vein
Superior Sagittal Sinus (rostral aspect)
Transverse Sinus (demonstrates late contrast opacification)
Great Vein of Galen and the Straight Sinus
Internal Cerebral Vein
Superior Sagittal Sinus (rostral aspect)

RIGHT AND LEFT CAROTID ANGIOGRAPHY IN A PATIENT WITH BILATERAL PERSISTENCE OF THE FETAL ORIGIN OF THE POSTERIOR CEREBRAL ARTERIES: VENOUS PHASES, TOWNE VARIANT OF A-P PROJECTION

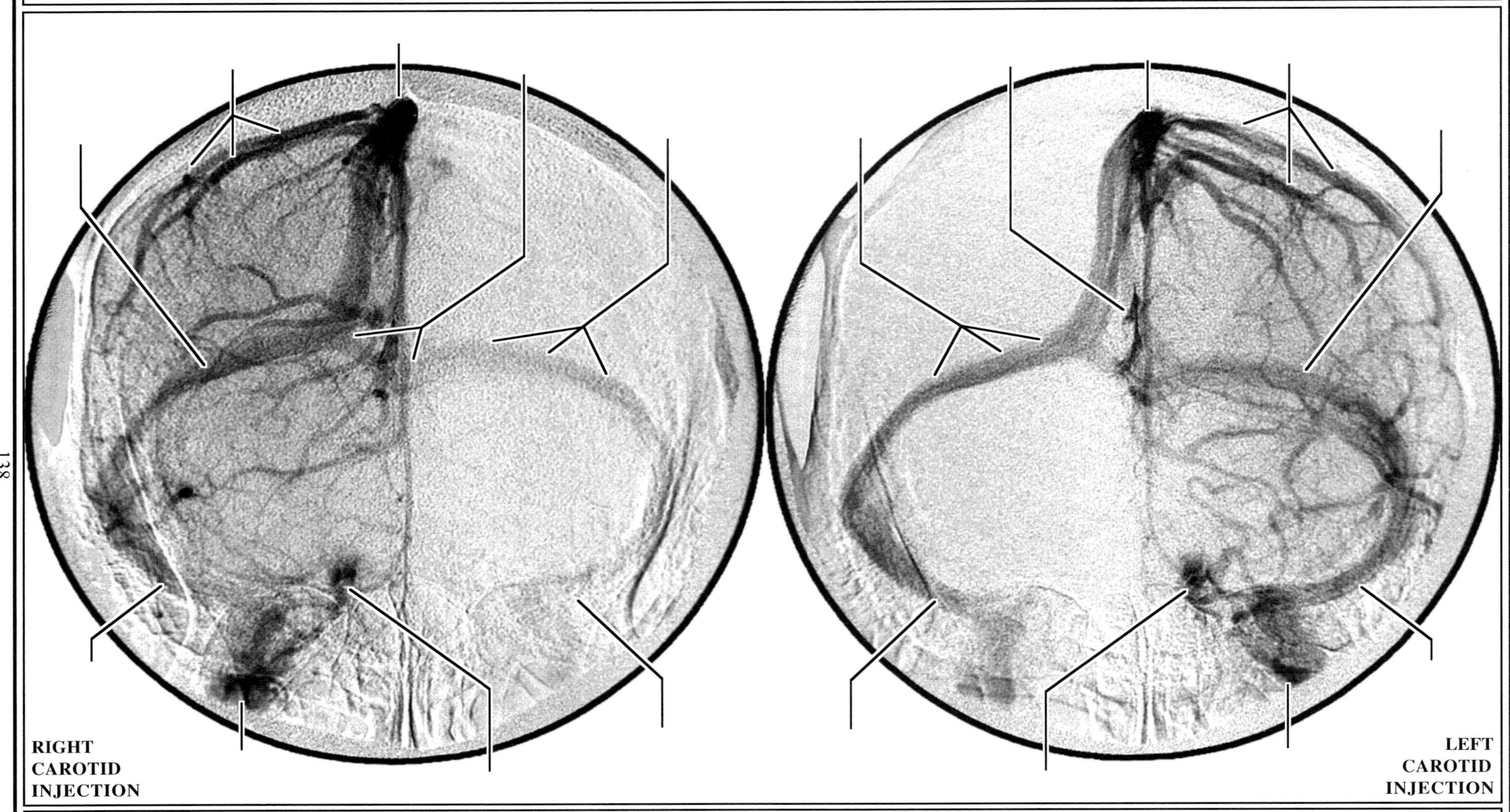

The confluence of sinuses (Torcular Herophili) represents the junction of the occipital sinus, the larger superior sagittal and straight sinuses, and the transverse sinuses. (The occipital sinus courses along the falx cerebelli and opens into the confluence.) Anatomic characteristics of the confluence are accompanied by an asymmetry in venous flow into the straight sinuses. The right transverse sinus is generally a continuation of the superior sagittal sinus. Blood flow from the straight sinus is directed into the left transverse sinus. The venous phase carotid angiograms (above) demonstrate this asymmetry. Blood flow from the superior cerebral veins of either hemisphere empties into the superior sagittal sinus, with subsequent flow directed into the right straight sinus.

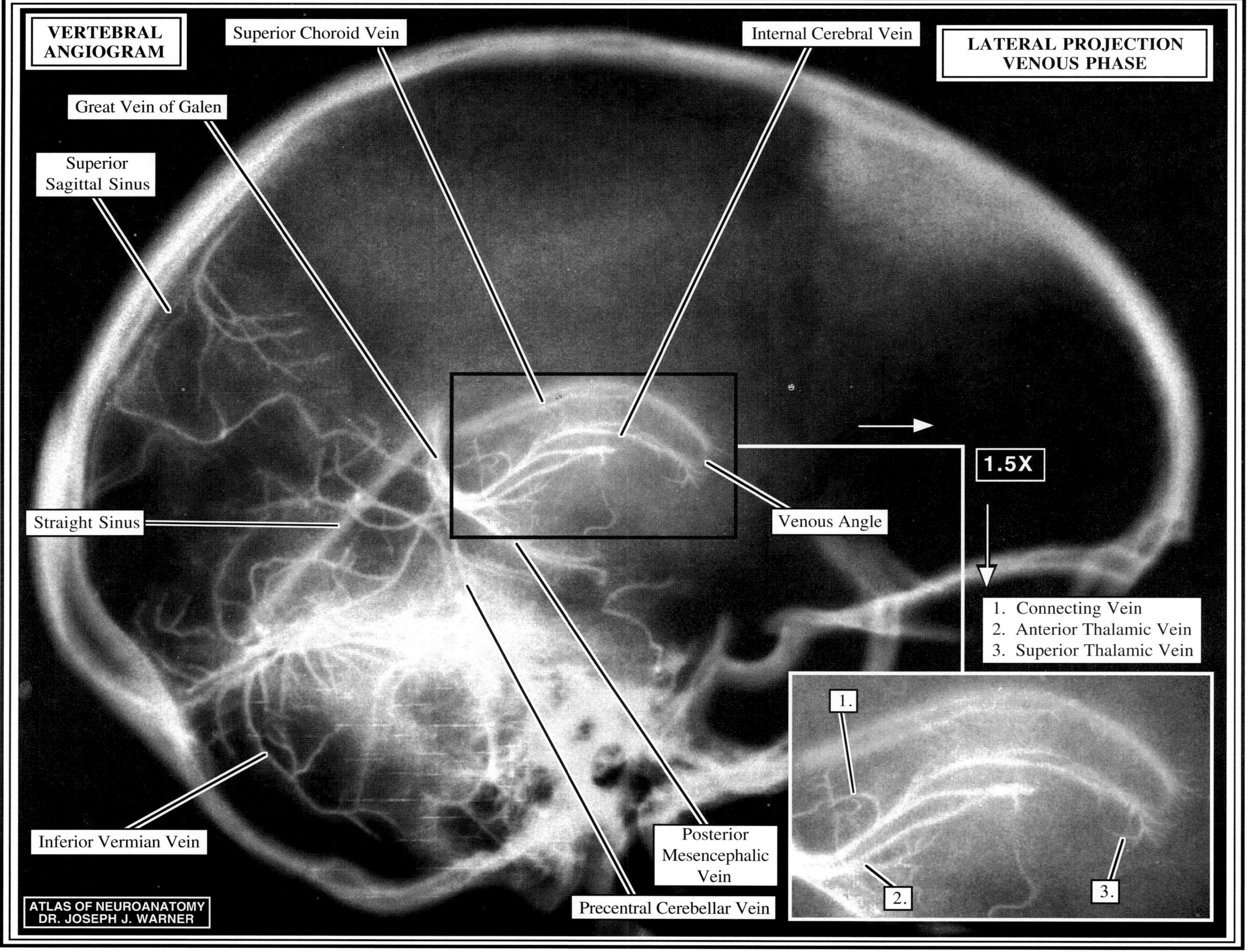

VERTEBRAL ANGIOGRAM
Superior Choroid Vein
Internal Cerebral Vein
LATERAL PROJECTION VENOUS PHASE
Great Vein of Galen
Superior Sagittal Sinus
Straight Sinus
Venous Angle
1.5X
1. Connecting Vein
2. Anterior Thalamic Vein
3. Superior Thalamic Vein
1.
2.
3.
Inferior Vermian Vein
Posterior Mesencephalic Vein
Precentral Cerebellar Vein
ATLAS OF NEUROANATOMY
DR. JOSEPH J. WARNER

VERTEBRAL ANGIOGRAM: TOWNE PROJECTION, VENOUS PHASE

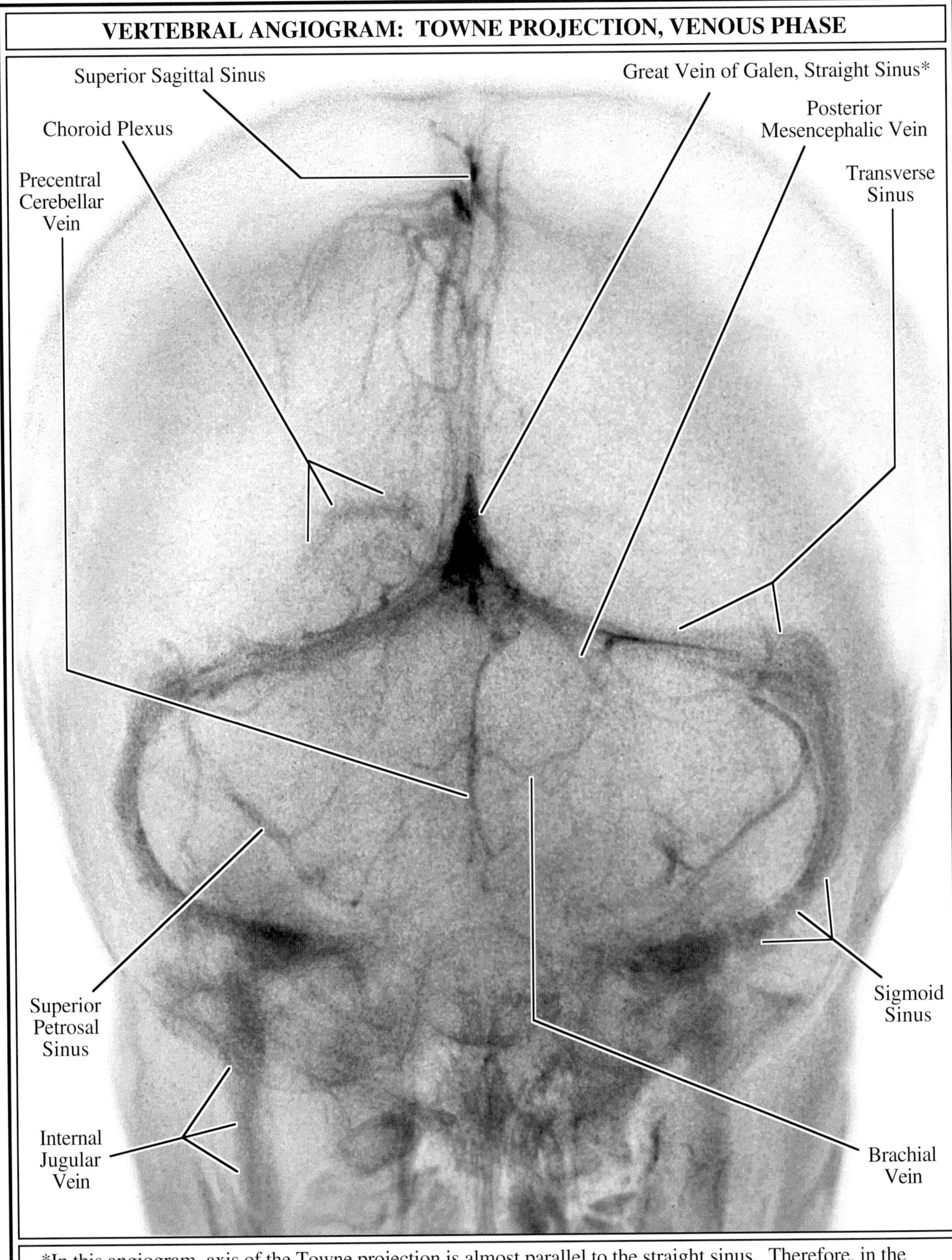

*In this angiogram, axis of the Towne projection is almost parallel to the straight sinus. Therefore, in the venous phase, contrast flow through the straight sinus is superimposed upon that of the Great Vein of Galen.

MAGNETIC RESONANCE ANGIOGRAPHY: AXIAL AND SAGITTAL ROTATIONAL IMAGING

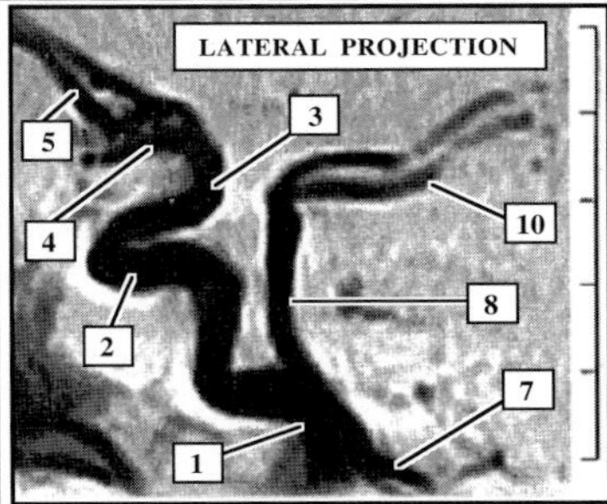

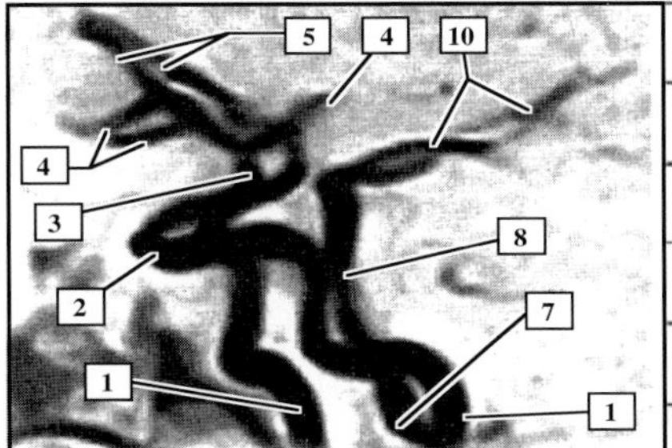

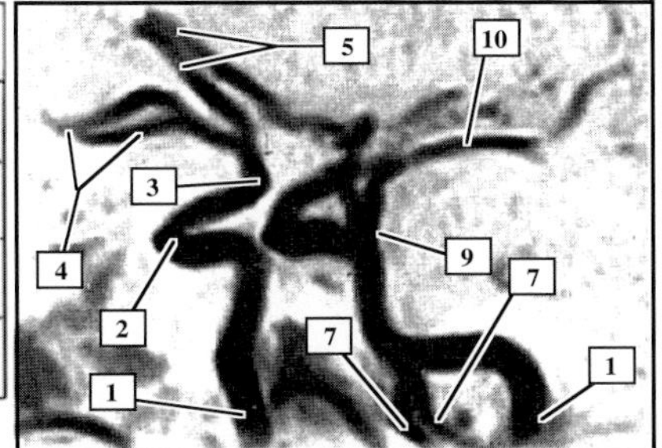

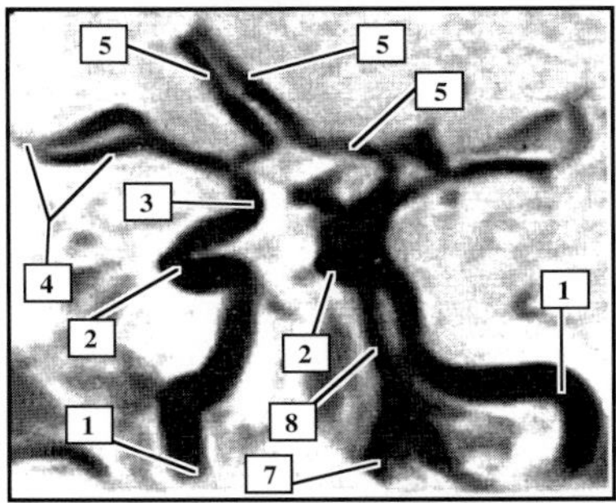

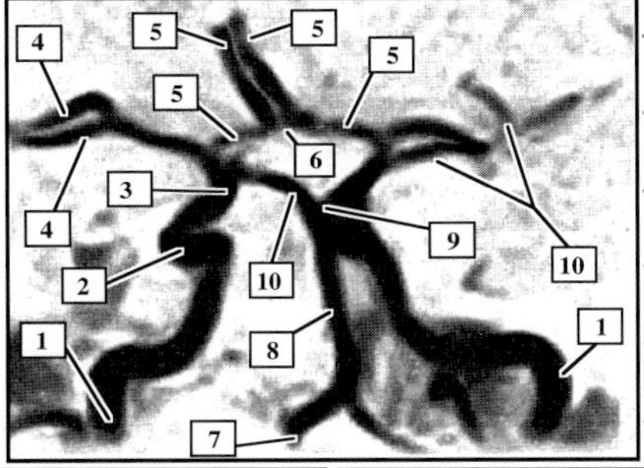

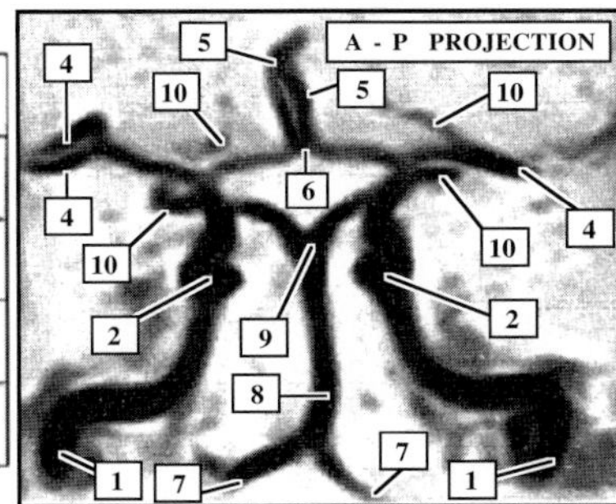

MAGNETIC RESONANCE ANGIOGRAPHY: AXIAL ROTATIONAL VIEWS OF THE CEREBROVASCULATURE

This is a magnetic resonance imaging study of the cerebrovasculature which applies a specific image reconstruction based on blood flow signal characteristics to a gadolinium-enhanced scan of the brain. Selection of the specific signal characteristics of the cerebrovasculature is used to generate a three-dimensional image of the blood supply to the brain. This image may be displayed in various rotational projections for examination of the anatomy of the vertebrobasilar and internal carotid arterial systems. In this study, the three-dimensional reconstruction is horizontally rotated about a vertical axis passing through the Circle of Willis.

KEY TO NUMBERED STRUCTURES

1. Extracranial segment of Internal Carotid Artery
2. Carotid Siphon
3. Supraclinoid segment of the Internal Carotid Artery
4. Middle Cerebral Artery
5. Anterior Cerebral Artery
6. Anterior Communicating Artery
7. Vertebral Artery
8. Basilar Artery
9. Basilar Bifurcation
10. Posterior Cerebral Artery

The Posterior Cerebral Artery may be distinguished from the Middle Cerebral Artery in A-P images by the characteristic course of the PCA as each passes laterally around the mesencephalon, then posteromedially (superior to the tentorium) toward the medial occipital lobe.

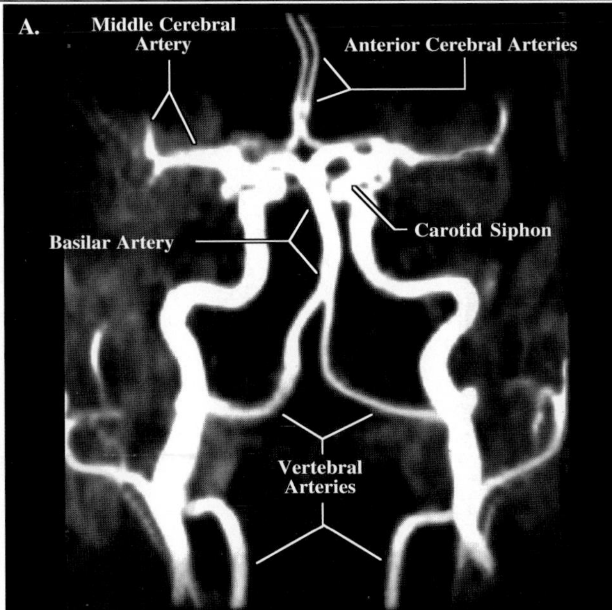

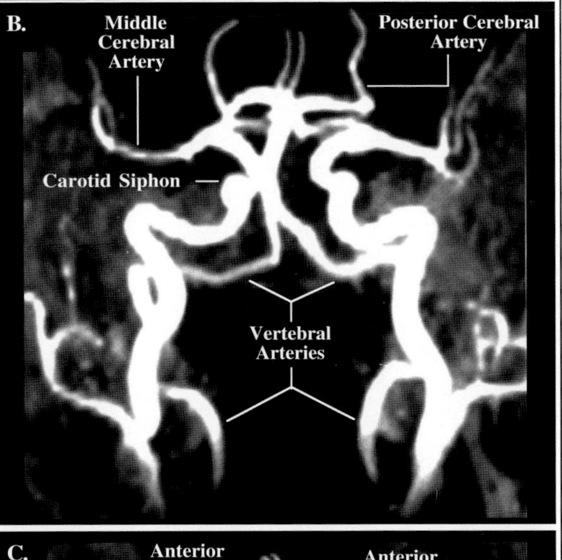

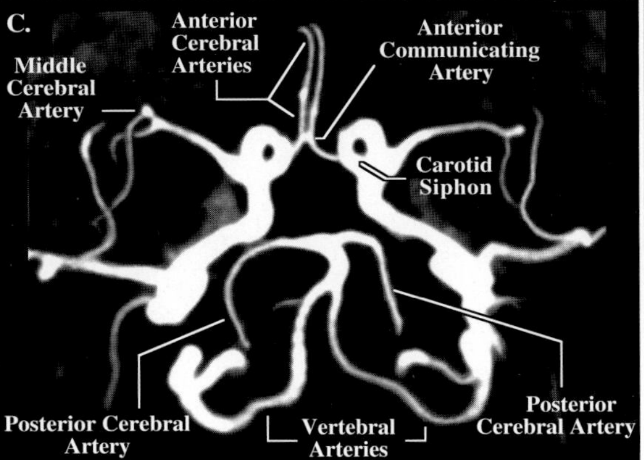

MAGNETIC RESONANCE ANGIOGRAPHY: SAGITTAL ROTATIONAL VIEWS OF THE CEREBROVASCULATURE

Images A-C were selected from a series in which the cerebrovasculature was reconstructed in incremental rotations along an axis perpendicular to the sagittal plane. One major advantage of this technique is to avoid bilateral superimposition of the vasculature while maintaining a symmetical view of the vessels. Various structures often superimposed in anterior-posterior or Towne projections may be viewed by specific rotations along this axis. Note the view of the vasculature provided in image C, which represents a projection along the dorsoventral axis of the cranium. This clearly demonstrates the anterior, middle, and posterior cerebral arteries as well as distinguishing the vertebrobasilar and carotid arterial systems. This series of rotational views is also used in the radiologic examination of the Circle of Willis.

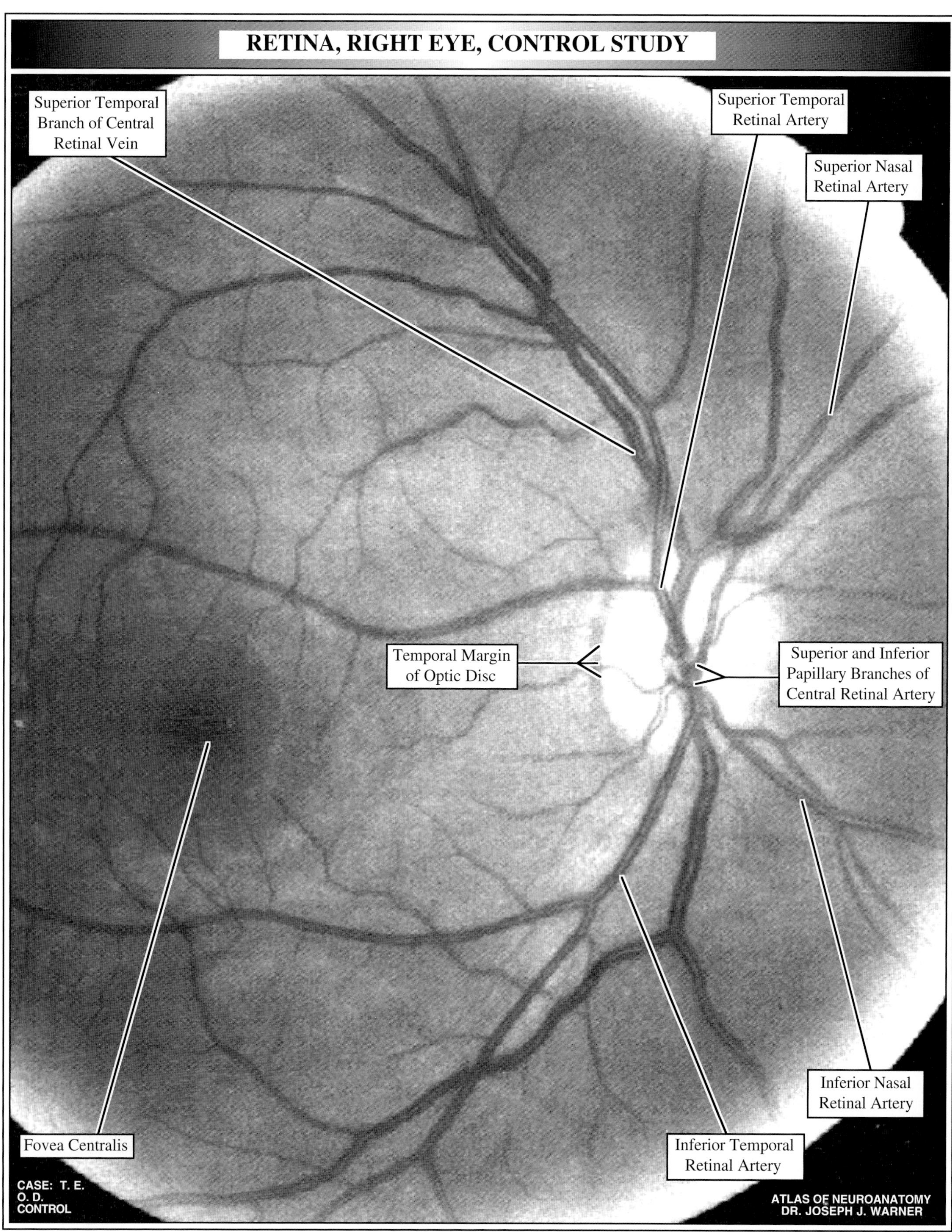
RETINA, RIGHT EYE, CONTROL STUDY
Superior Temporal Branch of Central Retinal Vein
Superior Temporal Retinal Artery
Superior Nasal Retinal Artery
Temporal Margin of Optic Disc
Superior and Inferior Papillary Branches of Central Retinal Artery
Fovea Centralis
Inferior Nasal Retinal Artery
Inferior Temporal Retinal Artery
CASE: T. E.
O. D.
CONTROL
ATLAS OF NEUROANATOMY
DR. JOSEPH J. WARNER

ANEURYSM AT THE JUNCTION OF THE POSTERIOR COMMUNICATING ARTERY AND THE INTERNAL CAROTID ARTERY: VENTRAL VIEW OF THE BRAIN

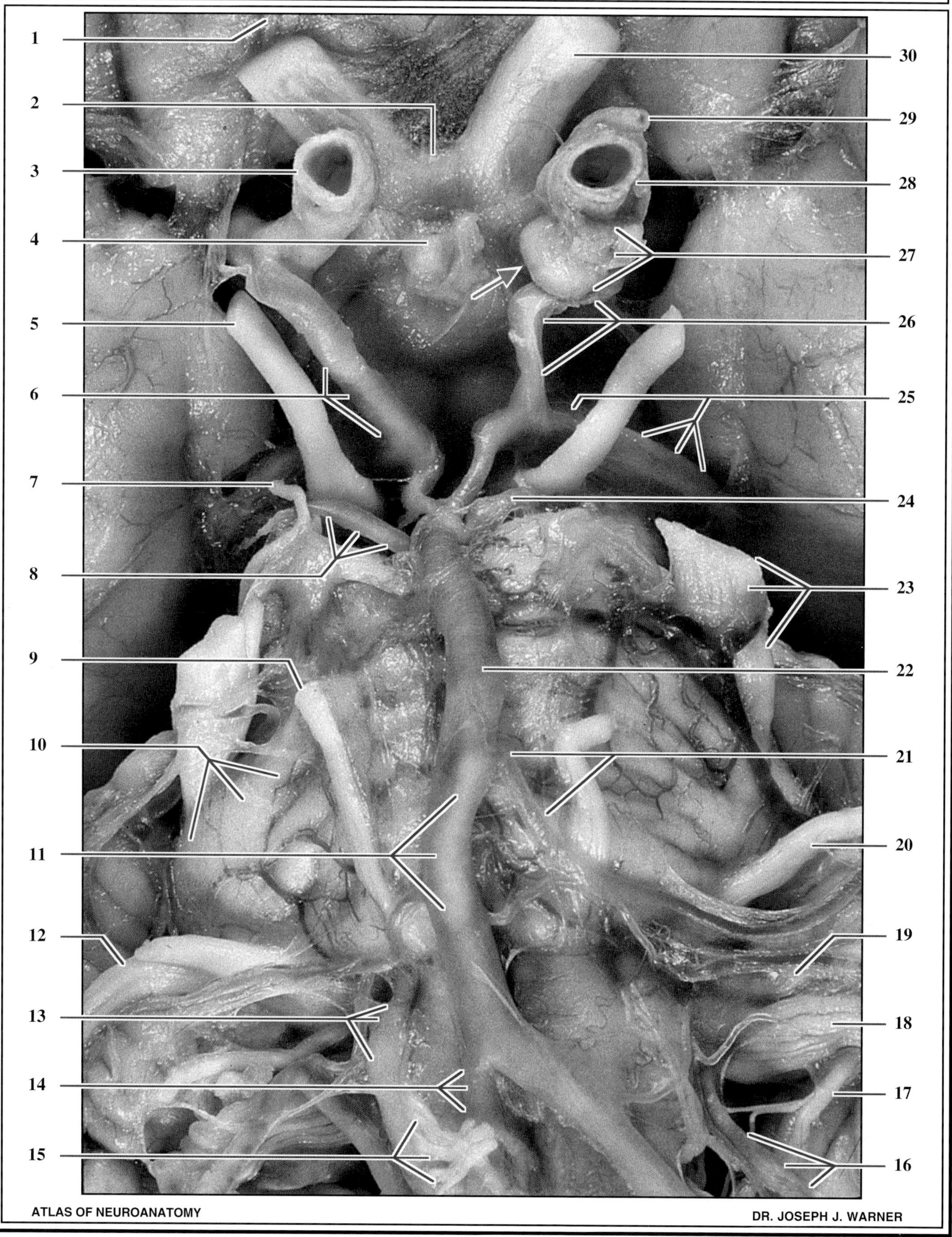

ANEURYSM AT THE JUNCTION OF THE POSTERIOR COMMUNICATING ARTERY AND THE INTERNAL CAROTID ARTERY: KEY TO NUMBERED STRUCTURES

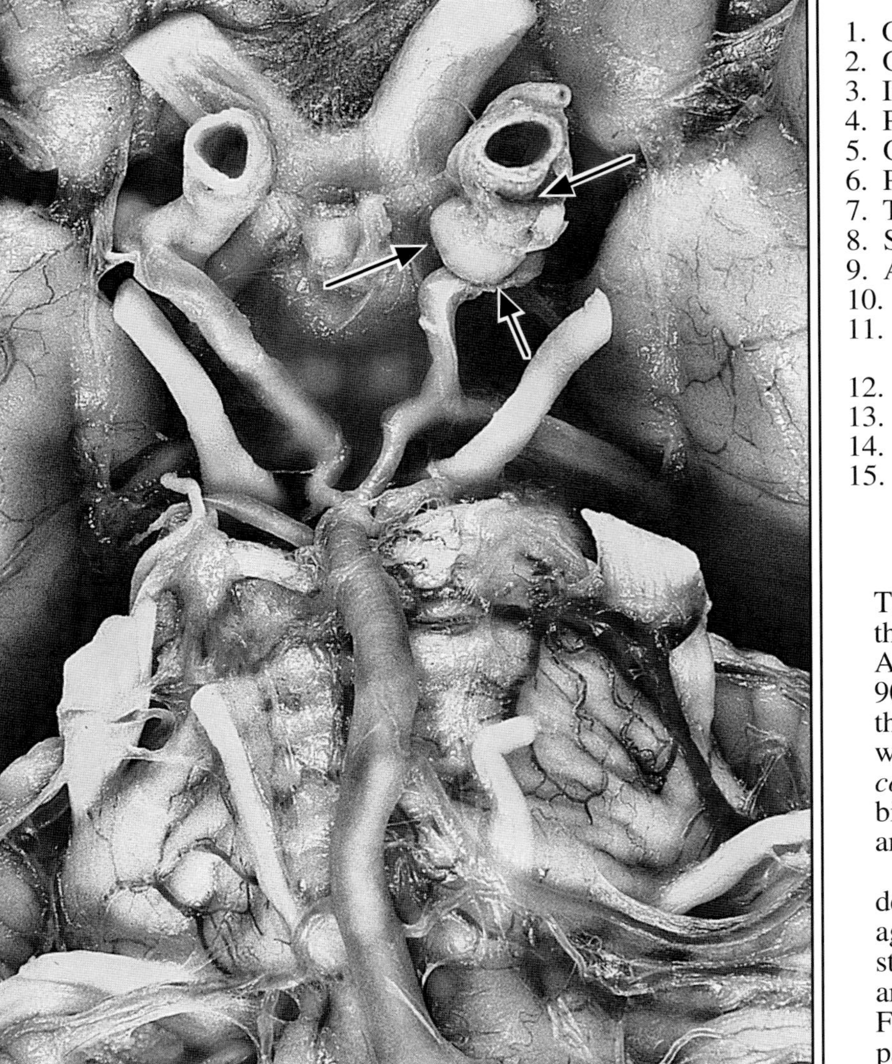

1. Olfactory Tract
2. Optic Chiasm
3. Internal Carotid Artery
4. Pituitary Stalk
5. Oculomotor (III) Nerve
6. Posterior Communicating Artery
7. Trochlear (IV) Nerve
8. Superior Cerebellar Artery
9. Abducens (VI) Nerve
10. Middle Cerebellar Peduncle
11. Atherosclerotic Plaque of the Basilar Artery
12. Vestibulocochlear (VIII) Nerve
13. Inferior Olive
14. Vertebral Artery
15. Fascicles of the Hypoglossal (XII) Nerve
16. Posterior Inferior Cerebellar Artery
17. Spinal Accessory (XI) Nerve
18. Vagus (X) Nerve
19. Glossopharyngeal (IX) Nerve
20. Facial (VII) Nerve
21. Anterior Inferior Cerebellar Artery
22. Basilar Artery
23. Trigeminal (V) Nerve
24. Superior Cerebellar Artery
25. Posterior Cerebral Artery
26. Posterior Communicating Artery
27. Lateral margin of the aneurysm
28. Internal Carotid Artery
29. Ophthalmic Artery
30. Optic (II) Nerve

This case is representative of the entity of saccular aneurysm. These lesions are characterized by thin-walled balloon-like formations that protrude from arteries of the circle of Willis or its branches. Aneurysms generally form at arterial bifurcations or branchings. Over 90% of saccular aneurysms are found on the anterior or rostral aspect of the circle of Willis. The four most common sites are (1) in association with the anterior communicating artery, (2) *the origin of the posterior communicating artery from the internal carotid artery*, (3) major bifurcation of the middle cerebral artery, and (4) the carotid origin of the anterior cerebral artery.

Theories with respect to pathogenesis include developmental defects in the media or elastic components of the arterial wall. However, age-related progression is suggested by postmortem neuropathologic studies, which support the hypothesis that developmental or acquired arterial defects may be important factors in aneurysmal formation. Fusiform or arteriosclerotic aneurysms appear to represent a separate pathogenetic entity. Saccular aneurysms have been associated with an increased incidence of other developmental abnormalities such as congenital polycystic kidney disease, coarctation of the aorta, and fibromuscular dysplasia.

CEREBRAL ARTERIOGRAM DEMONSTRATING AN ANEURYSM OF THE RIGHT INTERNAL CAROTID ARTERY

RIGHT INTERNAL CAROTID ARTERY INJECTION, LATERAL PROJECTION, ARTERIAL PHASE

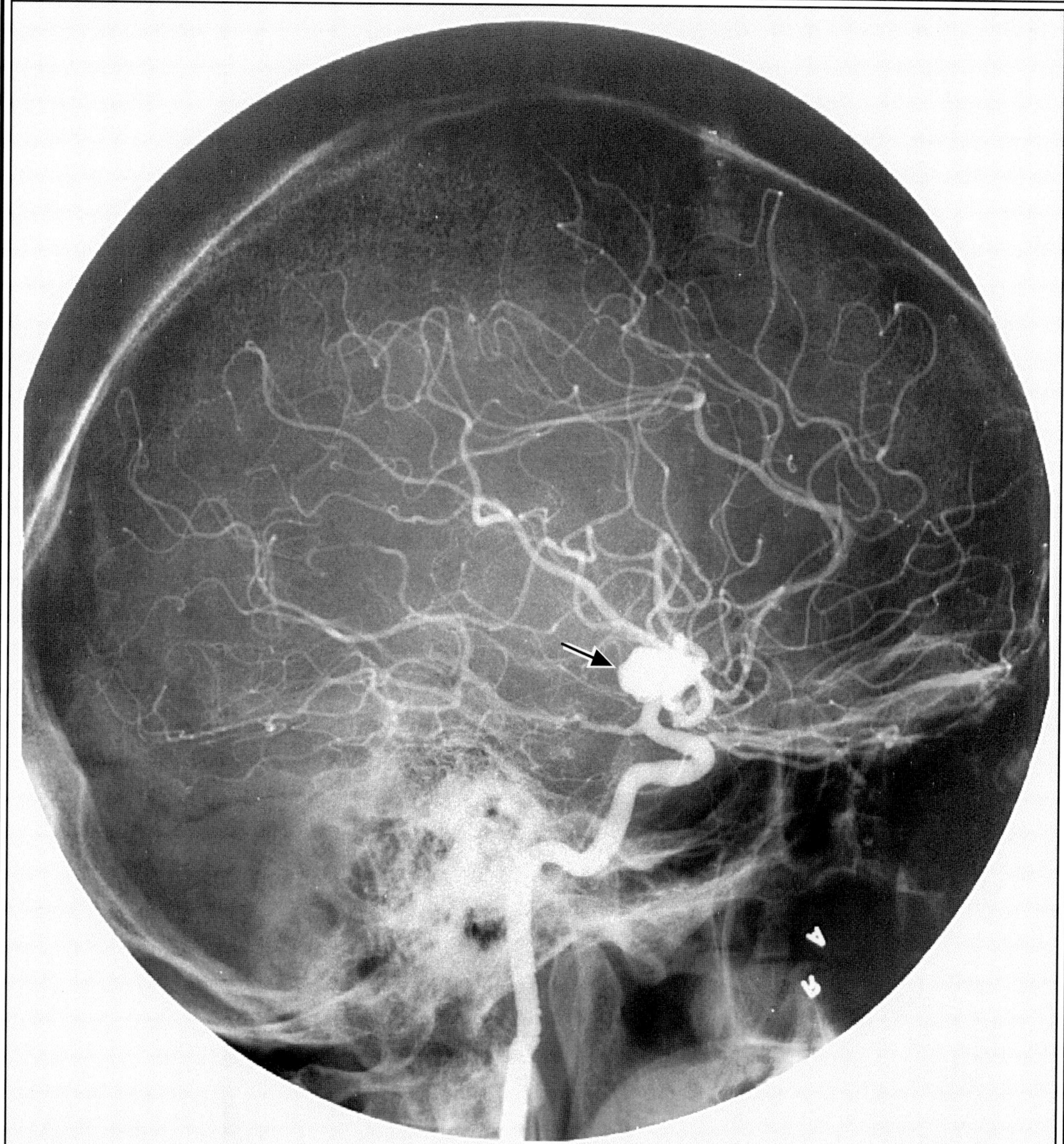

This angiogram demonstrates a large saccular aneurysm of the supraclinoid segment of the right internal carotid artery. Common locations for saccular aneurysms include the bifurcation of the internal carotid into the middle and anterior cerebral arteries and the carotid origin of the posterior communicating artery.

ANTERIOR COMMUNICATING ARTERY ANEURYSM: CAROTID ARTERIOGRAM (OBLIQUE PROJECTION) FOLLOWING SUBARACHNOID HEMORRHAGE WITH RIGHT FRONTAL INTRAPARENCHYMAL HEMATOMA

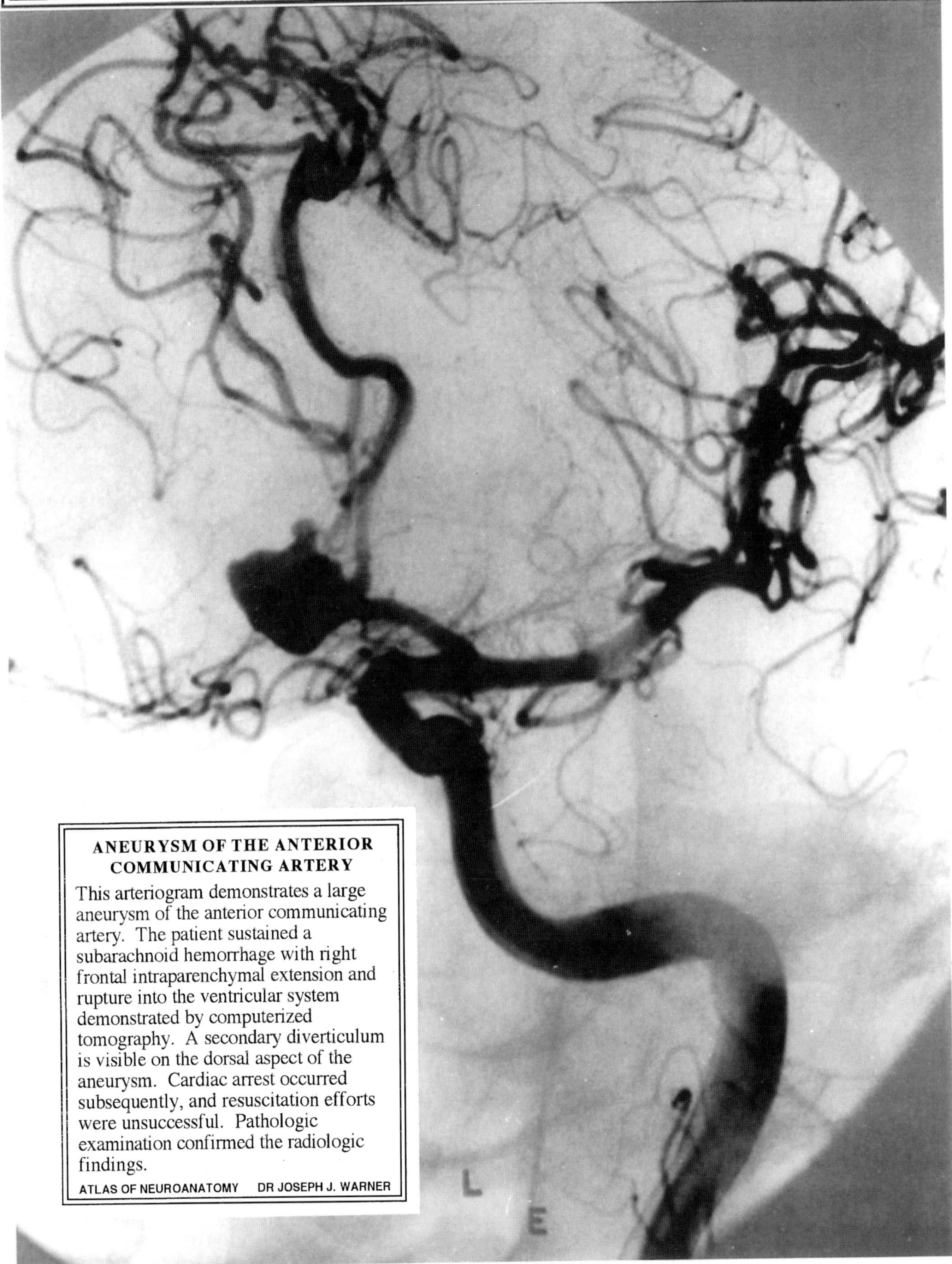

ANEURYSM OF THE ANTERIOR COMMUNICATING ARTERY

This arteriogram demonstrates a large aneurysm of the anterior communicating artery. The patient sustained a subarachnoid hemorrhage with right frontal intraparenchymal extension and rupture into the ventricular system demonstrated by computerized tomography. A secondary diverticulum is visible on the dorsal aspect of the aneurysm. Cardiac arrest occurred subsequently, and resuscitation efforts were unsuccessful. Pathologic examination confirmed the radiologic findings.

ATLAS OF NEUROANATOMY   DR JOSEPH J. WARNER

ANEURYSM OF THE ROSTRAL BASILAR ARTERY BIFURCATION

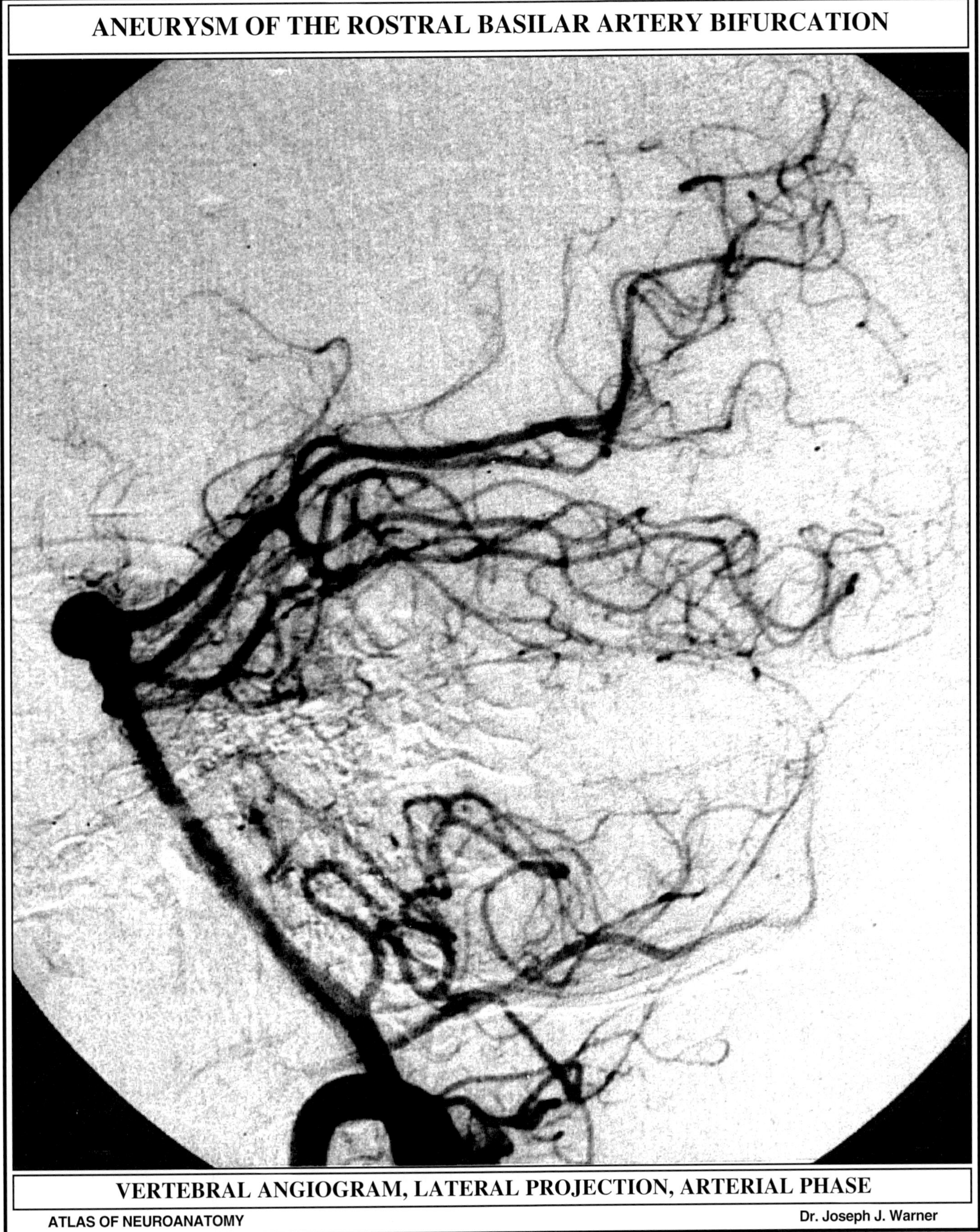

VERTEBRAL ANGIOGRAM, LATERAL PROJECTION, ARTERIAL PHASE

ANEURYSM OF THE ROSTRAL BASILAR ARTERY (BIFURCATION)

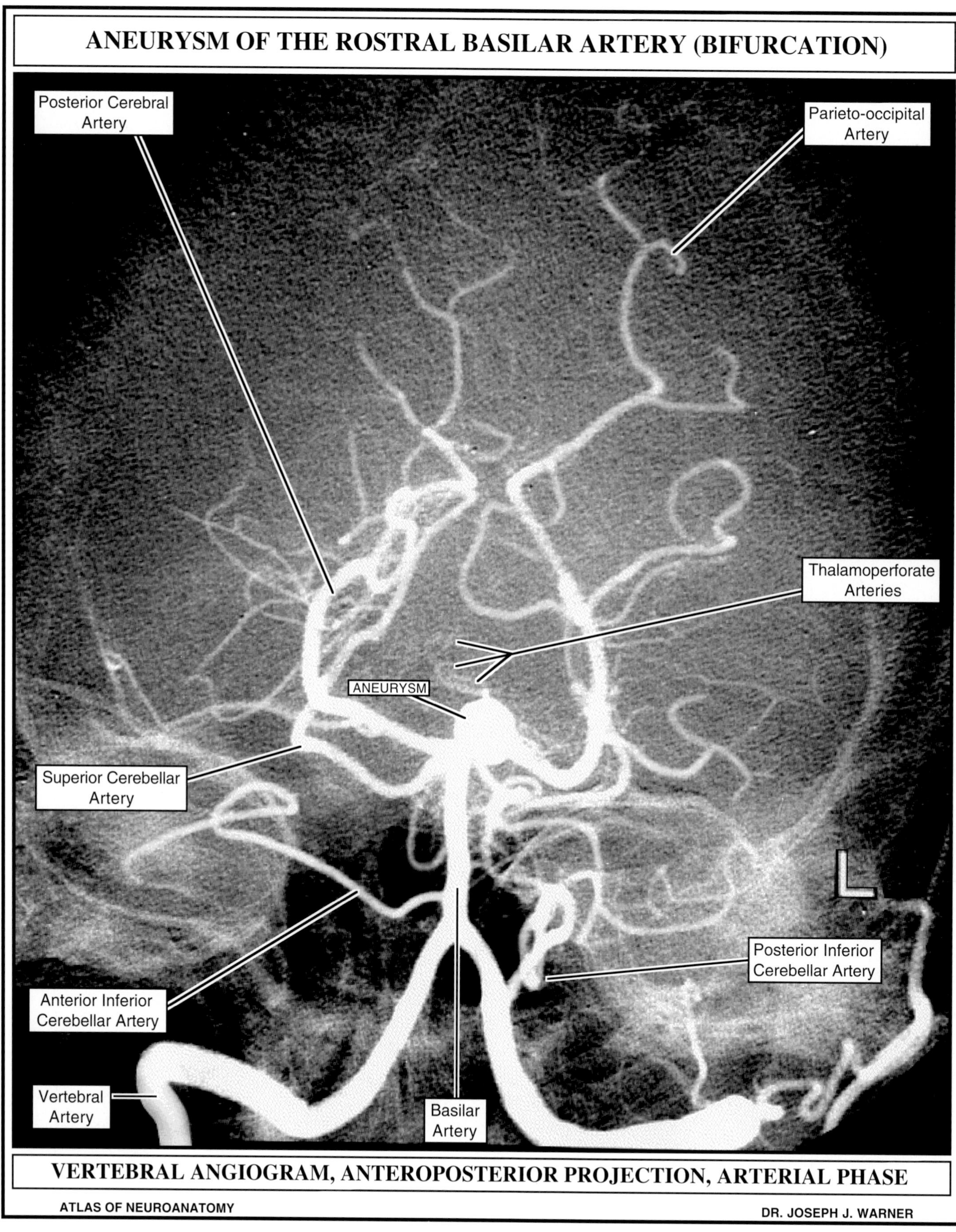

VERTEBRAL ANGIOGRAM, ANTEROPOSTERIOR PROJECTION, ARTERIAL PHASE

ANEURYSM OF THE BASILAR BIFURCATION, OBLIQUE PROJECTION

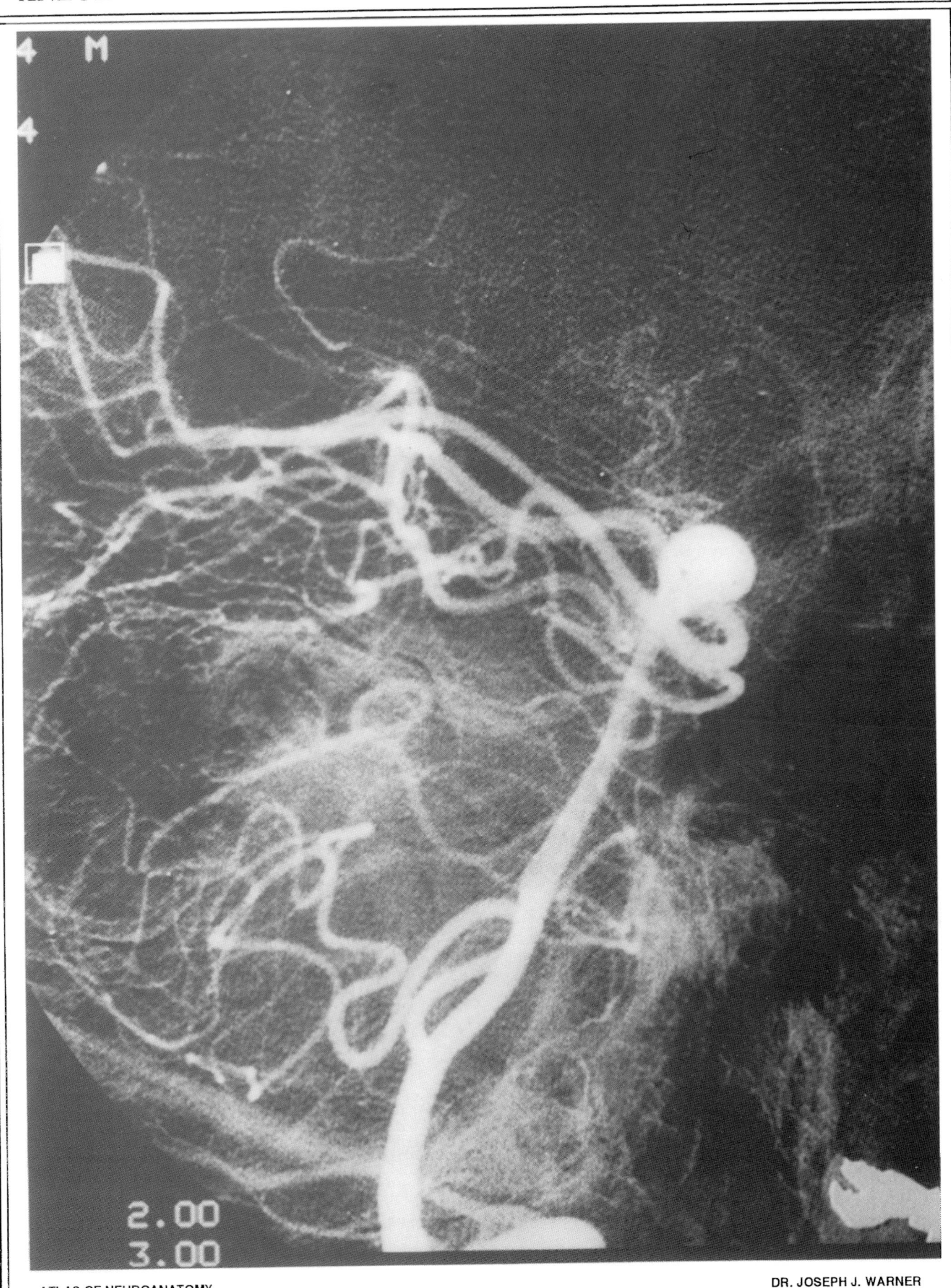

LEFT CAROTID ARTERIOGRAM IN A PATIENT WITH A LEFT MIDDLE CEREBRAL ARTERY EMBOLUS: DOUBLE SUBTRACTION STUDY DEMONSTRATING ARTERIAL AND VENOUS PHASES, LATERAL PROJECTION

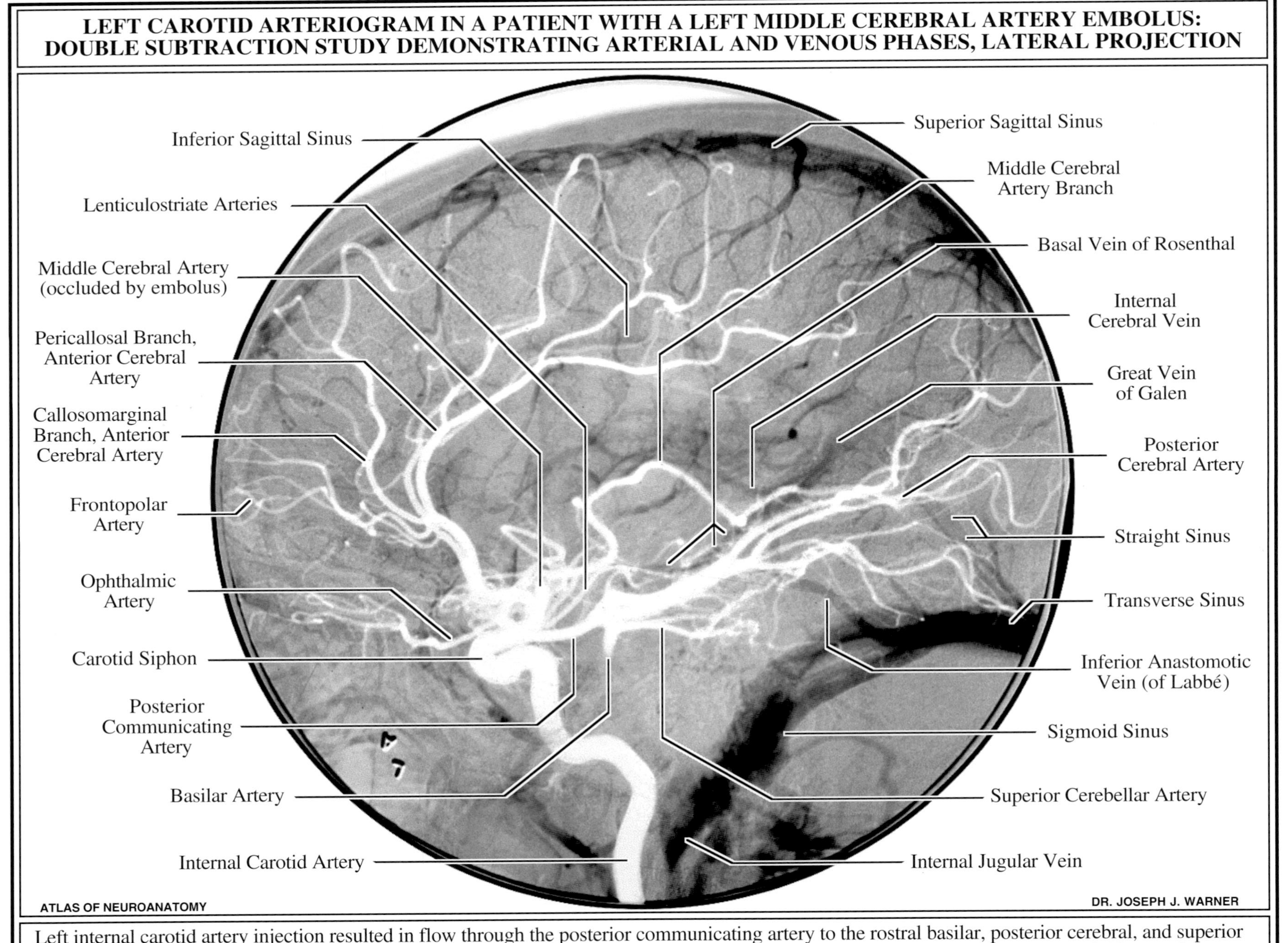

ATLAS OF NEUROANATOMY

DR. JOSEPH J. WARNER

Left internal carotid artery injection resulted in flow through the posterior communicating artery to the rostral basilar, posterior cerebral, and superior cerebellar arteries. The embolic occlusion of the proximal middle cerebral artery is evident, with no flow seen in distal branches of this vessel.

LEFT CAROTID ARTERIOGRAM IN A PATIENT WITH A LEFT MIDDLE CEREBRAL ARTERY EMBOLUS: A-P PROJECTION, ARTERIAL PHASE, DEMONSTRATING FLOW INTO THE POSTERIOR CEREBRAL ARTERIES

This projection demonstrates contrast flow from the internal carotid artery through the posterior communicating and posterior cerebral arteries.

Embolic occlusion of the middle cerebral artery is evident, with minimal or absent discernible contrast filling of distal branches.

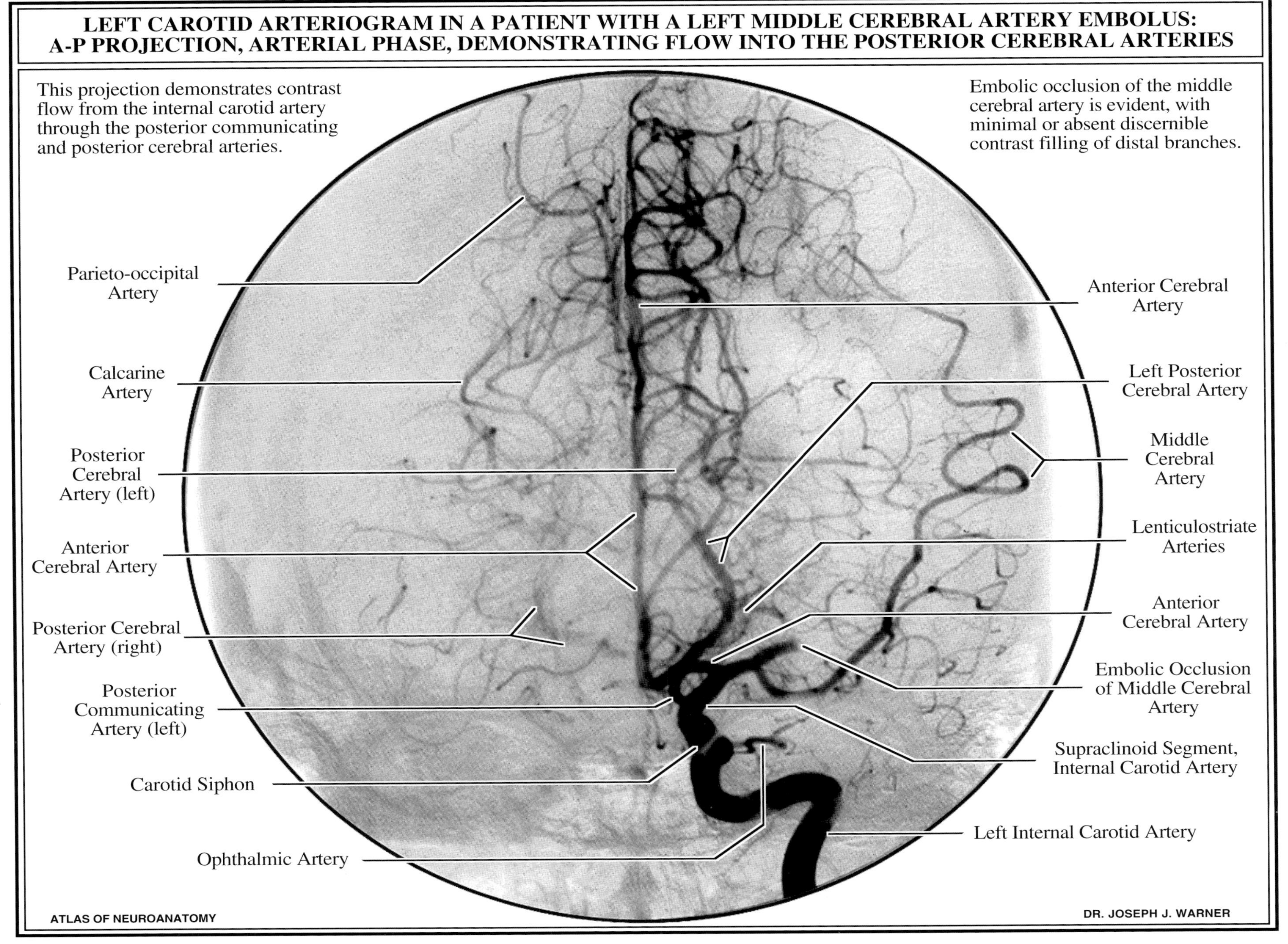

PART II: SECTIONAL NEUROANATOMY

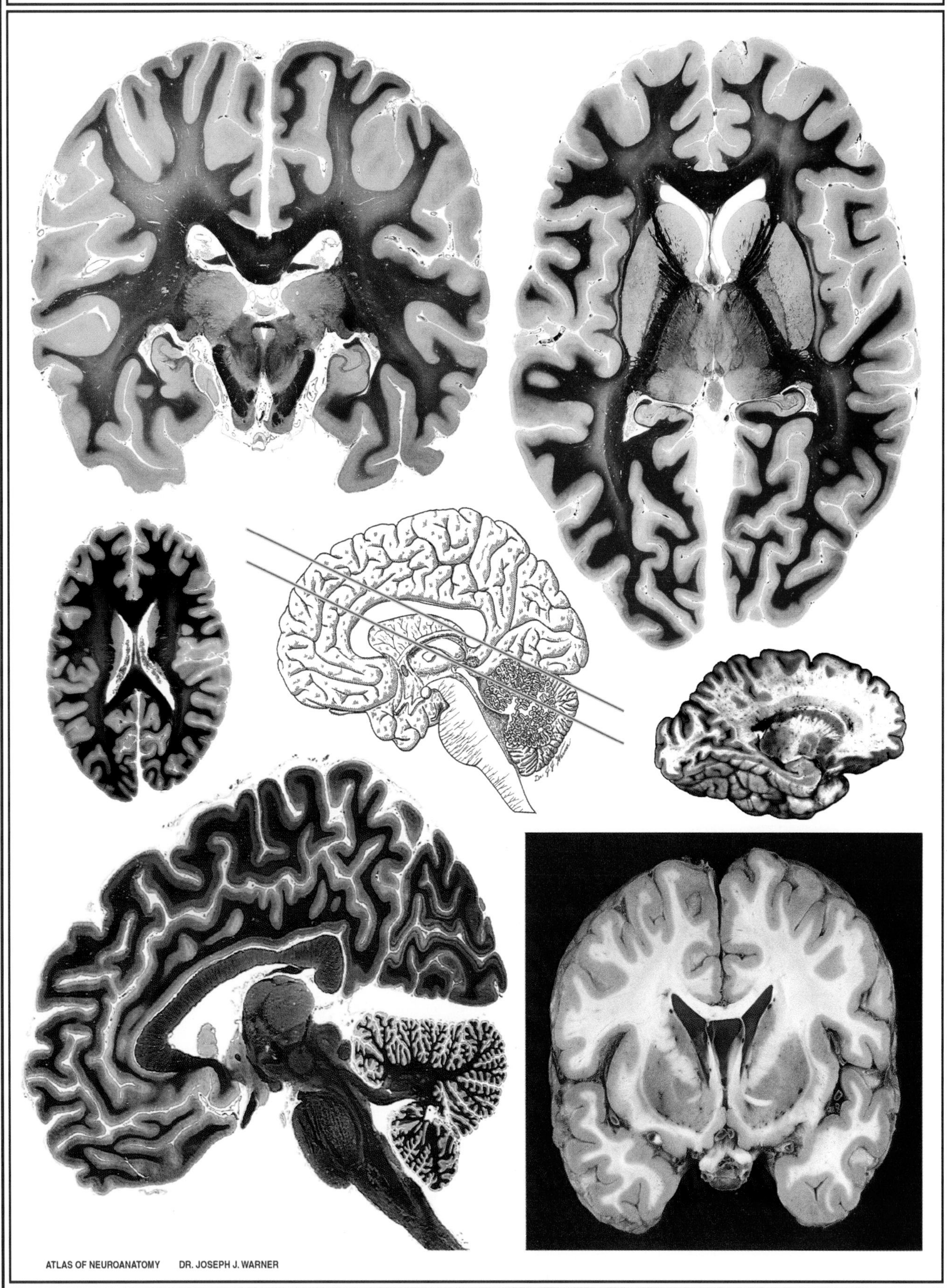

CORONAL SECTIONAL NEUROANATOMY

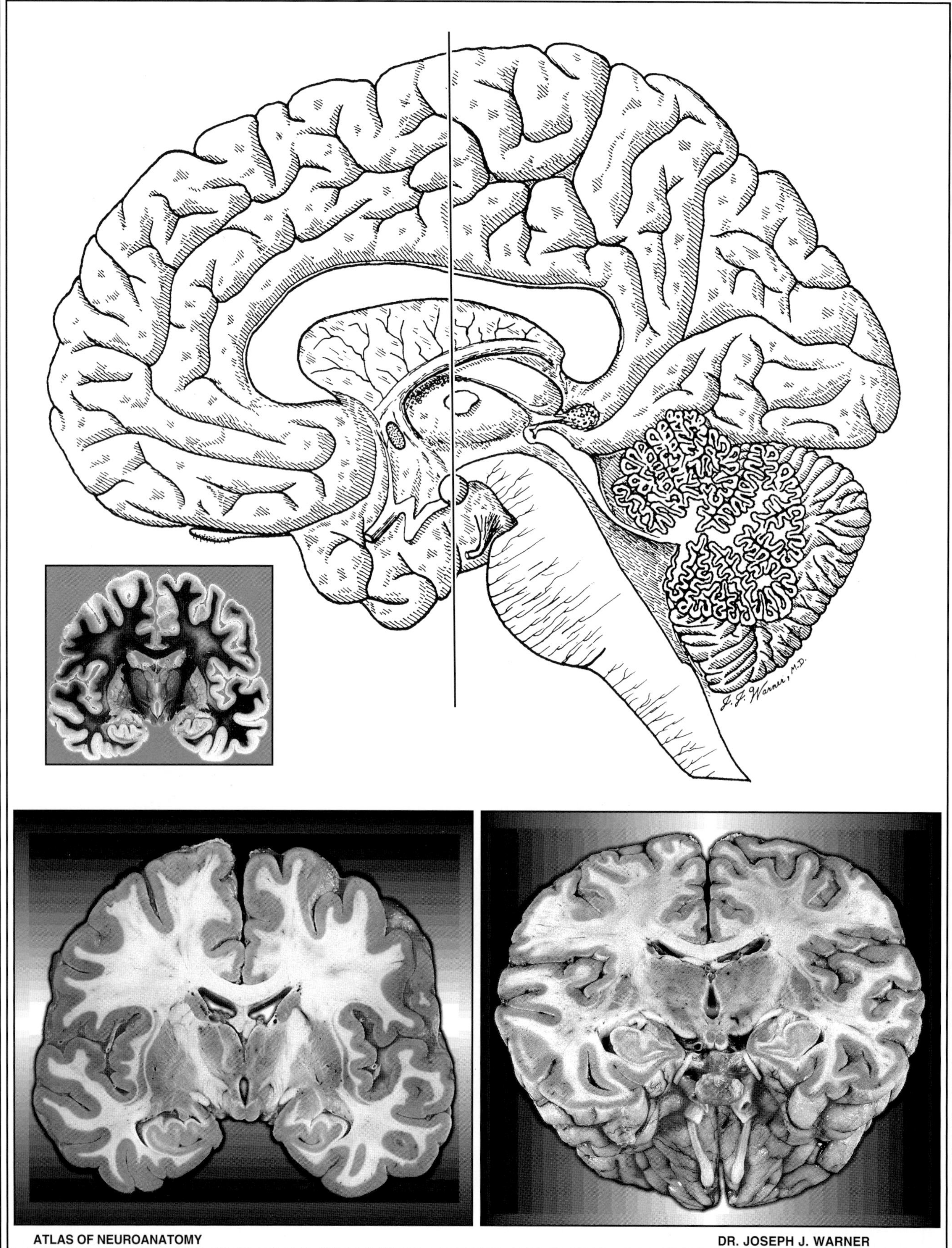

FRONTAL LOBES, ROSTRAL: COMPLETE CORONAL SECTION ROSTRAL TO CAUDAL PERSPECTIVE

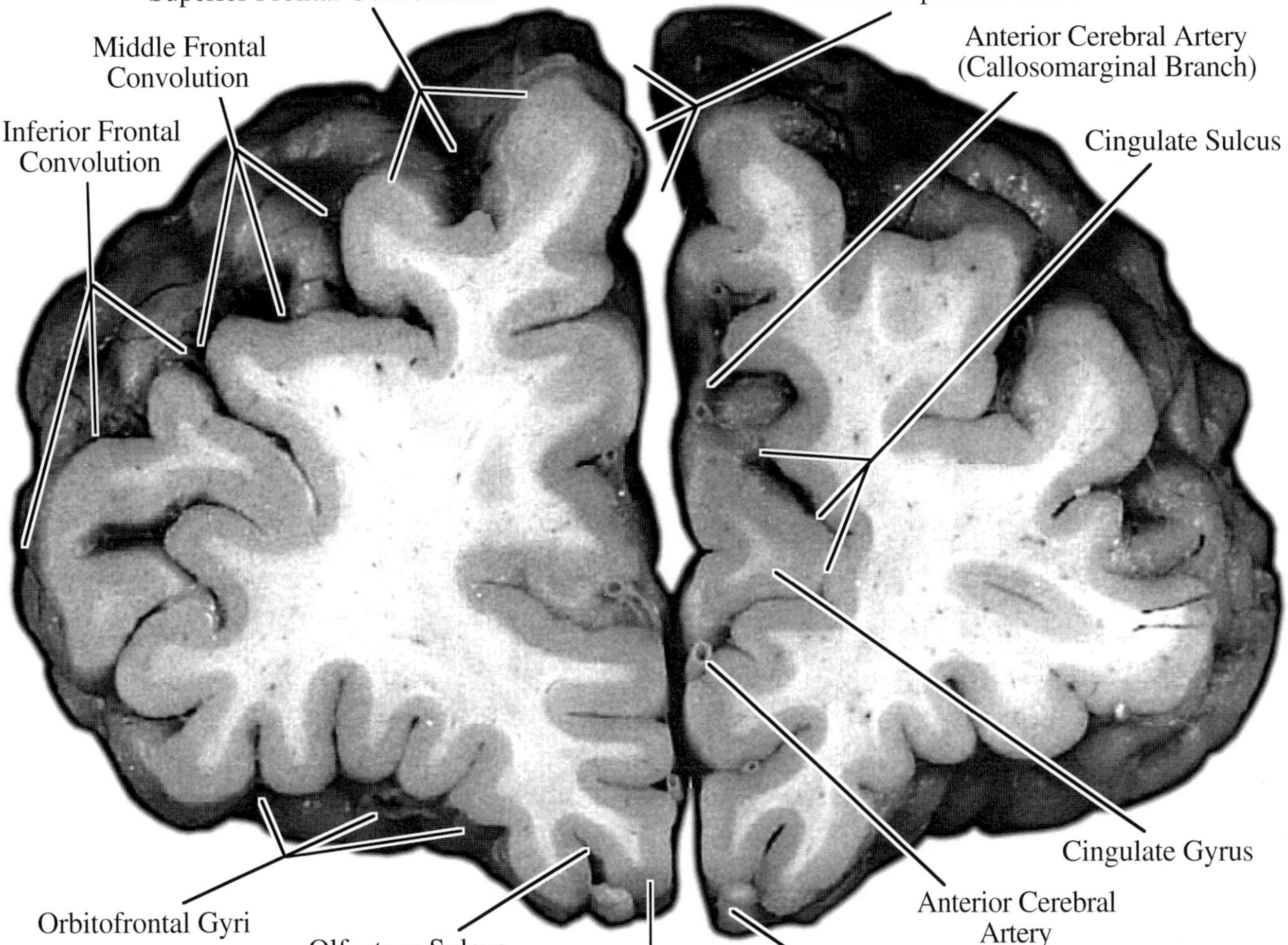

Superior Frontal Convolution
Middle Frontal Convolution
Inferior Frontal Convolution
Interhemispheric Fissure
Anterior Cerebral Artery (Callosomarginal Branch)
Cingulate Sulcus
Cingulate Gyrus
Anterior Cerebral Artery
Orbitofrontal Gyri
Olfactory Sulcus
Gyrus Rectus
Olfactory Tract

The plane of section passes through the rostral aspect of the cingulate gyrus as it curves circumferentially around the genu of the corpus callosum. The cingulate sulcus follows a parallel course, as do branches of the anterior cerebral artery. The callosomarginal branch of this artery frequently originates adjacent to the genu of the corpus callosum, coursing rostrally, then curving dorsally and caudally adjacent to the cingulate sulcus. The contour of the orbitofrontal gyri conforms to the floor of the anterior cranial fossa, comprised of the roof of the orbit, the olfactory groove, and the cribriform plate. Thus, the contour of the inferior surface of the frontal lobes is concave, with the medial aspect (including the gyrus rectus and olfactory tract) occupying a ventral position relative to the lateral aspect.

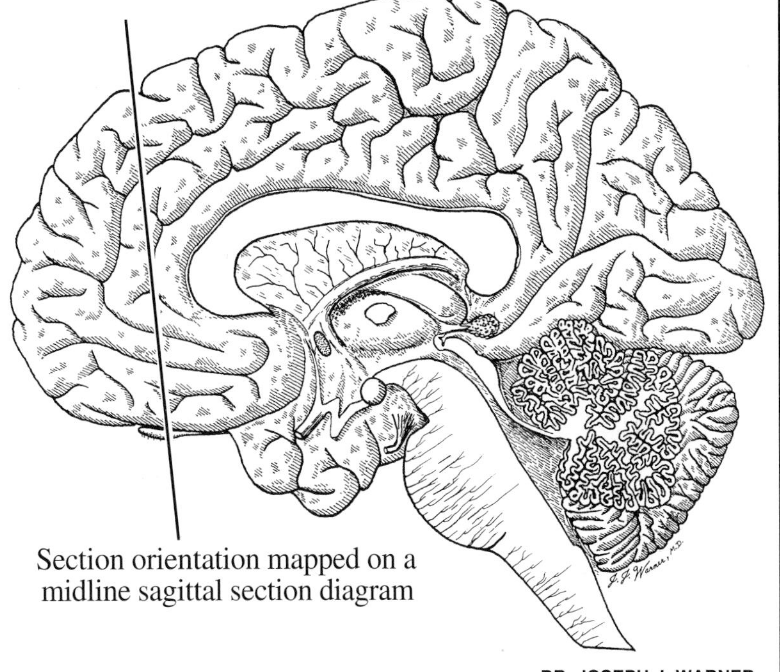

Section orientation mapped on a midline sagittal section diagram

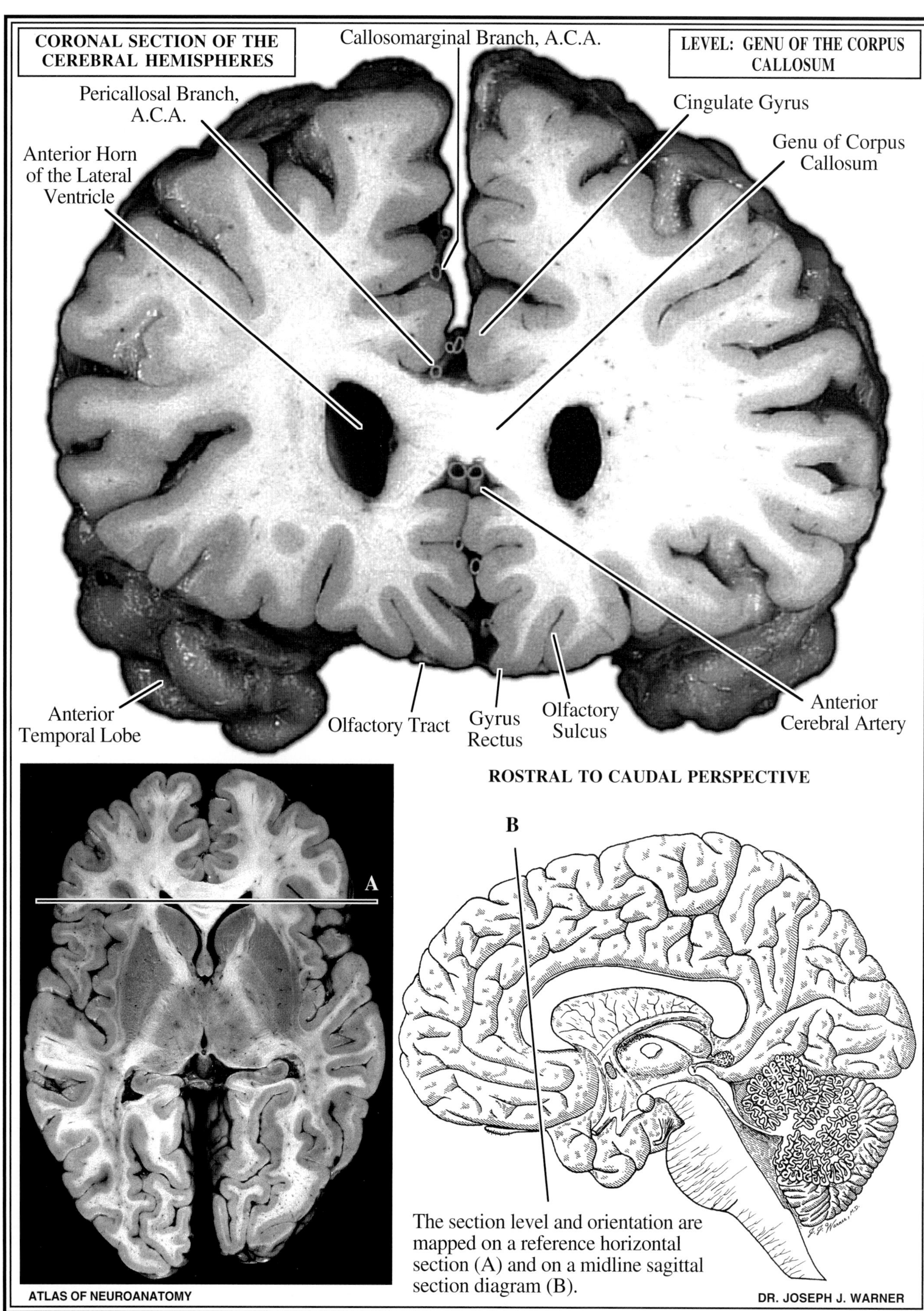

The section level and orientation are mapped on a reference horizontal section (A) and on a midline sagittal section diagram (B).

CORONAL SECTION OF THE BRAIN, COMPLETE; LEVEL OF THE HEAD OF THE CAUDATE NUCLEUS, ROSTRAL TO THE ANTERIOR LIMB OF THE INTERNAL CAPSULE: ROSTRAL TO CAUDAL PERSPECTIVE

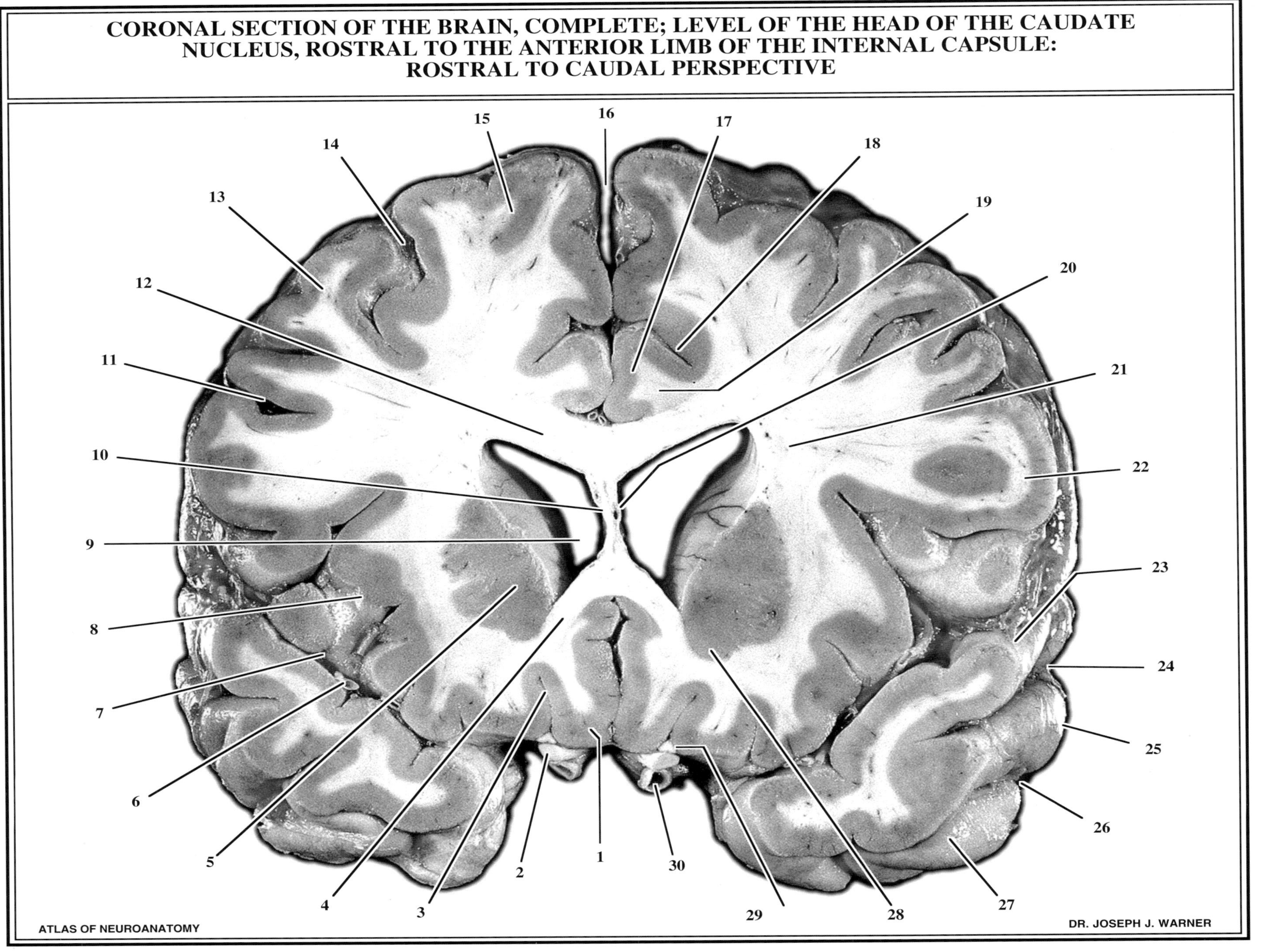

CORONAL SECTION OF THE BRAIN, COMPLETE; LEVEL OF THE HEAD OF THE CAUDATE NUCLEUS, ROSTRAL TO THE ANTERIOR LIMB OF THE INTERNAL CAPSULE: SECTION ORIENTATION AND KEY TO NUMBERED STRUCTURES

KEY TO NUMBERED STRUCTURES

1. Gyrus Rectus
2. Optic (II) Nerve
3. Olfactory Sulcus
4. Rostrum of the Corpus Callosum
5. Head of the Caudate Nucleus
6. Middle Cerebral Arterial Branch in the Sylvian Fissure
7. Sylvian Fissure
8. Insula
9. Anterior Horn of the Lateral Ventricle
10. Septum Pellucidum
11. Inferior Frontal Sulcus*
12. Body of the Corpus Callosum
13. Middle Frontal Convolution*
14. Superior Frontal Sulcus*
15. Superior Frontal Convolution*
16. Interhemispheric Fissure
17. Cingulate Cortex
18. Cingulate Sulcus
19. Cingulum
20. Septal Vein
21. Superior Longitudinal Fasciculus
22. Inferior Frontal Convolution*
23. Superior Temporal Gyrus
24. Superior Temporal Sulcus
25. Middle Temporal Gyrus
26. Middle Temporal Sulcus
27. Inferior Temporal Gyrus
28. Nucleus Accumbens (rostral aspect)
29. Olfactory Tract
30. Internal Carotid Artery

* Each frontal lobe, rostral to the precentral gyrus, is divided into three broad, longitudinally oriented convolutions. These convolutions exhibit considerable variability between different brains, and frequently appear discontinuous. The superior and middle frontal convolutions are divided by the superior frontal sulcus, whereas the middle and inferior frontal convolutions are divided by the inferior frontal sulcus.

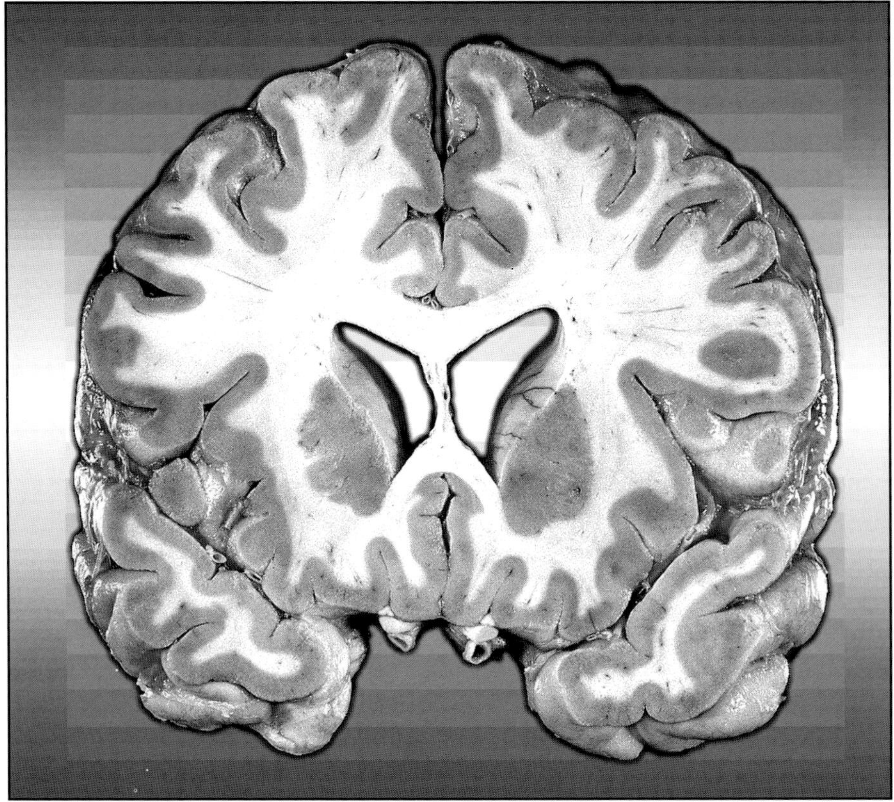

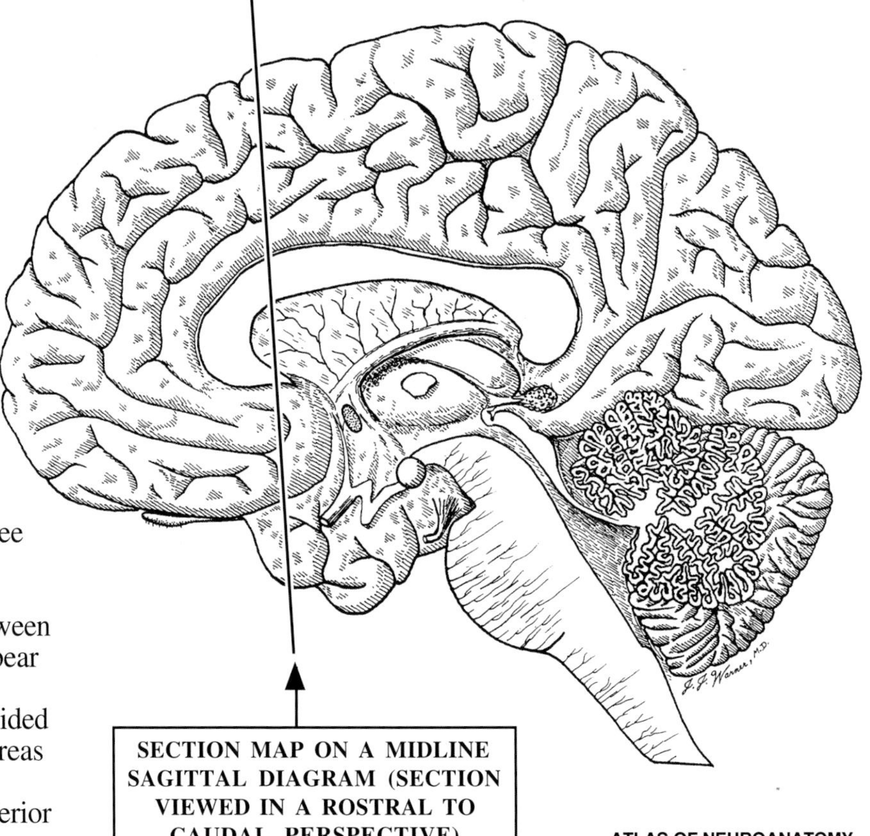

SECTION MAP ON A MIDLINE SAGITTAL DIAGRAM (SECTION VIEWED IN A ROSTRAL TO CAUDAL PERSPECTIVE)

ATLAS OF NEUROANATOMY
DR. JOSEPH J. WARNER

CORONAL SECTION OF THE BRAIN, COMPLETE; LEVEL OF THE NUCLEUS ACCUMBENS AND THE ROSTRAL FIBERS OF THE ANTERIOR LIMB OF THE INTERNAL CAPSULE: ROSTRAL TO CAUDAL PERSPECTIVE

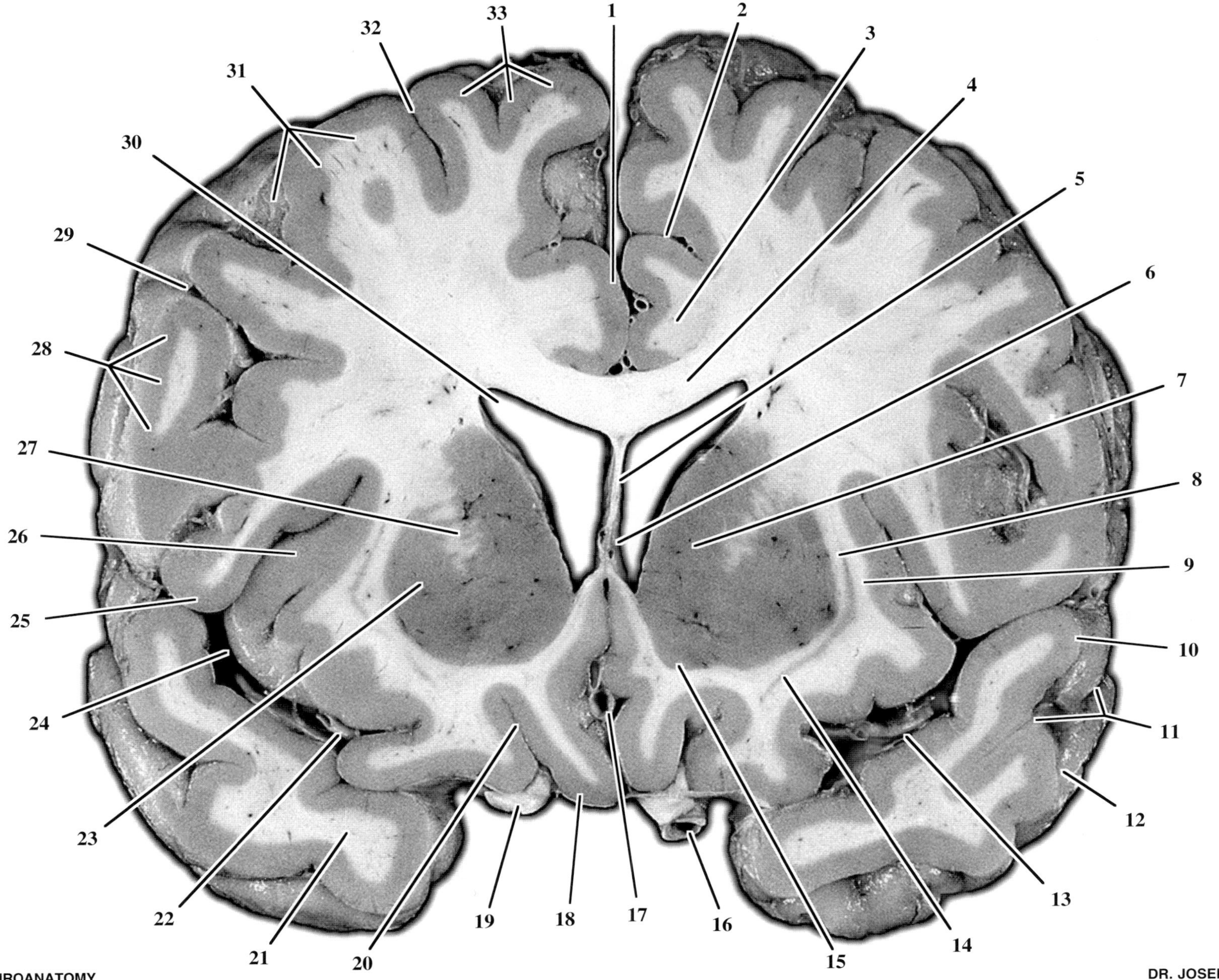
1
2
3
4
5
6
7
8
9
10
11
12
13
14
15
16
17
18
19
20
21
22
23
24
25
26
27
28
29
30
31
32
33

ATLAS OF NEUROANATOMY

DR. JOSEPH J. WARNER

CORONAL SECTION OF THE BRAIN, COMPLETE; LEVEL OF THE NUCLEUS ACCUMBENS AND THE ANTERIOR LIMB OF THE INTERNAL CAPSULE: SECTION ORIENTATION AND KEY TO NUMBERED STRUCTURES

KEY TO NUMBERED STRUCTURES

1. Cingulate Cortex
2. Cingulate Sulcus
3. Cingulum
4. Corpus Callosum
5. Septum Pellucidum
6. Septal Vein
7. Head of the Caudate Nucleus
8. External Capsule
9. Extreme Capsule
10. Superior Temporal Gyrus
11. Superior Temporal Sulcus
12. Middle Temporal Gyrus
13. Middle Cerebral Artery
14. Claustrum
15. Nucleus Accumbens*
16. Internal Carotid Artery
17. Anterior Cerebral Artery
18. Gyrus Rectus
19. Optic Nerve
20. Olfactory Sulcus
21. Anterior Temporal Lobe
22. Middle Cerebral Artery
23. Putamen
24. Sylvian Fissure
25. Frontal Opercular Region
26. Insular Cortex (rostral)
27. Anterior Limb of the Internal Capsule
28. Inferior Frontal Convolution
29. Inferior Frontal Sulcus
30. Anterior Horn of the Lateral Ventricle
31. Middle Frontal Convolution
32. Superior Frontal Sulcus
33. Superior Frontal Convolution

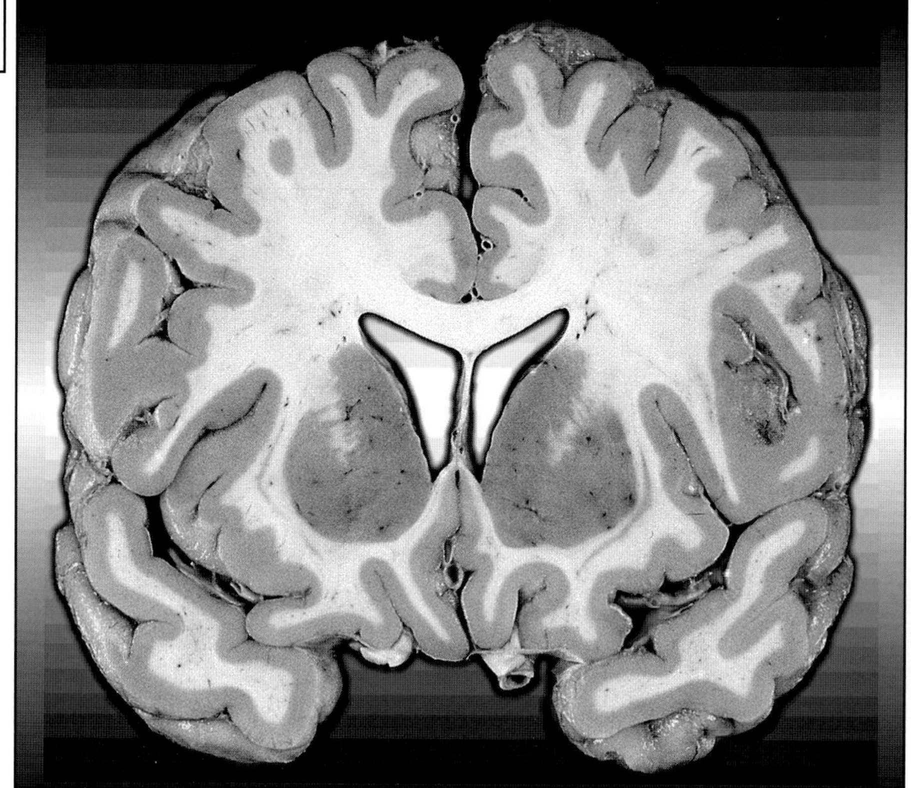

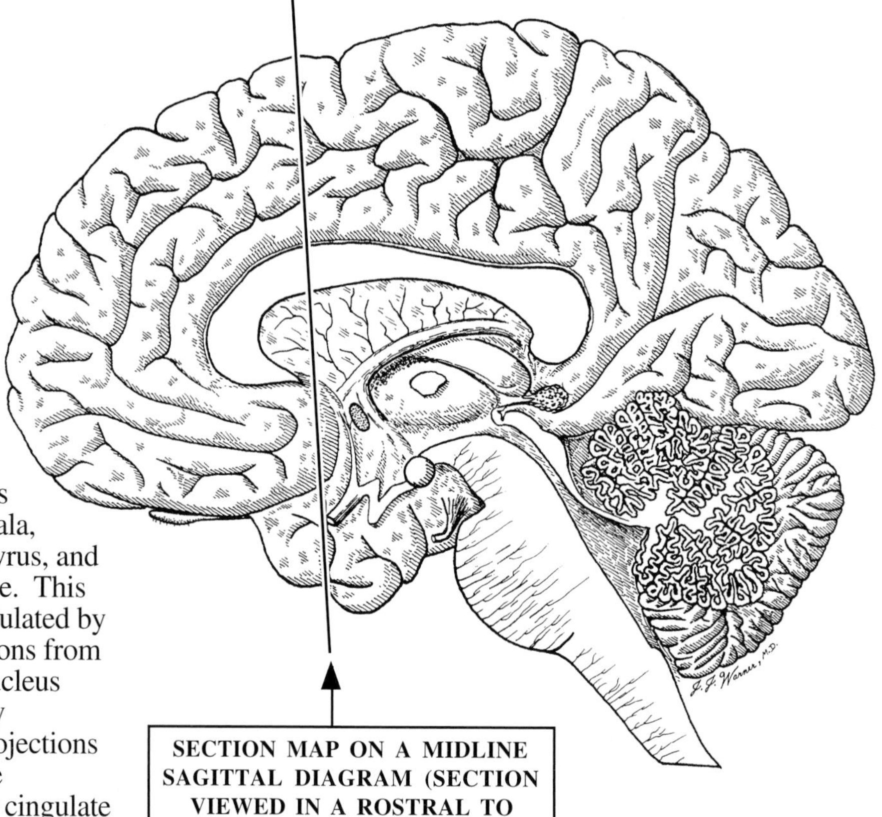

SECTION MAP ON A MIDLINE SAGITTAL DIAGRAM (SECTION VIEWED IN A ROSTRAL TO CAUDAL PERSPECTIVE)

* The nucleus accumbens receives convergent inputs from the amygdala, hippocampus, anterior cingulate gyrus, and certain regions of the temporal lobe. This convergent afferent activity is modulated by mesolimbic dopaminergic projections from the ventral tegmental area to the nucleus accumbens. Dopaminergic activity influences the activity of neural projections from the nucleus accumbens to the hypothalamus, septal area, anterior cingulate and frontal regions.

COMPLETE CORONAL SECTION OF A BRAIN WITH CAVUM SEPTUM PELLUCIDUM, PITUITARY INTACT: LEVEL OF THE NUCLEUS BASALIS OF MEYNERT, ROSTRAL TO CAUDAL PERSPECTIVE

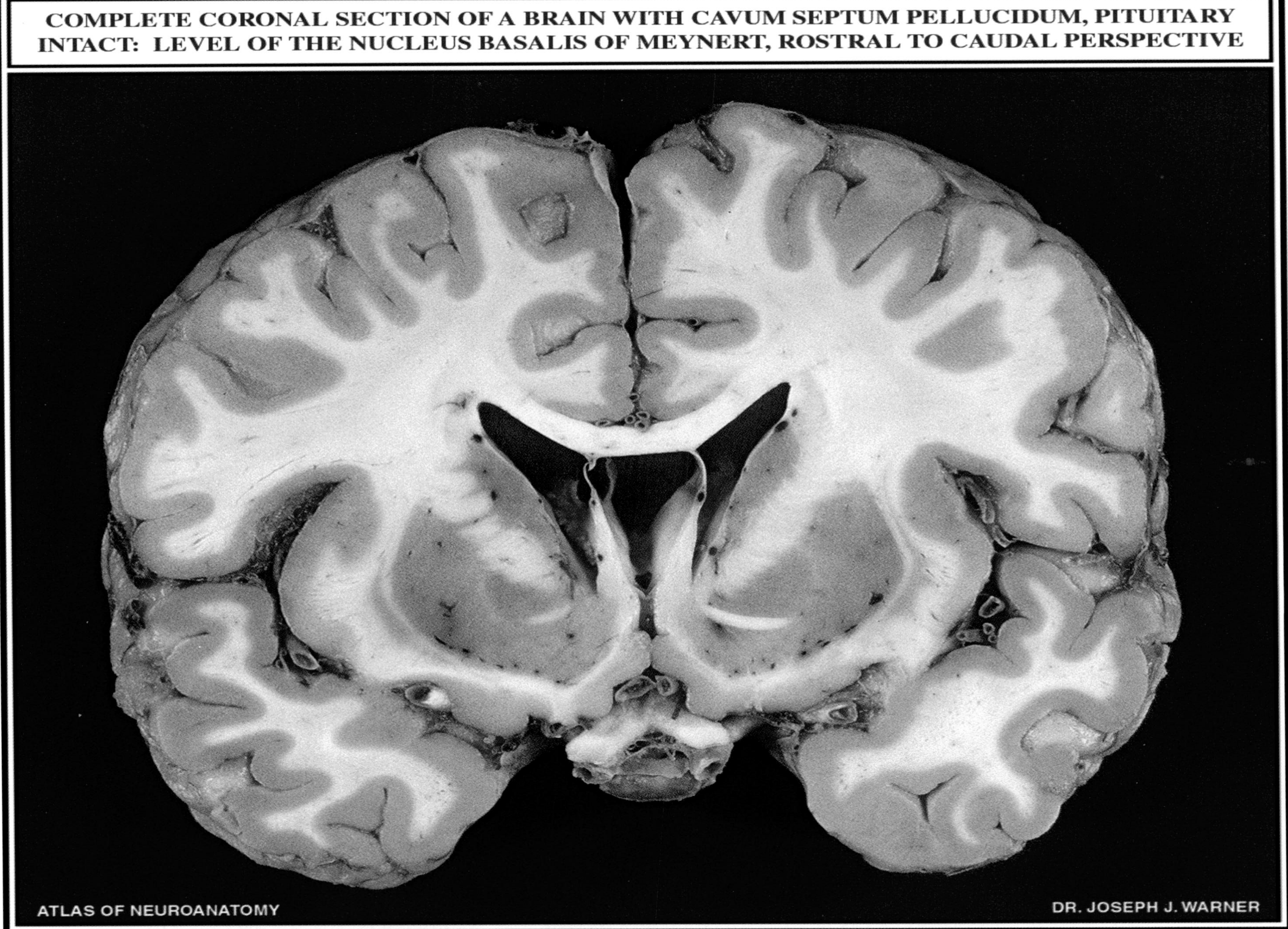

COMPLETE CORONAL SECTION OF A BRAIN WITH CAVUM SEPTUM PELLUCIDUM, PITUITARY INTACT: LEVEL OF THE NUCLEUS BASALIS OF MEYNERT, ROSTRAL TO CAUDAL PERSPECTIVE

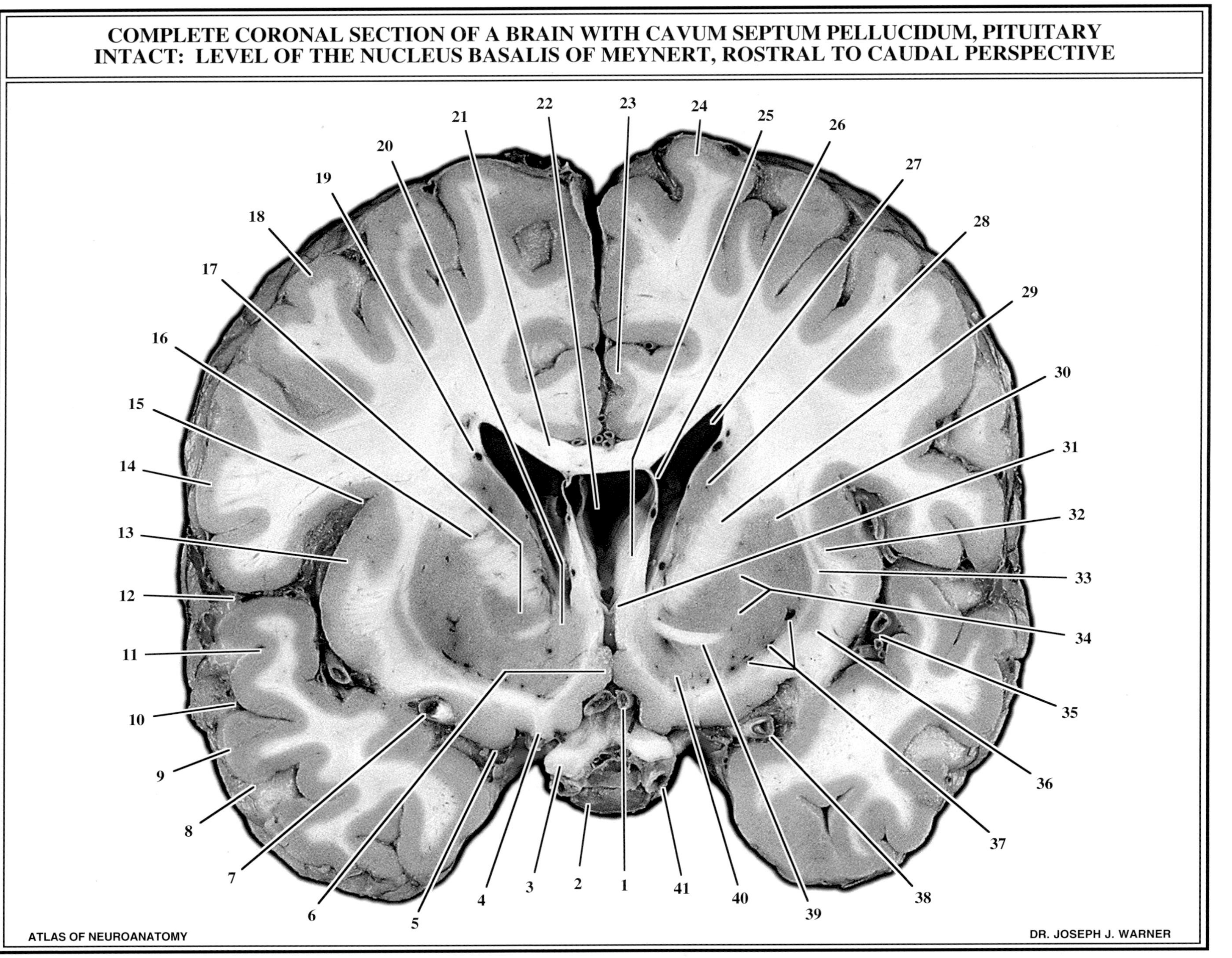

COMPLETE CORONAL SECTION OF A BRAIN WITH CAVUM SEPTUM PELLUCIDUM, PITUITARY INTACT: LEVEL OF THE NUCLEUS BASALIS OF MEYNERT, ROSTRAL TO CAUDAL PERSPECTIVE

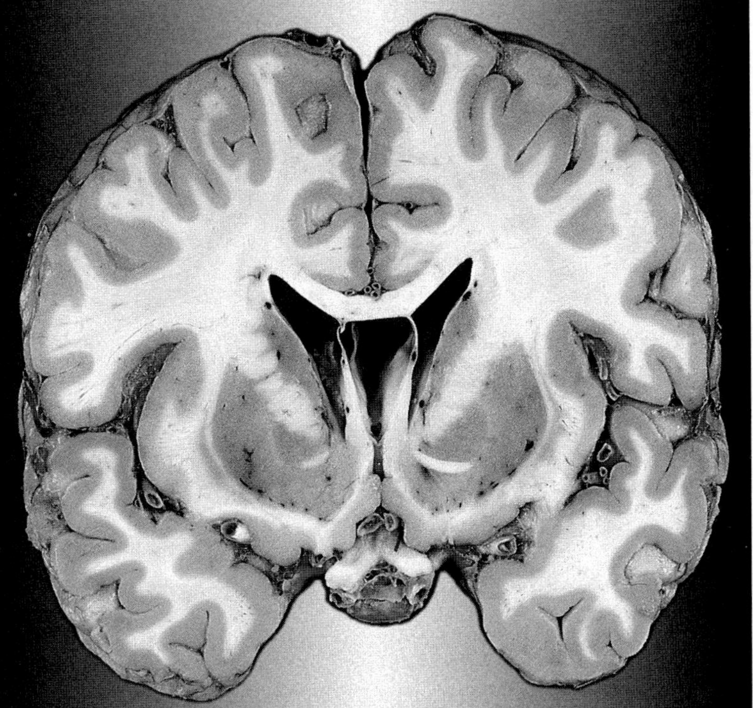

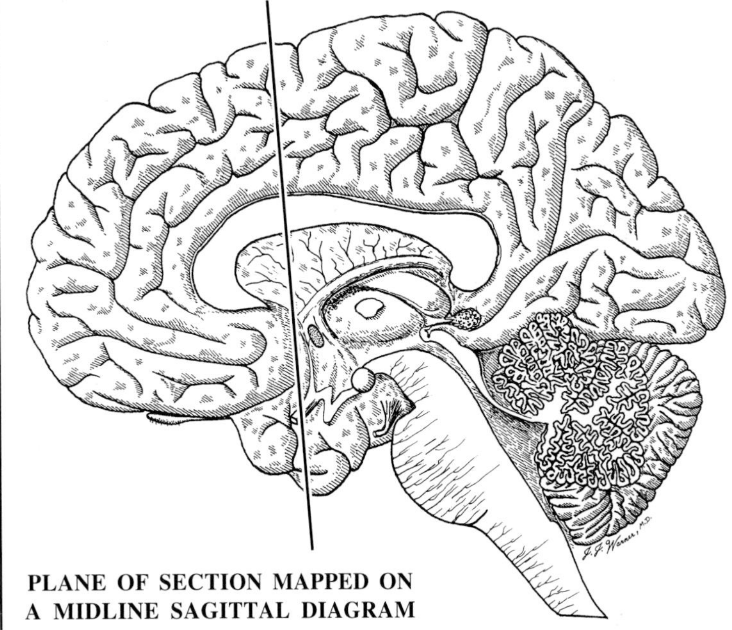

PLANE OF SECTION MAPPED ON A MIDLINE SAGITTAL DIAGRAM

KEY TO NUMBERED STRUCTURES

1. Anterior Cerebral Artery
2. Pituitary Gland
3. Optic Nerve
4. Termination of Olfactory Tract
5. Anterior Perforated Substance
6. Paraterminal Gyrus
7. Middle Cerebral Artery
8. Middle Temporal Sulcus
9. Middle Temporal Gyrus
10. Superior Temporal Sulcus
11. Superior Temporal Gyrus
12. Sylvian Fissure
13. Insular Cortex
14. Inferior Frontal Convolution
15. Circular Sulcus
16. Transcapsular Caudatolenticular Gray Stria
17. Globus Pallidus
18. Middle Frontal Convolution
19. Longitudinal Vein
20. Septal Nuclei
21. Corpus Callosum
22. Cavum Septum Pellucidum
23. Cingulate Gyrus
24. Superior Frontal Convolution
25. Fornix
26. Septum Pellucidum (dual structure on either side of the Cavum)
27. Body of the Lateral Ventricle
28. Caudate Nucleus
29. Anterior Limb of the Internal Capsule
30. Putamen
31. Lamina Terminalis
32. Extreme Capsule
33. External Capsule
34. External Medullary Lamina
35. Middle Cerebral Artery branches
36. Claustrum
37. Lenticulostriate Arteries arising from the Middle Cerebral Artery
38. Middle Cerebral Artery
39. Anterior Commissure
40. Nucleus Basalis of Meynert* (contiguous with the caudal aspect of the Nucleus Accumbens)
41. Supraclinoid segment of the Internal Carotid Artery

*Although the anatomic demarcation of the nucleus basalis of Meynert from the nucleus accumbens is not easily identified on gross sections, it may be clearly demonstrated using histochemical techniques. The nucleus basalis is adjacent to the anterior commissure, whereas the nucleus accumbens is more rostrally situated, ventral to the anterior limb of the internal capsule. The nucleus basalis of Meynert contains cholinergic neurons with widely distributed projections to the cerebral cortex. Neuronal loss in the nucleus basalis, accompanied by a decrease of choline acetyltransferase activity, has been observed in Alzheimer's disease.

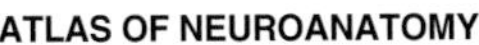

CORONAL SECTION OF THE BRAIN: MAGNIFIED ROSTRAL TO CAUDAL VIEW OF THE PITUITARY AND OF THE ANTERIOR CEREBRAL, MIDDLE CEREBRAL, AND INTERNAL CAROTID ARTERIES

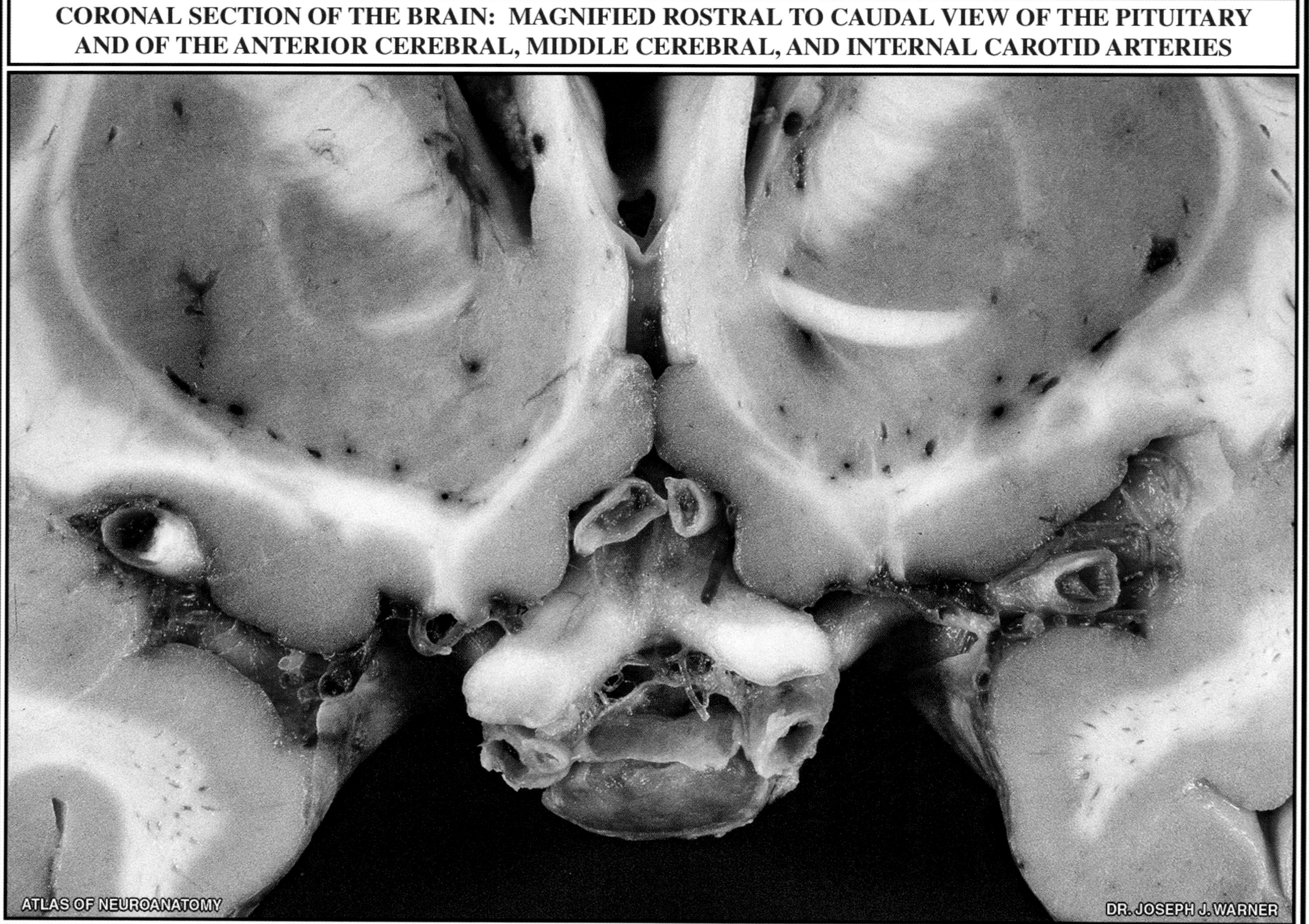

CORONAL SECTION OF A BRAIN WITH CAVUM SEPTUM PELLUCIDUM, PITUITARY INTACT: LEVEL OF THE NUCLEUS BASALIS OF MEYNERT; MAGNIFIED ROSTRAL TO CAUDAL VIEW DEMONSTRATING THE PITUITARY AND THE ANTERIOR CEREBRAL, MIDDLE CEREBRAL, AND INTERNAL CAROTID ARTERIES

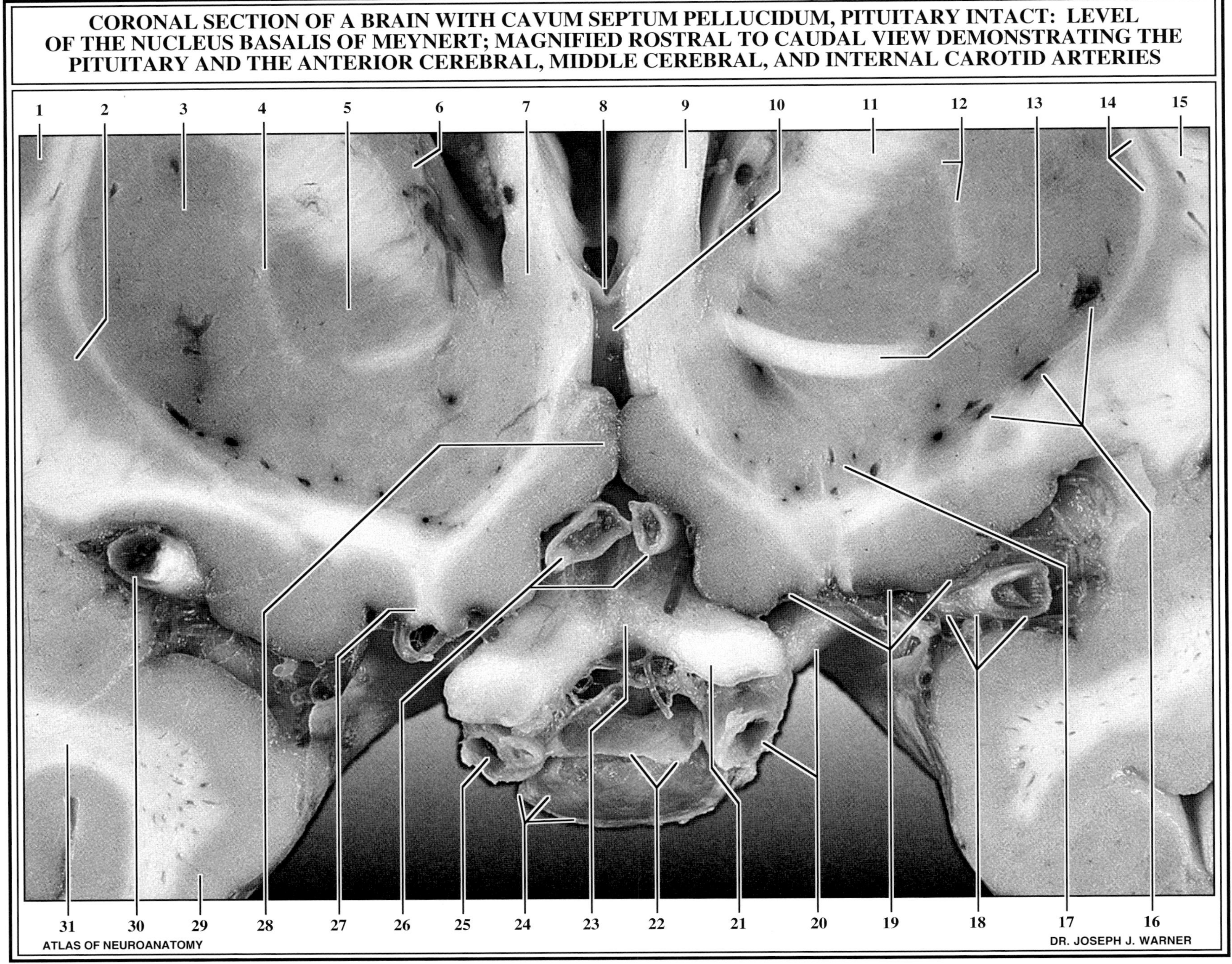

CORONAL SECTION OF A BRAIN WITH CAVUM SEPTUM PELLUCIDUM, PITUITARY INTACT: LEVEL OF THE NUCLEUS BASALIS OF MEYNERT, ROSTRAL TO CAUDAL VIEW DEMONSTRATING THE PITUITARY AND THE ANTERIOR CEREBRAL, MIDDLE CEREBRAL, AND INTERNAL CAROTID ARTERIES

KEY TO NUMBERED STRUCTURES

1. Insular Cortex
2. Claustrum
3. Putamen
4. External Medullary Lamina
5. Globus Pallidus
6. Caudate Nucleus
7. Septal Nuclei
8. Lamina Terminalis
9. Fornix (note relationship to dual Septum Pellucidum on either side of the Cavum)
10. Anterior Commissure (rostral contour)
11. Anterior Limb of the Internal Capsule
12. External Medullary Lamina
13. Anterior Commissure
14. External Capsule
15. Extreme Capsule
16. Lenticulostriate Arteries arising from the Middle Cerebral Artery
17. Nucleus Basalis of Meynert (contiguous with the caudal aspect of the Nucleus Accumbens)
18. Middle Cerebral Artery
19. Anterior Perforated Substance
20. Internal Carotid Artery (Supraclinoid segment)
21. Optic Nerve
22. Diaphragma Sellae
23. Optic Chiasm
24. Pituitary Gland
25. Internal Carotid Artery
26. Anterior Cerebral Arteries
27. Termination of the Olfactory Tract
28. Paraterminal Gyrus
29. Rostral aspect of the Parahippocampal Gyrus
30. Middle Cerebral Artery
31. White matter of the Temporal Pole

Relationships between the rostral aspect of the Circle of Willis, the pituitary gland, and the optic chiasm are demonstrated in this section. Each internal carotid artery courses lateral to the pituitary and continues dorsal to the sella turcica. The supraclinoid carotid artery gives rise to the posterior communicating and anterior cerebral arteries. This section demonstrates the anterior cerebral arteries dorsal to the optic chiasm. Lenticulostriate arteries originate from the middle cerebral arteries as the latter vessels course laterally toward the Sylvian fissure.

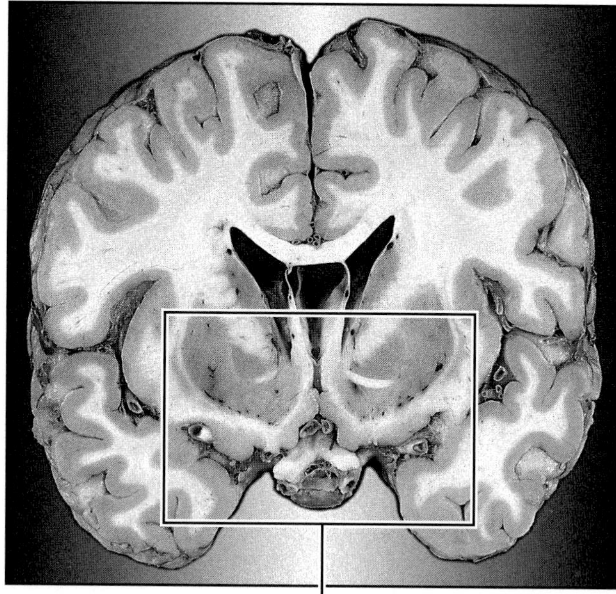

AREA OF MAGNIFIED VIEW

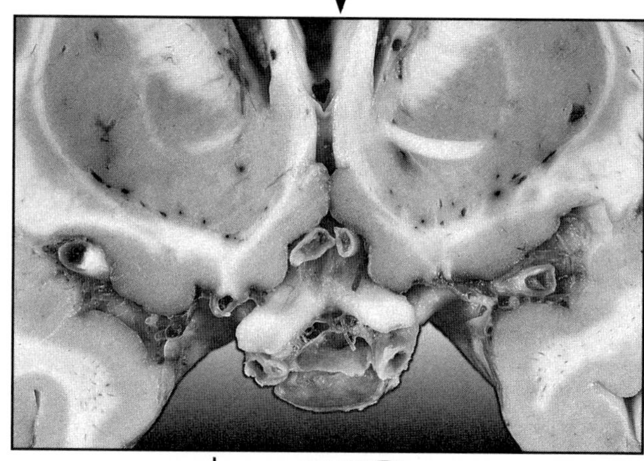

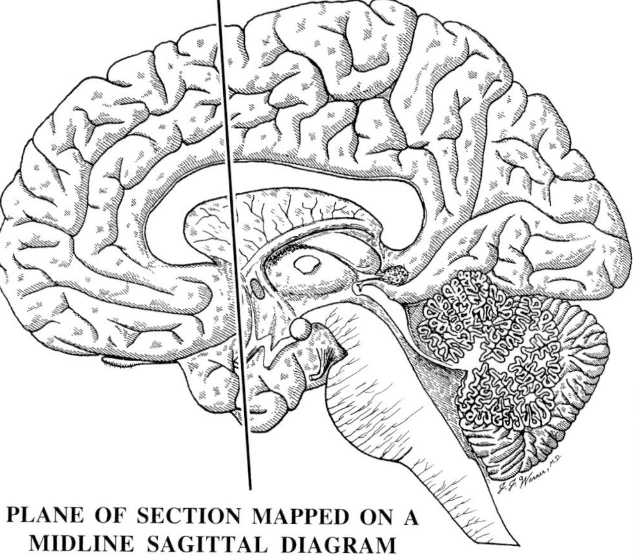

PLANE OF SECTION MAPPED ON A MIDLINE SAGITTAL DIAGRAM

CORONAL SECTION OF THE BRAIN, COMPLETE; LEVEL OF THE ANTERIOR COMMISSURE AND OPTIC CHIASM: CAUDAL TO ROSTRAL PERSPECTIVE

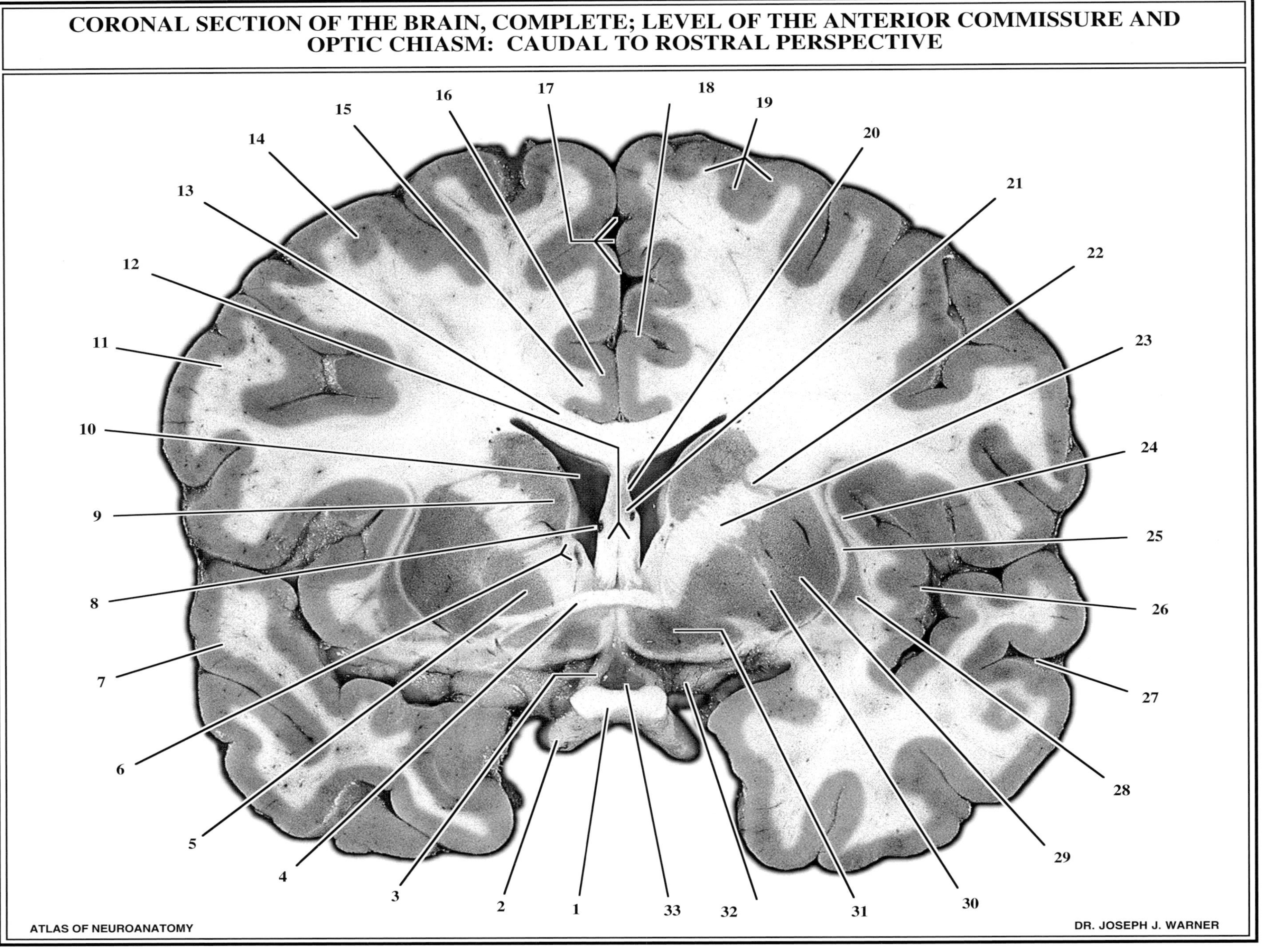

ATLAS OF NEUROANATOMY

DR. JOSEPH J. WARNER

CORONAL SECTION OF THE BRAIN, COMPLETE; LEVEL INCLUDING THE ANTERIOR COMMISSURE AND OPTIC CHIASM: SECTION ORIENTATION AND KEY TO NUMBERED STRUCTURES

KEY TO NUMBERED STRUCTURES

1. Optic Chiasm
2. Optic Nerve
3. Lamina Terminalis
4. Anterior Commissure
5. Globus Pallidus II
6. Stria Terminalis and rostral curve of Thalamostriate Vein (adjacent to venous angle)*
7. Superior Temporal Gyrus
8. Septal Vein
9. Head of the Caudate Nucleus
10. Anterior Horn of the Lateral Ventricle
11. Inferior Frontal Convolution
12. Fornices
13. Corpus Callosum
14. Middle Frontal Convolution
15. Cingulum
16. Cortex of the Cingulate Gyrus
17. Interhemispheric Fissure
18. Cingulate Sulcus
19. Superior Frontal Convolution
20. Septum Pellucidum
21. Septal Nuclei
22. Transcapsular Caudato-lenticular Gray Stria
23. Anterior Limb of the Internal Capsule
24. Extreme Capsule
25. External Capsule
26. Insular Cortex
27. Superior Temporal Sulcus
28. Claustrum
29. Putamen
30. External Medullary Lamina
31. Nucleus Basalis of Meynert
32. Ventral Surface of Anterior Perforated Substance
33. Supraoptic Recess of the Third Ventricle

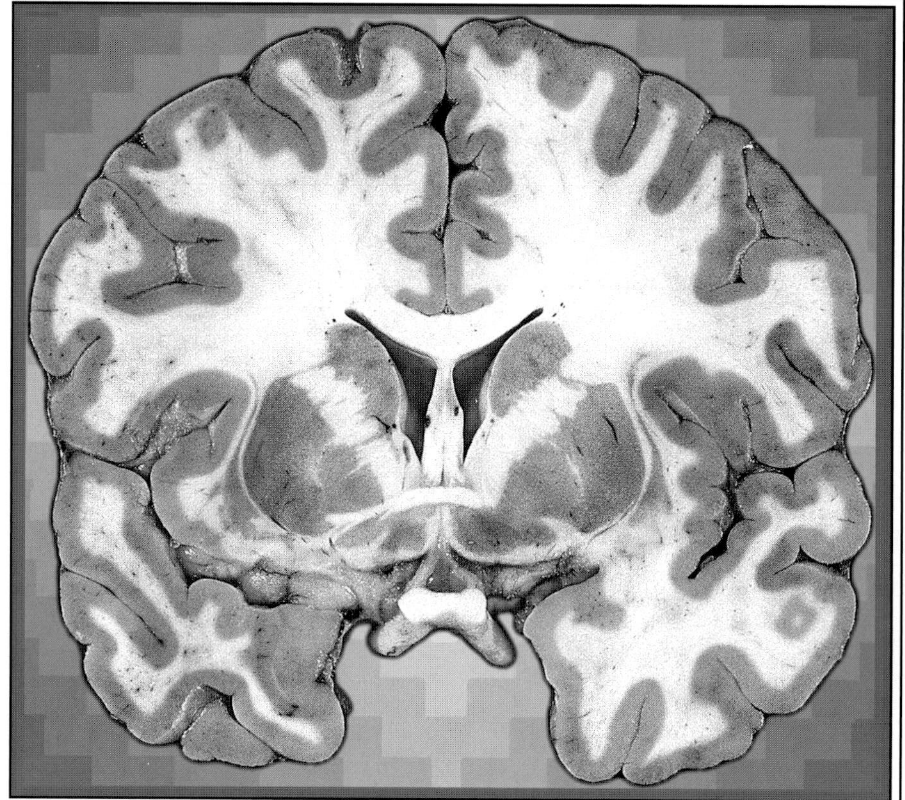

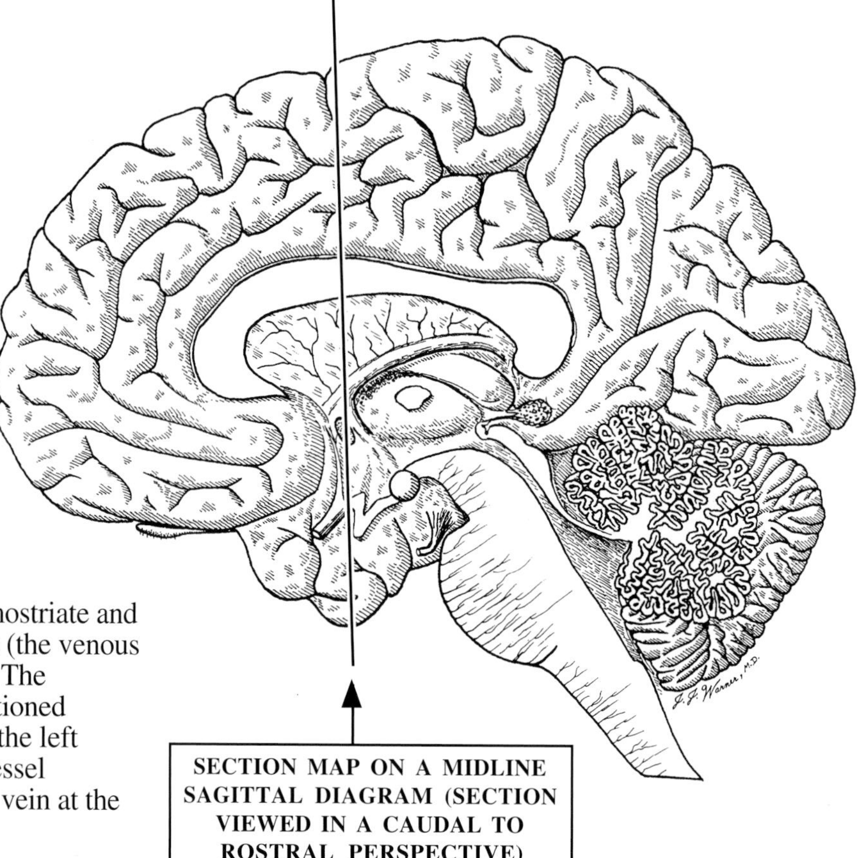

* Anatomic variations of the thalamostriate and septal veins and of their confluence (the venous angle) are frequently encountered. The thalamostriate vein is obliquely sectioned rostral to the foramen of Monro in the left hemisphere of this section. This vessel generally joins the ipsilateral septal vein at the foramen of Monro.

SECTION MAP ON A MIDLINE SAGITTAL DIAGRAM (SECTION VIEWED IN A CAUDAL TO ROSTRAL PERSPECTIVE)

CORONAL SECTION, LEVEL OF THE GENU AND ANTERIOR LIMB OF THE INTERNAL CAPSULE: MAGNIFIED VIEW INCLUDING THE CAUDATE, THE AMYGDALA, THE LENTICULAR NUCLEI (PUTAMEN AND GLOBUS PALLIDUS), AND THE ANSA LENTICULARIS

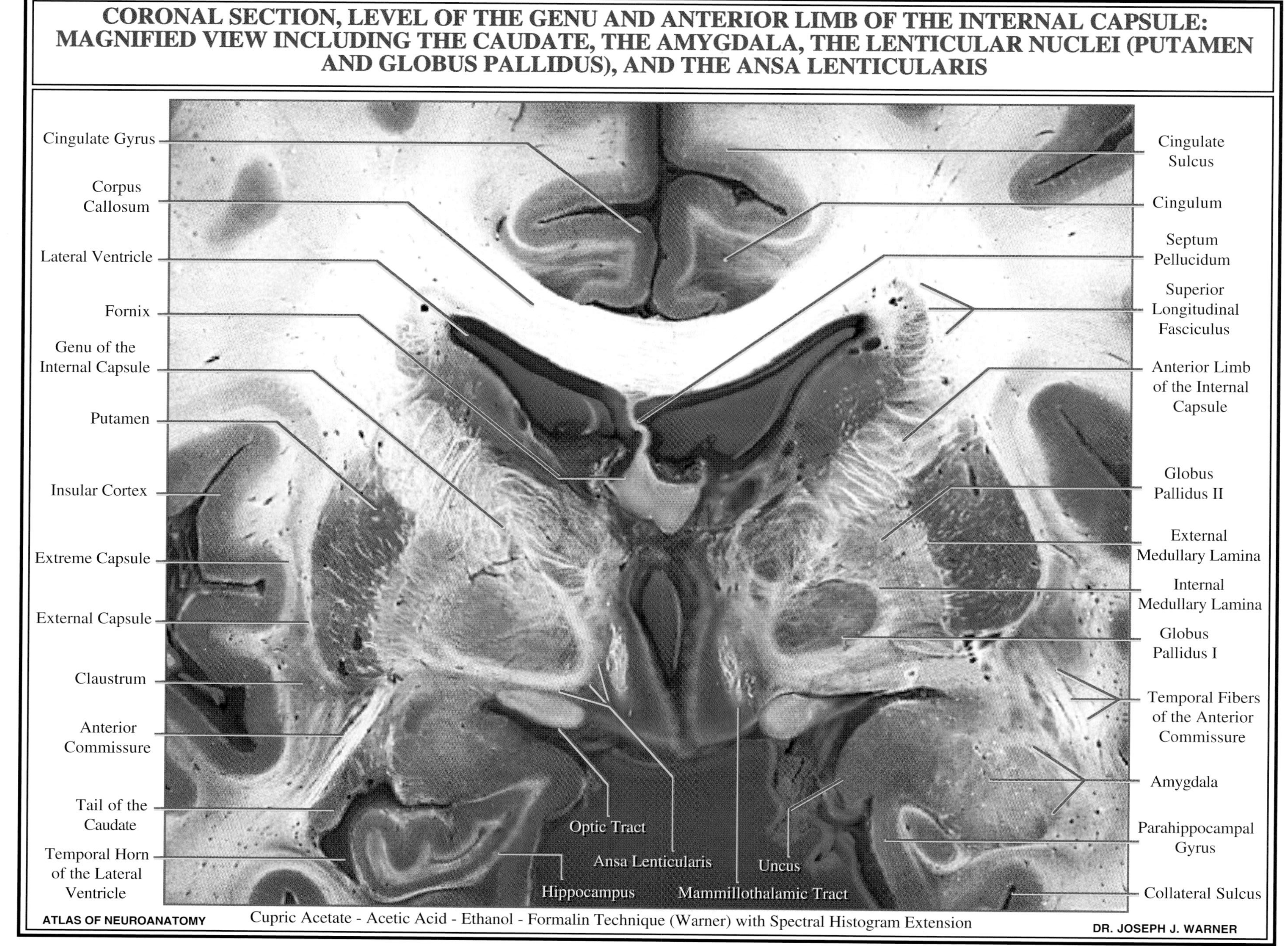

Cupric Acetate - Acetic Acid - Ethanol - Formalin Technique (Warner) with Spectral Histogram Extension

CORONAL SECTION OF THE BRAIN, COMPLETE: LEVEL OF THE MAMMILLARY BODIES AND THE ANTERIOR NUCLEUS OF THE THALAMUS, ROSTRAL TO CAUDAL PERSPECTIVE

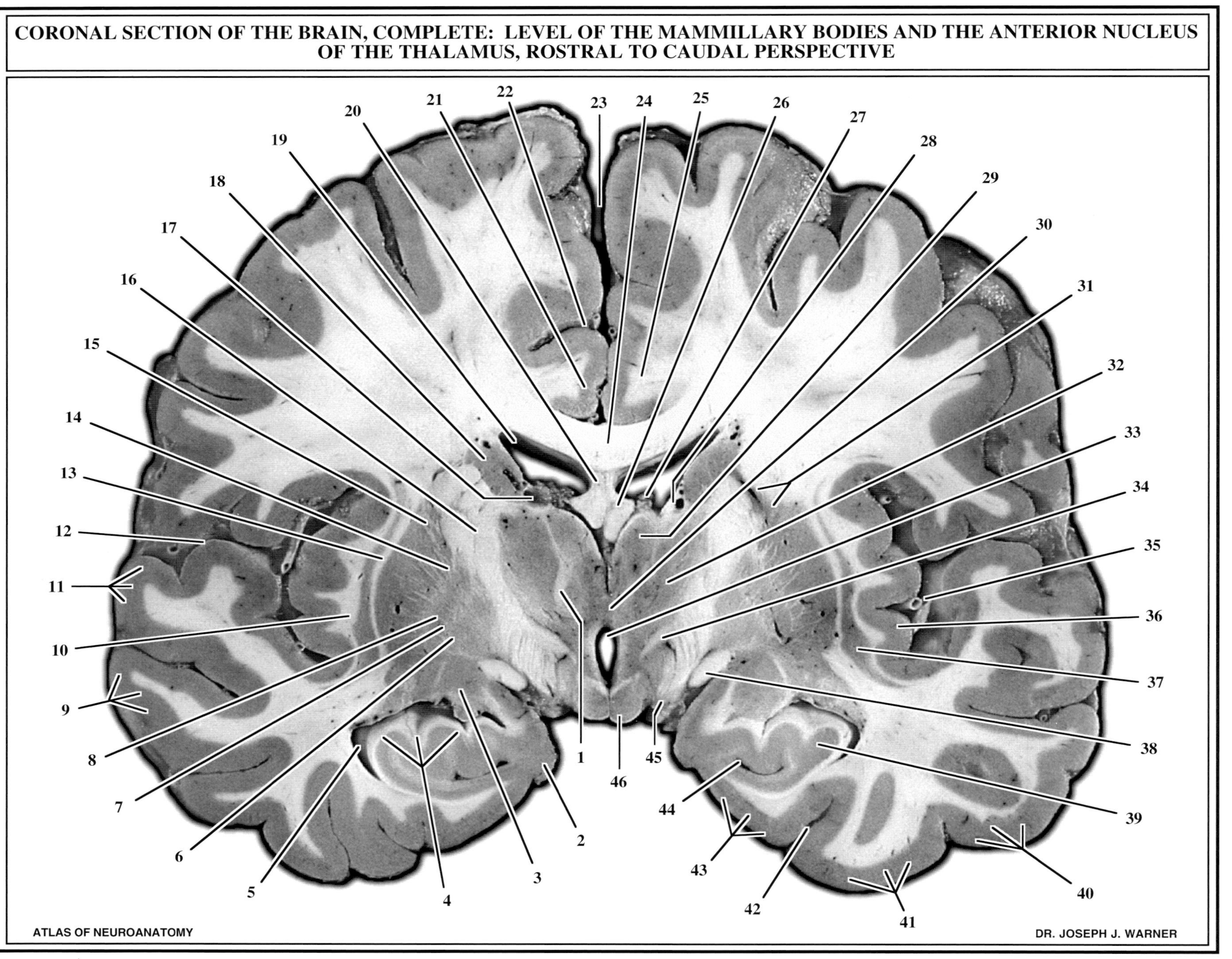

ATLAS OF NEUROANATOMY

DR. JOSEPH J. WARNER

CORONAL SECTION OF THE BRAIN, COMPLETE; LEVEL OF THE MAMMILLARY BODIES AND OF THE ANTERIOR NUCLEUS OF THE THALAMUS: SECTION ORIENTATION AND KEY TO NUMBERED STRUCTURES

KEY TO NUMBERED STRUCTURES

1. Mammillothalamic Tract
2. Uncus
3. Amygdala
4. Alveus
5. Temporal Horn of the Lateral Ventricle
6. Globus Pallidus I
7. Internal Medullary Lamina
8. Globus Pallidus II
9. Middle Temporal Gyrus
10. Extreme Capsule
11. Superior Temporal Gyrus
12. Sylvian Fissure
13. External Capsule
14. External Medullary Lamina
15. Putamen
16. Posterior Limb of the Internal Capsule
17. Thalamostriate Vein
18. Caudate Nucleus
19. Body of the Lateral Ventricle
20. Septum Pellucidum
21. Cingulate Cortex
22. Cingulate Sulcus
23. Interhemispheric Fissure
24. Corpus Callosum
25. Cingulum
26. Fornix
27. Choroid Plexus
28. Stria Terminalis and Thalamostriate Vein
29. Anterior Nucleus of the Thalamus
30. Massa Intermedia
31. Transcapsular Caudatolenticular Gray Stria
32. Ventroanterior Nucleus of the Thalamus
33. Third Ventricle
34. Lenticular Fasciculus
35. Middle Cerebral Artery
36. Insular Cortex
37. Claustrum
38. Optic Tract
39. Hippocampus
40. Inferior Temporal Gyrus
41. Fusiform Gyrus
42. Collateral Sulcus
43. Parahippocampal Gyrus
44. Hippocampal Fissure
45. Cerebral Peduncle
46. Mammillary Body

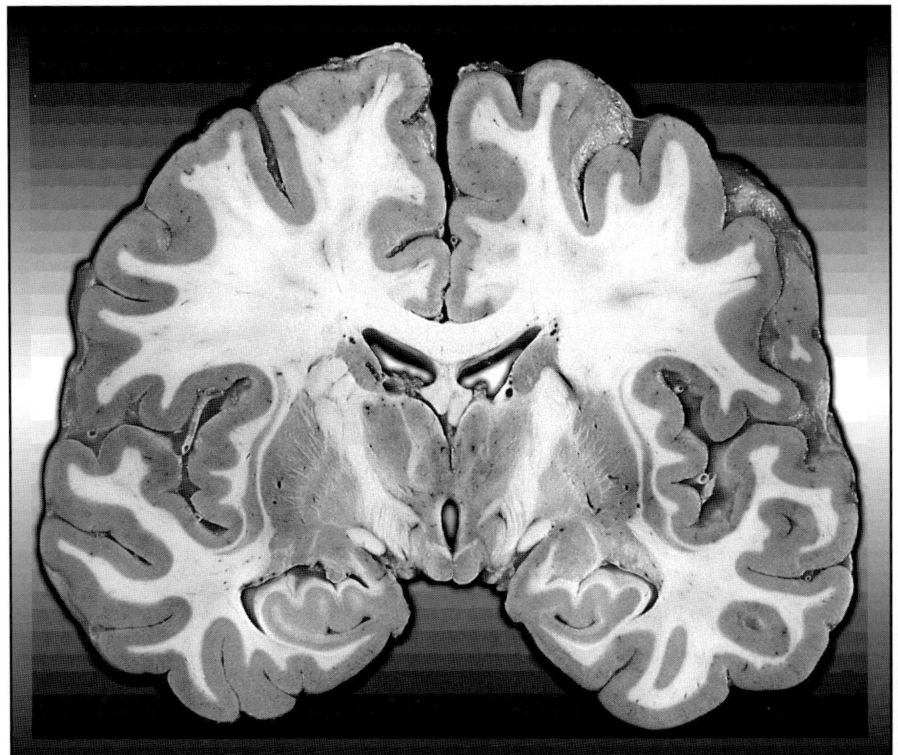

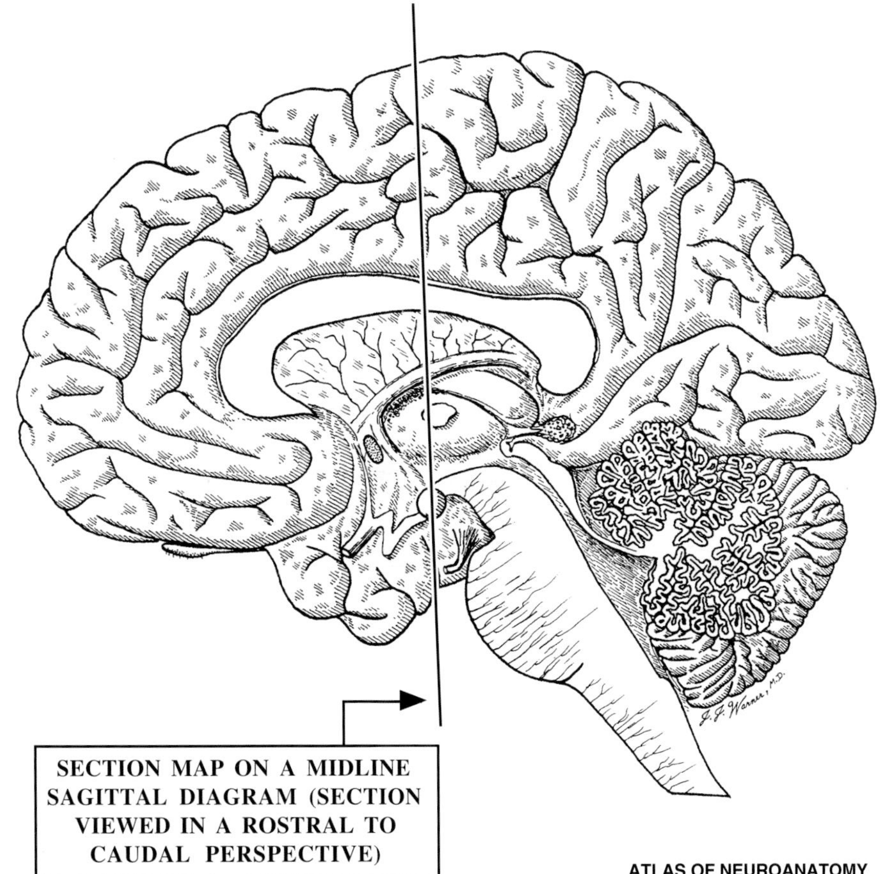

SECTION MAP ON A MIDLINE SAGITTAL DIAGRAM (SECTION VIEWED IN A ROSTRAL TO CAUDAL PERSPECTIVE)

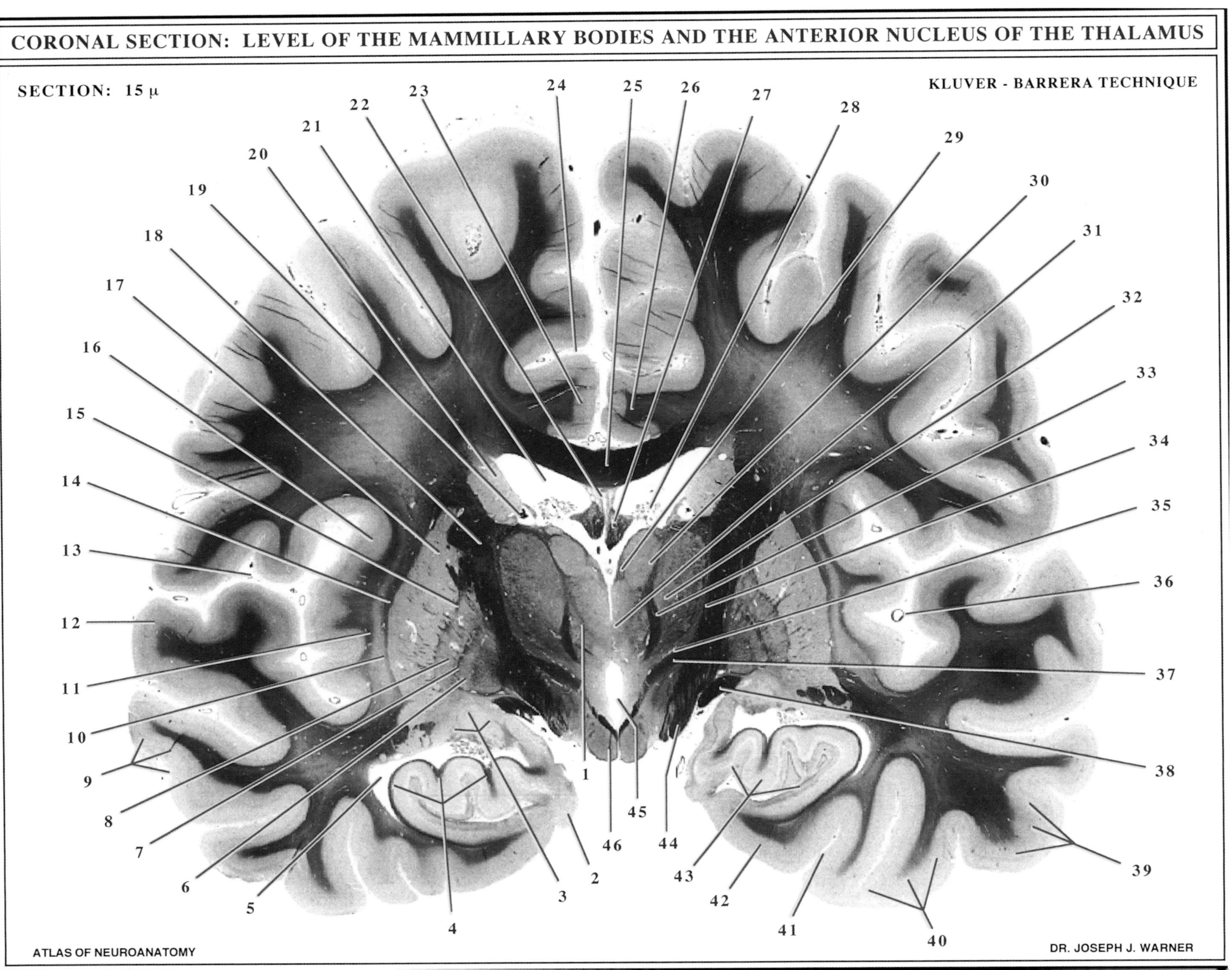
CORONAL SECTION: LEVEL OF THE MAMMILLARY BODIES AND THE ANTERIOR NUCLEUS OF THE THALAMUS
SECTION: 15 μ
KLUVER - BARRERA TECHNIQUE
1
2
3
4
5
6
7
8
9
10
11
12
13
14
15
16
17
18
19
20
21
22
23
24
25
26
27
28
29
30
31
32
33
34
35
36
37
38
39
40
41
42
43
44
45
46
ATLAS OF NEUROANATOMY
DR. JOSEPH J. WARNER

COMPLETE CORONAL SECTION OF THE BRAIN, LEVEL OF THE MAMMILLARY BODIES AND THE ANTERIOR NUCLEUS OF THE THALAMUS: 15μ, KLUVER - BARRERA TECHNIQUE

KEY TO NUMBERED STRUCTURES

1. Internal Medullary Lamina of the Thalamus
2. Uncus
3. Amygdala
4. Alveus (fibers of the Fornix)
5. Temporal Horn, Lateral Ventricle
6. Globus Pallidus I
7. Internal Medullary Lamina
8. Globus Pallidus II
9. Middle Temporal Gyrus
10. Claustrum
11. Extreme Capsule
12. Superior Temporal Gyrus
13. Sylvian Fissure
14. External Capsule
15. External Medullary Lamina
16. Insular Cortex
17. Putamen
18. Internal Capsule, Posterior Limb
19. Thalamostriate Vein (adjacent to Stria Terminalis)
20. Caudate Nucleus
21. Body of the Lateral Ventricle
22. Septum Pellucidum
23. Cingulate Cortex
24. Cingulate Sulcus
25. Corpus Callosum
26. Cingulum (White Matter)
27. Fornix
28. Choroid Plexus
29. Stria Medullaris
30. Anterior Nucleus of the Thalamus
31. Massa Intermedia
32. Ventroanterior Nucleus of the Thalamus
33. Mammillothalamic Tract
34. Reticular Nucleus of the Thalamus
35. Zona Incerta
36. Branch of the Middle Cerebral Artery
37. Lenticular Fasciculus
38. Optic Tract
39. Inferior Temporal Gyrus
40. Fusiform Gyrus
41. Collateral Sulcus
42. Parahippocampal Gyrus
43. Hippocampus (rostral aspect)
44. Cerebral Peduncle
45. Third Ventricle
46. Mammillary Body

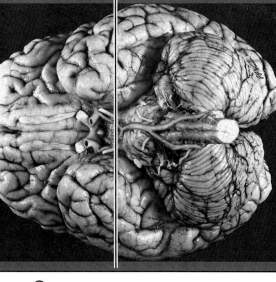

SECTION MAP ON VENTRAL ASPECT OF THE BRAIN

SECTION MAP ON MIDLINE SAGITTAL DIAGRAM

CORONAL SECTION OF THE BRAIN; LEVEL OF THE MAMMILLARY BODIES AND THE ANTERIOR NUCLEUS OF THE THALAMUS, ROSTRAL TO CAUDAL PERSPECTIVE: AREA OF MAGNIFIED VIEW

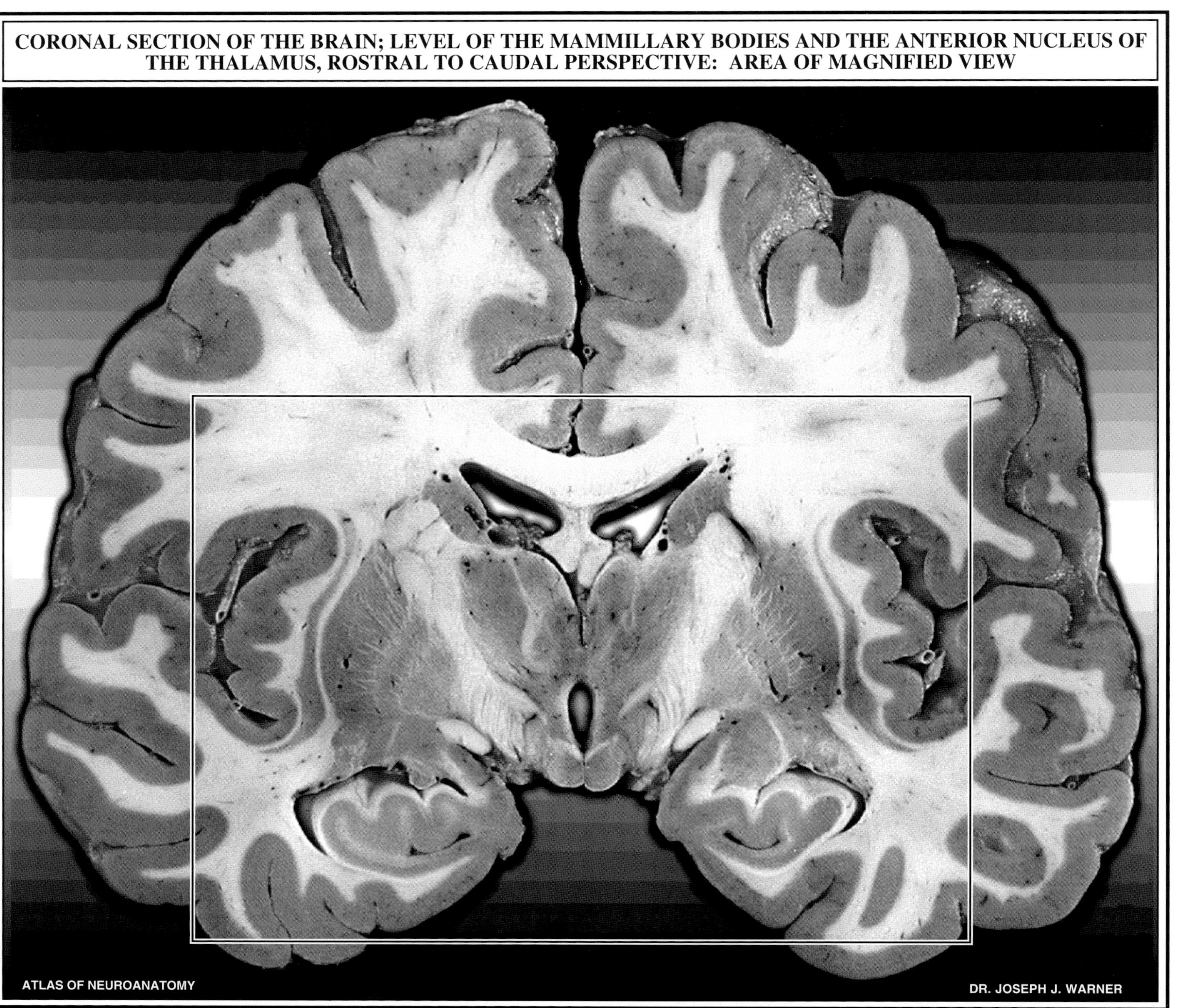

CORONAL SECTION, LEVEL OF THE ANTERIOR NUCLEUS OF THE THALAMUS AND THE MAMMILLARY BODIES

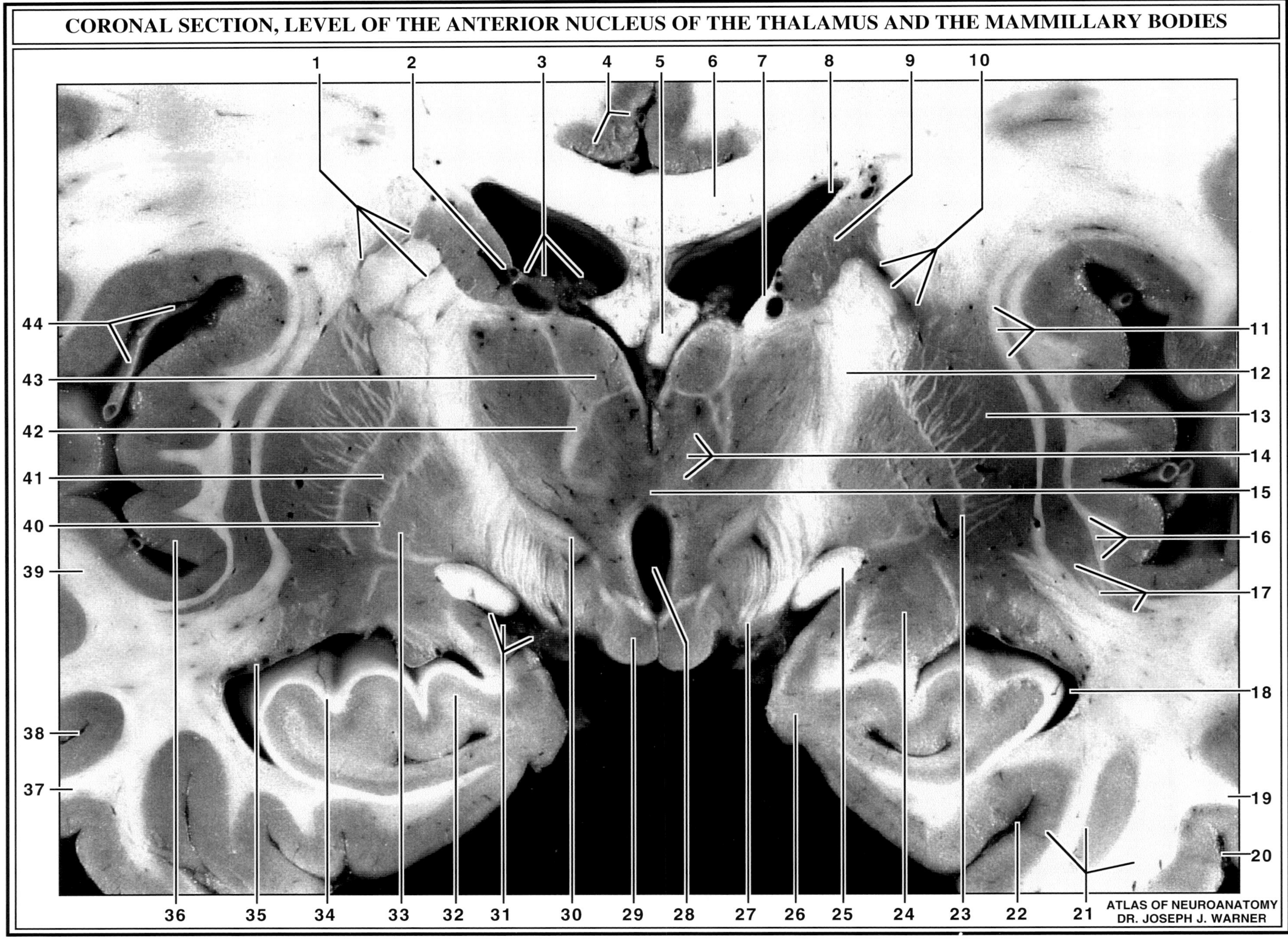

CORONAL SECTION OF THE BRAIN (MAGNIFIED VIEW), LEVEL OF THE ANTERIOR NUCLEUS OF THE THALAMUS AND THE MAMMILLARY BODIES: SECTION MAP AND KEY TO NUMBERED STRUCTURES

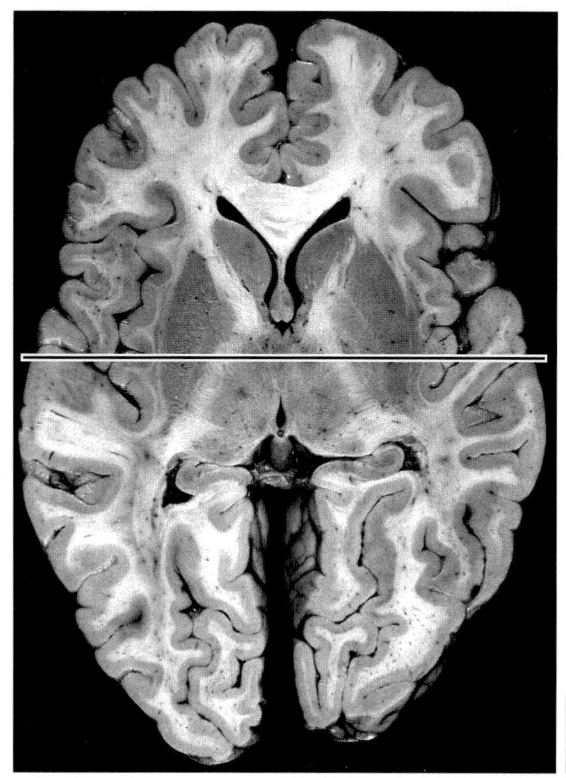

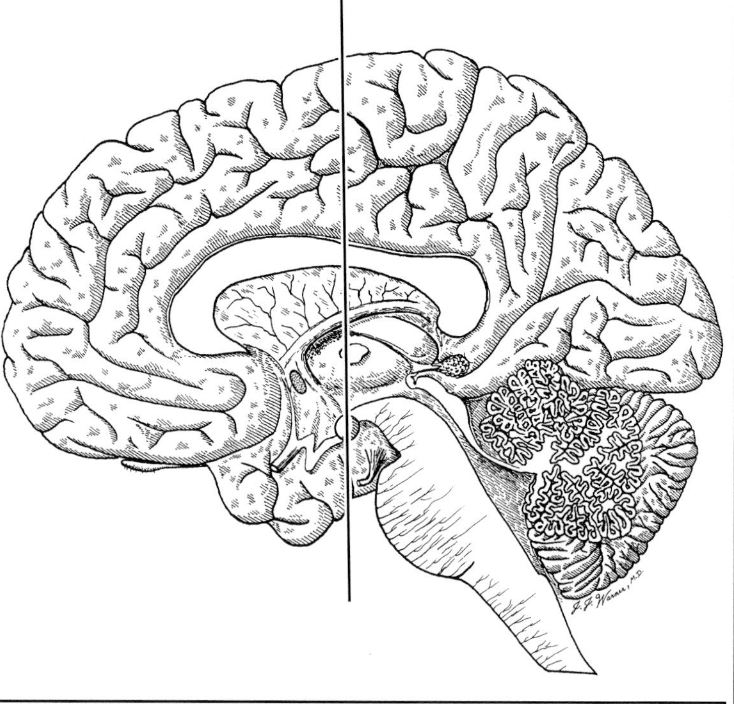

Coronal plane mapped in reference to a horizontal section (left) and to a midline sagittal diagram (above)

KEY TO NUMBERED STRUCTURES

1. Transcapsular Caudatolenticular Gray Striae
2. Thalamostriate Vein
3. Choroid Plexus
4. Cingulate Gyrus
5. Fornix
6. Corpus Callosum
7. Stria Terminalis
8. Lateral Ventricle
9. Caudate Nucleus
10. Transcapsular Caudatolenticular Gray Striae
11. External Capsule
12. Internal Capsule, Posterior Limb
13. Putamen
14. Internal Medullary Lamina of the Thalamus
15. Massa Intermedia
16. Extreme Capsule
17. Claustrum
18. Temporal Horn of the Lateral Ventricle
19. Inferior Temporal Gyrus
20. Inferior Temporal Sulcus
21. Fusiform Gyrus
22. Collateral Sulcus
23. External Medullary Lamina
24. Amygdala
25. Optic Tract
26. Uncus
27. Cerebral Peduncle
28. Third Ventricle
29. Mammillary Body
30. Lenticular Fasciculus
31. Choroidal Fissure (rostral aspect)
32. Hippocampal Formation
33. Globus Pallidus I
34. Alveus
35. Tail of the Caudate
36. Insular Cortex
37. Inferior Temporal Gyrus
38. Middle Temporal Sulcus
39. Superior Temporal Gyrus
40. Internal Medullary Lamina
41. Globus Pallidus II
42. Mammillothalamic Tract
43. Anterior Nucleus of the Thalamus
44. Middle Cerebral Artery (branch within the Sylvian Fissure)

CORONAL SECTION, LEVEL INCLUDING THE SUBTHALAMIC NUCLEUS (ROSTRAL ASPECT), MAMMILLARY BODIES, AND TRANSITION FROM THE ANTERIOR NUCLEUS TO THE LATERAL DORSAL NUCLEUS OF THE THALAMUS

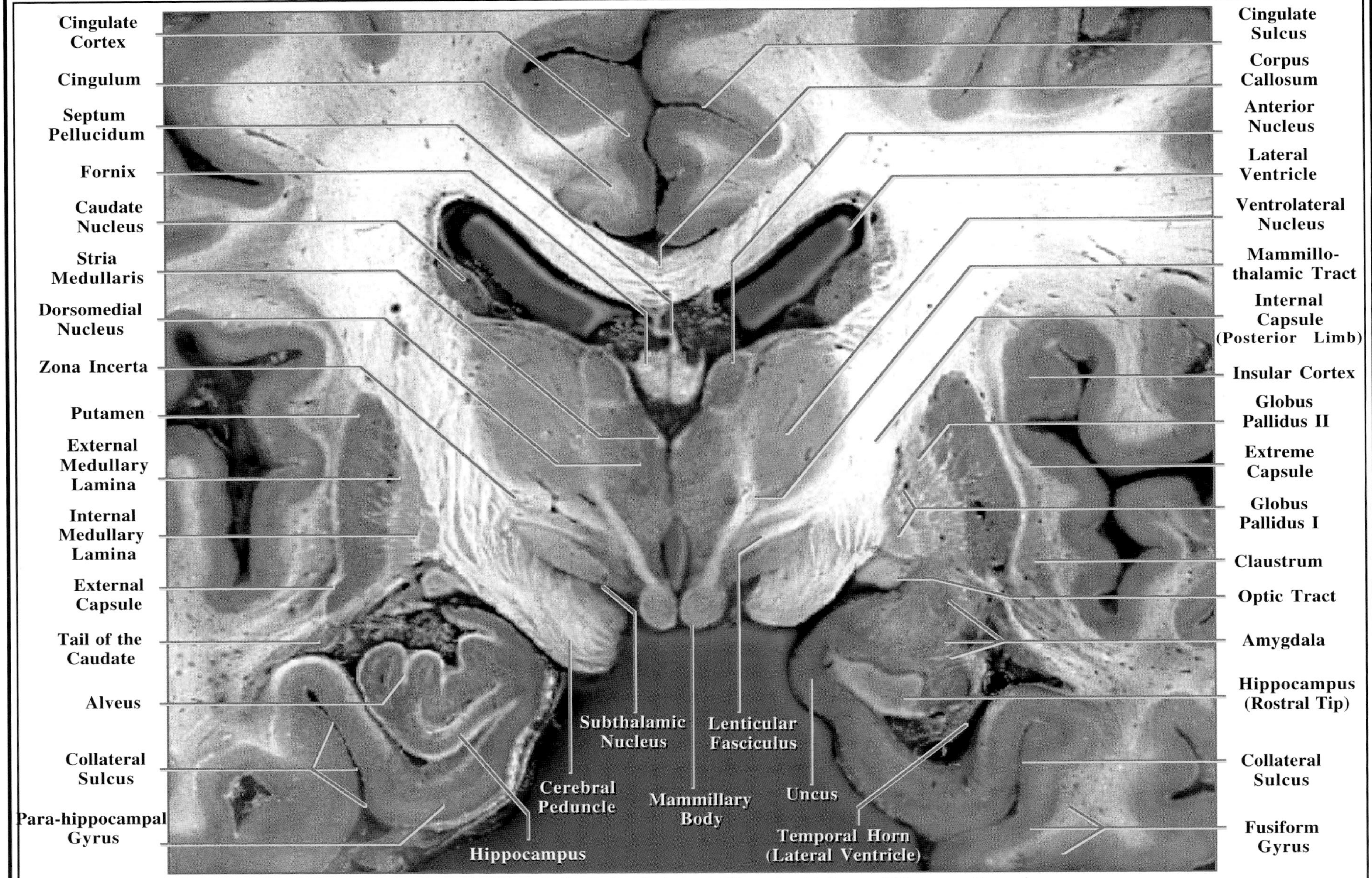

Cingulate Cortex
Cingulum
Septum Pellucidum
Fornix
Caudate Nucleus
Stria Medullaris
Dorsomedial Nucleus
Zona Incerta
Putamen
External Medullary Lamina
Internal Medullary Lamina
External Capsule
Tail of the Caudate
Alveus
Collateral Sulcus
Para-hippocampal Gyrus
Hippocampus
Cerebral Peduncle
Subthalamic Nucleus
Mammillary Body
Lenticular Fasciculus
Uncus
Temporal Horn (Lateral Ventricle)
Cingulate Sulcus
Corpus Callosum
Anterior Nucleus
Lateral Ventricle
Ventrolateral Nucleus
Mammillo-thalamic Tract
Internal Capsule (Posterior Limb)
Insular Cortex
Globus Pallidus II
Extreme Capsule
Globus Pallidus I
Claustrum
Optic Tract
Amygdala
Hippocampus (Rostral Tip)
Collateral Sulcus
Fusiform Gyrus

Cupric Acetate - Acetic Acid - Ethanol - Formalin Technique (Warner) with Spectral Histogram Extension

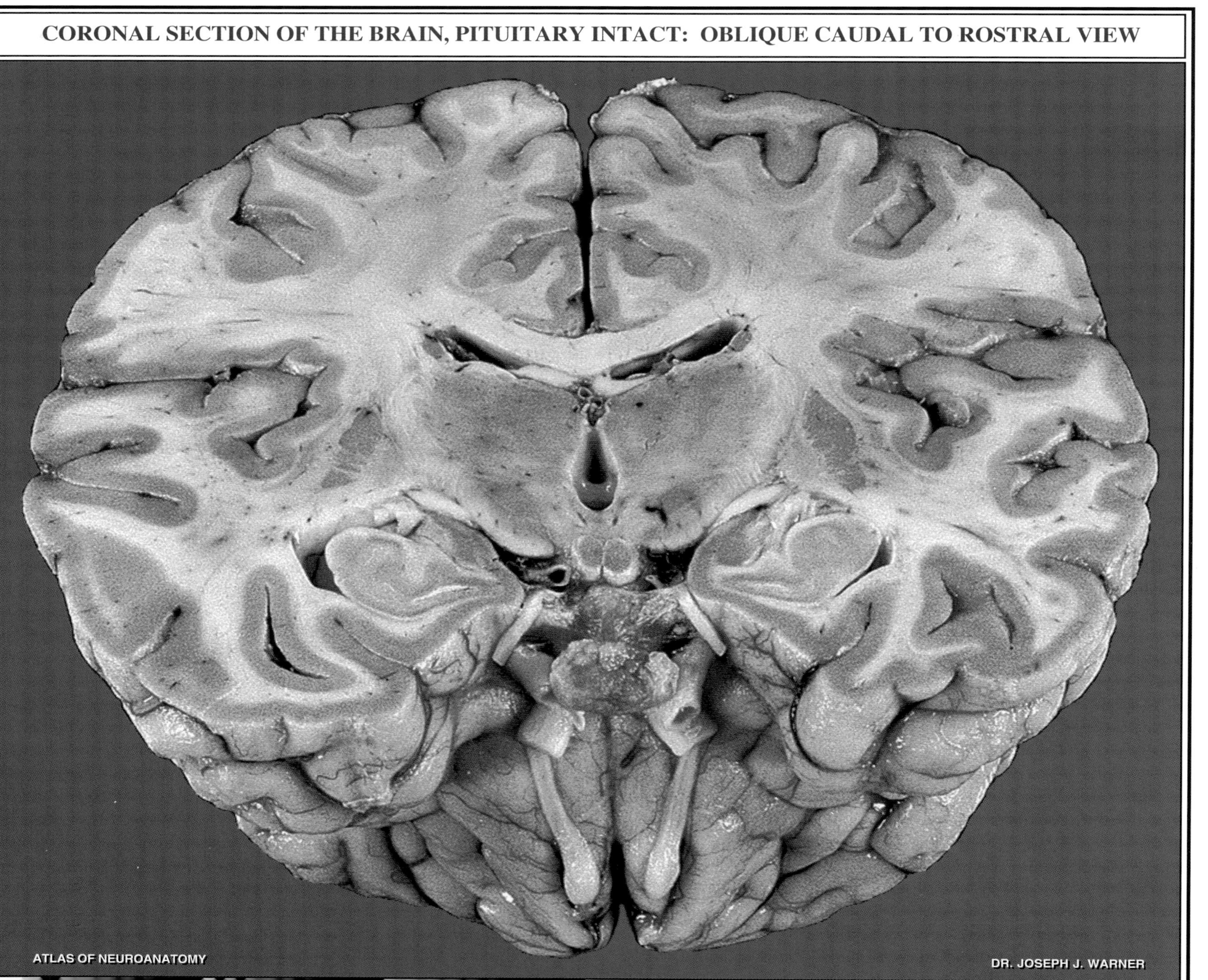
CORONAL SECTION OF THE BRAIN, PITUITARY INTACT: OBLIQUE CAUDAL TO ROSTRAL VIEW
ATLAS OF NEUROANATOMY
DR. JOSEPH J. WARNER

BRAIN SECTIONED IN THE CORONAL PLANE, LEVEL OF THE MAMMILLARY BODIES: OBLIQUE CAUDAL TO ROSTRAL PERSPECTIVE INCLUDING VENTRAL STRUCTURES

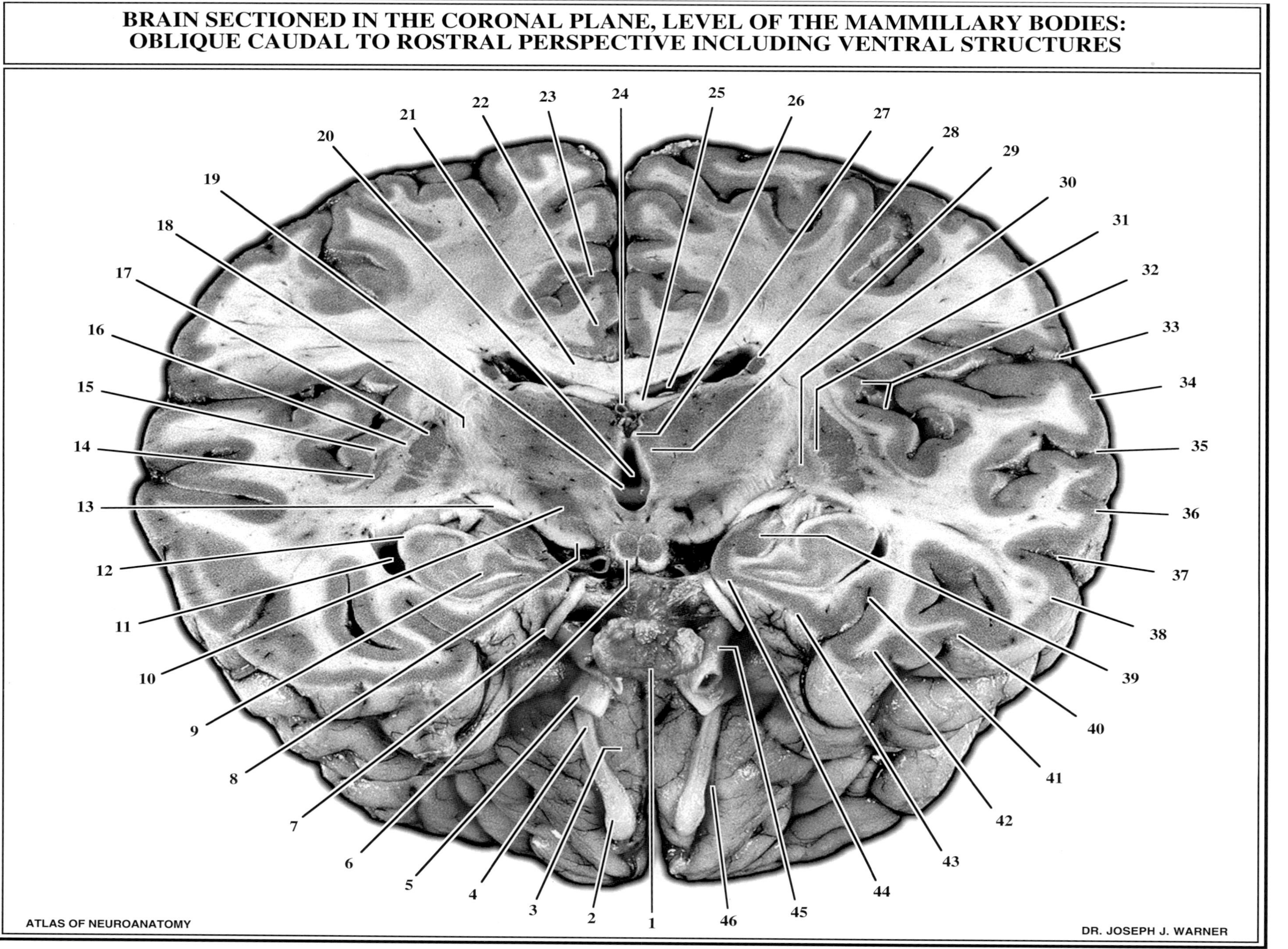

ATLAS OF NEUROANATOMY

DR. JOSEPH J. WARNER

BRAIN (WITH INTACT PITUITARY) SECTIONED IN THE CORONAL PLANE, LEVEL OF THE MAMMILLARY BODIES; VENTRAL OBLIQUE (CAUDAL TO ROSTRAL) PERSPECTIVE: SPECIMEN ORIENTATION

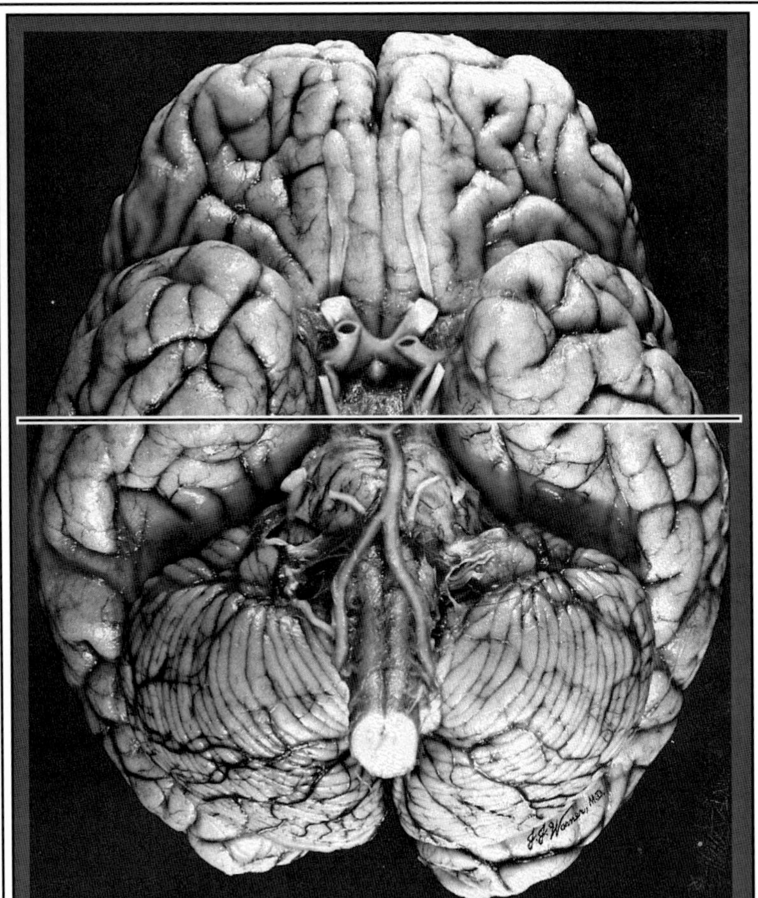

Examination of this type of dissection is essential to the achievement of a basic three-dimensional understanding of the relationships between structures that appear in sections and external anatomic landmarks. First, the position and orientation of the plane of section are approximated relative to the whole brain. The perspective or direction in which the specimen is viewed should then be established. Gyral and sulcal morphology may be studied by examination of the surface of the brain, then enhanced through the identification of these structures in sectioned specimens. The next step includes a careful study of the relationships between surface landmarks and subjacent neural and vascular structures. The position and appearance of specific structures should be made by cross-comparison with other planes of section. The process of examining three-dimensional neuroanatomic organization is facilitated by mapping the level and orientation of each section being examined on external views of the brain and on sections cut in different planes. This process avoids the "pattern recognition" method of learning (memorizing) certain planes of section.

The "pattern recognition" method of identifying structures on a given section is not conducive to the three-dimensional study of the brain. This method frequently results in structural misidentification due to anatomic variability between brains and variations in section orientation (e.g. not all coronal sections are created equal).

The plane of section of this specimen includes the caudal aspect of the mammillary bodies, the rostral aspect of the subthalamic nucleus, and the thalamus caudal to the massa intermedia. The configuration of the fornix (dorsal to the thalamus) in this section is flattened and juxtaposed to the inferior surface of the corpus callosum.

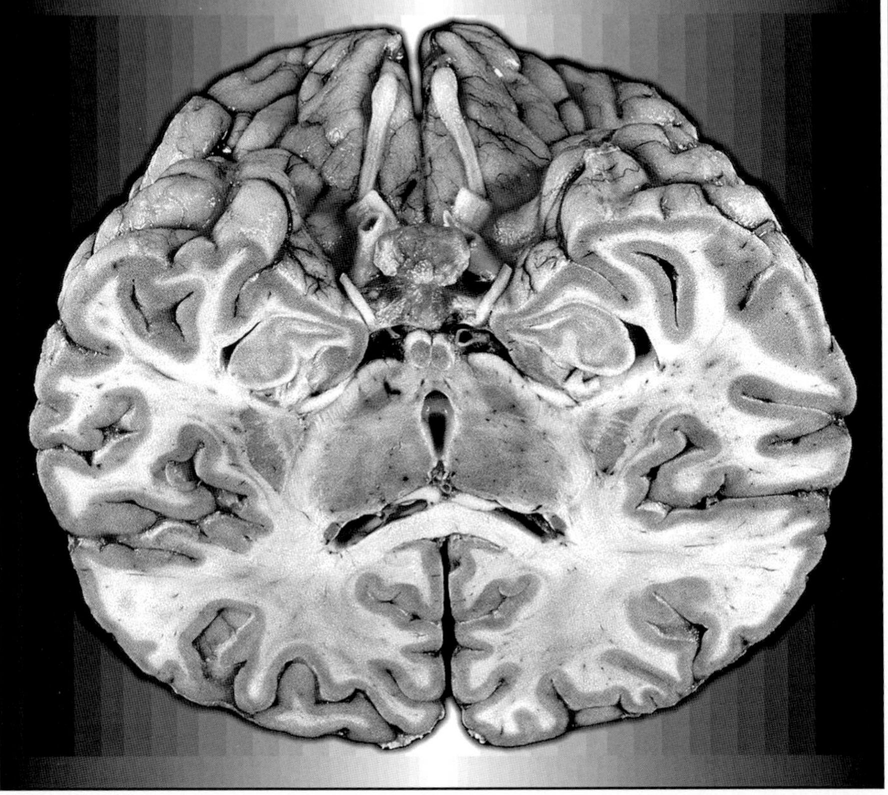

BRAIN (WITH INTACT PITUITARY) SECTIONED IN THE CORONAL PLANE, LEVEL OF THE MAMMILLARY BODIES; VENTRAL OBLIQUE (CAUDAL TO ROSTRAL) PERSPECTIVE: SPECIMEN ORIENTATION AND KEY TO NUMBERED STRUCTURES

KEY TO NUMBERED STRUCTURES

1. Pituitary Gland
2. Olfactory Bulb
3. Gyrus Rectus
4. Olfactory Tract
5. Optic (II) Nerve
6. Mammillary Body
7. Oculomotor (III) Nerve
8. Cerebral Peduncle
9. Hippocampus
10. Subthalamic Nucleus
11. Temporal Horn of the Lateral Ventricle
12. Alveus
13. Optic Tract
14. Claustrum
15. Extreme Capsule
16. External Capsule
17. Putamen
18. Posterior Limb of the Internal Capsule
19. Massa Intermedia
20. Third Ventricle
21. Body of the Corpus Callosum
22. Cingulate Cortex
23. Cingulate Sulcus
24. Internal Cerebral Vein
25. Fornix
26. Body of the Lateral Ventricle
27. Stria Medullaris
28. Caudate Nucleus
29. Dorsomedial Nucleus of the Thalamus
30. Globus Pallidus II
31. External Medullary Lamina
32. Insular Cortex
33. Sylvian Fissure
34. Superior Temporal Gyrus
35. Superior Temporal Sulcus
36. Middle Temporal Gyrus
37. Middle Temporal Sulcus
38. Inferior Temporal Gyrus
39. Amygdala
40. Inferior Temporal Sulcus
41. Collateral Fissure
42. Fusiform Gyrus
43. Parahippocampal Gyrus
44. Uncus
45. Internal Carotid Artery
46. Olfactory Sulcus

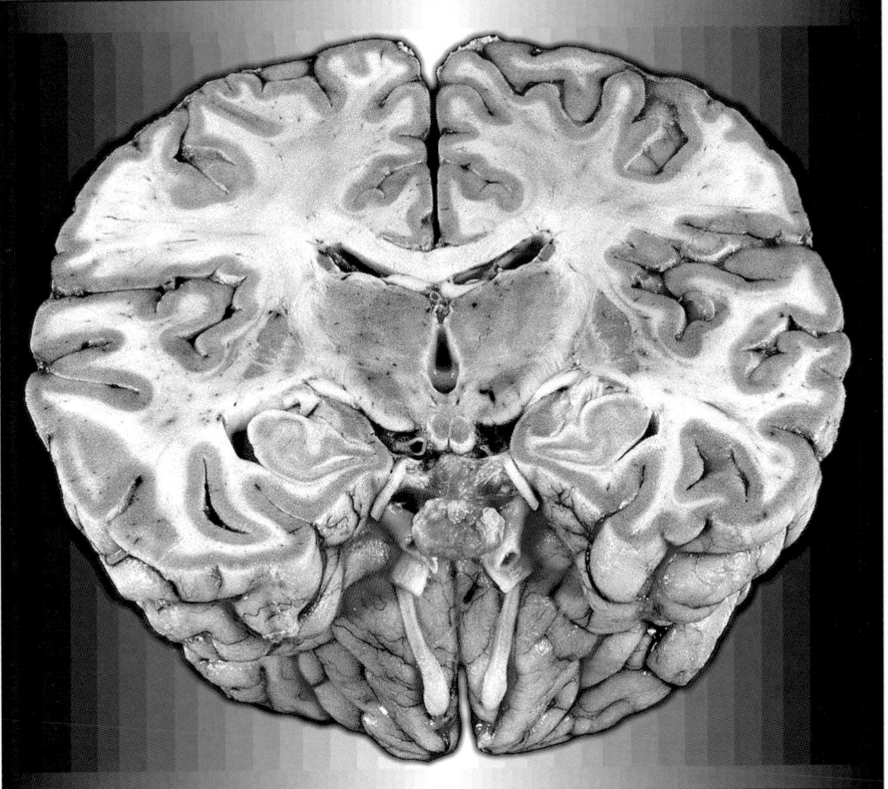

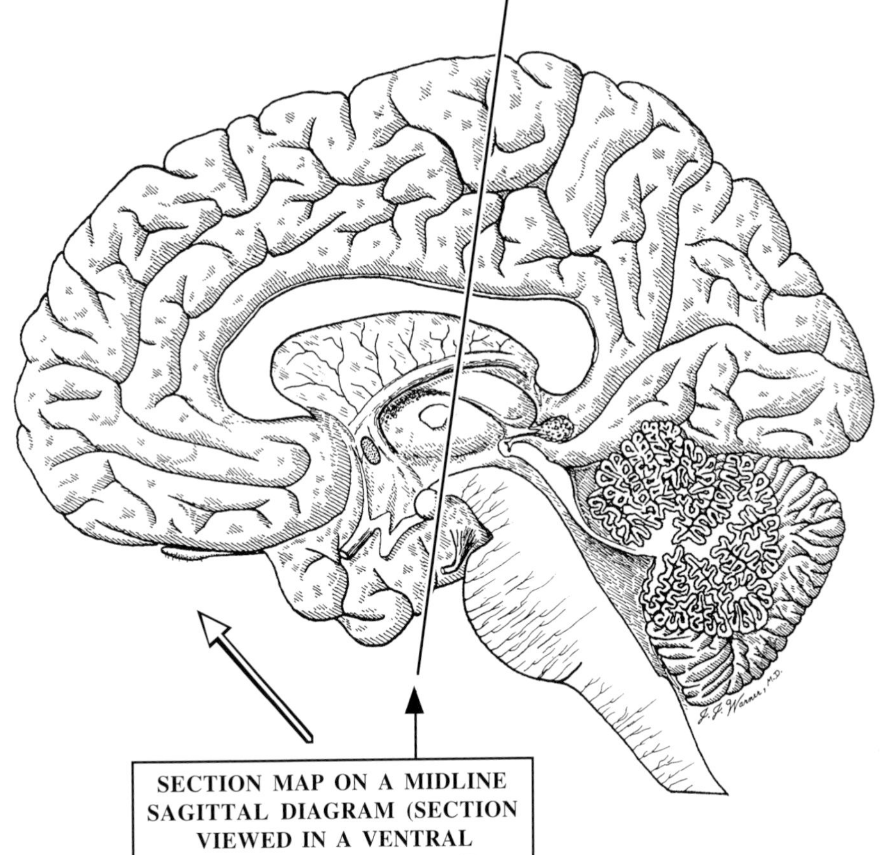

SECTION MAP ON A MIDLINE SAGITTAL DIAGRAM (SECTION VIEWED IN A VENTRAL OBLIQUE PERSPECTIVE)

CORONAL SECTION OF THE BRAIN; LEVEL INCLUDING THE SUBTHALAMIC NUCLEUS AND THE ROSTRAL ASPECT OF THE RED NUCLEUS: MAGNIFIED VIEW

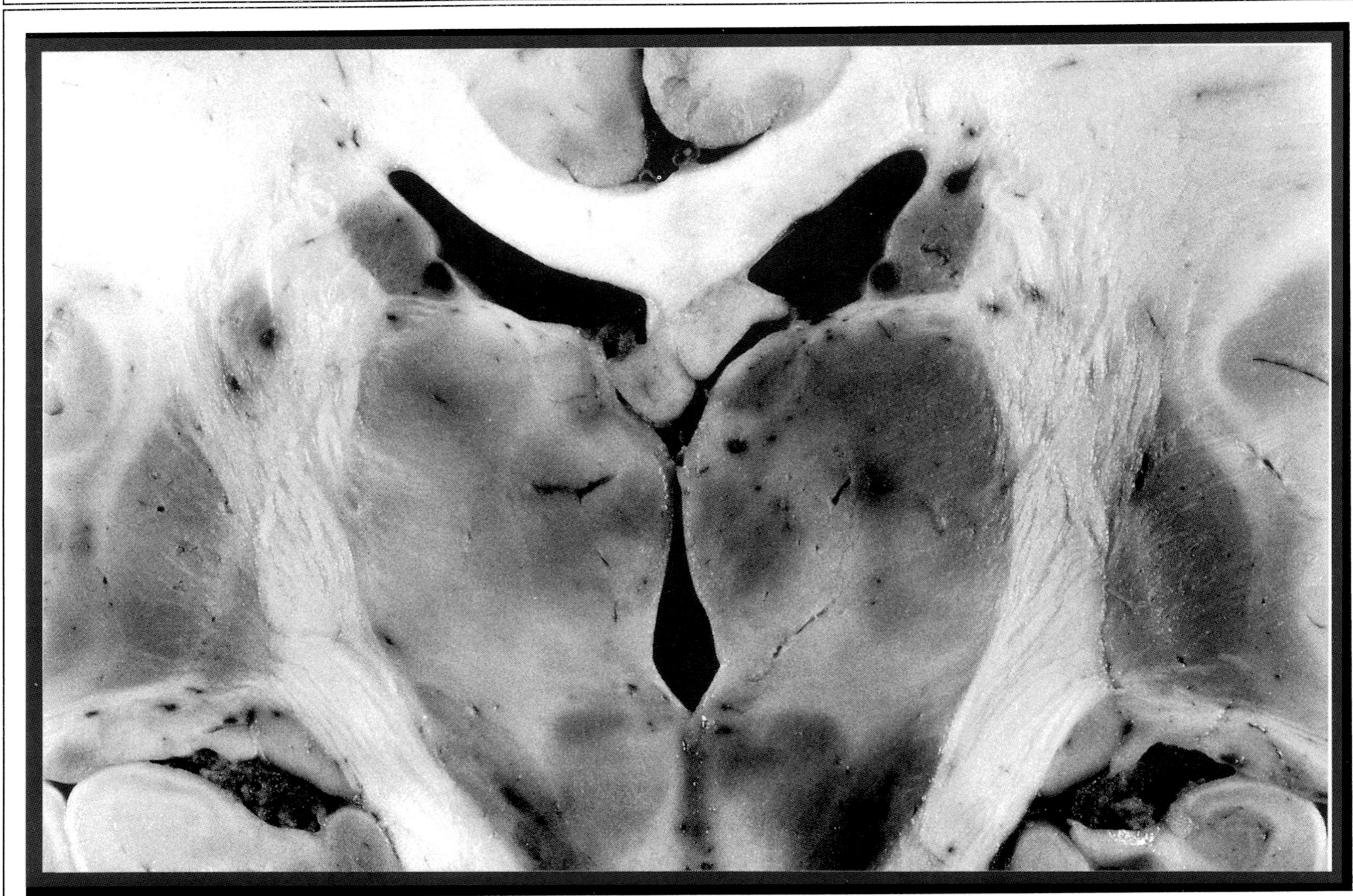

(REFER TO KLUVER - BARRERA STAINED HISTOLOGICAL SECTION FROM THIS SPECIMEN)

THALAMUS, SUBTHALAMIC NUCLEUS, ROSTRAL ASPECT OF RED NUCLEUS, CORONAL SECTION

KEY TO NUMBERED STRUCTURES

1. Hippocampus
2. Internal Medullary Lamina
3. External Medullary Lamina
4. Internal Medullary Lamina, Thalamus
5. Nucleus Reticularis
6. Dorsomedial Nucleus
7. Lateral Posterior Nucleus
8. Lateral Dorsal Nucleus
9. Stria Terminalis and Thalamostriate Vein
10. Corpus Callosum
11. Indusium Griseum
12. Fornix
13. Caudate Nucleus
14. Stria Medullaris
15. Ventroanterior, Ventrolateral Nucleus
16. Internal Capsule, Posterior Limb
17. Extreme Capsule
18. Claustrum
19. External Capsule
20. External Medullary Lamina, Thalamus
21. Putamen
22. Globus Pallidus II
23. Globus Pallidus I
24. Optic Tract
25. Zona Incerta
26. Subthalamic Nucleus
27. Fields of Forel
28. Habenulointer-peduncular Tract
29. Third Ventricle
30. Red Nucleus
31. Substantia Nigra
32. Cerebral Peduncle

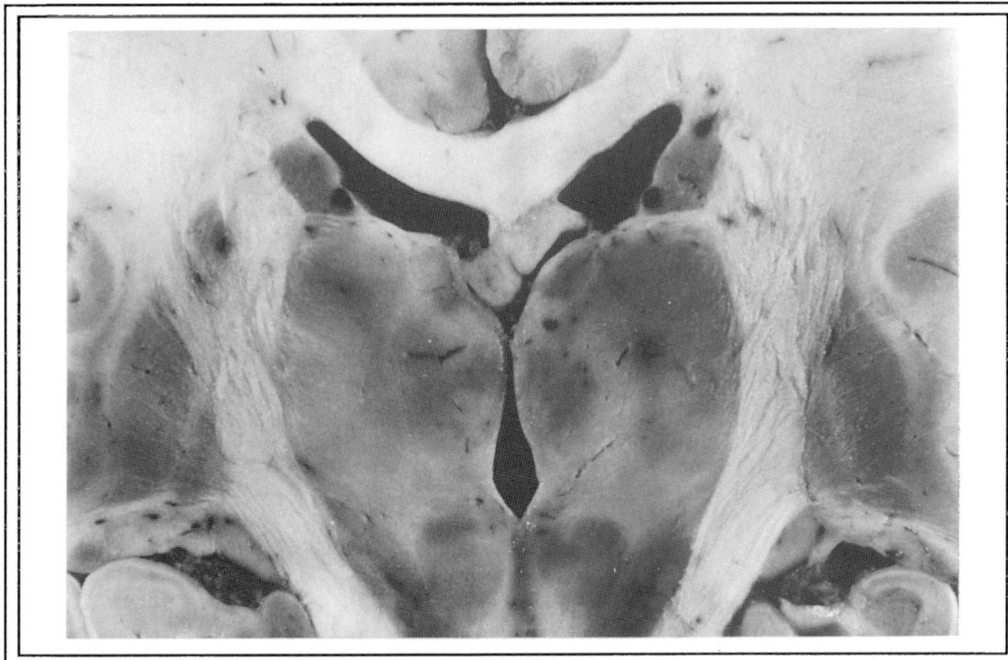

Unstained section, (above), same section Kluver-Barrera stained, 15μ (below)

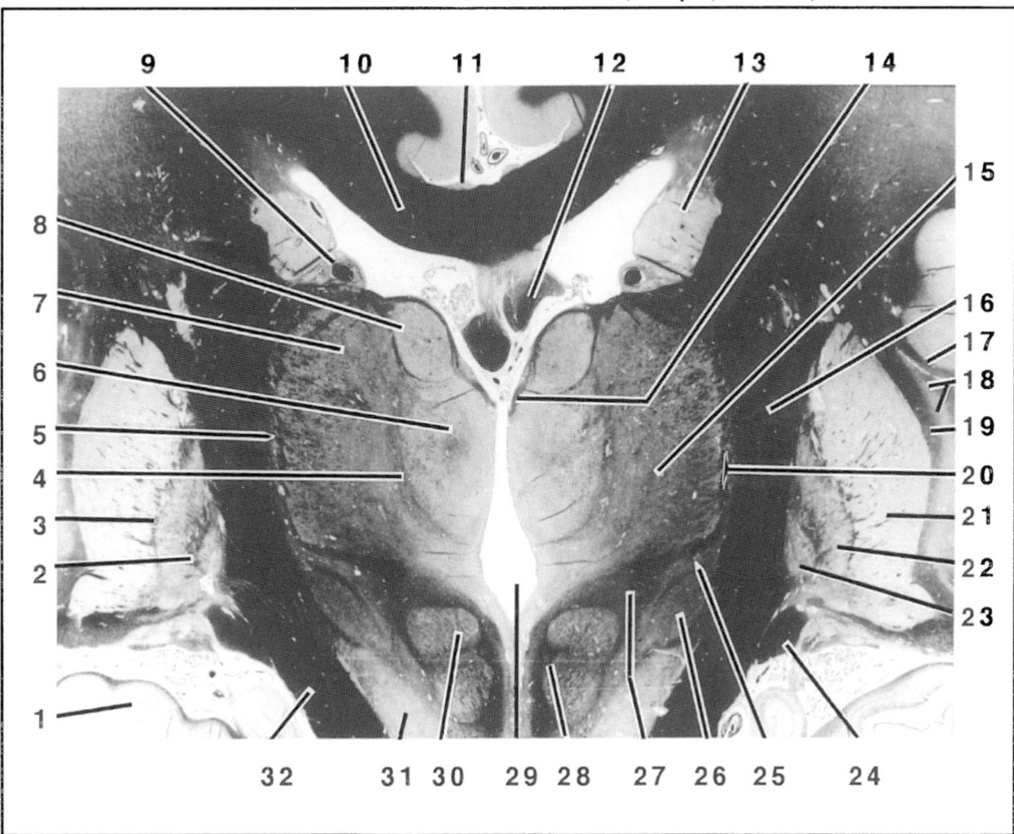

The anterior nucleus and the lateral dorsal nucleus are both situated on the dorsal aspect of the thalamus. The anterior nucleus is subjacent to the anterior tubercle of the thalamus, a prominent rostral and dorsal surface landmark. The caudal aspect of the anterior nucleus represents a transition to the lateral dorsal nucleus, which appears more flattened in coronal section. The mammillothalamic tract projects into the anterior nucleus, and is not seen ventral to the lateral dorsal nucleus. The mammillary bodies are ventral to the anterior nucleus, whereas the red nuclei are located ventral to the lateral dorsal nucleus.

CORONAL SECTION OF THE BRAIN, COMPLETE; LEVEL INCLUDING THE SUBSTANTIA NIGRA, THE LATERAL GENICULATE NUCLEI, AND THE VENTRAL ASPECT OF THE BASIS PONTIS: ROSTRAL TO CAUDAL PERSPECTIVE

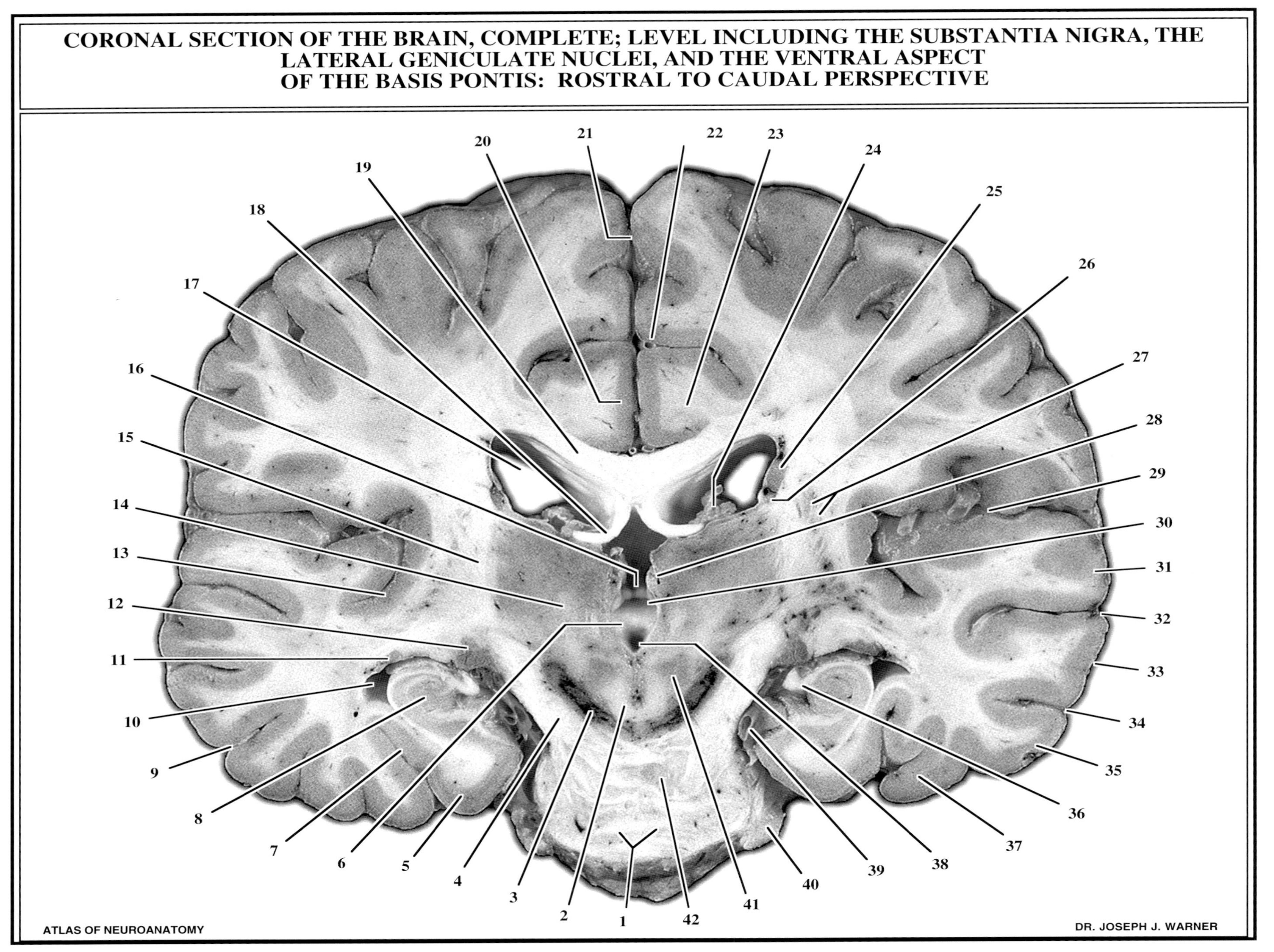

CORONAL SECTION OF THE BRAIN, COMPLETE; LEVEL OF THE SUBSTANTIA NIGRA, THE LATERAL GENICULATE NUCLEI, AND THE VENTRAL ASPECT OF THE BASIS PONTIS: SECTION ORIENTATION AND KEY TO NUMBERED STRUCTURES

KEY TO NUMBERED STRUCTURES

1. Transverse Pontocerebellar Fibers
2. Decussation of the Superior Cerebellar Peduncles
3. Substantia Nigra
4. Cerebral Peduncle
5. Parahippocampal Gyrus
6. Posterior Commissure
7. Collateral Sulcus
8. Hippocampus
9. Inferior Temporal Sulcus
10. Temporal Horn of the Lateral Ventricle
11. Tail of the Caudate Nucleus
12. Lateral Geniculate Nucleus
13. Insular Cortex
14. Centromedian Nucleus of the Thalamus
15. Caudal aspect of the Posterior Limb of the Internal Capsule
16. Habenulae and Habenular Commissure
17. Body of the Lateral Ventricle
18. Fornix
19. Corpus Callosum
20. Cingulate Cortex
21. Interhemispheric Fissure
22. Callosomarginal Branch of the Anterior Cerebral Artery
23. Cingulum
24. Choroid Plexus
25. Caudate Nucleus
26. Stria Terminalis and Thalamostriate Vein
27. Putamen, caudal aspect
28. Stria Medullaris
29. Sylvian Fissure
30. Third Ventricle
31. Superior Temporal Gyrus
32. Superior Temporal Sulcus
33. Middle Temporal Gyrus
34. Middle Temporal Sulcus
35. Inferior Temporal Gyrus
36. Fimbria of the Fornix
37. Fusiform Gyrus
38. Rostral Orifice of the Aqueduct of Sylvius
39. Posterior Cerebral Artery
40. Trigeminal (V) Nerve
41. Red Nucleus
42. Pontine Nuclei

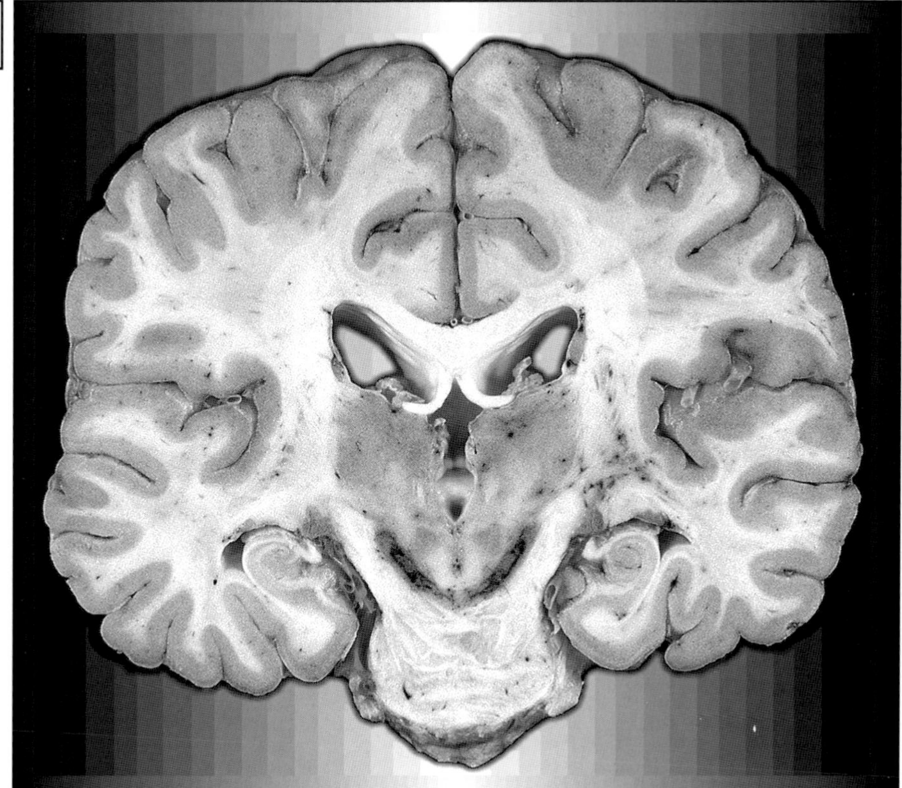

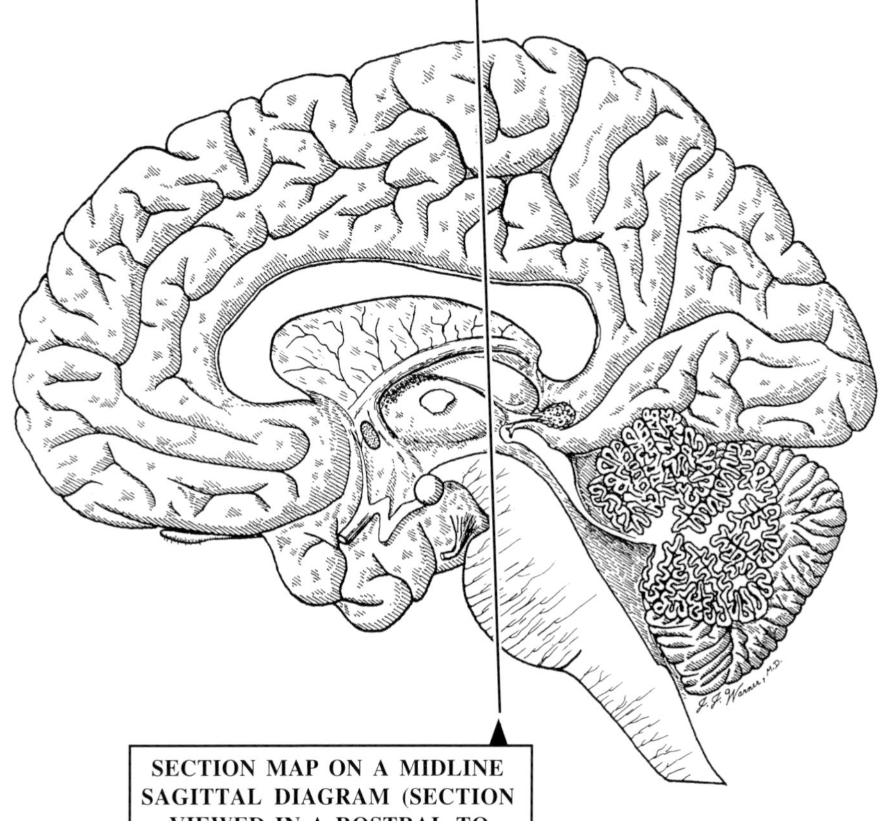

SECTION MAP ON A MIDLINE SAGITTAL DIAGRAM (SECTION VIEWED IN A ROSTRAL TO CAUDAL PERSPECTIVE)

ATLAS OF NEUROANATOMY
DR. JOSEPH J. WARNER

THE LATERAL GENICULATE NUCLEUS AND HIPPOCAMPUS: 12 μ CORONAL SECTION, LFB - PAS - HEMATOXYLIN

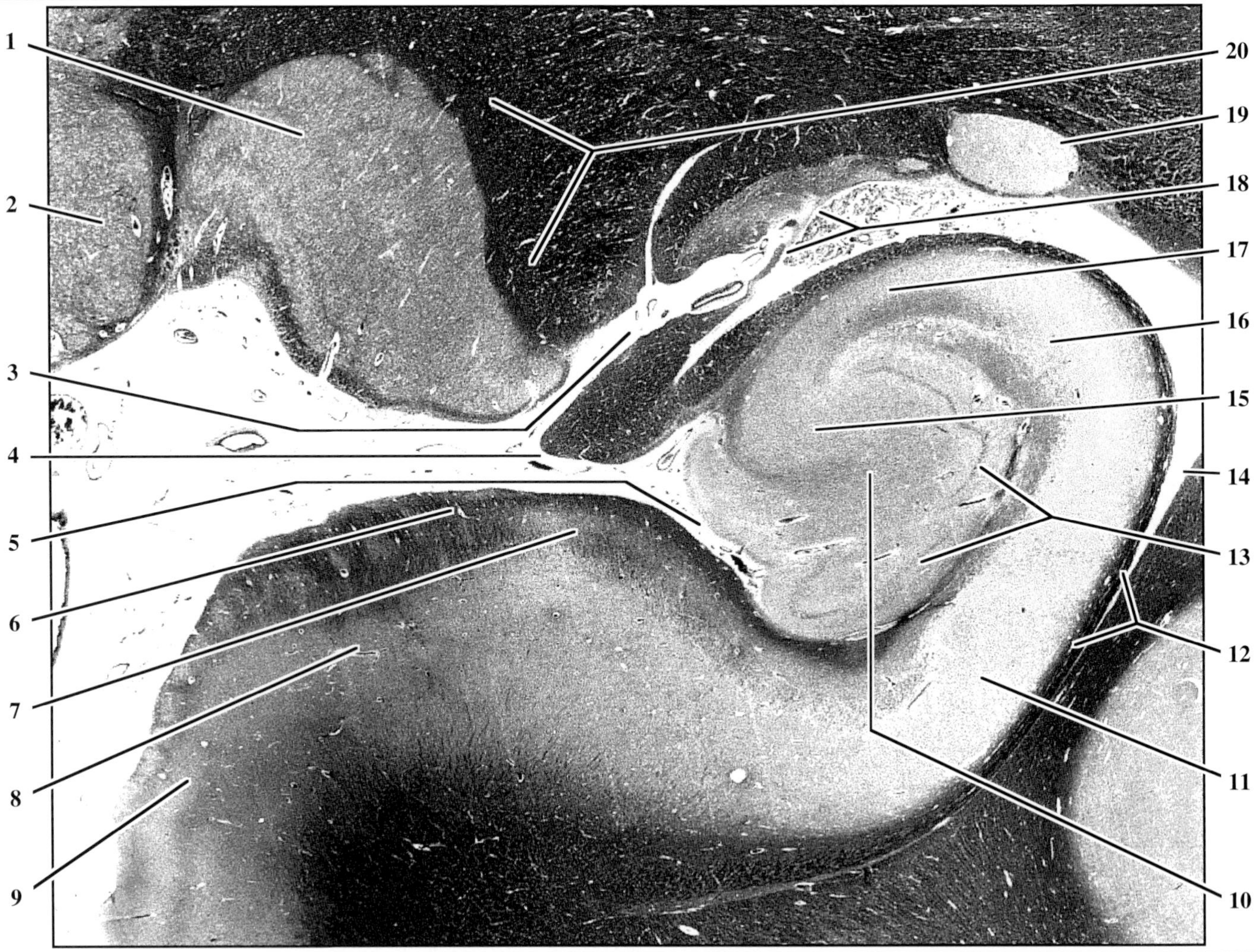

SECTION ORIENTATION AND KEY TO NUMBERED STRUCTURES

1. Lateral Geniculate Nucleus
2. Medial Geniculate Nucleus
3. Choroidal Fissure
4. Fimbria of the Fornix
5. Hippocampal Fissure
6. Superficial Medullary Stratum of the Subiculum
7. Prosubiculum
8. Subiculum
9. Presubiculum
10. CA 4 of the Hippocampus
11. Transition: Subiculum to Hippocampus
12. Alveus
13. Dentate Gyrus of the Hippocampus
14. Temporal Horn of the Lateral Ventricle
15. CA 3 of the Hippocampus
16. CA 1 of the Hippocampus
17. CA 2 of the Hippocampus
18. Tela Choroidea
19. Tail of the Caudate Nucleus
20. Geniculocalcarine Radiations

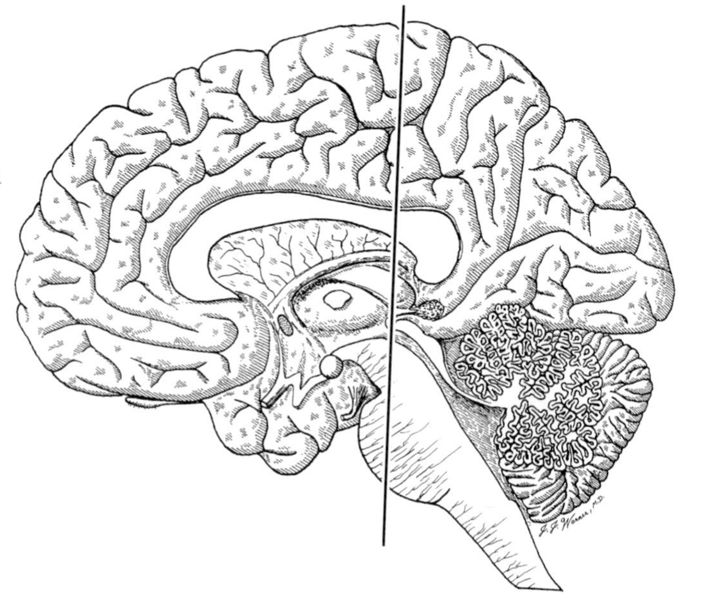

CORONAL SECTION, COMPLETE: LEVEL OF THE CAUDAL PULVINAR, THE MEDIAL GENICULATE NUCLEUS AND THE BRACHIUM OF THE SUPERIOR COLLICULUS

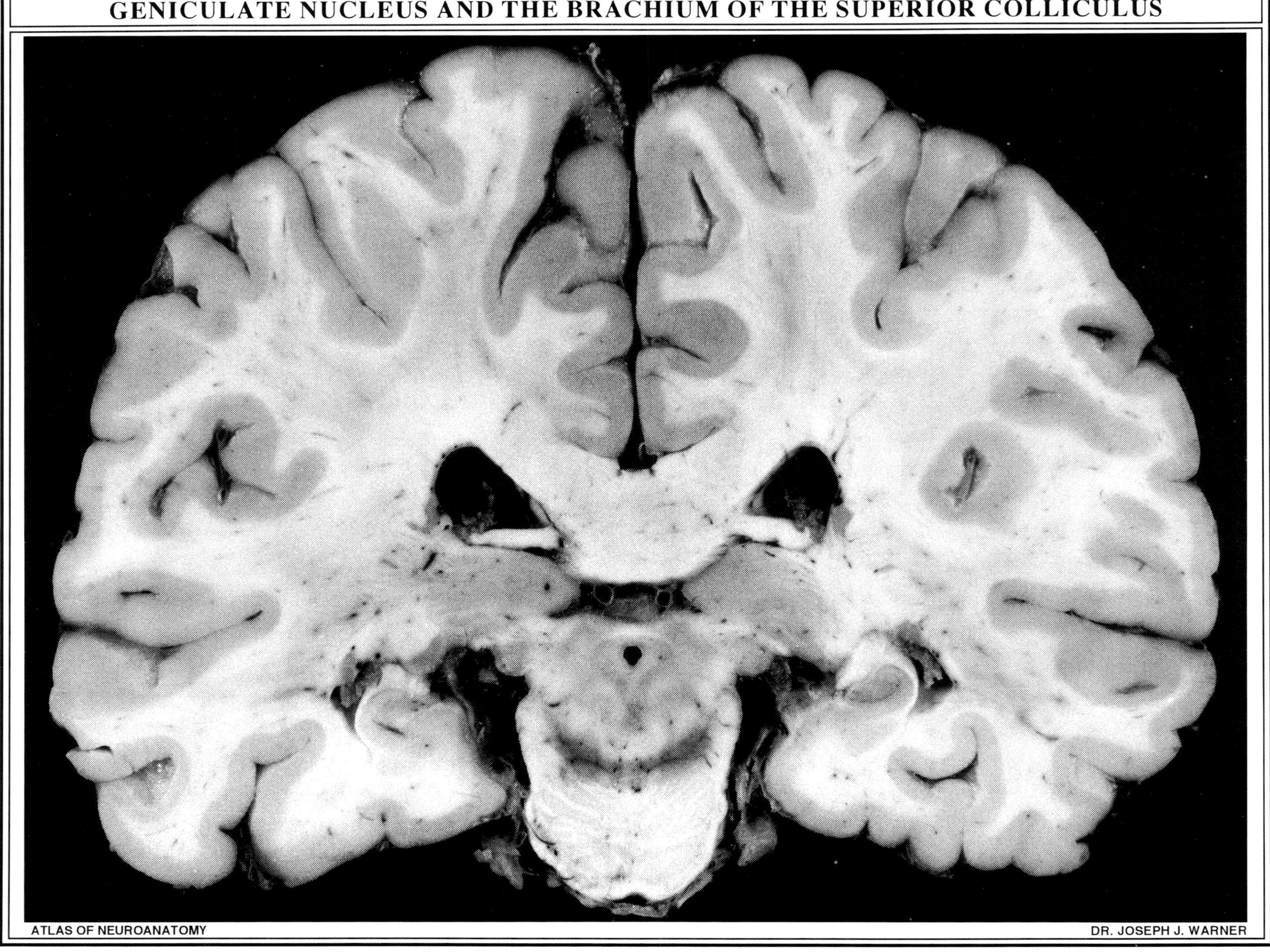

CORONAL SECTION: LEVEL OF THE CAUDAL PULVINAR NUCLEUS, THE MEDIAL GENICULATE NUCLEUS, AND THE BRACHIUM OF THE SUPERIOR COLLICULUS (MAGNIFIED VIEW)

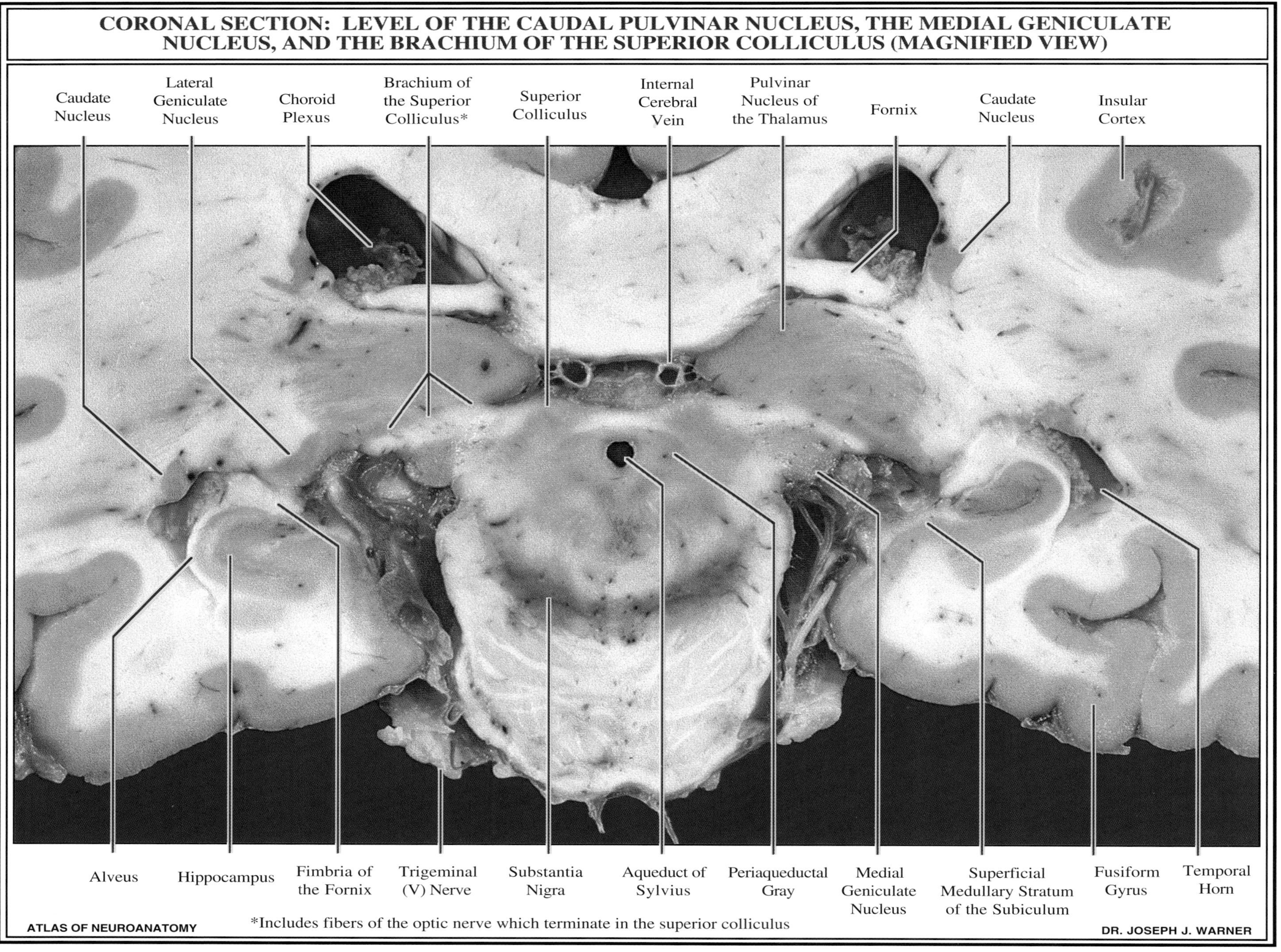

*Includes fibers of the optic nerve which terminate in the superior colliculus

CORONAL SECTION OF THE BRAIN, COMPLETE; LEVEL INCLUDING THE CAUDAL ASPECT OF THE PULVINAR NUCLEUS, THE INFERIOR COLLICULUS, AND THE TRIGEMINAL NERVE: ROSTRAL TO CAUDAL PERSPECTIVE

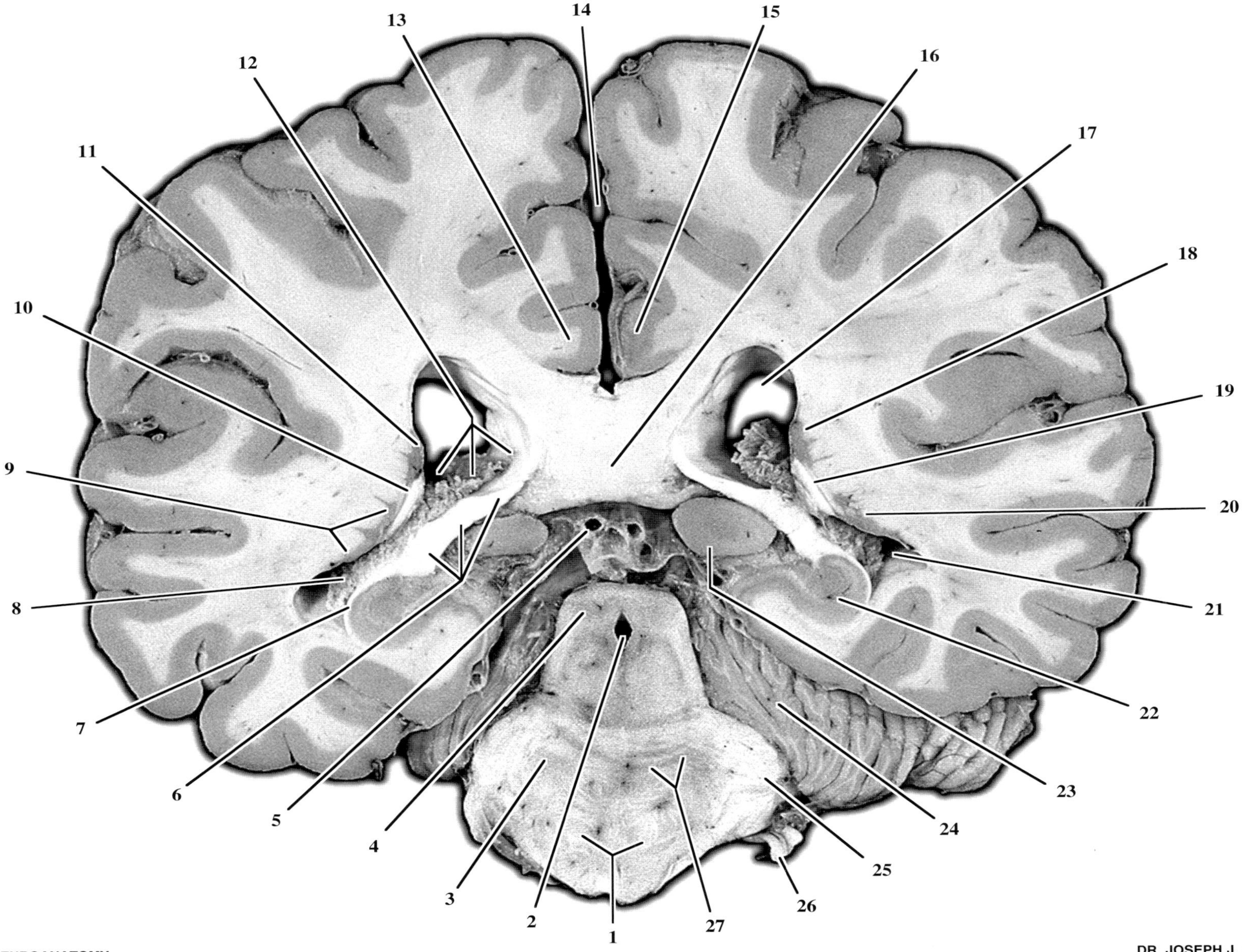

13 14 15
12 16
11 17
18
10
19
9
20
8
21
7
22
6
23
5 24
4 25
3 26
2 27
1

ATLAS OF NEUROANATOMY

DR. JOSEPH J. WARNER

CORONAL SECTION OF THE BRAIN, COMPLETE; LEVEL OF THE INFERIOR COLLICULUS AND OF THE CAUDAL ASPECT OF THE PULVINAR NUCLEUS: SECTION ORIENTATION AND KEY TO NUMBERED STRUCTURES

KEY TO NUMBERED STRUCTURES

1. Basis Pontis
2. Aqueduct of Sylvius
3. Pontine Nuclei
4. Inferior Colliculus
5. Internal Cerebral Vein
6. Fornix
7. Alveus
8. Choroid Plexus
9. Tail of the Caudate Nucleus
10. Stria Terminalis
11. Tail of the Caudate Nucleus
12. Atrium of the Lateral Ventricle
13. Cingulum
14. Interhemispheric Fissure
15. Cingulate Cortex
16. Splenium of the Corpus Callosum
17. Caudal extent of the Body of the Lateral Ventricle
18. Tail of the Caudate Nucleus
19. Stria Terminalis
20. Tail of the Caudate Nucleus
21. Temporal Horn of the Lateral Ventricle
22. Hippocampus
23. Caudal aspect of the Pulvinar Nucleus of the Thalamus
24. Anterior Lobe of the Cerebellum
25. Middle Cerebellar Peduncle
26. Trigeminal (V) Nerve
27. Transverse Pontocerebellar Fibers

The internal cerebral veins (clearly visible in this section) course ventral to the splenium of the corpus callosum. They are joined by the basal veins of Rosenthal, and merge to form the great vein of Galen. The coronal plane passes obliquely through the inferior colliculus, the aqueduct of Sylvius, and finally the pons. From the temporal lobe, the fornix,stria terminalis and tail of the Caudate course in a caudal, dorsomedial, then rostral direction. Each structure is tangentially sectioned at the caudal aspect of the loop thus formed.

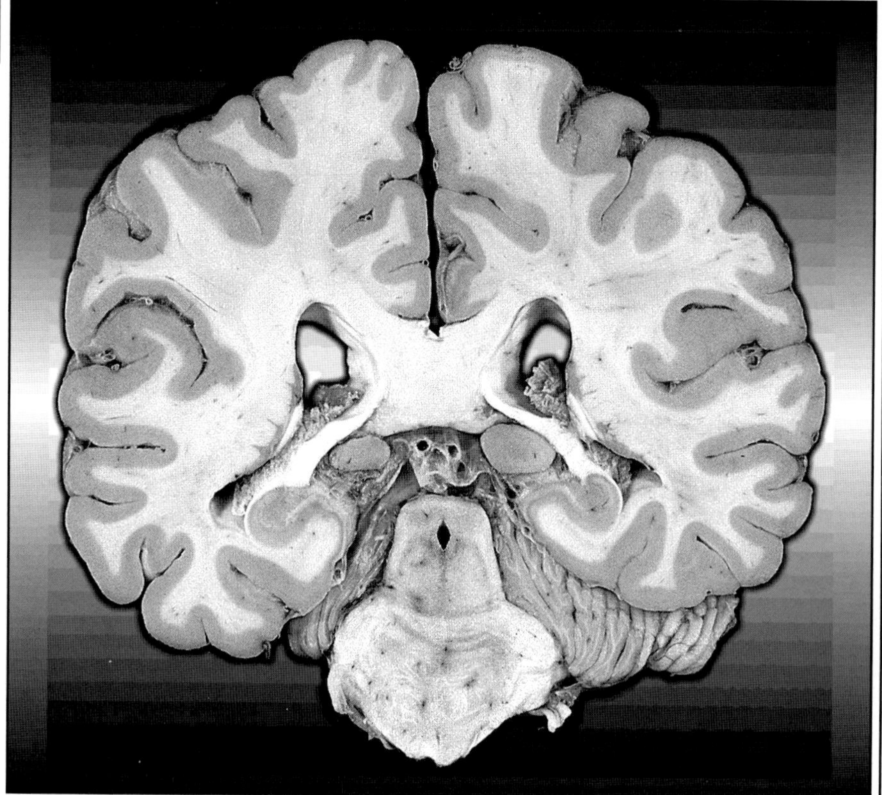

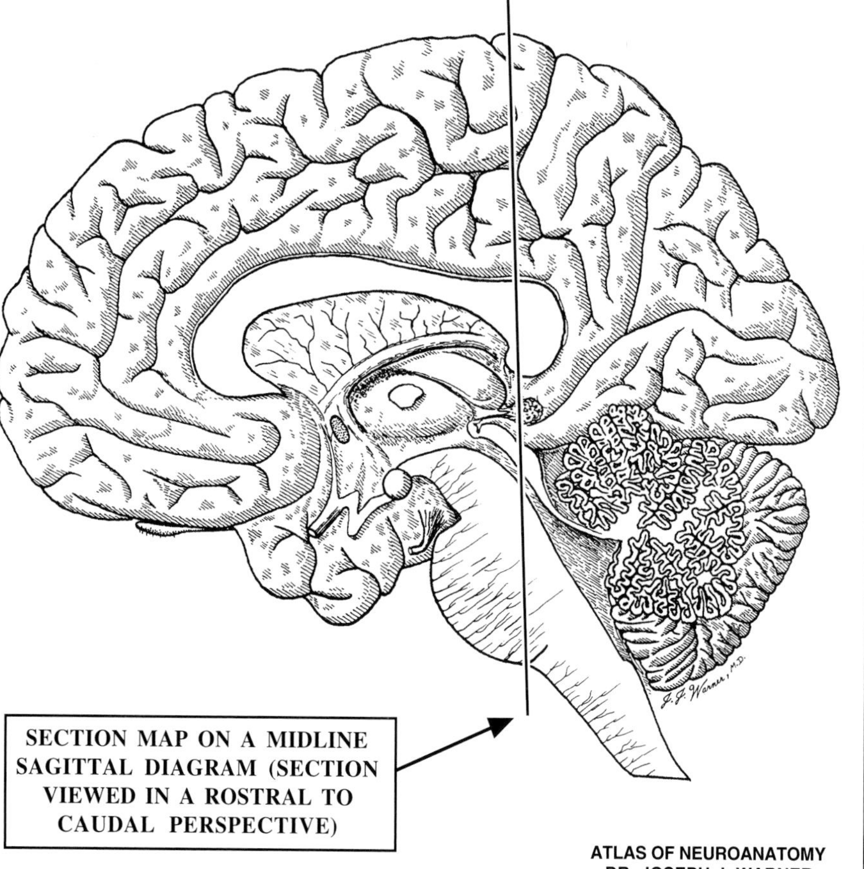

SECTION MAP ON A MIDLINE SAGITTAL DIAGRAM (SECTION VIEWED IN A ROSTRAL TO CAUDAL PERSPECTIVE)

CORONAL SECTION OF THE BRAIN, LEVEL INCLUDING THE CAUDAL ASPECT OF THE PULVINAR NUCLEUS AND THE INFERIOR COLLICULUS: MAGNIFIED VIEW, CAUDAL TO ROSTRAL PERSPECTIVE

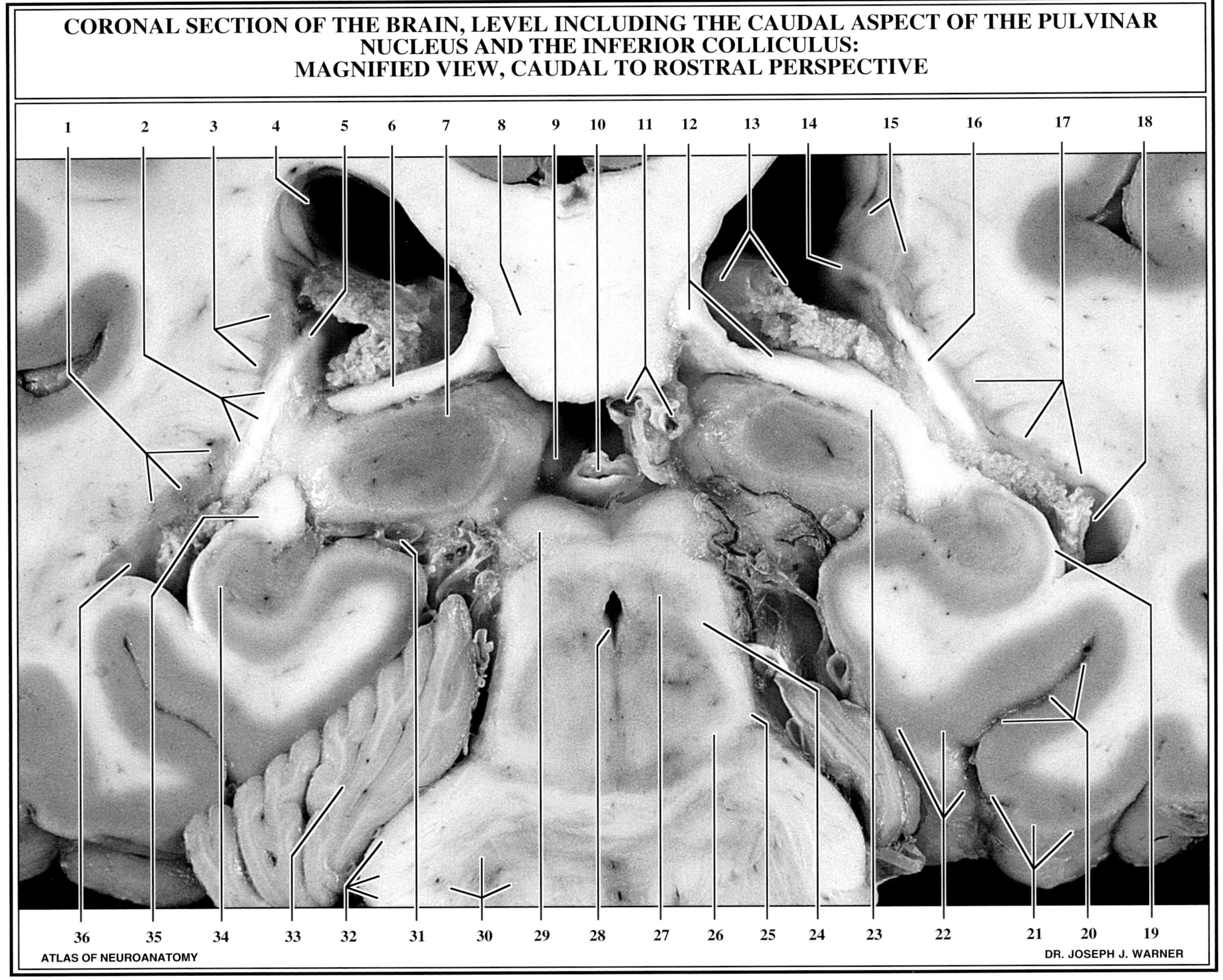

ATLAS OF NEUROANATOMY

DR. JOSEPH J. WARNER

CORONAL SECTION OF THE BRAIN, LEVEL OF THE INFERIOR COLLICULUS AND OF THE CAUDAL ASPECT OF THE PULVINAR NUCLEUS, MAGNIFIED VIEW: SECTION ORIENTATION AND KEY TO NUMBERED STRUCTURES

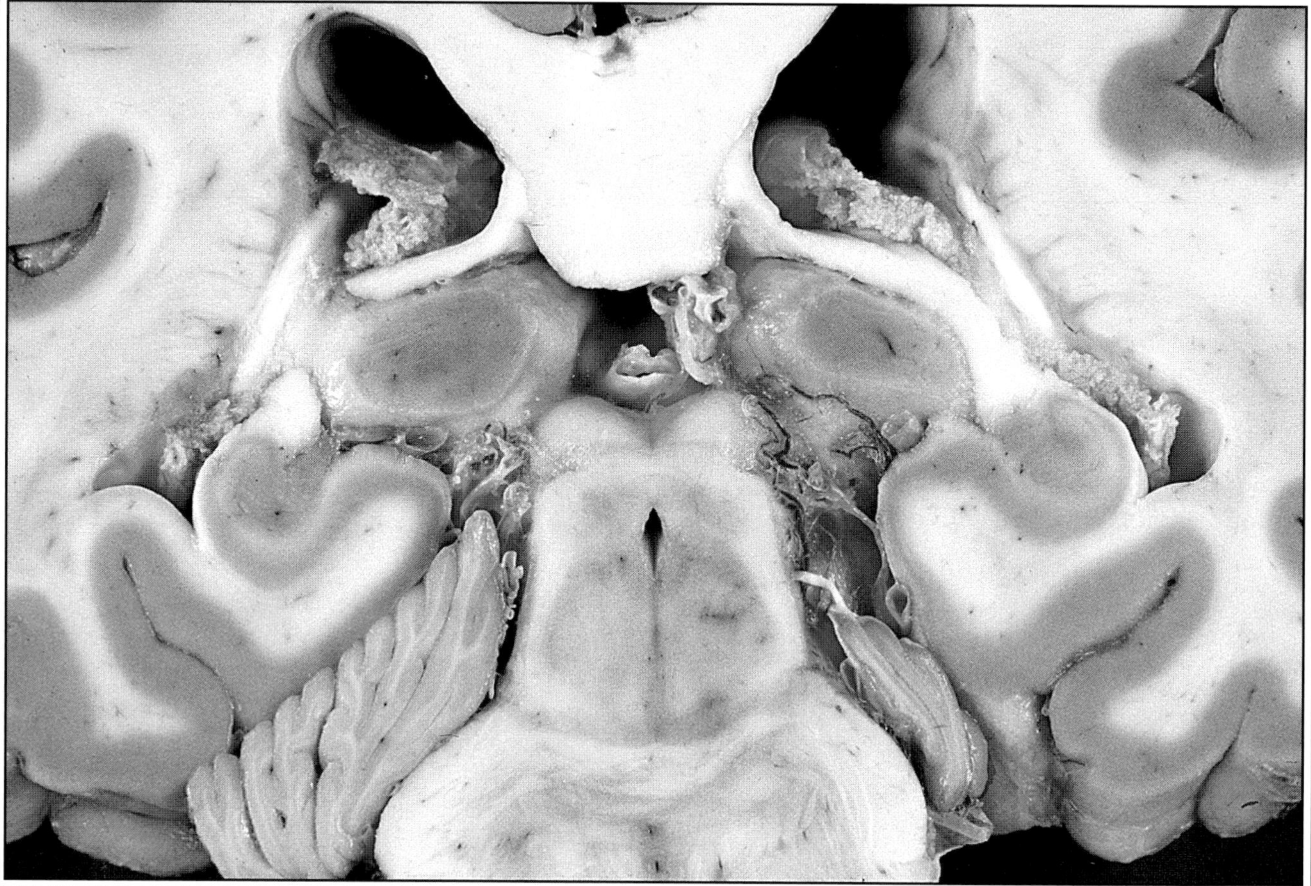

KEY TO NUMBERED STRUCTURES

1, 3, 15, 17: Tail of the Caudate Nucleus
2, 5, 14, 16: Stria Terminalis
4. Body of the Lateral Ventricle
6,12, 23, 35: Fornix
7. Pulvinar Nucleus of the Thalamus
8. Splenium of the Corpus Callosum
9. Habenula
10. Pineal Recess of the Third Ventricle
11. Internal Cerebral Veins
13, 18: Choroid Plexus
19. Alveus
20. Collateral Sulcus
21. Fusiform Gyrus
22. Parahippocampal Gyrus
24. Lateral Lemniscus
25. Spinothalamic Tract
26. Medial Lemniscus
27. Inferior Colliculus
28. Aqueduct of Sylvius
29. Superior Colliculus
30. Basis Pontis
31. Posterior Cerebral Artery
32. Middle Cerebellar Peduncle
33. Anterior Lobe of the Cerebellum
34. Hippocampus
36. Temporal Horn of the Lateral Ventricle

SECTION VIEWED FROM A CAUDAL TO ROSTRAL PERSPECTIVE

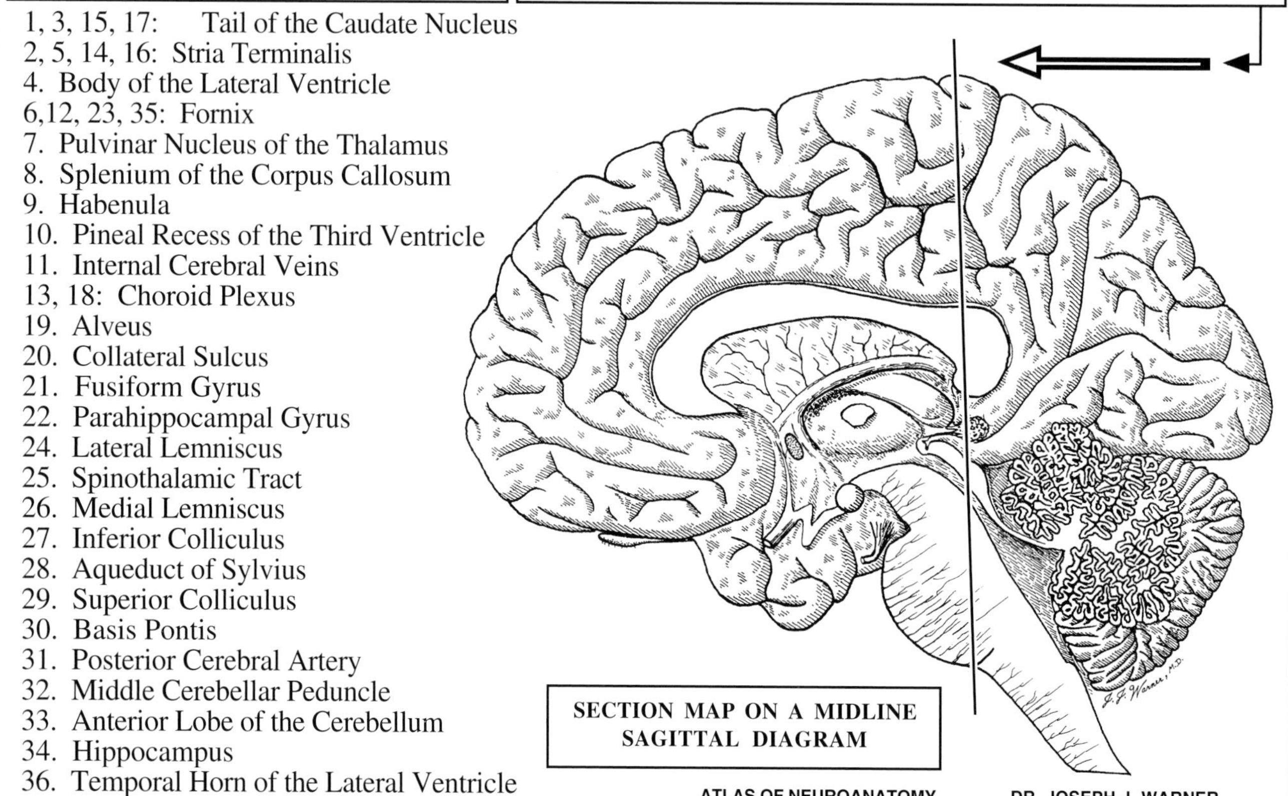

SECTION MAP ON A MIDLINE SAGITTAL DIAGRAM

CORONAL SECTION OF THE BRAIN, COMPLETE; LEVEL INCLUDING THE SPLENIUM OF THE CORPUS CALLOSUM, THE ATRIA OF THE LATERAL VENTRICLES, AND THE SUPERIOR CEREBELLAR PEDUNCLES: CAUDAL TO ROSTRAL PERSPECTIVE

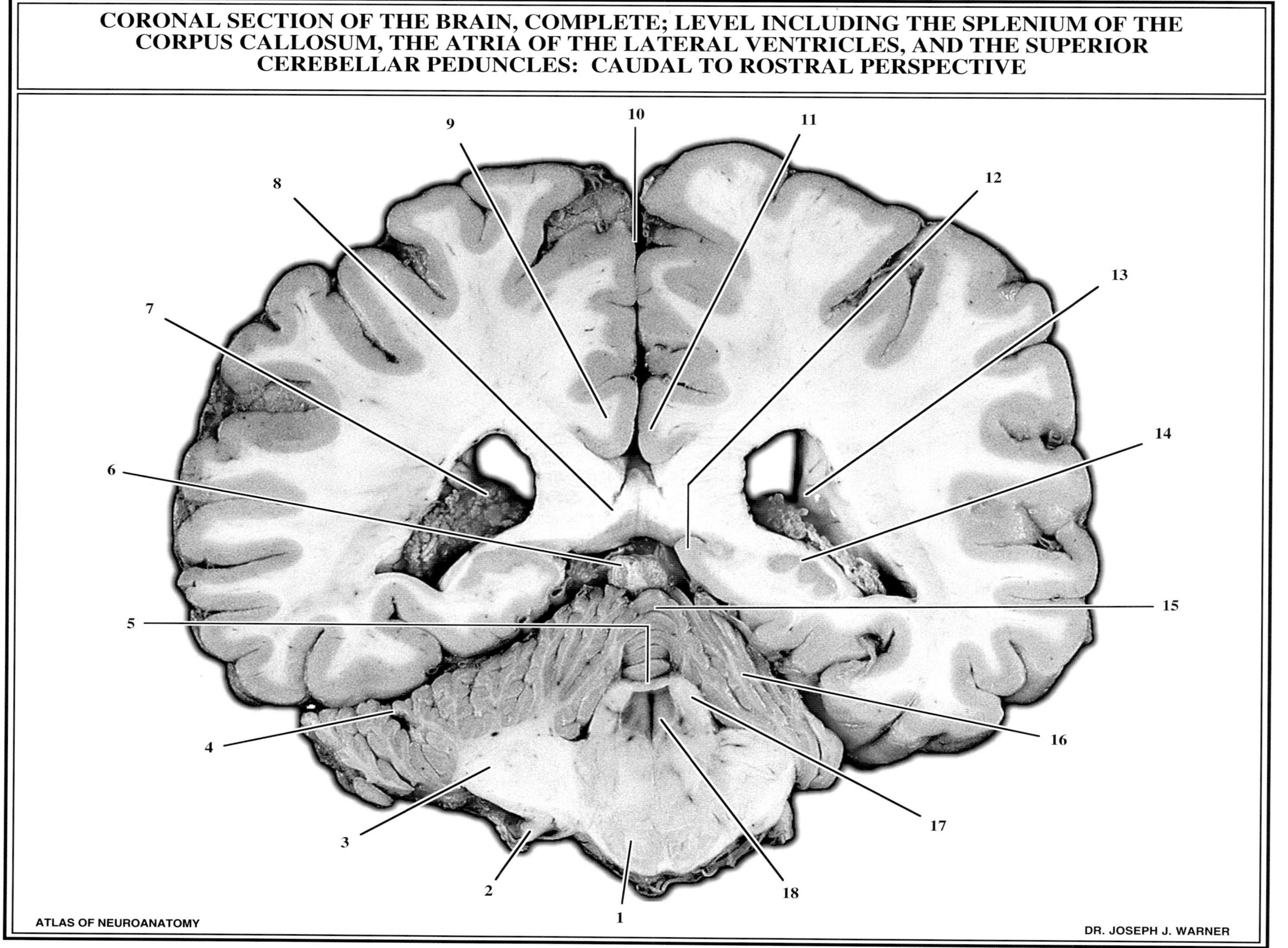

DR. JOSEPH J. WARNER

CORONAL SECTION OF THE BRAIN, COMPLETE; LEVEL OF THE SUPERIOR CEREBELLAR PEDUNCLES AND OF THE SPLENIUM OF THE CORPUS CALLOSUM : SECTION ORIENTATION AND KEY TO NUMBERED STRUCTURES

KEY TO NUMBERED STRUCTURES

1. Basis Pontis
2. Trigeminal (V) Nerve
3. Middle Cerebellar Peduncle
4. Primary Fissure of the Cerebellum
5. Anterior Medullary Velum
6. Pineal Body
7. Choroid Plexus within the Lateral Ventricle
8. Splenium of the Corpus Callosum
9. Cingulum
10. Interhemispheric Fissure
11. Cingulate Cortex
12. Isthmus of the Gyrus Fornicatus
13. Atrium of the Lateral Ventricle
14. Caudal extent of the Hippocampus
15. Superior Cerebellar Vermis
16. Anterior Lobe of the Cerebellum
17. Superior Cerebellar Peduncle
18. Fourth Ventricle

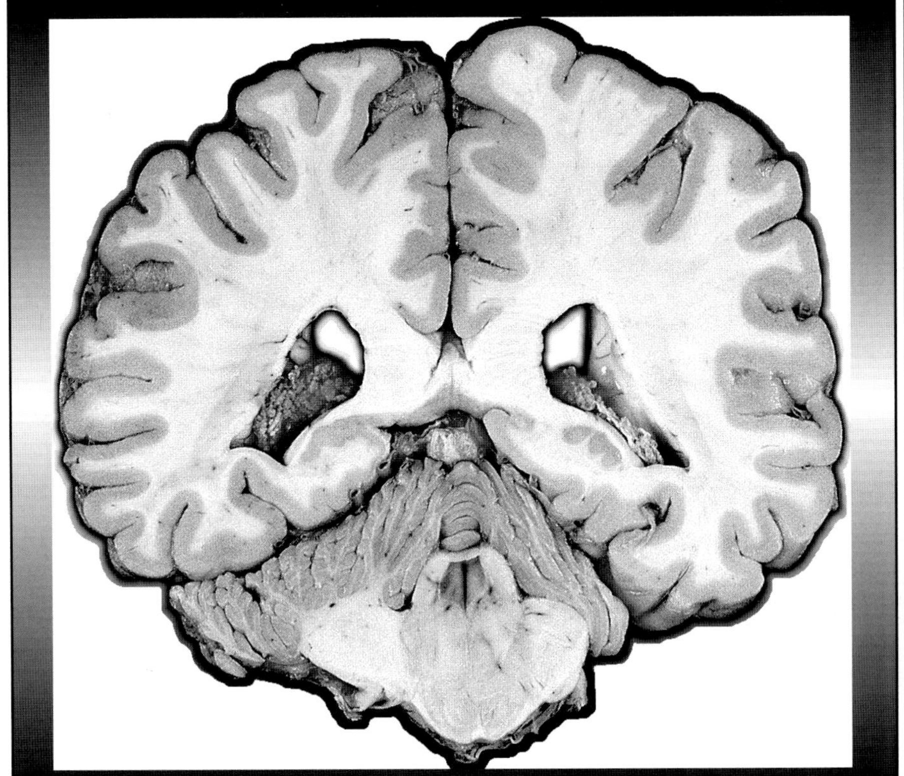

The inferior surface of the cerebral hemispheres caudal to the splenium of the corpus callosum assumes a contour that conforms to the tentorium and superior surface of the cerebellum. The ventrally biconvex contour contrasts with the configuration of the inferior frontal lobes. (Compare with rostral coronal sections.) Ventral to the splenium, the cerebral hemispheres diverge (in coronal section) at an angle of approximately 100°, with the apex corresponding to the location of the great vein of Galen and the straight sinus.
As the cingulate gyrus courses caudal to the splenium of the corpus callosum, it curves ventrolaterally as the isthmus of the gyrus fornicatus. The isthmus turns rostrally (parallel to the lingular gyrus) and continues as the parahippocampal gyrus.

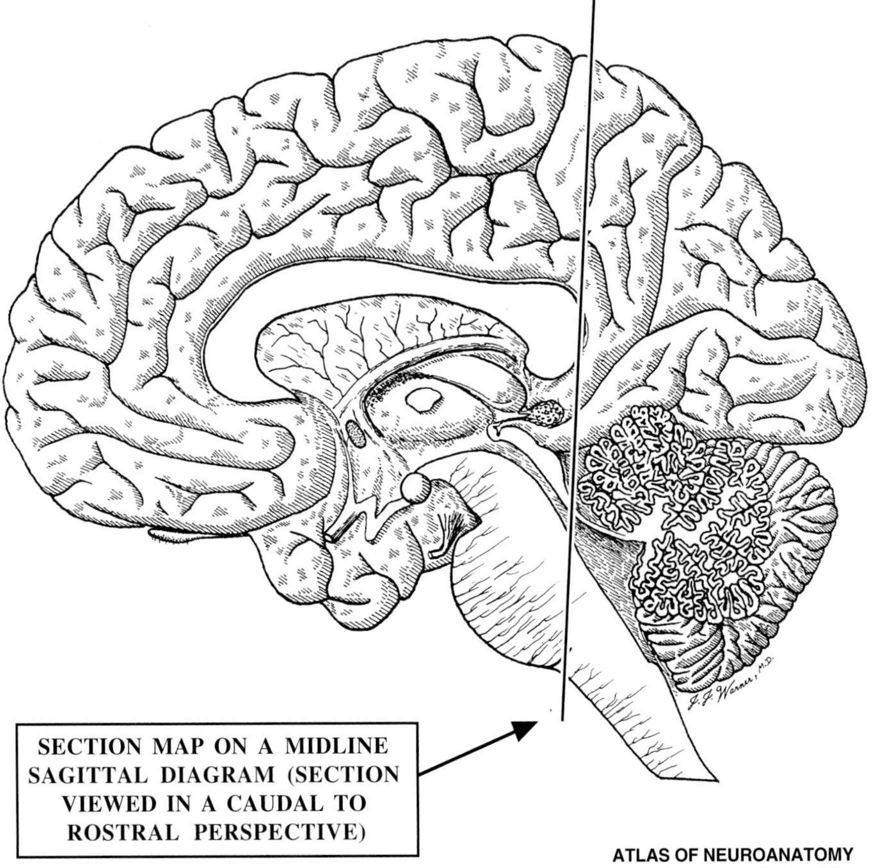

SECTION MAP ON A MIDLINE SAGITTAL DIAGRAM (SECTION VIEWED IN A CAUDAL TO ROSTRAL PERSPECTIVE)

CORONAL SECTION OF THE CEREBRAL HEMISPHERES: LEVEL OF THE CAUDAL EXTENT OF THE OCCIPITAL HORNS OF THE LATERAL VENTRICLES

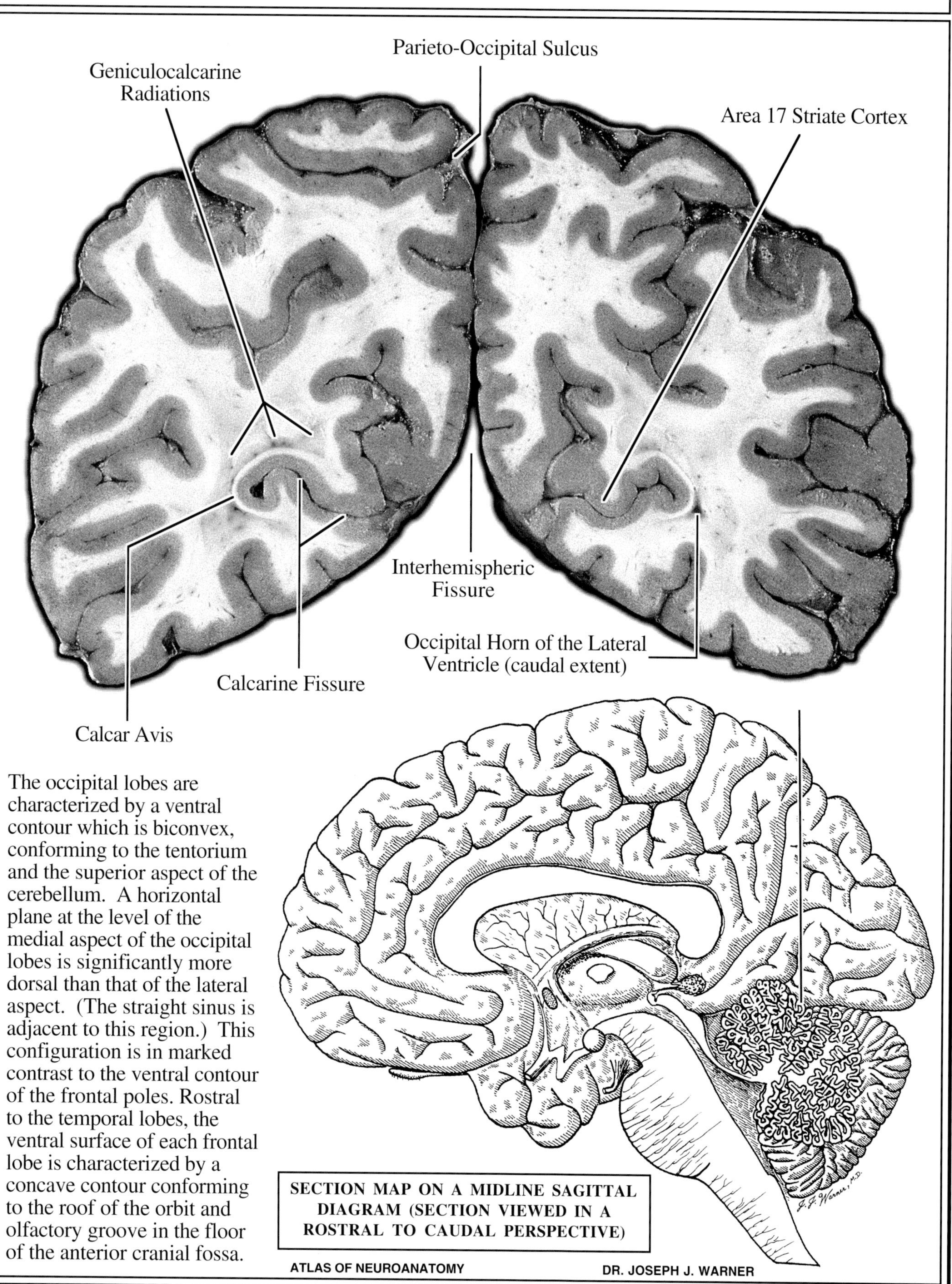

The occipital lobes are characterized by a ventral contour which is biconvex, conforming to the tentorium and the superior aspect of the cerebellum. A horizontal plane at the level of the medial aspect of the occipital lobes is significantly more dorsal than that of the lateral aspect. (The straight sinus is adjacent to this region.) This configuration is in marked contrast to the ventral contour of the frontal poles. Rostral to the temporal lobes, the ventral surface of each frontal lobe is characterized by a concave contour conforming to the roof of the orbit and olfactory groove in the floor of the anterior cranial fossa.

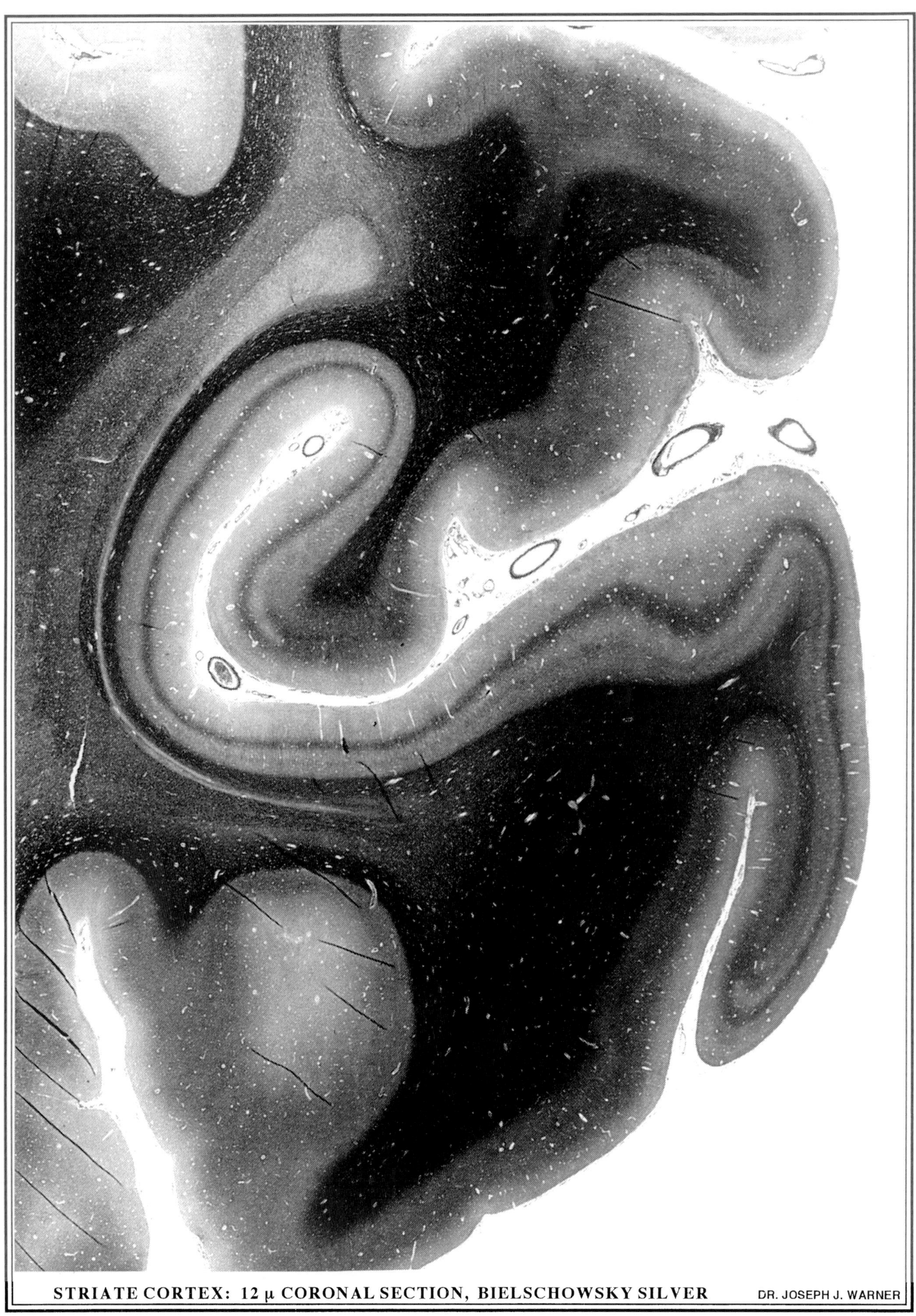

STRIATE CORTEX: 12 μ CORONAL SECTION, BIELSCHOWSKY SILVER DR. JOSEPH J. WARNER

HORIZONTAL SECTIONAL NEUROANATOMY

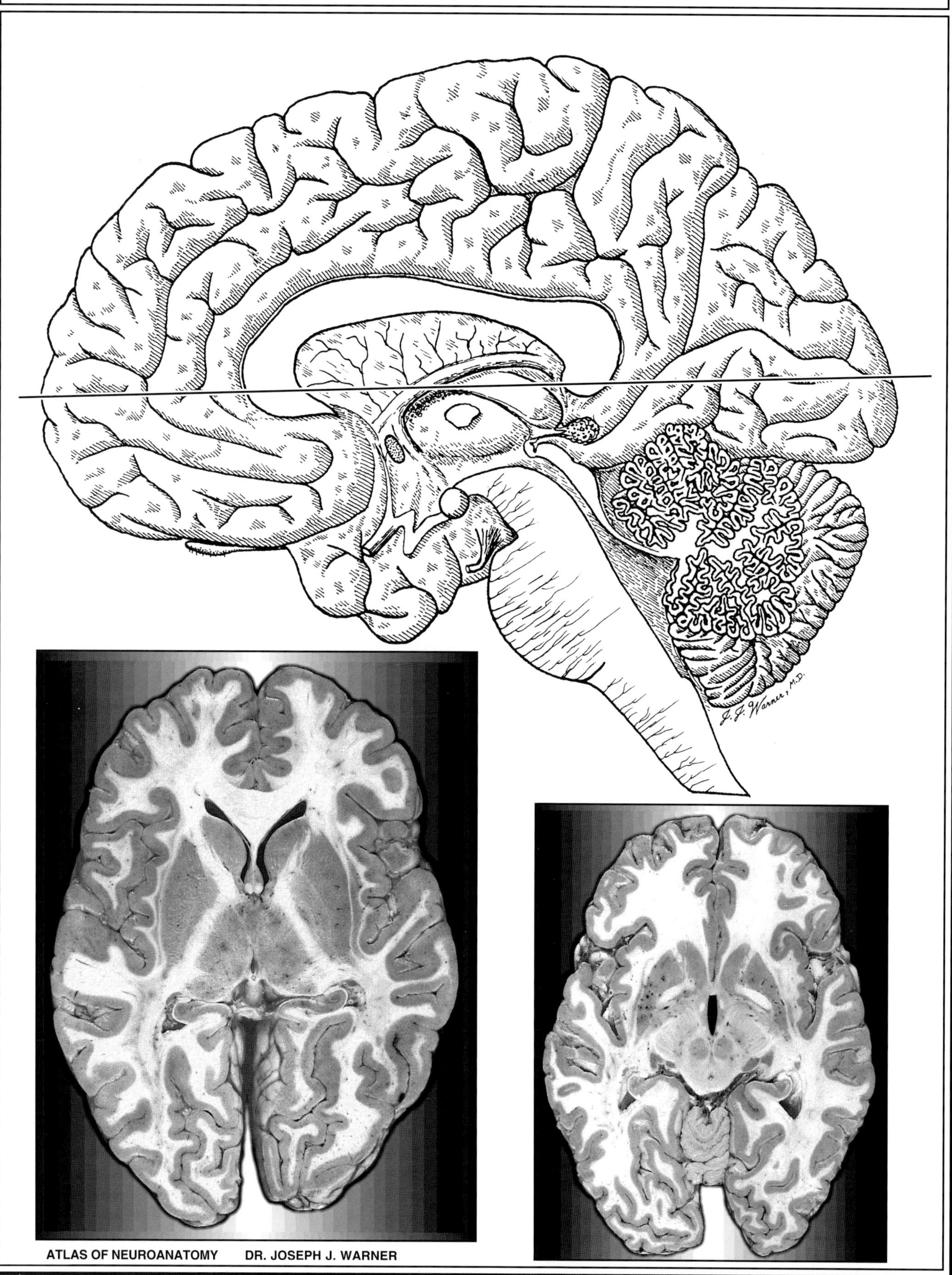

HORIZONTAL SECTION OF THE BRAIN, COMPLETE: LEVEL INCLUDING THE OPTIC CHIASM, INFUNDIBULUM, AMYGDALA, AND PONTOMESENCEPHALIC JUNCTION

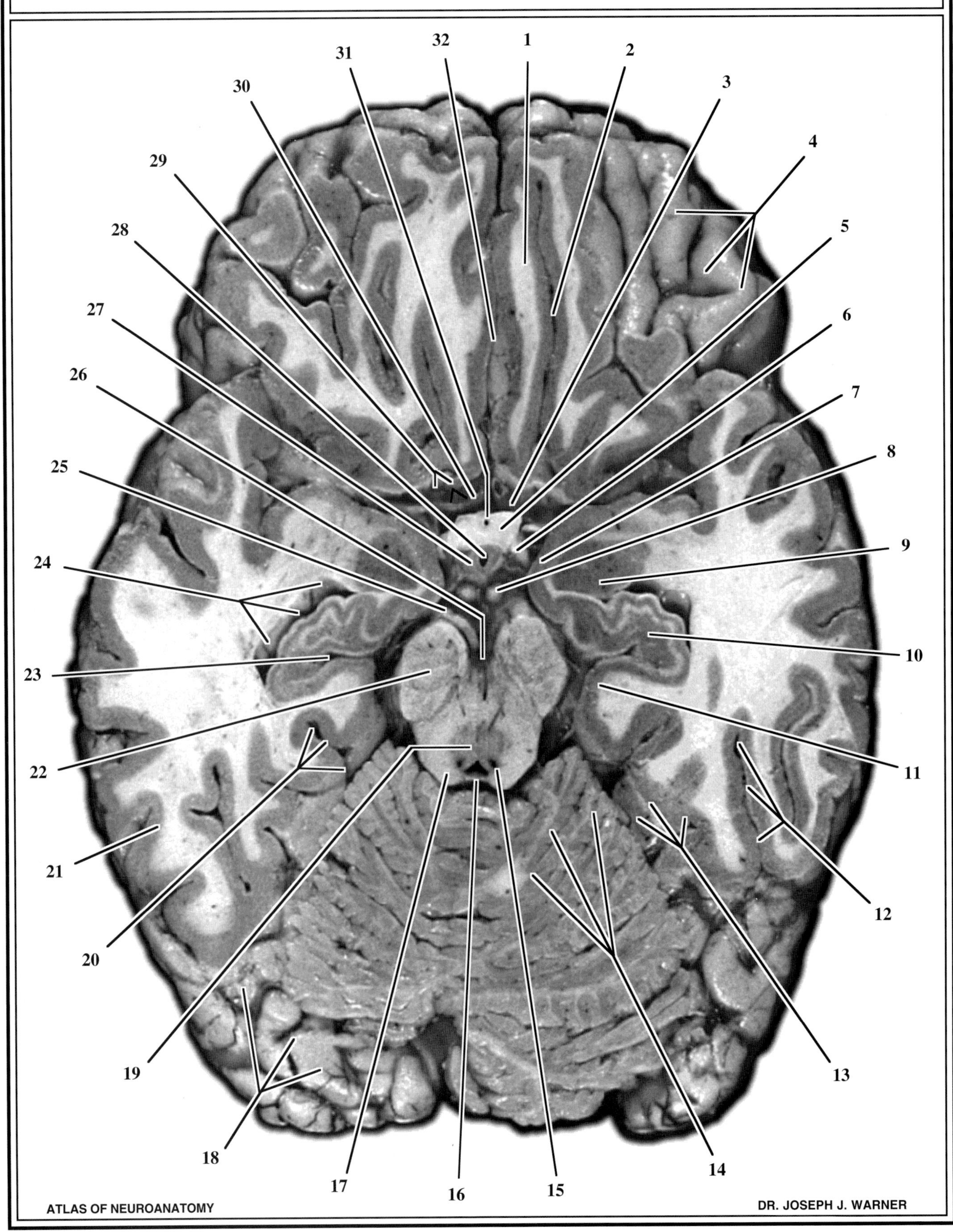

HORIZONTAL SECTION OF THE BRAIN, COMPLETE; LEVEL INCLUDING THE OPTIC CHIASM, INFUNDIBULUM, AMYGDALA, AND PONTOMESENCEPHALIC JUNCTION: SECTION ORIENTATION AND KEY TO NUMBERED STRUCTURES

KEY TO NUMBERED STRUCTURES

1. Gyrus Rectus
2. Olfactory Sulcus
3. Anterior Perforated Substance*
4. Orbitofrontal Gyri
5. Optic Chiasm
6. Optic Tract**
7. Uncus
8. Mammillary Body
9. Amygdala
10. Hippocampus
11. Parahippocampal Gyrus
12. Inferior Temporal Sulcus
13. Fusiform Gyrus
14. Anterior Lobe of the Cerebellum
15. Locus Coeruleus
16. Anterior Medullary Velum
17. Superior Cerebellar Peduncle
18. Inferior (tentorial) surface of the Occipital Lobe
19. Periaqueductal Gray
20. Collateral Sulcus
21. Inferior Temporal Gyrus
22. Cerebral Peduncle
23. Hippocampal Fissure
24. Temporal Horn of the Lateral Ventricle
25. Oculomotor Nerve
26. Interpeduncular Fossa
27. Infundibulum
28. Infundibular Recess (Third Ventricle)
29. Olfactory Trigone*
30. Anterior Cerebral Artery
31. Supraoptic Recess (Third Ventricle)
32. Interhemispheric Fissure

* The Anterior Perforated Substance is located caudal to the division of each Olfactory Tract into the Medial and Lateral Olfactory Striae (Olfactory Trigone). Ventral retraction of the Optic Nerves and Chiasm allows visualization of this region. Numerous small arteries, which arise from the rostral aspect of the Circle of Willis, course dorsally into the cerebral hemispheres. Resection of this vasculature reveals numerous perivascular spaces which appear as perforations on the ventral surface of the brain, hence the name of this region.

** Each Optic Tract courses caudally, dorsally, and laterally, circumferentially passing the lateral aspect of the cerebral peduncle to terminate in the Lateral Geniculate Nucleus.

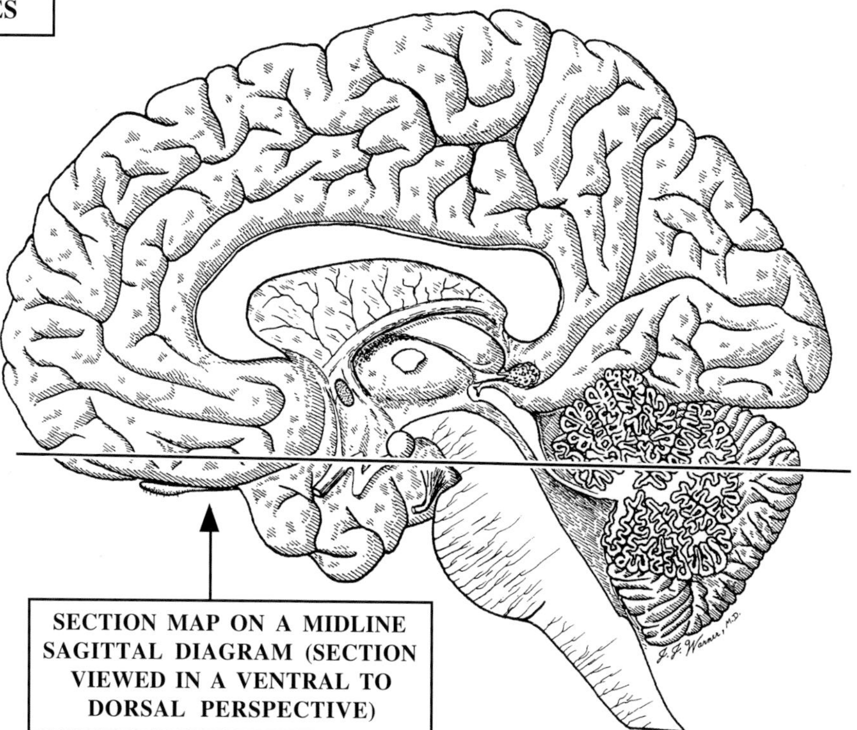

SECTION MAP ON A MIDLINE SAGITTAL DIAGRAM (SECTION VIEWED IN A VENTRAL TO DORSAL PERSPECTIVE)

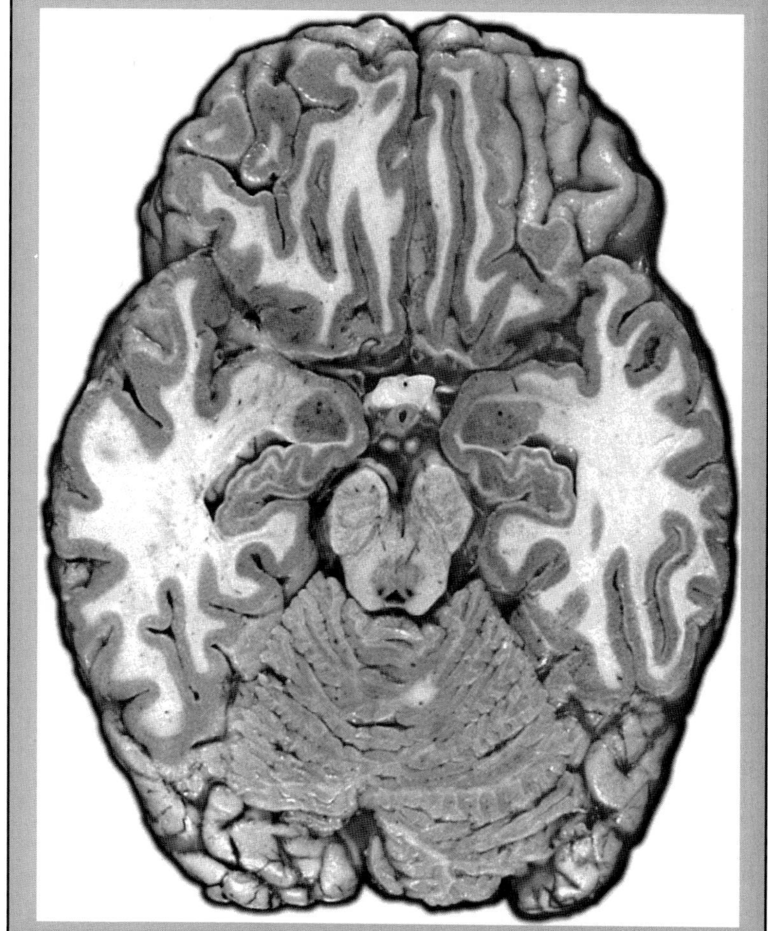

HORIZONTAL SECTION OF THE BRAIN, COMPLETE; LEVEL INCLUDING THE OPTIC CHIASM, INFUNDIBULUM, AMYGDALA, AND PONTOMESENCEPHALIC JUNCTION: MAGNIFIED VIEW, VENTRAL TO DORSAL PERSPECTIVE

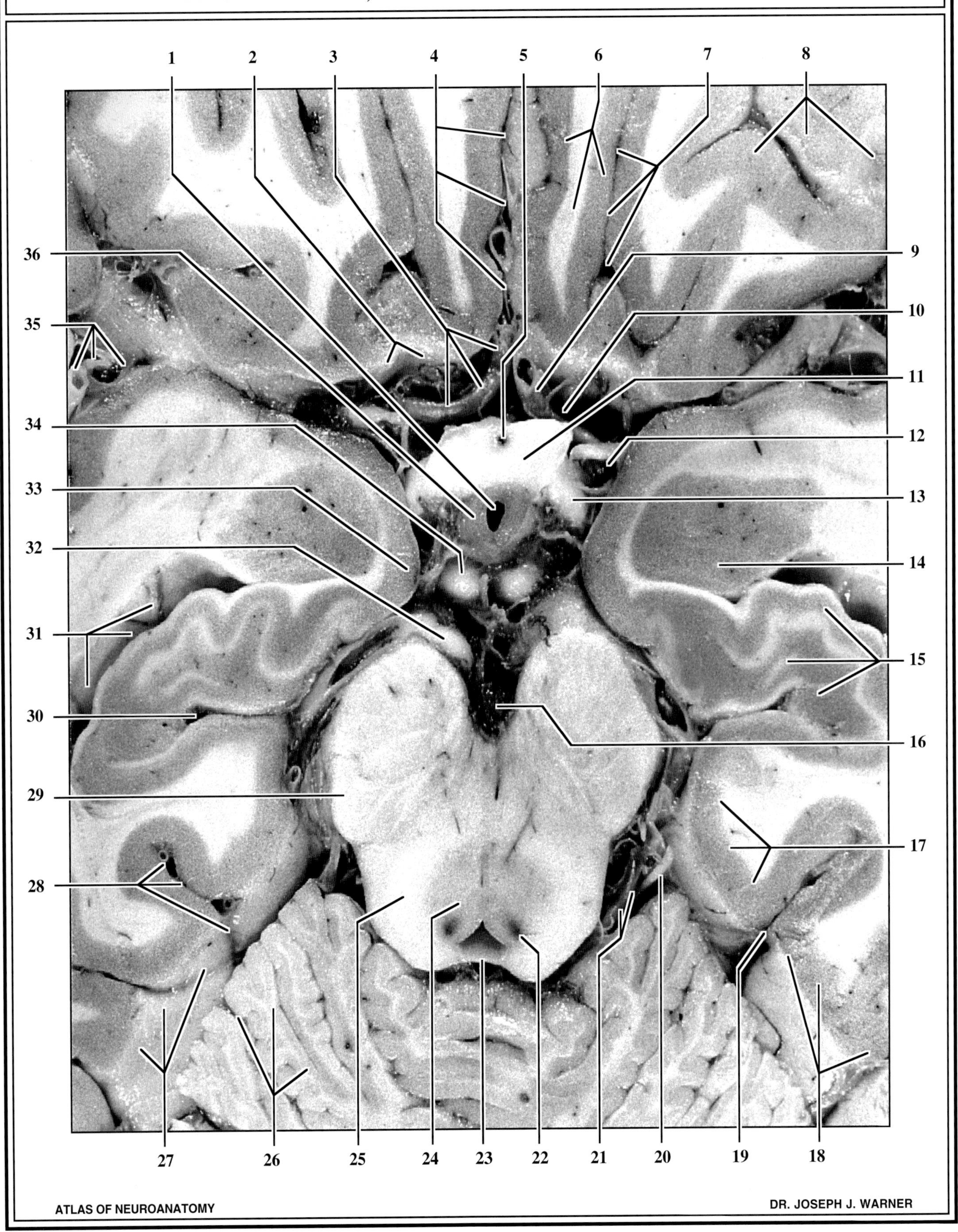

HORIZONTAL SECTION (MAGNIFIED VIEW); LEVEL INCLUDING THE OPTIC CHIASM, INFUNDIBULUM, AMYGDALA, AND PONTOMESENCEPHALIC JUNCTION: SECTION MAPS AND KEY TO NUMBERED STRUCTURES

KEY TO NUMBERED STRUCTURES

1. Infundibular Recess (Third Ventricle)
2. Olfactory Trigone
3. Anterior Cerebral Artery
4. Interhemispheric Fissure
5. Supraoptic Recess (Third Ventricle)
6. Gyrus Rectus
7. Olfactory Sulcus
8. Orbitofrontal Gyri
9. Anterior Cerebral Artery
10. Anterior Perforated Substance
11. Optic Chiasm
12. Internal Carotid Artery
13. Optic Tract
14. Amygdala*
15. Hippocampus*
16. Interpeduncular Fossa
17. Parahippocampal Gyrus
18. Fusiform Gyrus
19. Collateral Sulcus
20. Trochlear (IV) Nerve
21. Superior Cerebellar Artery
22. Locus Coeruleus
23. Anterior Medullary Velum
24. Periaqueductal Gray
25. Superior Cerebellar Peduncle
26. Anterior Lobe of the Cerebellum
27. Fusiform Gyrus
28. Collateral Sulcus
29. Cerebral Peduncle
30. Hippocampal Fissure
31. Temporal Horn of the Lateral Ventricle*
32. Oculomotor (III) Nerve
33. Uncus
34. Mammillary Body
35. Middle Cerebral Artery Trifurcation
36. Infundibulum

*Identification of the amygdala in various planes of section is facilitated by its relationship to major ventral brain structures. The amygdala is characterized by a rostrocaudal span from the level of the optic chiasm through the level of the mammillary bodies. A ventromedial curvature of the rostral aspect of the temporal horn of each lateral ventricle is intercalated between the amygdala and the rostral hippocampus.

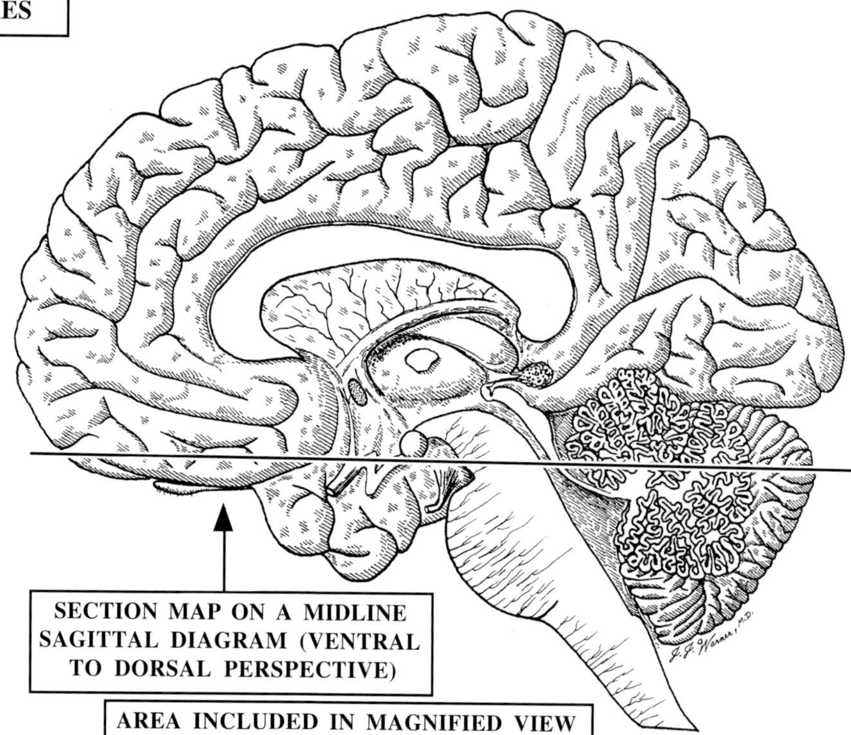

SECTION MAP ON A MIDLINE SAGITTAL DIAGRAM (VENTRAL TO DORSAL PERSPECTIVE)

AREA INCLUDED IN MAGNIFIED VIEW

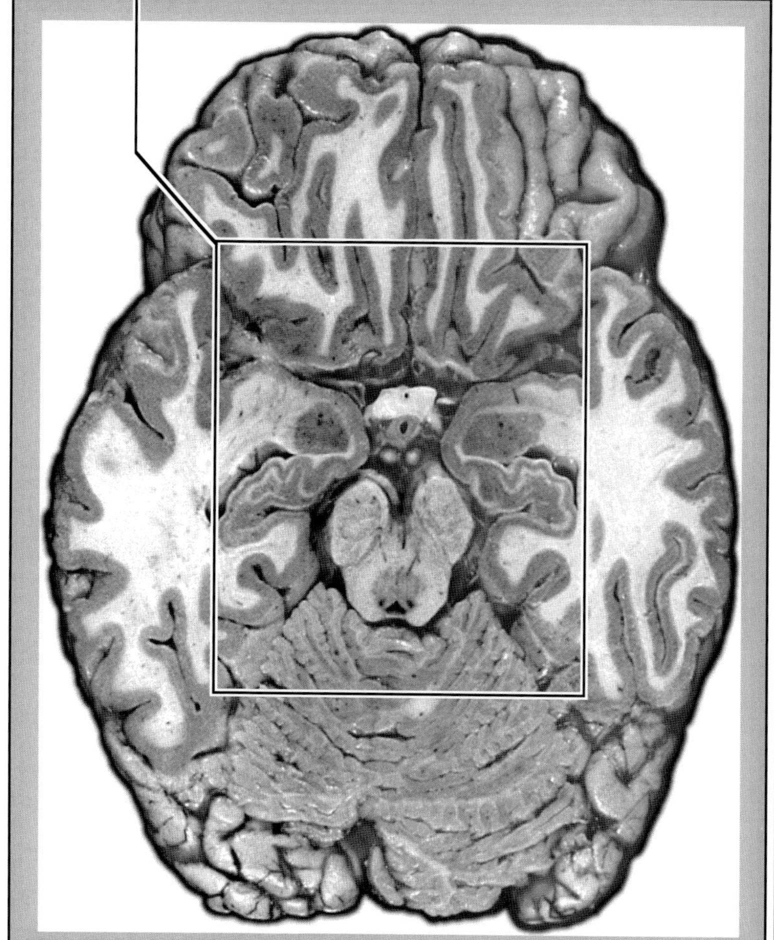

HORIZONTAL SECTION OF THE BRAIN, COMPLETE: LEVEL INCLUDING THE OPTIC CHIASM AND THE ROSTRAL OPTIC TRACTS

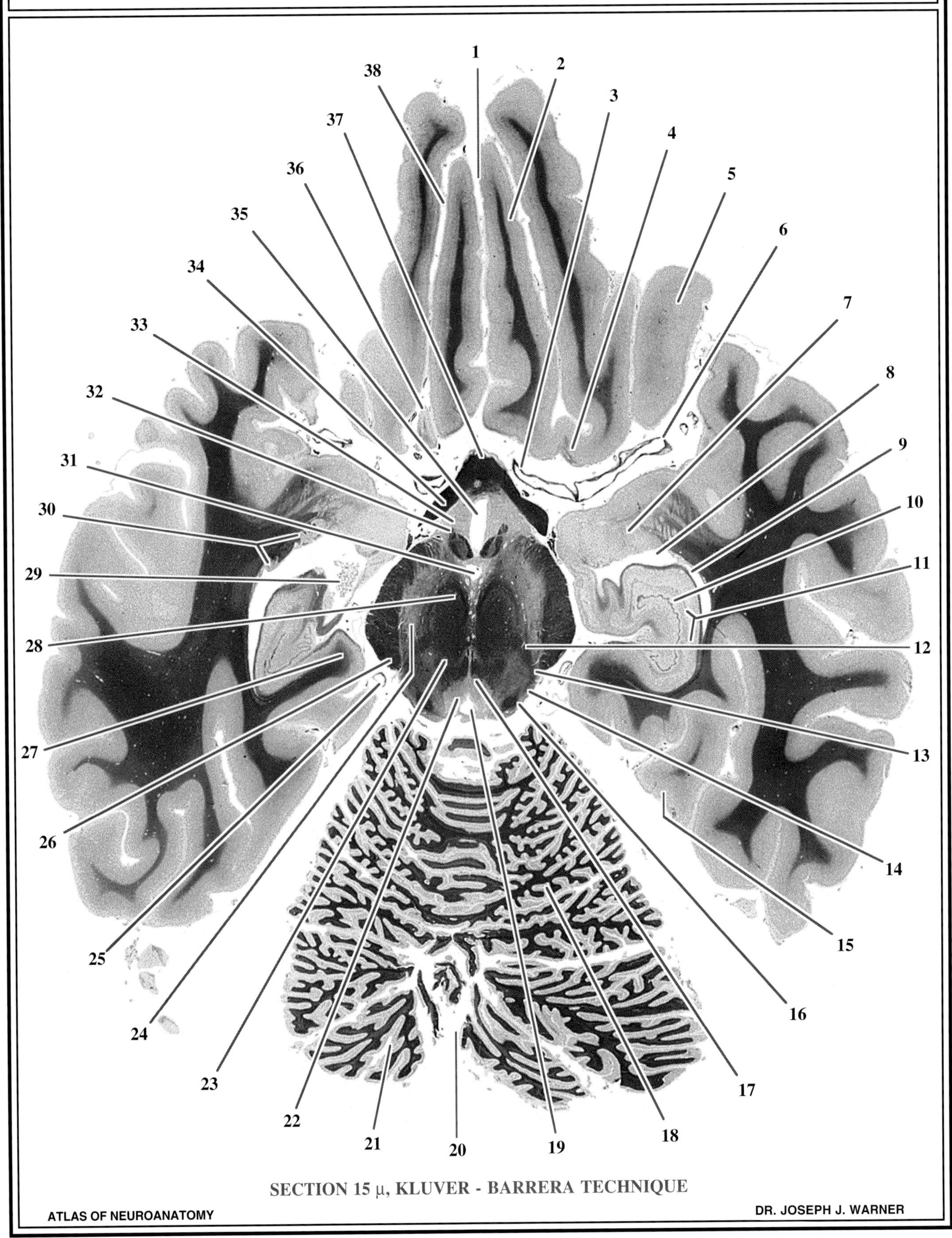

SECTION 15 μ, KLUVER - BARRERA TECHNIQUE

HORIZONTAL SECTION OF THE BRAIN, COMPLETE; LEVEL INCLUDING THE OPTIC CHIASM AND THE ROSTRAL OPTIC TRACTS: SECTION ORIENTATION AND KEY TO NUMBERED STRUCTURES

KEY TO NUMBERED STRUCTURES

1. Interhemispheric Fissure
2. Gyrus Rectus
3. Anterior Cerebral Artery
4. Lateral Olfactory Stria*
5. Orbitofrontal Gyri
6. Middle Cerebral Artery
7. Amygdala
8. Temporal Horn of the Lateral Ventricle
9. Alveus
10. Dentate Gyrus of the Hippocampus
11. Hippocampus
12. Medial Lemniscus
13. Spinothalamic and Trigeminothalamic Tracts
14. Lateral Lemniscus
15. Fusiform Gyrus
16. Caudal aspect of the Inferior Colliculus
17. Medial Longitudinal Fasciculus
18. Anterior Lobe of the Cerebellum
19. Aqueduct of Sylvius
20. Posterior Incisure
21. Posterior Lobe of the Cerebellum
22. Periaqueductal Gray
23. Central Tegmental Tract
24. Substantia Nigra
25. Posterior Cerebral Artery
26. Cerebral Peduncle
27. Parahippocampal Gyrus
28. Red Nucleus
29. Choroid Plexus
30. Tail of the Caudate Nucleus
31. Interpeduncular Fossa
32. Fibers of the Fornix and of the Principal Mammillary Fasciculus
33. Hypothalamus
34. Optic Tract**
35. Third Ventricle
36. Olfactory Tract (caudal aspect)*
37. Optic Chiasm
38. Olfactory Sulcus

*The olfactory tract divides into the medial and lateral olfactory striae (olfactory trigone).

**Each optic tract courses laterally to the hypothalamus, passing circumferentially in a caudal and dorsal direction. Thus, the caudal aspect of the optic tract is dorsal to the plane of section.

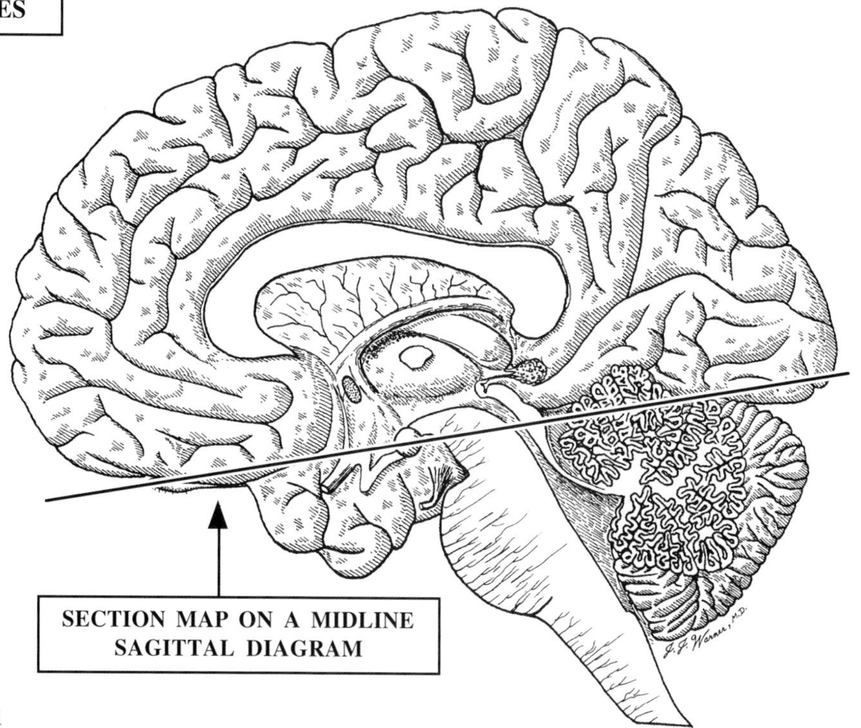

SECTION MAP ON A MIDLINE SAGITTAL DIAGRAM

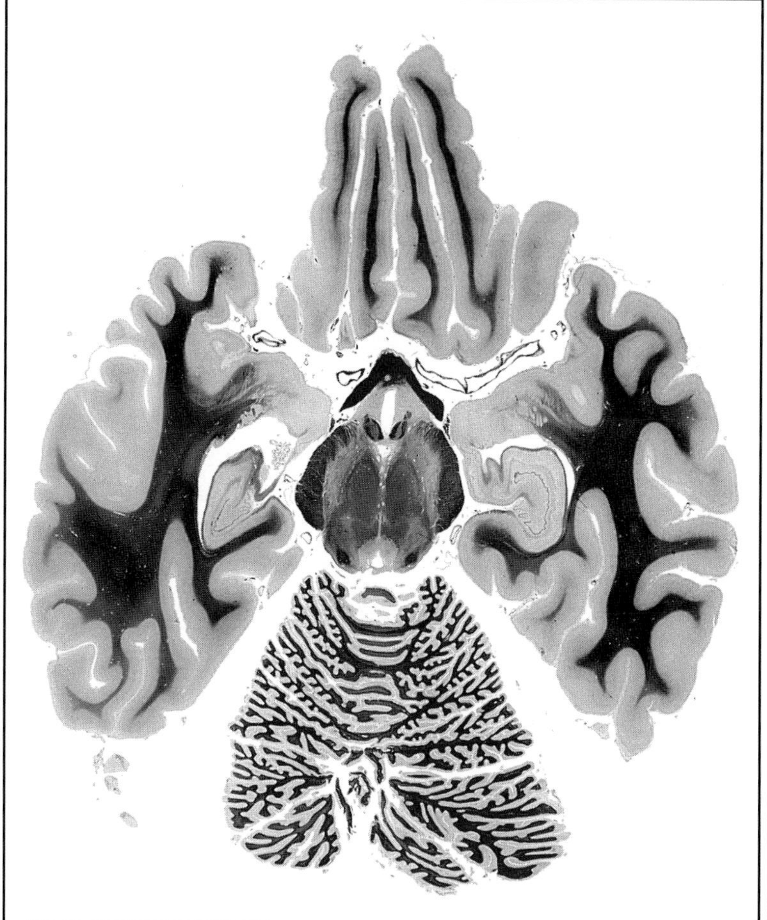

ATLAS OF NEUROANATOMY DR. JOSEPH J. WARNER

HORIZONTAL SECTION OF THE BRAIN, COMPLETE: LEVEL OF THE MESENCEPHALIC-DIENCEPHALIC JUNCTION, INCLUDING THE MEDIAL AND LATERAL GENICULATE NUCLEI

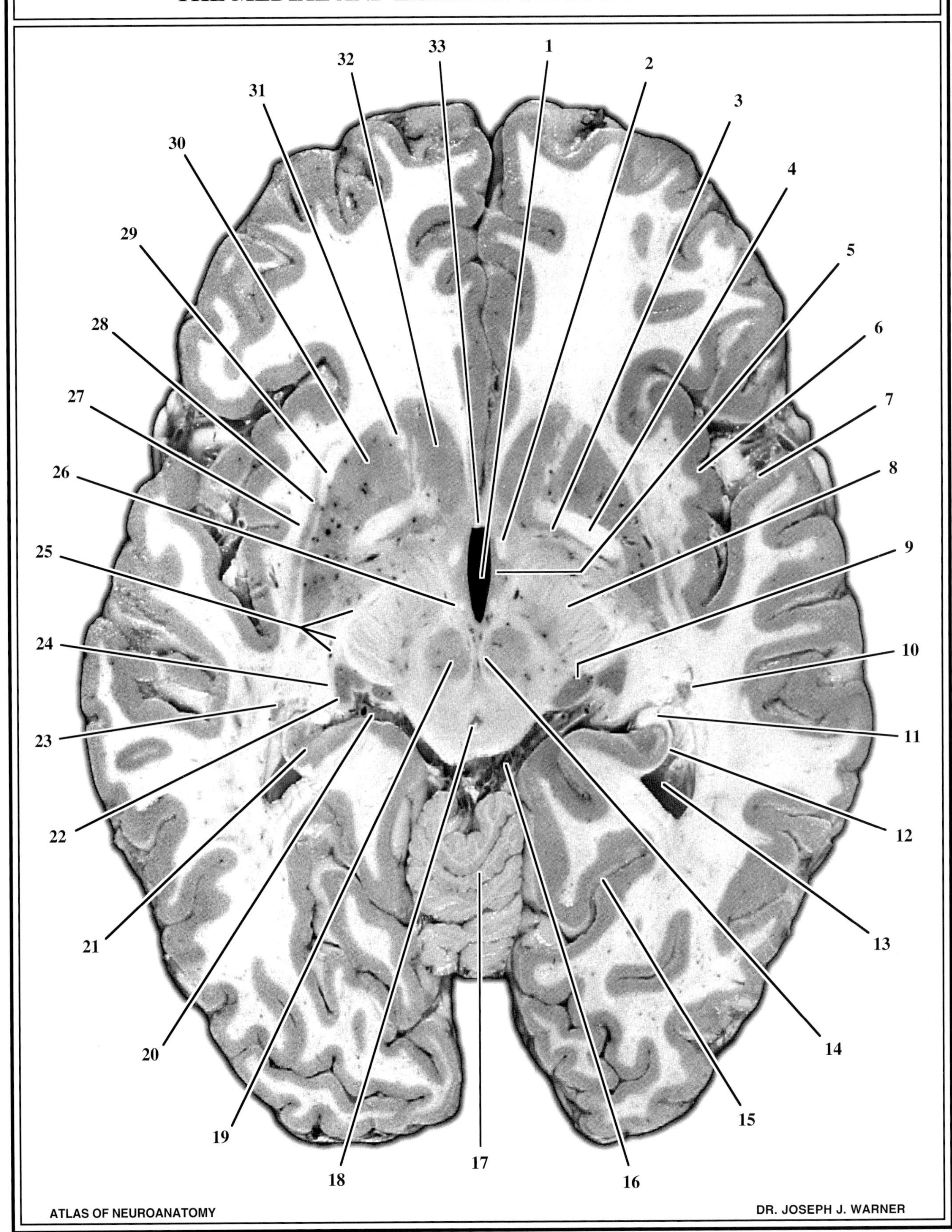

HORIZONTAL SECTION; LEVEL OF THE MESENCEPHALIC-DIENCEPHALIC JUNCTION, INCLUDING THE MEDIAL AND LATERAL GENICULATE NUCLEI: SECTION ORIENTATION AND KEY TO NUMBERED STRUCTURES

KEY TO NUMBERED STRUCTURES

1. Third Ventricle
2. Postcommissural Fibers of the Fornix
3. Globus Pallidus*
4. Anterior Commissure*
5. Hypothalamus
6. Insular Cortex
7. Sylvian Fissure
8. Cerebral Peduncle
9. Medial Geniculate Nucleus
10. Tail of the Caudate Nucleus
11. Fimbria of the Fornix
12. Alveus
13. Temporal Horn of the Lateral Ventricle
14. Fasciculus Retroflexus of Meynert (Habenulo-interpeduncular Tract)
15. Ventroanterior extension of Calcarine Fissure
16. Quadrigeminal Cistern
17. Superior Cerebellar Vermis
18. Aqueduct of Sylvius
19. Red Nucleus
20. Posterior Cerebral Artery
21. Hippocampus
22. Lateral Geniculate Nucleus
23. Tail of the Caudate Nucleus
24. Geniculocalcarine Radiations
25. Optic Tract*
26. Mammillothalamic Tract
27. Extreme Capsule
28. Claustrum
29. External Capsule
30. Putamen
31. Anterior Limb of the Internal Capsule
32. Head of the Caudate Nucleus
33. Anterior Commissure (dorsal to the plane of section)

*Reference to coronal and sagittal sections emphasizes the close anatomic proximity of the globus pallidus, optic tract, and anterior commissure. The globus pallidus, situated medial to the putamen, is located dorsal and anterolateral to the optic tract. The anterior commissure, included in this plane of section, passes through the ventral aspect of the globus pallidus. *Note that the anterior commissure crosses the midline dorsal to the level of its lateral fibers.*

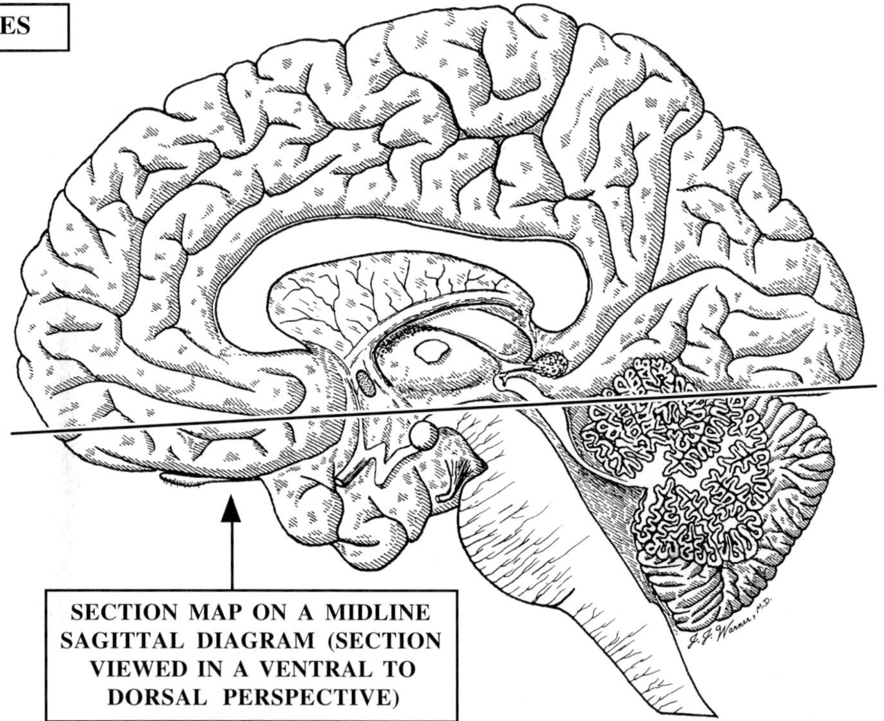

SECTION MAP ON A MIDLINE SAGITTAL DIAGRAM (SECTION VIEWED IN A VENTRAL TO DORSAL PERSPECTIVE)

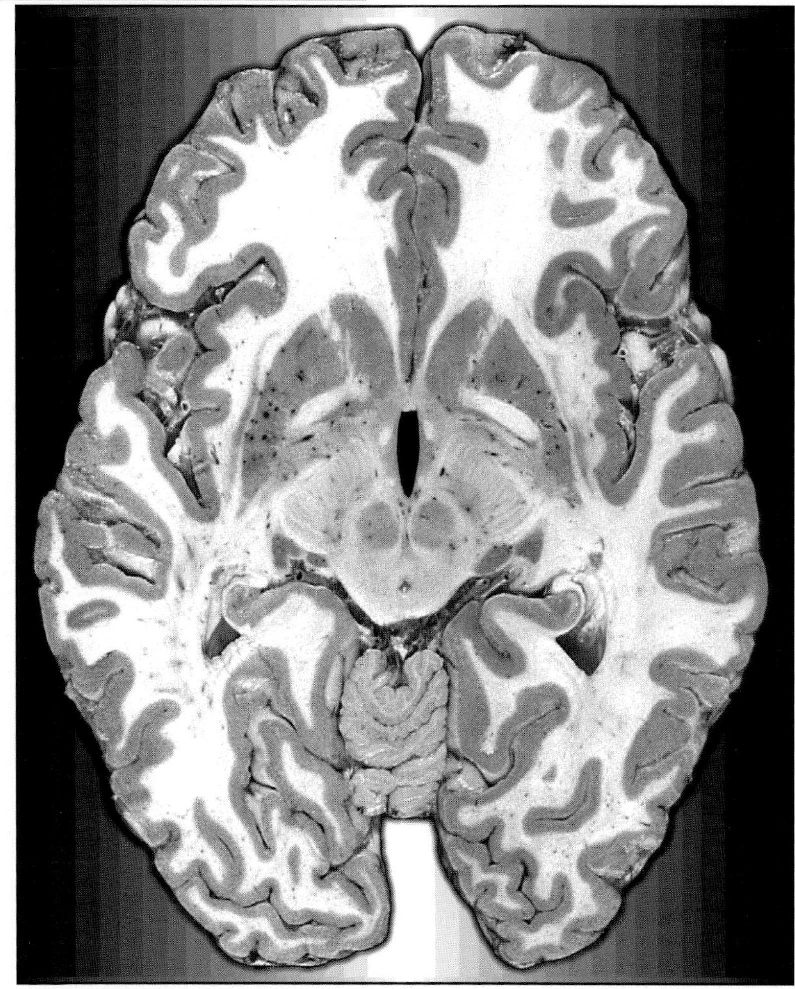

HORIZONTAL SECTION OF THE BRAIN; LEVEL OF THE MESENCEPHALIC-DIENCEPHALIC JUNCTION, INCLUDING THE MEDIAL AND LATERAL GENICULATE NUCLEI: MAGNIFIED VIEW, *DORSAL TO VENTRAL* PERSPECTIVE

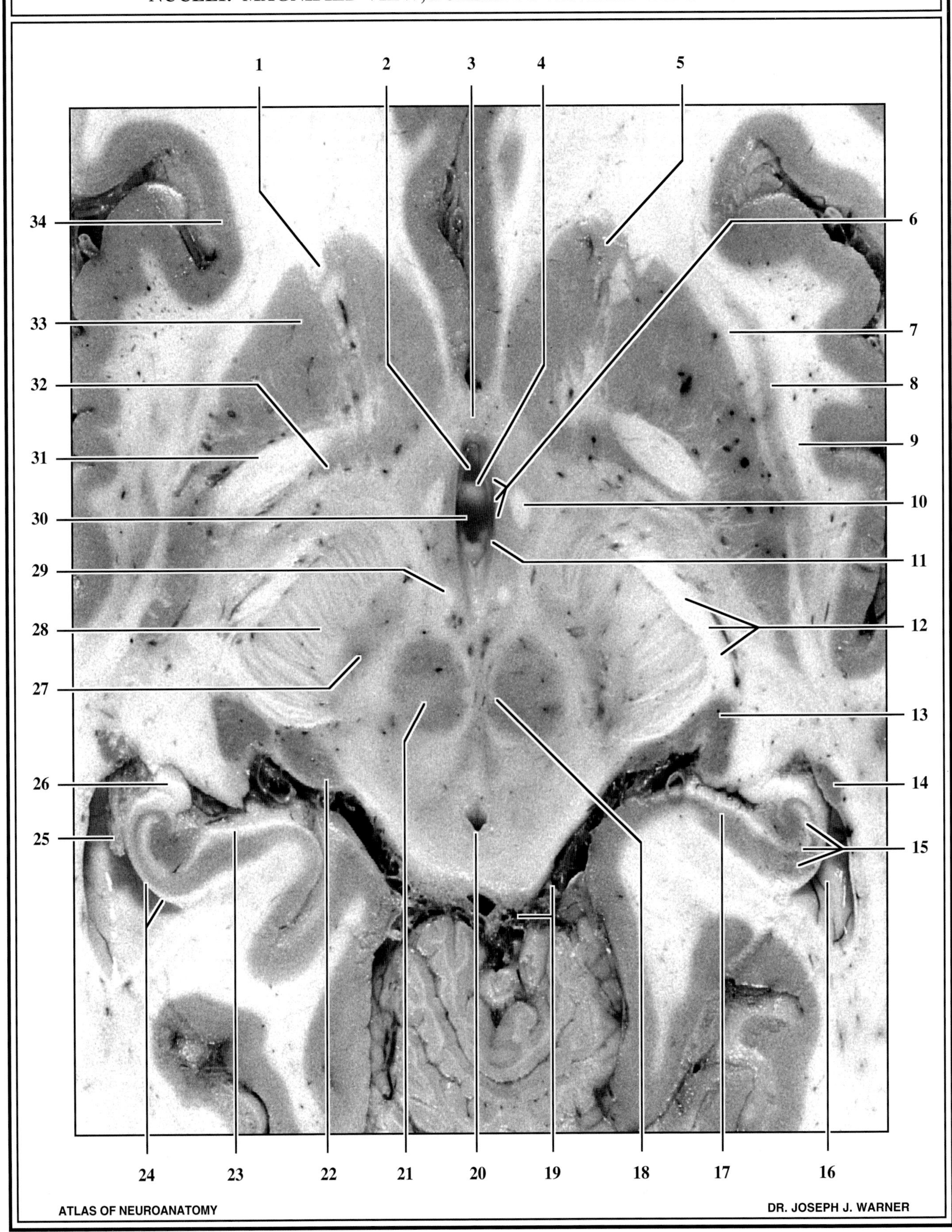

HORIZONTAL SECTION (MAGNIFIED VIEW); LEVEL OF THE MESENCEPHALIC-DIENCEPHALIC JUNCTION, INCLUDING THE MEDIAL AND LATERAL GENICULATE NUCLEI: SECTION MAP AND KEY TO NUMBERED STRUCTURES

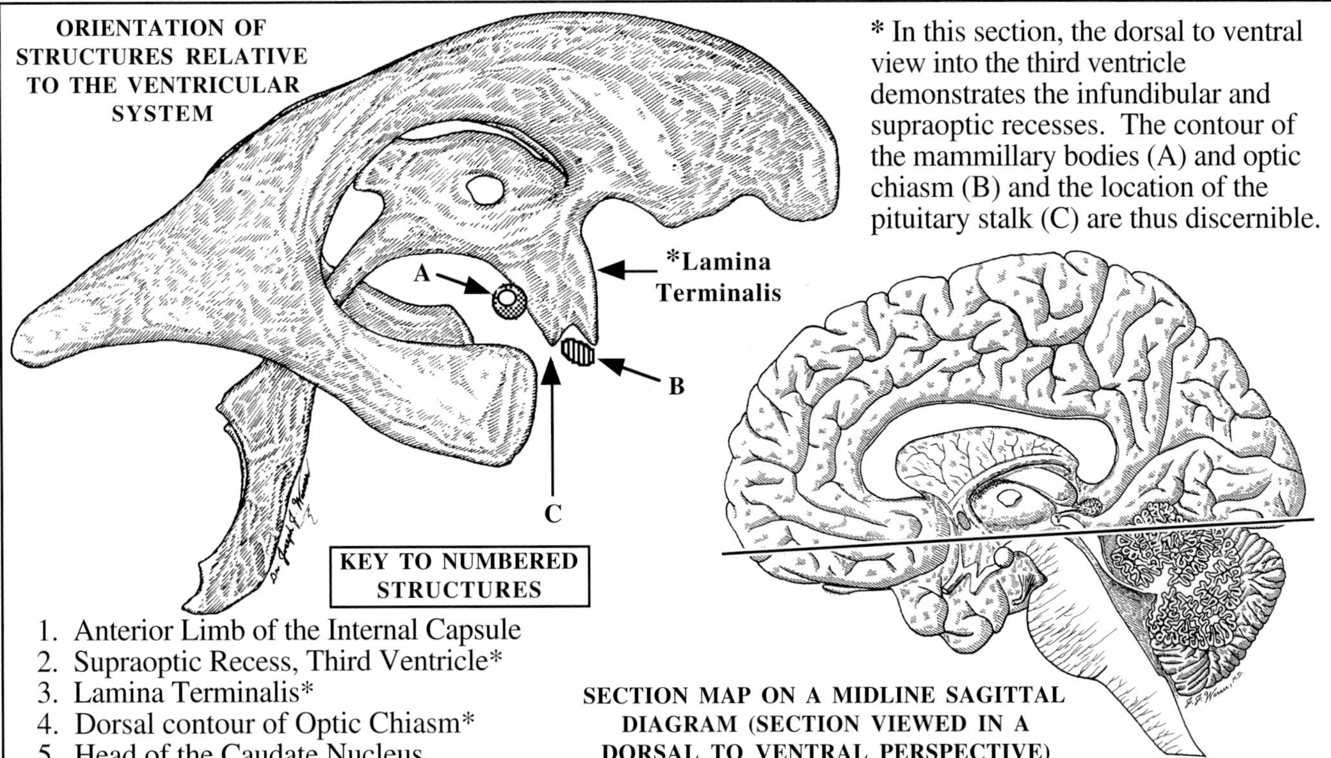

* In this section, the dorsal to ventral view into the third ventricle demonstrates the infundibular and supraoptic recesses. The contour of the mammillary bodies (A) and optic chiasm (B) and the location of the pituitary stalk (C) are thus discernible.

SECTION MAP ON A MIDLINE SAGITTAL DIAGRAM (SECTION VIEWED IN A DORSAL TO VENTRAL PERSPECTIVE)

KEY TO NUMBERED STRUCTURES

1. Anterior Limb of the Internal Capsule
2. Supraoptic Recess, Third Ventricle*
3. Lamina Terminalis*
4. Dorsal contour of Optic Chiasm*
5. Head of the Caudate Nucleus
6. Hypothalamus
7. External Capsule
8. Claustrum
9. Extreme Capsule
10. Postcommissural Fibers of the Fornix
11. Dorsomedial contour of the Mammillary Body*
12. Optic Tract
13. Lateral Geniculate Nucleus
14. Tail of the Caudate Nucleus
15. Hippocampus
16. Temporal Horn of the Lateral Ventricle
17. Subiculum
18. Habenulointerpeduncular Tract
19. Quadrigeminal Cistern
20. Aqueduct of Sylvius
21. Red Nucleus
22. Medial Geniculate Nucleus
23. Superficial Medullary Stratum of the Subiculum
24. Alveus
25. Choroid Plexus
26. Fimbria of the Fornix
27. Subthalamic Nucleus
28. Cerebral Peduncle
29. Mammillothalamic Tract
30. Infundibular Recess, Third Ventricle*
31. Anterior Commissure
32. Globus Pallidus
33. Putamen
34. Insular Cortex

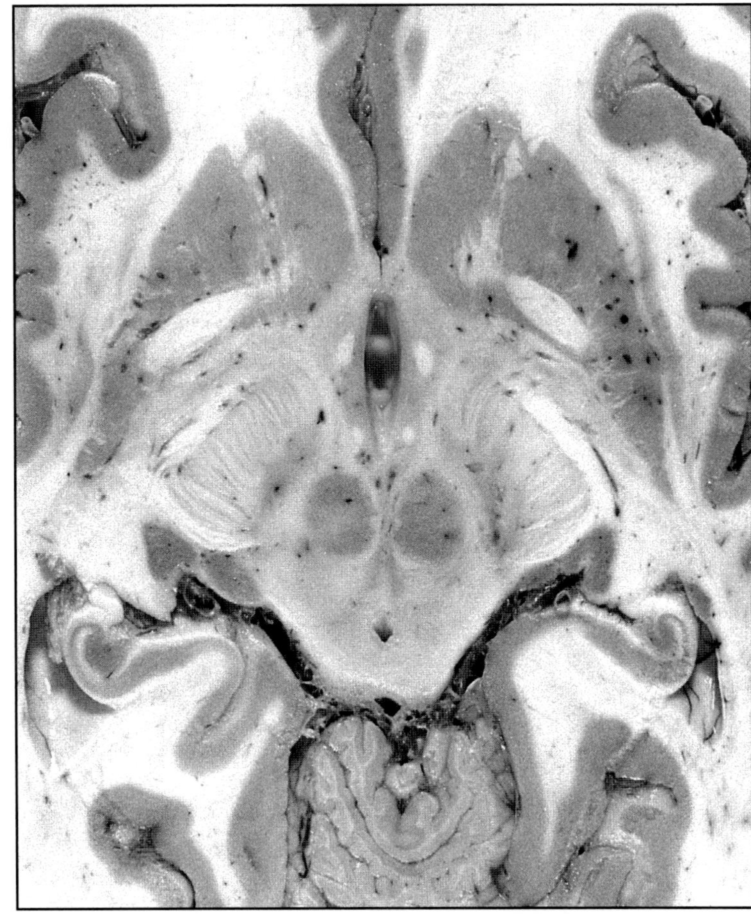

HORIZONTAL SECTION OF THE BRAIN, COMPLETE: LEVEL IMMEDIATELY DORSAL TO THE ANTERIOR COMMISSURE AND THE PINEAL BODY, VENTRAL TO DORSAL PERSPECTIVE

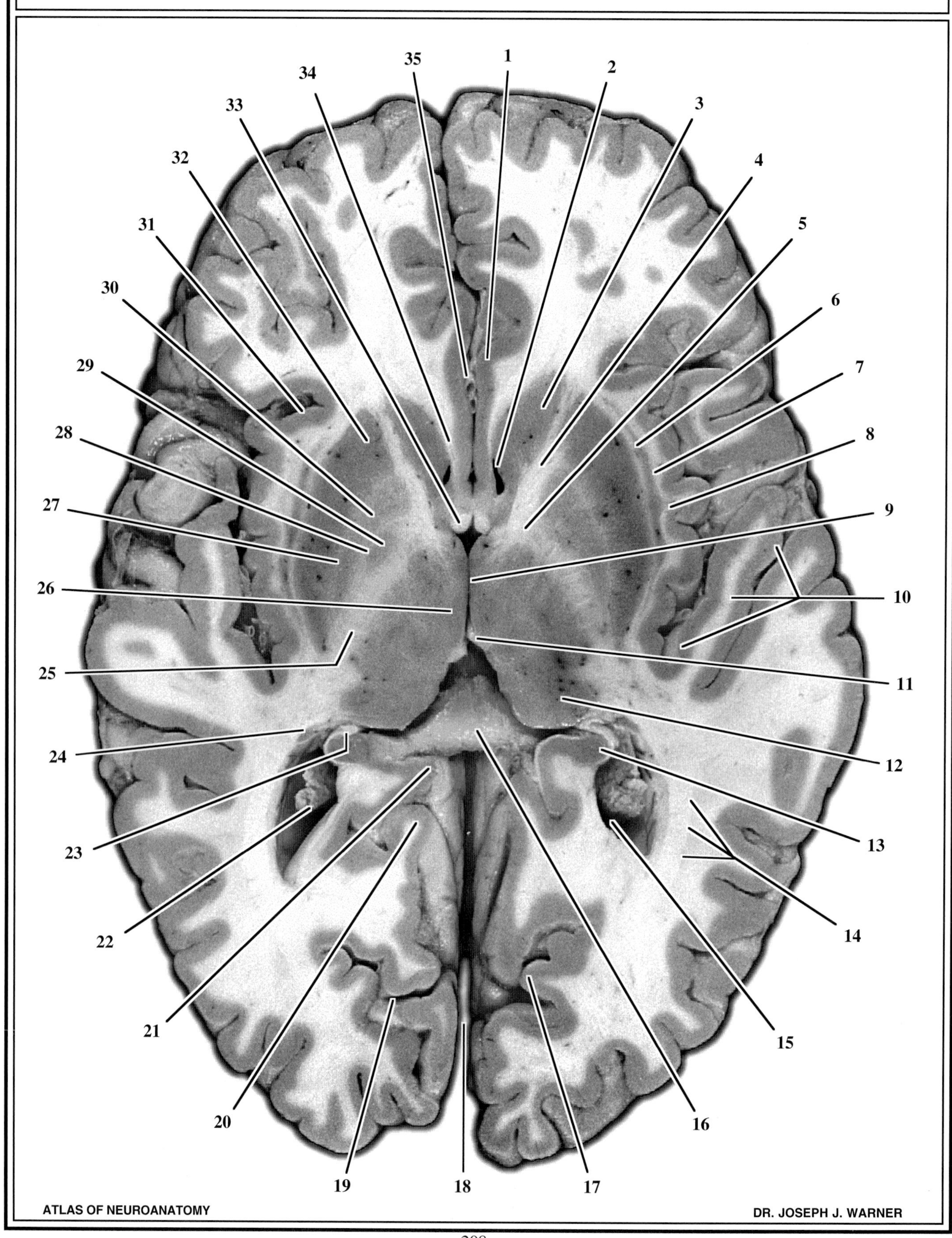

HORIZONTAL SECTION OF THE BRAIN, COMPLETE; LEVEL IMMEDIATELY DORSAL TO THE ANTERIOR COMMISSURE AND THE PINEAL BODY: SECTION ORIENTATION AND KEY TO NUMBERED STRUCTURES

KEY TO NUMBERED STRUCTURES

1. Cingulate Gyrus
2. Ventral extent of the Anterior Horn of the Lateral Ventricle
3. Head of the Caudate Nucleus
4. Anterior Limb of the Internal Capsule
5. Genu of the Internal Capsule
6. External Capsule
7. Claustrum
8. Extreme Capsule
9. Third Ventricle
10. Heschl's Gyrus*
11. Stria Medullaris
12. Pulvinar Nucleus of the Thalamus
13. Hippocampus
14. Optic Radiations
15. Atrium of the Lateral Ventricle
16. Splenium of the Corpus Callosum
17. Striate (Area 17) Cortex
18. Interhemispheric Fissure
19. Calcarine Fissure
20. Lingular Gyrus
21. Isthmus of the Gyrus Fornicatus
22. Choroid Plexus
23. Fimbria of the Fornix
24. Tail of the Caudate Nucleus
25. Posterior Limb of the Internal Capsule
26. Dorsomedial Nucleus of the Thalamus
27. External Medullary Lamina
28. Internal Medullary Lamina
29. Globus Pallidus I
30. Globus Pallidus II
31. Insular Cortex
32. Putamen
33. Fornix
34. Ventral Fibers of the Rostrum of the Corpus Callosum**
35. Anterior Cerebral Arteries

*Heschl's gyrus (Brodmann's Area 41) and the planum temporale are frequently characterized by morphologic asymmetries between the left and right hemispheres. A single, large Heschl's gyrus is often seen on the left, whereas a smaller, often doubled homologue characterizes the right temporal lobe. The left planum temporale is generally larger than that of the right hemisphere.
**Refer to morphology on coronal sections.

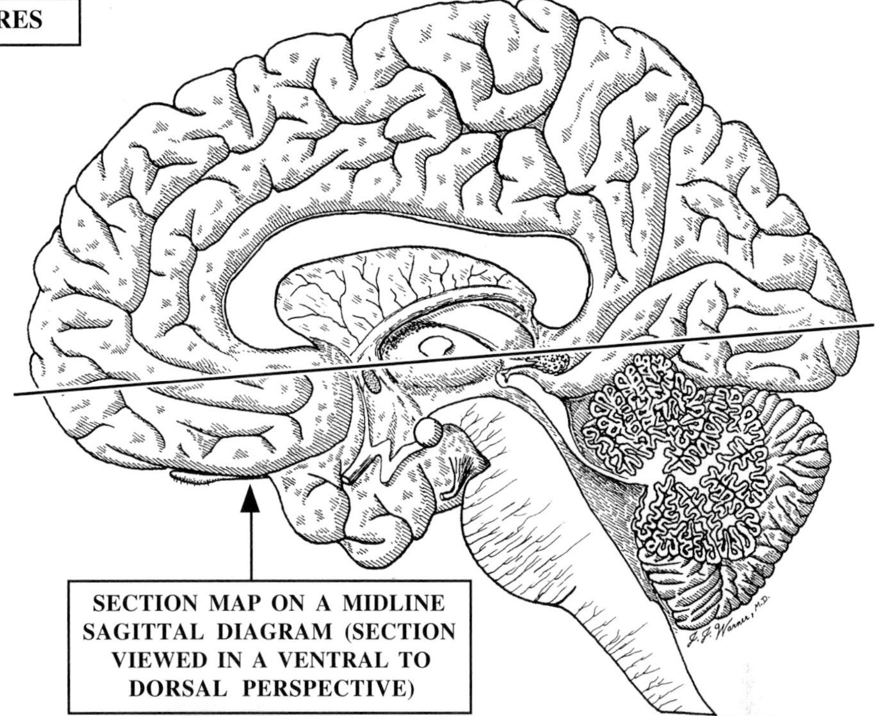

SECTION MAP ON A MIDLINE SAGITTAL DIAGRAM (SECTION VIEWED IN A VENTRAL TO DORSAL PERSPECTIVE)

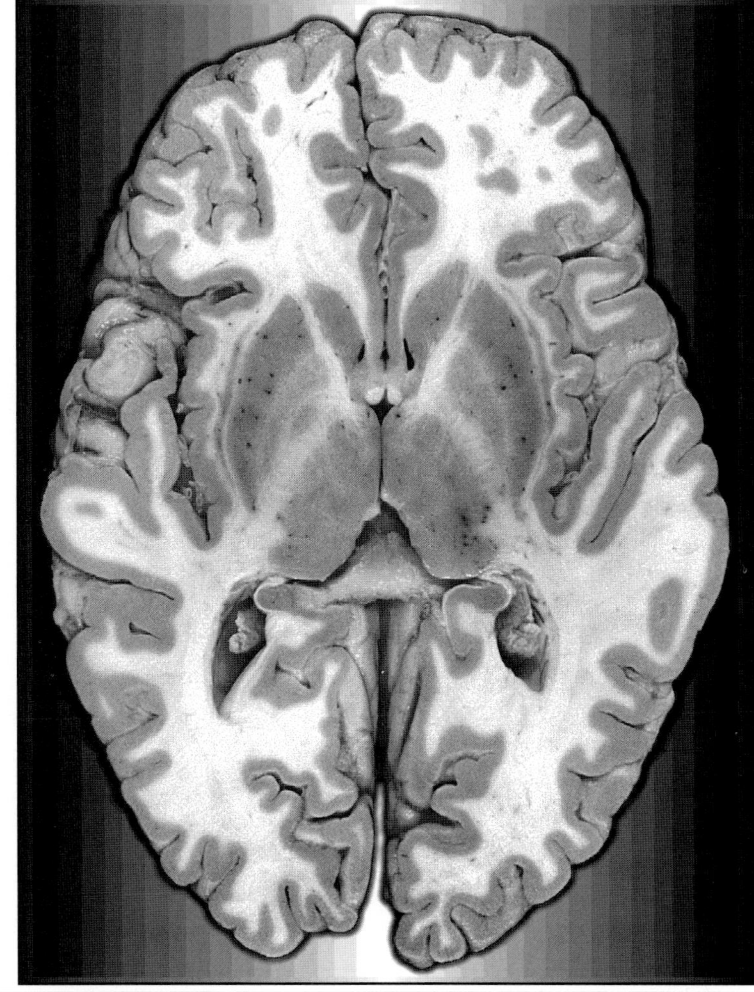

HORIZONTAL SECTION OF THE BRAIN; LEVEL IMMEDIATELY DORSAL TO THE ANTERIOR AND POSTERIOR COMMISSURES AND TO THE PINEAL BODY: MAGNIFIED VIEW, *DORSAL TO VENTRAL* PERSPECTIVE

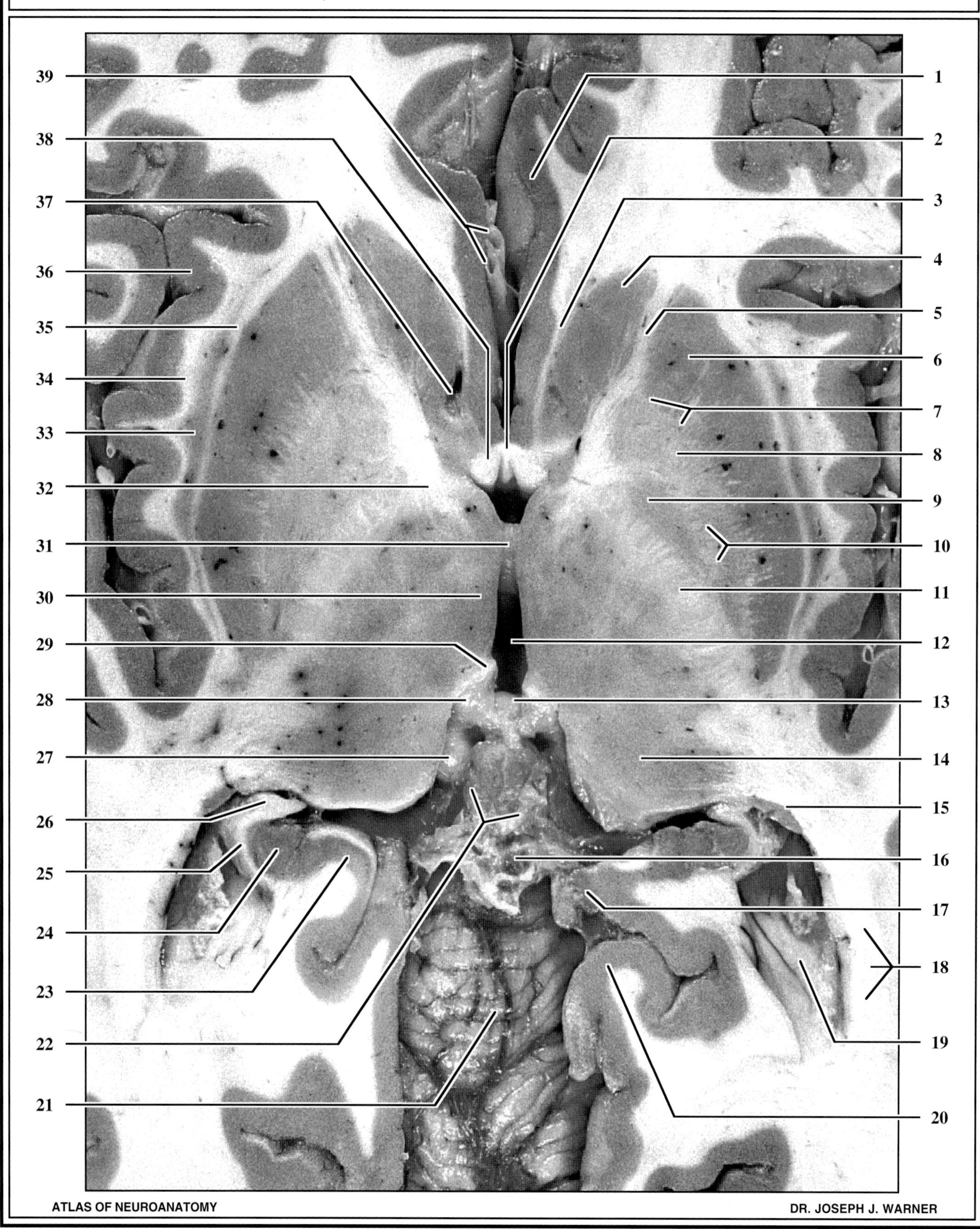

HORIZONTAL SECTION (MAGNIFIED DORSAL TO VENTRAL VIEW); LEVEL IMMEDIATELY DORSAL TO THE ANTERIOR AND POSTERIOR COMMISSURES AND TO THE PINEAL BODY: SECTION MAP AND KEY TO NUMBERED STRUCTURES

KEY TO NUMBERED STRUCTURES

1. Cingulate Gyrus
2. Anterior Commissure
3. Rostrum of the Corpus Callosum
4. Head of the Caudate Nucleus
5. Anterior Limb of the Internal Capsule
6. Putamen
7. External Medullary Lamina
8. Globus Pallidus II
9. Globus Pallidus I
10. Internal Medullary Lamina
11. Posterior Limb of the Internal Capsule
12. Third Ventricle
13. Posterior Commissure
14. Pulvinar Nucleus of the Thalamus
15. Tail of the Caudate Nucleus
16. Arachnoid subjacent to the Great Vein of Galen
17. Isthmus of the Gyrus Fornicatus
18. Optic (Geniculocalcarine) Radiations
19. Atrium of the Lateral Ventricle
20. Lingular Gyrus
21. Superior Cerebellar Vermis
22. Pineal Body
23. Subiculum
24. Hippocampus
25. Alveus
26. Fimbria of the Fornix
27. Superior Colliculus (ventral to the plane of section)
28. Habenula
29. Stria Medullaris
30. Dorsomedial Nucleus of the Thalamus
31. Massa Intermedia*
32. Genu of the Internal Capsule
33. Claustrum
34. Extreme Capsule
35. External Capsule
36. Insular Cortex
37. Ventral extent of the Anterior Horn of the Lateral Ventricle
38. Fornix
39. Anterior Cerebral Arteries

*Normal anatomic variability between brains accounts for the position of the massa intermedia ventral to the plane of this section, as opposed to the general position of that structure as mapped on the midline sagittal diagram.

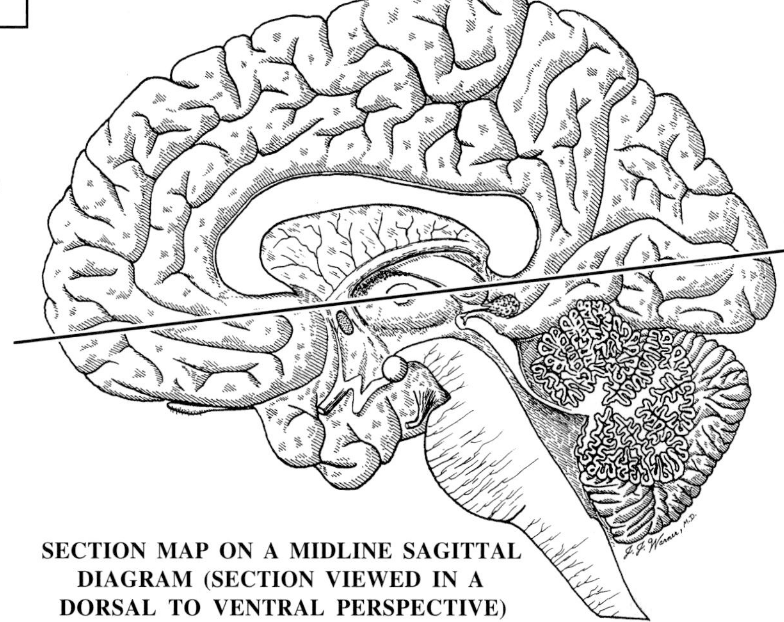

SECTION MAP ON A MIDLINE SAGITTAL DIAGRAM (SECTION VIEWED IN A DORSAL TO VENTRAL PERSPECTIVE)

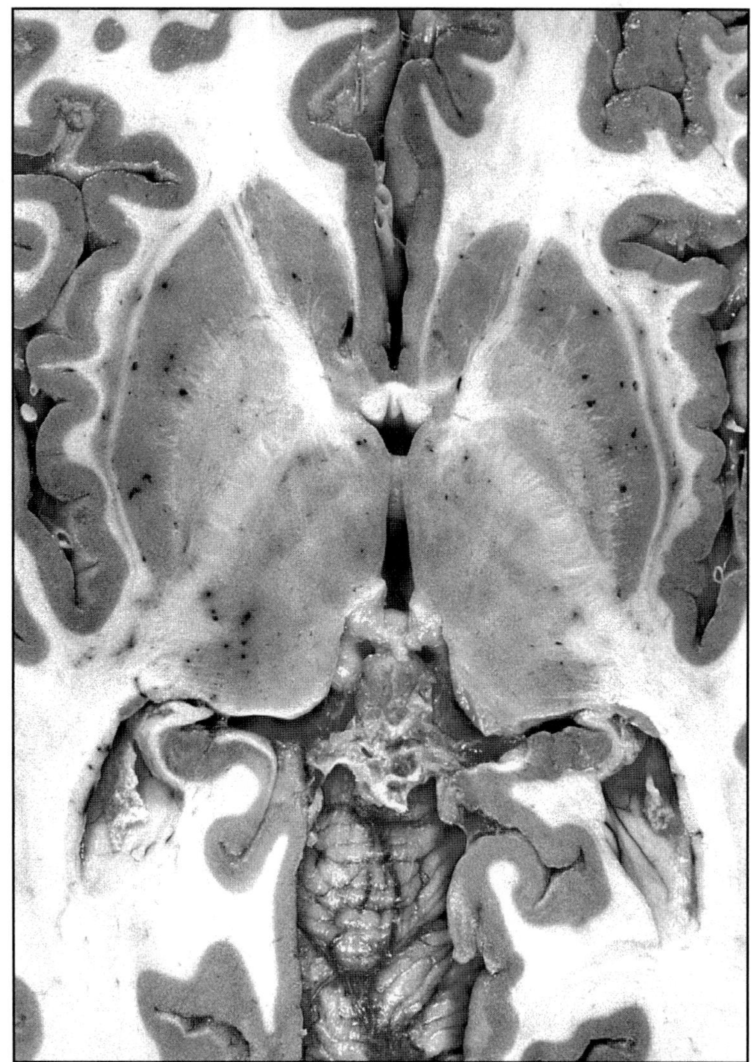

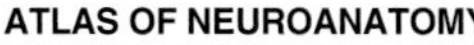

HORIZONTAL SECTION OF THE BRAIN; LEVEL OF THE FORAMEN OF MONRO, MASSA INTERMEDIA, AND THE PINEAL RECESS OF THE THIRD VENTRICLE: MAGNIFIED VIEW, *DORSAL TO VENTRAL* PERSPECTIVE

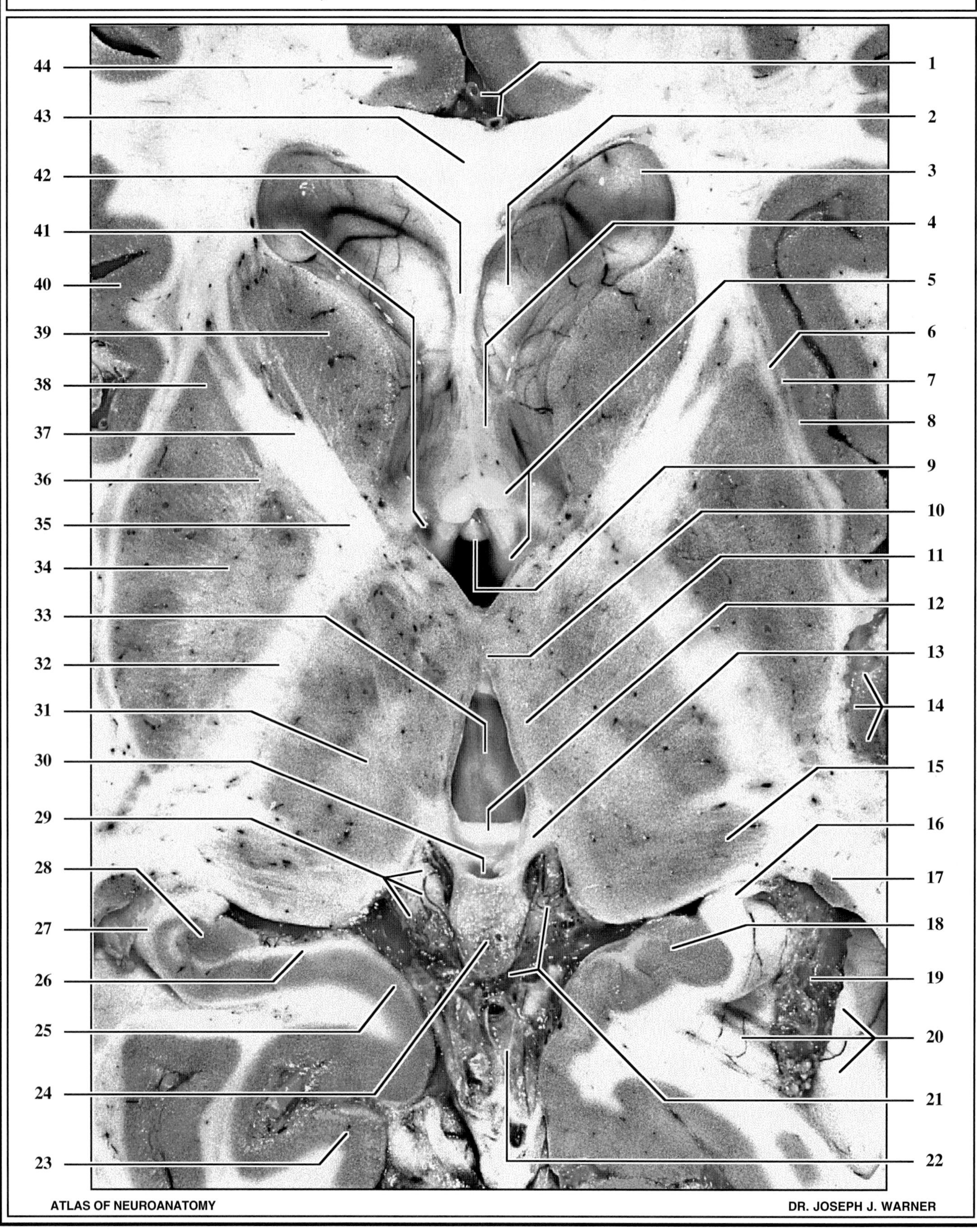

HORIZONTAL SECTION (MAGNIFIED DORSAL TO VENTRAL VIEW); LEVEL OF THE FORAMEN OF MONRO, MASSA INTERMEDIA, AND THE PINEAL RECESS OF THE THIRD VENTRICLE: SECTION MAP AND KEY TO NUMBERED STRUCTURES

KEY TO NUMBERED STRUCTURES

1. Anterior Cerebral Arteries
2. Rostrum of the Corpus Callosum*
3. Anterior Horn of the Lateral Ventricle*
4. Septal Nuclei
5. Fornix
6. External Capsule
7. Claustrum
8. Extreme Capsule
9. Anterior Commissure
10. Massa Intermedia
11. Dorsomedial Nucleus of the Thalamus
12. Posterior Commissure
13. Habenula
14. Infarction involving Middle Cerebral Artery branch distribution
15. Pulvinar Nucleus of the Thalamus
16. Fimbria of the Fornix
17. Tail of the Caudate Nucleus
18. Retrosplenial Gyrus of the Hippocampus
19. Choroid Plexus
20. Atrium of the Lateral Ventricle
21. Quadrigeminal Cistern
22. Ventral curve of the Great Vein of Galen
23. Lingular Gyrus
24. Pineal Body
25. Isthmus of the Gyrus Fornicatus
26. Superficial Medullary Stratum of the Subiculum
27. Alveus
28. Hippocampus
29. Superior Colliculus (ventral to the plane of section)
30. Pineal Recess of the Third Ventricle
31. Centromedian Nucleus of the Thalamus
32. Posterior Limb of the Internal Capsule
33. Floor of the Third Ventricle
34. Globus Pallidus II
35. Genu of the Internal Capsule
36. External Medullary Lamina
37. Anterior Limb of the Internal Capsule
38. Putamen
39. Head of the Caudate Nucleus
40. Insular Cortex
41. Foramen of Monro
42. Septum Pellucidum
43. Genu of the Corpus Callosum
44. Cingulum

* The rostrum of the corpus callosum forms the floor of the anterior horn of the lateral ventricles. This relationship is clearly shown on paramedian sagittal and rostral coronal sections.

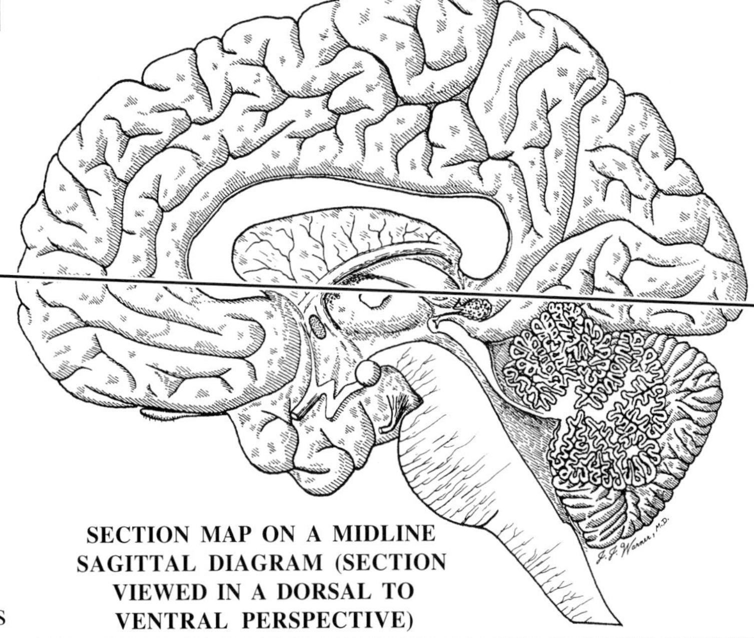

SECTION MAP ON A MIDLINE SAGITTAL DIAGRAM (SECTION VIEWED IN A DORSAL TO VENTRAL PERSPECTIVE)

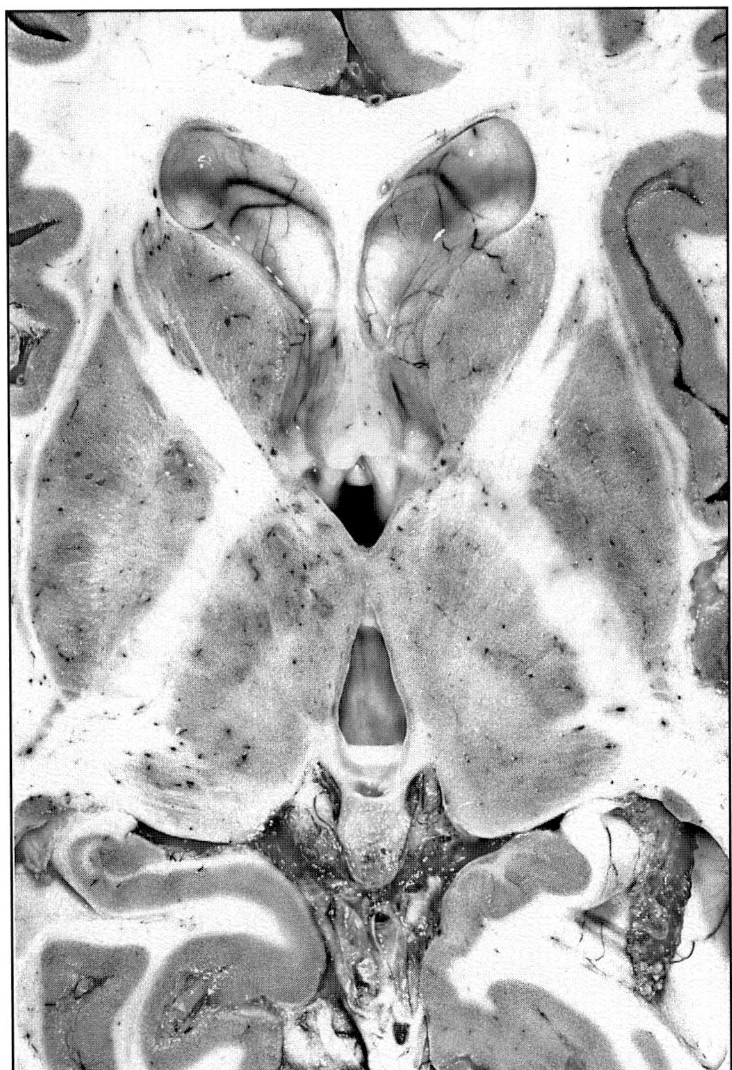

HORIZONTAL SECTION OF THE BRAIN, COMPLETE: LEVEL OF THE PINEAL BODY AND OF THE GENU TO ROSTRUM OF THE CORPUS CALLOSUM, VENTRAL TO DORSAL PERSPECTIVE

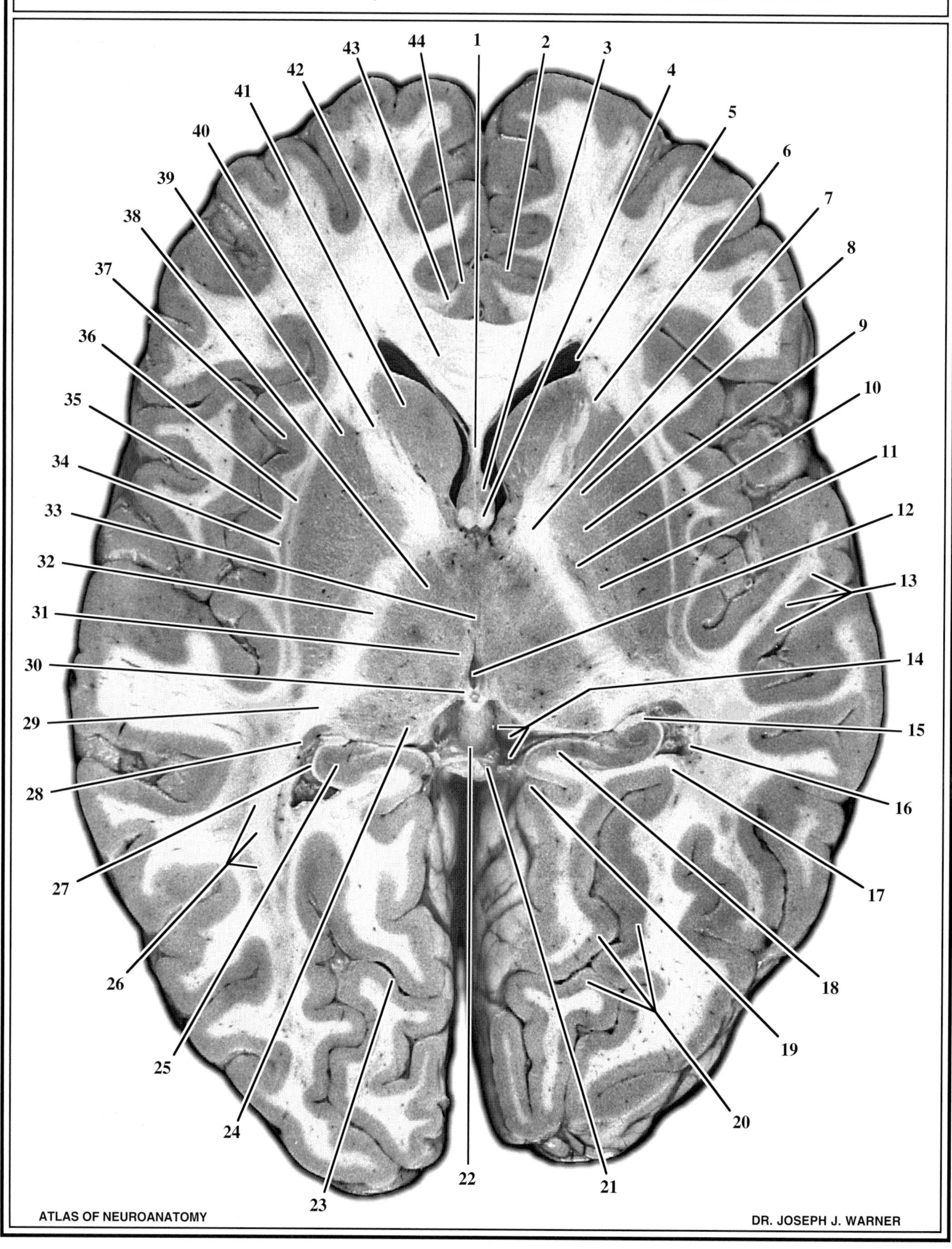

HORIZONTAL SECTION OF THE BRAIN, COMPLETE; LEVEL OF THE PINEAL BODY AND OF THE GENU TO ROSTRUM OF THE CORPUS CALLOSUM: SECTION ORIENTATION AND KEY TO NUMBERED STRUCTURES

KEY TO NUMBERED STRUCTURES

1. Septum Pellucidum
2. Cingulate Sulcus
3. Septal Nuclei
4. Fornix
5. Anterior Horn of the Lateral Ventricle
6. Transcapsular Caudatolenticular Gray Stria
7. Genu of the Internal Capsule
8. External Medullary Lamina
9. Globus Pallidus II
10. Globus Pallidus I
11. Internal Medullary Lamina
12. Third Ventricle
13. Heschl's Gyrus
14. Quadrigeminal Cistern
15. Fimbria of the Fornix
16. Atrium of the Lateral Ventricle
17. Calcar Avis
18. Subiculum
19. Lingular Gyrus
20. Area 17 Striate Cortex
21. Splenium of the Corpus Callosum
22. Pineal Body
23. Calcarine Fissure
24. Pulvinar Nucleus of the Thalamus
25. Hippocampus
26. Optic (Geniculocalcarine) Radiations
27. Alveus
28. Tail of the Caudate Nucleus
29. Retrolenticular component of the Posterior Limb of the Internal Capsule
30. Habenula
31. Dorsomedial Nucleus of the Thalamus
32. Posterior Limb of the Internal Capsule
33. Massa Intermedia
34. Claustrum
35. Extreme Capsule
36. External Capsule
37. Insular Cortex
38. Ventroanterior Nucleus of the Thalamus
39. Putamen
40. Anterior Limb of the Internal Capsule
41. Head of the Caudate Nucleus
42. Genu of the Corpus Callosum
43. Cingulum
44. Cingulate Cortex

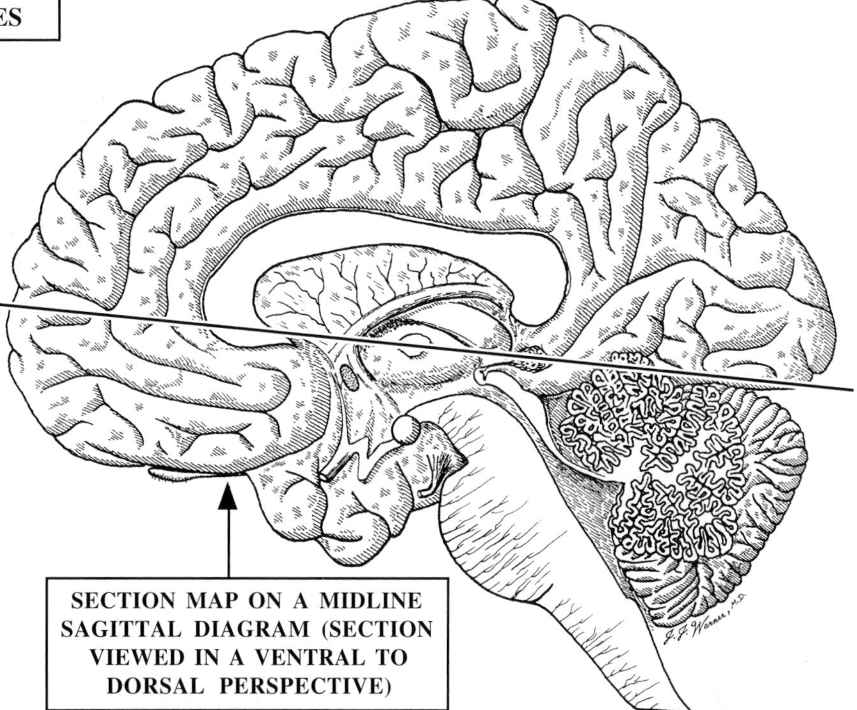

SECTION MAP ON A MIDLINE SAGITTAL DIAGRAM (SECTION VIEWED IN A VENTRAL TO DORSAL PERSPECTIVE)

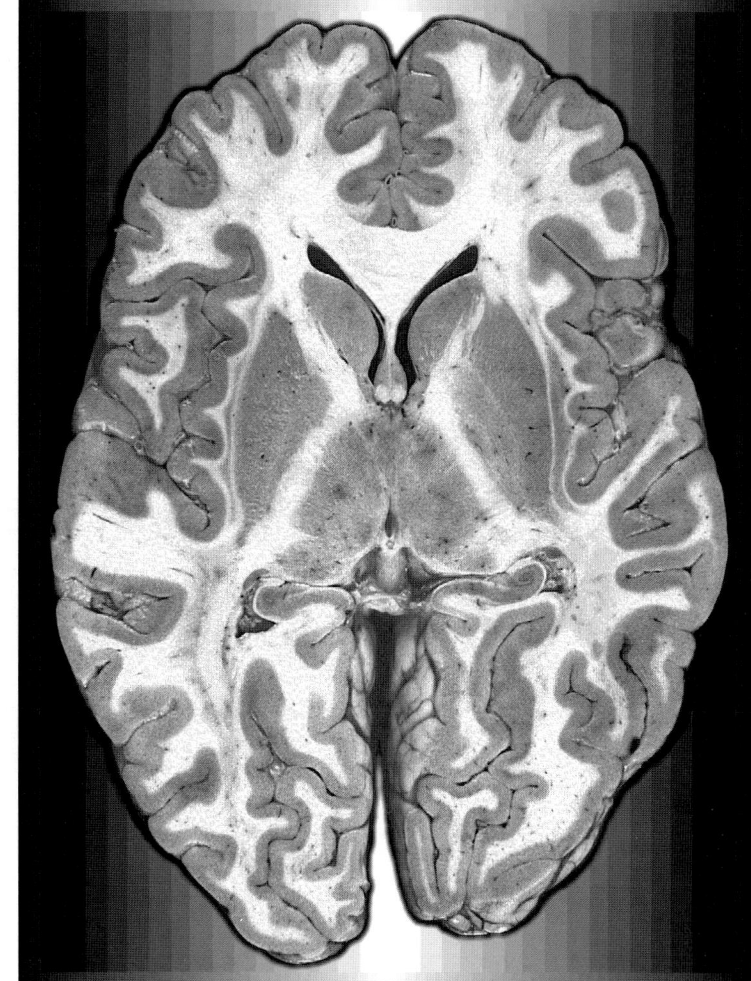

HORIZONTAL SECTION OF THE BRAIN, COMPLETE; LEVEL OF THE PINEAL BODY AND OF THE GENU OF THE CORPUS CALLOSUM: SECTION 15 μ, KLUVER - BARRERA TECHNIQUE

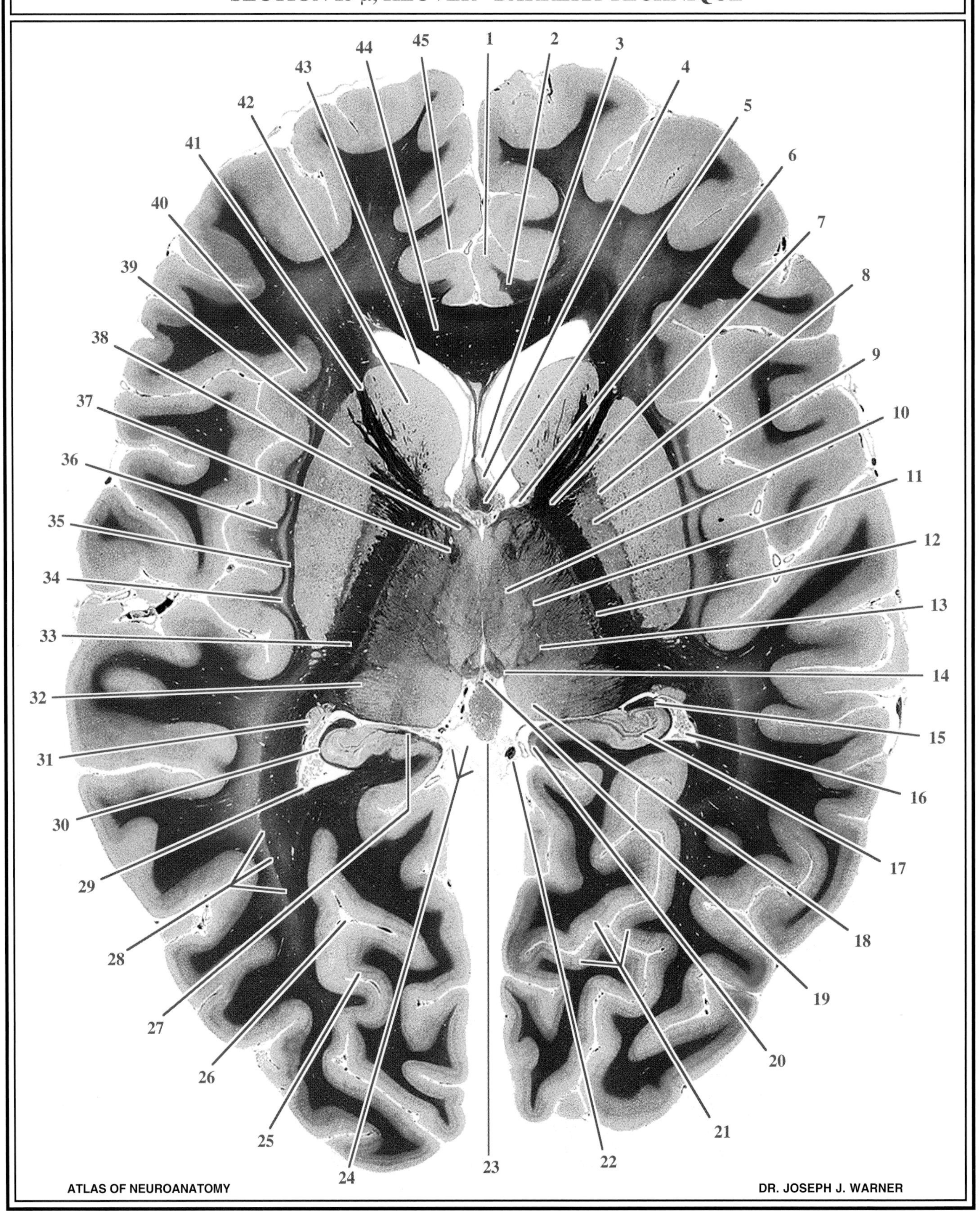

HORIZONTAL SECTION OF THE BRAIN, COMPLETE; LEVEL OF THE PINEAL BODY AND OF THE GENU OF THE CORPUS CALLOSUM: SECTION 15 μ, KLUVER-BARRERA TECHNIQUE

KEY TO NUMBERED STRUCTURES

1. Cingulate Gyrus
2. Cingulum
3. Septal Vein
4. Septal Nuclei
5. Fornix
6. Thalamostriate Vein
7. Genu of the Internal Capsule
8. External Medullary Lamina
9. Globus Pallidus II
10. Dorsomedial Nucleus of the Thalamus
11. Internal Medullary Lamina of the Thalamus
12. Nucleus Reticularis of the Thalamus
13. Centromedian Nucleus of the Thalamus
14. Habenula
15. Fimbria of the Fornix
16. Choroid Plexus
17. Hippocampal Formation
18. Medial Pulvinar Nucleus of the Thalamus
19. Pineal Recess of the Third Ventricle
20. Isthmus of the Gyrus Fornicatus
21. Area 17 Striate Cortex
22. Posterior Cerebral Artery
23. Pineal Body
24. Quadrigeminal Cistern and Arachnoid
25. Area 17 Striate Cortex
26. Calcarine Fissure
27. Superficial Medullary Stratum of the Subiculum
28. Optic (Geniculocalcarine) Radiations
29. Temporal Horn of the Lateral Ventricle
30. Alveus
31. Tail of the Caudate Nucleus
32. Lateral Pulvinar Nucleus of the Thalamus
33. Posterior Limb of the Internal Capsule
34. Claustrum
35. External Capsule
36. Extreme Capsule
37. Mammillothalamic Tract
38. Anterior Nucleus of the Thalamus (ventral aspect)
39. Putamen
40. Insular Cortex
41. Anterior Limb of the Internal Capsule
42. Head of the Caudate Nucleus
43. Anterior Horn of the Lateral Ventricle
44. Corpus Callosum
45. Cingulate Sulcus

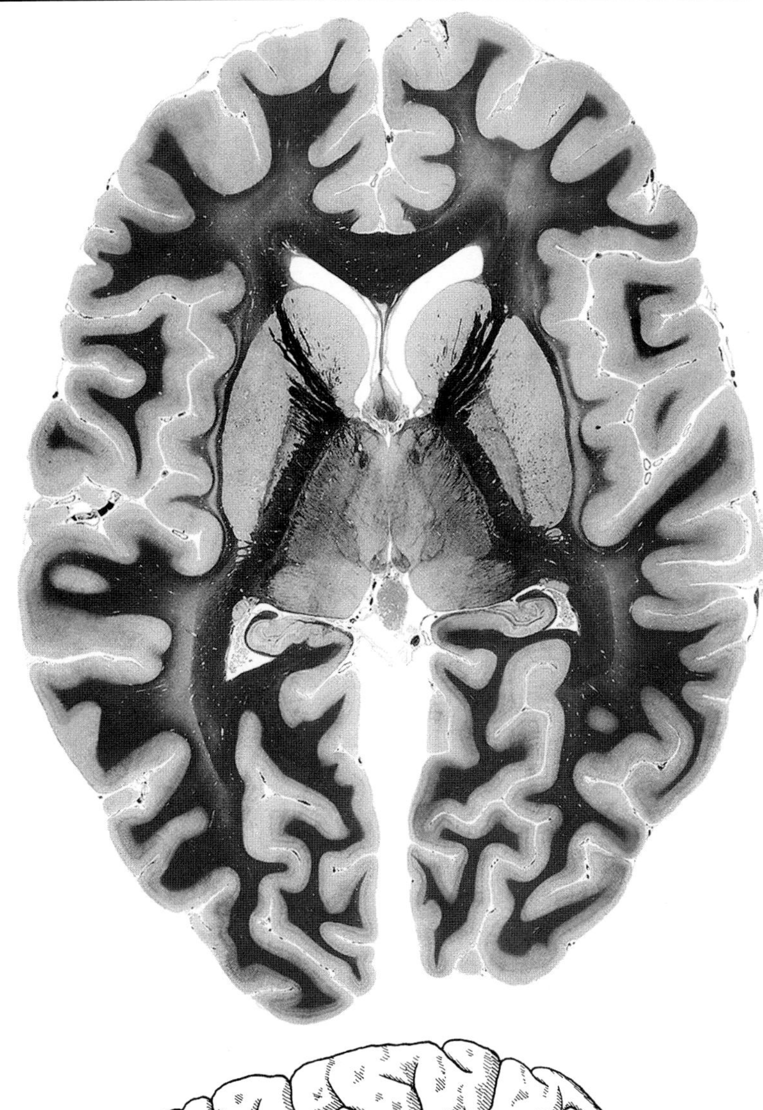

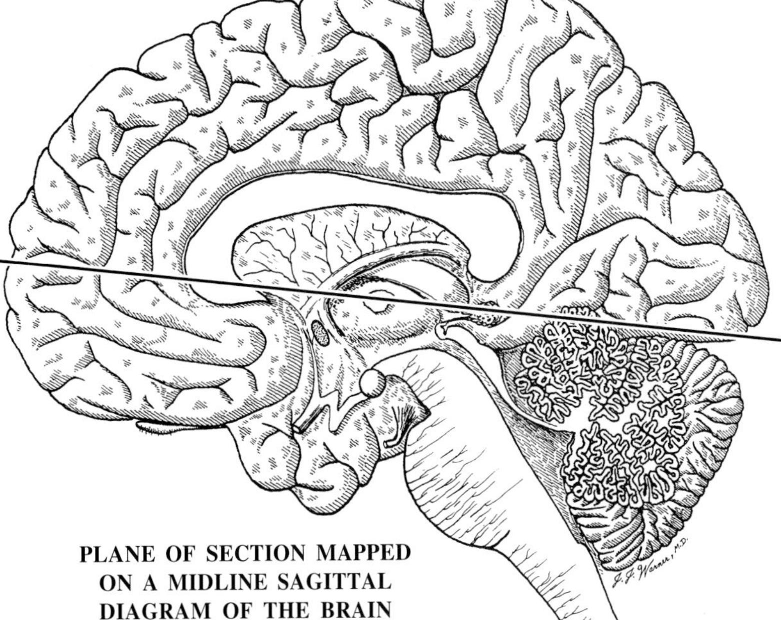

PLANE OF SECTION MAPPED ON A MIDLINE SAGITTAL DIAGRAM OF THE BRAIN

HORIZONTAL SECTION OF THE BRAIN, COMPLETE; LEVEL OF THE PINEAL BODY AND OF THE GENU OF THE CORPUS CALLOSUM: SECTION 15 μ, BIELSCHOWSKY SILVER TECHNIQUE

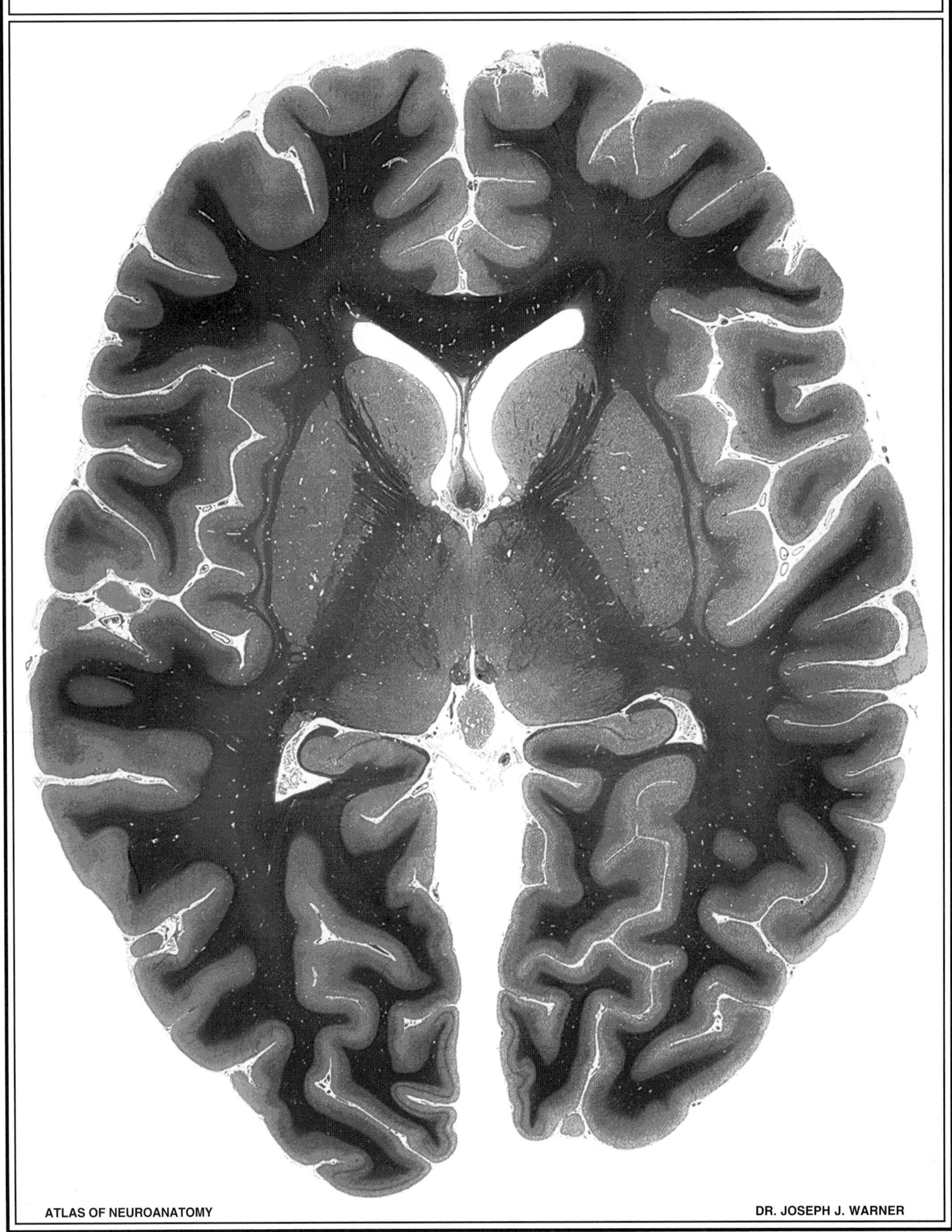

HORIZONTAL SECTION OF THE BRAIN: LEVEL INCLUDING THE CENTROMEDIAN NUCLEUS OF THE THALAMUS, THE PINEAL BODY, AND THE GENU OF THE CORPUS CALLOSUM KLUVER - BARRERA TECHNIQUE, 15 μ SECTION

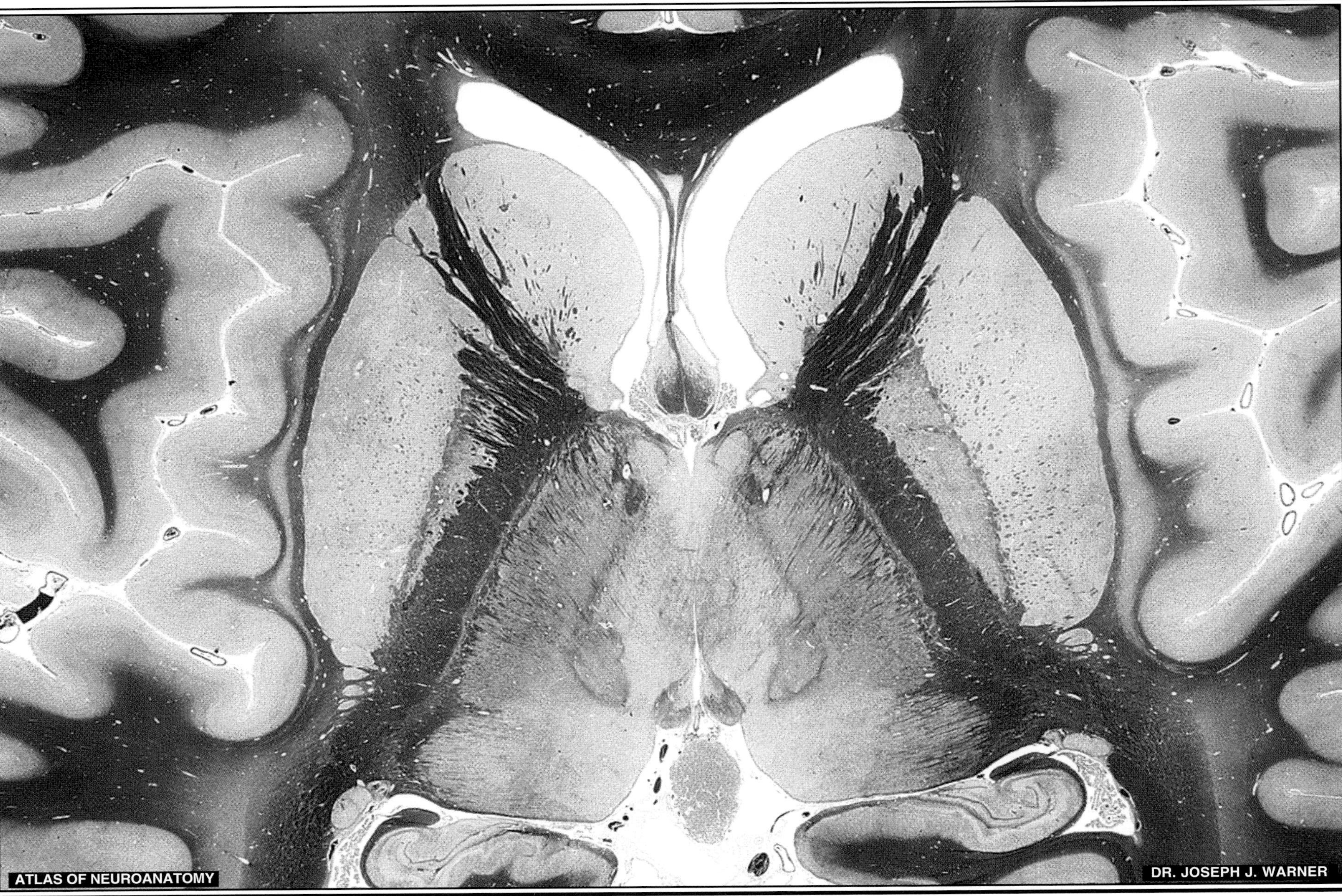

HORIZONTAL SECTION OF THE BRAIN: LEVEL INCLUDING THE CENTROMEDIAN NUCLEUS OF THE THALAMUS, THE PINEAL BODY, AND THE GENU OF THE CORPUS CALLOSUM

SECTION 15 μ, KLUVER-BARRERA TECHNIQUE

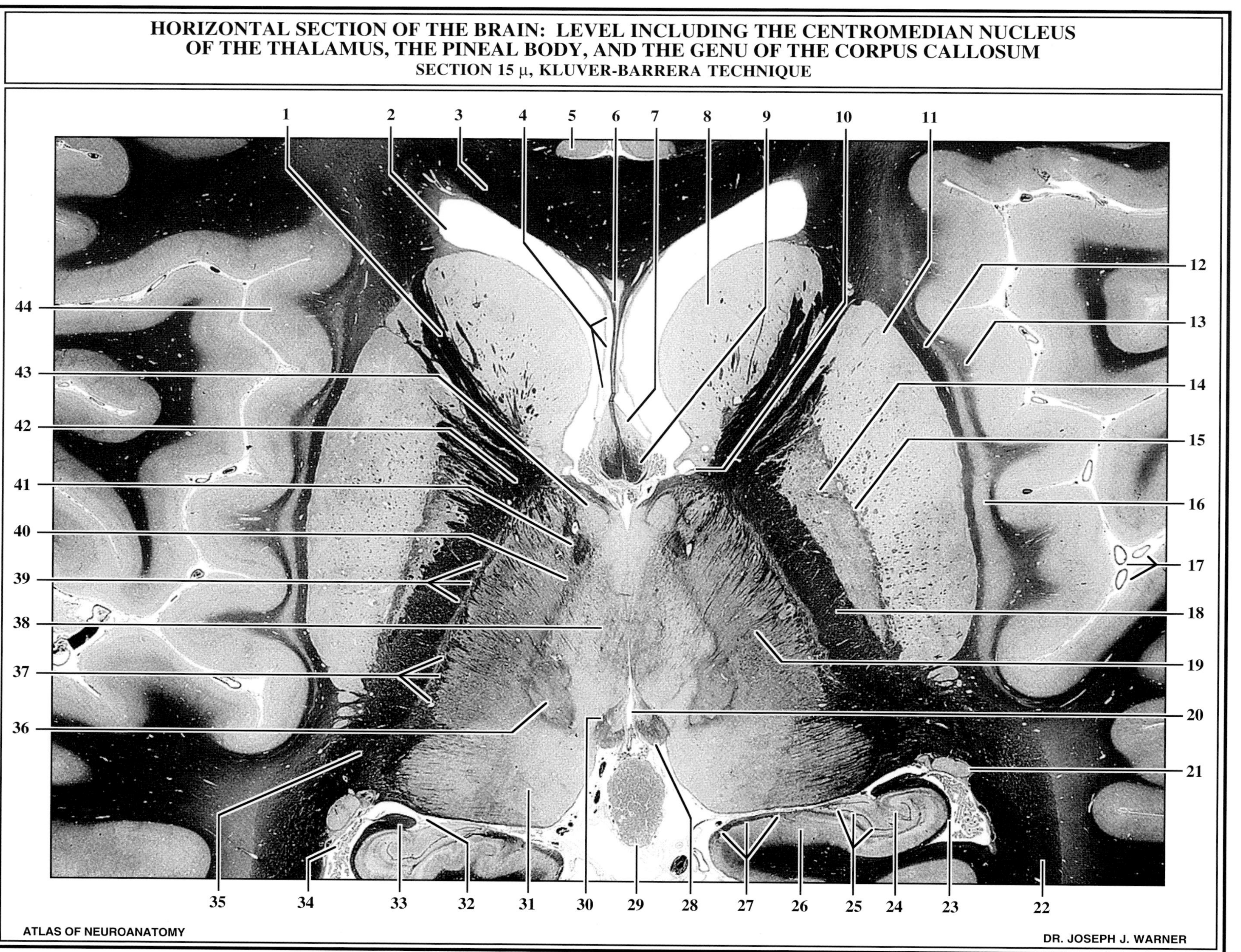

ATLAS OF NEUROANATOMY

DR. JOSEPH J. WARNER

HORIZONTAL SECTION OF THE BRAIN; LEVEL INCLUDING THE CENTROMEDIAN NUCLEUS OF THE THALAMUS, THE PINEAL BODY, AND THE GENU OF THE CORPUS CALLOSUM (MAGNIFIED VIEW): SECTION ORIENTATION AND KEY TO NUMBERED STRUCTURES

KEY TO NUMBERED STRUCTURES

1. Anterior Limb of the Internal Capsule
2. Anterior Horn of the Lateral Ventricle
3. Genu of the Corpus Callosum
4. Septal Vein
5. Cingulate Cortex
6. Septum Pellucidum
7. Septal Nuclei
8. Head of the Caudate Nucleus
9. Fornix
10. Thalamostriate Vein
11. Putamen
12. External Capsule
13. Extreme Capsule
14. Globus Pallidus II
15. External Medullary Lamina
16. Claustrum
17. Middle Cerebral Artery Branches
18. Posterior Limb of the Internal Capsule
19. Ventrolateral Nucleus of the Thalamus
20. Third Ventricle
21. Tail of the Caudate Nucleus
22. Geniculocalcarine Radiations
23. Alveus
24. Hippocampus
25. Dentate Gyrus of the Hippocampus
26. Subiculum
27. Superficial Medullary Stratum of the Subiculum
28. Habenula
29. Pineal Body
30. Stria Medullaris
31. Pulvinar Nucleus of the Thalamus
32. Choroidal Fissure
33. Fimbria of the Fornix
34. Temporal Horn of the Lateral Ventricle
35. Retrolenticular Fibers of the Internal Capsule
36. Centromedian Nucleus of the Thalamus
37. External Medullary Lamina of the Thalamus
38. Dorsomedial Nucleus of the Thalamus
39. Nucleus Reticularis of the Thalamus
40. Internal Medullary Lamina of the Thalamus
41. Mammillothalamic Tract
42. Genu of the Internal Capsule
43. Anterior Nucleus of the Thalamus
44. Insular Cortex

J. J. Warner, M.D.

SECTION MAP ON A MIDLINE SAGITTAL DIAGRAM

AREA OF MAGNIFIED VIEW

HISTOLOGICAL SECTION: 15 μ, KLUVER - BARRERA TECHNIQUE

HORIZONTAL SECTION OF THE BRAIN, COMPLETE; LEVEL INCLUDING THE GENU AND SPLENIUM OF THE CORPUS CALLOSUM: DORSAL TO VENTRAL PERSPECTIVE

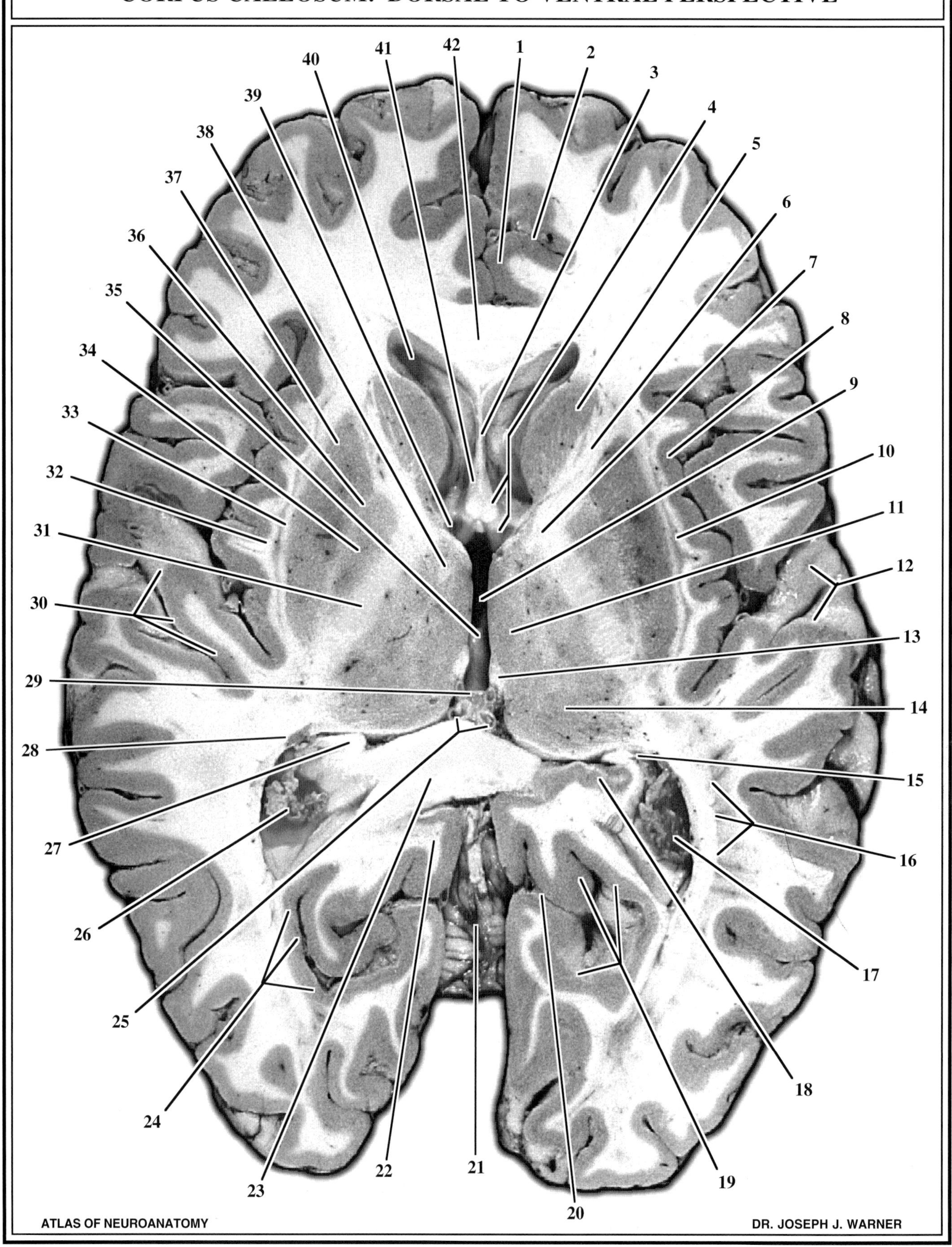

HORIZONTAL SECTION; LEVEL OF HESCHL'S GYRI AND OF THE GENU AND SPLENIUM OF THE CORPUS CALLOSUM: SECTION ORIENTATION AND KEY TO NUMBERED STRUCTURES

KEY TO NUMBERED STRUCTURES

1. Cingulate Cortex
2. Cingulate Sulcus
3. Septum Pellucidum
4. Fornix
5. Head of the Caudate Nucleus
6. Anterior Limb of the Internal Capsule
7. Genu of the Internal Capsule
8. Insular Cortex
9. Third Ventricle
10. Claustrum
11. Dorsomedial Nucleus of the Thalamus
12. Heschl's Gyri (Areas 41, 42)*
13. Stria Medullaris
14. Pulvinar Nucleus of the Thalamus
15. Fimbria of the Fornix
16. Optic (Geniculocalcarine) Radiations
17. Atrium of the Lateral Ventricle
18. Retrosplenial Gyri of the Hippocampus
19. Striate (Area 17) Cortex
20. Calcarine Fissure
21. Superior Cerebellar Vermis
22. Cingulum
23. Splenium of the Corpus Callosum
24. Striate (Area 17) Cortex
25. Internal Cerebral Veins
26. Choroid Plexus
27. Crus of the Fornix
28. Tail of the Caudate Nucleus
29. Posterior Commissure (ventral to the plane of section)
30. Heschl's Gyrus (Areas 41, 42)*
31. Posterior Limb of the Internal Capsule
32. Extreme Capsule
33. External Capsule
34. Globus Pallidus II
35. Massa Intermedia
36. Internal Medullary Lamina
37. Putamen
38. Mammillothalamic Tract
39. Foramen of Monro
40. Anterior Horn of the Lateral Ventricle
41. Septal Nuclei
42. Genu of the Corpus Callosum

* This brain is characterized by a single, large Heschl's gyrus on the left, with a smaller, doubled homologue over the superior aspect of the right temporal lobe. This specimen is from a right-handed male.

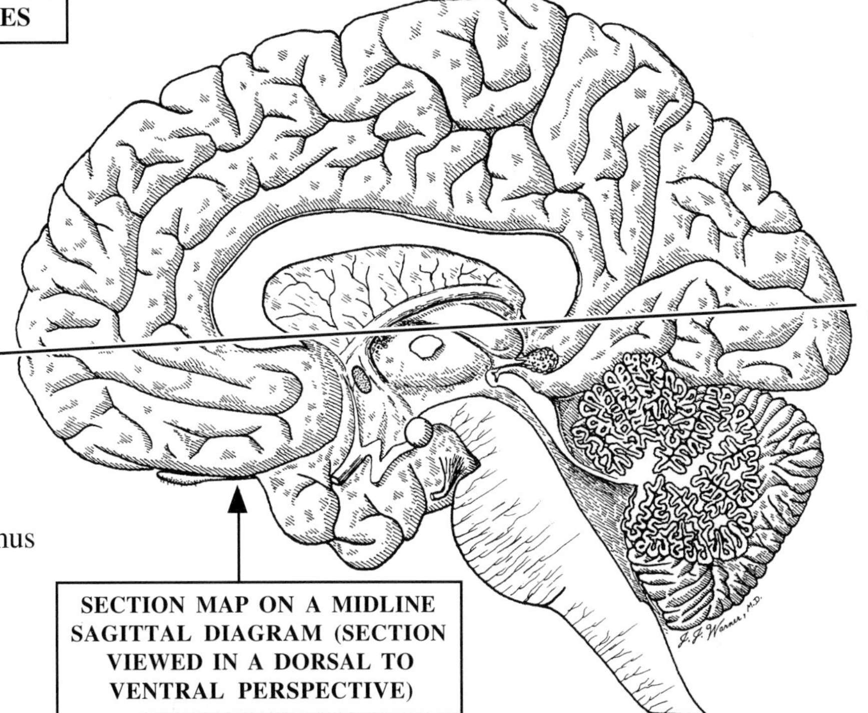

SECTION MAP ON A MIDLINE SAGITTAL DIAGRAM (SECTION VIEWED IN A DORSAL TO VENTRAL PERSPECTIVE)

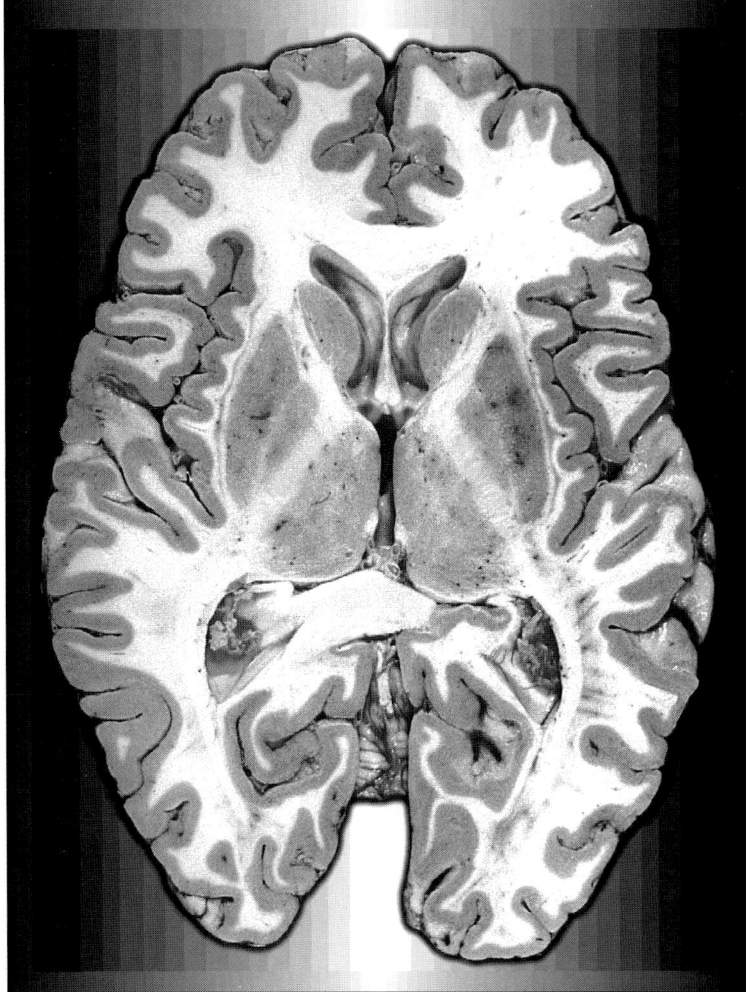

HORIZONTAL SECTION OF THE BRAIN, COMPLETE: LEVEL INCLUDING THE DORSAL THALAMUS AND THE LONGITUDINAL COURSE OF THE FORNIX, DORSAL TO VENTRAL PERSPECTIVE

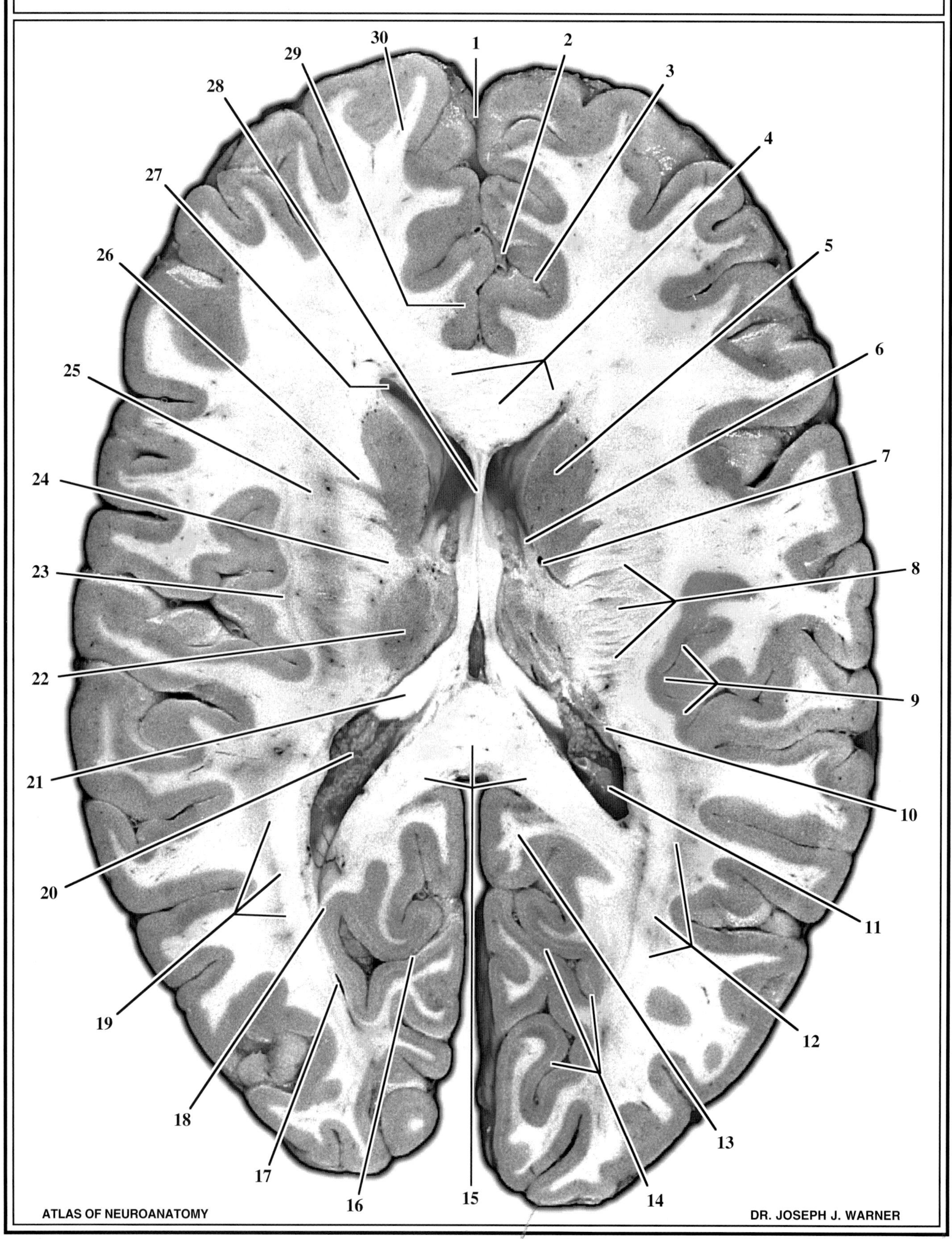

ATLAS OF NEUROANATOMY

DR. JOSEPH J. WARNER

HORIZONTAL SECTION OF THE BRAIN, COMPLETE; LEVEL INCLUDING THE DORSAL THALAMUS AND THE LONGITUDINAL COURSE OF THE FORNIX: SECTION ORIENTATION AND KEY TO NUMBERED STRUCTURES

KEY TO NUMBERED STRUCTURES

1. Interhemispheric Fissure
2. Anterior Cerebral Artery, Callosomarginal Branch
3. Cingulate Sulcus
4. Forceps Minor of the Corpus Callosum
5. Head of the Caudate Nucleus
6. Stria Terminalis
7. Thalamostriate Vein
8. Corona Radiata
9. Superior aspect of the Insular Cortex
10. Tail of the Caudate Nucleus
11. Atrium of the Lateral Ventricle
12. Optic (Geniculocalcarine) Radiations
13. Cingulum
14. Area 17 Striate Cortex
15. Forceps Major of the Corpus Callosum
16. Calcarine Fissure
17. Tangential section through the Occipital Horn of the Lateral Ventricle
18. Calcar Avis
19. Optic (Geniculocalcarine) Radiations
20. Choroid Plexus in the Lateral Ventricle
21. Crus of the Fornix
22. Thalamus (dorsal aspect)
23. Claustrum
24. Transition from the Internal Capsule to the Corona Radiata
25. Dorsal extent of the Putamen
26. Transcapsular Caudatolenticular Gray Stria
27. Anterior Horn of the Lateral Ventricle
28. Septum Pellucidum
29. Cingulate Cortex
30. Superior Frontal Convolution

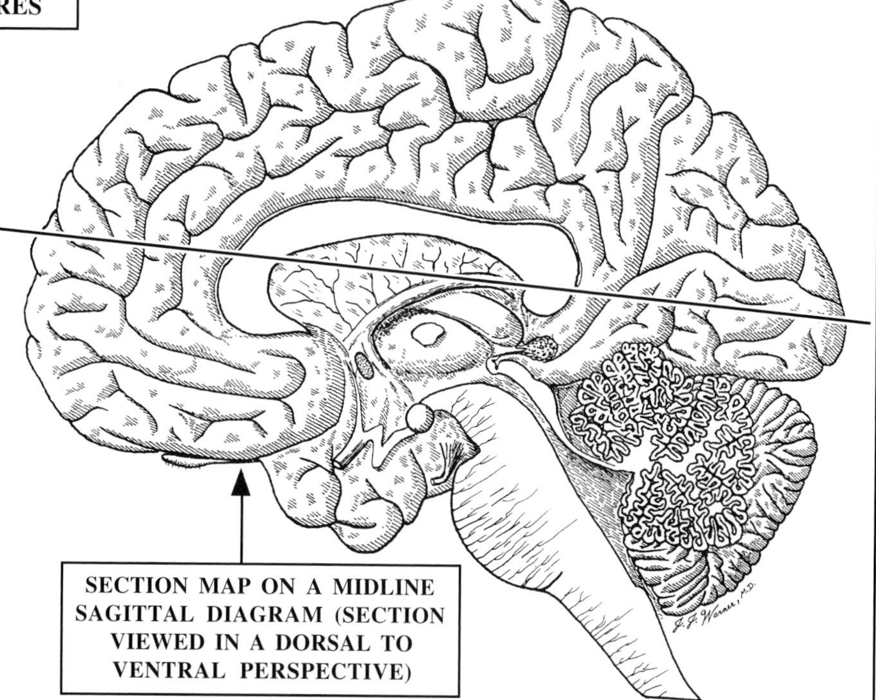

SECTION MAP ON A MIDLINE SAGITTAL DIAGRAM (SECTION VIEWED IN A DORSAL TO VENTRAL PERSPECTIVE)

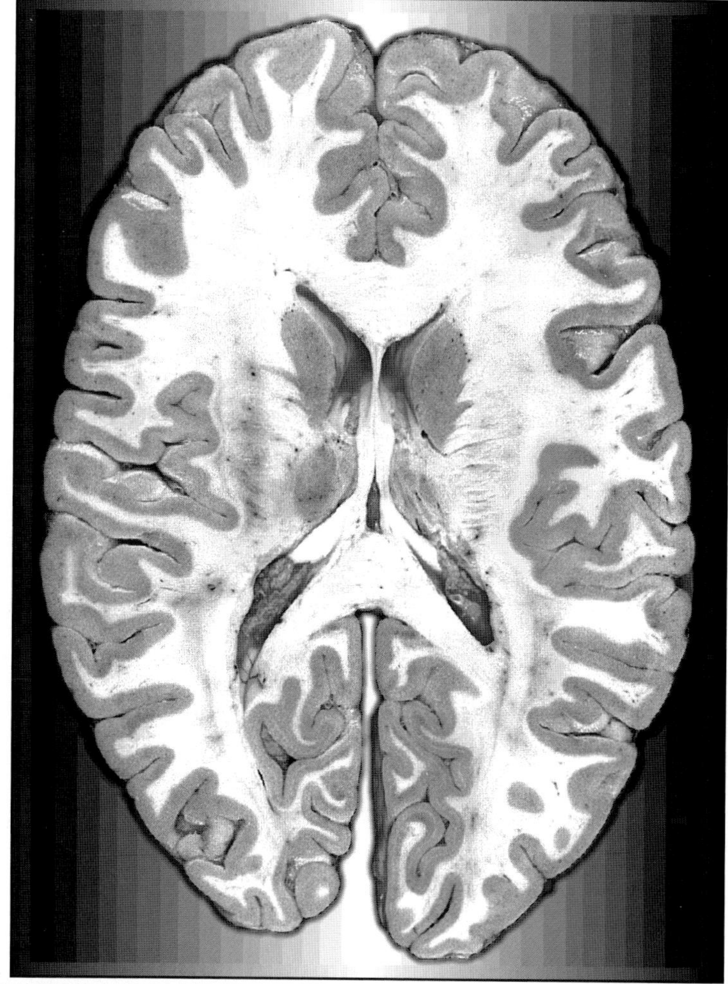

The course of the fornix, as it passes dorsal to the thalamus, is clearly demonstrated by the dorsal to ventral perspective of this plane of section. Each fornix courses dorsomedially from the ipsilateral hippocampus in close proximity to the corpus callosum toward a paramedian position.The fornices then continue rostrally along a longitudinally oriented course dorsal to the thalamus, with a subsequent ventral curvature. The post-commissural component of the fornix terminates in the ipsilateral mammillary body.

HORIZONTAL SECTION OF THE BRAIN, COMPLETE: LEVEL DORSAL TO THE PARAMEDIAN LONGITUDINAL COURSE OF THE FORNIX, DORSAL TO VENTRAL PERSPECTIVE

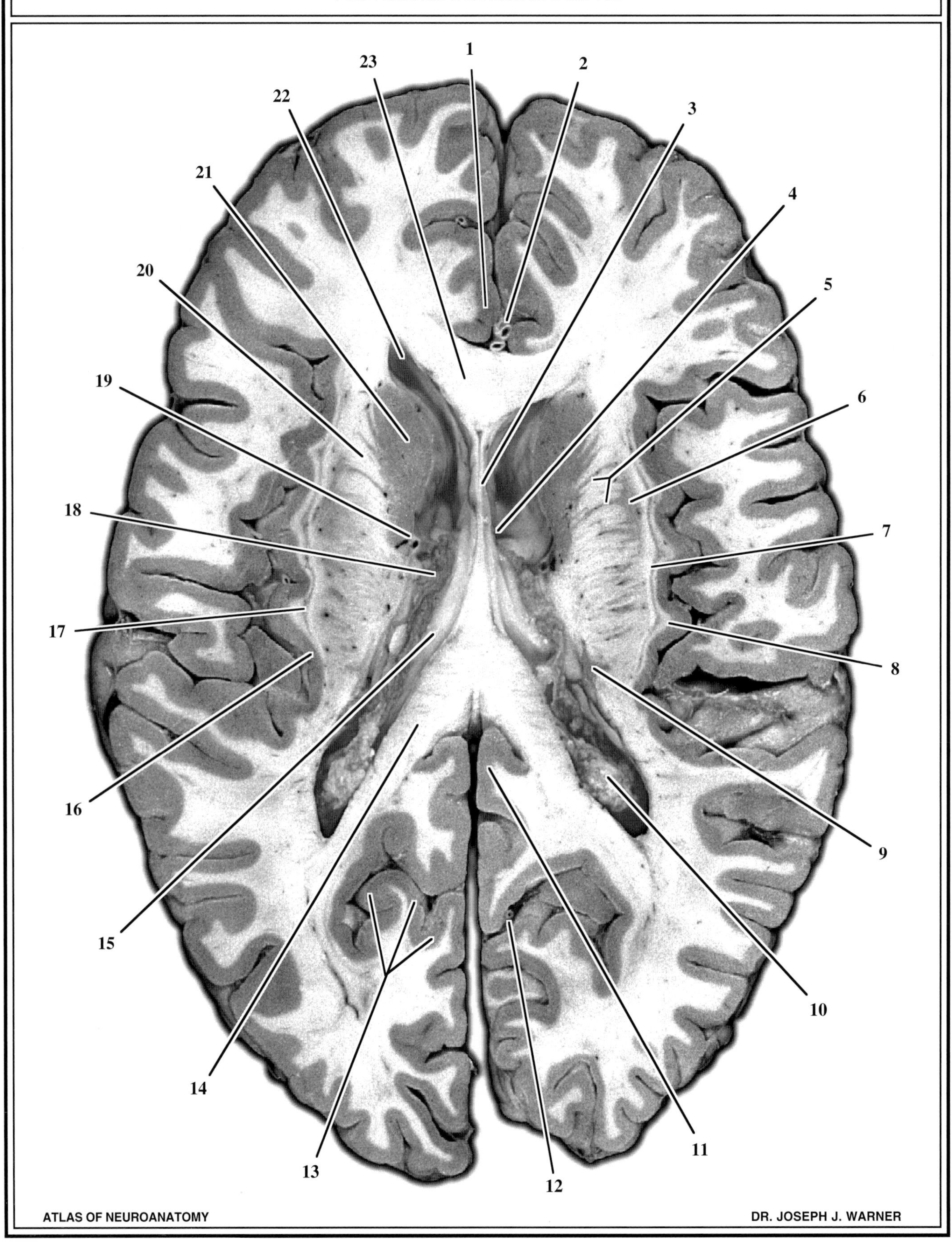

HORIZONTAL SECTION OF THE BRAIN, COMPLETE; LEVEL DORSAL TO THE PARAMEDIAN LONGITUDINAL COURSE OF THE FORNIX: SECTION ORIENTATION AND KEY TO NUMBERED STRUCTURES

KEY TO NUMBERED STRUCTURES

1. Cingulate Cortex
2. Anterior Cerebral Arteries
3. Septum Pellucidum
4. Foramen of Monro (ventral to the plane of section)*
5. Transcapsular Caudatolenticular Gray Striae
6. Dorsal extent of the Putamen
7. External Capsule
8. Extreme Capsule
9. Tail of the Caudate Nucleus
10. Choroid Plexus
11. Cingulate Cortex
12. Calcarine Fissure
13. Area 17 Striate Cortex
14. Forceps Major of the Corpus Callosum
15. Fornix
16. Insula
17. Claustrum
18. Body of the Lateral Ventricle
19. Thalamostriate Vein
20. Transition of the Internal Capsule to the Corona Radiata
21. Head of the Caudate Nucleus
22. Anterior Horn of the Lateral Ventricle
23. Forceps Minor of the Corpus Callosum

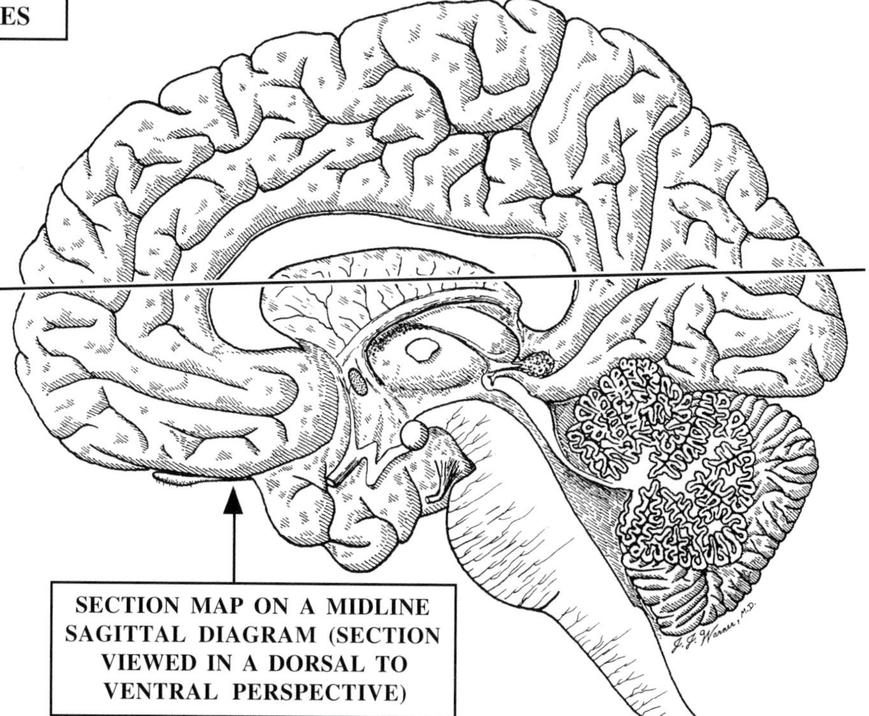

SECTION MAP ON A MIDLINE SAGITTAL DIAGRAM (SECTION VIEWED IN A DORSAL TO VENTRAL PERSPECTIVE)

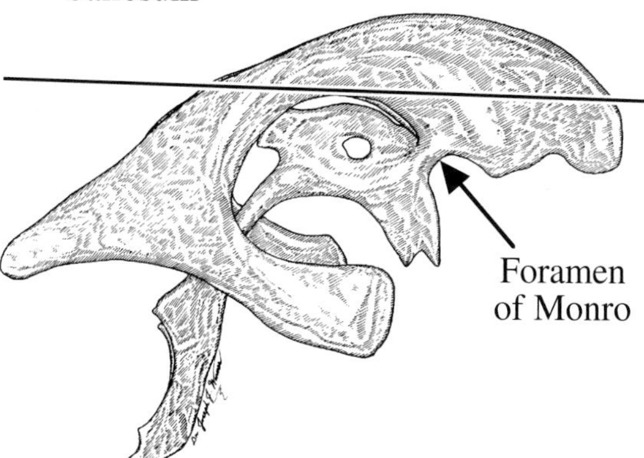

PLANE OF SECTION MAPPED ON A LATERAL DIAGRAM OF THE VENTRICULAR SYSTEM

*In this dorsal to ventral perspective, the foramen of Monro is visible bilaterally. The orifice is ventral to the plane of section, adjacent to the sharp ventral curvature of the fornix. The third ventricle is not visible, covered by the taenia thalami, tela choroidea, choroid plexus, and the fornix as it passes dorsal to the thalamus.

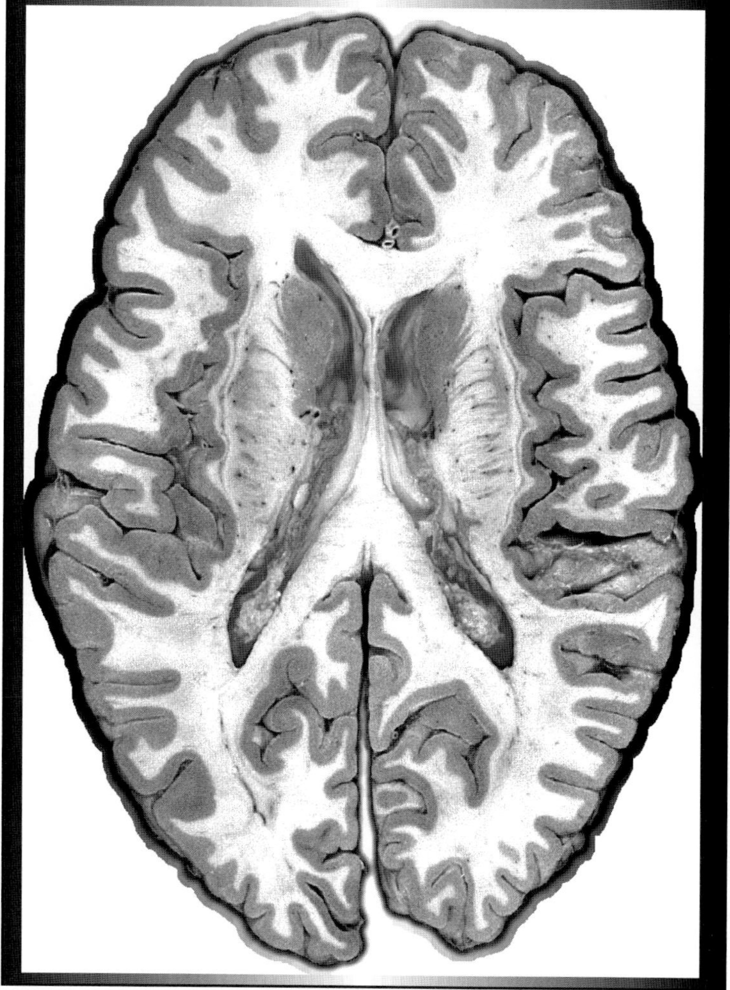

HORIZONTAL SECTION OF THE BRAIN, COMPLETE: LEVEL DORSAL TO THE PARAMEDIAN LONGITUDINAL COURSE OF THE FORNIX *VENTRAL TO DORSAL* PERSPECTIVE

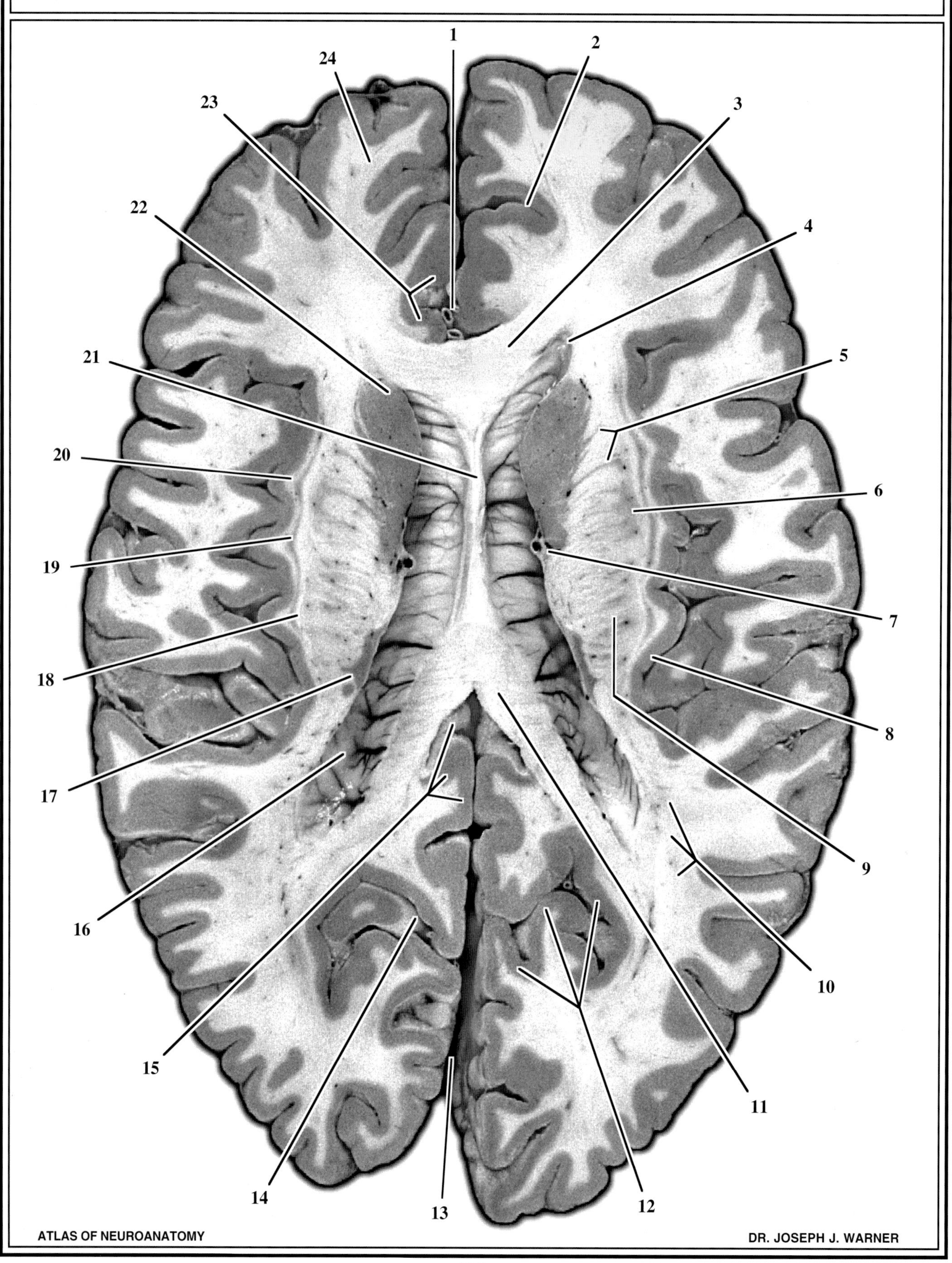

HORIZONTAL SECTION OF THE BRAIN, COMPLETE; LEVEL DORSAL TO THE PARAMEDIAN LONGITUDINAL COURSE OF THE FORNIX: SECTION ORIENTATION AND KEY TO NUMBERED STRUCTURES

KEY TO NUMBERED STRUCTURES

1. Anterior Cerebral Arteries
2. Cingulate Sulcus
3. Forceps Minor (Corpus Callosum)
4. Anterior Horn, Lateral Ventricle
5. Caudatolenticular Gray Striae
6. Dorsal extent of the Putamen
7. Thalamostriate Vein
8. Insular Cortex
9. Corona Radiata
10. Geniculocalcarine Radiations
11. Forceps Major
12. Area 17 Striate Cortex
13. Interhemispheric Fissure
14. Calcarine Fissure
15. Cingulate Gyrus
16. Body of the Lateral Ventricle
17. Tail of the Caudate Nucleus
18. External Capsule
19. Claustrum
20. Extreme Capsule
21. Septum Pellucidum
22. Head of the Caudate Nucleus
23. Cingulate Gyrus
24. Superior Frontal Convolution

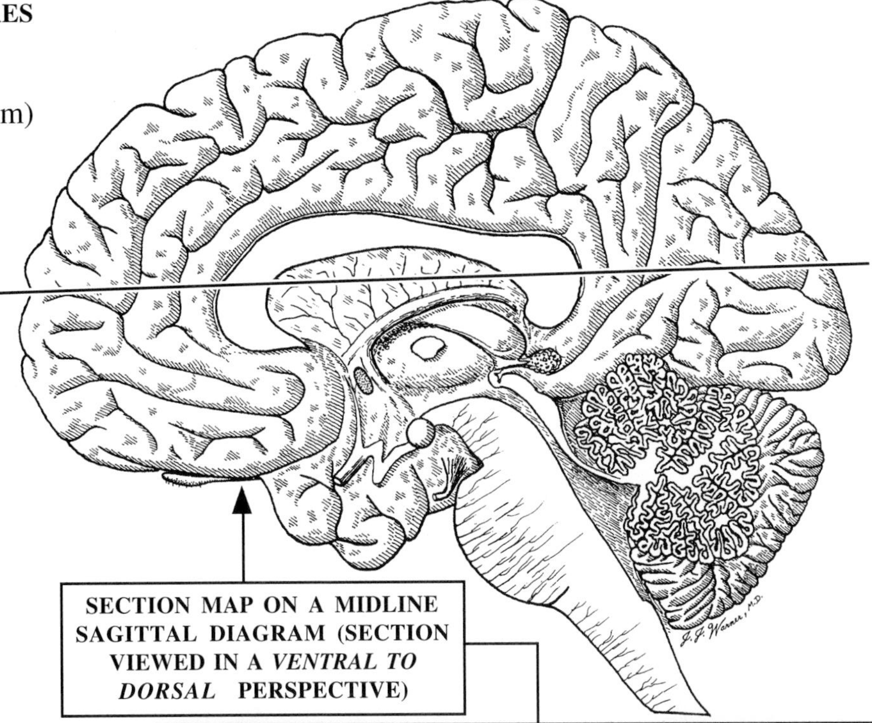

SECTION MAP ON A MIDLINE SAGITTAL DIAGRAM (SECTION VIEWED IN A *VENTRAL TO DORSAL* PERSPECTIVE)

These two specimens share the same section plane. The ventral to dorsal view from this plane demonstrates the corpus callosum forming the roof of the lateral ventricles.

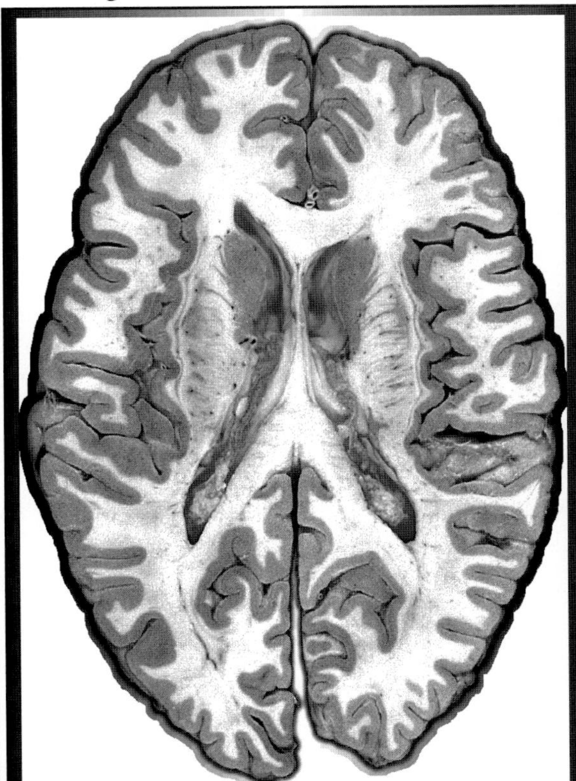

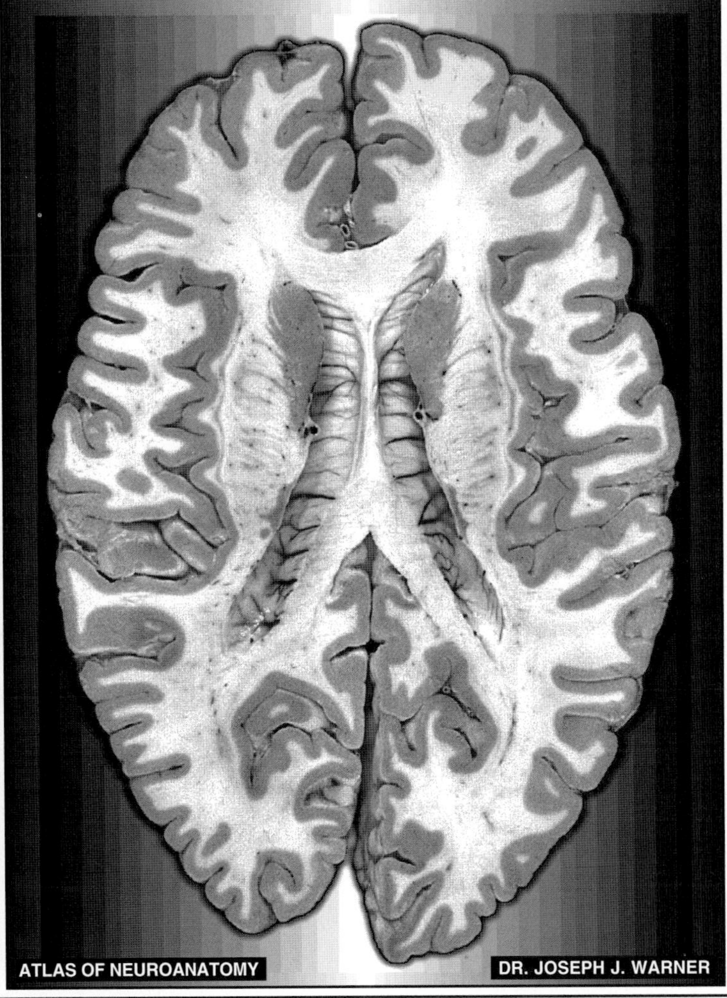

HORIZONTAL SECTION OF THE BRAIN, COMPLETE: LEVEL OF THE CORONA RADIATA, THE DORSAL ASPECT OF THE CAUDATE NUCLEUS AND THE BODIES OF THE LATERAL VENTRICLES

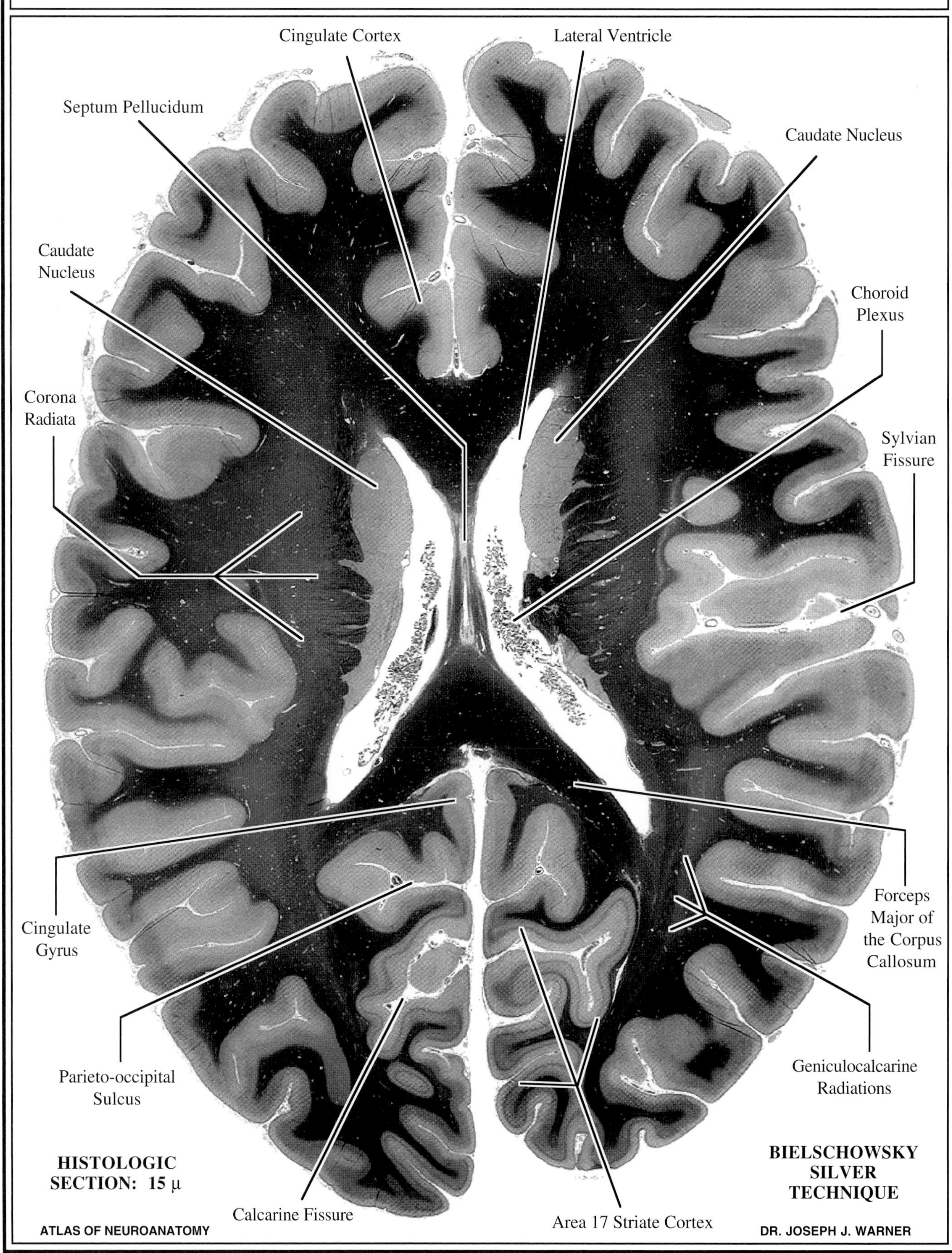

SAGITTAL SECTIONAL NEUROANATOMY

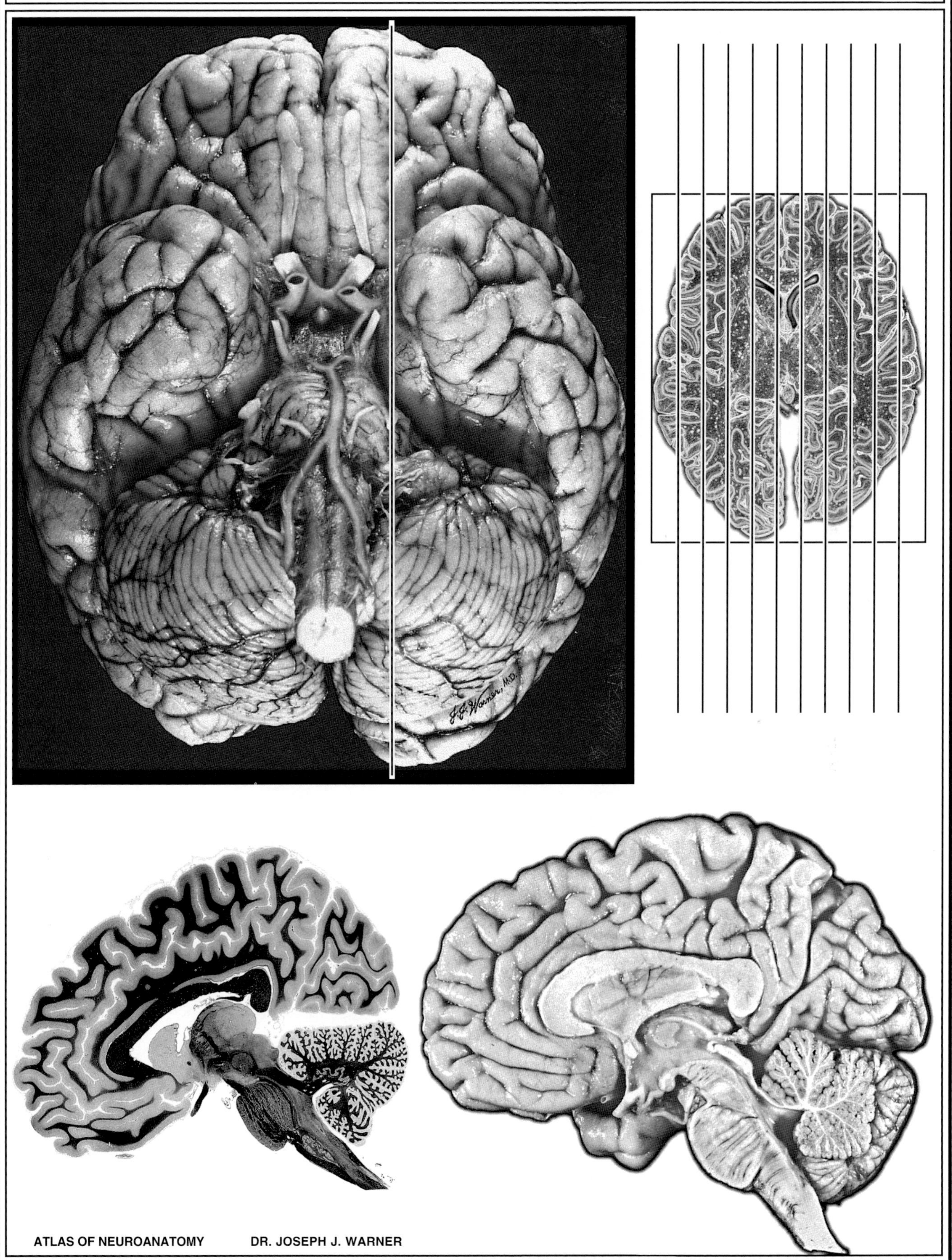

MIDLINE SAGITTAL SECTION OF THE BRAIN, VIEW OF RIGHT HEMISPHERE

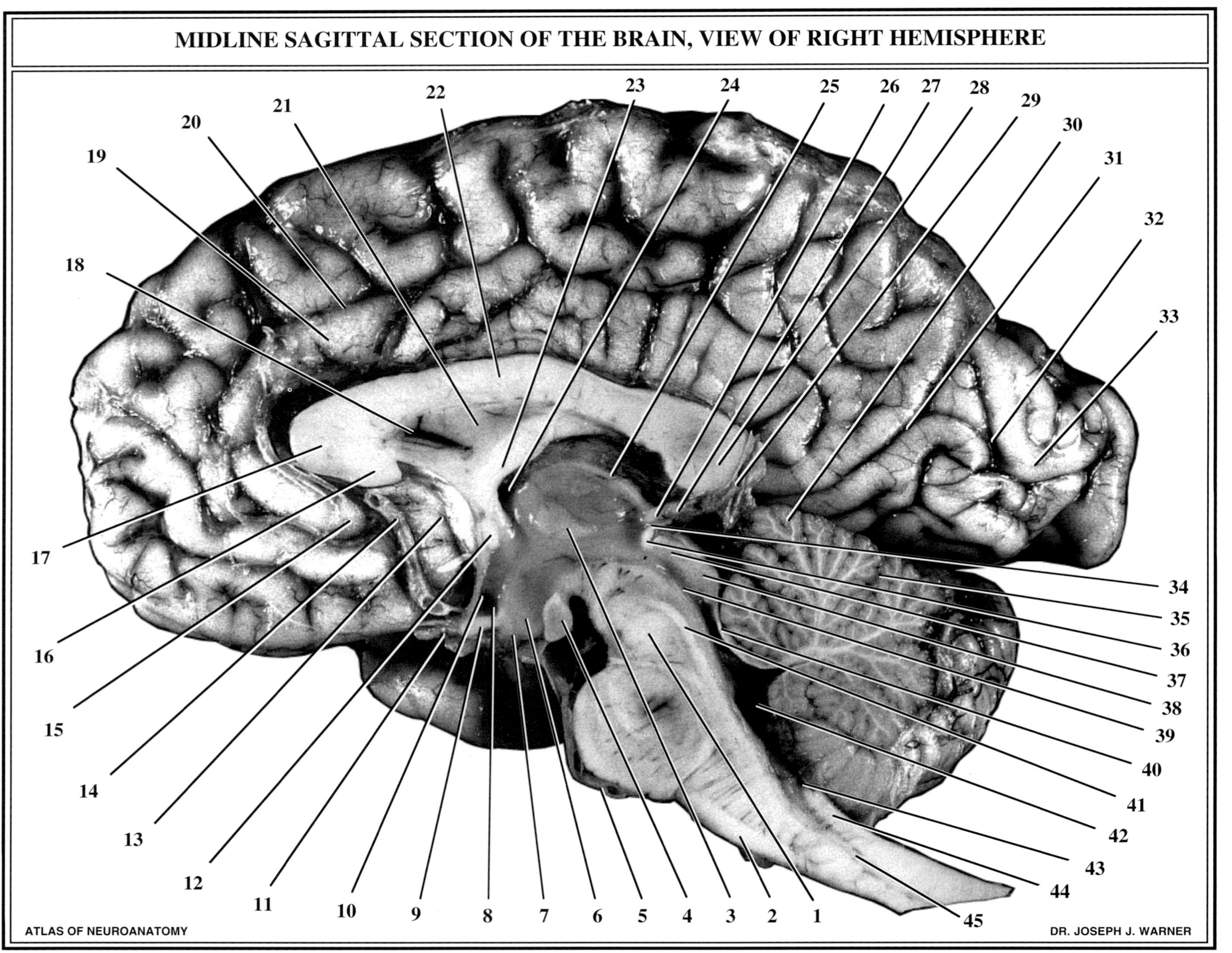

ATLAS OF NEUROANATOMY

DR. JOSEPH J. WARNER

MIDLINE SAGITTAL SECTION OF THE BRAIN: KEY TO NUMBERED STRUCTURES

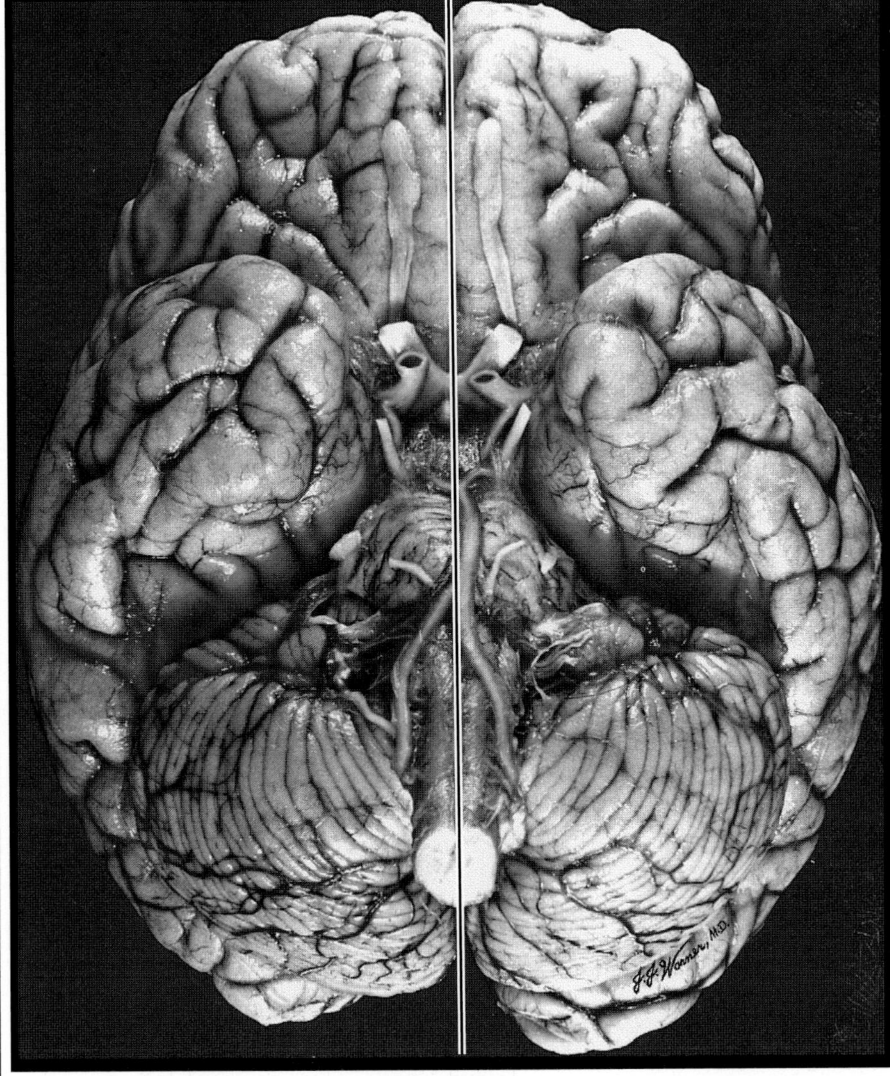

MIDLINE SAGITTAL SECTION: MAP IN REFERENCE TO THE VENTRAL ASPECT OF THE BRAIN

This section plane demonstrates a well-visualized septal vein, anterior commissure, fornix, foramen of Monro, supraoptic and pineal recesses of the third ventricle, stria medullaris and habenula. The posterior commissure is a landmark for the rostral opening of the aqueduct of Sylvius, which courses ventral to the corpora quadrigemina (superior and inferior colliculi) to open into the fourth ventricle. A medial structure, the frenulum, arises from the caudal aspect of the inferior colliculi and continues as the rostral aspect of the anterior or superior medullary velum, a component of the roof of the fourth ventricle. The medial longitudinal fasciculus is clearly discerned dorsal to the decussation of the superior cerebellar peduncles. (The medial longitudinal fasciculus is often not discernible in sections through the midline of the brainstem, as this white matter tract assumes its maximum diameter approx. 1+ mm lateral to the midline.) The rostral cervical spinal cord is included in the specimen, demonstrating the relationship of the central canal to the fourth ventricle and foramen of Monro. The ventral structures on the sagittal section should be identified on the ventral view of the brain (shown above) for spatial orientation.

1. Decussation of Superior Cerebellar Peduncle
2. Pyramidal Tract
3. Massa Intermedia
4. Mammillary Body
5. Basilar Artery
6. Infundibular Recess of Third Ventricle
7. Infundibulum
8. Supraoptic Recess of Third Ventricle
9. Optic Chiasm
10. Lamina Terminalis
11. Optic Nerve
12. Anterior Commissure
13. Paraterminal Gyrus
14. Anterior Cerebral Artery
15. Subcallosal Gyrus
16. Rostrum of Corpus Callosum
17. Genu of Corpus Callosum
18. Septal Vein
19. Cingulate Gyrus
20. Cingulate Sulcus
21. Septum Pellucidum
22. Body of Corpus Callosum
23. Fornix
24. Foramen of Monro
25. Stria Medullaris
26. Habenula
27. Pineal Body
28. Splenium of Corpus Callosum
29. Great Vein of Galen
30. Superior Cerebellar Vermis
31. Parieto-Occipital Sulcus
32. Calcarine Fissure
33. Area 17 Striate Cortex
34. Pineal Recess of Third Ventricle
35. Primary Fissure of Cerebellum
36. Posterior Commissure
37. Superior Colliculus
38. Inferior Colliculus
39. Aqueduct of Sylvius
40. Anterior (Superior) Medullary Velum
41. Medial Longitudinal Fasciculus
42. Fourth Ventricle
43. Foramen of Magendie
44. Fasciculus and Nucleus Gracilis
45. Central Canal

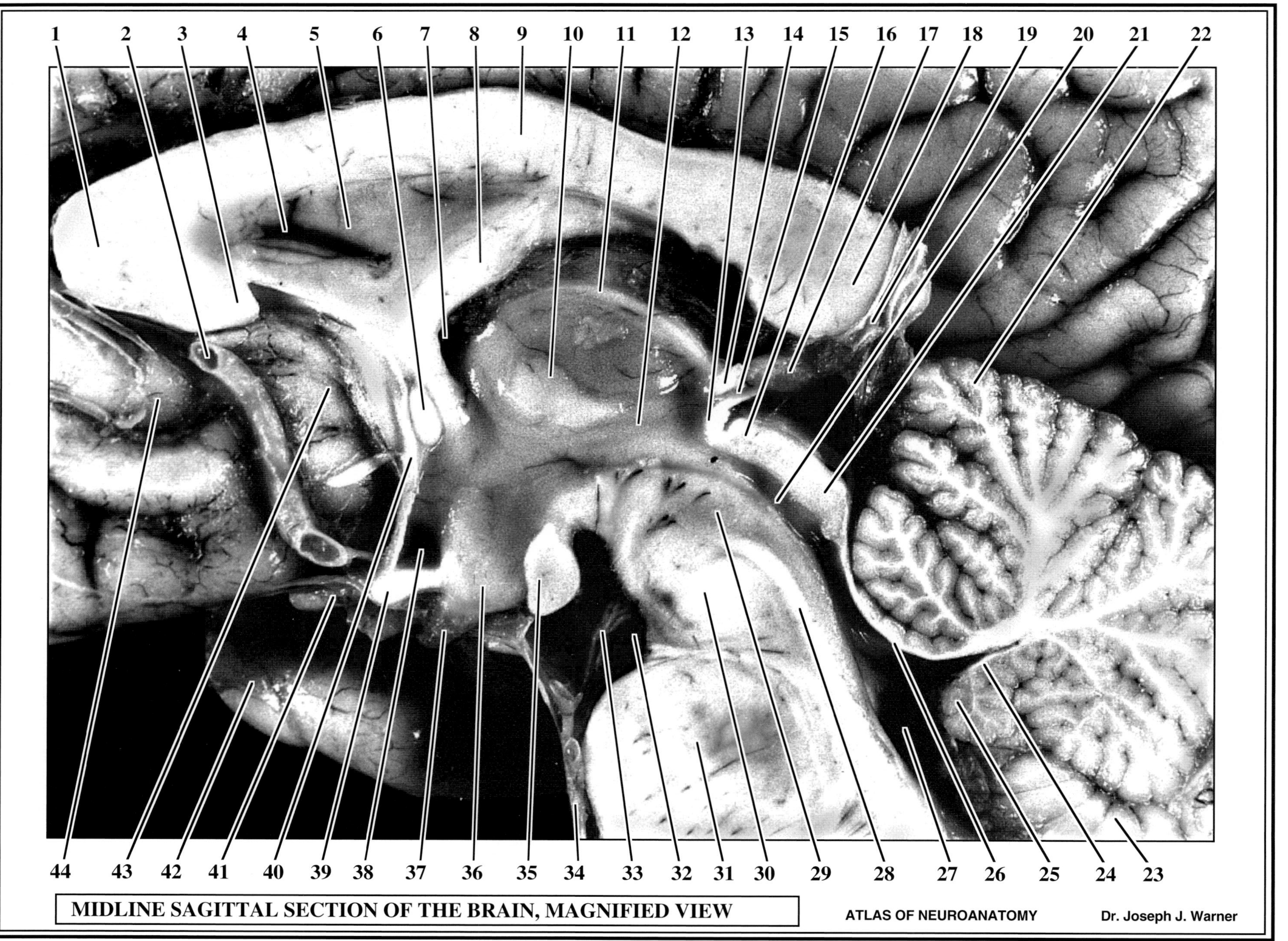
1
2
3
4
5
6
7
8
9
10
11
12
13
14
15
16
17
18
19
20
21
22
44
43
42
41
40
39
38
37
36
35
34
33
32
31
30
29
28
27
26
25
24
23
MIDLINE SAGITTAL SECTION OF THE BRAIN, MAGNIFIED VIEW
ATLAS OF NEUROANATOMY
Dr. Joseph J. Warner

MIDLINE SAGITTAL SECTION OF THE BRAIN: KEY TO NUMBERED STRUCTURES

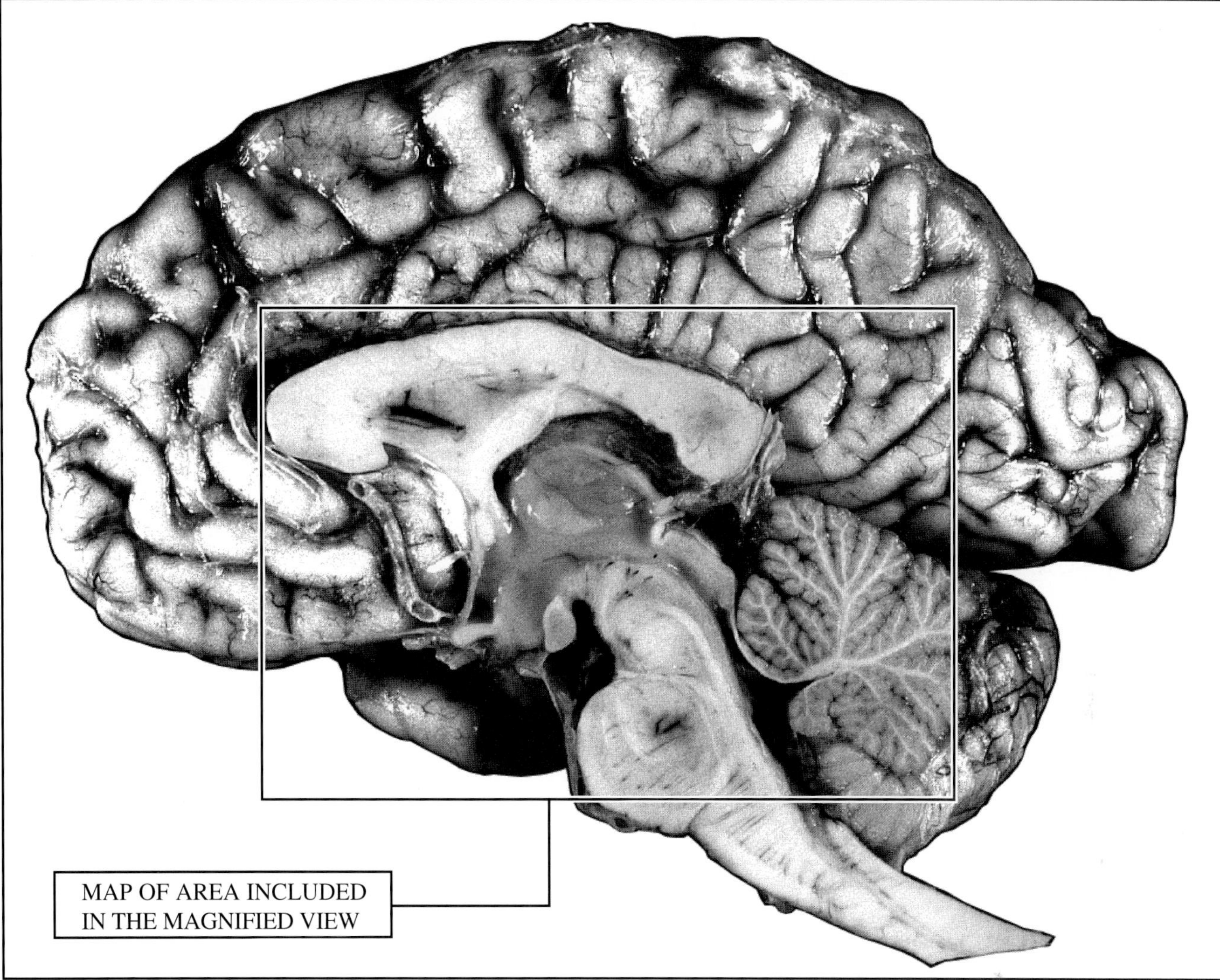

1. Genu of Corpus Callosum
2. Anterior Cerebral Artery
3. Rostrum of Corpus Callosum
4. Septal Vein
5. Septum Pellucidum
6. Anterior Commissure
7. Foramen of Monro
8. Fornix
9. Body of Corpus Callosum
10. Massa Intermedia
11. Stria Medullaris
12. Hypothalamic Sulcus
13. Posterior Commissure
14. Habenula
15. Pineal Recess of Third Ventricle
16. Superior Colliculus
17. Pineal Body
18. Splenium of Corpus Callosum
19. Great Vein of Galen
20. Aqueduct of Sylvius
21. Inferior Colliculus
22. Superior Cerebellar Vermis
23. Cerebellar Tonsil
24. Posterior (Inferior) Medullary Velum
25. Nodulus of Cerebellum
26. Anterior (Superior) Medullary Velum
27. Fourth Ventricle
28. Medial Longitudinal Fasciculus
29. Mesencephalic Tegmentum
30. Decussation of Superior Cerebellar Peduncle
31. Pons
32. Interpeduncular Fossa
33. Oculomotor Nerve
34. Basilar Artery
35. Mammillary Body
36. Infundibular Recess of Third Ventricle
37. Infundibulum
38. Supraoptic Recess of Third Ventricle
39. Optic Chiasm
40. Lamina Terminalis
41. Optic Nerve
42. Anterior Temporal Lobe
43. Paraterminal Gyrus
44. Subcallosal Gyrus

COMPLETE MIDLINE SAGITTAL SECTION OF THE BRAIN

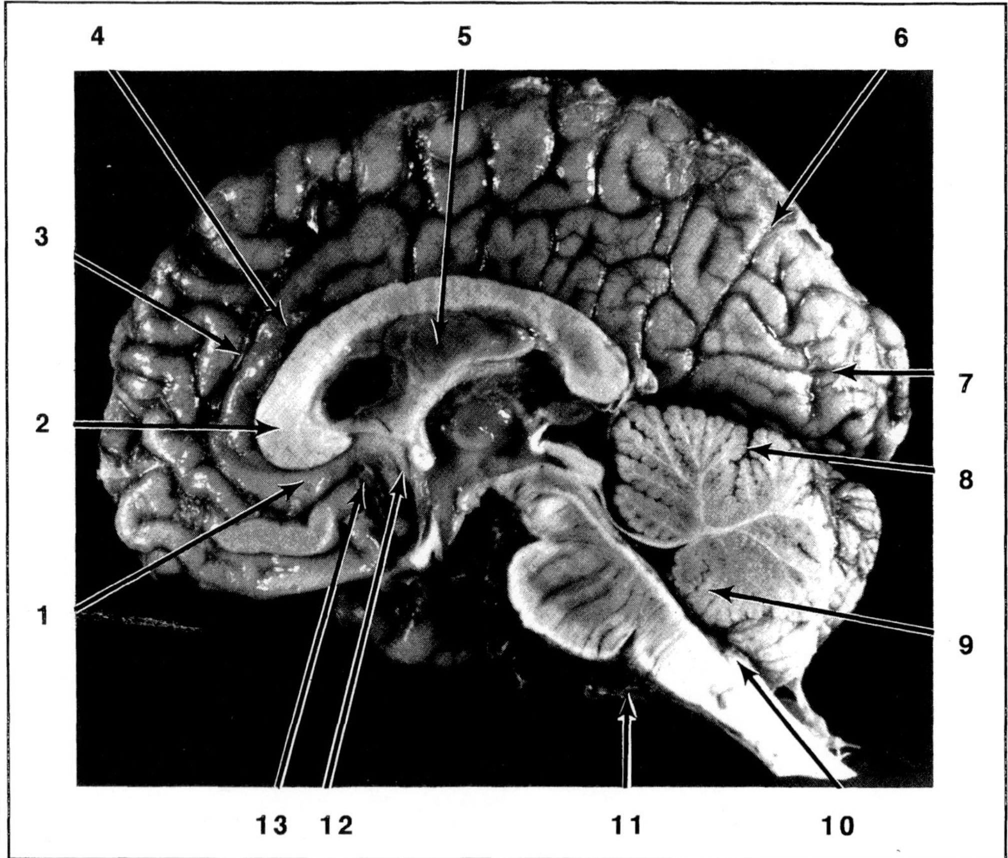

MIDLINE SAGITTAL SECTION, MAGNIFIED VIEW

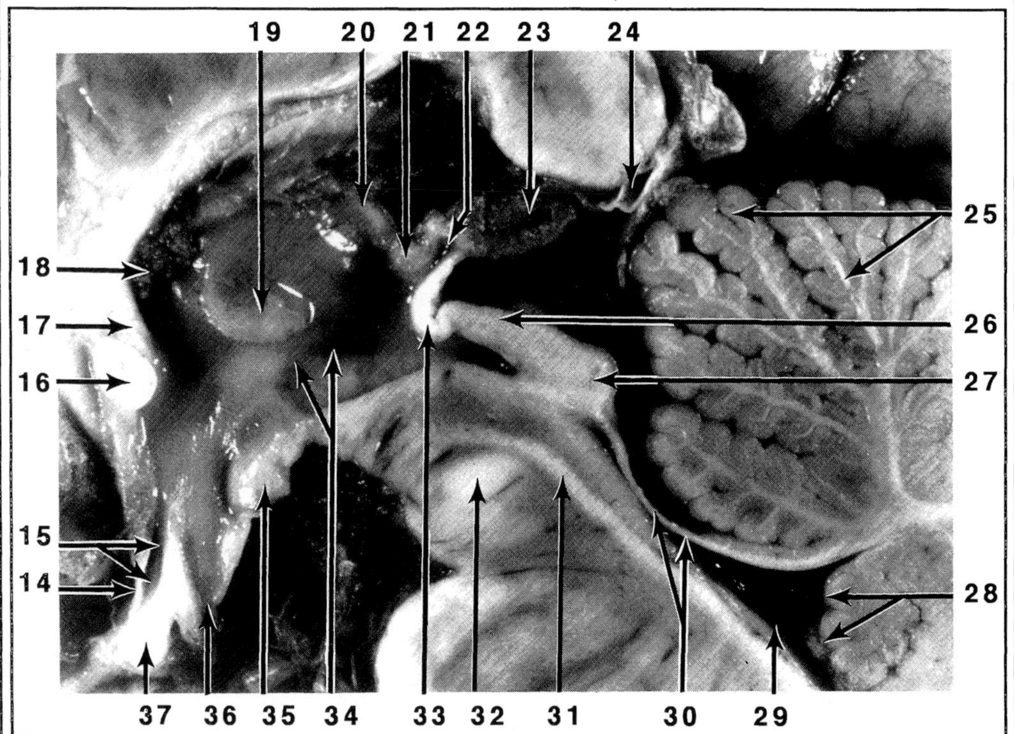

Comparison of midline sagittal sections through various specimens reveals the normal anatomic variations characteristic of the human brain. Note the configuration of the corpus callosum, cerebellum, and the relative positions of midline diencephalic structures in such comparisons.

KEY TO NUMBERED STRUCTURES

1. Subcallosal Gyrus
2. Genu of Corpus Callosum
3. Anterior Cerebral Artery, Calloso-marginal branch
4. Cingulate Gyrus
5. Septum Pellucidum
6. Parieto-occipital Sulcus
7. Calcarine Fissure
8. Primary Fissure of Cerebellum
9. Cerebellar Nodulus
10. Gracile Tubercle
11. Vertebral Artery
12. Paraterminal Gyrus
13. Anterior Cerebral Artery
14. Lamina Terminalis
15. Supraoptic Recess, Third Ventricle
16. Anterior Commissure
17. Fornix
18. Foramen of Monro
19. Massa Intermedia
20. Stria Medullaris
21. Habenula
22. Pineal Recess, Third Ventricle
23. Pineal body
24. Great Vein of Galen
25. Anterior Lobe, Cerebellum
26. Superior Colliculus
27. Inferior Colliculus
28. Cerebellar Nodulus
29. Fourth Ventricle
30. Anterior (superior) Medullary Velum
31. Medial Longitudinal Fasciculus
32. Decussation of Superior Cerebellar Peduncle
33. Posterior Commissure
34. Hypothalamic Sulcus
35. Mammillary Body
36. Infundibular Recess, Third Ventricle
37. Optic Chiasm

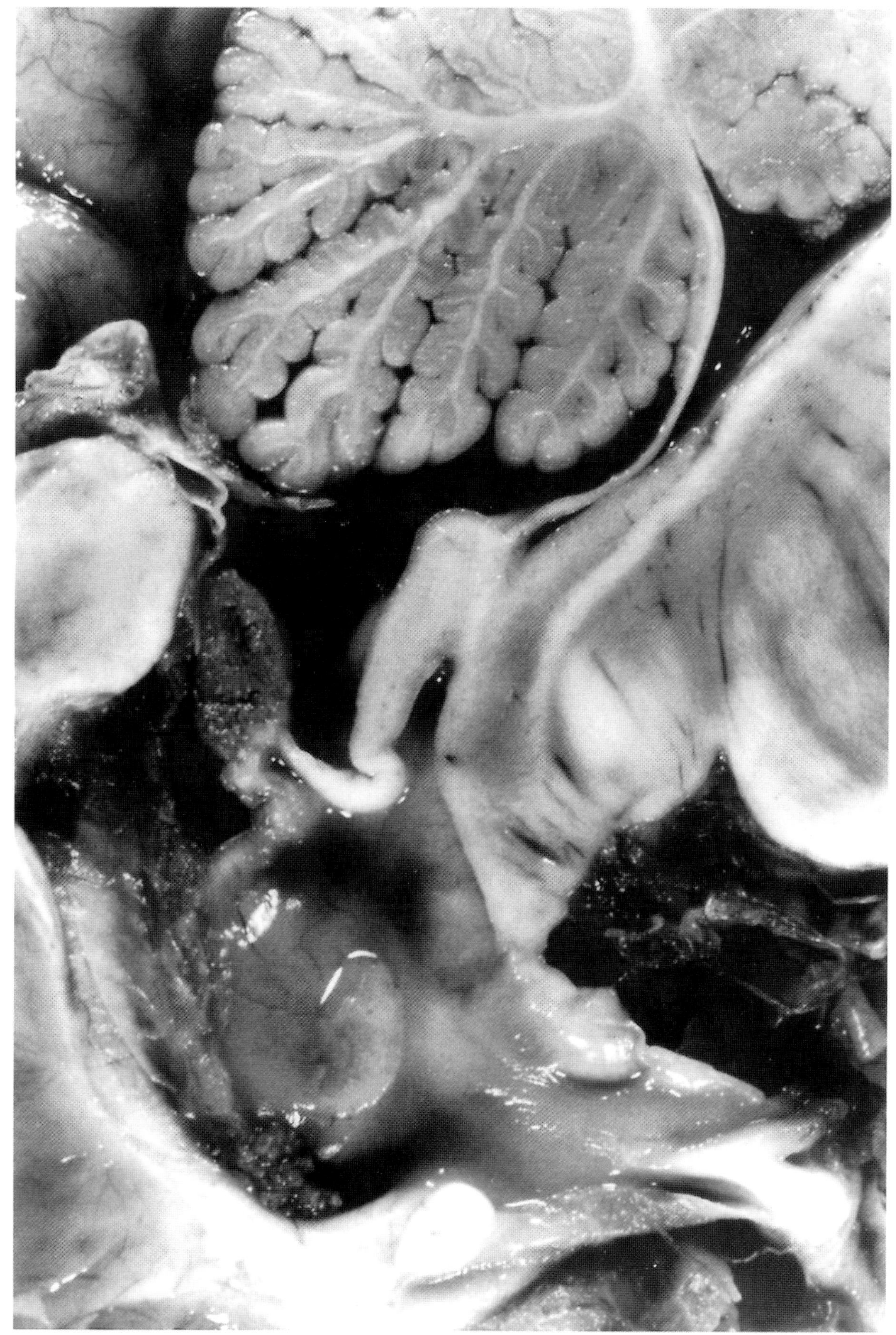

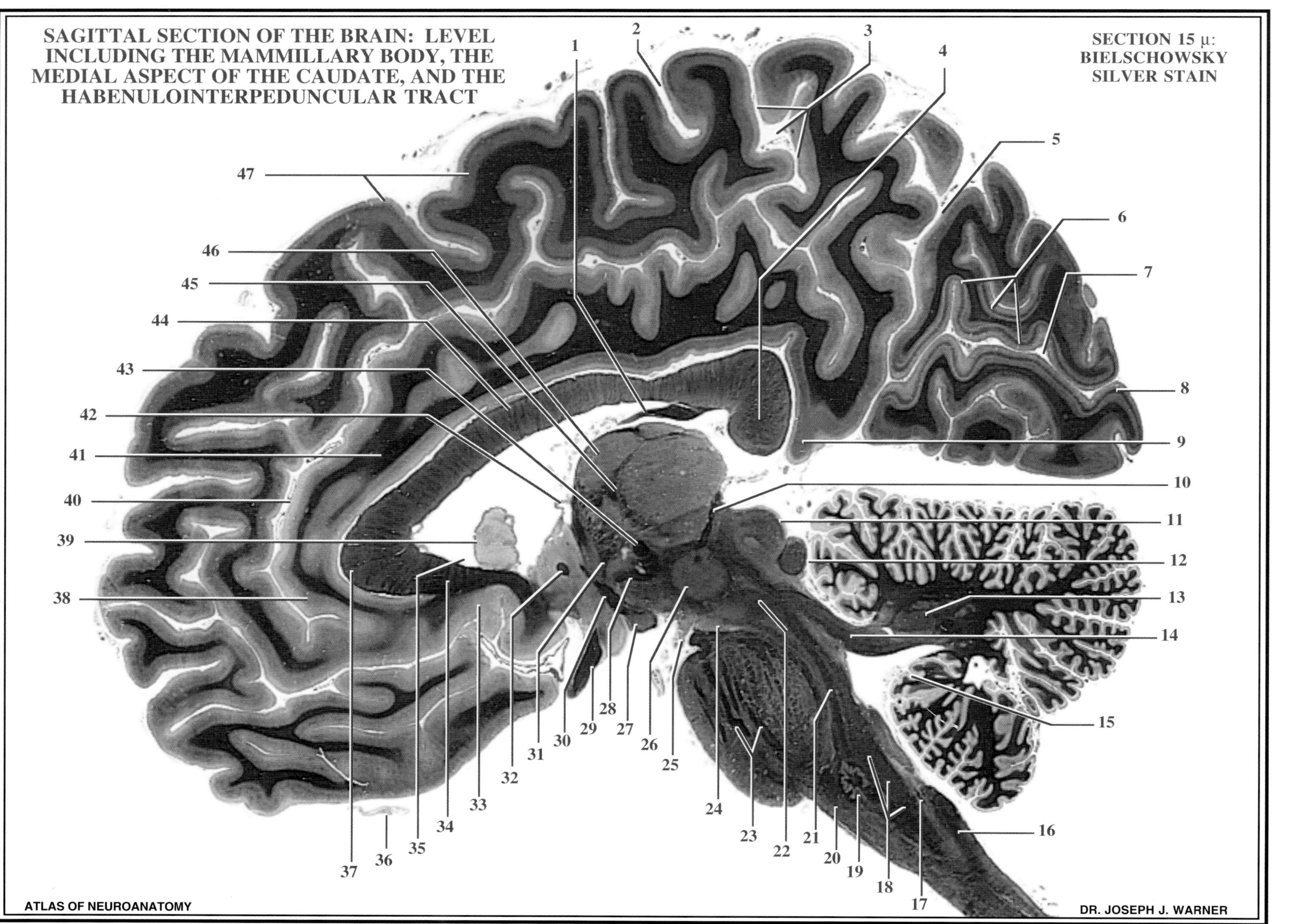
SAGITTAL SECTION OF THE BRAIN: LEVEL INCLUDING THE MAMMILLARY BODY, THE MEDIAL ASPECT OF THE CAUDATE, AND THE HABENULOINTERPEDUNCULAR TRACT
SECTION 15 μ: BIELSCHOWSKY SILVER STAIN
1
2
3
4
5
6
7
8
9
10
11
12
13
14
15
16
17
18
19
20
21
22
23
24
25
26
27
28
29
30
31
32
33
34
35
36
37
38
39
40
41
42
43
44
45
46
47
ATLAS OF NEUROANATOMY
DR. JOSEPH J. WARNER

SAGITTAL SECTION OF THE BRAIN; LEVEL INCLUDING THE MAMMILLARY BODY, THE MEDIAL ASPECT OF THE CAUDATE NUCLEUS, AND THE HABENULOINTERPEDUNCULAR TRACT (15 μ, BIELSCHOWSKY SILVER STAIN): SECTION MAP AND KEY TO NUMBERED STRUCTURES

KEY TO NUMBERED STRUCTURES

1. Fornix
2. Rolandic Fissure
3. Pars Marginalis, (extension of the Cingulate Sulcus)
4. Splenium of the Corpus Callosum
5. Parieto-occipital Sulcus
6. Area 17 Striate Cortex
7. Calcarine Fissure
8. Area 17 Striate Cortex, inferior bank of Calcarine Fissure
9. Isthmus of the Gyrus Fornicatus
10. Habenulointerpeduncular Tract (Fasciculus Retroflexus of Meynert)
11. Superior Colliculus
12. Inferior Colliculus
13. Nucleus Interpositus
14. Superior Cerebellar Peduncle
15. Nodulus
16. Fasciculus Gracilis
17. Nucleus and Tractus Solitarius
18. Medial Lemniscus
19. Inferior Olivary Nucleus
20. Medullary Pyramid
21. Central Tegmental Tract
22. Decussation of the Superior Cerebellar Peduncle
23. Corticobulbar and Corticospinal Tracts
24. Substantia Nigra
25. Oculomotor (III) Nerve
26. Red Nucleus
27. Mammillary Body
28. Lenticular Fasciculus
29. Optic Chiasm
30. Postcommissural Fornix
31. Inferior Thalamic Peduncle
32. Anterior Commissure
33. Subcallosal Gyrus
34. Rostrum of the Corpus Callosum
35. Anterior Horn of the Lateral Ventricle
36. Olfactory Bulb
37. Genu of the Corpus Callosum
38. Cingulate Cortex
39. Head of the Caudate Nucleus
40. Cingulate Sulcus
41. Cingulum
42. Thalamostriate Vein
43. Mammillothalamic Tract
44. Body of the Corpus Callosum
45. Internal Medullary Lamina of the Thalamus
46. Anterior Nucleus of the Thalamus
47. Superior Frontal Convolution

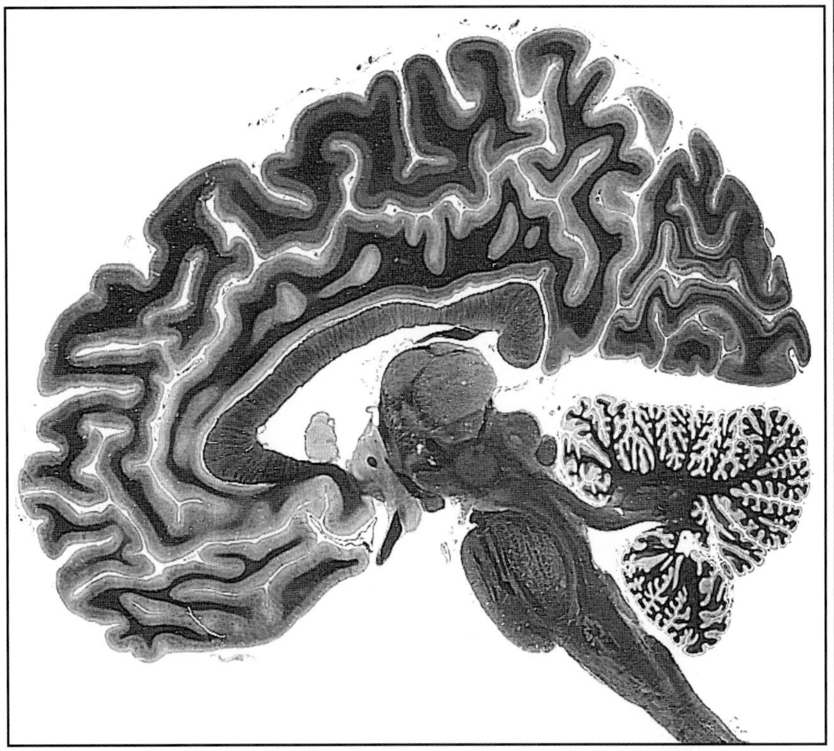

SECTION MAPPED ON VENTRAL VIEW OF THE BRAIN

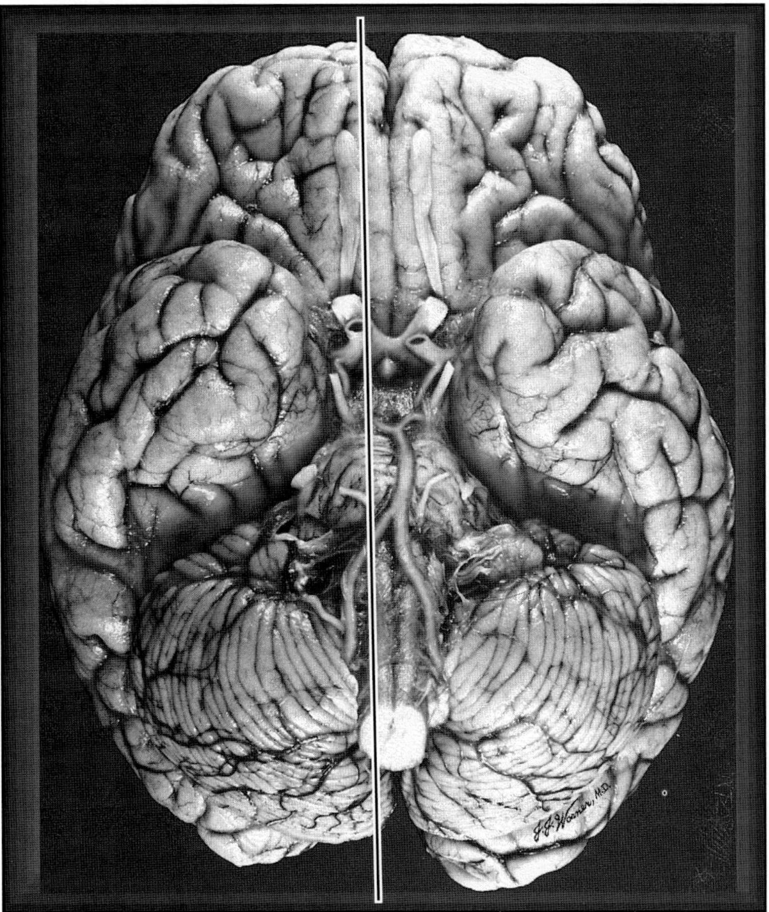

SAGITTAL SECTION OF THE BRAIN, COMPLETE: LEVEL OF THE MAMMILLOTHALAMIC TRACT AND THE ROSTRAL TERMINATION OF THE LATERAL LEMNISCUS

HISTOLOGIC SECTION, 15 μ:
KLUVER - BARRERA TECHNIQUE

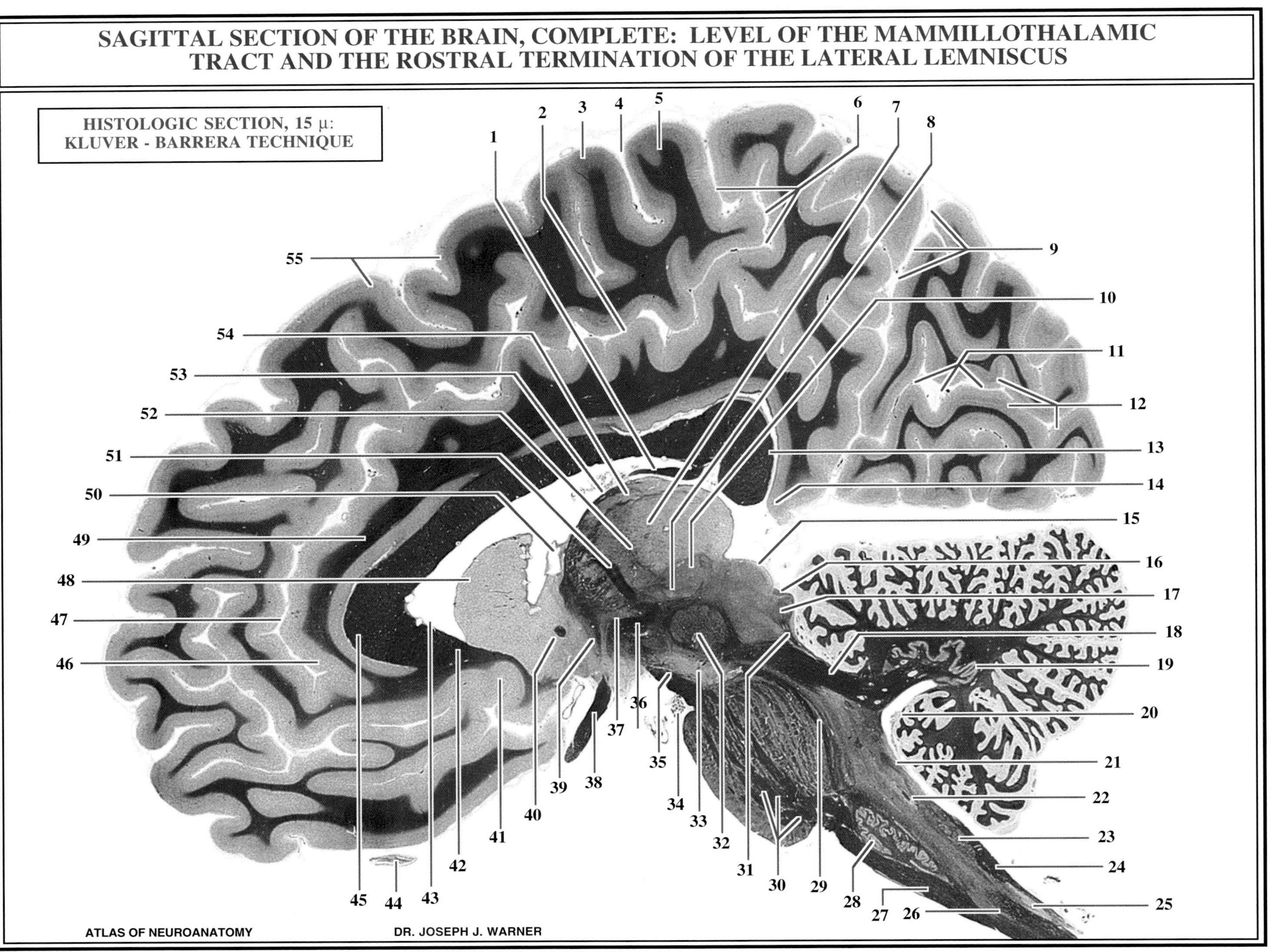

SAGITTAL SECTION OF THE BRAIN, COMPLETE; LEVEL OF THE MAMMILLOTHALAMIC TRACT AND THE ROSTRAL TERMINATION OF THE LATERAL LEMNISCUS (15 μ, KLUVER - BARRERA TECHNIQUE): SECTION MAP AND KEY TO NUMBERED STRUCTURES

KEY TO NUMBERED STRUCTURES

1. Fornix
2. Cingulate Sulcus
3. Precentral Gyrus
4. Rolandic Fissure
5. Postcentral Gyrus
6. Pars Marginalis (extension of the Cingulate Sulcus)
7. Dorsomedial Nucleus of the Thalamus*
8. Ventroposteromedial Nucleus (VPM) of the Thalamus
9. Parieto-Occipital Sulcus
10. Centromedian Nucleus of the Thalamus*
11. Calcarine Fissure
12. Area 17 Striate Cortex
13. Splenium of the Corpus Callosum
14. Isthmus of the Gyrus Fornicatus
15. Superior Colliculus
16. Brachium of the Inferior Colliculus
17. Inferior Colliculus
18. Superior Cerebellar Peduncle
19. Dentate Nucleus of the Cerebellum
20. Inferior Medullary Velum
21. Genu of the Facial Nerve
22. Nucleus and Tractus Solitarius
23. Nucleus Cuneatus
24. Fasciculus Cuneatus
25. Spinal Nucleus of the Trigeminal Nerve
26. Pyramidal Decussation and Lateral Corticospinal Tract
27. Medullary Pyramid
28. Inferior Olivary Nucleus
29. Medial Lemniscus
30. Corticobulbar, Corticospinal Tracts
31. Lateral Lemniscus
32. Red Nucleus
33. Substantia Nigra
34. Oculomotor (III) Nerve
35. Cerebral Peduncle
36. Lenticular Fasciculus
37. Zona Incerta
38. Optic Chiasm
39. Inferior Thalamic Peduncle
40. Anterior Commissure
41. Paraolfactory Area
42. Rostrum of the Corpus Callosum
43. Anterior Horn of the Lateral Ventricle*
44. Olfactory Bulb

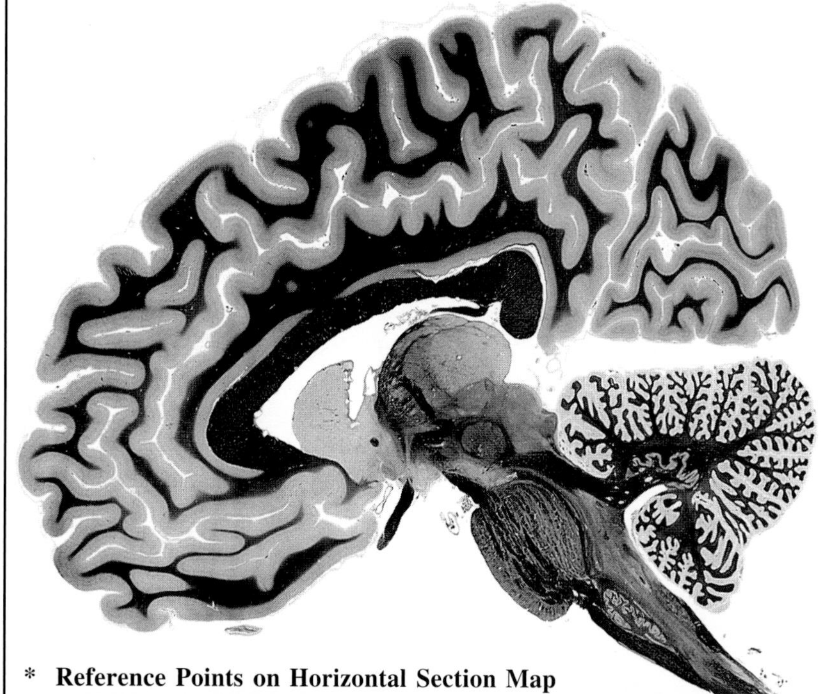

* **Reference Points on Horizontal Section Map**

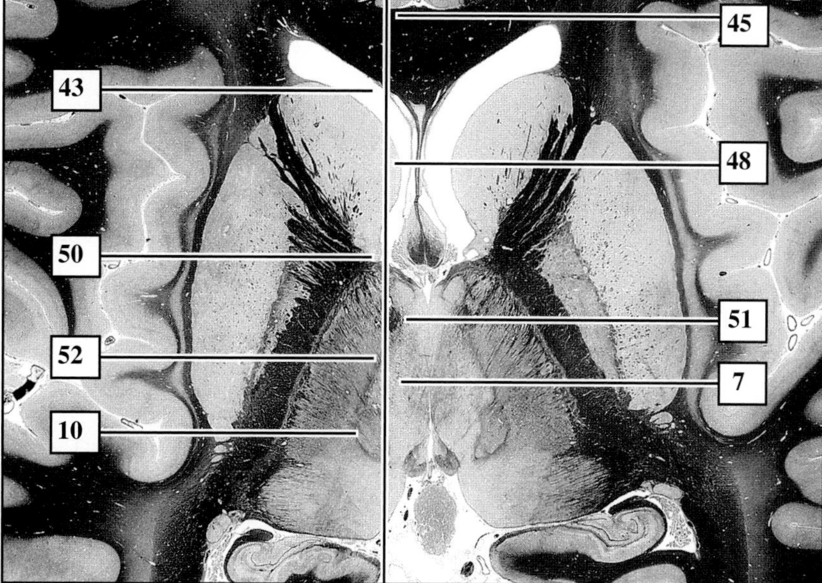

SAGITTAL PLANE MAPPED ON A HORIZONTAL SECTION AT THE LEVEL OF THE CENTROMEDIAN NUCLEUS OF THE THALAMUS

45. Genu of the Corpus Callosum*
46. Cingulate Cortex
47. Cingulate Sulcus
48. Head of the Caudate Nucleus*
49. Cingulum
50. Thalamostriate Vein*
51. Mammillothalamic Tract*
52. Internal Medullary Lamina of the Thalamus*
53. Dorsomedial extension of the External Medullary Lamina of the Thalamus
54. Lateral Dorsal Nucleus
55. Superior Frontal Convolution

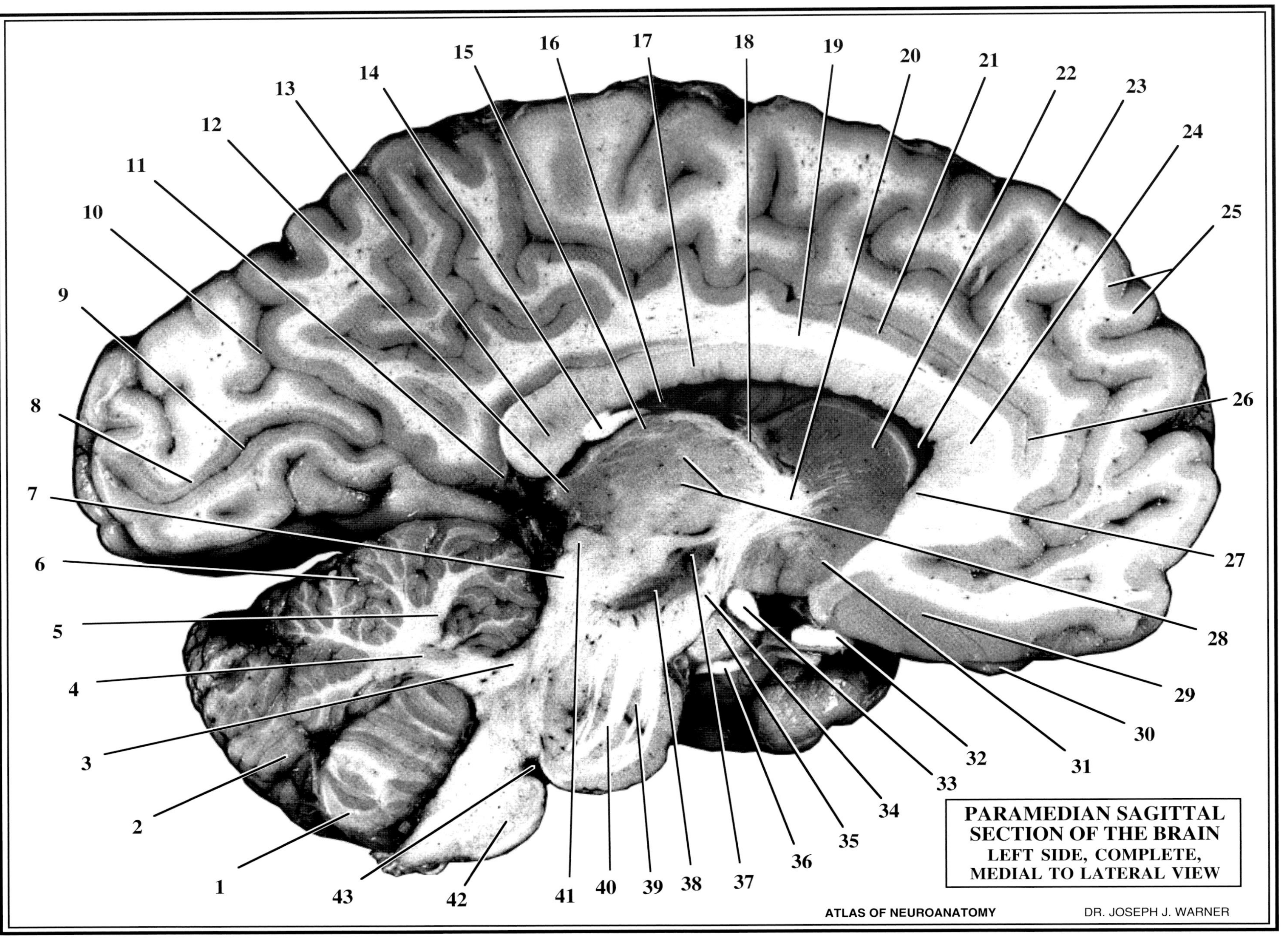
PARAMEDIAN SAGITTAL
SECTION OF THE BRAIN
LEFT SIDE, COMPLETE,
MEDIAL TO LATERAL VIEW
ATLAS OF NEUROANATOMY
DR. JOSEPH J. WARNER
1
2
3
4
5
6
7
8
9
10
11
12
13
14
15
16
17
18
19
20
21
22
23
24
25
26
27
28
29
30
31
32
33
34
35
36
37
38
39
40
41
42
43

BRAIN, PARAMEDIAN SAGITTAL SECTION, LEFT, MEDIAL TO LATERAL VIEW

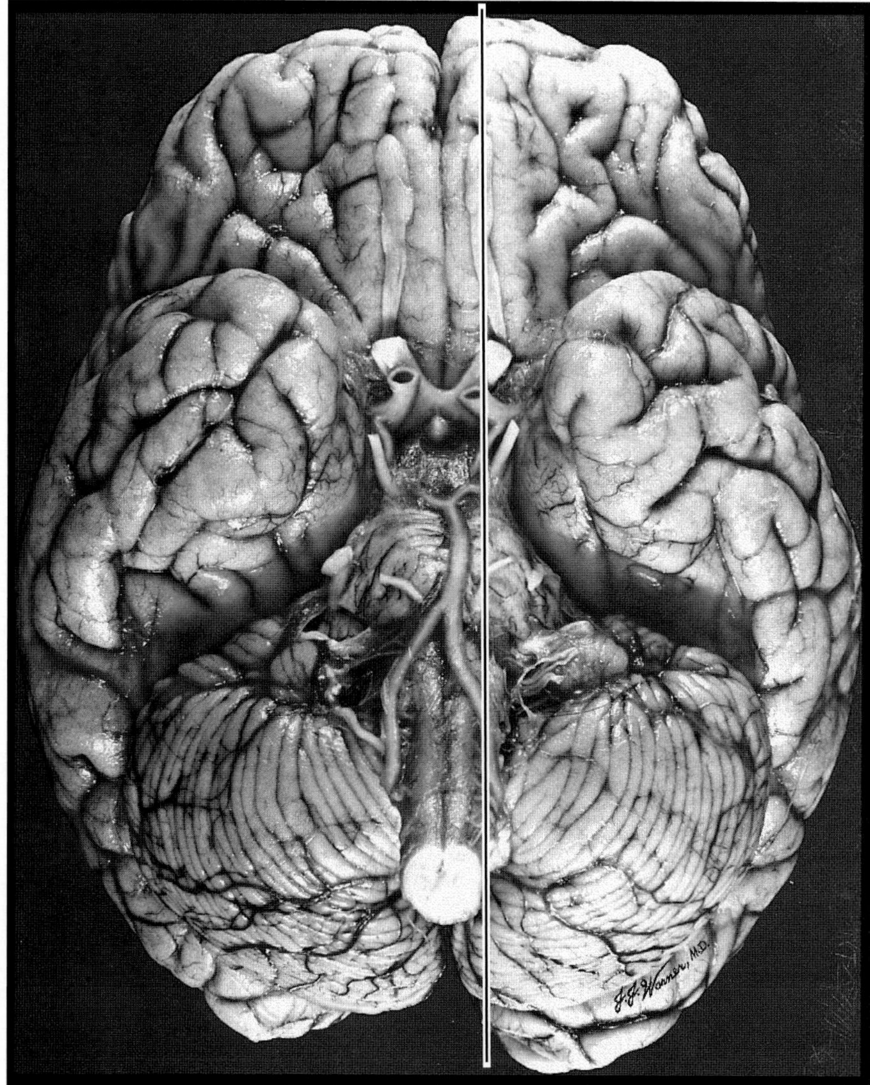

PARAMEDIAN SAGITTAL SECTION, LEVEL OF THE SUBSTANTIA NIGRA AND SUBTHALAMIC NUCLEUS

Note the appearance of the lateral aspect of the cervicomedullary junction, caudal to which is the prominence of the inferior olivary nucleus. Lateral to the fourth ventricle, the section passes through the cerebellar tonsil and the superior cerebellar peduncle. This left hemispheric section (viewed from medial to lateral) demonstrates the rostral medial temporal lobe, with the medial aspect of the uncus included in the plane of section. The head of the caudate nucleus is demonstrated in cut section. The caudate nucleus is seen in the lateral aspect of the lateral ventricle. Note the prominent corticobulbar and corticospinal fibers coursing from the cerebral peduncle longitudinally through the base of the pons. Rostral to the cerebral peduncle, the contiguous relationship of the optic tract is seen. The optic chiasm, medial to the plane of section, is not visualized. However, the plane of section passes through the optic nerve as it courses rostrally and laterally. The crus of the fornix is clearly discerned, located just ventral to the corpus callosum. The cingulum (white matter) is exposed by this section, subjacent to the cortex of the cingulate gyrus.

KEY TO NUMBERED STRUCTURES

1. Cerebellar Tonsil
2. Posterior Lobe of the Cerebellum
3. Superior Cerebellar Peduncle
4. Nucleus Interpositus
5. Anterior Lobe, Cerebellum
6. Primary Fissure of the Cerebellum
7. Inferior Colliculus
8. Area 17 Striate Cortex
9. Calcarine Fissure
10. Parieto-Occipital Sulcus
11. Isthmus of the Gyrus Fornicatus
12. Pulvinar Nucleus
13. Splenium of Corpus Callosum
14. Crus of the Fornix
15. Lateral Dorsal Nucleus
16. Body of Lateral Ventricle
17. Body of Corpus Callosum
18. Stria Terminalis and Thalamostriate Vein
19. Cingulum
20. Genu of Internal Capsule
21. Cingulate Gyrus
22. Head of Caudate Nucleus
23. Anterior Horn of Lateral Ventricle
24. Genu of Corpus Callosum
25. Superior Frontal Convolution
26. Cingulate Sulcus
27. Rostrum, Corpus Callosum
28. Internal Medullary Lamina of the Thalamus
29. Gyrus Rectus
30. Olfactory Bulb
31. Nucleus Accumbens
32. Optic Nerve
33. Optic Tract
34. Cerebral Peduncle
35. Uncus
36. Oculomotor Nerve
37. Subthalamic Nucleus
38. Substantia Nigra
39. Pontine Nuclei
40. Corticobulbar and Corticospinal Tracts
41. Superior Colliculus
42. Inferior Olivary Nucleus
43. Pontomedullary Sulcus

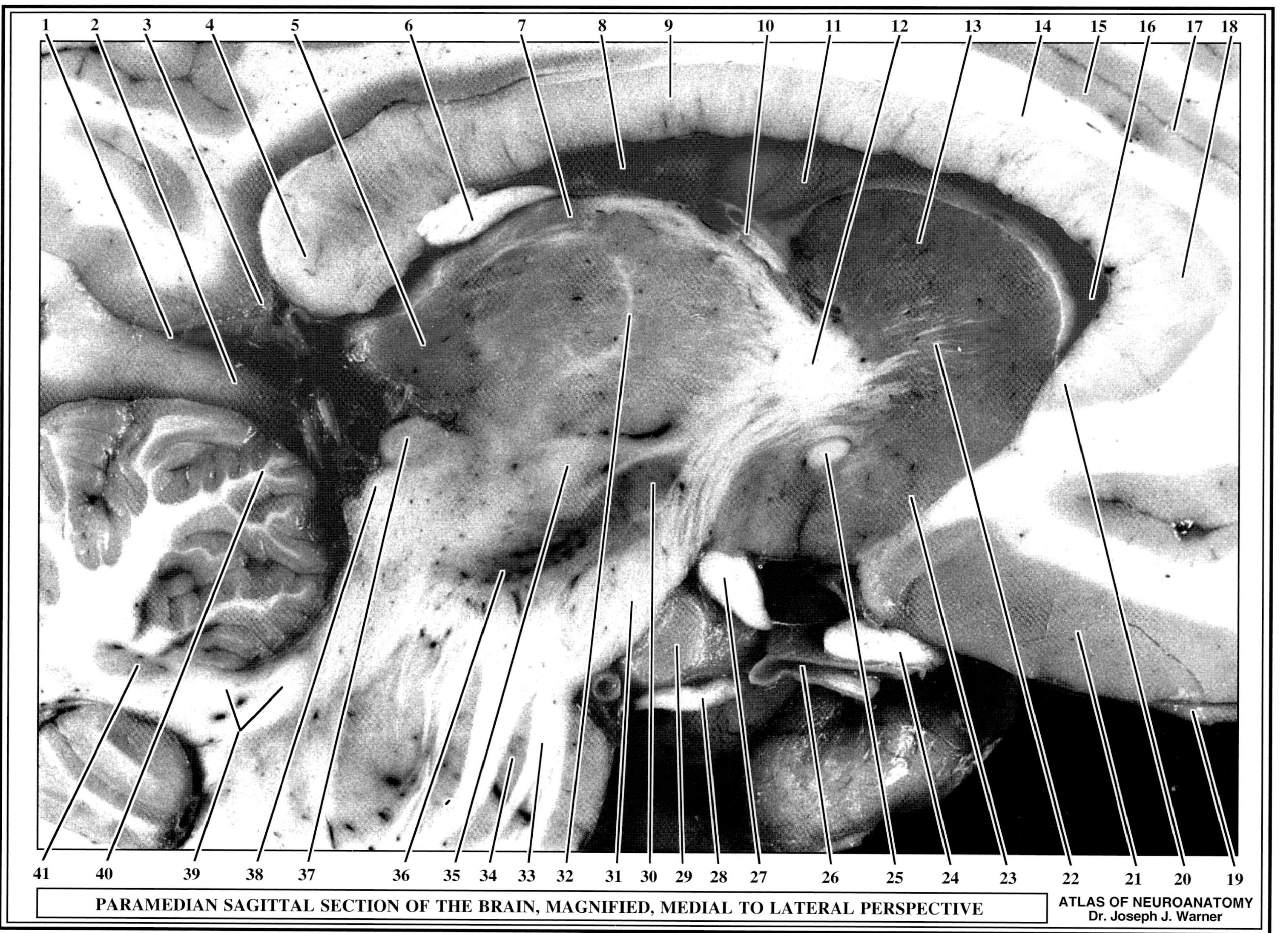

PARAMEDIAN SAGITTAL SECTION OF THE BRAIN, MAGNIFIED, MEDIAL TO LATERAL PERSPECTIVE

PARAMEDIAN SAGITTAL SECTION OF THE BRAIN, LEFT: MAGNIFIED VIEW

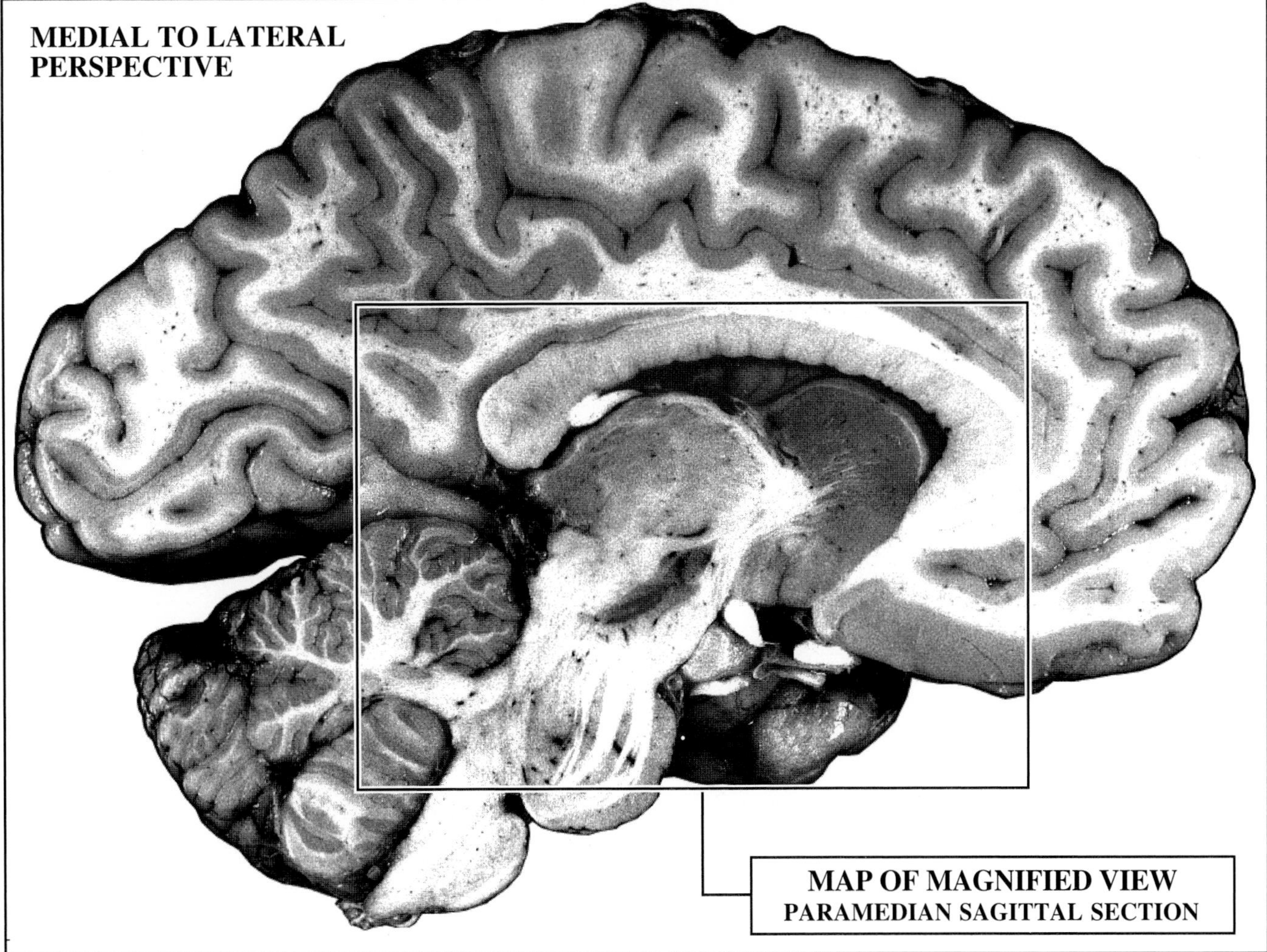

KEY TO NUMBERED STRUCTURES

1. Rostral extent, Parieto-Occipital Sulcus
2. Lingular Gyrus
3. Isthmus of Gyrus Fornicatus
4. Splenium of Corpus Callosum
5. Pulvinar
6. Crus of the Fornix
7. Lateral Dorsal Nucleus
8. Body of Lateral Ventricle
9. Body of Corpus Callosum
10. Stria Terminalis and Thalamostriate Vein
11. Caudate (lateral wall of Lateral Ventricle)
12. Genu of Internal Capsule
13. Head of the Caudate Nucleus
14. Cingulum (subjacent to Cingulate Cortex)
15. Cingulate Cortex
16. Anterior Horn of Lateral Ventricle
17. Cingulate Sulcus
18. Genu of Corpus Callosum
19. Olfactory Bulb
20. Rostrum of Corpus Callosum
21. Gyrus Rectus
22. Fibers of Anterior Limb of Internal Capsule
23. Nucleus Accumbens
24. Optic Nerve
25. Anterior Commissure
26. Terminal segment of Internal Carotid Artery
27. Optic Tract
28. Oculomotor Nerve
29. Uncus
30. Subthalamic Nucleus
31. Cerebral Peduncle
32. Internal Medullary Lamina of the Thalamus
33. Corticospinal and Corticobulbar Fibers (Corticobulbar Fibers generally course dorsally)
34. Pontine Nuclei
35. Fields of Forel
36. Substantia Nigra
37. Superior Colliculus
38. Inferior Colliculus (Gray Matter) and Brachium of Inferior Colliculus (White Matter extending rostrolaterally)
39. Superior Cerebellar Peduncle
40. Anterior Lobe of Cerebellum
41. Nucleus Interpositus

COMPLETE PARASAGITTAL SECTION, LEVEL OF THE MEDIAL GENICULATE NUCLEUS

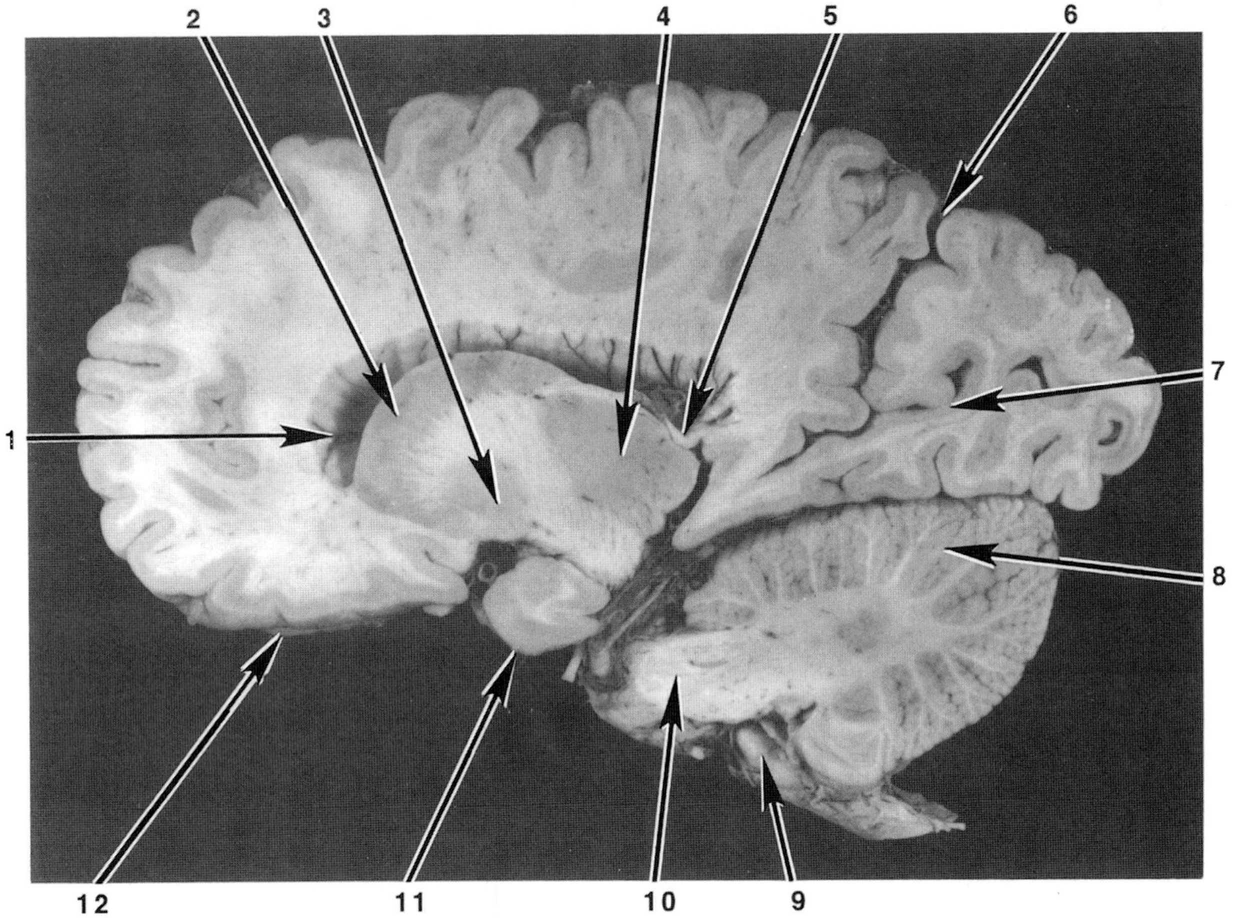

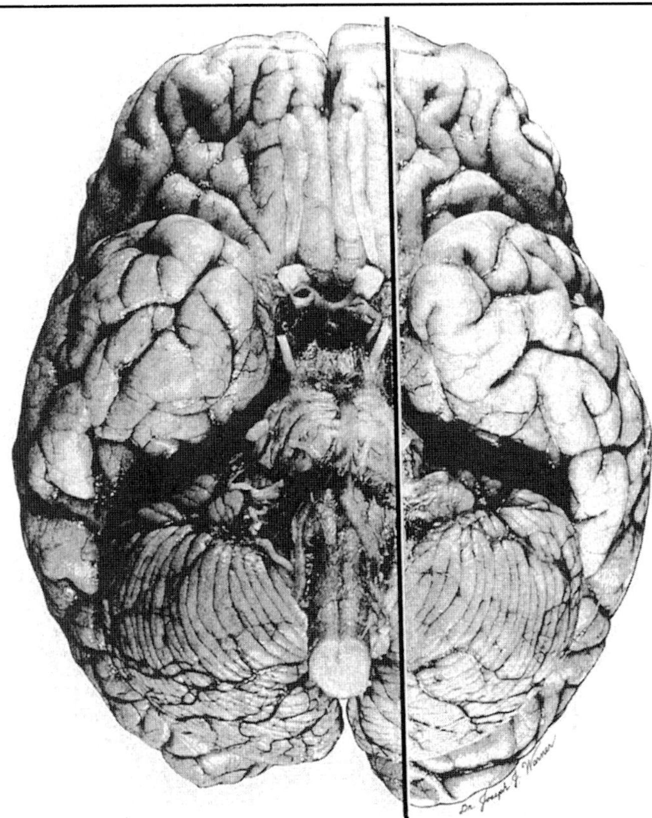

This section passes through the anterior limb, genu, and posterior limb of the internal capsule (refer to the description of the geometry of the internal capsule and its appearance in sagittal section). The medial geniculate nucleus is included in the plane of section, as is the uncus and a small area of medial temporal lobe white matter. This section through the left hemisphere is viewed from a lateral to a medial direction, thus the lateral aspect of the brainstem is visible rostral and caudal to the cut surface of the middle cerebellar peduncle and cerebellar hemisphere.

KEY TO NUMBERED STRUCTURES

1. Anterior Horn, Lateral Ventricle
2. Caudate Nucleus
3. Globus Pallidus
4. Thalamus
5. Fornix
6. Parieto-occipital Sulcus
7. Striate Cortex
8. Primary Fissure, Cerebellum
9. Inferior Olive
10. Middle Cerebellar Peduncle
11. Uncus
12. Olfactory Bulb

PARASAGITTAL SECTION, LEVEL OF THE MEDIAL GENICULATE NUCLEUS, MAGNIFIED VIEW

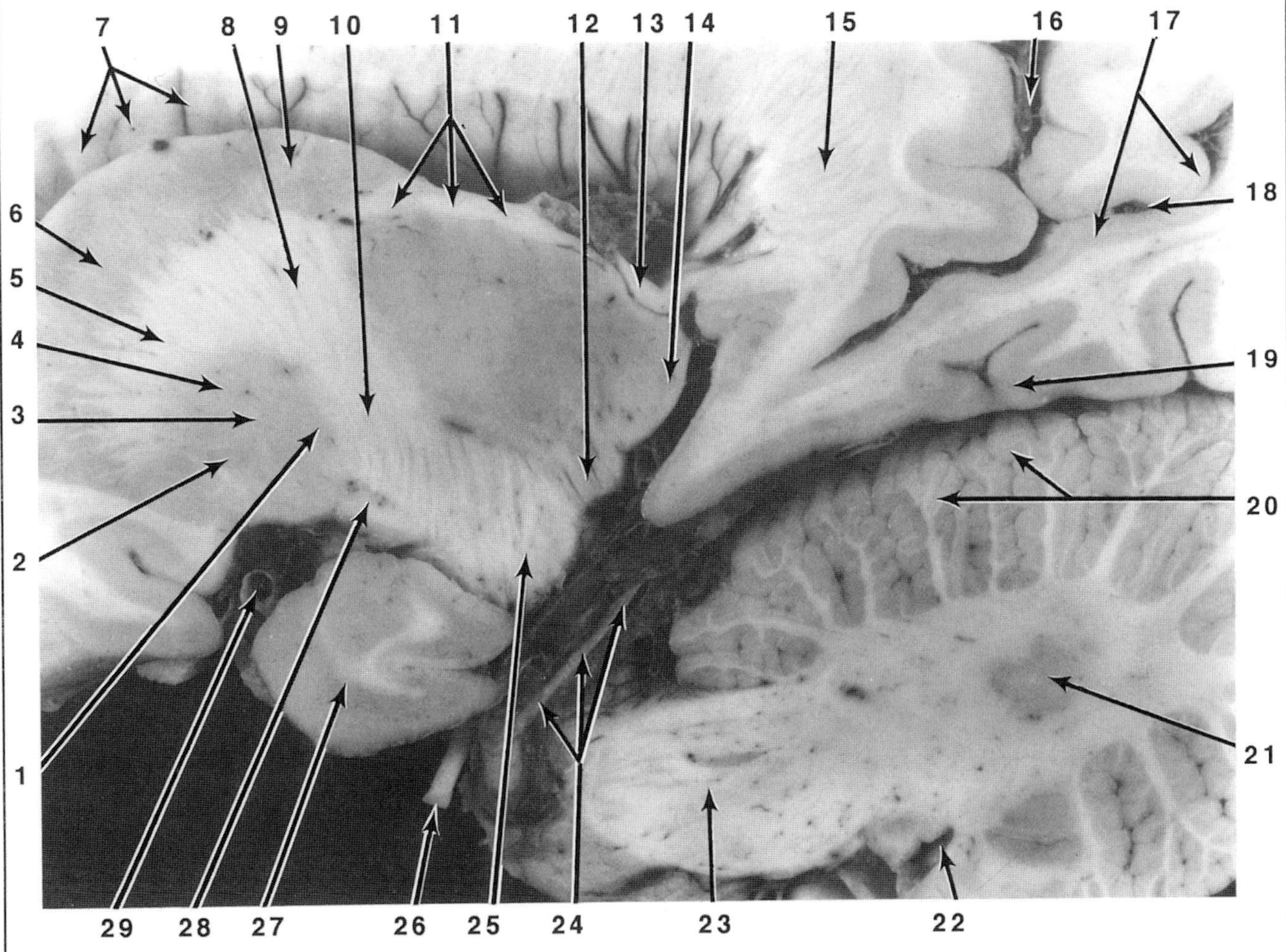

KEY TO NUMBERED STRUCTURES

1. Globus Pallidus I
2. Anterior Commissure
3. Internal Medullary Lamina
4. Globus Pallidus II
5. Anterior Limb, Internal Capsule
6. Head of Caudate Nucleus
7. Body of Lateral Ventricle
8. Genu, Internal Capsule
9. Caudate Nucleus
10. Posterior Limb, Internal Capsule
11. Stria Terminalis and External Medullary Lamina of the Thalamus
12. Medial Geniculate Nucleus
13. Fornix
14. Pulvinar Nucleus of the Thalamus
15. Splenium of Corpus Callosum
16. Parieto-occipital Sulcus
17. Striate Cortex (Area 17)
18. Calcarine Fissure
19. Tentorial (inferior) surface of Occipital Lobe
20. Anterior Lobe, Cerebellum
21. Dentate Nucleus of the Cerebellum
22. Foramen of Luschka
23. Middle Cerebellar Peduncle
24. Trochlear (IV) Nerve
25. Cerebral Peduncle
26. Oculomotor (III) Nerve
27. Uncus (and white matter of Parahippocampal Gyrus)
28. Optic Tract
29. Middle Cerebral Artery

PARASAGITTAL SECTION, LEVEL OF THE MEDIAL GENICULATE NUCLEUS: MAGNIFIED MEDIAL TO LATERAL VIEW

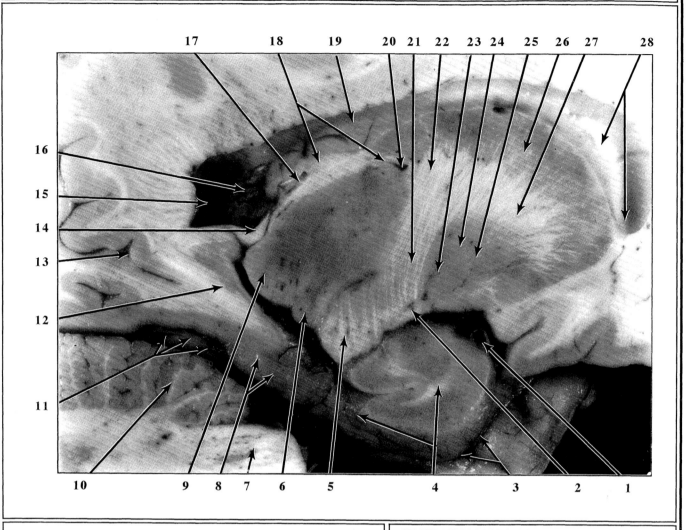

KEY TO NUMBERED STRUCTURES

1. Middle Cerebral Artery
2. Optic Tract
3. Rhinal Fissure
4. Parahippocampal Gyrus
5. Cerebral Peduncle
6. Medial Geniculate Nucleus
7. Middle Cerebral Peduncle
8. Parahippocampal Gyrus
9. Pulvinar Nucleus of the Thalamus
10. Anterior Lobe of the Cerebellum
11. Fusiform Gyrus
12. Isthmus of the Gyrus Fornicatus
13. Calcarine Fissure
14. Fornix
15. Atrium of the Lateral Ventricle
16. Choroid Plexus
17. External Medullary Lamina of the Thalamus
18. Stria Terminalis
19. Body of Lateral Ventricle
20. Thalamostriate Vein
21. Posterior Limb of the Internal Capsule
22. Genu of the Internal Capsule
23. Globus Pallidus I
24. Internal Medullary Lamina
25. Globus Pallidus II
26. Caudate Nucleus
27. Anterior Limb of the Internal Capsule
28. Anterior Horn of the Lateral Ventricle

SECTION MAPPED ON VENTRAL VIEW OF THE BRAIN

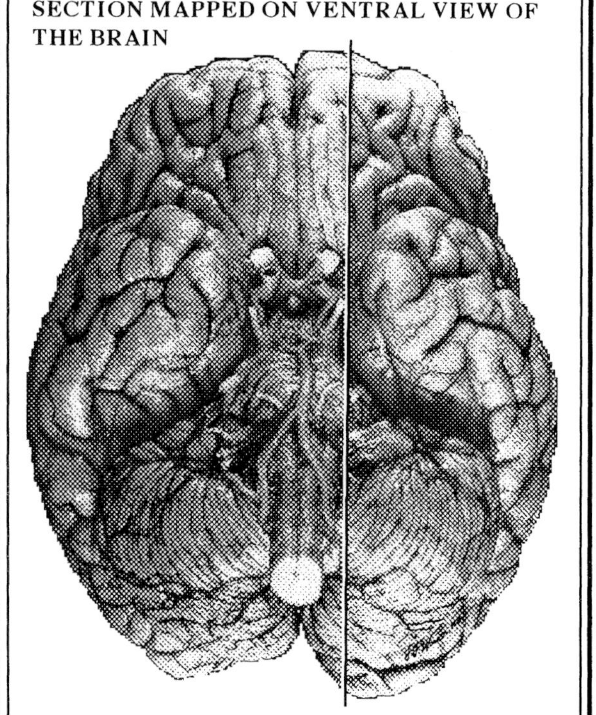

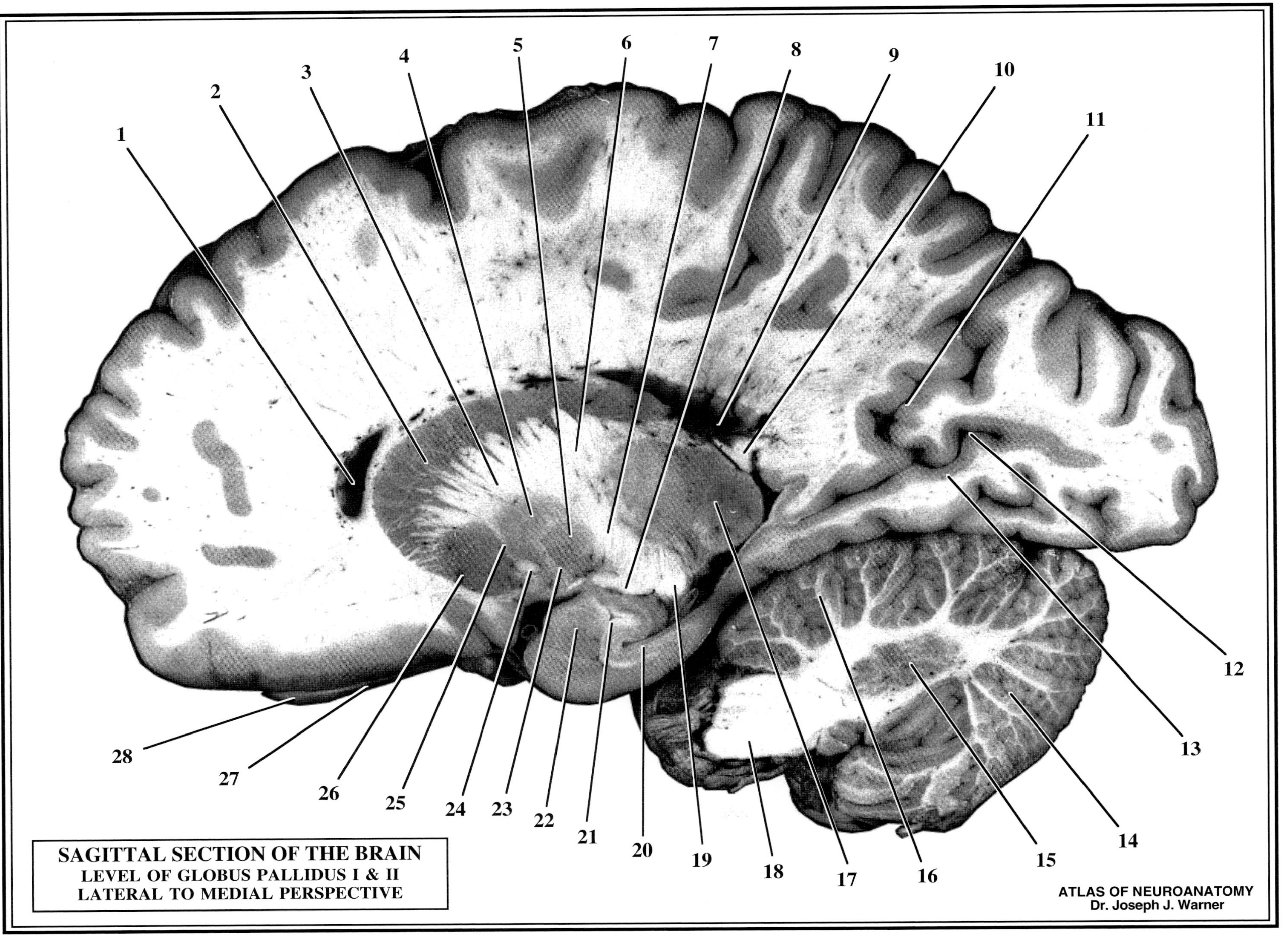

SAGITTAL SECTION OF THE BRAIN
LEVEL OF GLOBUS PALLIDUS I & II
LATERAL TO MEDIAL PERSPECTIVE

BRAIN, COMPLETE SAGITTAL SECTION AT LEVEL OF GLOBUS PALLIDUS, LEFT

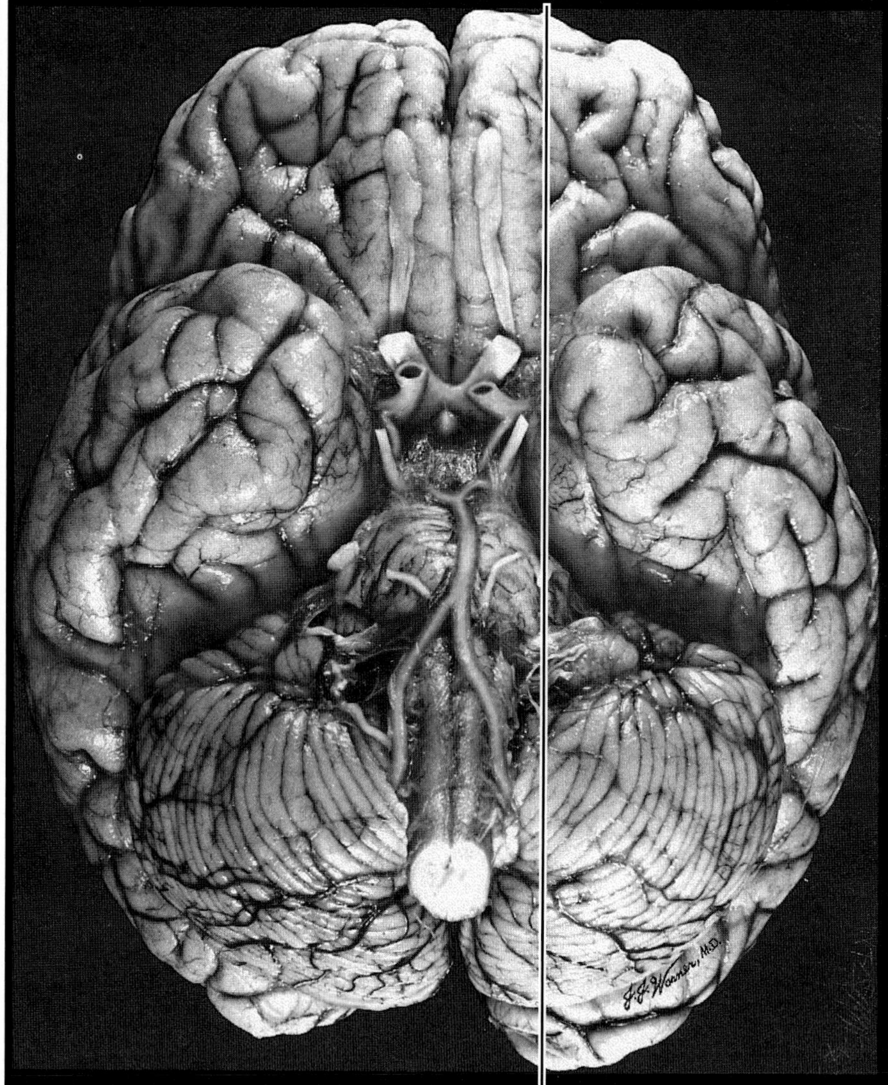

LATERAL TO MEDIAL PERSPECTIVE

KEY TO NUMBERED STRUCTURES

1. Anterior Horn of Lateral Ventricle
2. Head of the Caudate Nucleus
3. Anterior Limb of Internal Capsule
4. Globus Pallidus II
5. Globus Pallidus I
6. Genu of Internal Capsule
7. Posterior Limb of Internal Capsule
8. Optic Tract
9. Body of Lateral Ventricle
10. Fornix
11. Parieto-Occipital Sulcus
12. Calcarine Fissure
13. Area 17 Striate Cortex
14. Posterior Lobe, Cerebellum
15. Dentate Nucleus
16. Anterior Lobe, Cerebellum
17. Thalamus
18. Middle Cerebellar Peduncle
19. Cerebral Peduncle
20. Hippocampus
21. Temporal Horn of the Lateral Ventricle, (rostral extent)
22. Amygdala
23. Internal Medullary Lamina
24. Anterior Commissure
25. External Medullary Lamina
26. Putamen
27. Olfactory Tract
28. Olfactory Bulb

This section demonstrates the close proximity of the optic tract to the globus pallidus (G.P. I, internal segment). One of the serious clinical risks of pallidotomy for Parkinson's disease is contralateral homonymous hemianopsia due to involvement of the optic tract. The optic tract continues its course caudally and laterally around the cerebral peduncle, then terminates at the lateral geniculate nucleus.

Ventral to the anterior limb of the internal capsule, the head of the caudate nucleus and the putamen appear to merge into a region of gray matter, the nucleus accumbens. The gross anatomic delineation of this structure is indistinct. When studying the relationship of the putamen, caudate, and nucleus accumbens in sagittal sections, it is important to cross-reference these nuclei on a coronal section, examining their relative positions to each other and to the anterior limb of the internal capsule. The external medullary lamina is intercalated between the external segment of the globus pallidus and the putamen, demonstrated on this sagittal section.

As shown in this section, the anterior commissure passes through the ventral aspect of the globus pallidus as it courses laterally. Medially, it passes dorsal to the nucleus basalis of Meynert. The anterior commissure crosses the midline rostral to the postcommissural fibers of the fornix. Examination of the medial temporal lobe in this section demonstrates the intercalation of the rostral aspect of the temporal horn of the lateral ventricle between the amygdala and the rostral hippocampus. Cross-referencing to the horizontal plane of section and to cast models of the ventricular system, the rostral tip of the temporal horn turns medially. The hippocampus is located ventromedial to the temporal horn along its course. Where the abrupt medial curve occurs, the temporal horn separates the rostral hippocampus from the amygdala.

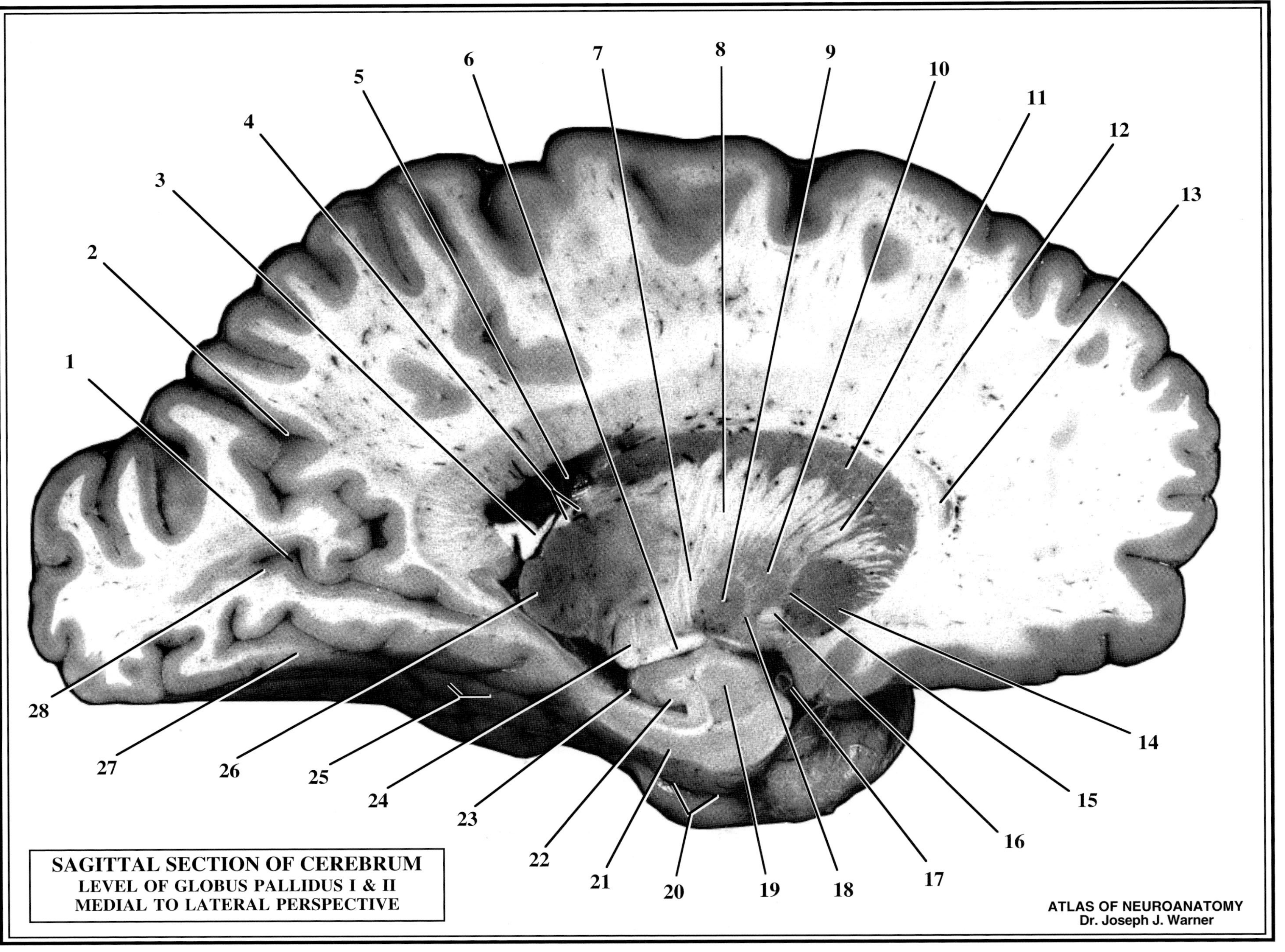
1
2
3
4
5
6
7
8
9
10
11
12
13
14
15
16
17
18
19
20
21
22
23
24
25
26
27
28
SAGITTAL SECTION OF CEREBRUM
LEVEL OF GLOBUS PALLIDUS I & II
MEDIAL TO LATERAL PERSPECTIVE
ATLAS OF NEUROANATOMY
Dr. Joseph J. Warner

CEREBRAL HEMISPHERE, SAGITTAL SECTION, LEVEL OF GLOBUS PALLIDUS

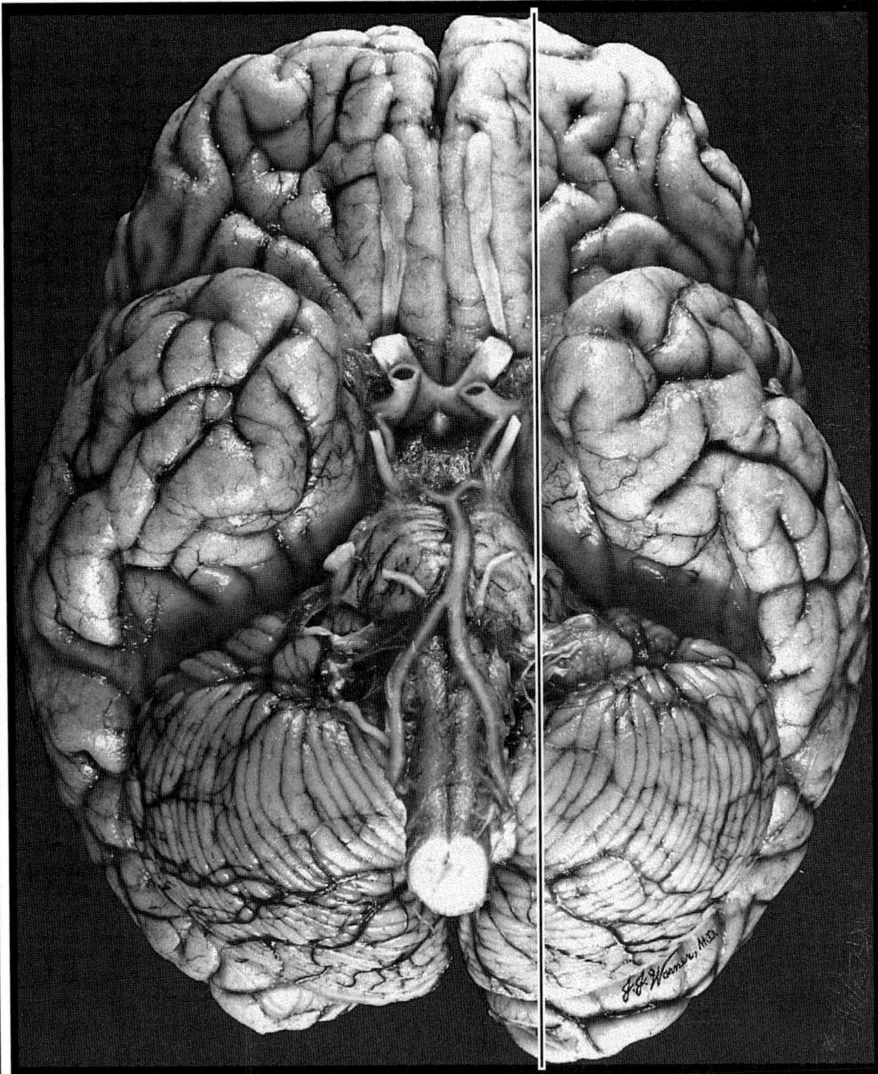

The plane of section is mapped above, however, the cerebellum has been removed, exposing the gyri on the ventral aspect of the temporal, parietal, and occipital regions. This specimen consists of the entire left cerebral hemisphere from the level of the globus pallidus laterally, and is shown in that perspective. The subsequent figure is a view of the same specimen dorsolaterally rotated to emphasize the relationships between the hippocampal formation, parahippocampal gyrus, and fusiform gyrus.

LEFT, MEDIAL TO LATERAL PERSPECTIVE

KEY TO NUMBERED STRUCTURES

1. Calcarine Fissure
2. Parieto-Occipital sulcus
3. Fornix
4. Stria Terminalis and Thalamostriate Vein
5. Body of Lateral Ventricle
6. Optic Tract
7. Posterior Limb, Internal Capsule
8. Genu, Internal Capsule
9. Globus Pallidus I
10. Globus Pallidus II
11. Caudate Nucleus
12. Anterior Limb, Internal Capsule
13. Anterior Horn, Lateral Ventricle
14. Nucleus Accumbens
15. External Medullary Lamina
16. Anterior Commissure
17. Middle Cerebral Artery
18. Internal Medullary Lamina
19. Amygdala
20. Collateral Sulcus
21. Parahippocampal Gyrus
22. Hippocampal Formation
23. Hippocampal Fissure
24. Cerebral Peduncle
25. Fusiform Gyrus
26. Pulvinar
27. Fusiform Gyrus
28. Area 17 Striate Cortex

The hippocampal fissure and parahippocampal gyrus pass circumferentially around the cerebral peduncle. The hippocampal fissure, an extension of the subarachnoid space, should not be misidentified as the temporal horn of the lateral ventricle in the sagittal plane of section. The section is parallel to a major segment of the hippocampal fissure. In this plane, the parahippocampal gyrus has been longitudinally sectioned. Subjacent to the parahippocampal cortex and white matter, the amygdala and hippocampus are exposed.

In this plane, the rostral tip of the temporal horn is visible, intercalated between the rostral hippocampus and the amygdala. However, the major portion of the temporal horn is lateral to this plane of section. Cross-reference to coronal and horizontal sections clarifies the contiguity of the optic tract, the cerebral peduncle, and the subarachnoid space of the perimesencephalic cisterns, distinct from the temporal horn of the lateral ventricle. The hippocampal fissure is thus readily distinguished from the temporal horn when exposed in sagittal sections.

LEFT CEREBRAL HEMISPHERE, SAGITTAL SECTION, MEDIAL TO LATERAL PERSPECTIVE DORSAL ASPECT OF SPECIMEN EXTERNALLY ROTATED

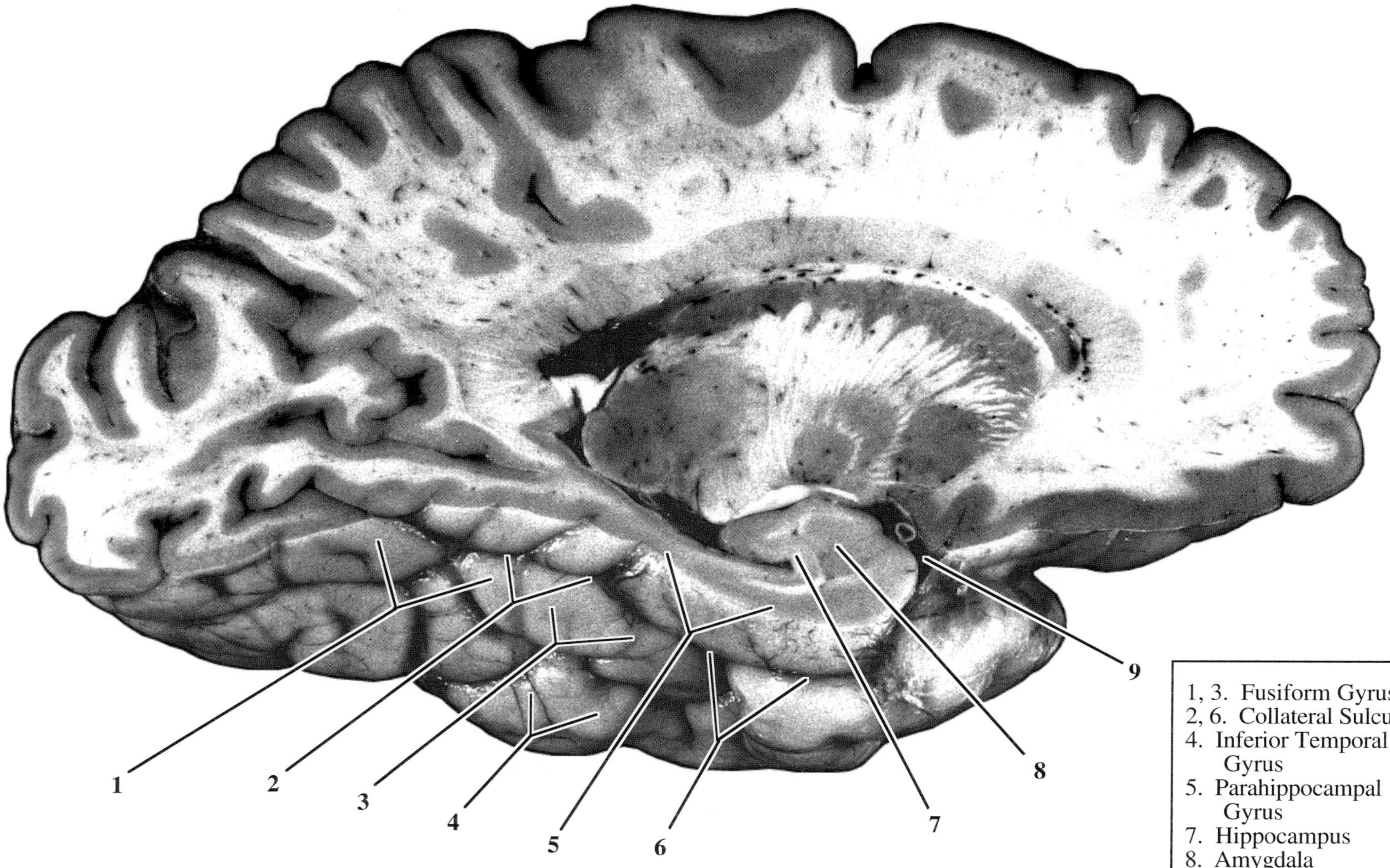

1 2 3 4 5 6 7 8 9

1, 3. Fusiform Gyrus
2, 6. Collateral Sulcus
4. Inferior Temporal Gyrus
5. Parahippocampal Gyrus
7. Hippocampus
8. Amygdala
9. Sylvian Fissure

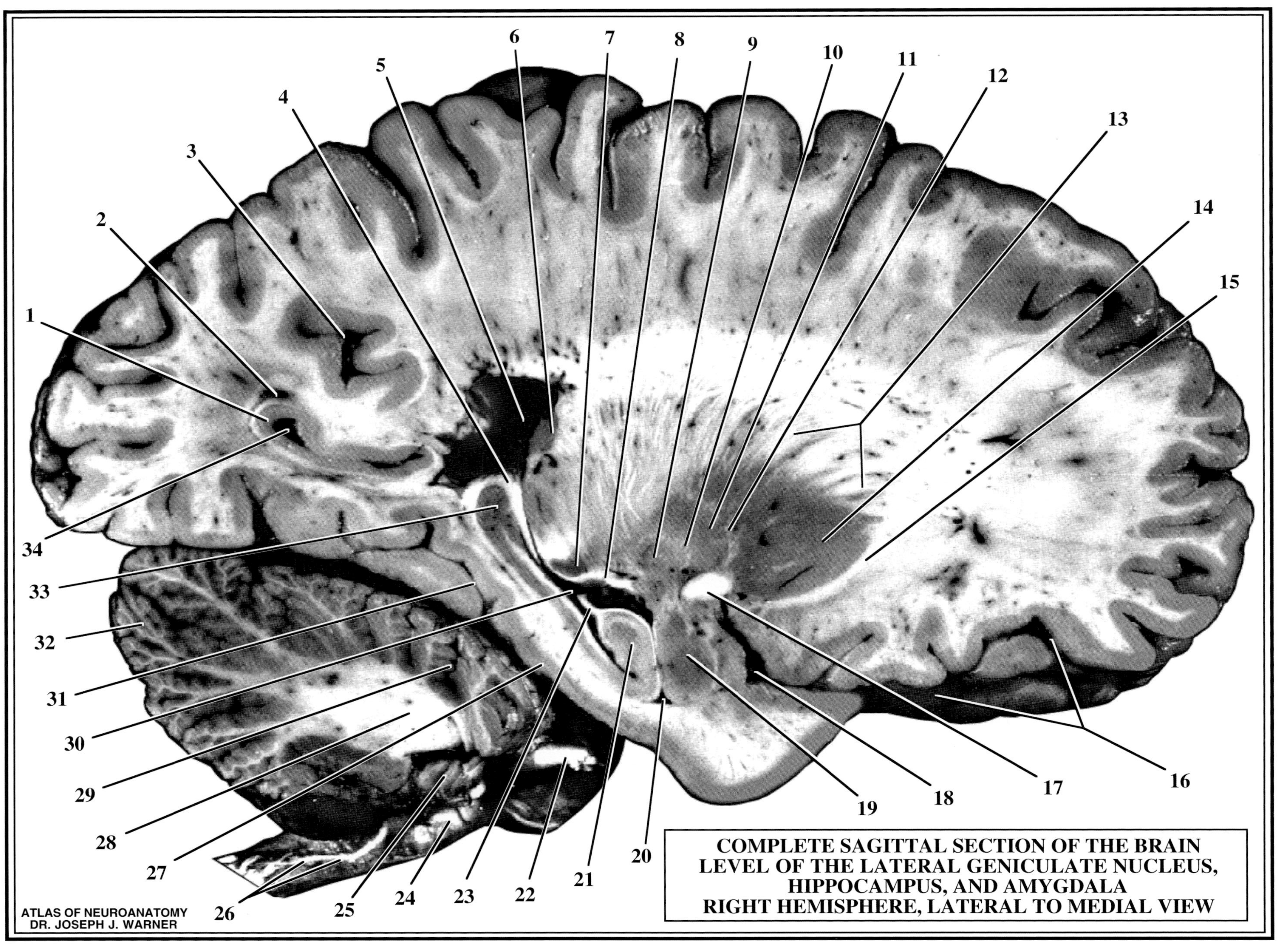

COMPLETE SAGITTAL SECTION OF THE BRAIN
LEVEL OF THE LATERAL GENICULATE NUCLEUS,
HIPPOCAMPUS, AND AMYGDALA
RIGHT HEMISPHERE, LATERAL TO MEDIAL VIEW

MAP OF SAGITTAL SECTION OF THE BRAIN AT THE LEVEL OF THE LATERAL GENICULATE NUCLEUS, HIPPOCAMPUS, AND AMYGDALA

REFERENCED TO A HORIZONTAL SECTION, LEVEL OF THE MESENCEPHALIC-DIENCEPHALIC TRANSITION (15μ, KLUVER-BARRERA TECHNIQUE)

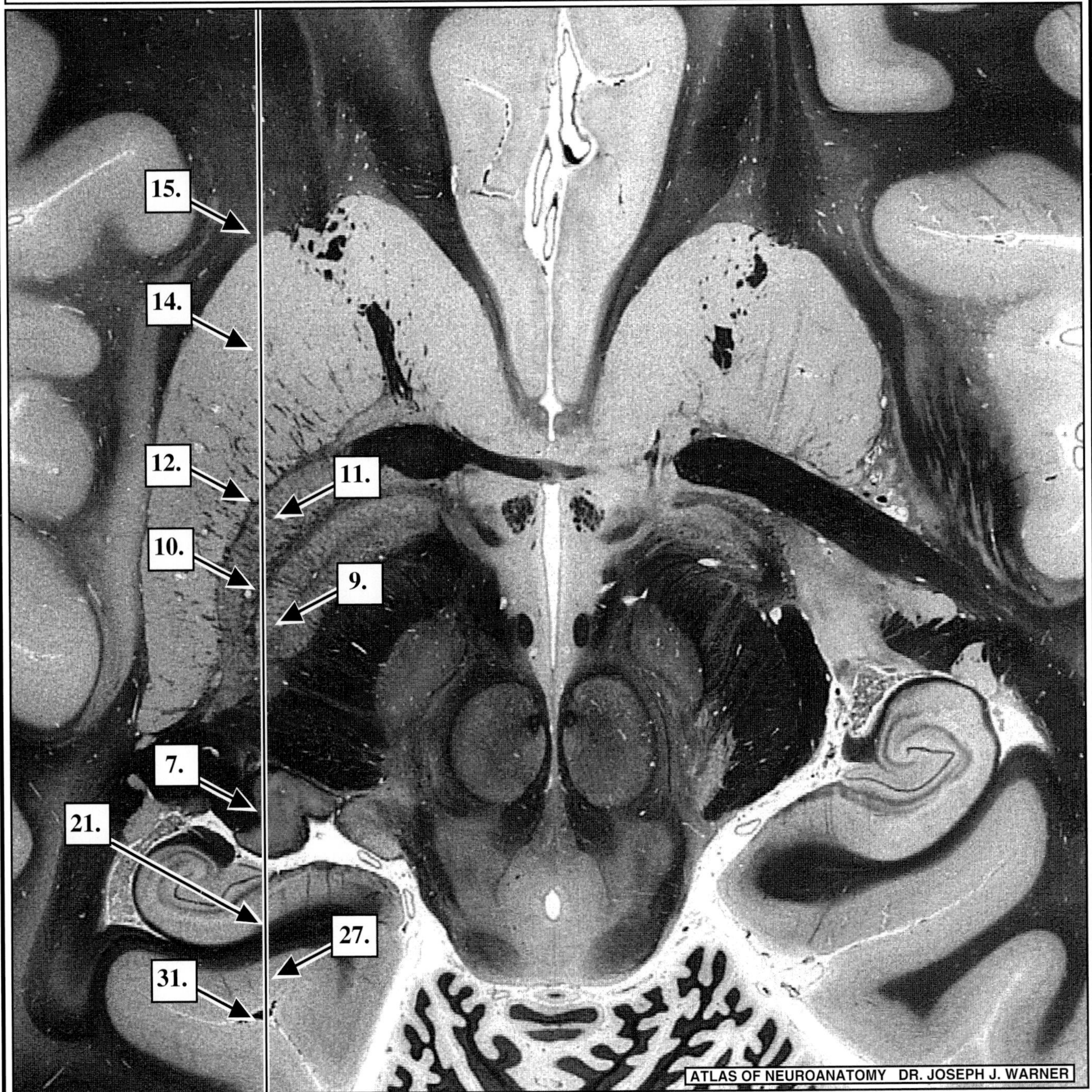

KEY TO NUMBERED STRUCTURES:

1. Area 17 Striate Cortex
2. Occipital Horn, Lateral Ventricle
3. Parieto-occipital Sulcus
4. Fornix
5. Atrium of Lateral Ventricle
6. Tail of the Caudate Nucleus
7. Lateral Geniculate Nucleus*
8. Lateral fibers of Optic Tract
9. Globus Pallidus I*
10. Internal Medullary Lamina*
11. Globus Pallidus II*
12. External Medullary Lamina*
13. Corona Radiata
14. Putamen*
15. External Capsule*
16. Orbitofrontal Gyri
17. Anterior Commissure
18. Sylvian Fissure
19. Amygdala
20. Temporal Horn, Lateral Ventricle
21. Hippocampus*
22. Trigeminal Nerve
23. Fornix
24. Inferior Olive
25. Flocculus
26. Spinal Accessory Nerve
27. Parahippocampal Gyrus*
28. Middle Cerebellar Peduncle
29. Anterior Lobe, Cerebellum*
30. Temporal Horn of Lateral Ventricle
31. Collateral Sulcus*
32. Posterior Lobe, Cerebellum
33. Hippocampus
34. Calcarine Fissure

*** Reference intersection points on this horizontal section**

PARASAGITTAL SECTION, LEVEL OF THE HIPPOCAMPUS

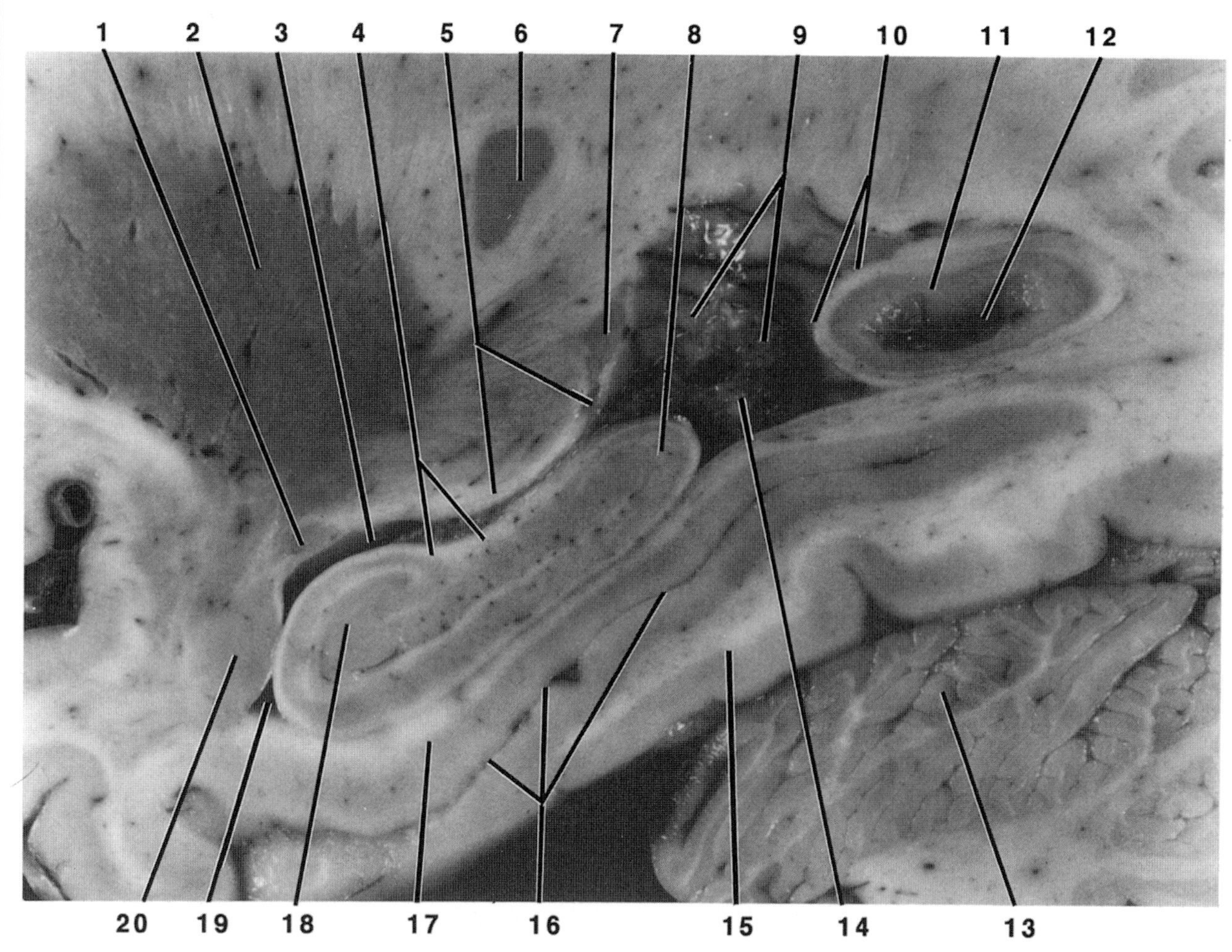

KEY TO NUMBERED STRUCTURES

1. Tail of the Caudate
2. Putamen
3. Temporal (Inferior) Horn of the Lateral Ventricle
4. Alveus (and Fimbria of the Fornix)
5. Stria Terminalis and Thalamostriate Vein
6. Insular Cortex
7. Tail of the Caudate
8. Caudal aspect of the Hippocampus
9. Atrium of the Lateral Ventricle
10. Calcar Avis
11. Striate Cortex
12. Calcarine Fissure
13. Anterior Lobe of the Cerebellum
14. Choroid Plexus
15. Fusiform Gyrus
16. Collateral Sulcus
17. Parahippocampal Gyrus
18. Rostral aspect of Hippocampus
19. Temporal Horn of the Lateral Ventricle
20. Amygdala

The temporal horn of the lateral ventricle passes ventrally and rostrally in the medial temporal lobe. The hippocampus is located ventral and medial to the temporal horn (refer to coronal sections to examine this relationship). The temporal horn continues rostrally, then curves medially between the amygdala and the rostral hippocampus. This is clearly shown on horizontal sections, and in sections parallel to the Sylvian Fissure (refer to the illustrations of sections in these orientations). This sagittal section demonstrates the spatial orientation of the hippocampus with respect to the temporal horn, and the separation of the rostral hippocampus from the amygdala by the rostral tip of the temporal horn of the lateral ventricle. The occipital pole of the lateral ventricle is indented by a deep extension of the striate cortex and calcarine fissure into the occipital lobe. The calcar avis, which forms this contour, is shown in the section.

SAGITTAL SECTION OF THE BRAIN, LEVEL OF THE HIPPOCAMPUS AND PUTAMEN LEFT CEREBRAL AND CEREBELLAR HEMISPHERE, LATERAL TO MEDIAL PERSPECTIVE

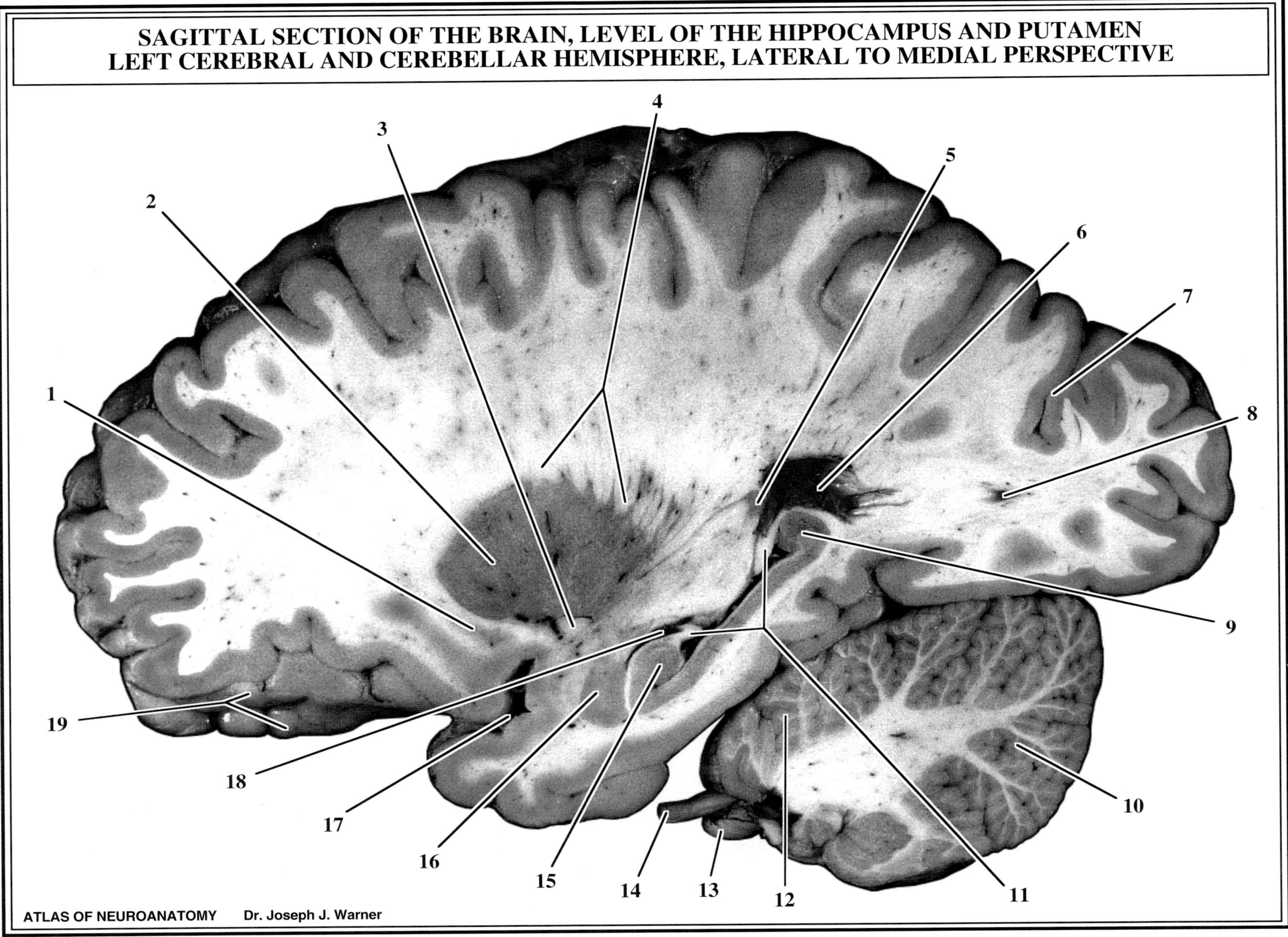

ATLAS OF NEUROANATOMY Dr. Joseph J. Warner

SAGITTAL SECTION OF THE BRAIN, LEVEL OF HIPPOCAMPUS AND PUTAMEN

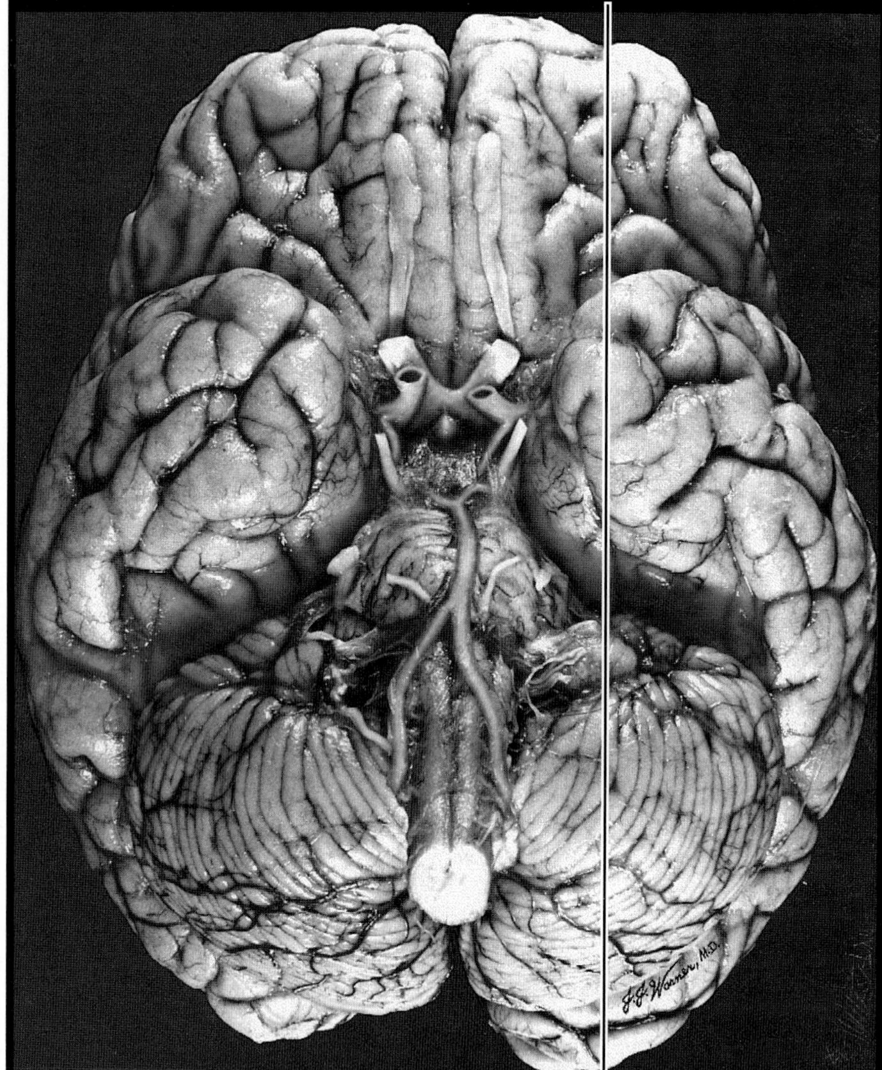

LEFT, LATERAL TO MEDIAL PERSPECTIVE

KEY TO NUMBERED STRUCTURES

1. Claustrum
2. Putamen
3. Anterior Commissure
4. Corona Radiata
5. Tail of the Caudate Nucleus
6. Atrium of the Lateral Ventricle
7. Parieto-Occipital Sulcus
8. Occipital Pole of the Lateral Ventricle
9. Hippocampus
10. Posterior Lobe of the Cerebellum
11. Fornix
12. Anterior Lobe of the Cerebellum
13. Middle Cerebellar Peduncle
14. Trigeminal Nerve
15. Hippocampus
16. Amygdala
17. Sylvian Fissure
18. Temporal (Inferior) Horn of the Lateral Ventricle
19. Orbitofrontal Gyri

COMPLETE SAGITTAL SECTION, LEVEL OF THE HIPPOCAMPUS, PUTAMEN, AND AMYGDALA, LATERAL TO MEDIAL VIEW:

Note the configuration of the fornix as it passes through the plane of section twice, in contiguity to the longitudinally oriented hippocampus. The curvature of the hippocampal formation accounts for this appearance. The orbitofrontal and dorsolateral frontal cortical surfaces are visible, thus indicating a lateral to medial perspective. This plane of section is lateral to the anterior horn and body of the lateral ventricle. The section does, however, pass through the atrium, the temporal (inferior) horn, and the medial tip of the occipital (posterior) horn of the lateral ventricle. As demonstrated previously, fibers of the anterior commissure course in a mediolateral direction along the ventral aspect of the globus pallidus. The anterior commissure then continues laterally, and is transected in this plane of section as it passes ventral to the putamen into the temporal lobe.

Adjacent to the ventral aspect of the cerebellum, the lateral surface of the middle cerebellar peduncle is discerned. The trigeminal nerve exits the mid-pons through the ventral aspect of the middle cerebellar peduncle, and is thus visible in this section as it passes rostrally from the pons toward the floor of the middle cranial fossa. This plane of section is lateral to the deep cerebellar nuclei.

SAGITTAL SECTION OF THE BRAIN, LEVEL OF DEEP INSULAR CORTEX AND CLAUSTRUM, LEFT CEREBRAL AND CEREBELLAR HEMISPHERE, LATERAL TO MEDIAL PERSPECTIVE

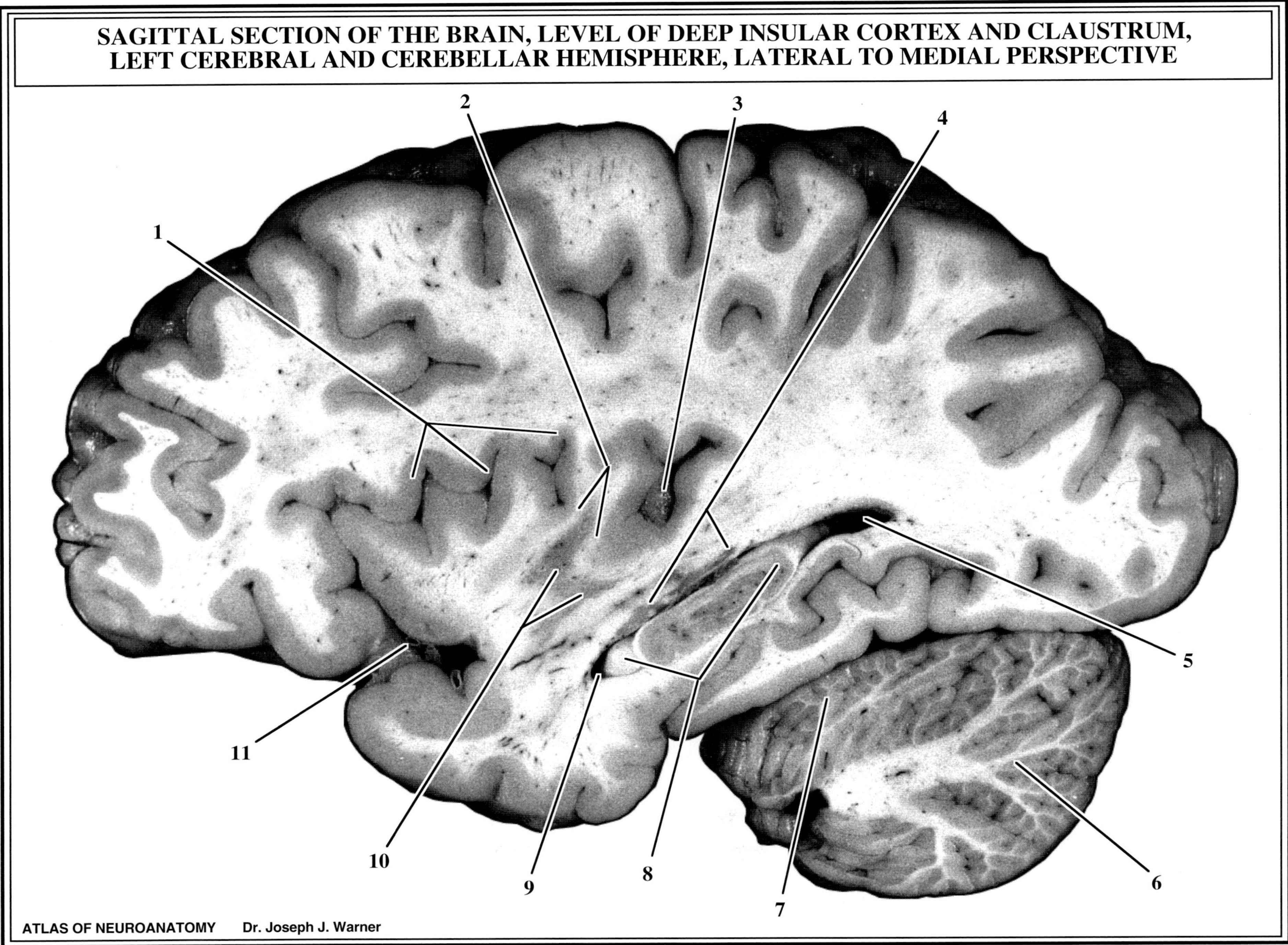

ATLAS OF NEUROANATOMY Dr. Joseph J. Warner

SAGITTAL SECTION OF THE BRAIN, LEVEL OF THE DEEP INSULAR CORTEX

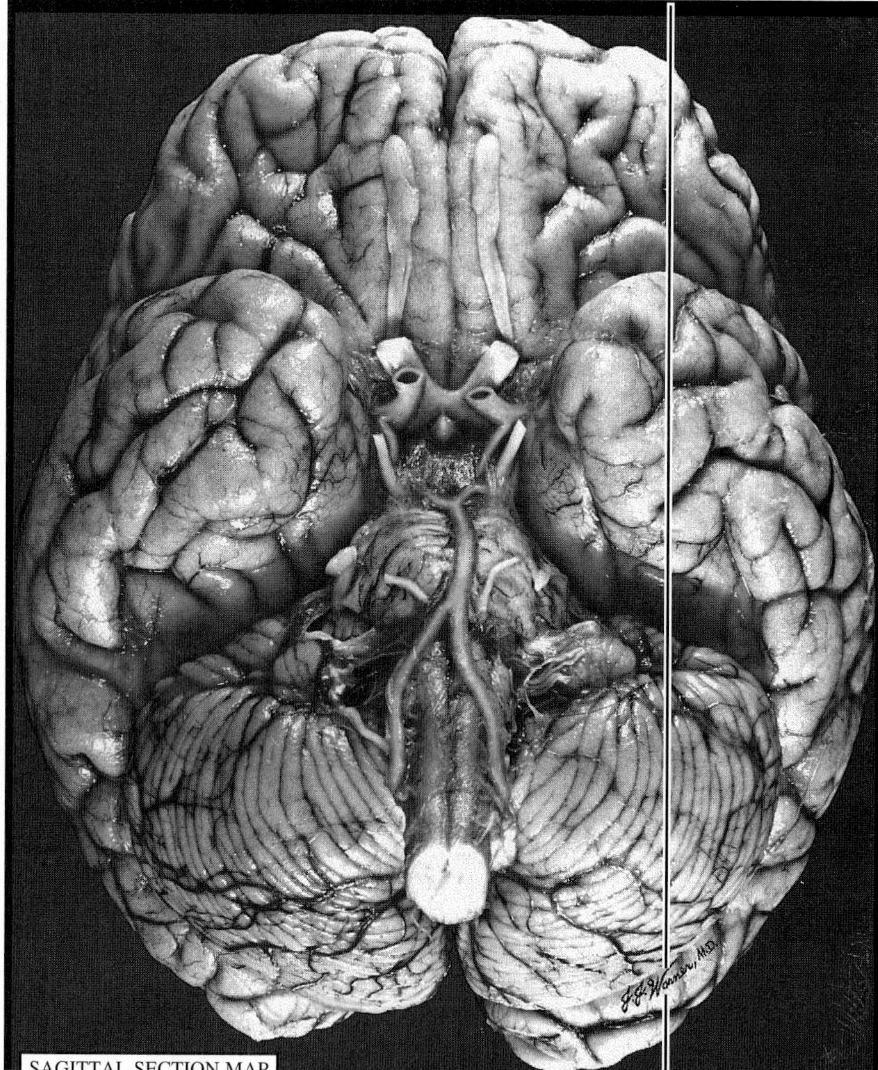

SAGITTAL SECTION MAP

LEFT, LATERAL TO MEDIAL PERSPECTIVE

KEY TO NUMBERED STRUCTURES

1. Insular Cortex
2. Extreme Capsule
3. Surface of the Deep Insular Cortex
4. Tail of the Caudate Nucleus
5. Temporal (Inferior) Horn of the Lateral Ventricle
6. Posterior Lobe of the Cerebellum
7. Anterior Lobe of the Cerebellum
8. Hippocampus
9. Temporal Horn of the Lateral Ventricle
10. Claustrum
11. Sylvian Fissure

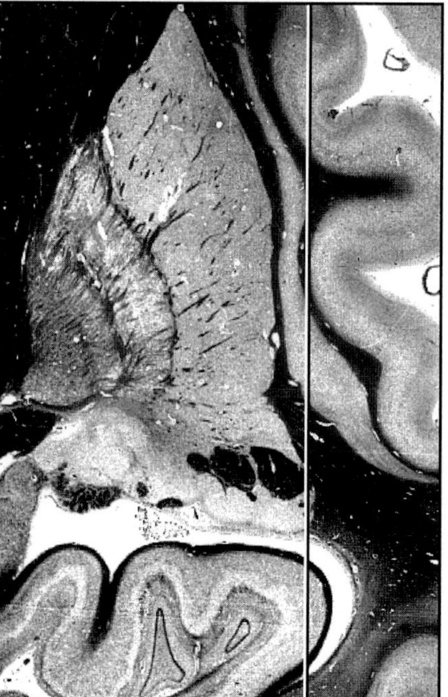

MAP OF THIS SAGITTAL PLANE ON A CORONAL SECTION, LEVEL OF THE MAMMILLARY BODIES

COMPLETE SAGITTAL SECTION, LEVEL OF THE DEEP INSULAR CORTEX, CLAUSTRUM, AND LATERAL ASPECT OF THE HIPPOCAMPUS, LEFT

The claustrum and extreme capsule are clearly discernible, subjacent to the deep insular gyri. Reference to horizontal and coronal sections clarifies the mediolateral relationship between the claustrum, extreme capsule, and insula. (Refer to coronal section at right.) This plane of section is lateral to the putamen and external capsule. The claustrum appears as an irregular sheet of gray matter at this plane, separated from the insular cortex by the extreme capsule.

The tail of the caudate nucleus is visible along the dorsal surface of the temporal horn of the lateral ventricle. The caudate nucleus is located in the lateral wall of the body of the lateral ventricle. This structure turns ventrally then rostrally as it is traced from the anterior horn through the atrium of the lateral ventricle. As this curvature is followed, the tail of the caudate nucleus assumes a position along the dorsal aspect of the temporal (inferior) horn. The caudate continues rostrally and terminates as it becomes contiguous to the amygdala.

Examination of this plane of section reveals the lateral aspect of the hippocampus. The medially concave curvature of the hippocampus accounts for the "double contour" appearance on more medial sagittal sections. The hippocampal formation forms the ventromedial contour of the temporal horn of the lateral ventricle (demonstrable on ventricular cast models and in coronal sections through these structures).

PARASAGITTAL SECTION, LEVEL OF THE INSULA, LEFT HEMISPHERE

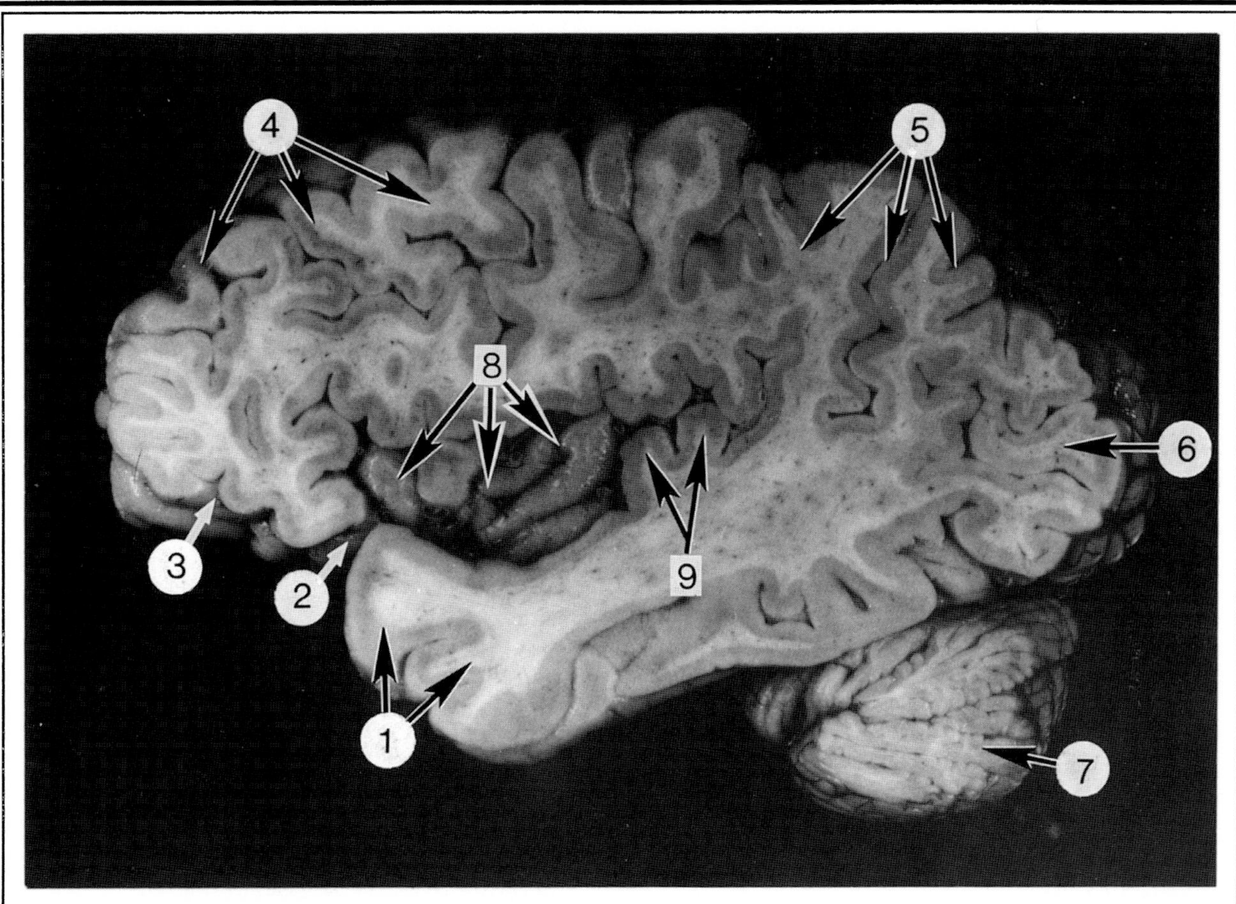

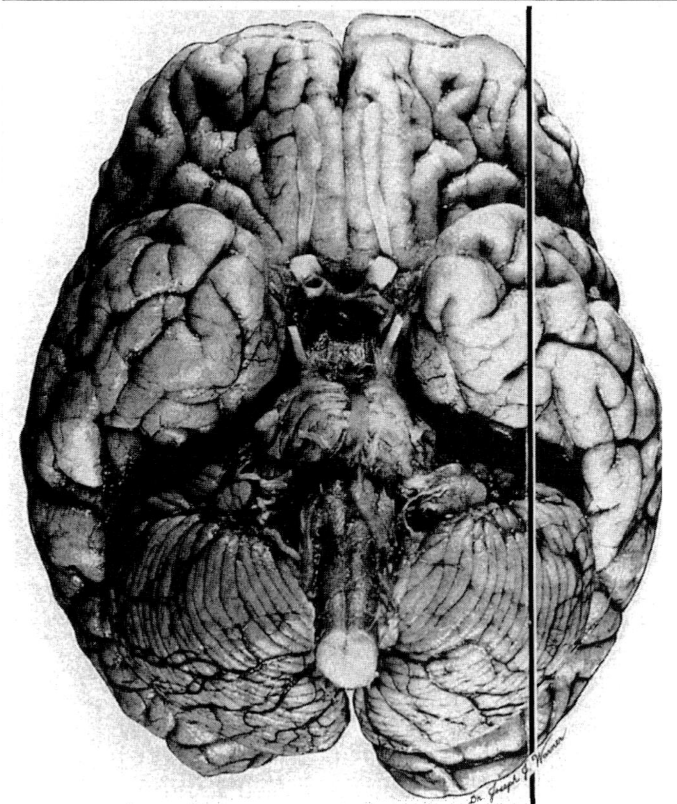

KEY TO NUMBERED STRUCTURES

1. Rostral Temporal Lobe
2. Sylvian Fissure
3. Orbitofrontal Cortex
4. Dorsolateral Frontal Lobe
5. Parietal Lobe
6. Occipital Lobe
7. Posterior Lobe of Cerebellum
8. Insular Gyri
9. Transverse Temporal Gyri of Heschl

[Refer to the magnified view of this section and accompanying lateral projection of Internal Carotid angiogram.]

Level of this section through the left hemisphere is mapped on the accompanying illustration of the ventral aspect of the brain.

PARASAGITTAL SECTION, LEVEL OF THE INSULA, LEFT HEMISPHERE, MAGNIFIED VIEW

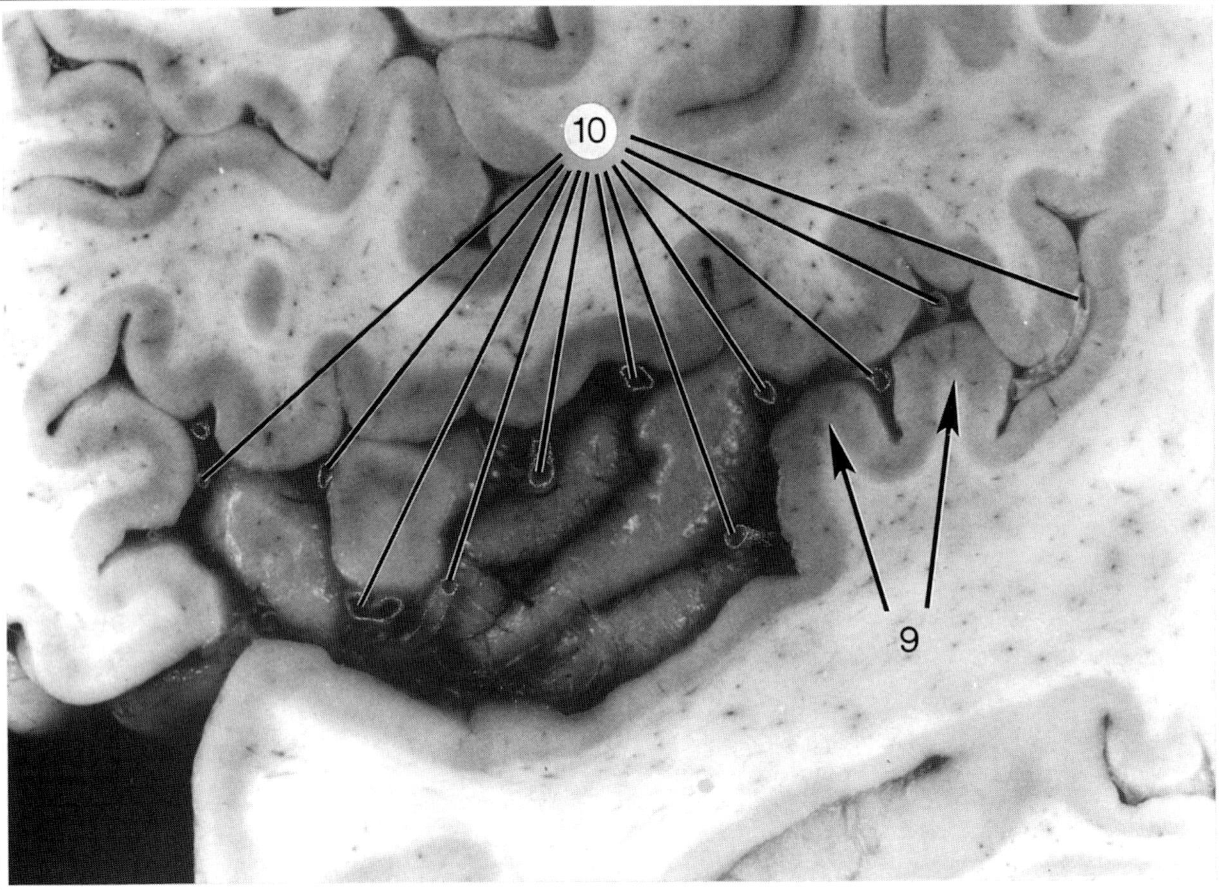

KEY TO NUMBERED STRUCTURES

9. Transverse Temporal Gyri of Heschl
10. Branches of Middle Cerebral Artery within the Sylvian Fissure.

The Transverse Gyri of Heschl, primary auditory cortex (Brodmann's Areas 41, 42) are located on the superior aspect of the temporal lobe. The morphology of this area in the left hemisphere differs from that of the right, including a greater size and complexity of the left transverse temporal gyri in most cases.

Examination of the magnified section above reveals numerous branches of the Middle Cerebral Artery as they course through the Sylvian Fissure adjacent to the insula. The accompanying carotid arteriogram shows these vessels. Arrows mark these vessels as they course through the Sylvian fissure to the cerebral convexities.

COURSE OF MIDDLE CEREBRAL ARTERIAL BRANCHES THROUGH THE SYLVIAN FISSURE
(CAROTID ARTERIOGRAM, LATERAL PROJECTION)

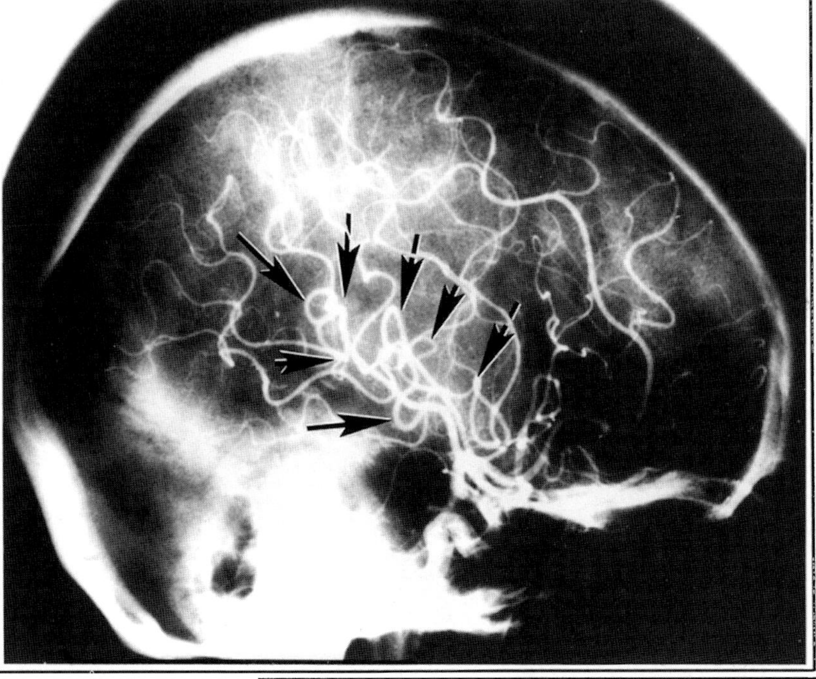

NEUROANATOMY OF SECTIONS PARALLEL TO THE LONGITUDINAL AXIS OF THE BRAINSTEM

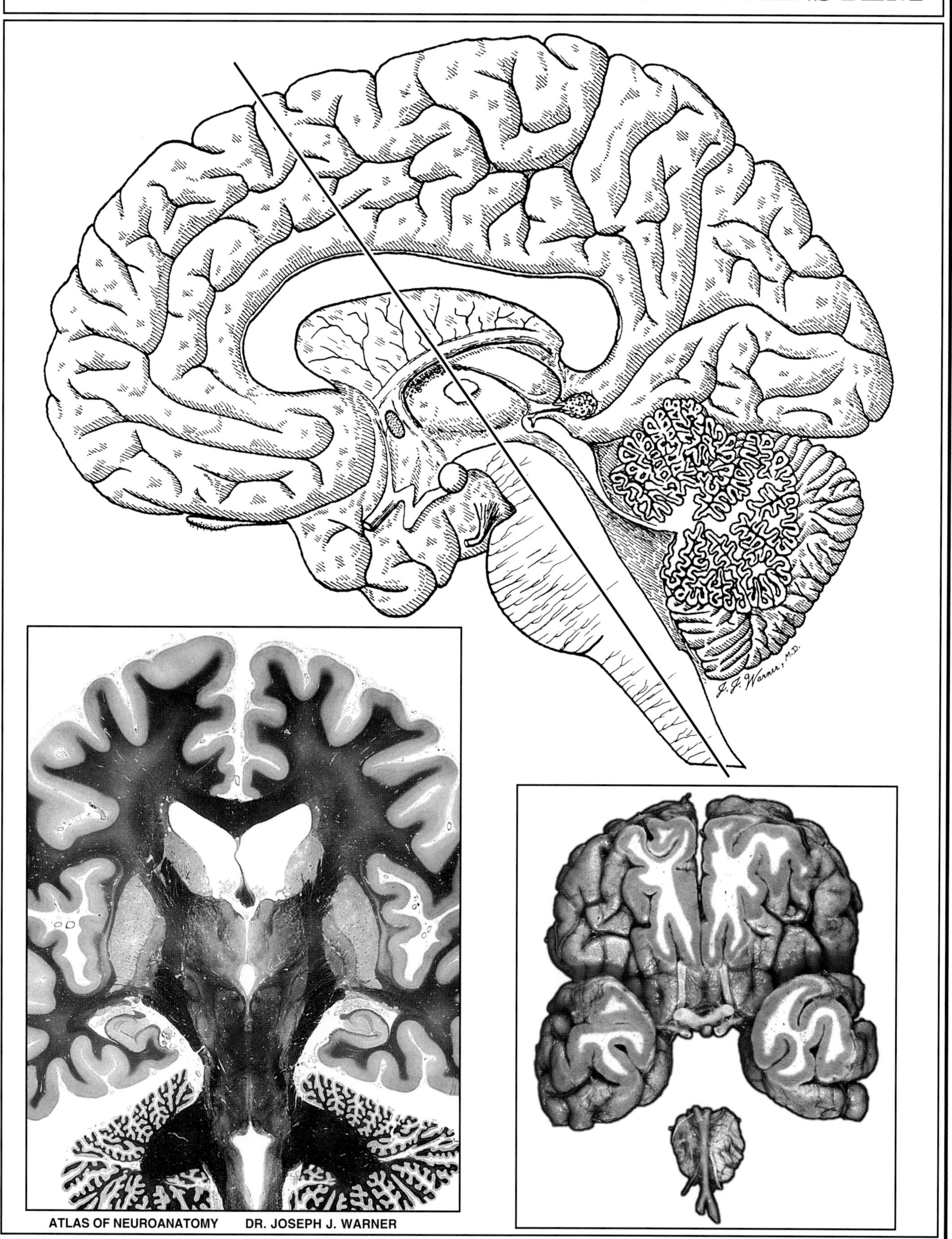

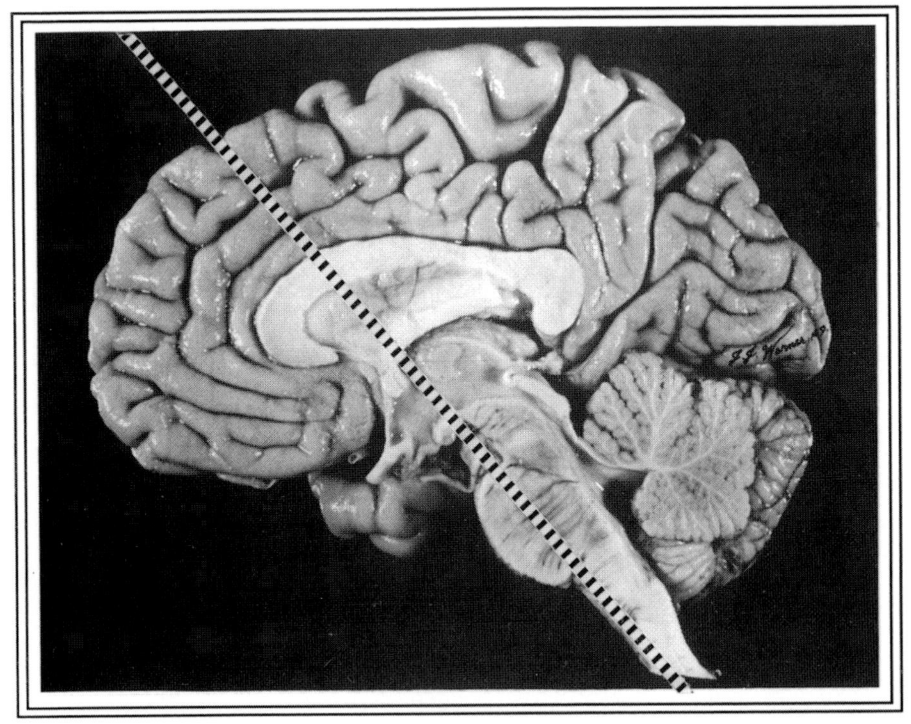

Midline sagittal section of the brain, upon which the plane of section (parallel to the longitudinal axis of the brainstem) is mapped. Note that this orientation is characterized by inclusion of rostral telencephalic structures at its most dorsal aspect, with passage through more caudal structures as the section continues through the ventral telencephalon, diencephalon, and brainstem.

This section, parallel to the longitudinal axis of the brainstem, is viewed toward the caudal aspect of the telencephalon. Thus, the cerebellum is visualized caudal and dorsal to the cut surface.

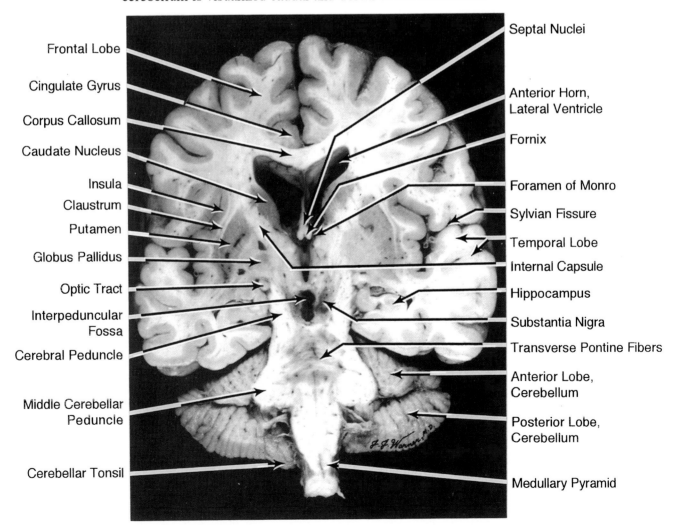

Frontal Lobe
Cingulate Gyrus
Corpus Callosum
Caudate Nucleus
Insula
Claustrum
Putamen
Globus Pallidus
Optic Tract
Interpeduncular Fossa
Cerebral Peduncle
Middle Cerebellar Peduncle
Cerebellar Tonsil

Septal Nuclei
Anterior Horn, Lateral Ventricle
Fornix
Foramen of Monro
Sylvian Fissure
Temporal Lobe
Internal Capsule
Hippocampus
Substantia Nigra
Transverse Pontine Fibers
Anterior Lobe, Cerebellum
Posterior Lobe, Cerebellum
Medullary Pyramid

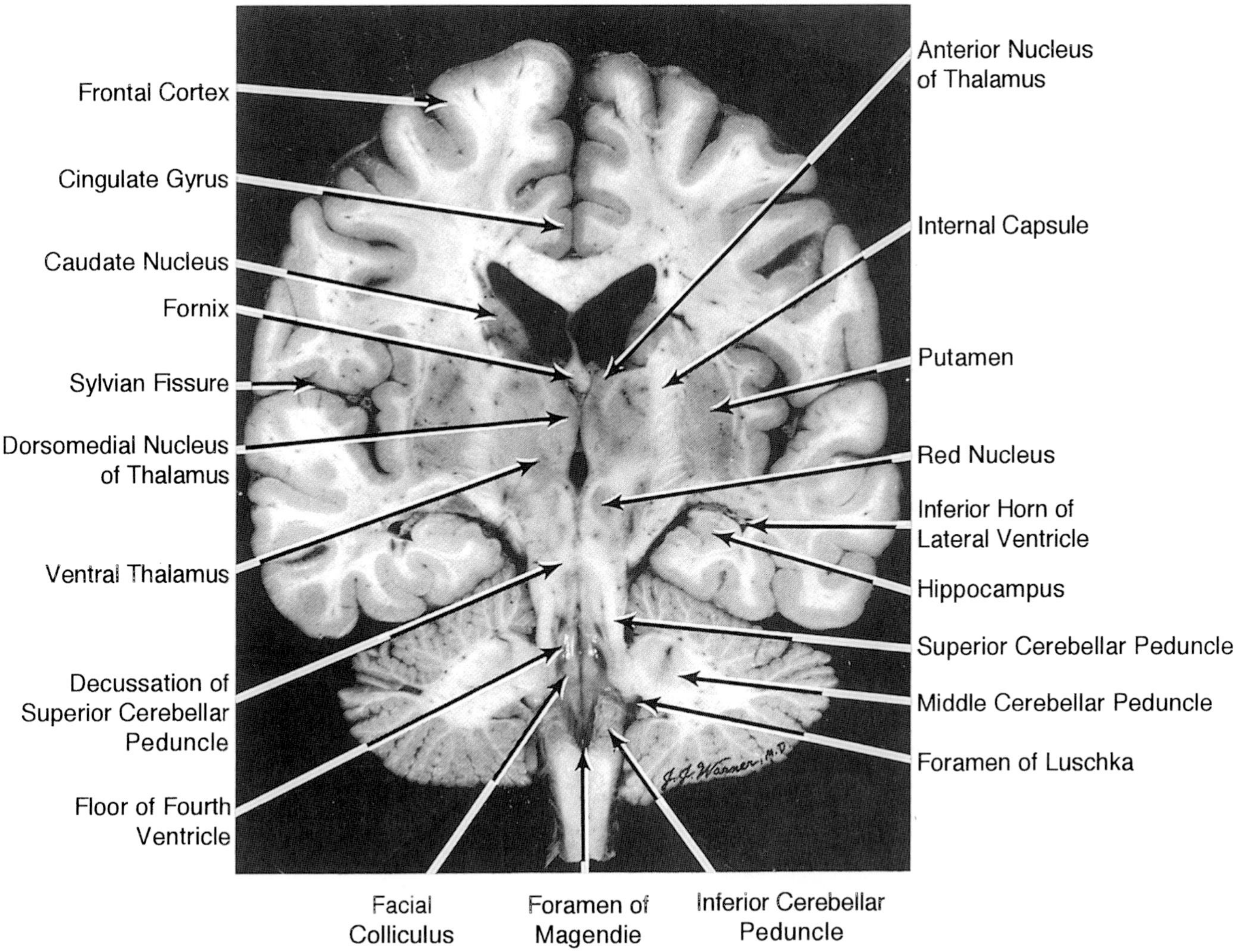

Frontal Cortex
Cingulate Gyrus
Caudate Nucleus
Fornix
Sylvian Fissure
Dorsomedial Nucleus of Thalamus
Ventral Thalamus
Decussation of Superior Cerebellar Peduncle
Floor of Fourth Ventricle
Anterior Nucleus of Thalamus
Internal Capsule
Putamen
Red Nucleus
Inferior Horn of Lateral Ventricle
Hippocampus
Superior Cerebellar Peduncle
Middle Cerebellar Peduncle
Foramen of Luschka
Facial Colliculus
Foramen of Magendie
Inferior Cerebellar Peduncle

This section, parallel to the longitudinal axis of the brainstem, passes through frontal cortex,body of the corpus callosum, anterior nucleus of the thalamus, red nucleus, decussation of the superior cerebellar peduncle, and dorsal to the floor of the fourth ventricle. (Refer to orientation of section as mapped on the midline sagittal diagram, line A).

All three cerebellar peduncles are well-visualized in this plane of section, as well as their relationship to the fourth ventricle. The superior cerebellar peduncle may be traced rostrally from the cerebellum to its decussation ventral to the Aqueduct of Sylvius in the caudal mesencephalon. Fibers then continue toward the red nucleus, also visualized in this section. (A significant proportion of these fibers continue to their termination in VL in the ventral tier of thalamic nuclei).

The section corresponding to the orientation mapped with Line B is presented subsequently.

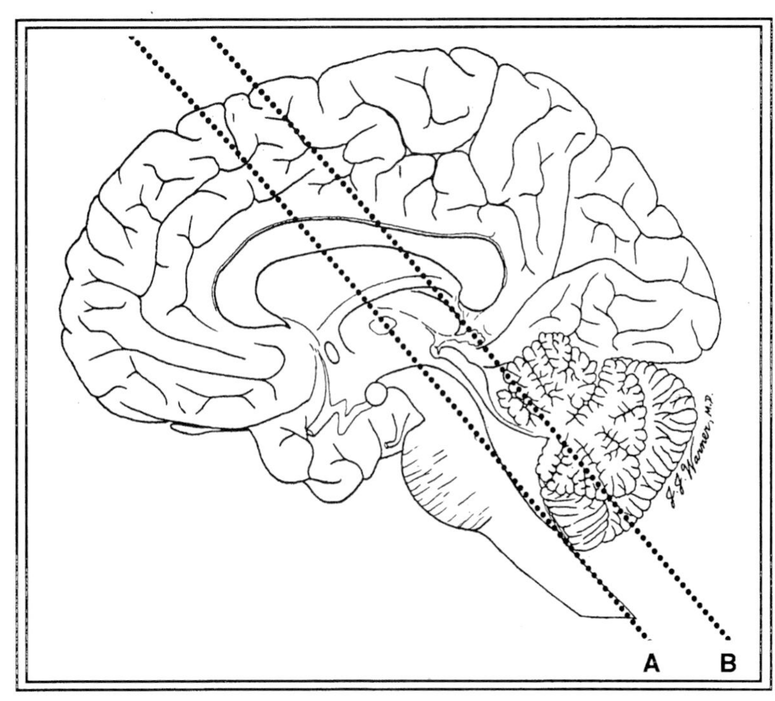

HISTOLOGIC SECTION OF THE BRAIN, PLANE PARALLEL TO THE LONGITUDINAL AXIS OF THE BRAINSTEM: LEVEL INCLUDING THE SUBTHALAMIC NUCLEUS AND THE ANTERIOR NUCLEUS OF THE THALAMUS

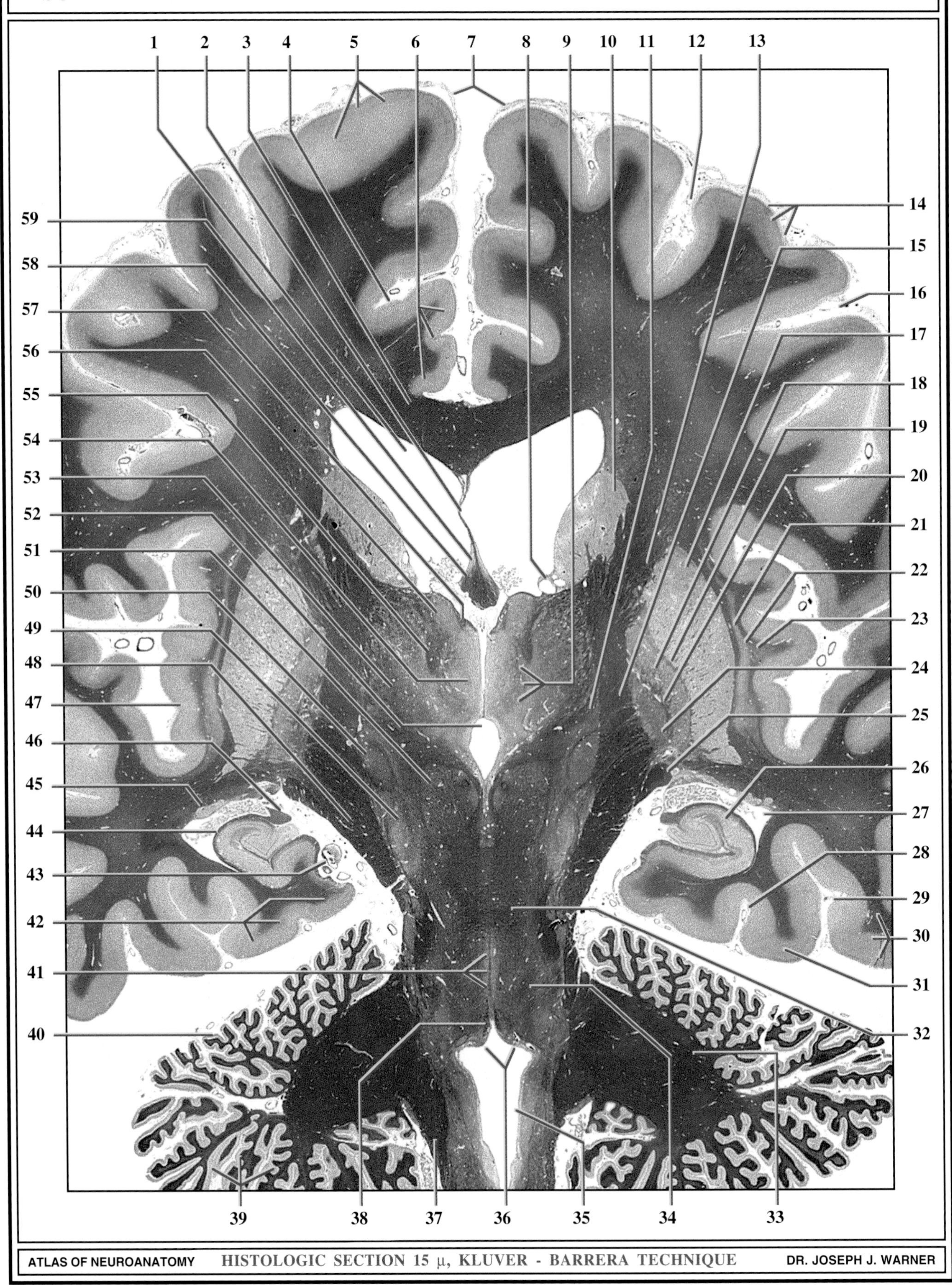

HISTOLOGIC SECTION OF THE BRAIN, PLANE PARALLEL TO THE LONGITUDINAL AXIS OF THE BRAINSTEM; LEVEL INCLUDING THE SUBTHALAMIC NUCLEUS AND THE ANTERIOR NUCLEUS OF THE THALAMUS: SECTION ORIENTATION AND KEY TO NUMBERED STRUCTURES

1. Body of the Lateral Ventricle
2. Septum Pellucidum
3. Body of the Corpus Callosum
4. Cingulate Sulcus
5. Superior Frontal Convolution
6. Cingulate Cortex
7. Arachnoid Granulations
8. Stria Terminalis and the Thalamostriate Vein
9. Internal Medullary Lamina of the Thalamus
10. Caudate Nucleus
11. Lenticular Fasciculus
12. Superior Frontal Sulcus
13. Anterior Limb of the Internal Capsule
14. Middle Frontal Convolution
15. Posterior Limb of the Internal Capsule
16. Inferior Frontal Sulcus
17. Putamen
18. Globus Pallidus II
19. External Medullary Lamina
20. Internal Medullary Lamina
21. External Capsule
22. Claustrum
23. Extreme Capsule
24. Globus Pallidus I
25. Optic Tract
26. Hippocampus
27. Temporal Horn of the Lateral Ventricle
28. Collateral Sulcus
29. Inferior Temporal Sulcus
30. Inferior Temporal Gyrus
31. Fusiform Gyrus
32. Decussation of the Superior Cerebellar Peduncle
33. Middle Cerebellar Peduncle
34. Central Tegmental Tract
35. Fourth Ventricle
36. Facial Colliculi
37. Inferior Cerebellar Peduncle
38. Medial Longitudinal Fasciculus
39. Posterior Lobe of the Cerebellum
40. Anterior Lobe of the Cerebellum
41. Median Raphe Nuclei
42. Parahippocampal Gyri
43. Posterior Cerebral Artery
44. Alveus
45. Tail of the Caudate Nucleus
46. Fimbria of the Fornix
47. Insula
48. Cerebral Peduncle
49. Substantia Nigra
50. Subthalamic Nucleus
51. Red Nucleus
52. Third Ventricle
53. Ventrolateral Nucleus of the Thalamus
54. Dorsomedial Nucleus of the Thalamus
55. Mammillothalamic Tract
56. Anterior Nucleus of the Thalamus
57. Stria Medullaris
58. Fornix
59. Septal Nuclei

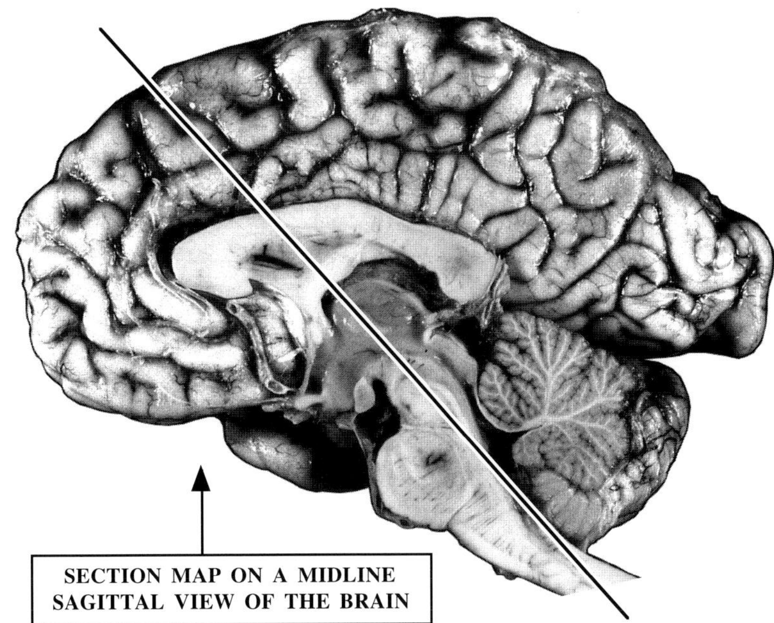

SECTION MAP ON A MIDLINE SAGITTAL VIEW OF THE BRAIN

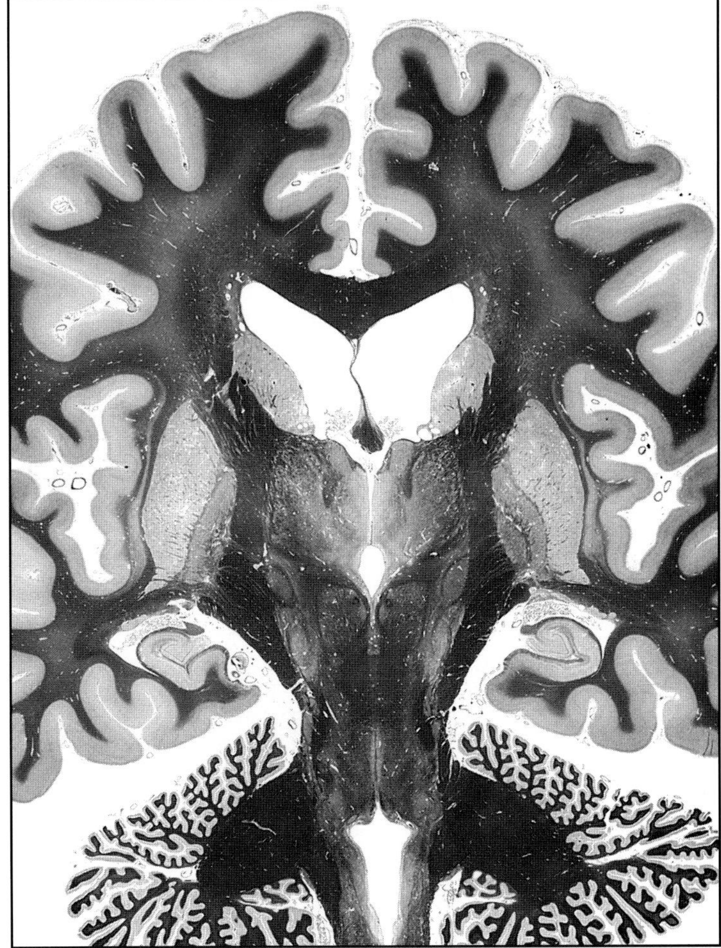

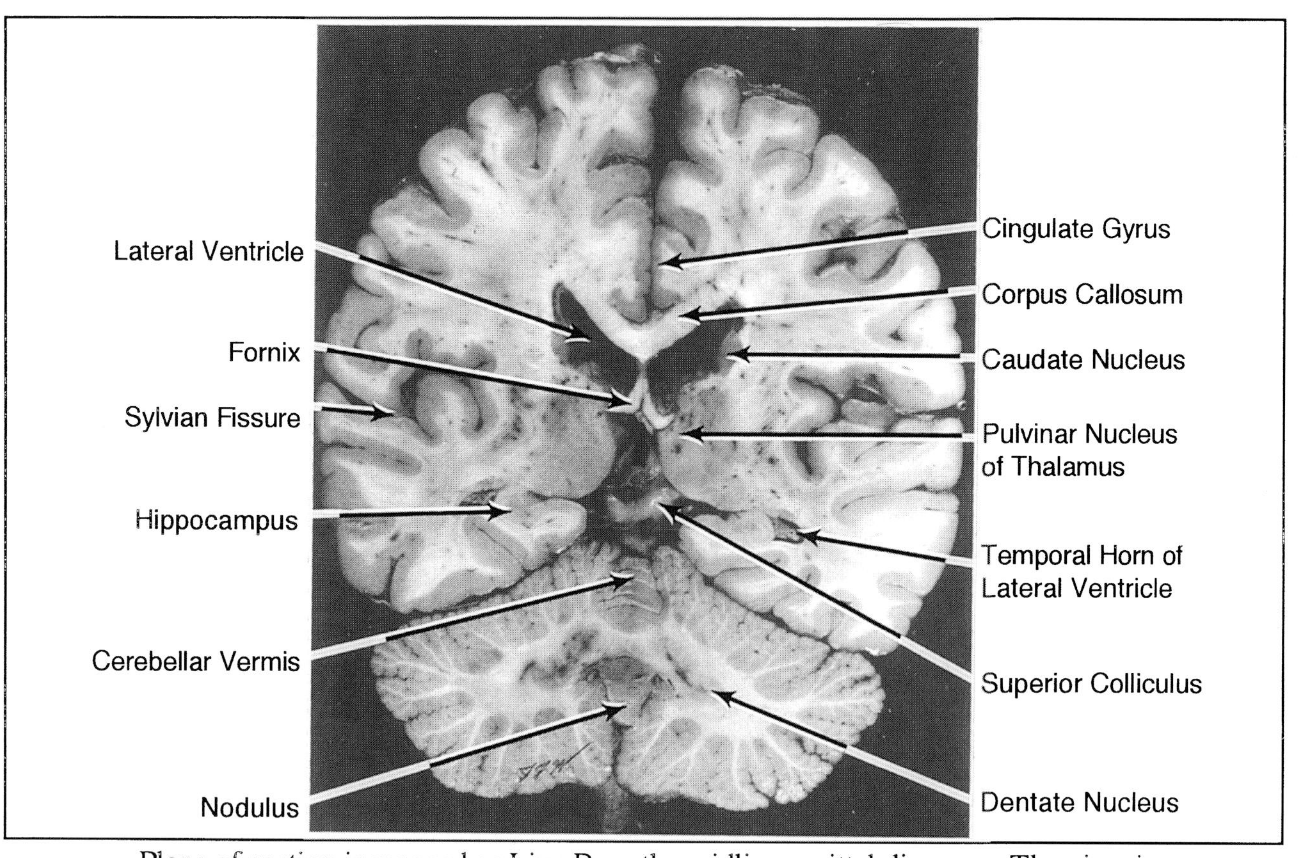

Plane of section is mapped as Line B on the midline sagittal diagram. The view is toward the rostral and ventral direction from the dorsal and caudal aspect of the section.

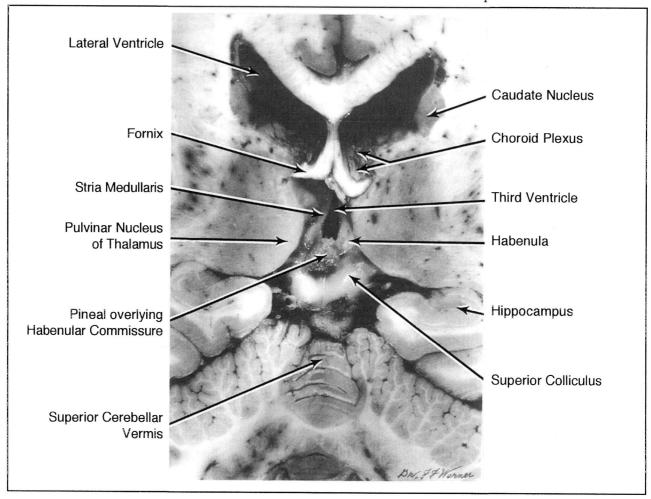

Lateral Ventricle
Caudate Nucleus
Fornix
Choroid Plexus
Stria Medullaris
Third Ventricle
Pulvinar Nucleus of Thalamus
Habenula
Pineal overlying Habenular Commissure
Hippocampus
Superior Colliculus
Superior Cerebellar Vermis

COMPLETE SECTION OF THE BRAIN, PLANE PARALLEL TO THE LONGITUDINAL AXIS OF THE BRAINSTEM: LEVEL INCLUDING THE PARASAGITTAL ASPECT OF THE ROLANDIC FISSURE

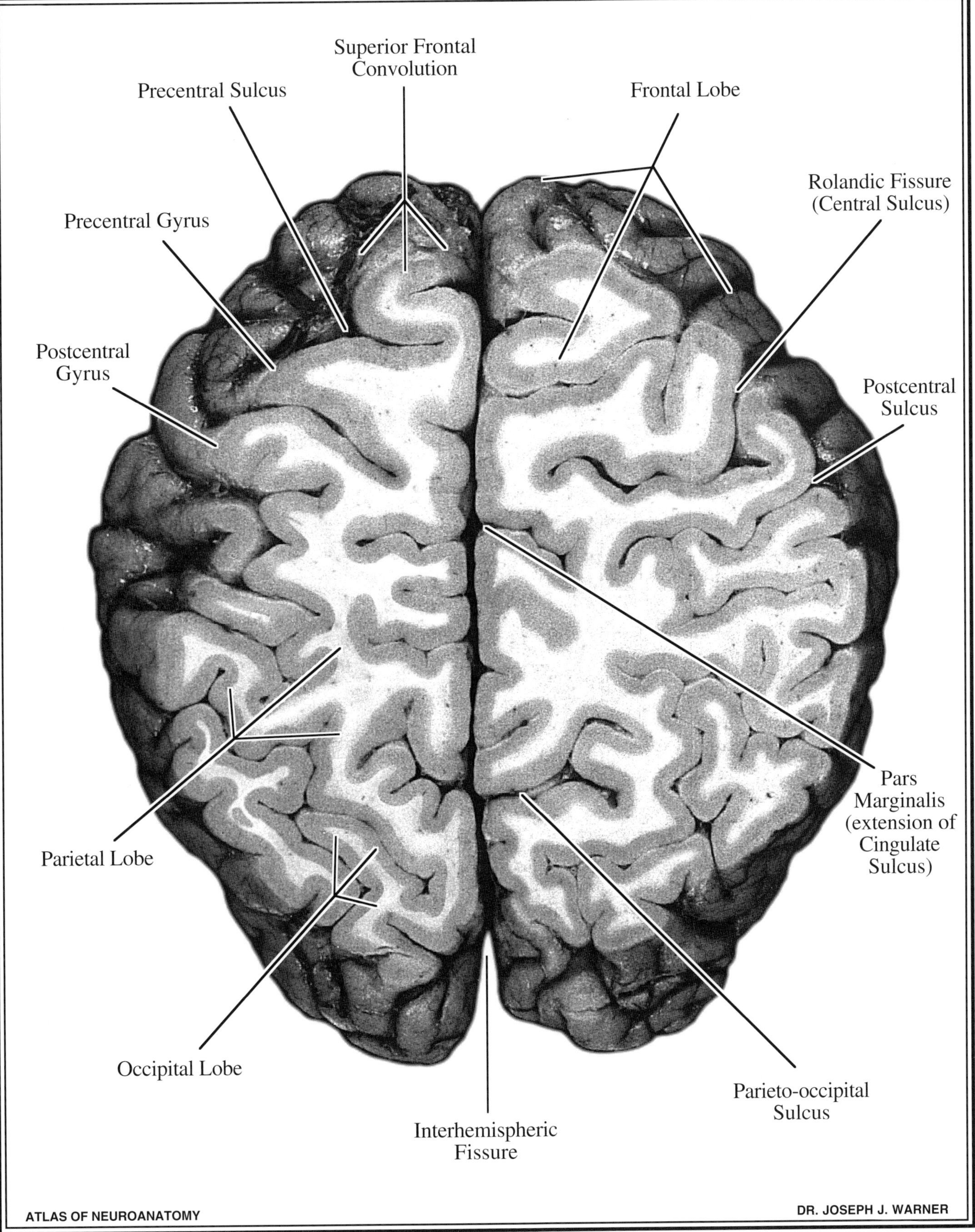

COMPLETE SECTION OF THE BRAIN, PLANE PARALLEL TO THE LONGITUDINAL AXIS OF THE BRAINSTEM: LEVEL OF SUBCORTICAL WHITE MATTER DORSAL TO THE CORPUS CALLOSUM

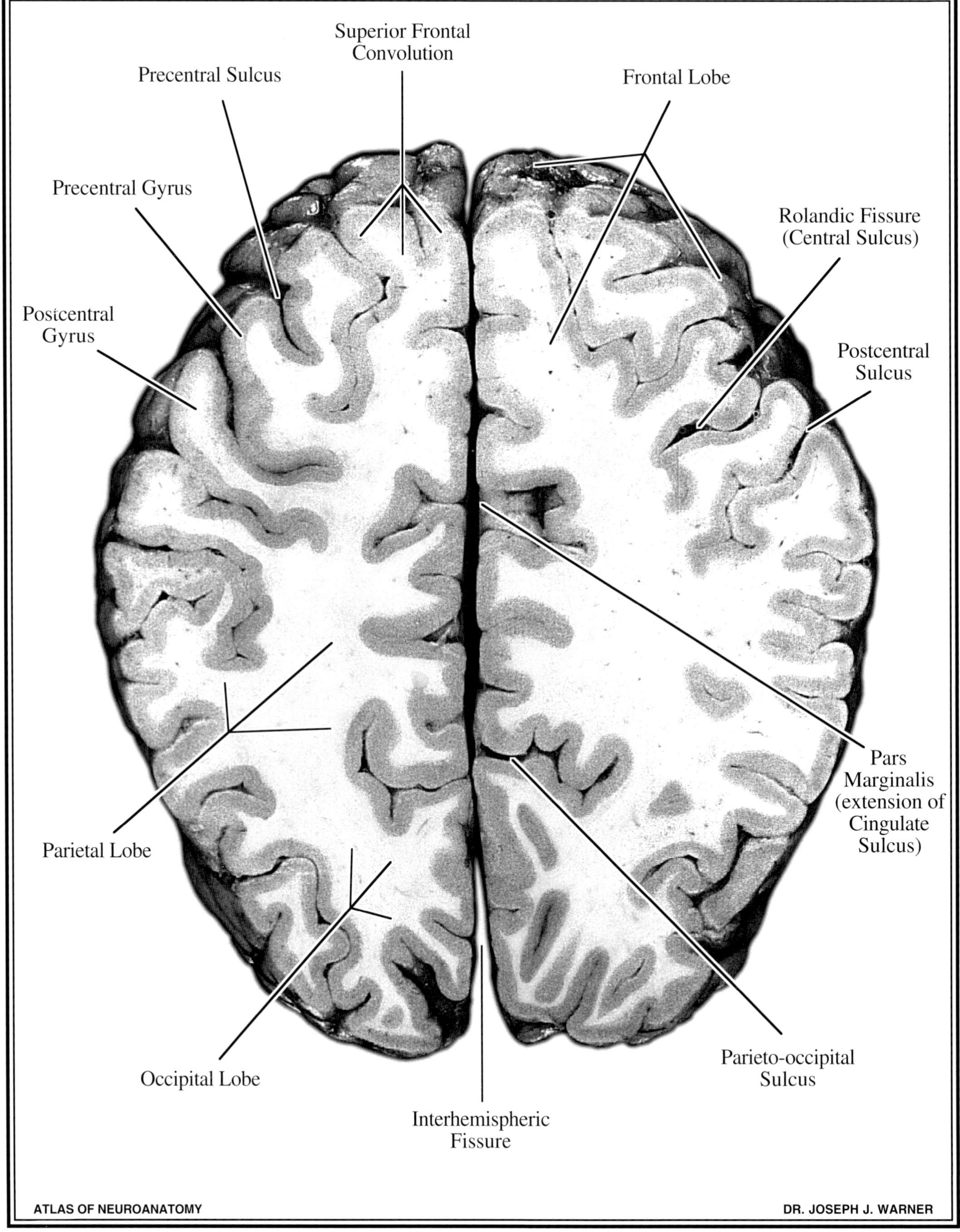

COMPLETE SECTIONS OF THE BRAIN PARALLEL TO THE LONGITUDINAL AXIS OF THE BRAINSTEM, LEVELS OF THE PARASAGITTAL ASPECT OF THE ROLANDIC FISSURE AND OF THE SUBCORTICAL WHITE MATTER DORSAL TO THE CORPUS CALLOSUM: KEY TO SECTION LEVELS AND ORIENTATIONS

A.

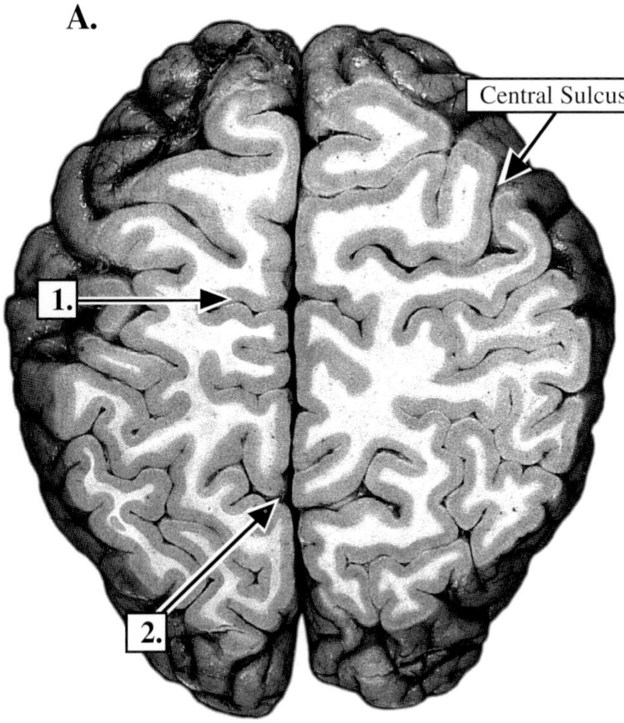

Level including the parasagittal aspect of the Rolandic Fissure (Central Sulcus)

B.

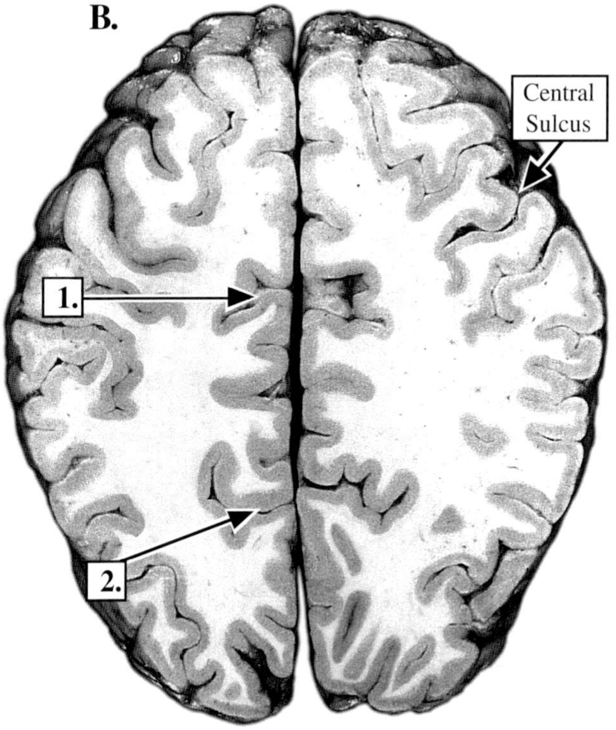

Level of the Subcortical White Matter dorsal to the Corpus Callosum

Major reference points include (1) the pars marginalis, which continues in a caudal and dorsal direction from the cingulate sulcus, and (2) the parieto-occipital sulcus.

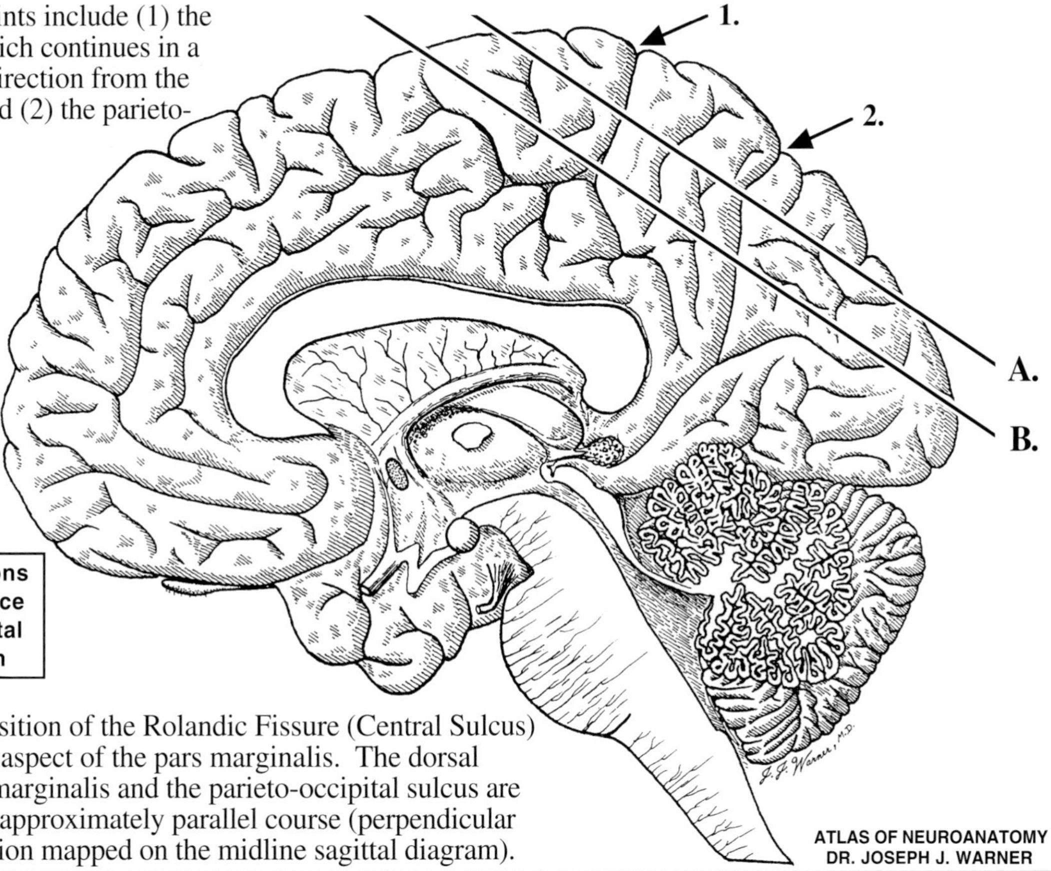

Section orientations mapped in reference to a Midline Sagittal Section Diagram

Note the relative position of the Rolandic Fissure (Central Sulcus) rostral to the dorsal aspect of the pars marginalis. The dorsal aspects of the pars marginalis and the parieto-occipital sulcus are characterized by an approximately parallel course (perpendicular to the planes of section mapped on the midline sagittal diagram).

ATLAS OF NEUROANATOMY
DR. JOSEPH J. WARNER

COMPLETE SECTION OF THE BRAIN, PLANE PARALLEL TO THE LONGITUDINAL AXIS OF THE BRAINSTEM: LEVEL INCLUDING THE ATRIUM OF THE LATERAL VENTRICLES

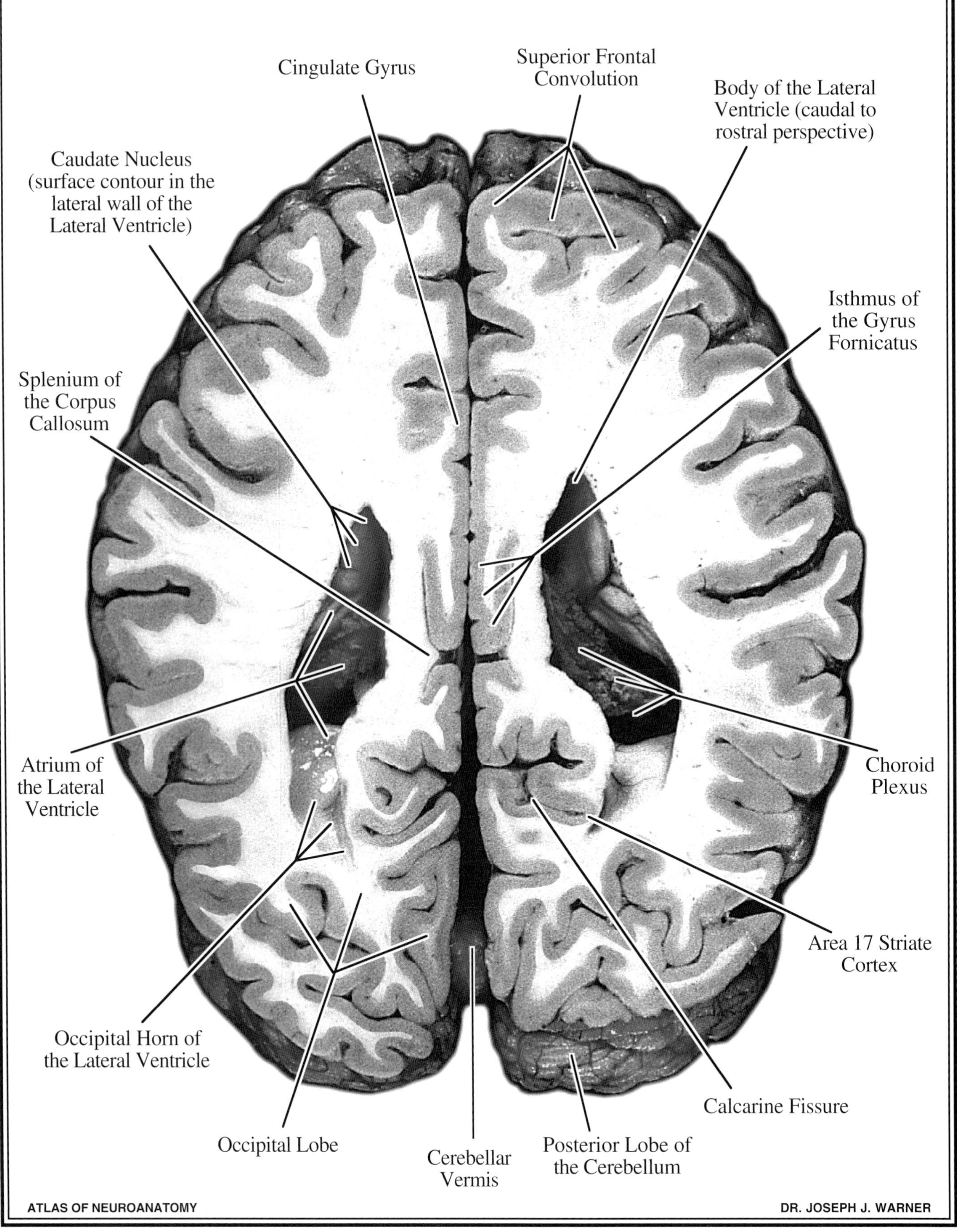

COMPLETE SECTION OF THE BRAIN, PLANE PARALLEL TO THE LONGITUDINAL AXIS OF THE BRAINSTEM: LEVEL OF THE CRUS OF THE FORNIX AND CAUDAL ASPECT OF THE PULVINAR NUCLEUS

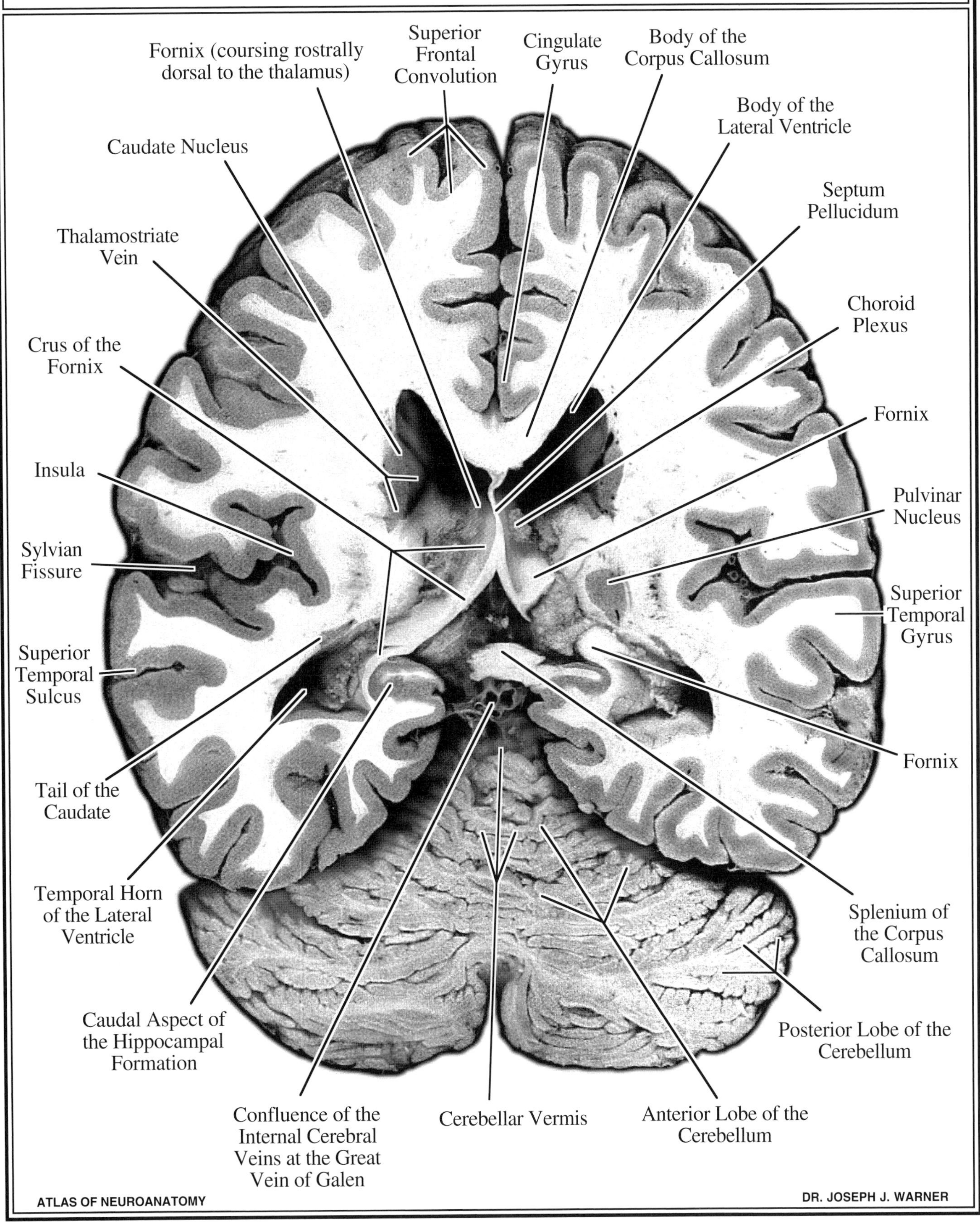

COMPLETE SECTIONS OF THE BRAIN PARALLEL TO THE LONGITUDINAL AXIS OF THE BRAINSTEM, LEVELS OF THE ATRIUM OF THE LATERAL VENTRICLES AND OF THE CRUS OF THE FORNIX: KEY TO SECTION LEVELS AND ORIENTATIONS

A.

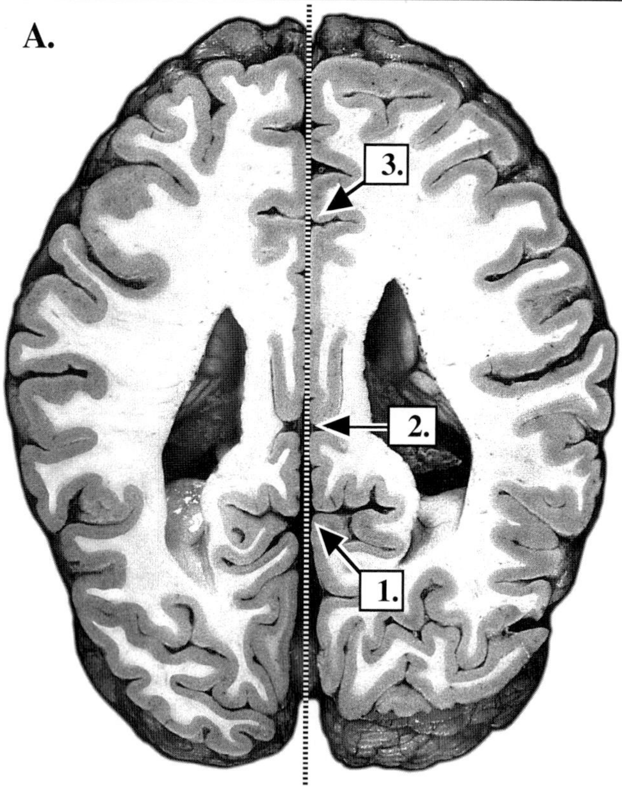

Level of the Atrium of the Lateral Ventricles

B.

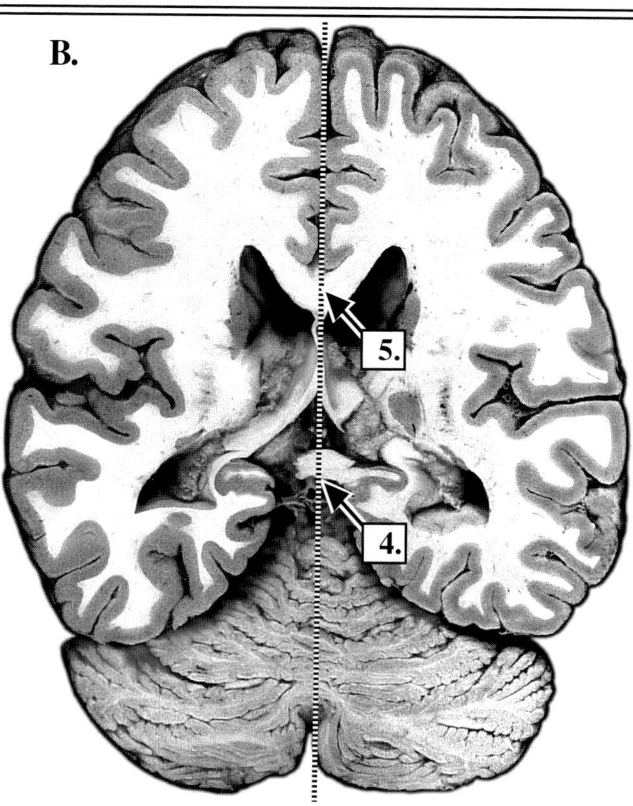

Level of the Crus of the Fornix and Caudal Putamen

1. Intersection of the Calcarine Fissure and the Parieto-Occipital Sulcus
2. Transition of Cingulate Gyrus to the Isthmus of the Gyrus Fornicatus
3. Cingulate Sulcus
4. Splenium of the Corpus Callosum (ventral aspect)
5. Body of the Corpus Callosum

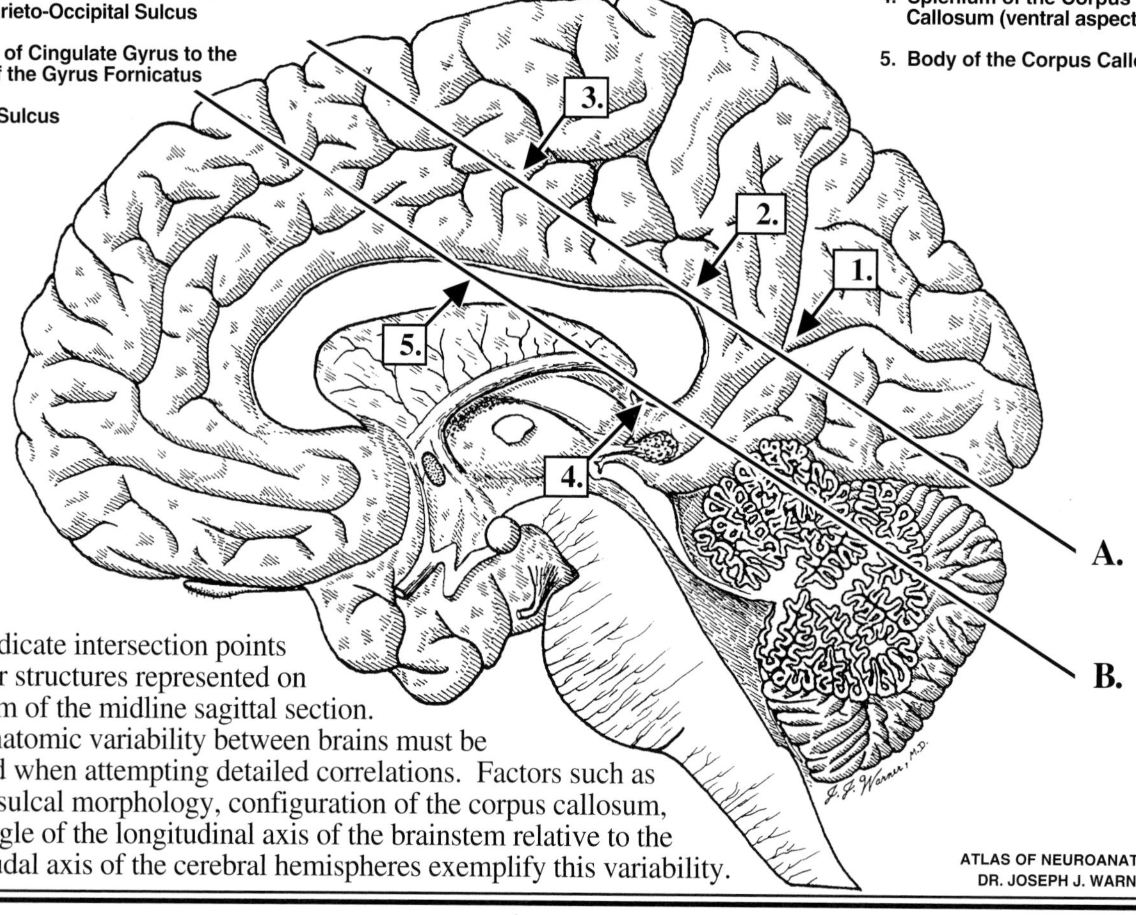

Arrows indicate intersection points with major structures represented on the diagram of the midline sagittal section. Normal anatomic variability between brains must be considered when attempting detailed correlations. Factors such as gyral and sulcal morphology, configuration of the corpus callosum, and the angle of the longitudinal axis of the brainstem relative to the rostral-caudal axis of the cerebral hemispheres exemplify this variability.

ATLAS OF NEUROANATOMY
DR. JOSEPH J. WARNER

COMPLETE SECTION OF THE BRAIN, PLANE PARALLEL TO THE LONGITUDINAL AXIS OF THE BRAINSTEM: LEVEL OF THE LATERAL AND MEDIAL GENICULATE NUCLEI

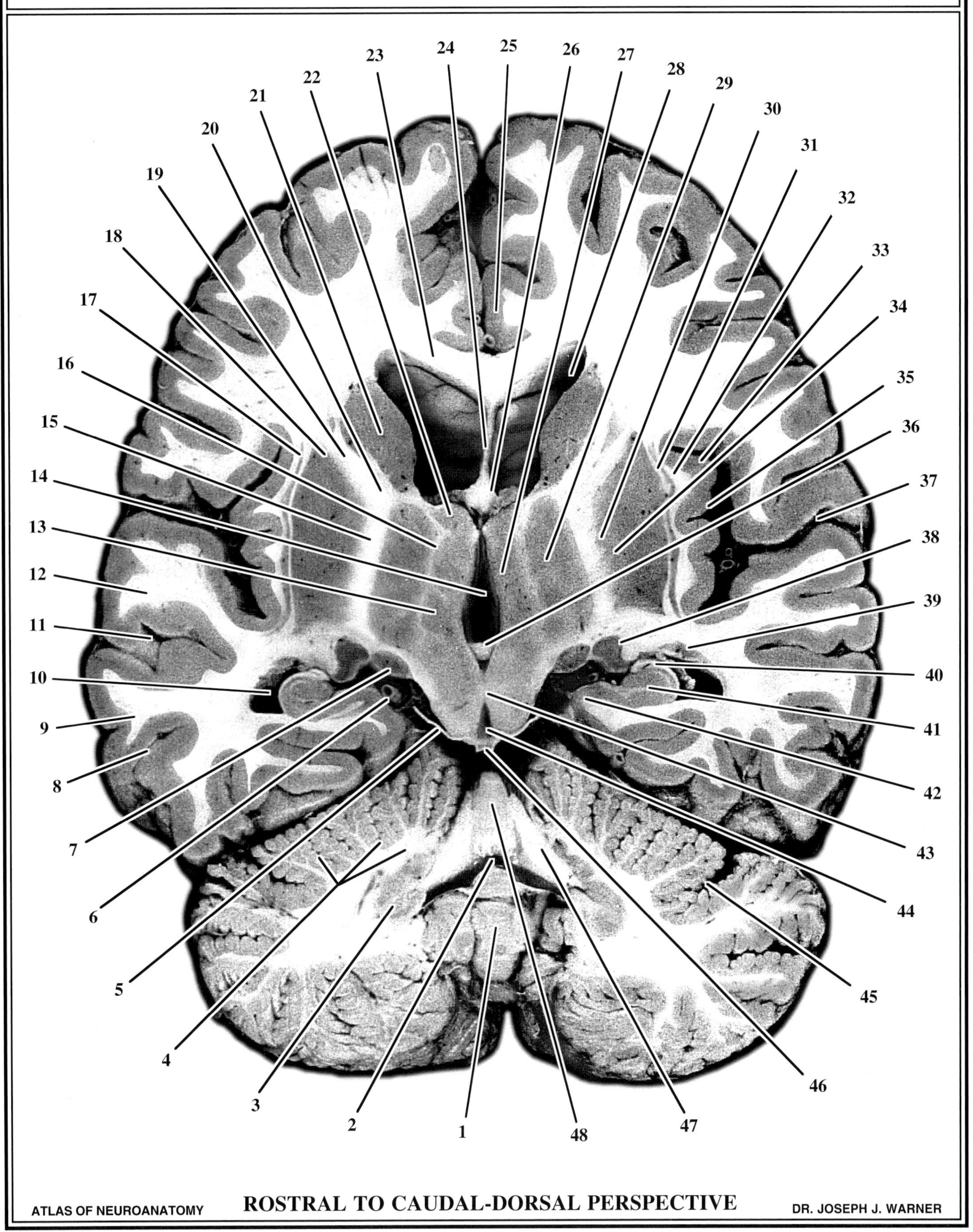

ATLAS OF NEUROANATOMY

ROSTRAL TO CAUDAL-DORSAL PERSPECTIVE

DR. JOSEPH J. WARNER

COMPLETE SECTION OF THE BRAIN PARALLEL TO THE LONGITUDINAL AXIS OF THE BRAINSTEM, LEVEL OF THE LATERAL AND MEDIAL GENICULATE NUCLEI; ROSTRAL TO CAUDAL-DORSAL PERSPECTIVE: KEY TO SECTION ORIENTATION AND SPECIFIC STRUCTURES

A key point in examining sections oriented in a specific plane include the anatomic direction in which the specimen is being viewed. Although sections on either side of a given plane share the same dissection surface, the anatomic structures demonstrated by each are quite different.

KEY TO NUMBERED STRUCTURES

1. Cerebellar Vermis
2. Fourth Ventricle
3. Dentate Nucleus
4. Anterior Lobe of the Cerebellum
5. Trochlear (IV) Nerve
6. Posterior Cerebral Artery
7. Medial Geniculate Nucleus
8. Middle Temporal Sulcus
9. Middle Temporal Gyrus
10. Temporal Horn of the Lateral Ventricle
11. Superior Temporal Sulcus
12. Superior Temporal Gyrus
13. Centromedian Nucleus of the Thalamus
14. Third Ventricle
15. Posterior Limb of the Internal Capsule
16. Internal Medullary Lamina of the Thalamus
17. Claustrum
18. Putamen
19. Anterior Limb of the Internal Capsule
20. Genu of the Internal Capsule
21. Caudate Nucleus
22. Anterior Nucleus of the Thalamus
23. Corpus Callosum
24. Septum Pellucidum
25. Cingulate Gyrus
26. Fornix
27. Dorsomedial Nucleus of the Thalamus
28. Body of the Lateral Ventricle
29. Ventroanterior, Ventrolateral Thalamic Nuclei
30. Globus Pallidus II
31. External Capsule
32. Extreme Capsule
33. Insular Cortex
34. External Medullary Lamina
35. Insular Cortex
36. Posterior Commissure
37. Sylvian Fissure
38. Lateral Geniculate Nucleus
39. Tail of the Caudate
40. Fimbria of the Fornix
41. Hippocampus
42. Parahippocampal Gyrus
43. Periaqueductal Gray
44. Aqueduct of Sylvius
45. Primary Fissure of the Cerebellum
46. Frenulum of the Anterior Medullary Velum
47. Superior Cerebellar Peduncle
48. Anterior Medullary Velum

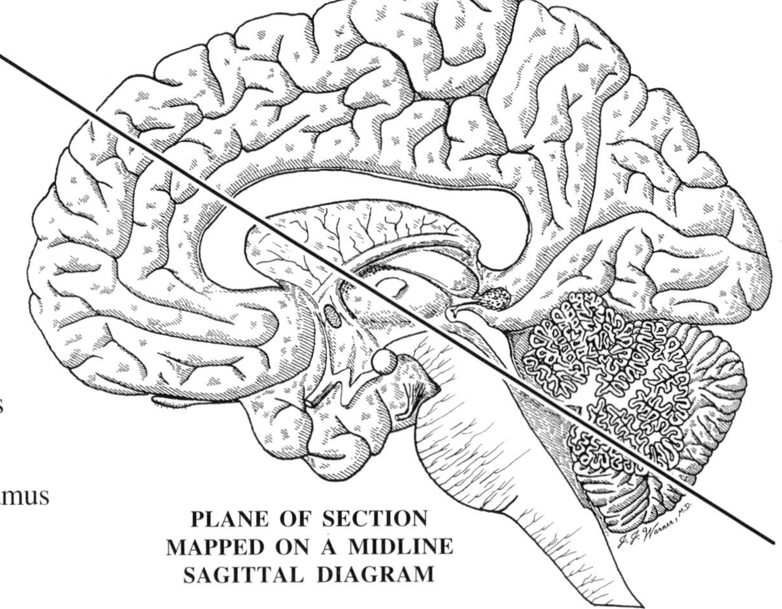

PLANE OF SECTION MAPPED ON A MIDLINE SAGITTAL DIAGRAM

For this section (viewed in the rostral to caudal perspective), major neuroanatomic landmarks include the Posterior Commissure, the Anterior Medullary Velum, and the Trochlear Nerves.

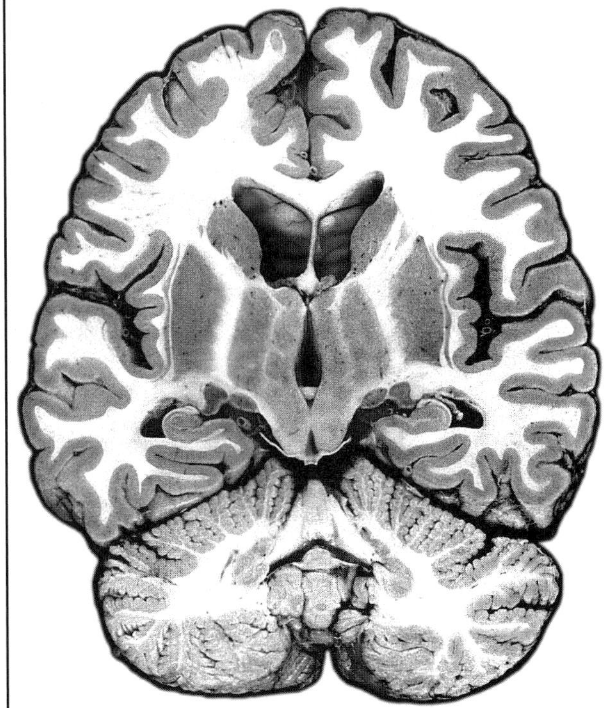

ATLAS OF NEUROANATOMY DR. JOSEPH J. WARNER

COMPLETE SECTION OF THE BRAIN (MAGNIFIED VIEW), PLANE PARALLEL TO THE LONGITUDINAL AXIS OF THE BRAINSTEM: LEVEL OF THE LATERAL AND MEDIAL GENICULATE NUCLEI (ROSTRAL TO CAUDAL-DORSAL PERSPECTIVE)

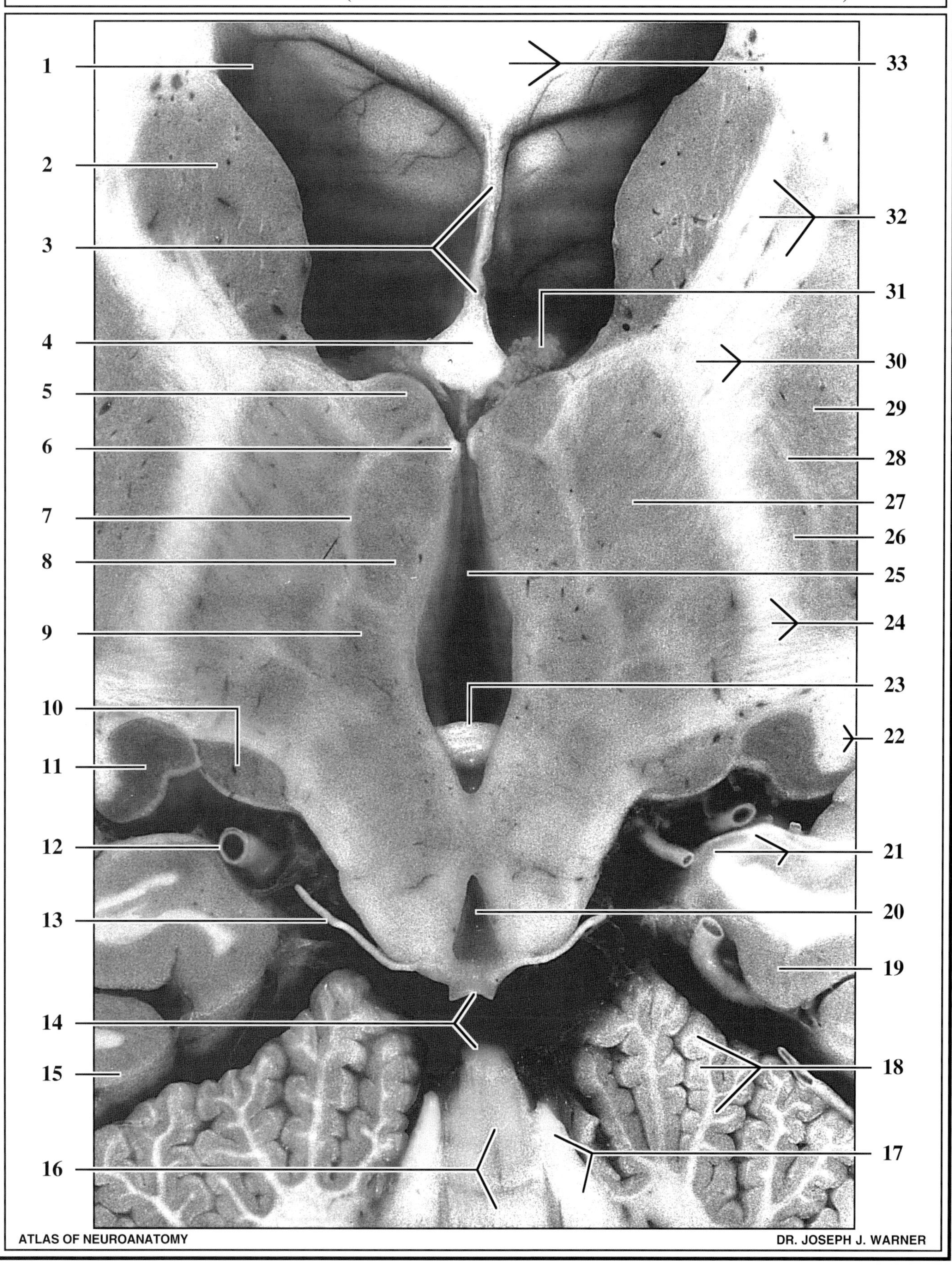

SECTION OF THE BRAIN PARALLEL TO THE LONGITUDINAL AXIS OF THE BRAINSTEM, LEVEL OF THE LATERAL AND MEDIAL GENICULATE NUCLEI; MAGNIFIED VIEW, ROSTRAL TO CAUDAL-DORSAL PERSPECTIVE: KEY TO SECTION ORIENTATION AND SPECIFIC STRUCTURES

KEY TO NUMBERED STRUCTURES

1. Body of the Lateral Ventricle
2. Caudate Nucleus
3. Septum Pellucidum
4. Fornix
5. Anterior Nucleus of the Thalamus
6. Stria Medullaris
7. Internal Medullary Lamina of the Thalamus
8. Dorsomedial Nucleus of the Thalamus
9. Centromedian Nucleus of the Thalamus
10. Medial Geniculate Nucleus
11. Lateral Geniculate Nucleus
12. Posterior Cerebral Artery
13. Trochlear (IV) Nerve
14. Anterior Medullary Velum* (the Frenulum is located rostromedially, adjacent to the Inferior Colliculi)
15. Fusiform Gyrus
16. Roof of the Fourth Ventricle
17. Superior Cerebellar Peduncle
18. Anterior Lobe of the Cerebellum
19. Parahippocampal Gyrus
20. Aqueduct of Sylvius
21. Presubiculum and Subiculum
22. Geniculocalcarine Radiations
23. Posterior Commissure
24. Posterior Limb of the Internal Capsule
25. Third Ventricle
26. Globus Pallidus II
27. Ventroanterior and Ventrolateral Thalamic Nuclei
28. External Medullary Lamina
29. Putamen
30. Genu of the Internal Capsule
31. Choroid Plexus
32. Anterior Limb of the Internal Capsule
33. Corpus Callosum

*The Anterior Medullary Velum has been separated by the plane of section, which has crossed the ventrally convex curvature of this structure.

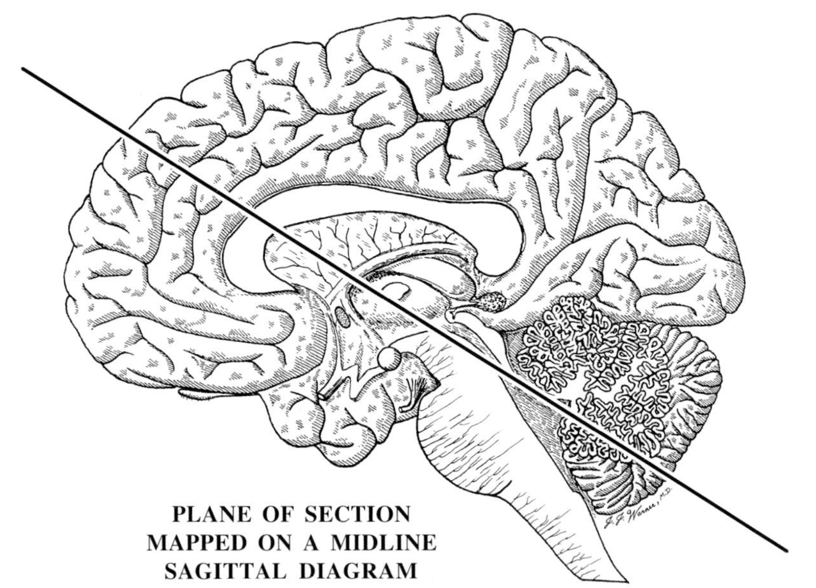

PLANE OF SECTION MAPPED ON A MIDLINE SAGITTAL DIAGRAM

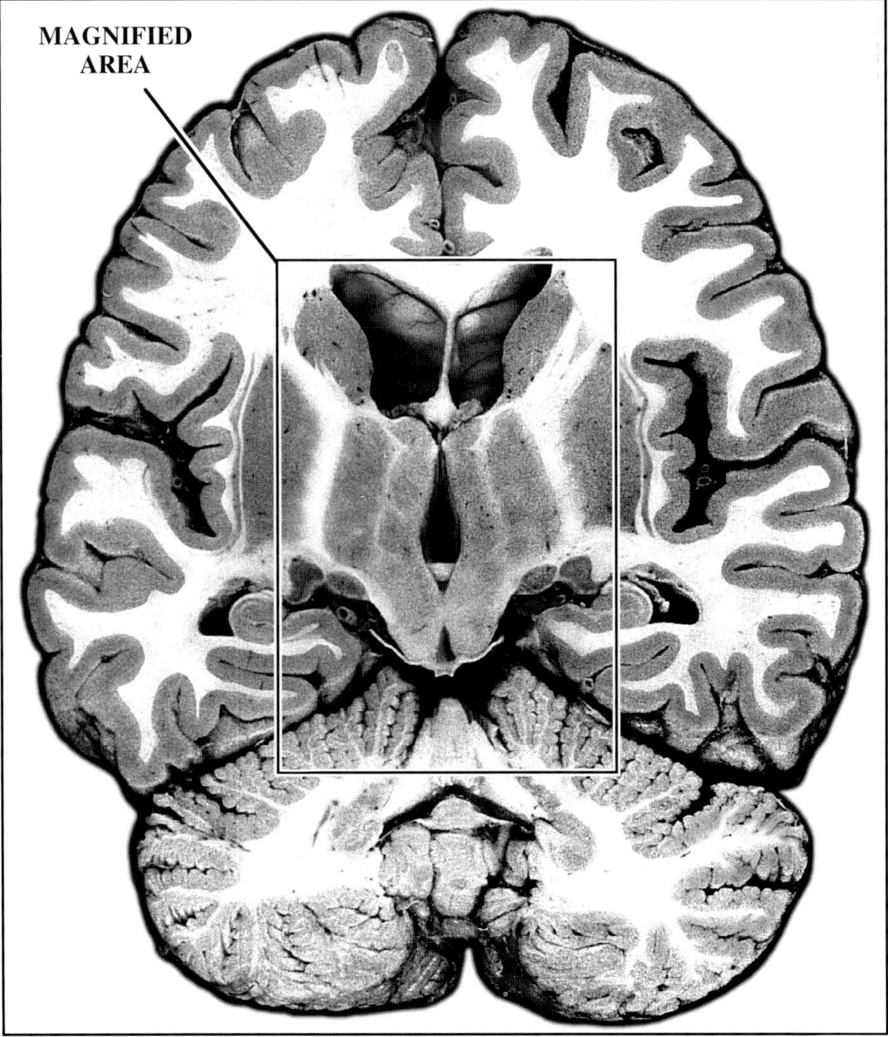

COMPLETE SECTION OF THE BRAIN, PLANE PARALLEL TO THE LONGITUDINAL AXIS OF THE BRAINSTEM: LEVEL OF THE LATERAL AND MEDIAL GENICULATE NUCLEI

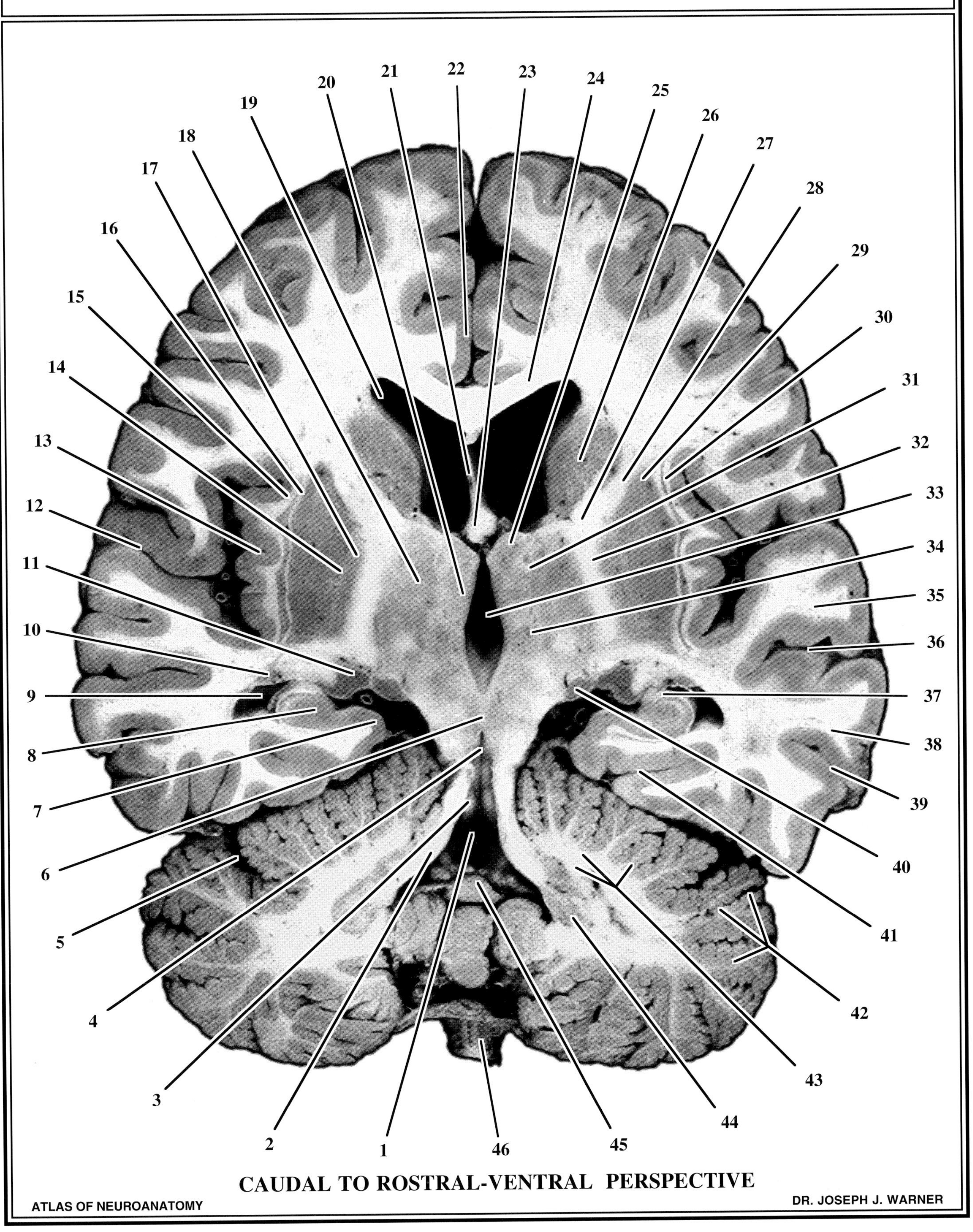

CAUDAL TO ROSTRAL-VENTRAL PERSPECTIVE

DR. JOSEPH J. WARNER

SECTION OF THE BRAIN PARALLEL TO THE LONGITUDINAL AXIS OF THE BRAINSTEM, LEVEL OF THE LATERAL AND MEDIAL GENICULATE NUCLEI; CAUDAL TO ROSTRAL-VENTRAL PERSPECTIVE: KEY TO SECTION ORIENTATION AND SPECIFIC STRUCTURES

KEY TO NUMBERED STRUCTURES

1. Fourth Ventricle
2. Superior Cerebellar Peduncle
3. Facial Colliculus
4. Aqueduct of Sylvius
5. Primary Fissure of the Cerebellum
6. Periaqueductal Gray
7. Parahippocampal Gyrus
8. Hippocampus
9. Temporal Horn of the Lateral Ventricle
10. Tail of the Caudate
11. Lateral Geniculate Nucleus
12. Sylvian Fissure
13. Insular Cortex
14. External Medullary Lamina
15. Extreme Capsule
16. External Capsule
17. Globus Pallidus II
18. Ventroanterior and Ventrolateral Thalamic Nuclei
19. Body of the Lateral Ventricle
20. Dorsomedial Nucleus of the Thalamus
21. Septum Pellucidum
22. Cingulate Gyrus
23. Fornix
24. Corpus Callosum
25. Anterior Nucleus of the Thalamus
26. Caudate Nucleus
27. Genu of the Internal Capsule
28. Anterior Limb of the Internal Capsule
29. Putamen
30. Claustrum
31. Internal Medullary Lamina of the Thalamus
32. Posterior Limb of the Internal Capsule
33. Third Ventricle
34. Centromedian Nucleus of the Thalamus
35. Superior Temporal Gyrus
36. Superior Temporal Sulcus
37. Fimbria of the Fornix
38. Middle Temporal Gyrus
39. Middle Temporal Sulcus
40. Medial Geniculate Nucleus
41. Collateral Sulcus
42. Posterior Lobe of the Cerebellum
43. Anterior Lobe of the Cerebellum
44. Dentate Nucleus
45. Nodulus
46. Dorsal Aspect of Cervicomedullary Junction

PLANE OF SECTION MAPPED ON A MIDLINE SAGITTAL DIAGRAM

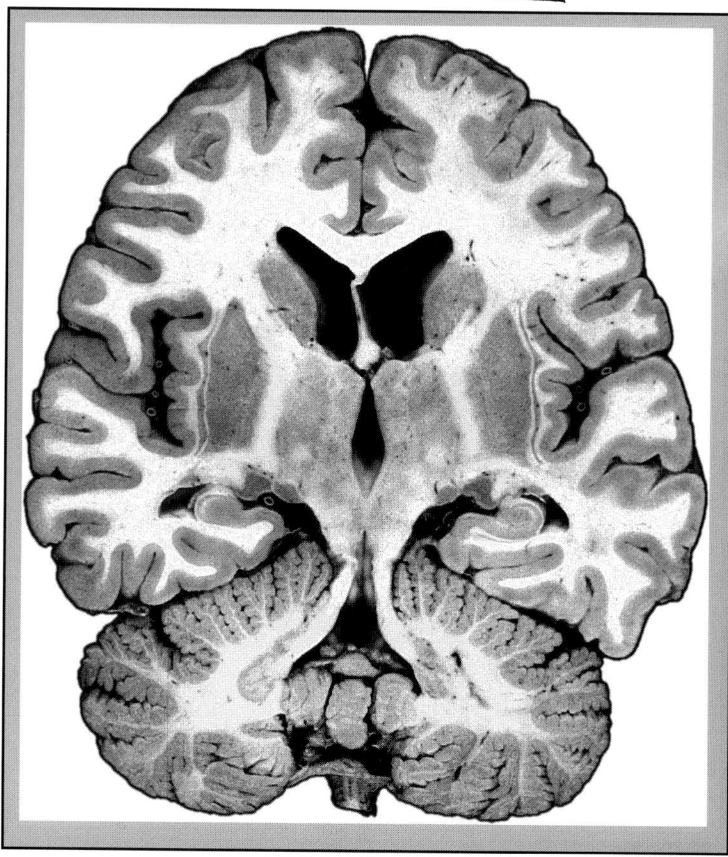

COMPLETE SECTION OF THE BRAIN (MAGNIFIED VIEW), PLANE PARALLEL TO THE LONGITUDINAL AXIS OF THE BRAINSTEM: LEVEL OF THE LATERAL AND MEDIAL GENICULATE NUCLEI (CAUDAL TO ROSTRAL-VENTRAL PERSPECTIVE)

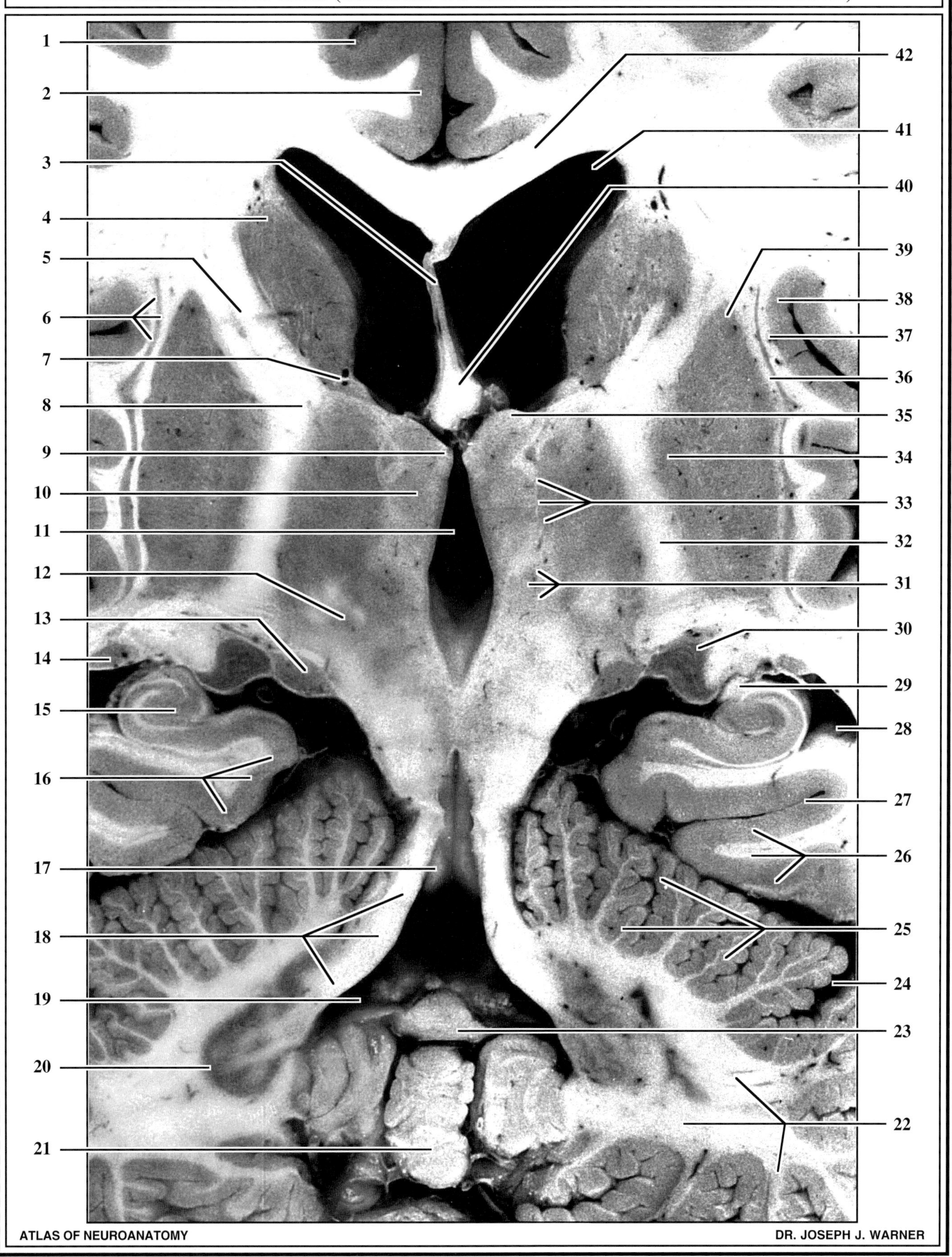

ATLAS OF NEUROANATOMY DR. JOSEPH J. WARNER

SECTION OF THE BRAIN PARALLEL TO THE LONGITUDINAL AXIS OF THE BRAINSTEM, LEVEL OF THE LATERAL AND MEDIAL GENICULATE NUCLEI; MAGNIFIED VIEW, CAUDAL TO ROSTRAL-VENTRAL PERSPECTIVE: KEY TO SECTION ORIENTATION AND SPECIFIC STRUCTURES

KEY TO NUMBERED STRUCTURES

1. Cingulate Sulcus
2. Cingulate Gyrus
3. Septum Pellucidum
4. Caudate Nucleus
5. Anterior Limb of the Internal Capsule
6. Claustrum
7. Stria Terminalis and Thalamostriate Vein
8. Genu of the Internal Capsule
9. Stria Medullaris
10. Dorsomedial Nucleus of the Thalamus
11. Third Ventricle
12. Ventroposteromedial (VPM) Nucleus of the Thalamus
13. Medial Geniculate Nucleus
14. Tail of the Caudate Nucleus
15. Hippocampus
16. Parahippocampal Gyrus
17. Facial Colliculus
18. Superior Cerebellar Peduncle
19. Lateral Recess of the Fourth Ventricle
20. Dentate Nucleus
21. Inferior Aspect of the Cerebellar Vermis
22. Posterior Lobe of the Cerebellum
23. Nodulus
24. Primary Fissure
25. Anterior Lobe of the Cerebellum
26. Fusiform Gyrus
27. Collateral Sulcus
28. Temporal Horn of the Lateral Ventricle
29. Fimbria of the Fornix
30. Lateral Geniculate Nucleus
31. Centromedian Nucleus of the Thalamus
32. Posterior Limb of the Internal Capsule
33. Internal Medullary Lamina of the Thalamus
34. Globus Pallidus II
35. Anterior Nucleus of the Thalamus
36. External Capsule
37. Extreme Capsule
38. Insular Cortex
39. Putamen
40. Fornix
41. Body of the Lateral Ventricle
42. Corpus Callosum

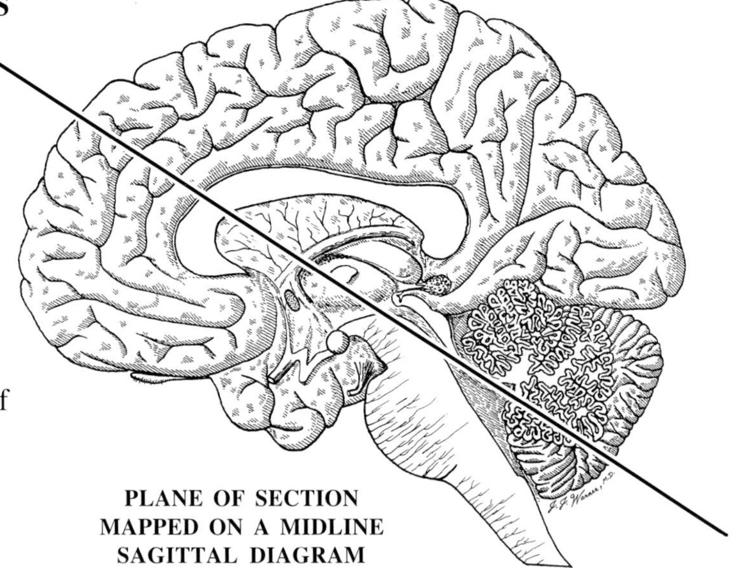

PLANE OF SECTION MAPPED ON A MIDLINE SAGITTAL DIAGRAM

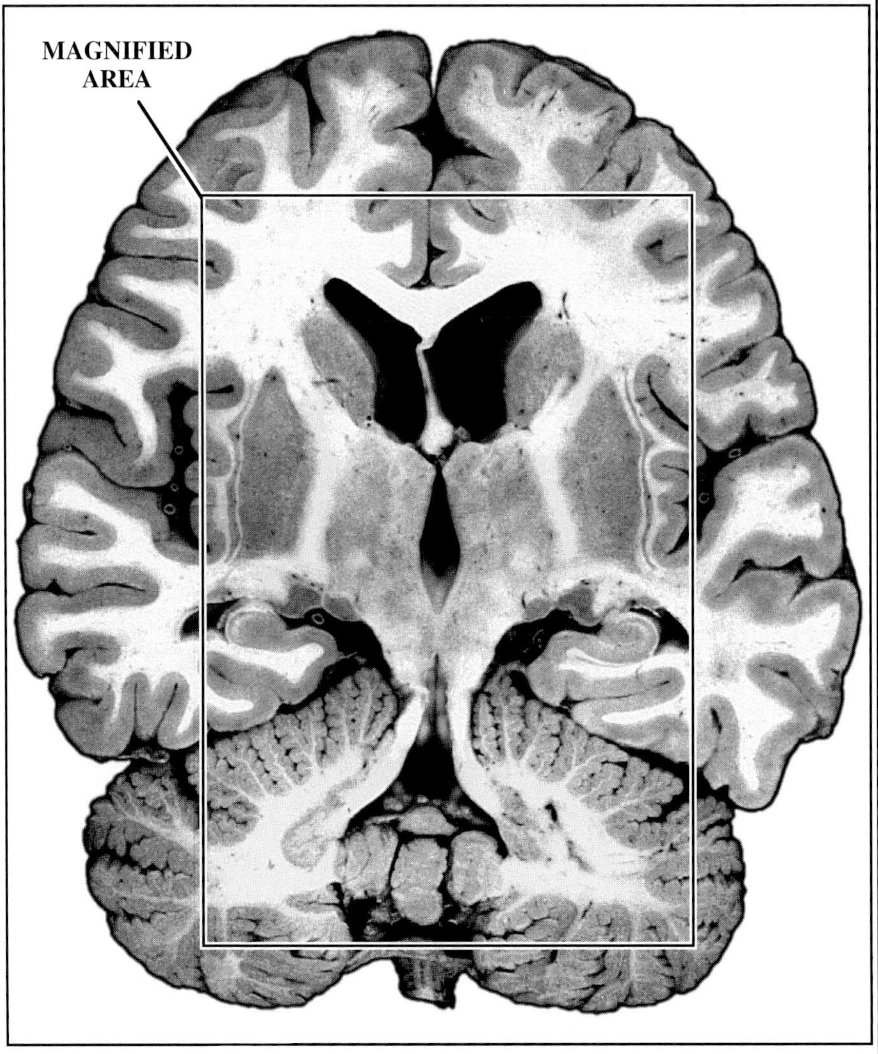

COMPLETE SECTION OF THE BRAIN, PLANE PARALLEL TO THE LONGITUDINAL AXIS OF THE BRAINSTEM: LEVEL OF THE ANTERIOR COMMISSURE (CAUDAL TO ROSTRAL - VENTRAL PERSPECTIVE)

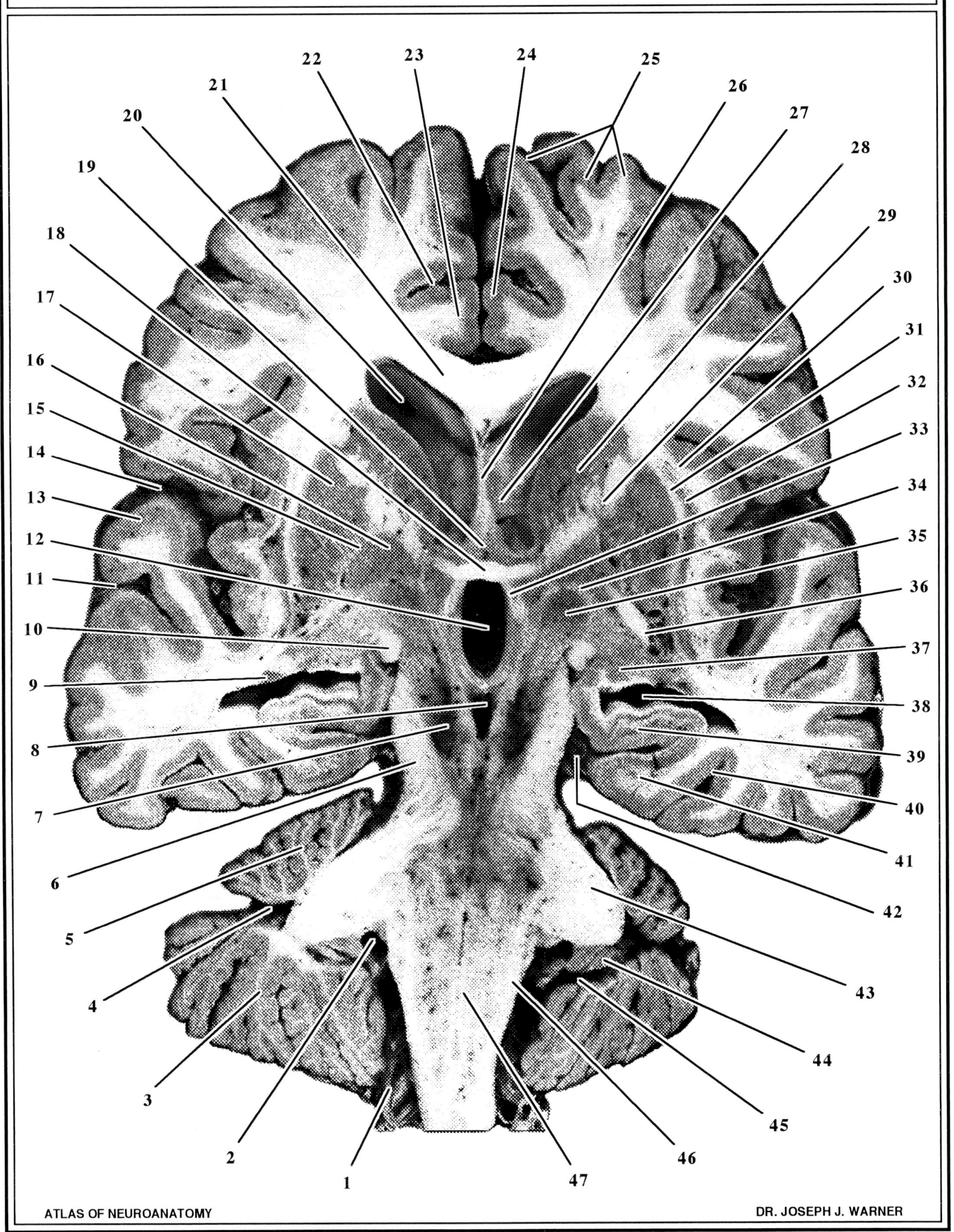

ATLAS OF NEUROANATOMY

DR. JOSEPH J. WARNER

SECTION OF THE BRAIN PARALLEL TO THE LONGITUDINAL AXIS OF THE BRAINSTEM, LEVEL OF THE ANTERIOR COMMISSURE; CAUDAL TO ROSTRAL-VENTRAL PERSPECTIVE: KEY TO SECTION ORIENTATION AND SPECIFIC STRUCTURES

KEY TO NUMBERED STRUCTURES

1. Spinal Accessory (XI) Nerve
2. Foramen of Luschka
3. Posterior Lobe of the Cerebellum (anterior-inferior aspect)
4. Primary Fissure
5. Anterior Lobe of the Cerebellum
6. Cerebral Peduncle
7. Substantia Nigra
8. Interpeduncular Fossa
9. Tail of the Caudate Nucleus
10. Optic Tract
11. Superior Temporal Sulcus
12. Third Ventricle
13. Superior Temporal Gyrus
14. Sylvian Fissure
15. External Medullary Lamina
16. Globus Pallidus II
17. Putamen
18. Anterior Commissure
19. Septal Nuclei
20. Anterior Horn of the Lateral Ventricle
21. Corpus Callosum
22. Cingulate Sulcus
23. Cingulum
24. Cingulate Gyrus
25. Superior Frontal Convolution
26. Septum Pellucidum
27. Ventricular Surface of the Genu of the Corpus Callosum
28. Head of the Caudate Nucleus
29. Anterior Limb of the Internal Capsule
30. Extreme Capsule
31. External Capsule
32. Claustrum
33. Fornix
34. Internal Medullary Lamina
35. Globus Pallidus I
36. Anterior Commissure
37. Amygdala
38. Temporal Horn of the Lateral Ventricle
39. Hippocampus
40. Collateral Sulcus
41. Parahippocampal Gyrus
42. Posterior Cerebral Artery
43. Middle Cerebellar Peduncle
44. Flocculus
45. Posterolateral Fissure
46. Inferior Cerebellar Peduncle
47. Medial Longitudinal Fasciculus and Tectospinal Tract

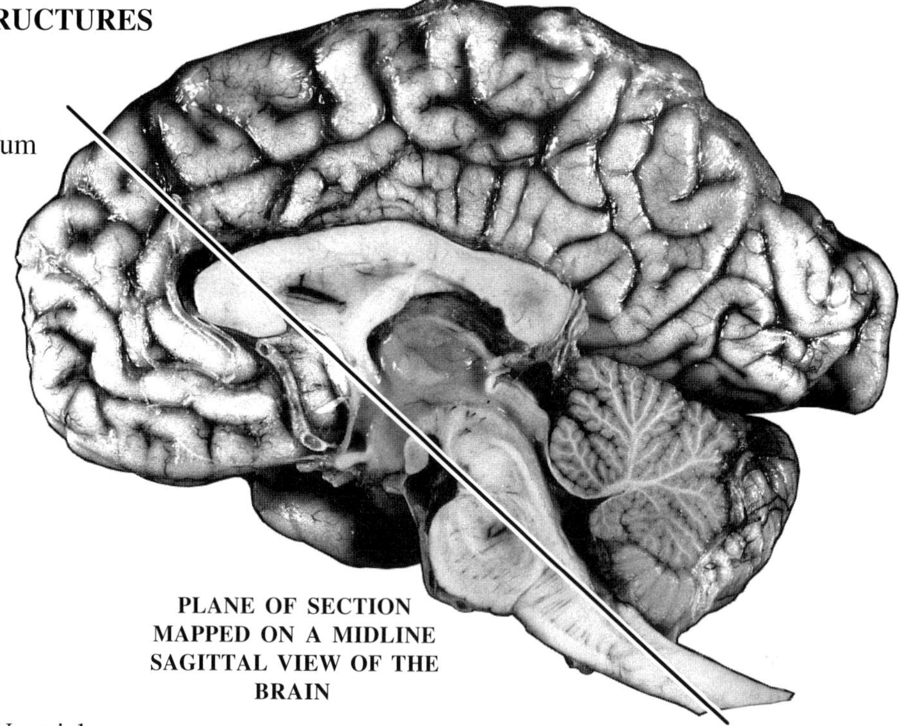

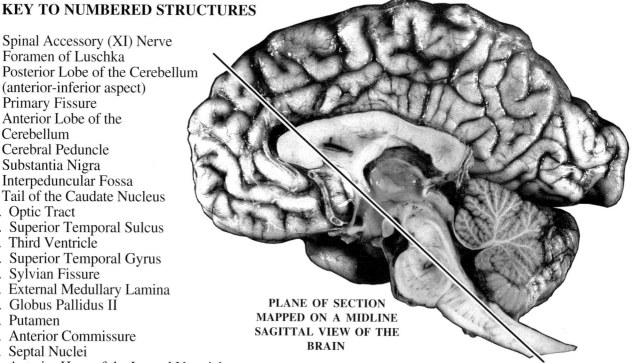

PLANE OF SECTION MAPPED ON A MIDLINE SAGITTAL VIEW OF THE BRAIN

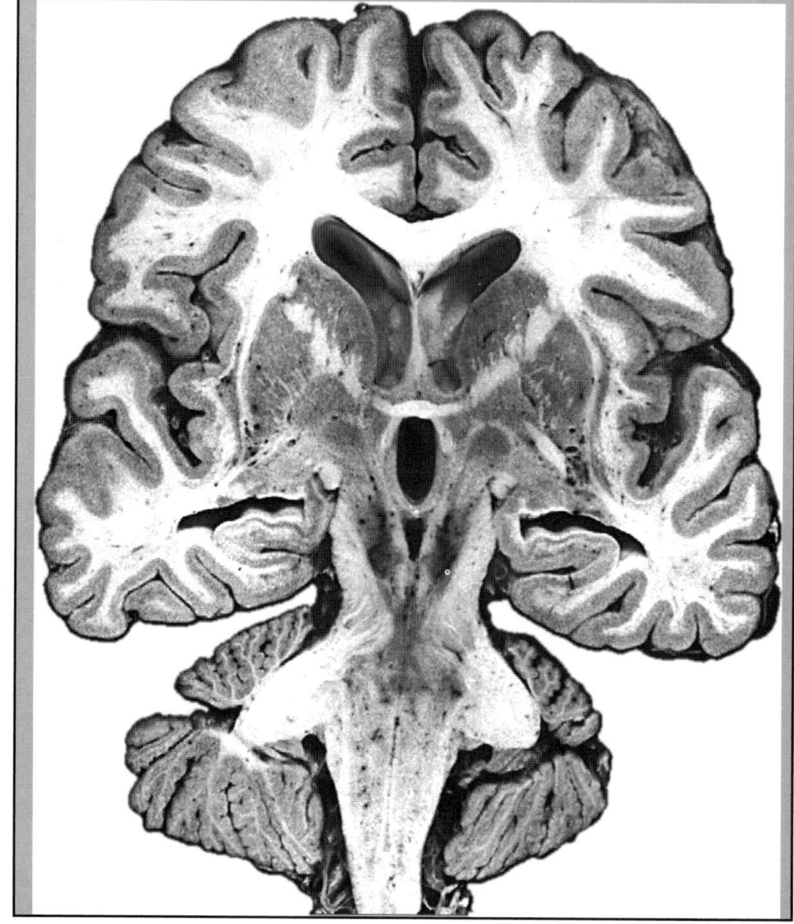

COMPLETE SECTION OF THE BRAIN (MAGNIFIED VIEW), PLANE PARALLEL TO THE LONGITUDINAL AXIS OF THE BRAINSTEM: LEVEL OF THE ANTERIOR COMMISSURE (CAUDAL TO ROSTRAL - VENTRAL PERSPECTIVE)

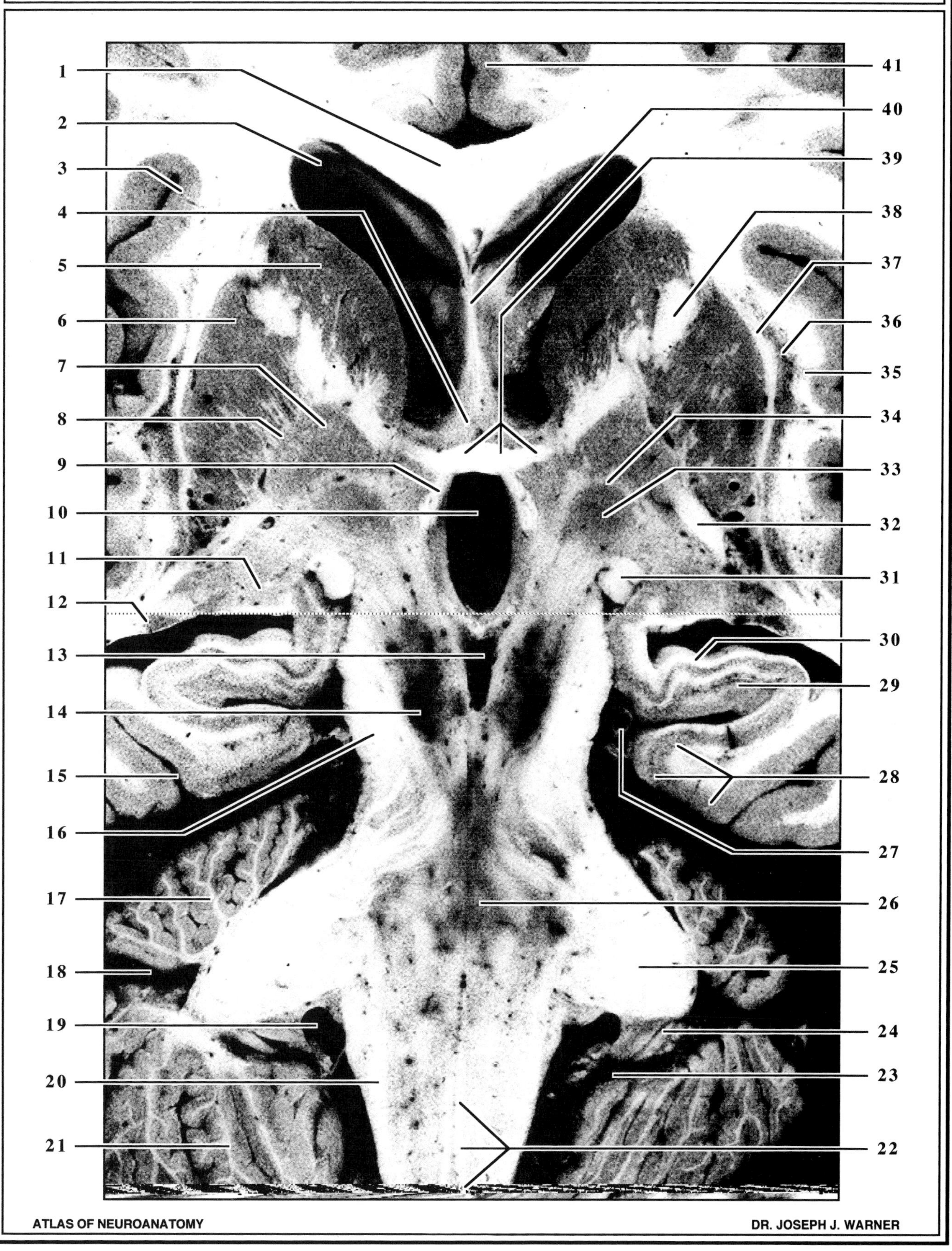

SECTION OF THE BRAIN PARALLEL TO THE LONGITUDINAL AXIS OF THE BRAINSTEM, LEVEL OF THE ANTERIOR COMMISSURE; MAGNIFIED VIEW, CAUDAL TO ROSTRAL-VENTRAL PERSPECTIVE: KEY TO SECTION ORIENTATION AND SPECIFIC STRUCTURES

KEY TO NUMBERED STRUCTURES

1. Corpus Callosum
2. Anterior Horn of the Lateral Ventricle
3. Insular Cortex
4. Septal Nuclei
5. Head of the Caudate Nucleus
6. Putamen
7. Globus Pallidus II
8. External Medullary Lamina
9. Fornix
10. Third Ventricle
11. Amygdala
12. Tail of the Caudate Nucleus
13. Interpeduncular Fossa
14. Substantia Nigra
15. Collateral Sulcus
16. Cerebral Peduncle
17. Anterior Lobe of the Cerebellum
18. Primary Fissure
19. Foramen of Luschka
20. Inferior Cerebellar Peduncle
21. Posterior Lobe of the Cerebellum
22. Medial Longitudinal Fasciculus, Tectospinal Tract, and Dorsal Fibers of the Medial Lemniscus
23. Posterolateral Fissure
24. Flocculus
25. Middle Cerebellar Peduncle
26. Pontine Tegmentum
27. Posterior Cerebral Artery
28. Parahippocampal Gyrus
29. Hippocampus
30. Alveus
31. Optic Tract
32. Anterior Commissure
33. Globus Pallidus I
34. Internal Medullary Lamina
35. Extreme Capsule
36. Claustrum
37. External Capsule
38. Anterior Limb of the Internal Capsule
39. Anterior Commissure
40. Septum Pellucidum
41. Cingulate Gyrus

At this level, important intersection points for cross-referencing to the midline sagittal section include the Anterior Commissure, the Third Ventricle, and the Interpeduncular Fossa.

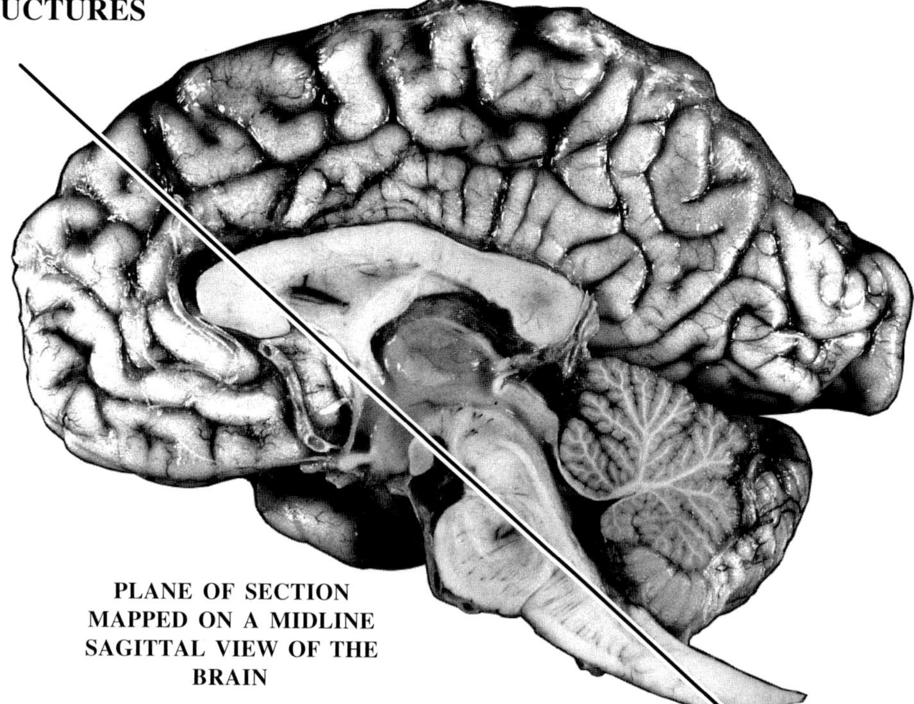

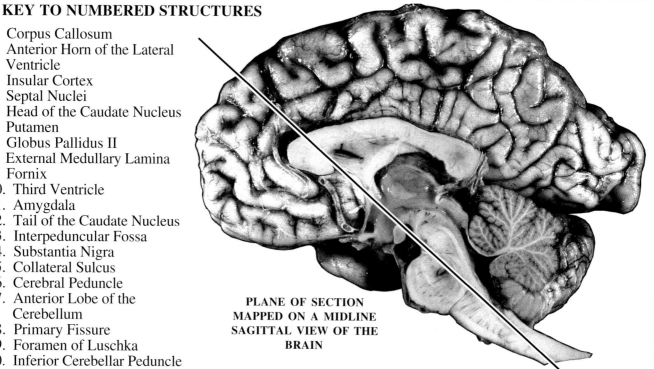

PLANE OF SECTION MAPPED ON A MIDLINE SAGITTAL VIEW OF THE BRAIN

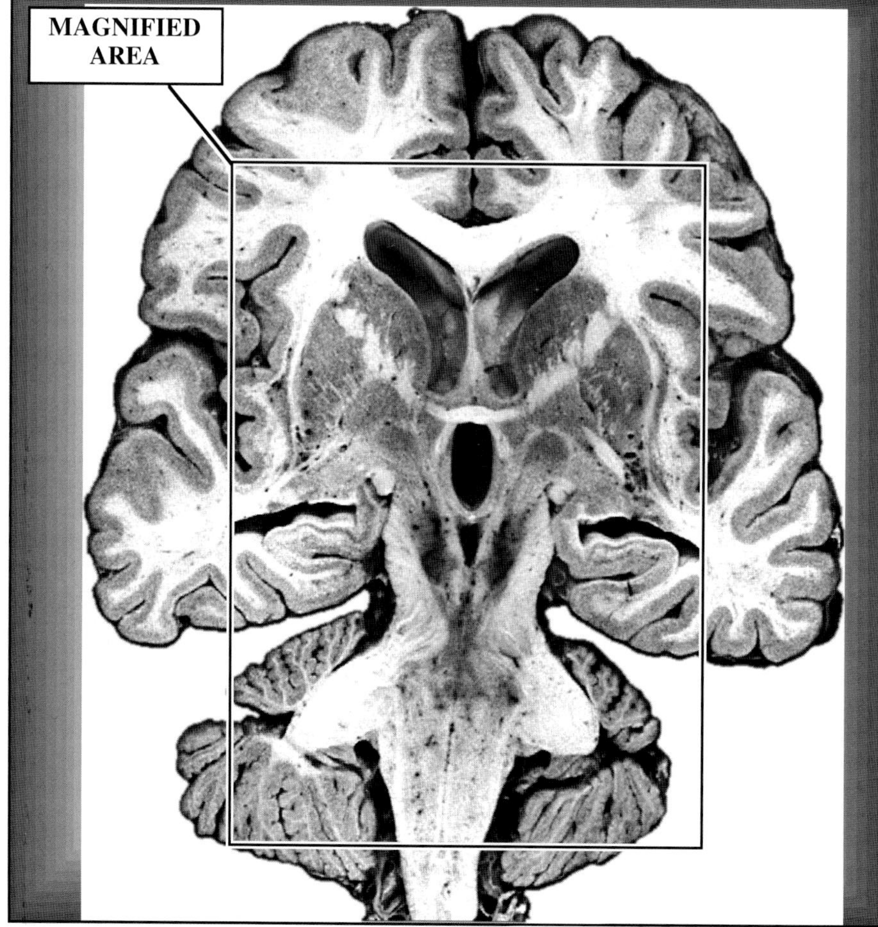

COMPLETE SECTION OF THE BRAIN, PLANE PARALLEL TO THE LONGITUDINAL AXIS OF THE BRAINSTEM: LEVEL OF THE OPTIC CHIASM AND BASIS PONTIS (ROSTRAL TO CAUDAL-DORSAL PERSPECTIVE)

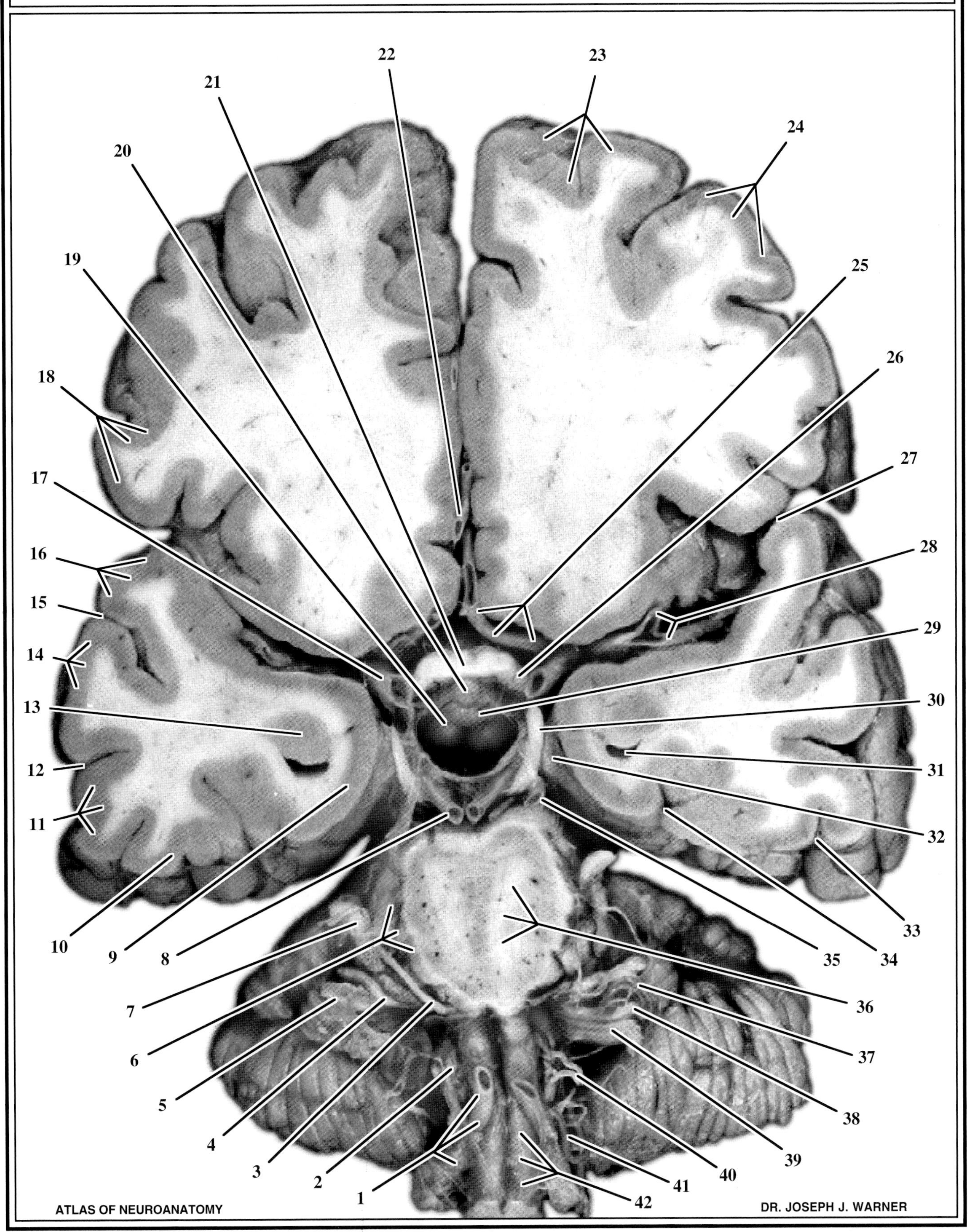

SECTION OF THE BRAIN PARALLEL TO THE LONGITUDINAL AXIS OF THE BRAINSTEM, LEVEL OF THE OPTIC CHIASM AND BASIS PONTIS; ROSTRAL TO CAUDAL-DORSAL PERSPECTIVE: KEY TO SECTION ORIENTATION AND SPECIFIC STRUCTURES

KEY TO NUMBERED STRUCTURES

1. Vertebral Artery
2. Inferior Olive
3. Abducens (VI) Nerve
4. Facial (VII) Nerve
5. Vestibulocochlear (VIII) Nerve
6. Middle Cerebellar Peduncle
7. Trigeminal (V) Nerve
8. Posterior Cerebral Artery
9. Parahippocampal Gyrus
10. Fusiform Gyrus
11. Inferior Temporal Gyrus
12. Middle Temporal Sulcus
13. Amygdala
14. Middle Temporal Gyrus
15. Superior Temporal Sulcus
16. Superior Temporal Gyrus
17. Internal Carotid Artery
18. Inferior Frontal Convolution
19. Mammillary Body
20. Pituitary Stalk
21. Optic Chiasm
22. Anterior Cerebral Artery
23. Superior Frontal Convolution
24. Middle Frontal Convolution
25. Anterior Cerebral Artery
26. Optic Tract
27. Sylvian Fissure
28. Middle Cerebral Arteries
29. Median Eminence
30. Oculomotor (III) Nerve
31. Temporal Horn of the Lateral Ventricle
32. Uncus
33. Inferior Temporal Sulcus
34. Collateral Sulcus
35. Superior Cerebellar Artery
36. Corticobulbar and Corticospinal Tracts
37. Anterior Inferior Cerebellar Artery
38. Glossopharyngeal (IX) Nerve
39. Vagus (X) Nerve
40. Hypoglossal (XII) Nerve
41. Posterior Inferior Cerebellar Artery
42. Medullary Pyramid

At this level, intersection points for cross-referencing to the midline sagittal section include the optic chiasm, the basis pontis, and anterior cerebral and anterior communicating arteries.

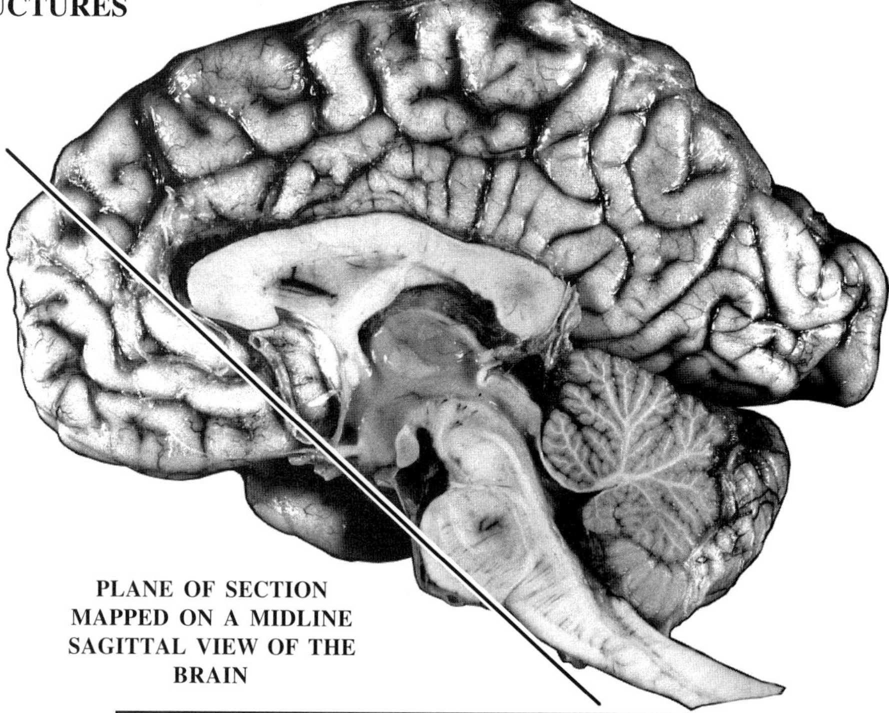

PLANE OF SECTION MAPPED ON A MIDLINE SAGITTAL VIEW OF THE BRAIN

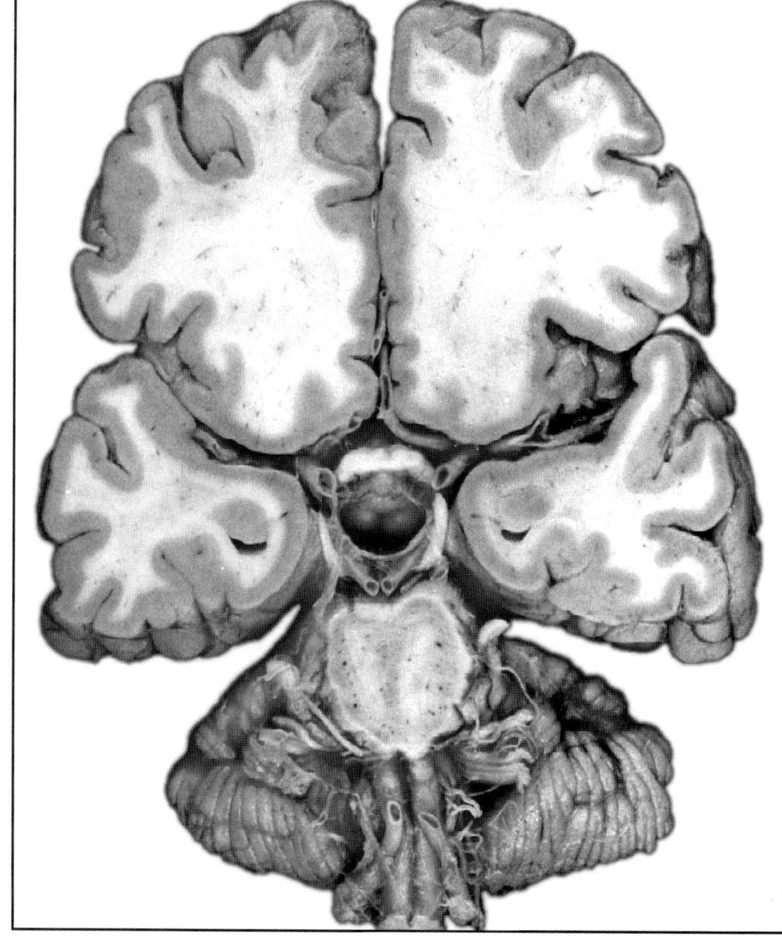

COMPLETE SECTION OF THE BRAIN (MAGNIFIED VIEW), PLANE PARALLEL TO THE LONGITUDINAL AXIS OF THE BRAINSTEM: LEVEL OF THE OPTIC CHIASM AND BASIS PONTIS (ROSTRAL TO CAUDAL-DORSAL PERSPECTIVE)

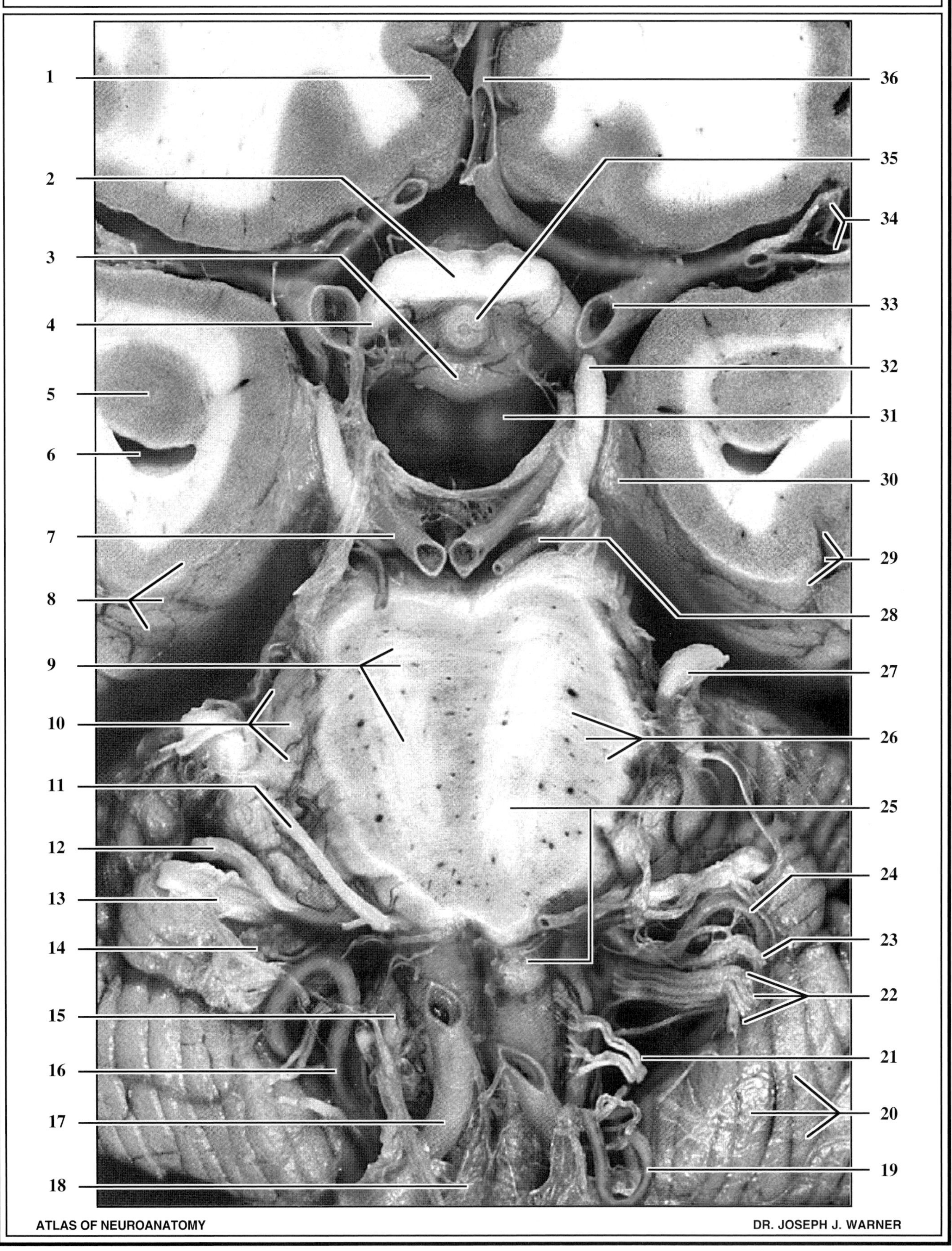

SECTION OF THE BRAIN PARALLEL TO THE LONGITUDINAL AXIS OF THE BRAINSTEM, LEVEL OF THE OPTIC CHIASM AND BASIS PONTIS; MAGNIFIED VIEW, ROSTRAL TO CAUDAL-DORSAL PERSPECTIVE: KEY TO SECTION ORIENTATION AND SPECIFIC STRUCTURES

KEY TO NUMBERED STRUCTURES

1. Medial Aspect, Frontal Lobe
2. Optic Chiasm
3. Median Eminence
4. Optic Tract
5. Amygdala
6. Temporal Horn of the Lateral Ventricle
7. Posterior Cerebral Artery*
8. Parahippocampal Gyrus
9. Corticobulbar and Corticospinal Tracts
10. Middle Cerebellar Peduncle
11. Abducens (VI) Nerve
12. Facial (VII) Nerve
13. Vestibulocochlear (VIII) Nerve
14. Choroid Plexus (adjacent to Lateral Recess of Fourth Ventricle and Foramen of Luschka)
15. Inferior Olive
16. Posterior Inferior Cerebellar Artery
17. Vertebral Artery
18. Caudal Medulla
19. Posterior Inferior Cerebellar Artery
20. Posterior Lobe of the Cerebellum
21. Hypoglossal (XII) Nerve
22. Vagus (X) Nerve
23. Glossopharyngeal (IX) Nerve
24. Anterior Inferior Cerebellar Artery
25. Corticobulbar and Corticospinal Tracts, with caudal continuation of the Corticospinal Tract into the ipsilateral Medullary Pyramid
26. Transverse (Pontocerebellar) Fibers
27. Trigeminal (V) Nerve
28. Superior Cerebellar Artery*
29. Collateral Sulcus
30. Uncus
31. Mammillary Body
32. Oculomotor (III) Nerve*
33. Internal Carotid Artery
34. Middle Cerebral Arteries
35. Pituitary Stalk
36. Anterior Cerebral Artery

*The posterior cerebral artery (at the basilar bifurcation) passes rostral and dorsal to the oculomotor nerve, whereas the superior cerebellar artery courses infratentorially, caudal to the oculomotor nerve

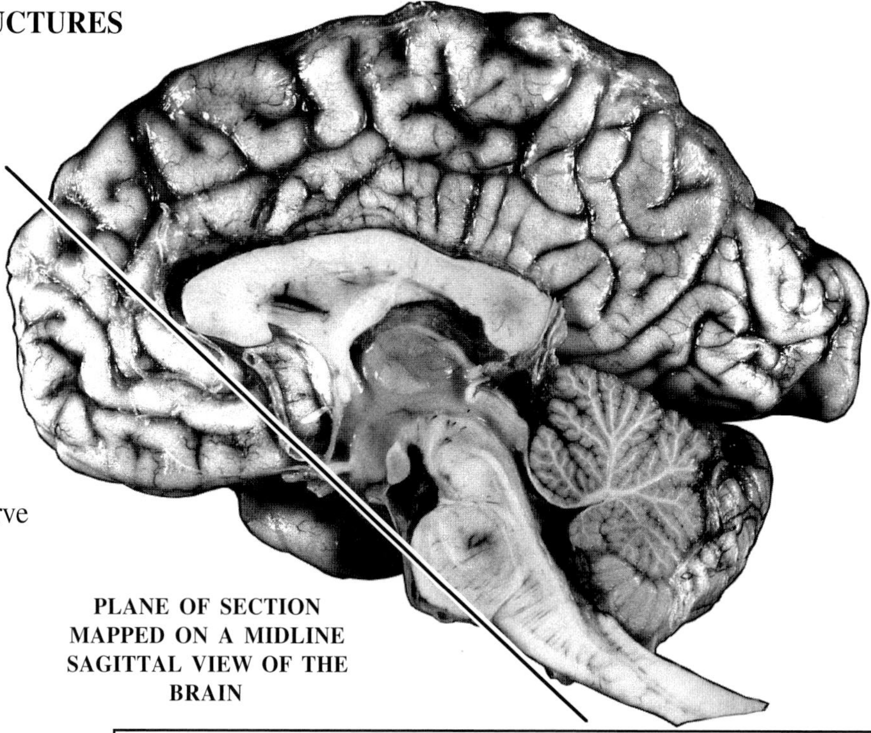

PLANE OF SECTION MAPPED ON A MIDLINE SAGITTAL VIEW OF THE BRAIN

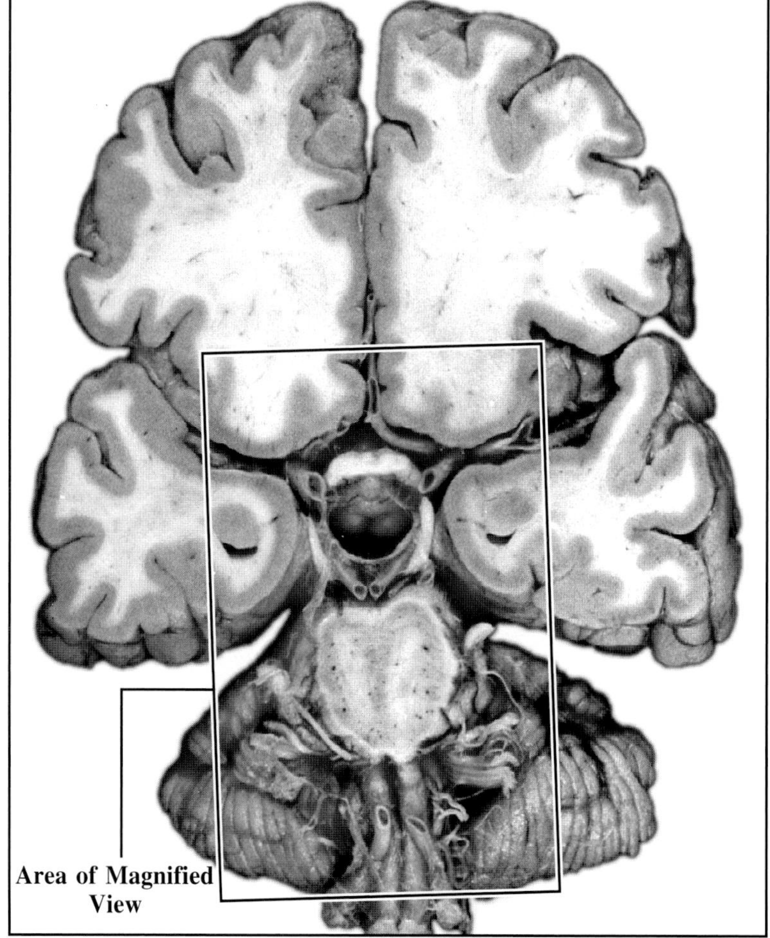

COMPLETE SECTION OF THE BRAIN, PLANE PARALLEL TO THE LONGITUDINAL AXIS OF THE BRAINSTEM: LEVEL INCLUDING THE OLFACTORY TRACTS AND THE ROSTRAL ASPECT OF THE FRONTAL AND TEMPORAL LOBES (ROSTRAL TO CAUDAL-DORSAL PERSPECTIVE)

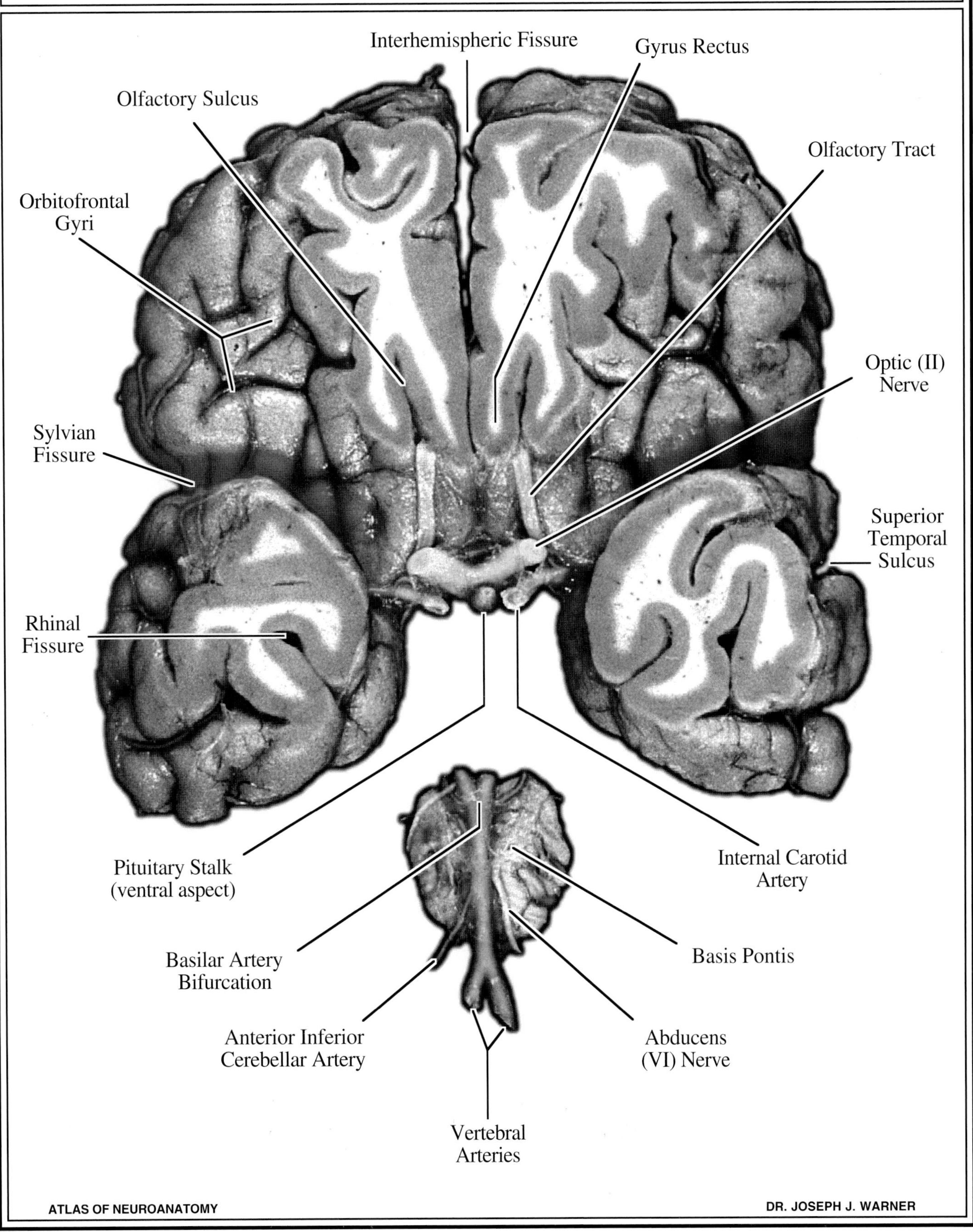

SECTION OF THE BRAIN, PLANE PARALLEL TO THE LONGITUDINAL AXIS OF THE BRAINSTEM: CAUDAL TO ROSTRAL PERSPECTIVE

ATLAS OF NEUROANATOMY

DR. JOSEPH J. WARNER

1. Rostral Cervical Spinal Cord
2. Gracile Tubercle
3. Hypoglossal Trigone
4. Median Fissure
5. Posterior Lobe of the Cerebellum
6. Middle Cerebellar Peduncle
7. Locus Coeruleus
8. Superior Cerebellar Peduncle
9. Decussation of the Superior Cerebellar Peduncle
10. Parahippocampal Gyrus
11. Inferior Temporal Gyrus
12. Middle Temporal Sulcus
13. Temporal Horn of the Lateral Ventricle
14. Middle Temporal Gyrus
15. Superior Temporal Sulcus
16. Superior Temporal Gyrus
17. Lateral Geniculate Nucleus
18. Branches of the Middle Cerebral Artery in the Sylvian Fissure
19. Insular Cortex
20. Extreme Capsule
21. External Capsule
22. Putamen
23. Posterior Limb of the Internal Capsule
24. Caudate Nucleus
25. Thalamostriate Vein
26. Dorsomedial Nucleus of the Thalamus
27. Cingulate Gyrus
28. Septum Pellucidum
29. Fornix
30. Anterior Nucleus of the Thalamus
31. Internal Medullary Lamina of the Thalamus
32. Transcapsular Caudatolenticular Gray Striae
33. Red Nucleus
34. Claustrum
35. External Medullary Lamina
36. Globus Pallidus
37. Subthalamic Nucleus
38. Substantia Nigra
39. Tail of the Caudate Nucleus
40. Hippocampal Formation
41. Cerebral Peduncle
42. Collateral Sulcus
43. Fusiform Gyrus
44. Primary Fissure of the Cerebellum
45. Anterior Lobe of the Cerebellum
46. Lateral Lemniscus
47. Facial Colliculus
48. Foramen of Luschka
49. Surface Contour of the Inferior Cerebellar Peduncle
50. Cerebellar Tonsil
51. Vagal Trigone

NEUROANATOMY OF SECTIONS PERPENDICULAR TO THE LONGITUDINAL AXIS OF THE BRAINSTEM OR PARALLEL TO THE PARIETO-OCCIPITAL SULCUS

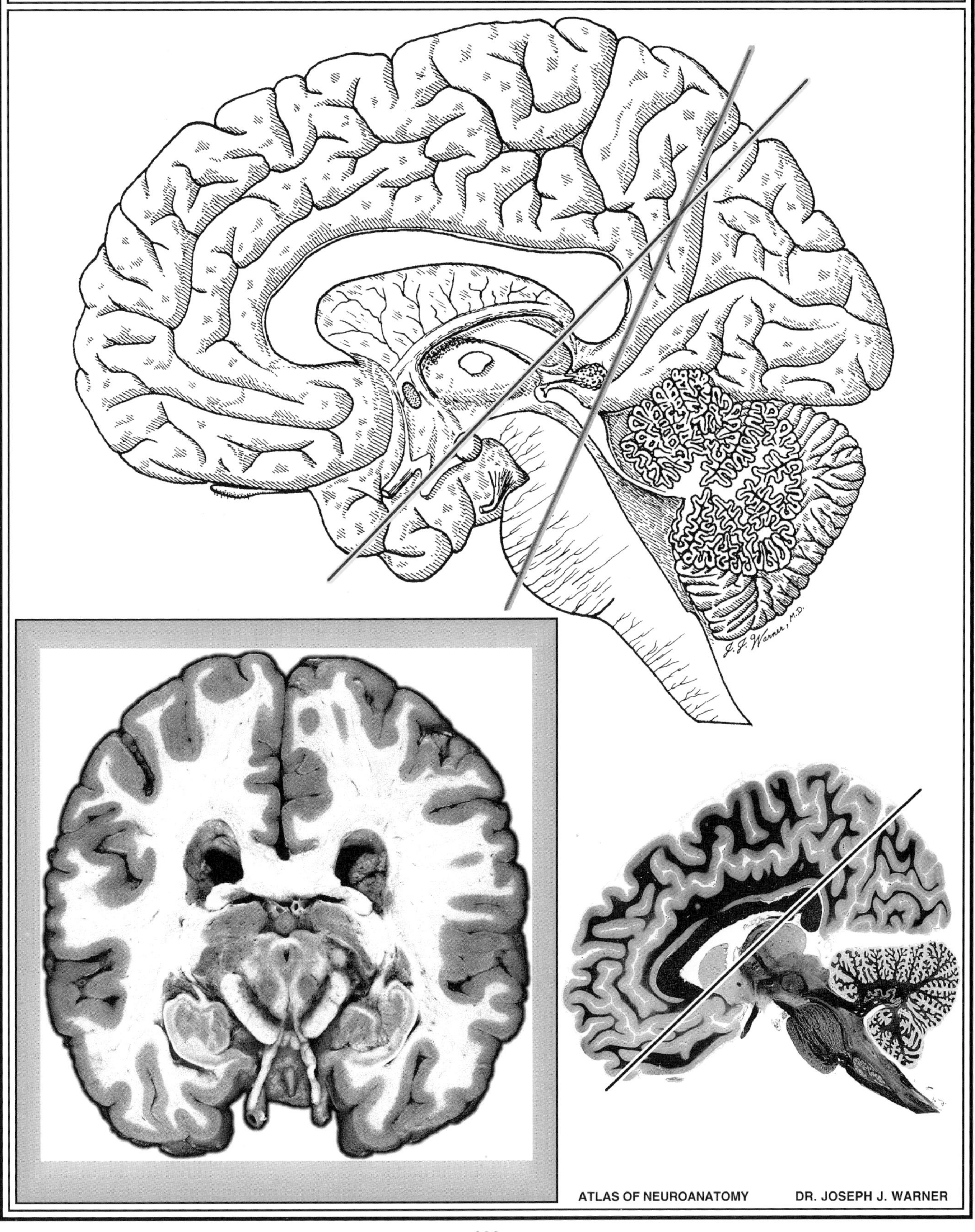

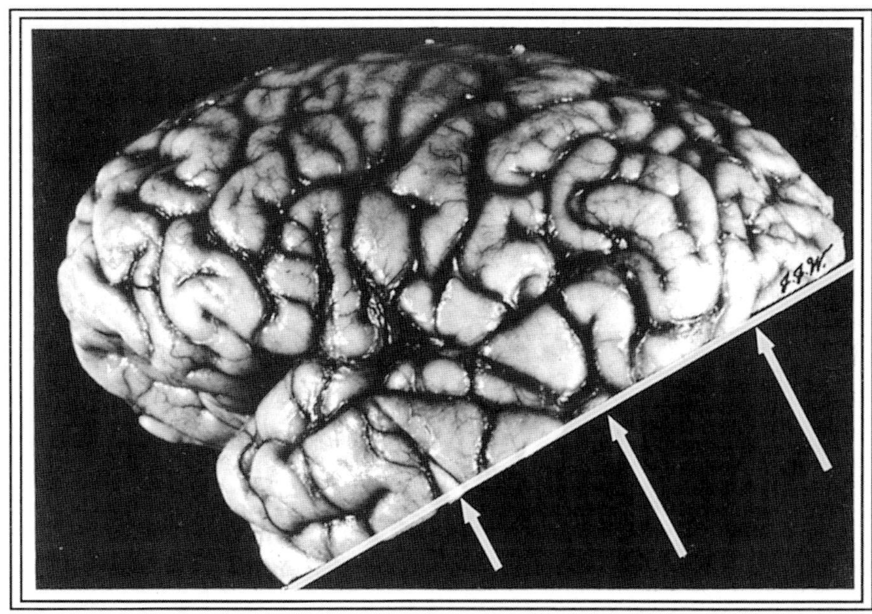

Lateral view of brain specimen cut in a plane perpendicular to the longitudinal axis of the brainstem. The cut surface of this specimen is shown below, with a view in the direction indicated by the white arrows, from the caudal inferior aspect of the section to the rostral and dorsal direction.

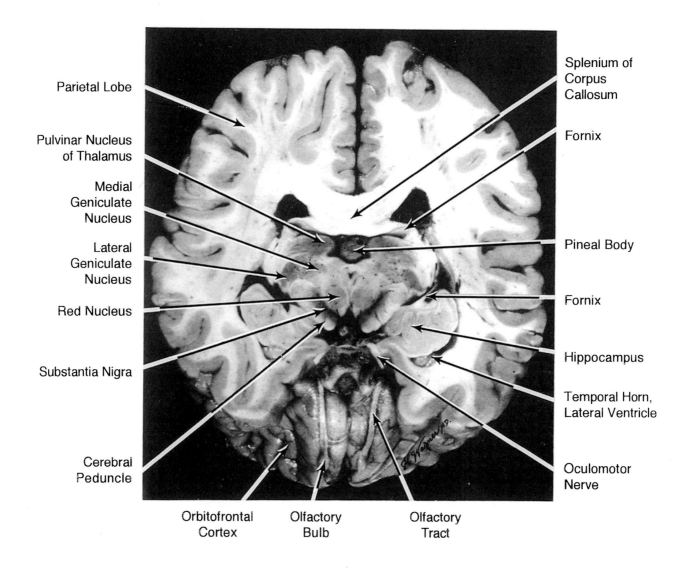

Parietal Lobe

Pulvinar Nucleus of Thalamus

Medial Geniculate Nucleus

Lateral Geniculate Nucleus

Red Nucleus

Substantia Nigra

Cerebral Peduncle

Splenium of Corpus Callosum

Fornix

Pineal Body

Fornix

Hippocampus

Temporal Horn, Lateral Ventricle

Oculomotor Nerve

Orbitofrontal Cortex

Olfactory Bulb

Olfactory Tract

This magnified view of the above section (perpendicular to the longitudinal axis of the brainstem) demonstrates the close spatial relationship of the hippocampus to the mesencephalon. Note the relative positions of the fornix, lateral geniculate, medial geniculate, and pulvinar nuclei. This view also clearly shows the course of the caudate nucleus as it follows the lateral wall of the lateral ventricle, recurving ventrally and rostrally into the roof of the temporal horn of the lateral ventricle. Fibers of the optic radiations, emanating from the lateral geniculate nucleus, pass into the temporal lobe, medial to the tail of the caudate nucleus, indenting the temporal horn of the lateral ventricle. This group of fibers, Meyer's Loop, then recurves caudally toward the occipital lobe to terminate in the ipsilateral primary visual cortex (Brodmann's area 17). This plane of section also passes through the fornix as it emanates from the hippocampus, and again as it approaches the midline as the crus of the fornix. Observe the close spatial relationship of the medial caudal aspect of the pulvinar nuclei, dorsal mesencephalon, pineal body, and internal cerebral veins, all bordering the subarachnoid space ventral to the splenium of the corpus callosum.

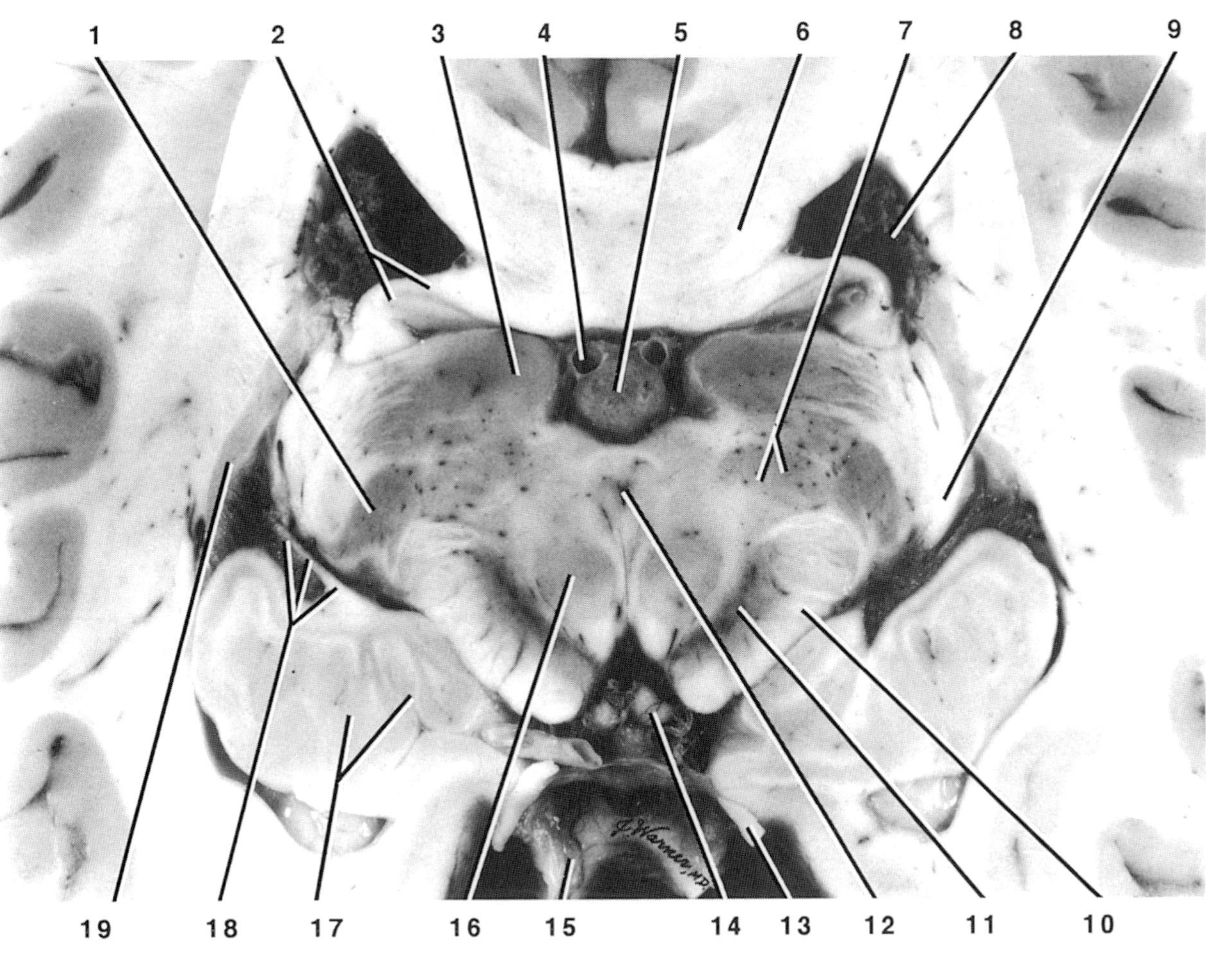

1. Lateral Geniculate Nucleus
2. Crus of the Fornix
3. Pulvinar Nucleus
4. Internal Cerebral Vein
5. Pineal Body
6. Splenium, Corpus Callosum
7. Medial Geniculate Nucleus
8. Lateral Ventricle
9. Optic radiations, Meyer's Loop
10. Cerebral Peduncle
11. Substantia Nigra
12. Aqueduct of Sylvius
13. Oculomotor Nerve
14. Mammillary Body
15. Optic Nerve
16. Red Nucleus
17. Hippocampus
18. Fornix
19. Tail of the Caudate Nucleus

COMPLETE SECTION OF THE BRAIN, PLANE PERPENDICULAR TO THE LONGITUDINAL AXIS OF THE BRAINSTEM, LEVEL OF THE MESENCEPHALON: CAUDAL TO ROSTRAL PERSPECTIVE

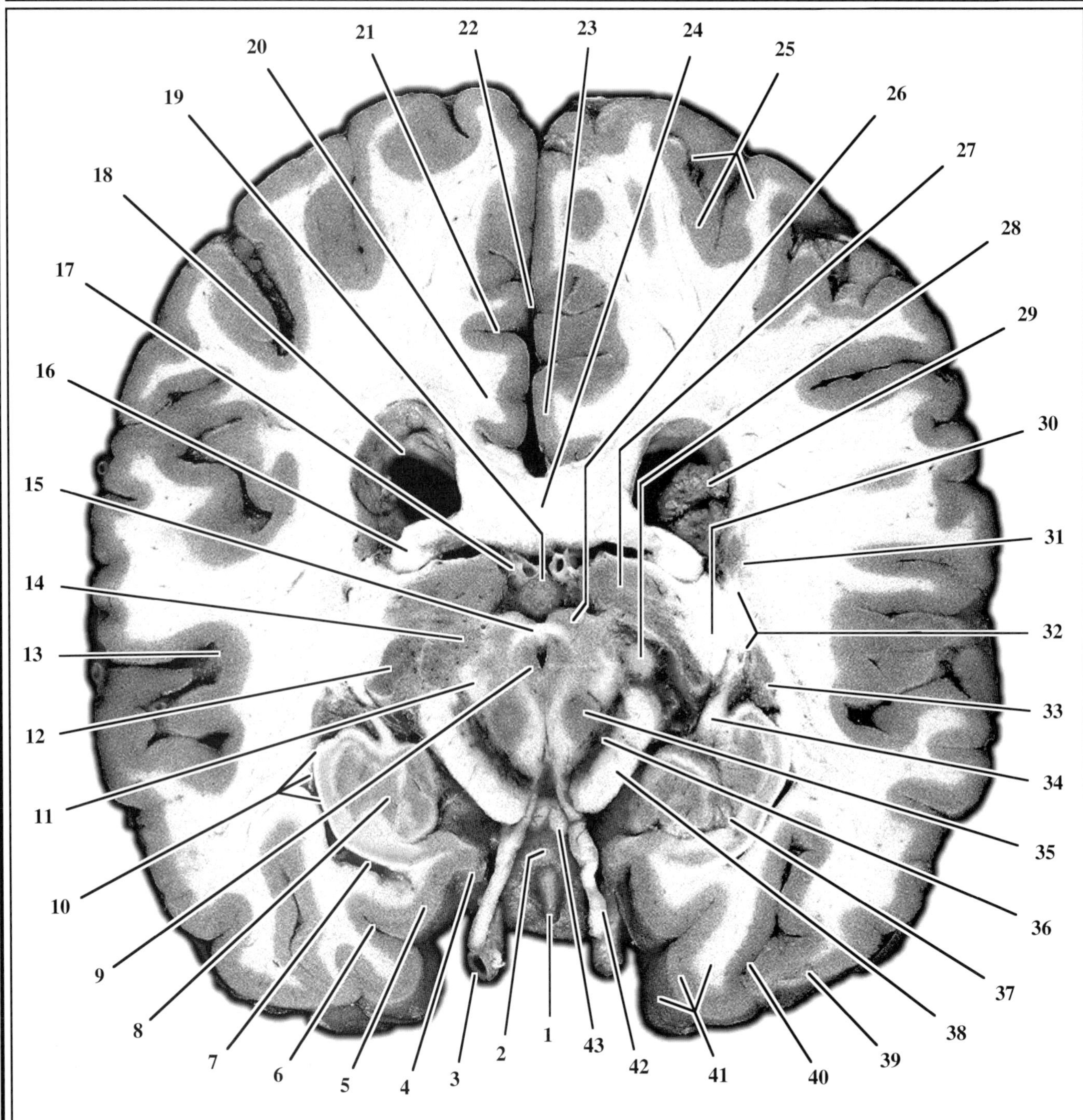

This plane of section, perpendicular to the longitudinal axis of the brainstem, includes a transverse section of the mesencephalon. The caudal to rostral perspective demonstrates surrounding diencephalic and telencephalic structures. The contiguous relationship of the medial and lateral geniculate nuclei and the pulvinar nucleus of the thalamus, adjacent to the dorsolateral mesencephalon, is clearly demonstrated. The lateral geniculate nucleus and the tail of the caudate are two gray matter structures in proximity to the hippocampus. The caudate is laterally situated as it follows the dorsolateral surface of the temporal horn of the lateral ventricle. The lateral geniculate nucleus, in contrast, borders on the subarachnoid space rather than the ventricle, is medial to the choroidal fissure, and is lateral to the cerebral peduncle. The medial geniculate nucleus is juxtaposed to the dorsolateral aspect of the mesencephalon, ventral to the pulvinar nucleus.

COMPLETE SECTION OF THE BRAIN, PLANE PERPENDICULAR TO THE LONGITUDINAL AXIS OF THE BRAINSTEM, LEVEL OF THE MESENCEPHALON: CAUDAL TO ROSTRAL PERSPECTIVE SECTION ORIENTATION AND KEY TO NUMBERED STRUCTURES

KEY TO NUMBERED STRUCTURES

1. Pituitary Stalk
2. Median Eminence
3. Internal Carotid Artery
4. Uncus
5. Parahippocampal Gyrus
6. Collateral Sulcus
7. Temporal Horn of the Lateral Ventricle
8. Hippocampus
9. Periaqueductal Gray
10. Alveus
11. Medial Lemniscus
12. Lateral Geniculate Nucleus
13. Insular Cortex
14. Medial Geniculate Nucleus
15. Posterior Commissure
16. Fornix*
17. Internal Cerebral Vein
18. Atrium of the Lateral Ventricle
19. Pineal Body
20. Cingulum
21. Cingulate Sulcus
22. Interhemispheric Fissure
23. Cingulate Cortex
24. Splenium of the Corpus Callosum
25. Posterior Parietal Lobe
26. Superior Colliculus
27. Pulvinar
28. Medial Geniculate Nucleus
29. Choroid Plexus
30. Geniculocalcarine Radiations
31. Tail of the Caudate Nucleus*
32. Stria Terminalis and Thalamostriate Vein*
33. Tail of the Caudate Nucleus*
34. Fornix*
35. Red Nucleus
36. Substantia Nigra
37. Hippocampal Fissure
38. Cerebral Peduncle
39. Inferior Temporal Gyrus
40. Inferior Temporal Sulcus
41. Fusiform Gyrus
42. Oculomotor (III) Nerve
43. Mammillary Body

*The stria terminalis and thalamostriate vein course parallel to the tail of the caudate from the body of the lateral ventricle into the temporal horn. The fornix is also characterized by a gradual 180+ degree curve. Thus, these structures pass twice through the plane of section.

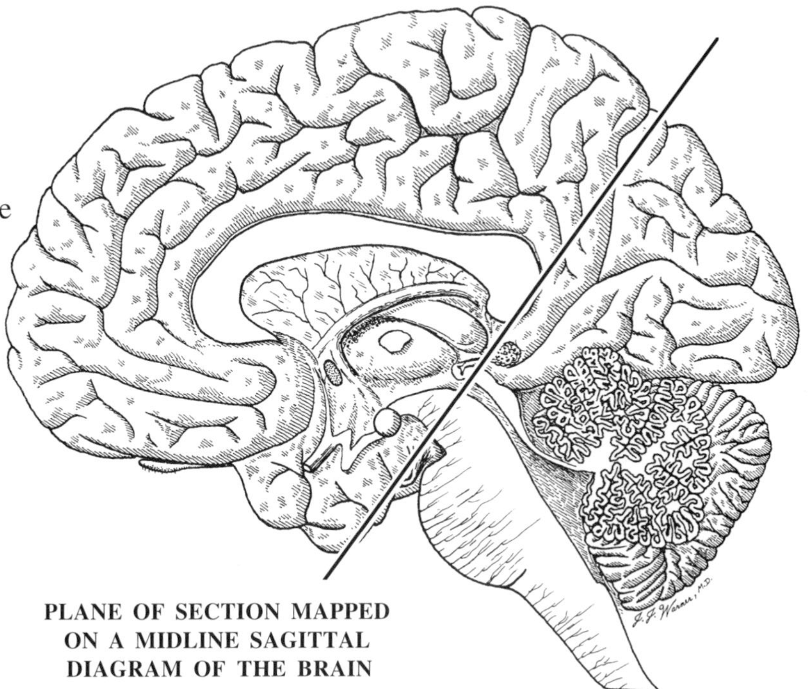

PLANE OF SECTION MAPPED ON A MIDLINE SAGITTAL DIAGRAM OF THE BRAIN

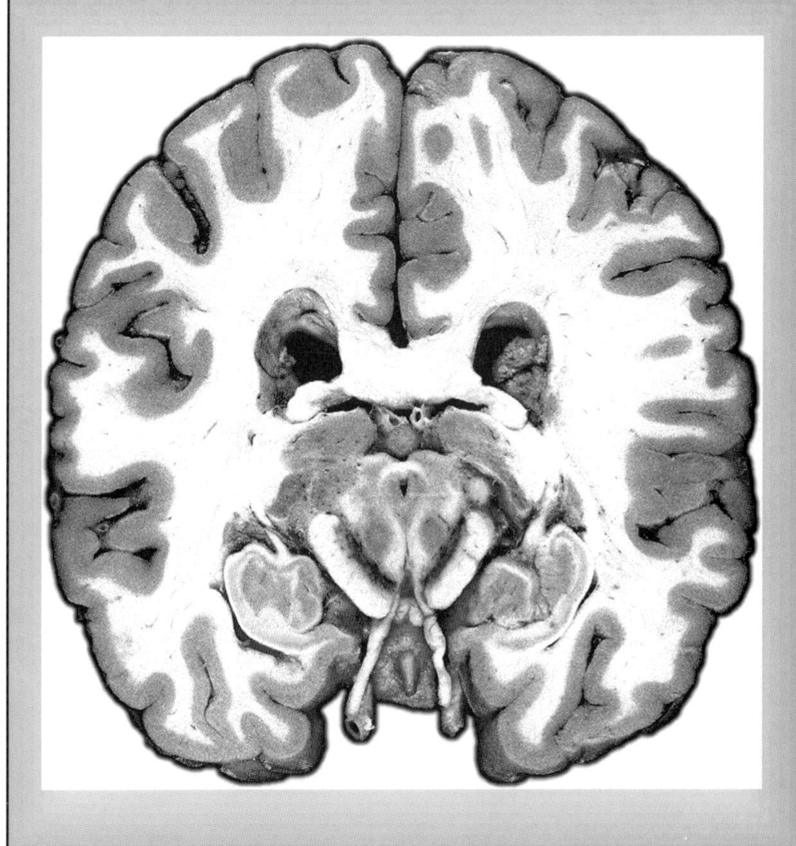

SECTION OF THE BRAIN PERPENDICULAR TO THE LONGITUDINAL AXIS OF THE BRAINSTEM, LEVEL OF THE MESENCEPHALON, CAUDAL TO ROSTRAL PERSPECTIVE: MAGNIFIED VIEW

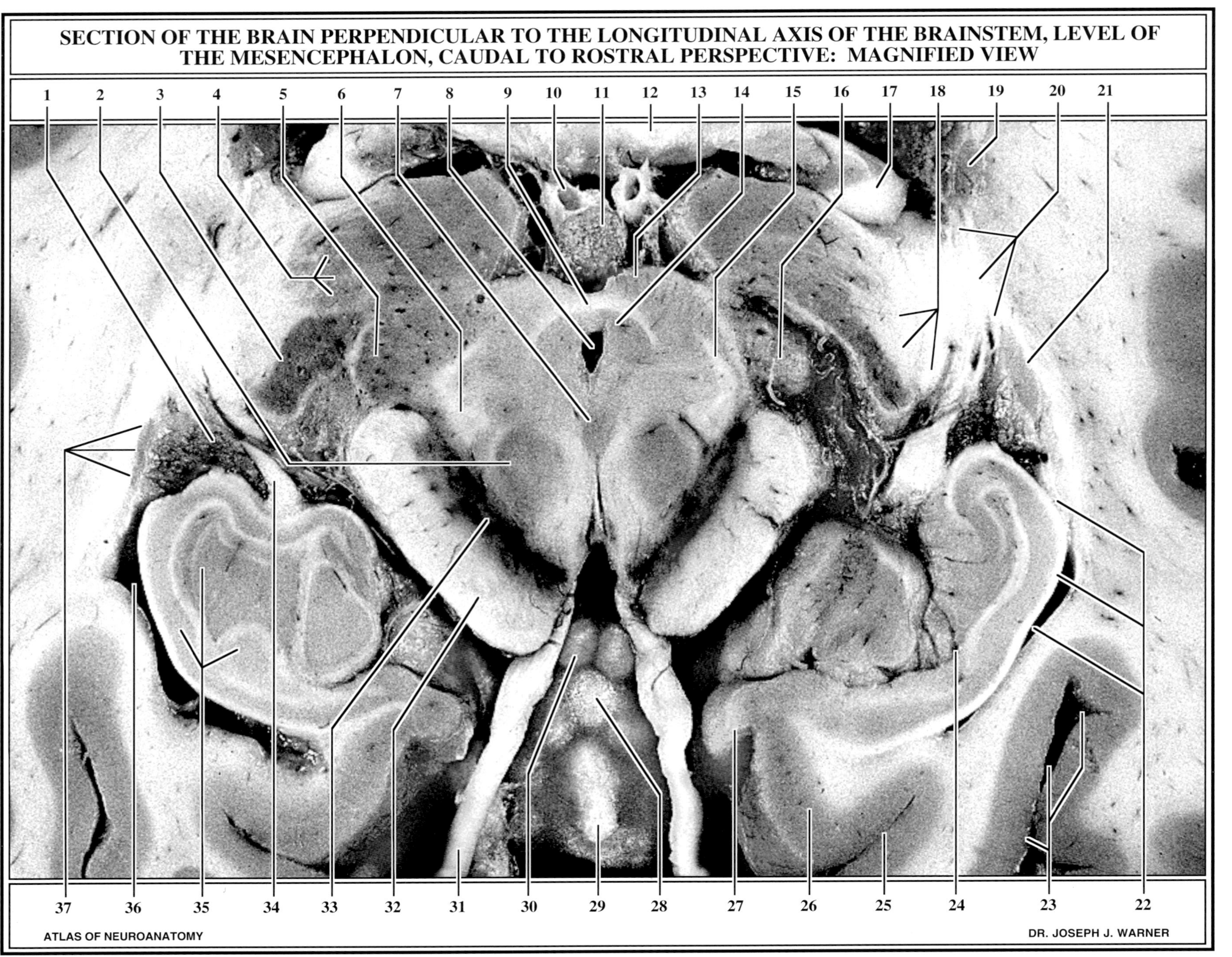

ATLAS OF NEUROANATOMY

DR. JOSEPH J. WARNER

SECTION OF THE BRAIN PERPENDICULAR TO THE LONGITUDINAL AXIS OF THE BRAINSTEM, LEVEL OF THE MESENCEPHALON: MAGNIFIED VIEW, CAUDAL TO ROSTRAL PERSPECTIVE
SECTION ORIENTATION AND KEY TO NUMBERED STRUCTURES

KEY TO NUMBERED STRUCTURES

1. Choroid Plexus of the Temporal Horn
2. Red Nucleus
3. Lateral Geniculate Nucleus
4. Pulvinar Nucleus of the Thalamus
5. Medial Geniculate Nucleus
6. Medial Lemniscus
7. Oculomotor (III) Nuclear Complex
8. Aqueduct of Sylvius
9. Caudal Aspect of the Posterior Commissure
10. Internal Cerebral Vein
11. Pineal Body
12. Splenium of the Corpus Callosum
13. Superior Colliculus
14. Periaqueductal Gray
15. Spinothalamic Tract
16. Medial Geniculate Nucleus
17. Fornix
18. Geniculocalcarine Radiations
19. Tail of the Caudate Nucleus
20. Stria Terminalis and Thalamostriate Vein
21. Tail of the Caudate Nucleus
22. Alveus
23. Inferior Temporal Sulcus
24. Hippocampal Fissure
25. Collateral Sulcus
26. Parahippocampal Gyrus
27. Uncus
28. Median Eminence
29. Pituitary Stalk
30. Mammillary Body
31. Oculomotor (III) Nerve
32. Cerebral Peduncle
33. Substantia Nigra
34. Fimbria of the Fornix
35. Hippocampus
36. Temporal Horn of the Lateral Ventricle
37. Tail of the Caudate Nucleus

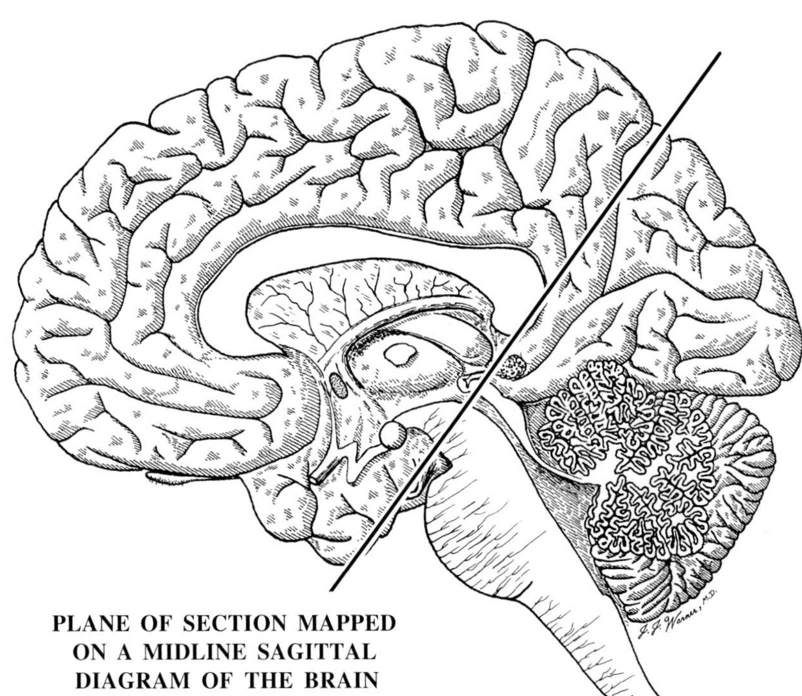

PLANE OF SECTION MAPPED ON A MIDLINE SAGITTAL DIAGRAM OF THE BRAIN

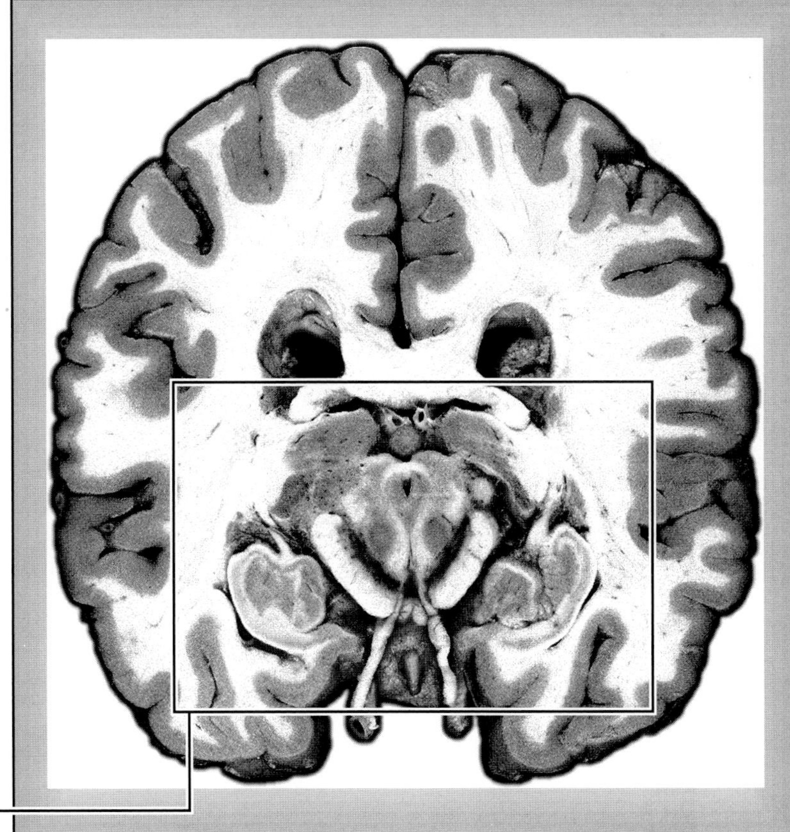

AREA OF MAGNIFIED VIEW MAPPED ON COMPLETE SECTION

COMPLETE SECTION OF THE BRAIN PARALLEL TO THE PARIETO-OCCIPITAL SULCUS: PLANE INCLUDING THE ANTERIOR PERFORATED SUBSTANCE, GLOBUS PALLIDUS, AND DORSOMEDIAL NUCLEUS OF THE THALAMUS

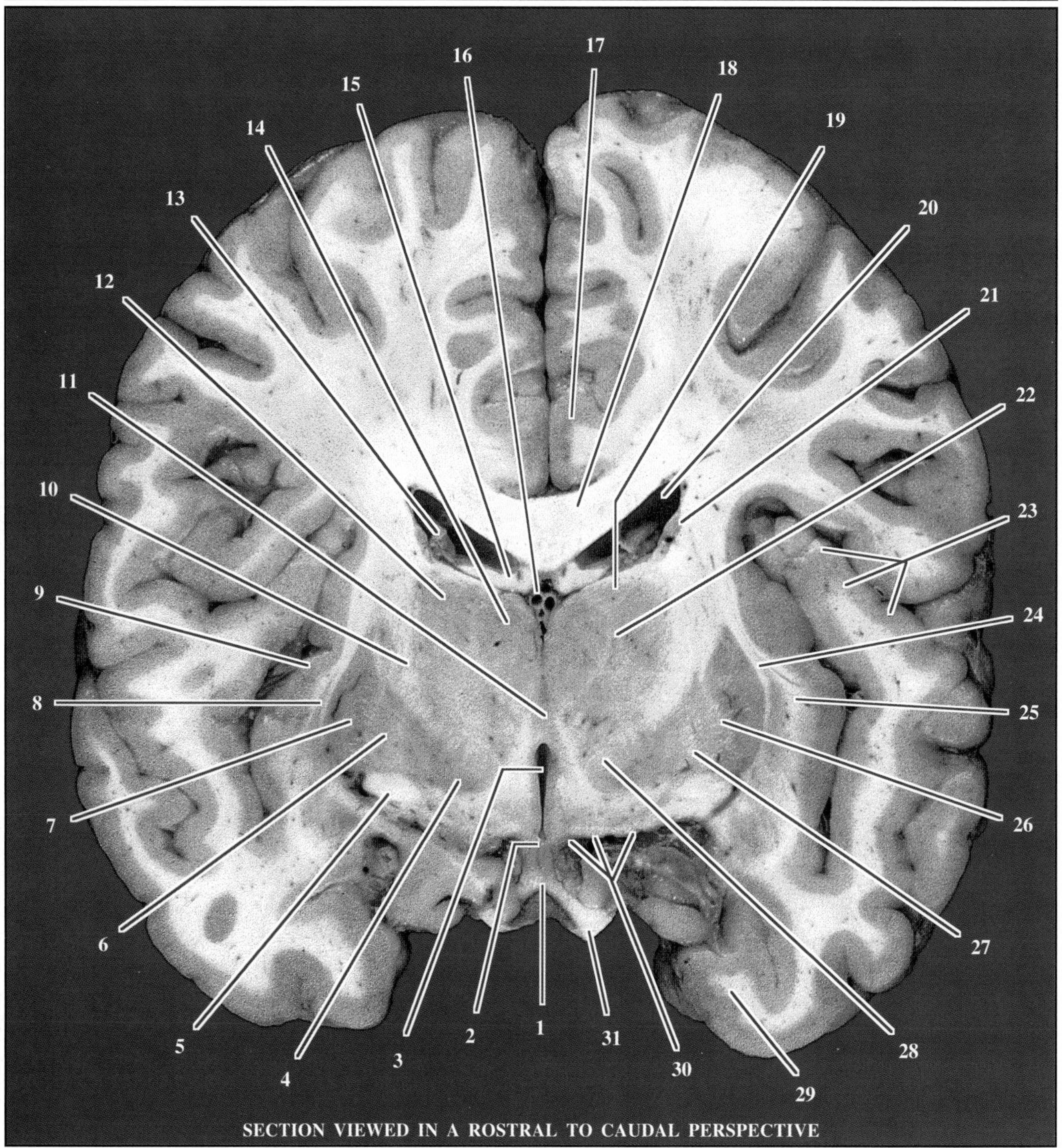

SECTION VIEWED IN A ROSTRAL TO CAUDAL PERSPECTIVE

The orientation of this plane of section provides visualization of relatively rostral structures ventrally, including the anterior perforated substance and the lamina terminalis forming the rostral wall of the supraoptic recess of the third ventricle. The optic nerves are oriented toward the observer. The anterior commissure passes through the section plane twice, as it crosses the midline rostral and dorsal to its lateral course. The plane of section demonstrates the transverse gyrus of Heschl and the planum temporale. The dorsal aspect of the section passes through relatively caudal structures, including the lateral dorsal nucleus and the lateral posterior nucleus of the thalamus. The flat, ribbon-like morphology of the fornix is characteristic of this structure as it courses dorsal to the thalamus.

COMPLETE SECTION OF THE BRAIN PARALLEL TO THE PARIETO-OCCIPITAL SULCUS; PLANE INCLUDING THE ANTERIOR PERFORATED SUBSTANCE, GLOBUS PALLIDUS, AND DORSOMEDIAL NUCLEUS OF THE THALAMUS: ORIENTATION AND KEY TO NUMBERED STRUCTURES

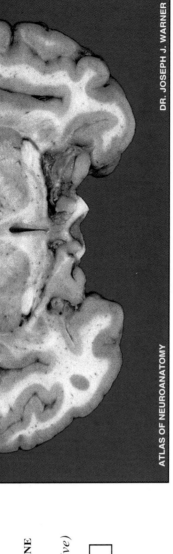

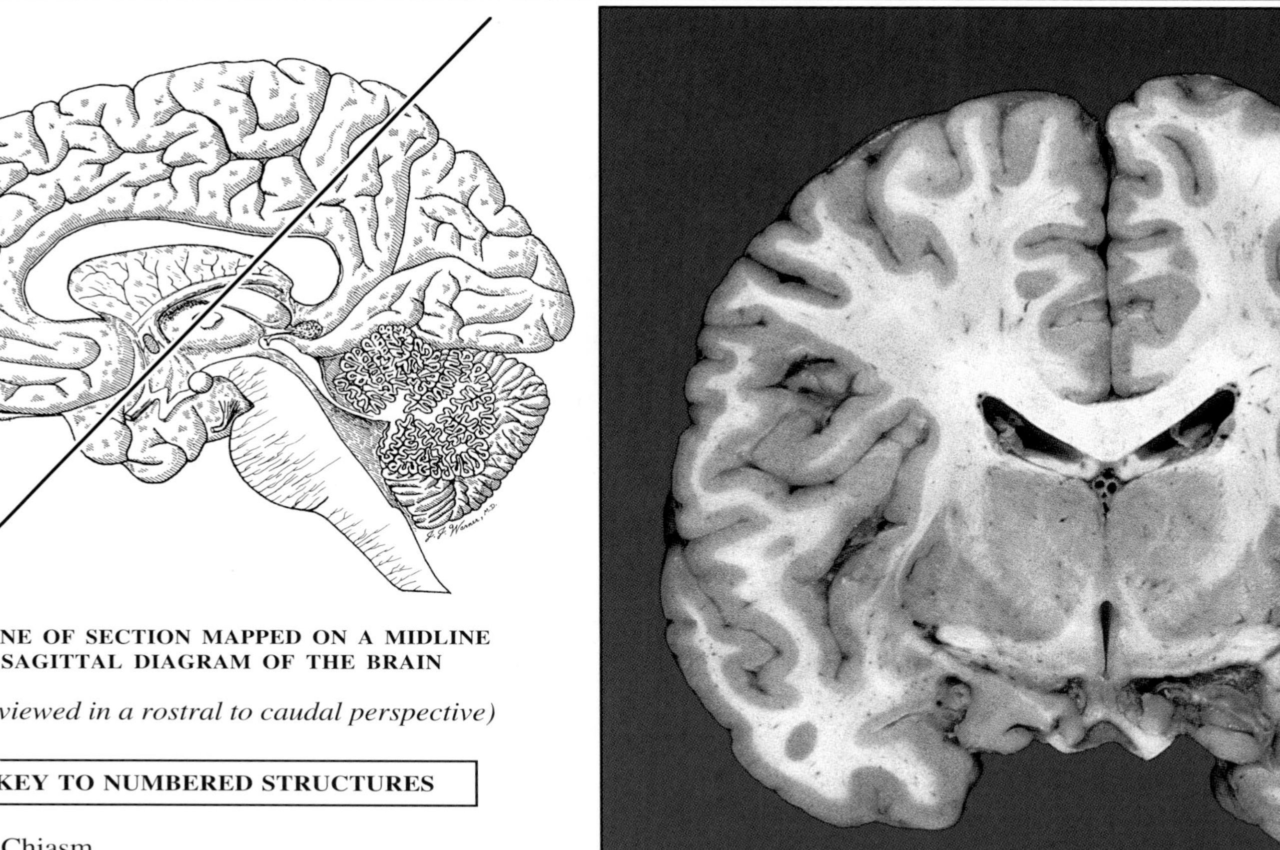

PLANE OF SECTION MAPPED ON A MIDLINE SAGITTAL DIAGRAM OF THE BRAIN

(Section viewed in a rostral to caudal perspective)

KEY TO NUMBERED STRUCTURES

1. Optic Chiasm
2. Lamina Terminalis
3. Third Ventricle
4. Globus Pallidus I
5. Anterior Commissure
6. Globus Pallidus II
7. Putamen
8. Claustrum
9. Insular Cortex
10. Posterior Limb of the Internal Capsule
11. Massa Intermedia
12. Lateral Posterior Nucleus of the Thalamus
13. Choroid Plexus
14. Dorsomedial Nucleus of the Thalamus
15. Fornix
16. Internal Cerebral Vein
17. Cingulate Gyrus
18. Body of the Corpus Callosum
19. Lateral Dorsal Nucleus of the Thalamus
20. Body of the Lateral Ventricle
21. Caudate Nucleus
22. Internal Medullary Lamina of the Thalamus
23. Transverse Gyrus of Heschl
24. External Capsule
25. Extreme Capsule
26. External Medullary Lamina
27. Internal Medullary Lamina
28. Genu of the Internal Capsule
29. Parahippocampal Gyrus
30. Anterior Perforated Substance
31. Optic Nerve

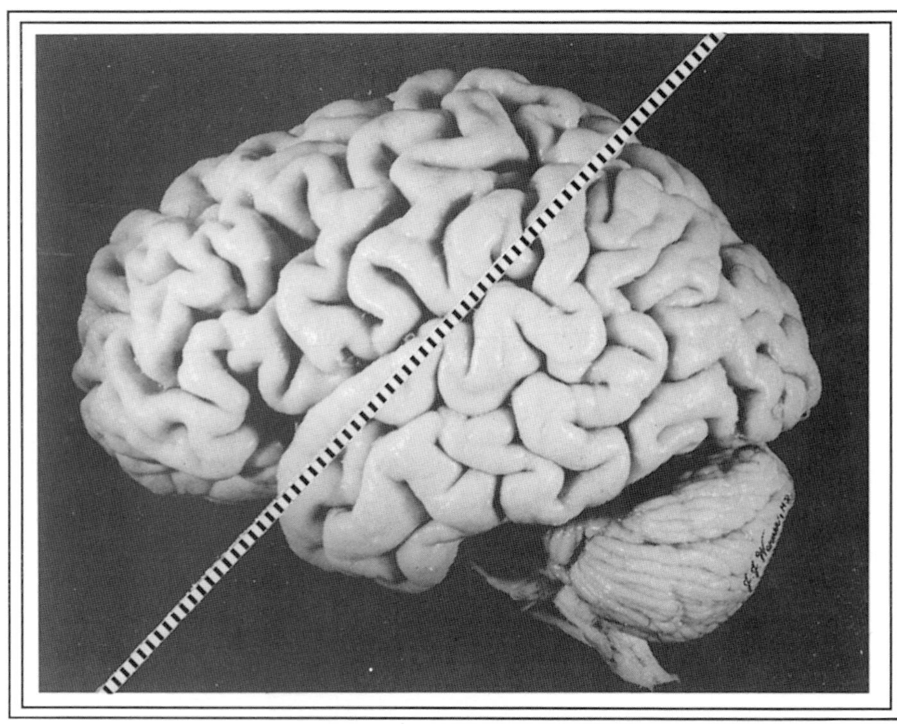

Lateral view of the brain, upon which is mapped the orientation of the section below. The plane of section is approximately perpendicular to the longitudinal axis of the brainstem.

This orientation includes rostral telencephalic structures ventrally, and more caudal structures dorsally. The rostral aspect of the superior temporal gyrus comprises most of the temporal lobe included in this section.

Note the extensive course of the Sylvian fissure demonstrated by this plane of section. The parietal lobe constitutes the upper half of the telencephalon visible in this orientation. Passing through the basal forebrain and structures ventral to the rostrum of the corpus callosum, this plane includes the caudal aspect of the orbitofrontal gyri.

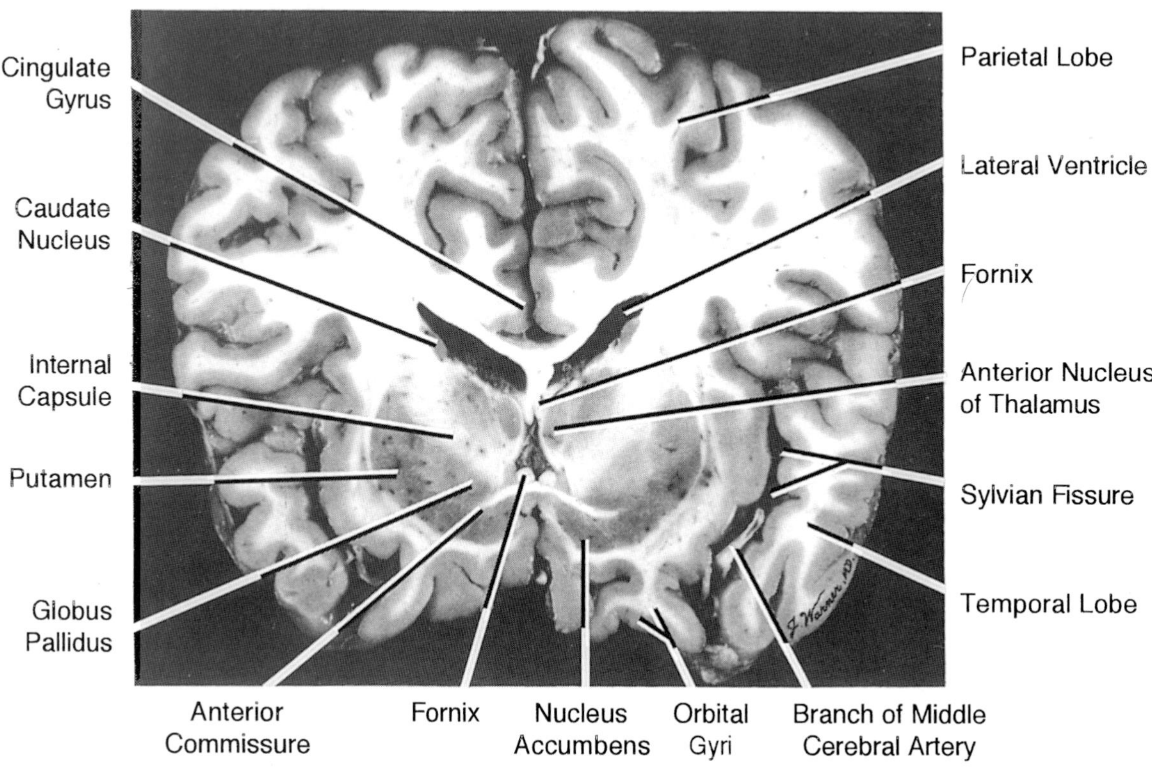

The following is a magnified view of the previous section. In this plane of section, the fornix appears as it courses over the anterior nucleus of the thalamus, and again as the post-commissural fibers recurve, adjacent to the anterior commissure, in a ventral and caudal direction toward the mammillary bodies. Reference to the map of this section on a diagram of the midline sagittal section (see figure) clarifies this anatomic relationship. The morphology of the fornix is characterized by a flat, ribbon-like structure dorsal and caudal to the thalamus. Rostrally, however, the fibers approach midline and assume a cylindrical shape as they curve ventrally.

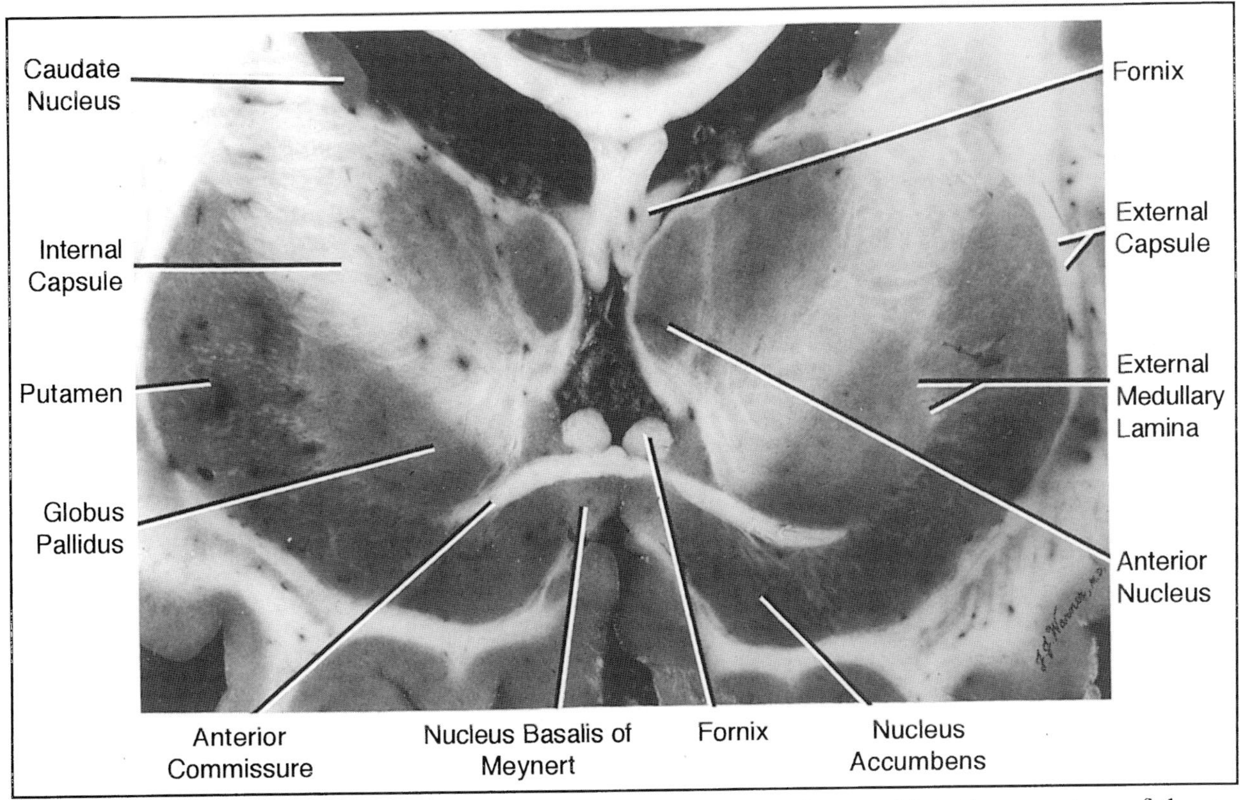

This section also includes a major portion of the anterior commissure. Note the curvature of these fibers as they cross the midline, concave toward the ventral and rostral telencephalon. As the fibers pass the ventral aspect of the globus pallidus, they recurve in the opposite direction. Thus, in conventional coronal or horizontal sections, the actual crossing of the anterior commissure is in a different plane from its lateral course.

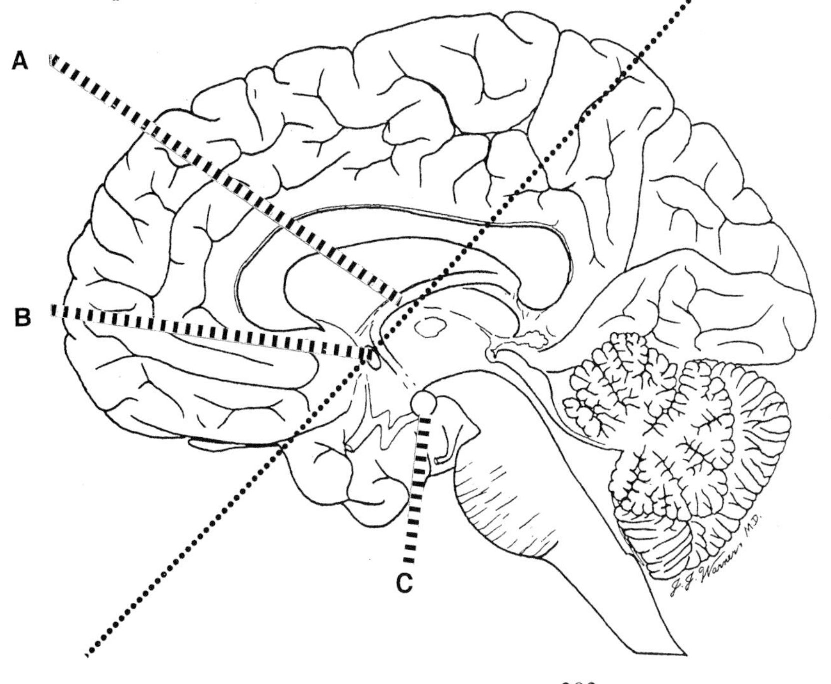

The plane of section is mapped on a midline sagittal diagram. Note the spatial relationships between the fornix (1), anterior commissure (2), and mammillary bodies (3). As shown by the diagram, this section crosses the fornix dorsal to the thalamus and again as it recurves caudal to the anterior commissure.

COMPLETE SECTION OF THE BRAIN, PLANE PARALLEL TO THE PARIETO-OCCIPITAL SULCUS: LEVEL OF THE PONTOMESENCEPHALIC JUNCTION (CAUDAL TO ROSTRAL PERSPECTIVE)

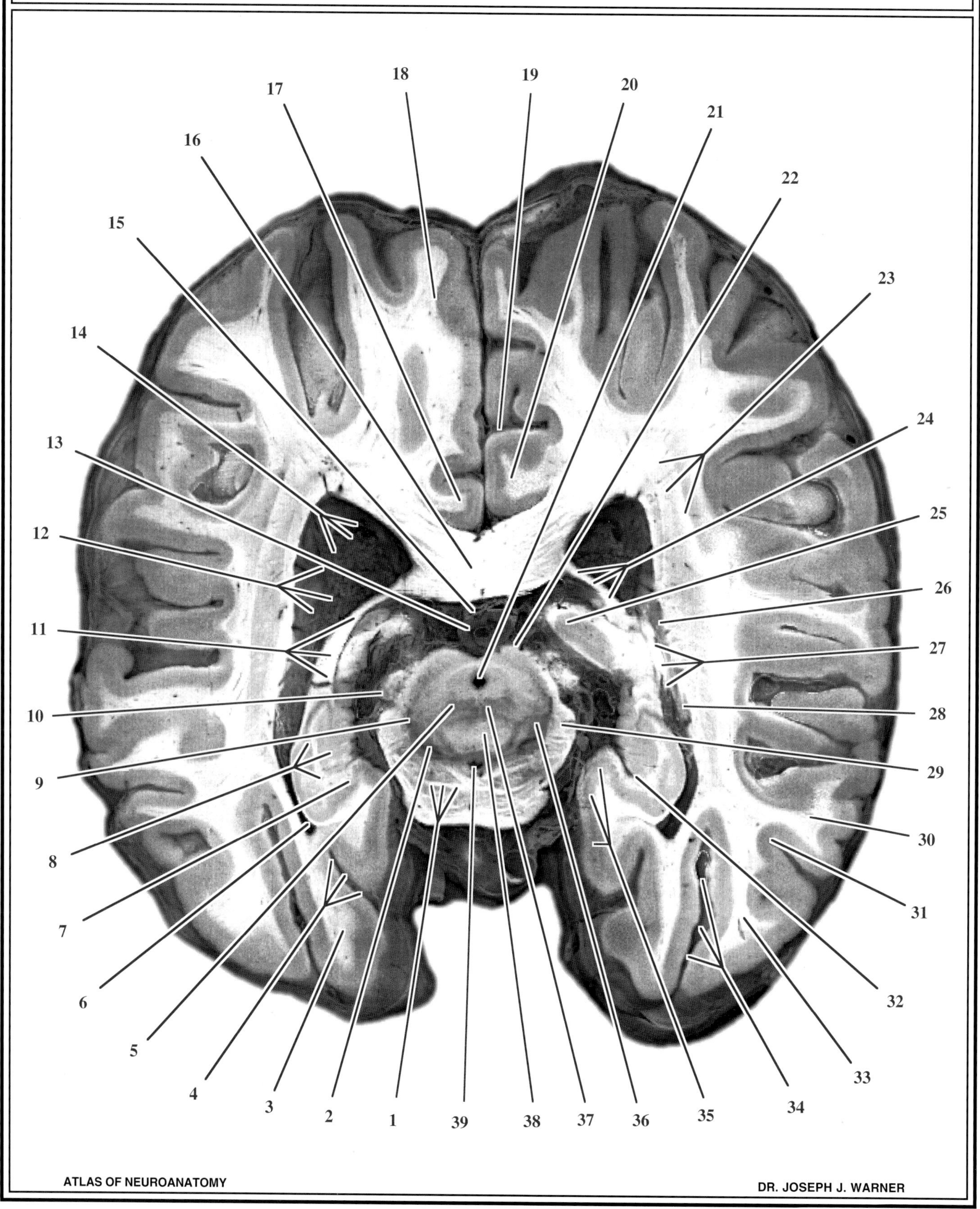

COMPLETE SECTION OF THE BRAIN, PLANE PARALLEL TO THE PARIETO-OCCIPITAL SULCUS: LEVEL OF THE PONTOMESENCEPHALIC JUNCTION (CAUDAL TO ROSTRAL PERSPECTIVE) SECTION MAP AND KEY TO NUMBERED STRUCTURES

KEY TO NUMBERED STRUCTURES

1. Transverse (Pontocerebellar) Fibers
2. Substantia Nigra
3. Fusiform Gyrus
4. Collateral Sulcus
5. Central Tegmental Tract
6. Temporal Horn of the Lateral Ventricle
7. Subiculum
8. Hippocampus
9. Spinothalamic Tract
10. Medial Geniculate Nucleus
11. Fornix
12. Atrium of the Lateral Ventricle
13. Pineal Recess of the Third Ventricle
14. Choroid Plexus
15. Pineal Body (rostral aspect)
16. Splenium of the Corpus Callosum
17. Cingulum (white matter tract)
18. Parietal Lobe
19. Cingulate Sulcus
20. Cingulate Gyrus
21. Aqueduct of Sylvius
22. Superior Colliculus
23. Optic Radiations
24. Fornix
25. Pulvinar Nucleus of the Thalamus
26. Tail of the Caudate Nucleus
27. Stria Terminalis
28. Tail of the Caudate Nucleus
29. Cerebral Peduncle
30. Middle Temporal Gyrus
31. Middle Temporal Sulcus
32. Hippocampal Fissure
33. Inferior Temporal Gyrus
34. Inferior Temporal Sulcus
35. Parahippocampal Gyrus
36. Medial Lemniscus
37. Medial Longitudinal Fasciculus
38. Decussation of the Superior Cerebellar Peduncles
39. Interpeduncular Fossa

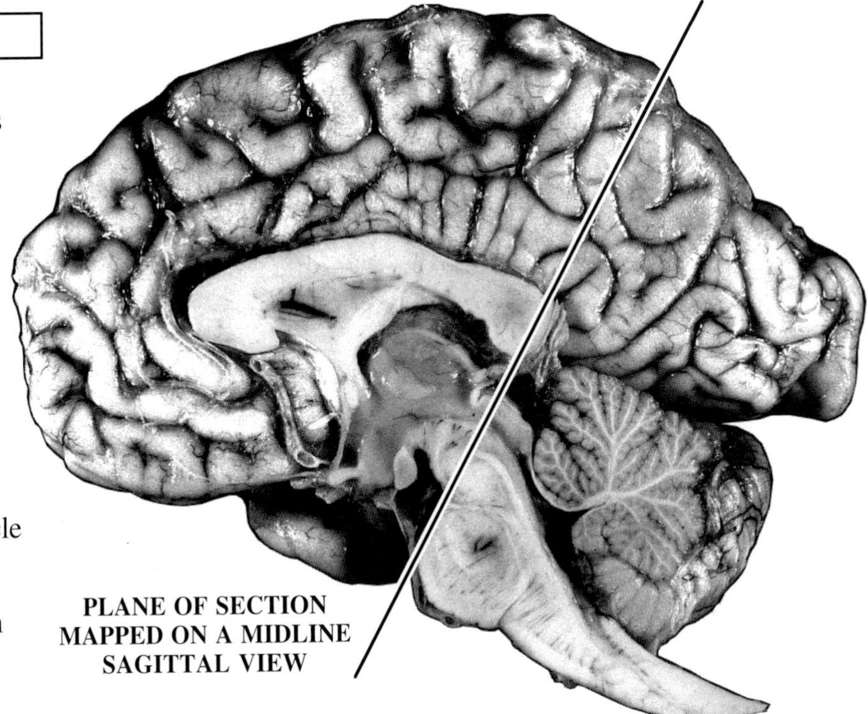

PLANE OF SECTION MAPPED ON A MIDLINE SAGITTAL VIEW

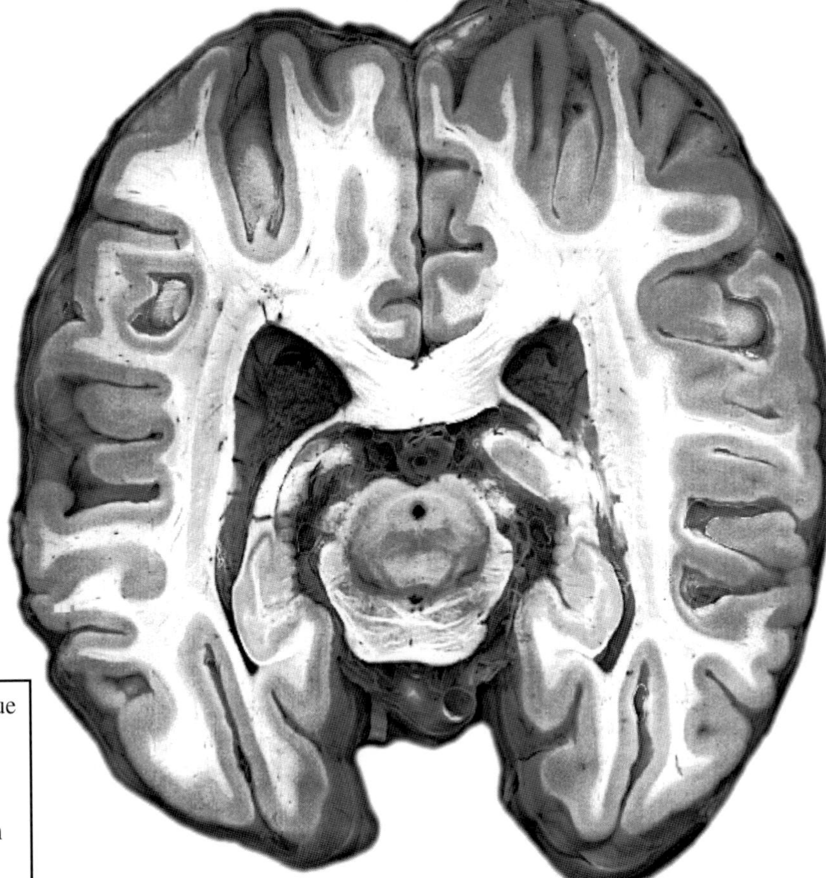

With the image histogram enhancement technique used in this section, transversely sectioned fiber tracts in the brainstem appear darker than those tracts with obliquely or longitudinally sectioned fibers. These tracts should not be confused with gray matter structures.

COMPLETE SECTION OF THE BRAIN; PLANE PARALLEL TO THE PARIETO-OCCIPITAL SULCUS: LEVEL INCLUDING THE POSTERIOR COMMISSURE AND THE LATERAL AND MEDIAL GENICULATE NUCLEI

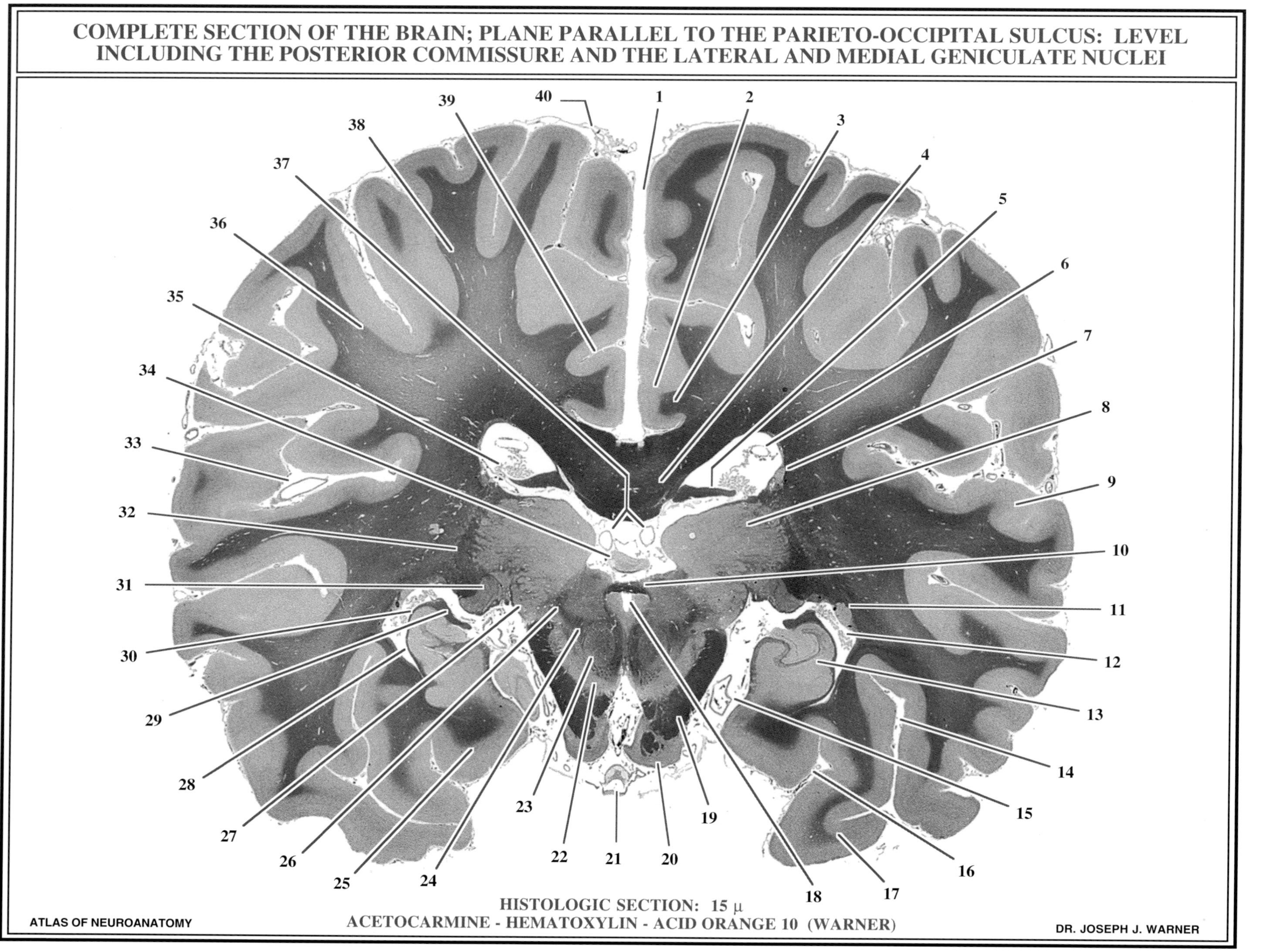

HISTOLOGIC SECTION: 15 μ
ACETOCARMINE - HEMATOXYLIN - ACID ORANGE 10 (WARNER)

DR. JOSEPH J. WARNER

COMPLETE SECTION OF THE BRAIN, PLANE PARALLEL TO THE PARIETO-OCCIPITAL SULCUS; LEVEL INCLUDING THE POSTERIOR COMMISSURE AND THE LATERAL AND MEDIAL GENICULATE NUCLEI: SECTION ORIENTATION AND KEY TO NUMBERED STRUCTURES

KEY TO NUMBERED STRUCTURES

1. Interhemispheric Fissure
2. Cingulate Cortex
3. Cingulum
4. Splenium of the Corpus Callosum
5. Fornix
6. Vein of the Choroid Plexus
7. Tail of the Caudate Nucleus
8. Pulvinar Nucleus of the Thalamus
9. Superior Temporal Gyrus
10. Posterior Commissure
11. Tail of the Caudate Nucleus
12. Choroid Plexus
13. Hippocampus
14. Inferior Temporal Sulcus
15. Posterior Cerebral Artery
16. Collateral Sulcus
17. Fusiform Gyrus
18. Aqueduct of Sylvius
19. Cerebral Peduncle
20. Basis Pontis and Pontine Gray
21. Basilar Artery
22. Substantia Nigra
23. Red Nucleus
24. Medial Lemniscus
25. Parahippocampal Gyrus
26. Spinothalamic and Trigeminothalamic Tracts
27. Medial Geniculate Nucleus
28. Temporal Horn of the Lateral Ventricle
29. Fimbria of the Fornix
30. Alveus
31. Lateral Geniculate Nucleus
32. Geniculocalcarine (Optic) Radiations
33. Middle Cerebral Artery
34. Pineal Body
35. Choroid Plexus in the Body of the Lateral Ventricle
36. Inferior Parietal Lobule
37. Internal Cerebral Veins
38. Superior Parietal Lobule
39. Cingulate Sulcus
40. Arachnoid Granulations

This plane of section clearly demonstrates the juxtaposition of the mesencephalon, metathalamus, thalamus, and epithalamus. The hippocampus surrounds the mesencephalic-diencephalic junction.

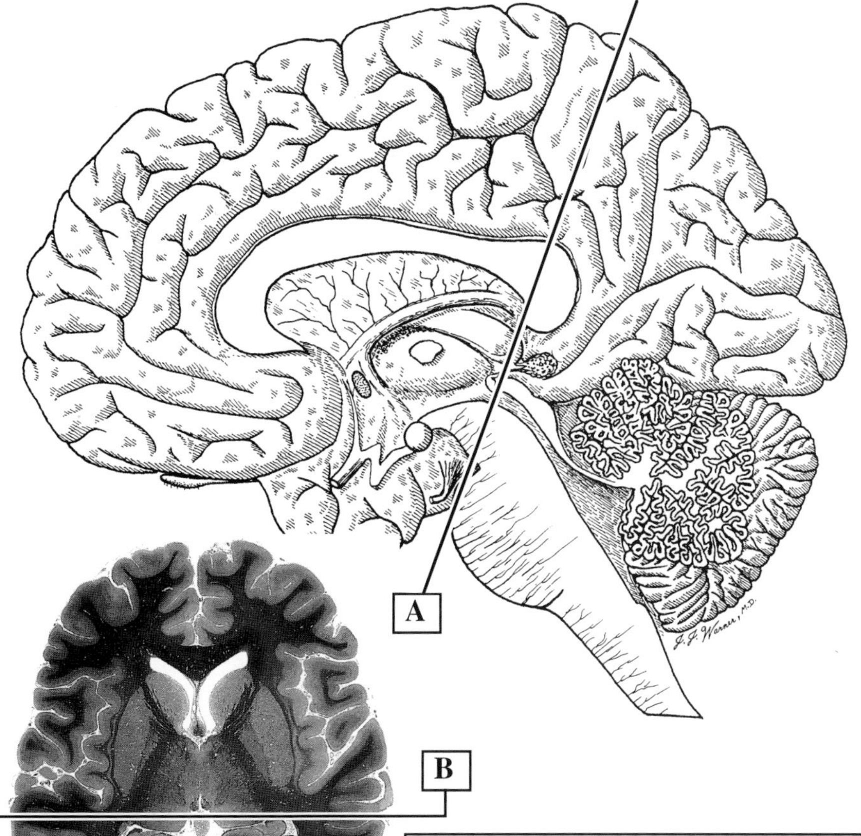

THE PLANE OF SECTION IS MAPPED IN REFERENCE TO (A) A MIDLINE SAGITTAL DIAGRAM, AND (B) A HORIZONTAL SECTION (LEVEL OF THE GENU OF THE CORPUS CALLOSUM AND THE PINEAL BODY)

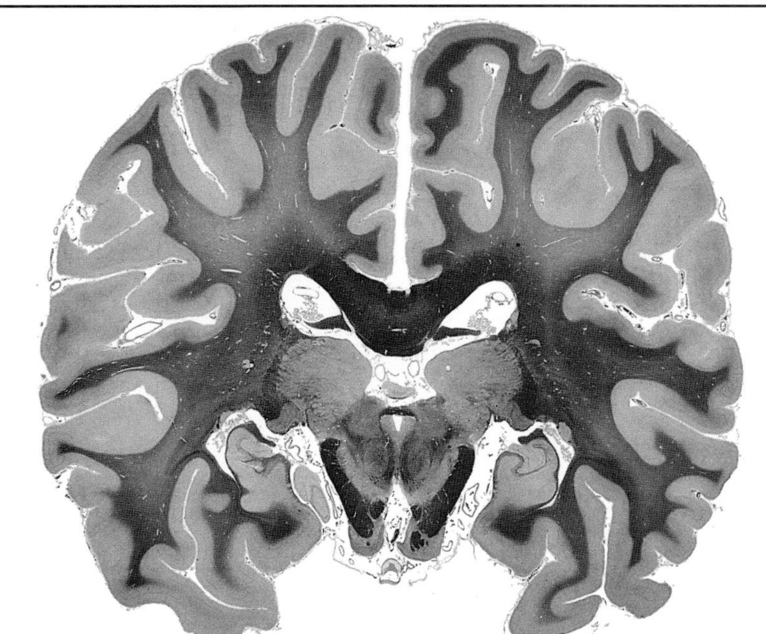

COMPARATIVE NEUROANATOMY: CORONAL SECTION OF THE FELINE BRAIN, LEVEL OF THE MESENCEPHALIC-DIENCEPHALIC TRANSITION

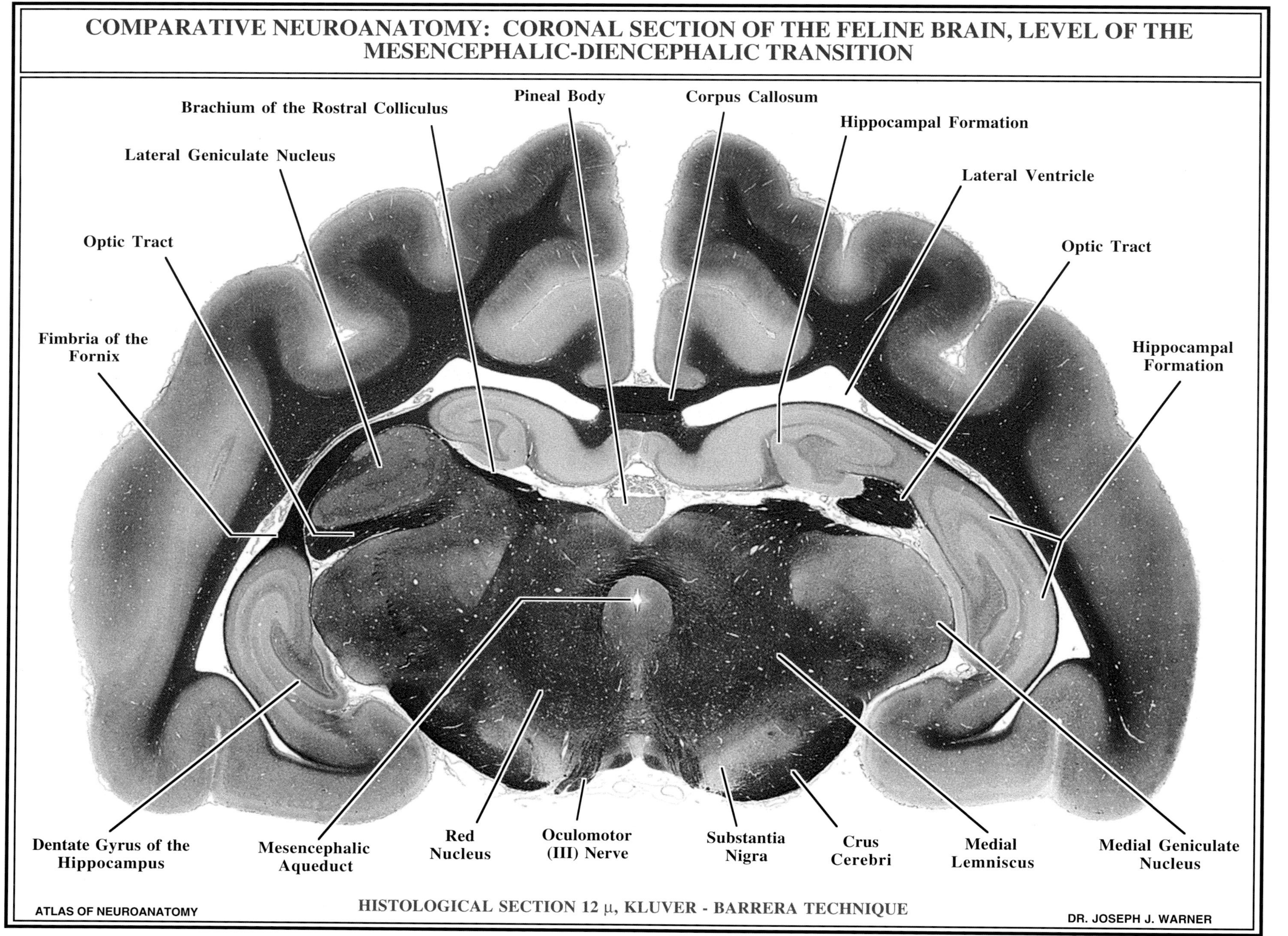

HISTOLOGICAL SECTION 12 μ, KLUVER - BARRERA TECHNIQUE

DR. JOSEPH J. WARNER

COMPARISON OF COMPLETE SECTIONS OF THE BRAIN OF THE CAT (A) AND HUMAN (B): PLANE INCLUDING THE MESENCEPHALON, HIPPOCAMPAL FORMATION, PINEAL BODY, AND THE LATERAL AND MEDIAL GENICULATE NUCLEI

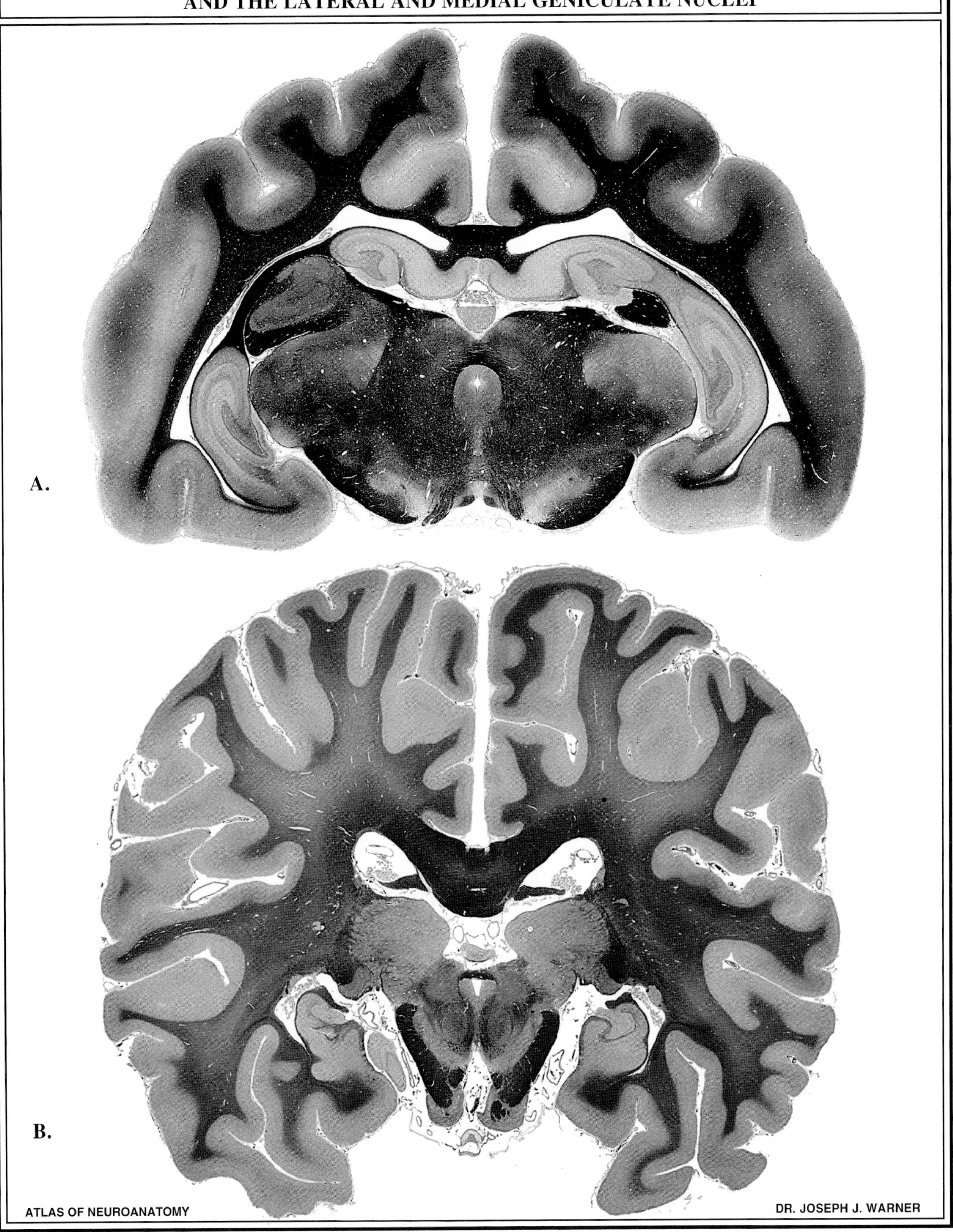

COMPLETE SECTION OF THE BRAIN, PLANE PARALLEL TO THE PARIETO-OCCIPITAL SULCUS: LEVEL OF THE CENTROMEDIAN NUCLEUS OF THE THALAMUS AND OF THE SUBTHALAMIC NUCLEUS (ROSTRAL TO CAUDAL PERSPECTIVE)

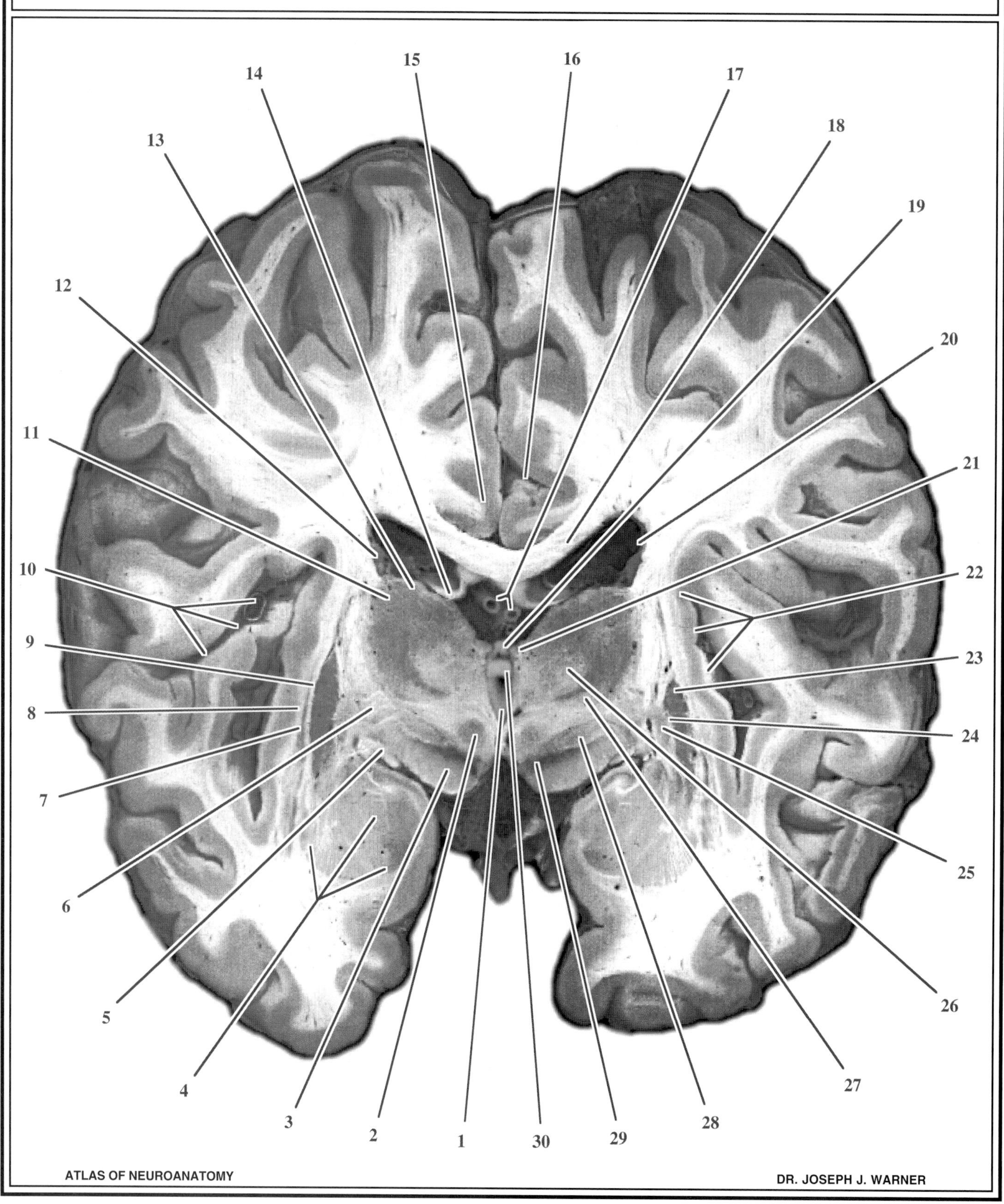

COMPLETE SECTION OF THE BRAIN, PLANE PARALLEL TO THE PARIETO-OCCIPITAL SULCUS: LEVEL OF THE CENTROMEDIAN NUCLEUS OF THE THALAMUS AND OF THE SUBTHALAMIC NUCLEUS (ROSTRAL TO CAUDAL PERSPECTIVE) SECTION MAP AND KEY TO NUMBERED STRUCTURES

KEY TO NUMBERED STRUCTURES

1. Third Ventricle
2. Red Nucleus
3. Cerebral Peduncle
4. Amygdala
5. Optic Tract
6. Internal Capsule, Posterior Limb
7. Claustrum
8. Extreme Capsule
9. External Capsule
10. Sylvian Fissure
11. Lateral Posterior Nucleus of the Thalamus
12. Tail of the Caudate
13. Lateral Dorsal Nucleus of the Thalamus
14. Fornix
15. Cingulate Gyrus
16. Cingulate Sulcus
17. Internal Cerebral Veins
18. Corpus Callosum
19. Habenular Commissure
20. Body of the Lateral Ventricle
21. Habenula
22. Insular Cortex
23. Putamen
24. External Medullary Lamina
25. Globus Pallidus II
26. Centromedian Nucleus of the Thalamus
27. Ventroposteromedial Nucleus of the Thalamus
28. Subthalamic Nucleus
29. Substantia Nigra
30. Posterior Commissure

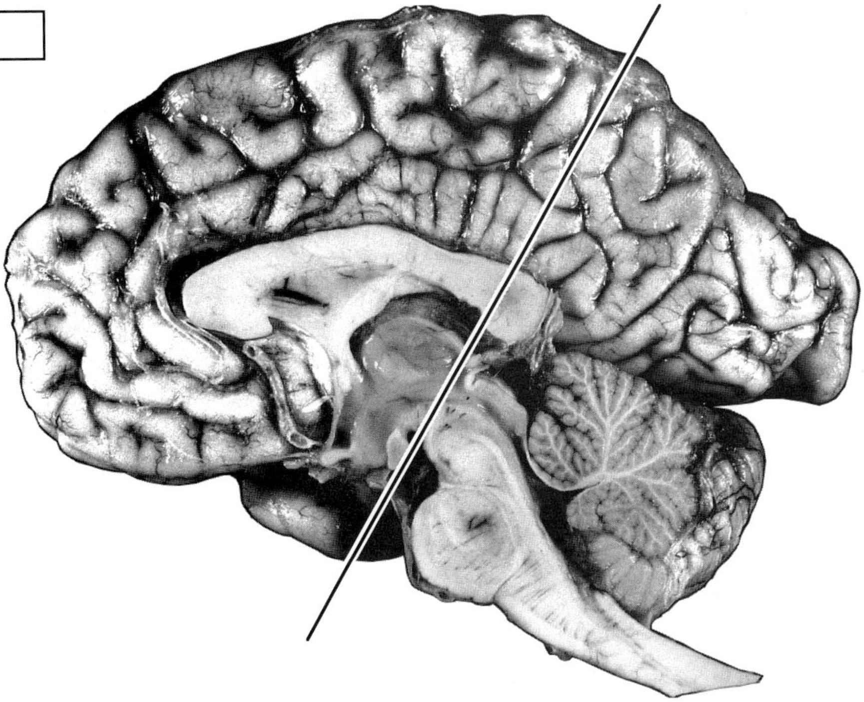

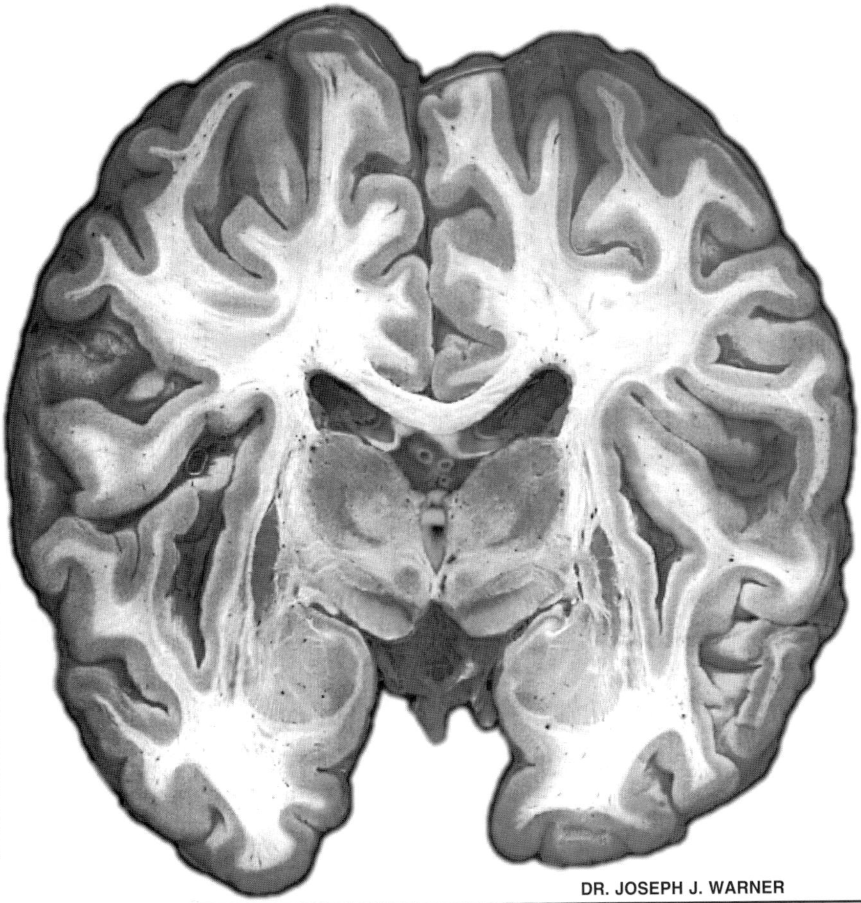

*The centromedian and ventroposteromedial nuclei of the thalamus are often characterized by a different hue than that of surrounding nuclei in gross sections. This difference has been enhanced in the image histogram redistribution, resulting in a lighter appearance (not to be confused with white matter). With the image histogram enhancement technique used in this section, transversely sectioned fiber tracts in the brainstem appear darker than those tracts with obliquely or longitudinally sectioned fibers. These tracts should not be confused with gray matter structures.

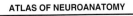

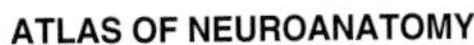

COMPLETE SECTION OF THE BRAIN, PLANE PARALLEL TO THE PARIETO-OCCIPITAL SULCUS: LEVEL OF THE ANTERIOR NUCLEUS OF THE THALAMUS (CAUDAL TO ROSTRAL PERSPECTIVE)

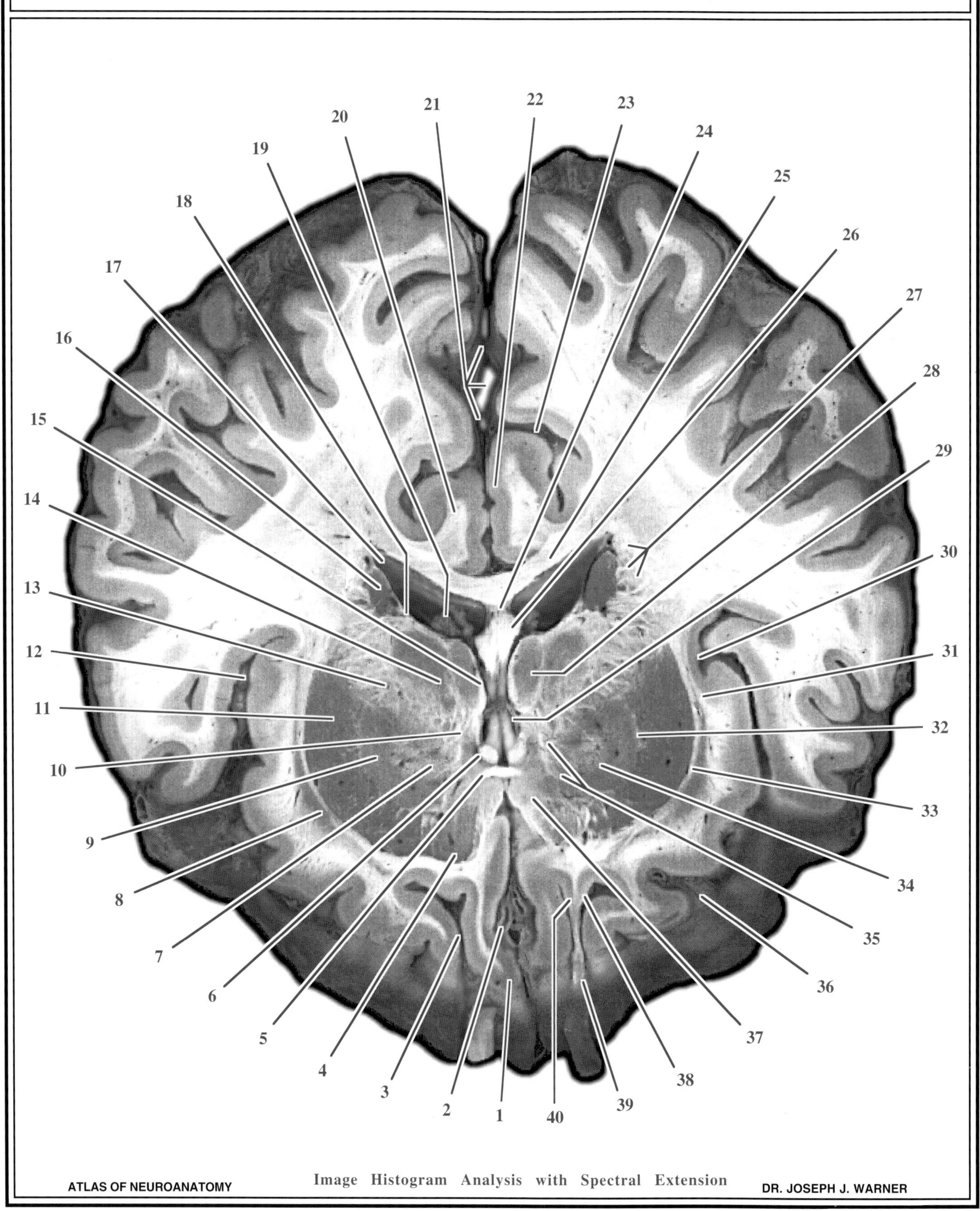

 Image Histogram Analysis with Spectral Extension

COMPLETE SECTION OF THE BRAIN, PLANE PARALLEL TO THE PARIETO-OCCIPITAL SULCUS: LEVEL OF THE ANTERIOR NUCLEUS OF THE THALAMUS (CAUDAL TO ROSTRAL PERSPECTIVE) SECTION MAP AND KEY TO NUMBERED STRUCTURES

KEY TO NUMBERED STRUCTURES

1. Gyrus Rectus
2. Anterior Cerebral Artery
3. Olfactory Sulcus
4. Nucleus Accumbens
5. Anterior Commissure
6. Postcommissural Fornix
7. Globus Pallidus I
8. Claustrum
9. Globus Pallidus II
10. Genu of the Internal Capsule
11. Putamen
12. Sylvian Fissure
13. Posterior Limb of the Internal Capsule
14. Ventroanterior, Ventrolateral Nuclei of the Thalamus
15. Stria Medullaris
16. Caudate Nucleus
17. Lateral Ventricle
18. Stria Terminalis and Thalamo-striate Vein
19. Choroid Plexus
20. Cingulum
21. Interhemispheric Fissure
22. Cortex of the Cingulate Gyrus
23. Cingulate Sulcus
24. Septum Pellucidum
25. Corpus Callosum
26. Fornix
27. Superior Longitudinal Fasciculus
28. Anterior Nucleus of the Thalamus
29. Choroid Plexus adjacent to Foramen of Monro (note curvature of the Fornix)
30. Insular Cortex
31. Extreme Capsule
32. External Medullary Lamina
33. External Capsule
34. Internal Medullary Lamina
35. Ansa Lenticularis
36. Orbitofrontal Gyri
37. Nucleus Basalis of Meynert
38. Lateral Olfactory Stria*
39. Olfactory Tract
40. Medial Olfactory Stria*

* The medial and lateral olfactory striae diverge at the olfactory trigone, thus forming the rostral demarcation of the anterior perforated substance.

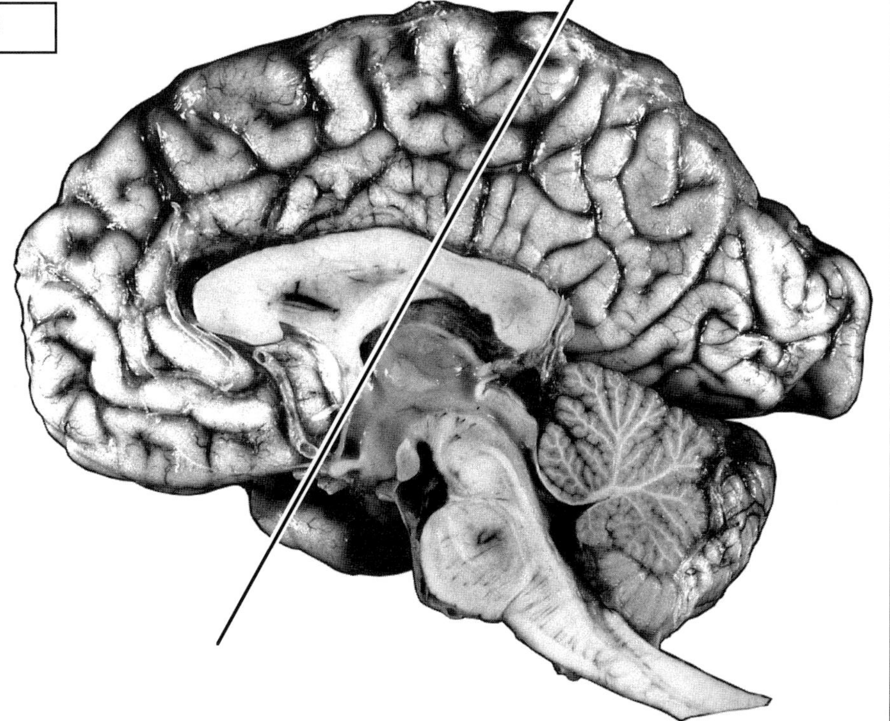

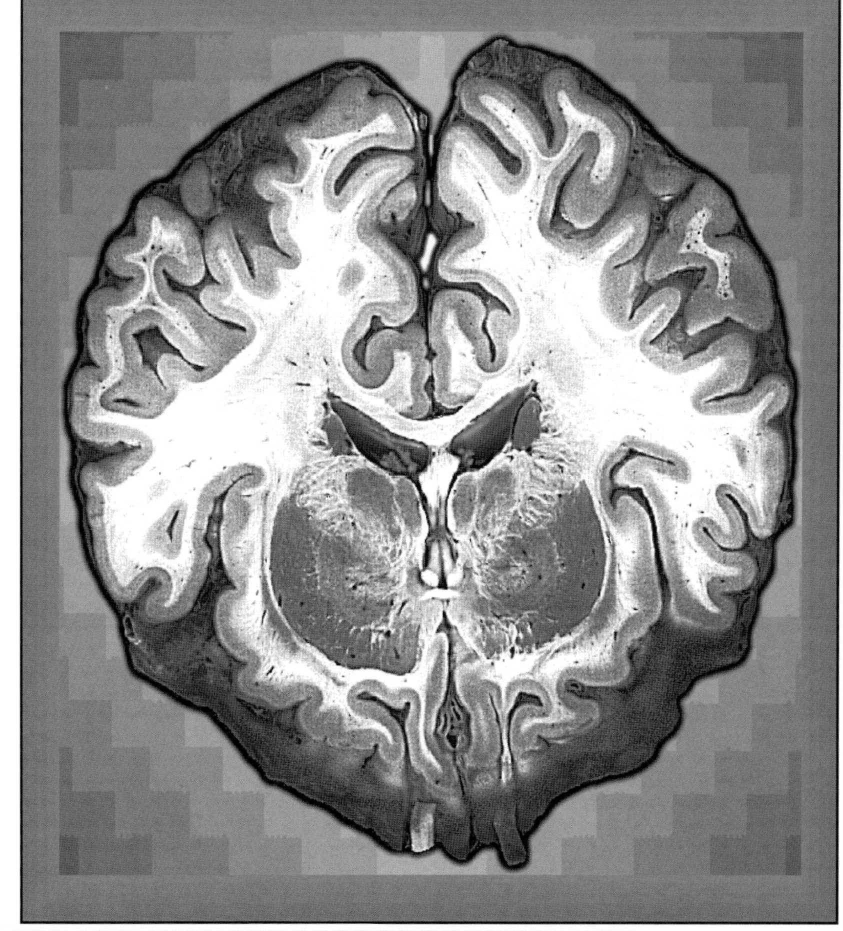

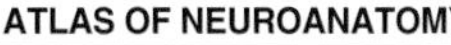

COMPLETE SECTION OF THE BRAIN, PLANE PARALLEL TO THE PARIETO-OCCIPITAL SULCUS: LEVEL OF THE HEAD OF THE CAUDATE NUCLEUS (CAUDAL TO ROSTRAL PERSPECTIVE)

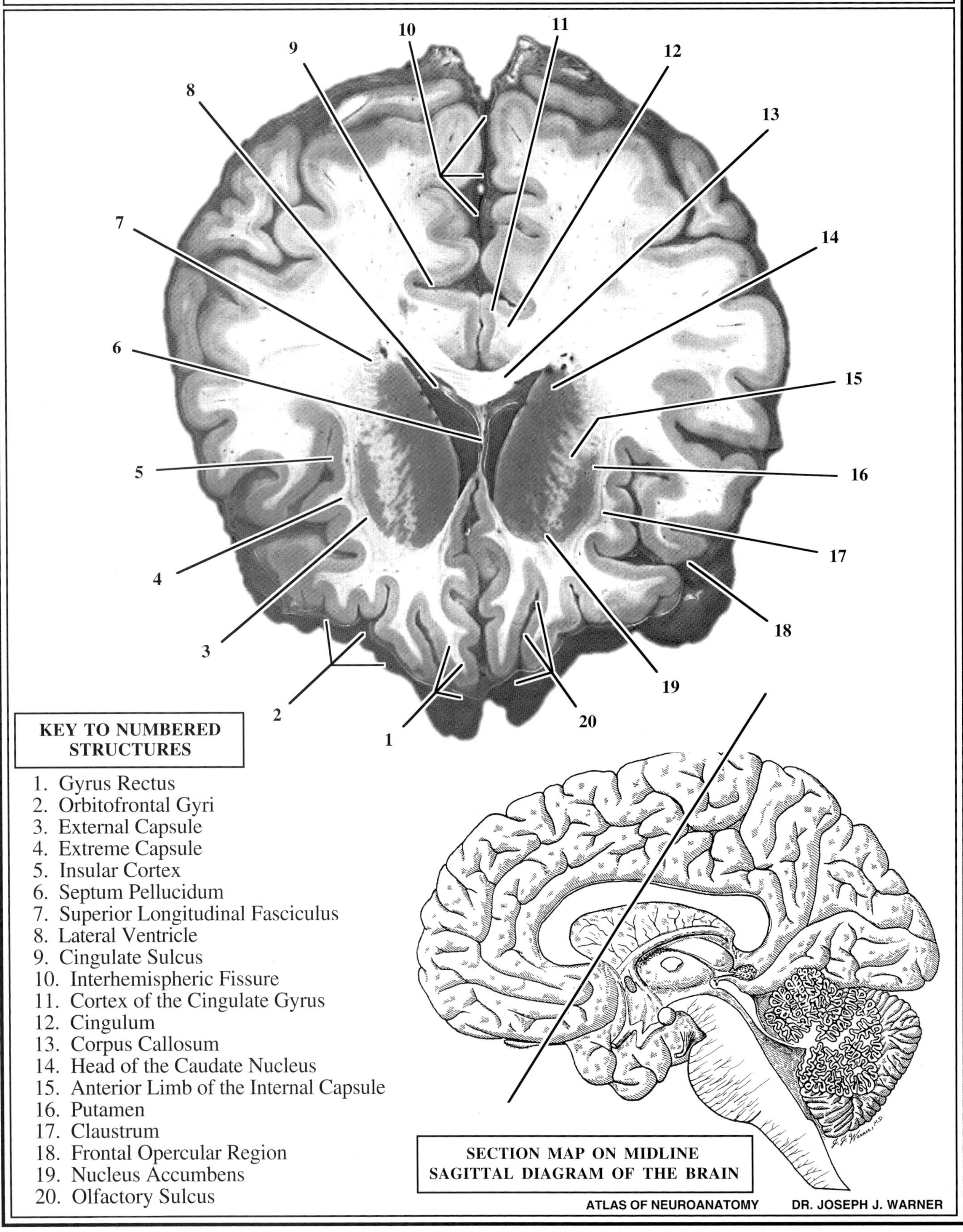

KEY TO NUMBERED STRUCTURES

1. Gyrus Rectus
2. Orbitofrontal Gyri
3. External Capsule
4. Extreme Capsule
5. Insular Cortex
6. Septum Pellucidum
7. Superior Longitudinal Fasciculus
8. Lateral Ventricle
9. Cingulate Sulcus
10. Interhemispheric Fissure
11. Cortex of the Cingulate Gyrus
12. Cingulum
13. Corpus Callosum
14. Head of the Caudate Nucleus
15. Anterior Limb of the Internal Capsule
16. Putamen
17. Claustrum
18. Frontal Opercular Region
19. Nucleus Accumbens
20. Olfactory Sulcus

PART III: NEUROHISTOLOGY

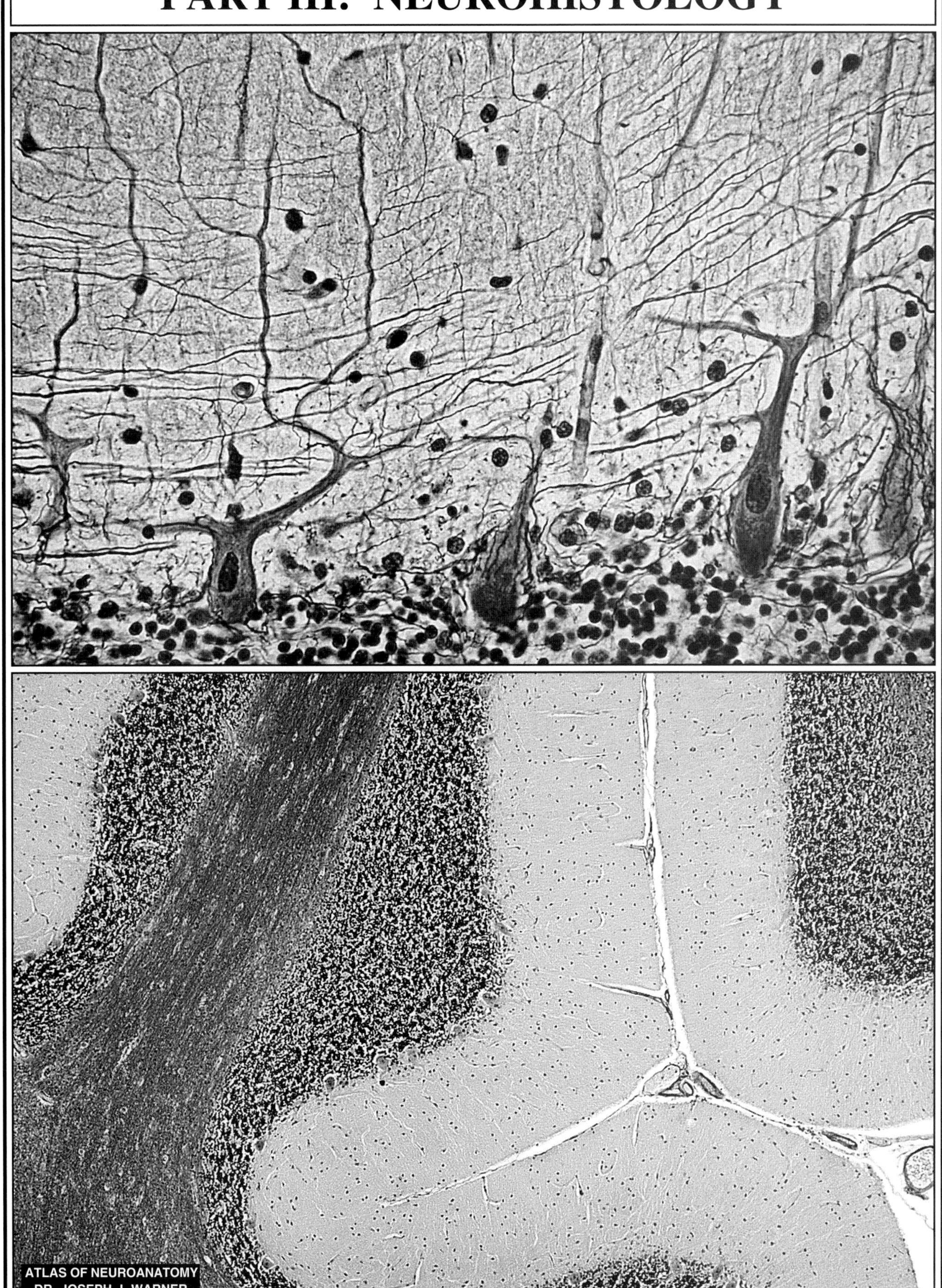

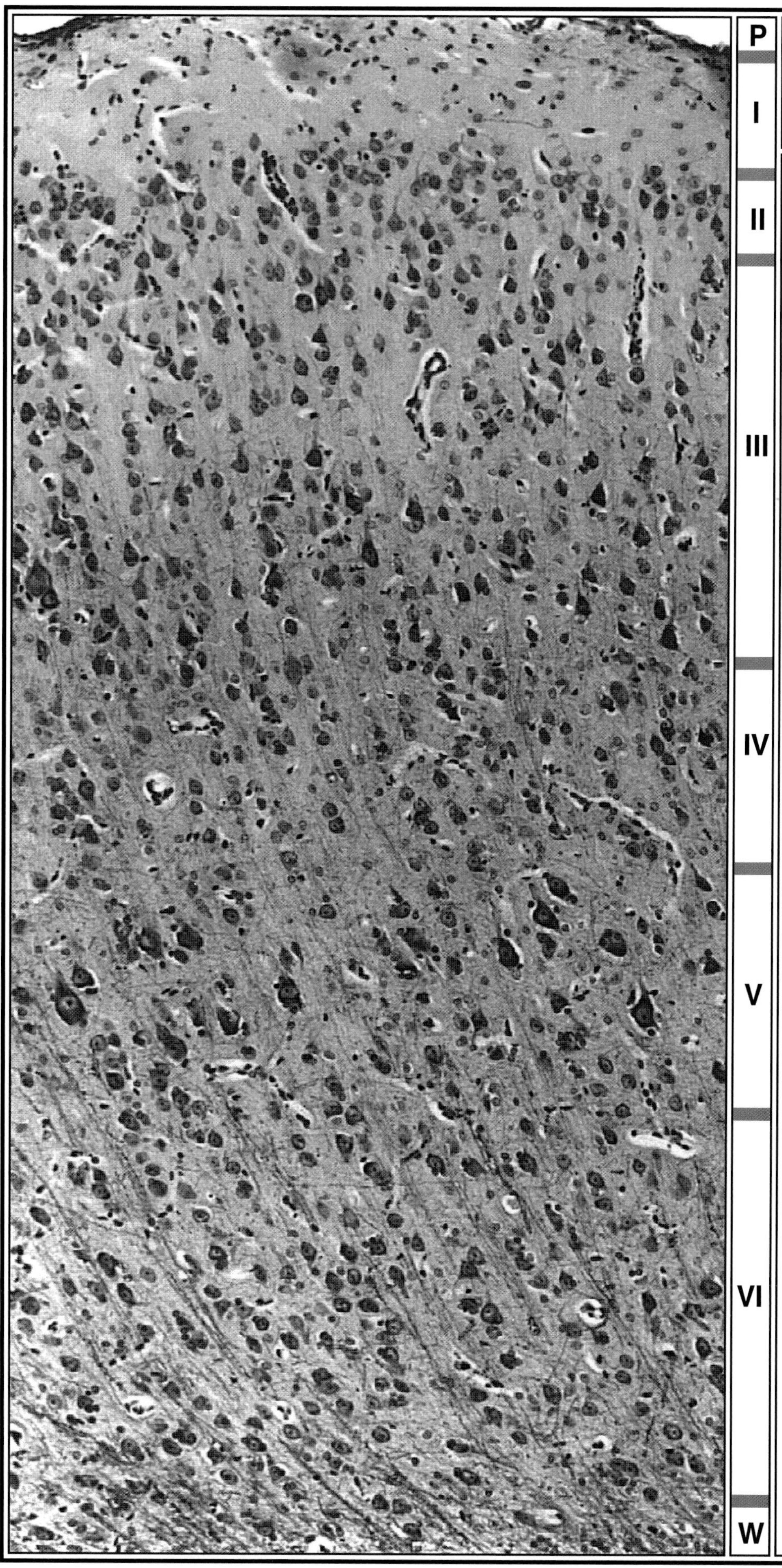

CEREBRAL CORTEX
AREA 3A TRANSITIONAL SENSORIMOTOR, 12 μ SECTION, KLUVER-BARRERA TECHNIQUE

P: Pial surface of cortex

I: Molecular or Plexiform layer; is comprised of cells with horizontal axons, Golgi type II cells, and terminal dendritic processes of pyramidal cells, fusiform cells, and axons of Martinotti cells. These fibers form a dense plexus in this layer.

II: External Granular layer; consists of granule cells with apical dendrites that terminate in the molecular layer.

III: External Pyramidal layer; consists of pyramidal neurons with apical dendrites which ascend to the molecular layer, and axons which descend into the white matter primarily as association or commissural fibers. Granule cells and Martinotti cells are also found in this layer.

IV: Internal Granular layer; is comprised of stellate cells and receives the main specific afferent projections. This layer is best developed in primary sensory cortical areas.

V: Internal Pyramidal layer; contains medium and large sized pyramidal cells. The apical dendrites of larger pyramidal cells ascend to the molecular layer, and their axons descend as projection fibers. Apical dendrites of the smaller pyramidal cells ascend to layer IV or terminate within layer V, and their axons enter the white matter as callosal fibers. Granule and Martinotti cells are also present.

VI: Polymorphic, Multiform, or Fusiform Cell layer; contains spindle-shaped cells oriented perpendicular to the cortical surface. Deep stellate cells of Layer VI send processes as short arcuate association fibers which connect adjacent gyri.

W: White matter

ATLAS OF NEUROANATOMY
DR. JOSEPH J. WARNER

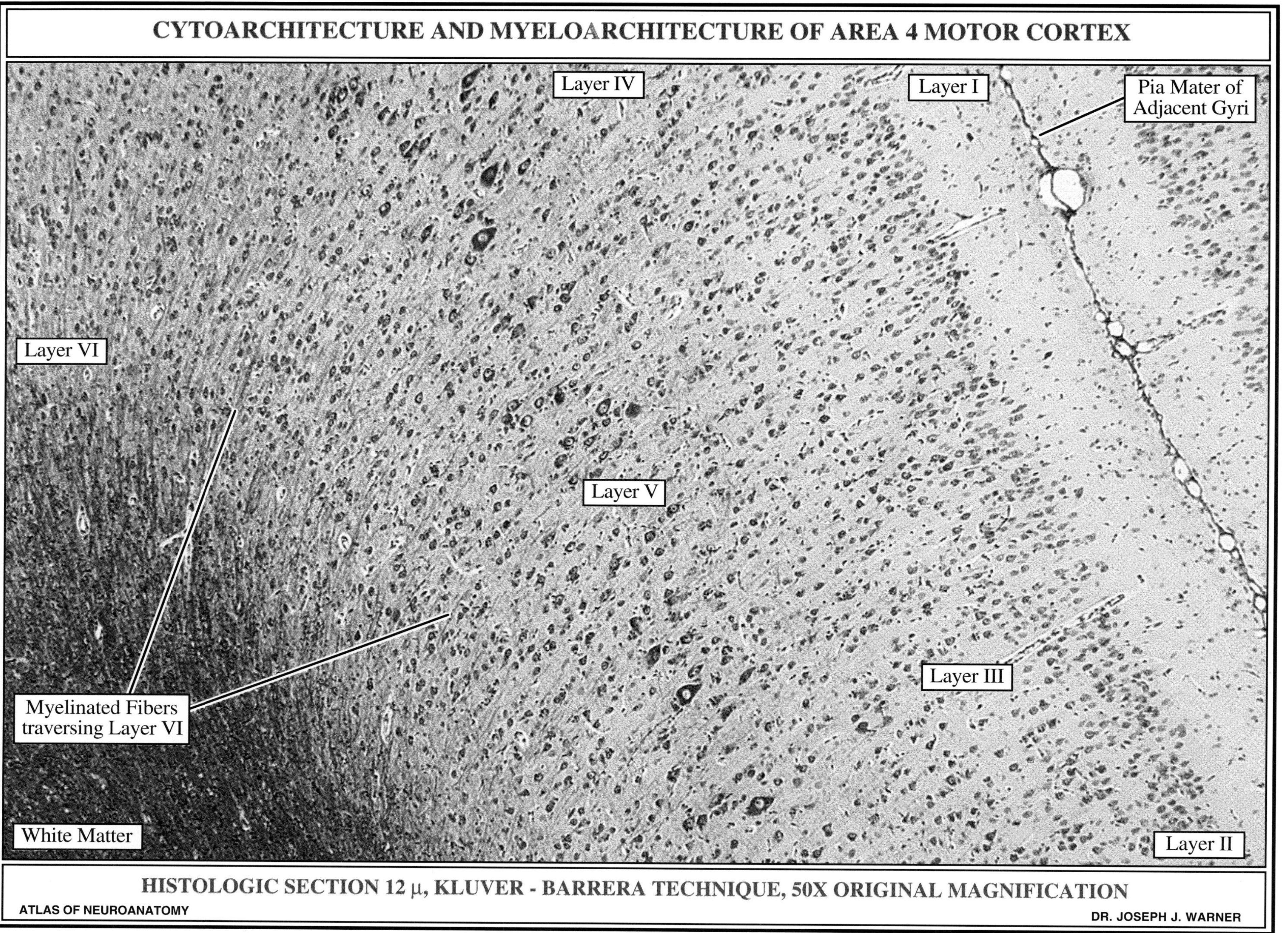
CYTOARCHITECTURE AND MYELOARCHITECTURE OF AREA 4 MOTOR CORTEX
Layer IV
Layer I
Pia Mater of Adjacent Gyri
Layer VI
Layer V
Layer III
Myelinated Fibers traversing Layer VI
White Matter
Layer II
HISTOLOGIC SECTION 12 μ, KLUVER - BARRERA TECHNIQUE, 50X ORIGINAL MAGNIFICATION
ATLAS OF NEUROANATOMY
DR. JOSEPH J. WARNER

CEREBRAL CORTEX, PRECENTRAL GYRUS: CYTOARCHITECTURE, NEURONS AND GLIA

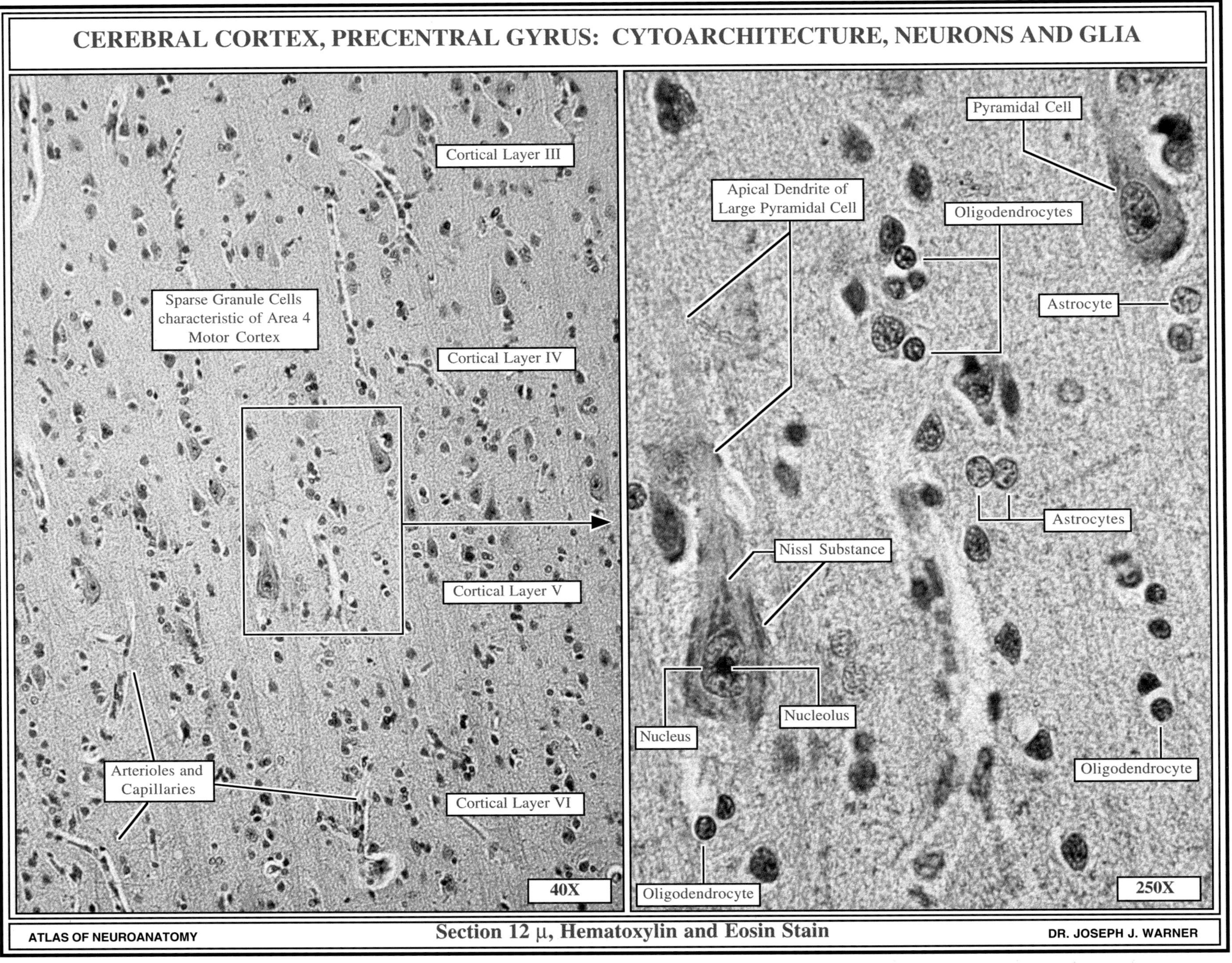

Section 12 μ, Hematoxylin and Eosin Stain

CEREBRAL CORTEX, PRECENTRAL GYRUS: PYRAMIDAL CELL
COMPARISON OF (A) NISSL AND (B) BODIAN SILVER PROTEINATE TECHNIQUES

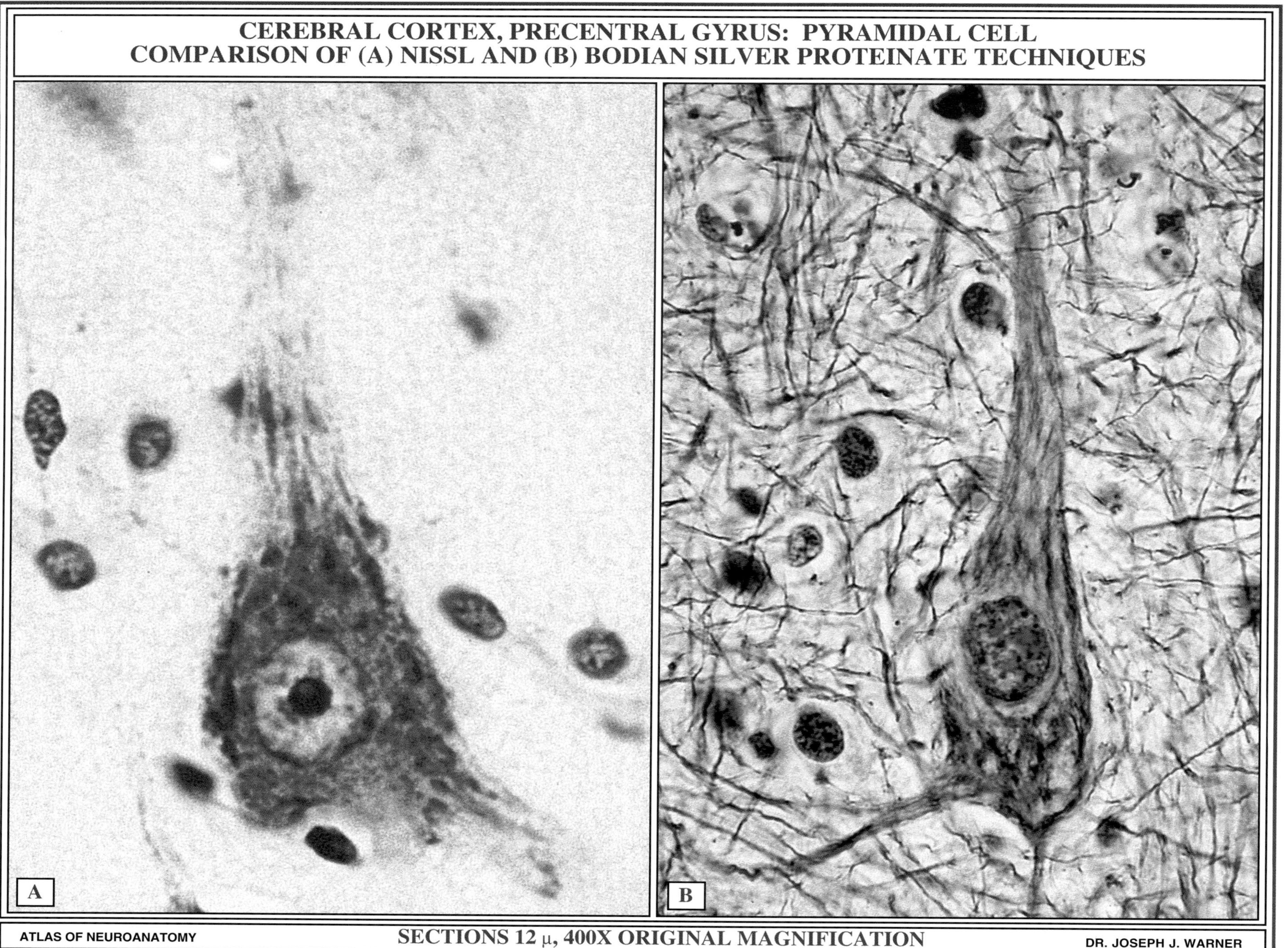

SECTIONS 12 μ, 400X ORIGINAL MAGNIFICATION

CEREBRAL CORTEX: PARASAGITTAL REGION OF THE PRECENTRAL GYRUS

BODIAN SILVER PROTEINATE PROCEDURE, 12 μ SECTION, 100X ORIGINAL MAGNIFICATION

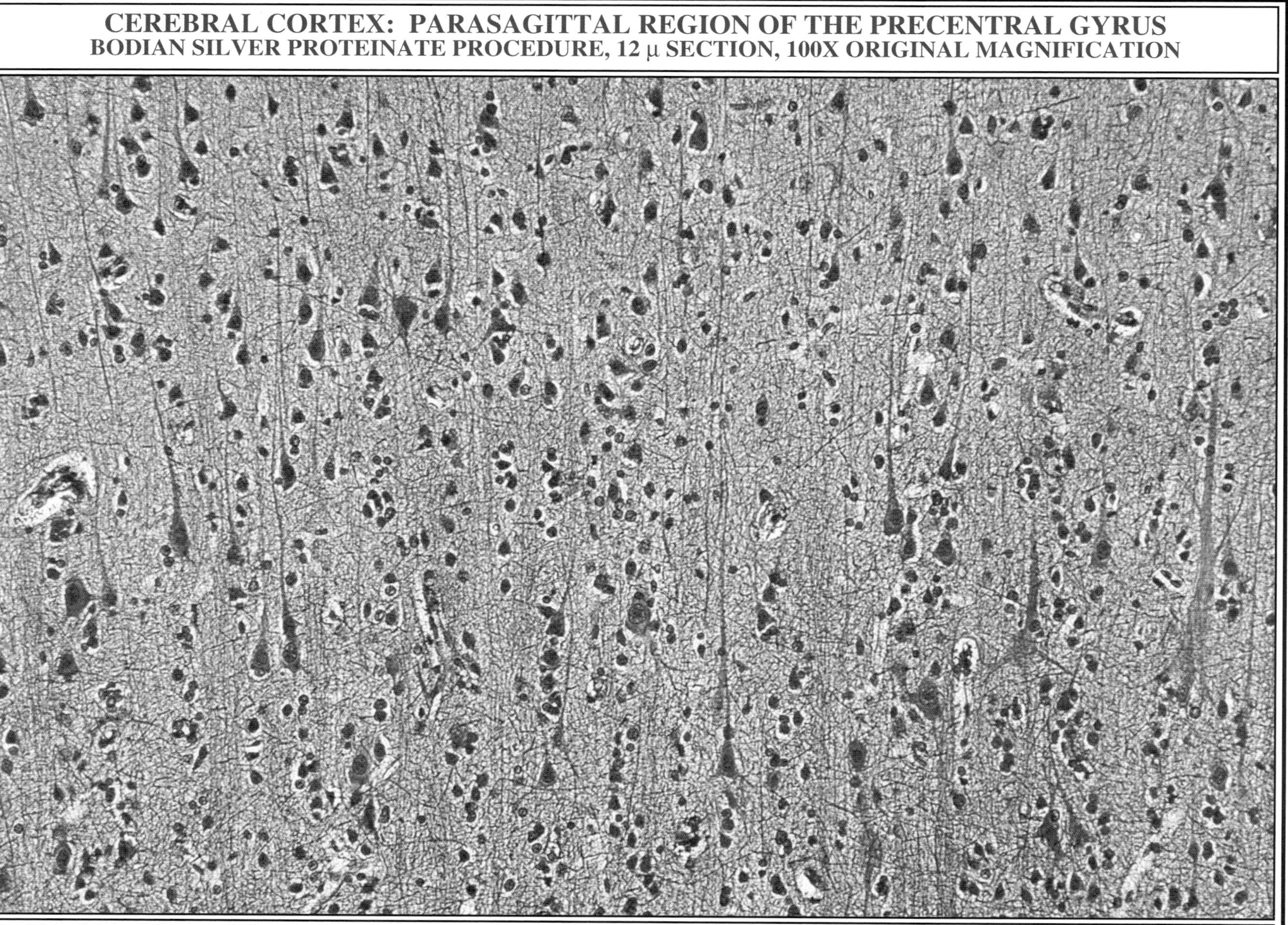

This field of view includes Cortical Layer V (the Inner Pyramidal Layer). Betz cells are found in Layer V of parasagittal motor cortex, which includes the somatotopic representation of the lower extremities. Axons of these large pyramidal cells descend in the corticospinal tracts and terminate in the contralateral spinal gray.

ATLAS OF NEUROANATOMY DR. JOSEPH J. WARNER

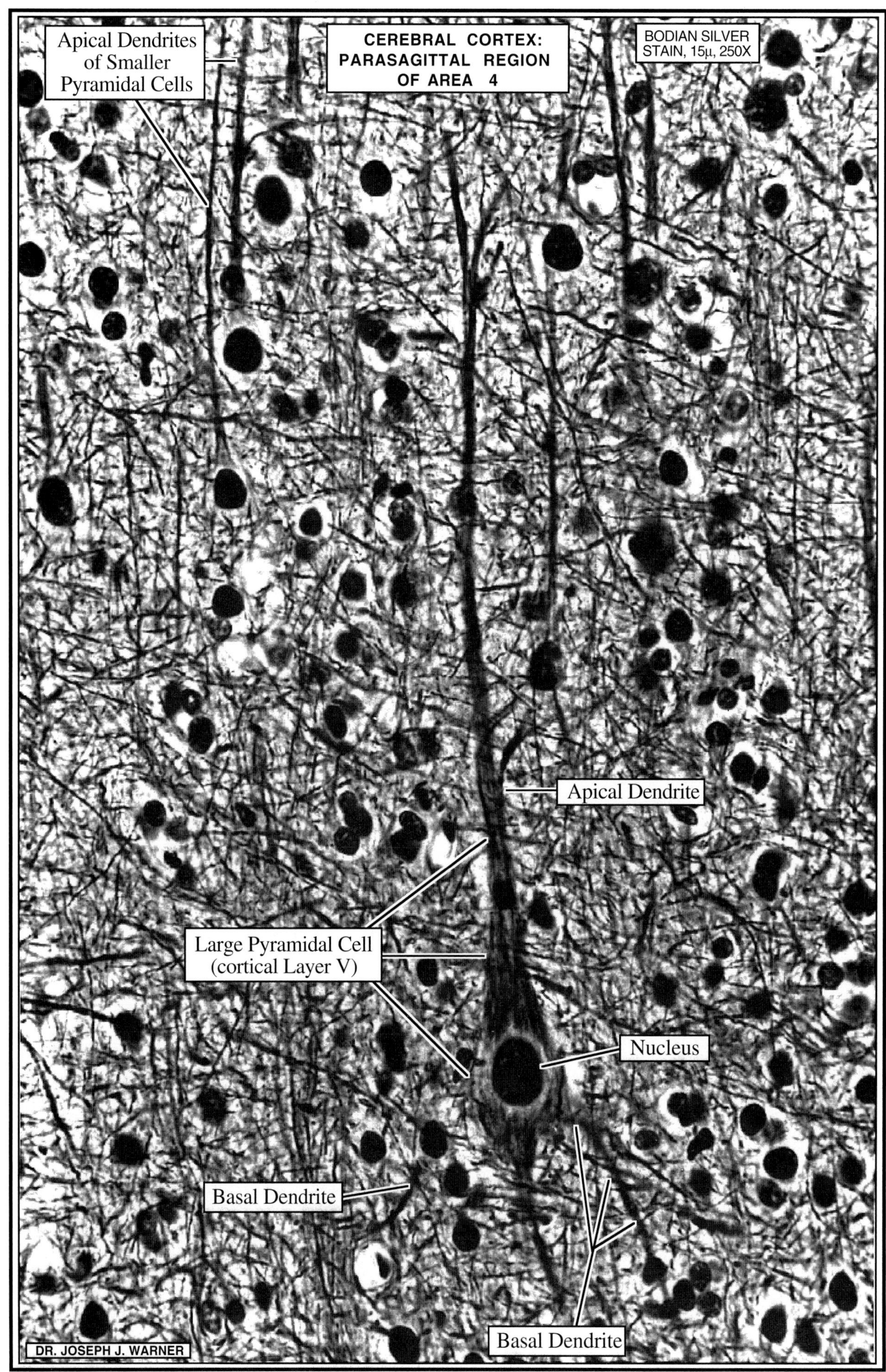
CEREBRAL CORTEX:
PARASAGITTAL REGION
OF AREA 4
BODIAN SILVER
STAIN, 15µ, 250X
Apical Dendrites
of Smaller
Pyramidal Cells
Apical Dendrite
Large Pyramidal Cell
(cortical Layer V)
Nucleus
Basal Dendrite
Basal Dendrite
DR. JOSEPH J. WARNER

CEREBRAL CORTEX: LAYER V (INNER PYRAMIDAL LAYER)

GOLGI SILVER TECHNIQUE: 250X MAGNIFICATION

SUBSTANTIA NIGRA, PARS COMPACTA: DOPAMINERGIC NEURONS DEMONSTRATING CYTOPLASMIC NEUROMELANIN

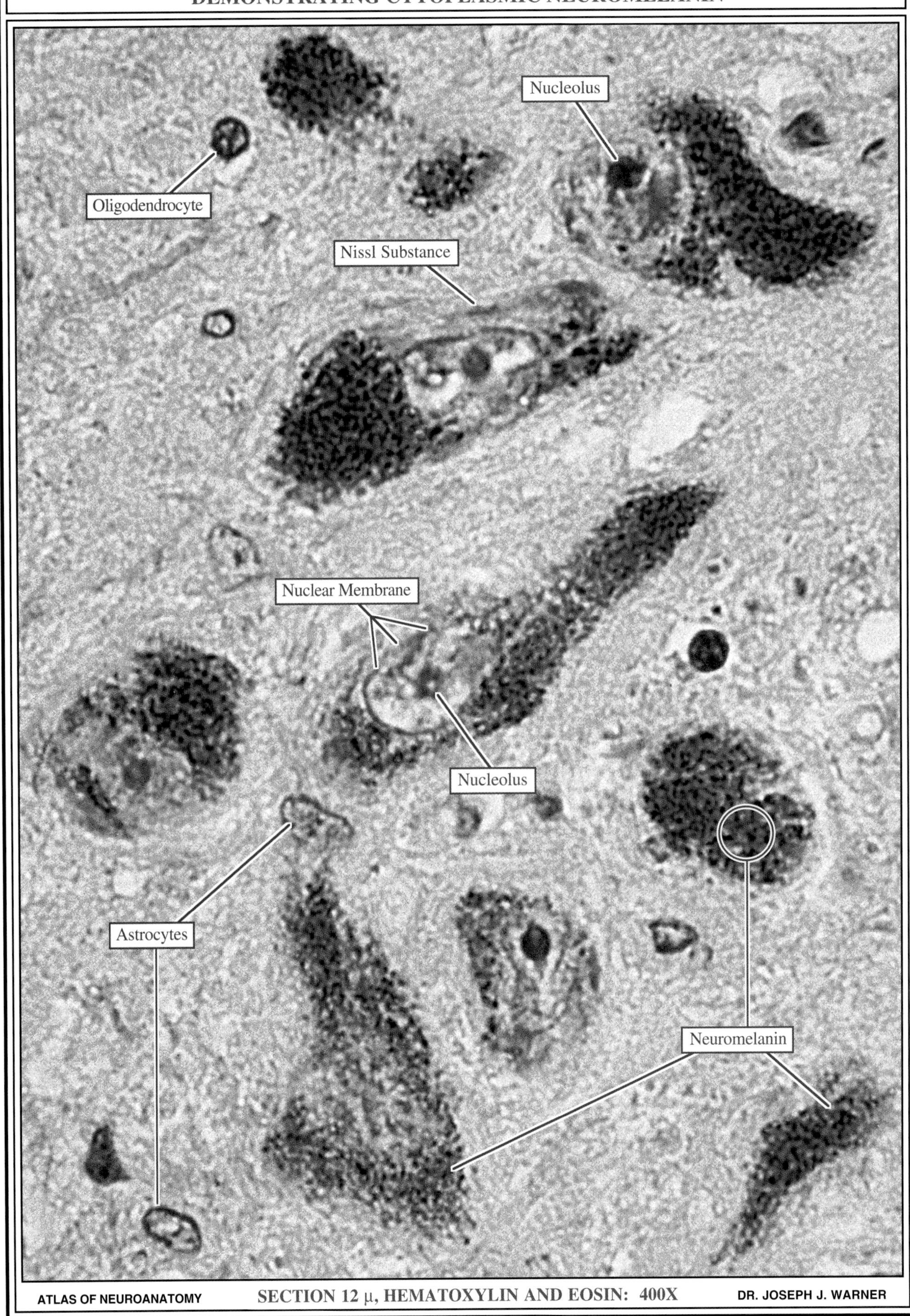

SECTION 12 μ, HEMATOXYLIN AND EOSIN: 400X

NEUROHISTOLOGY: (1) CHOROID PLEXUS (2) SUBCORTICAL WHITE MATTER

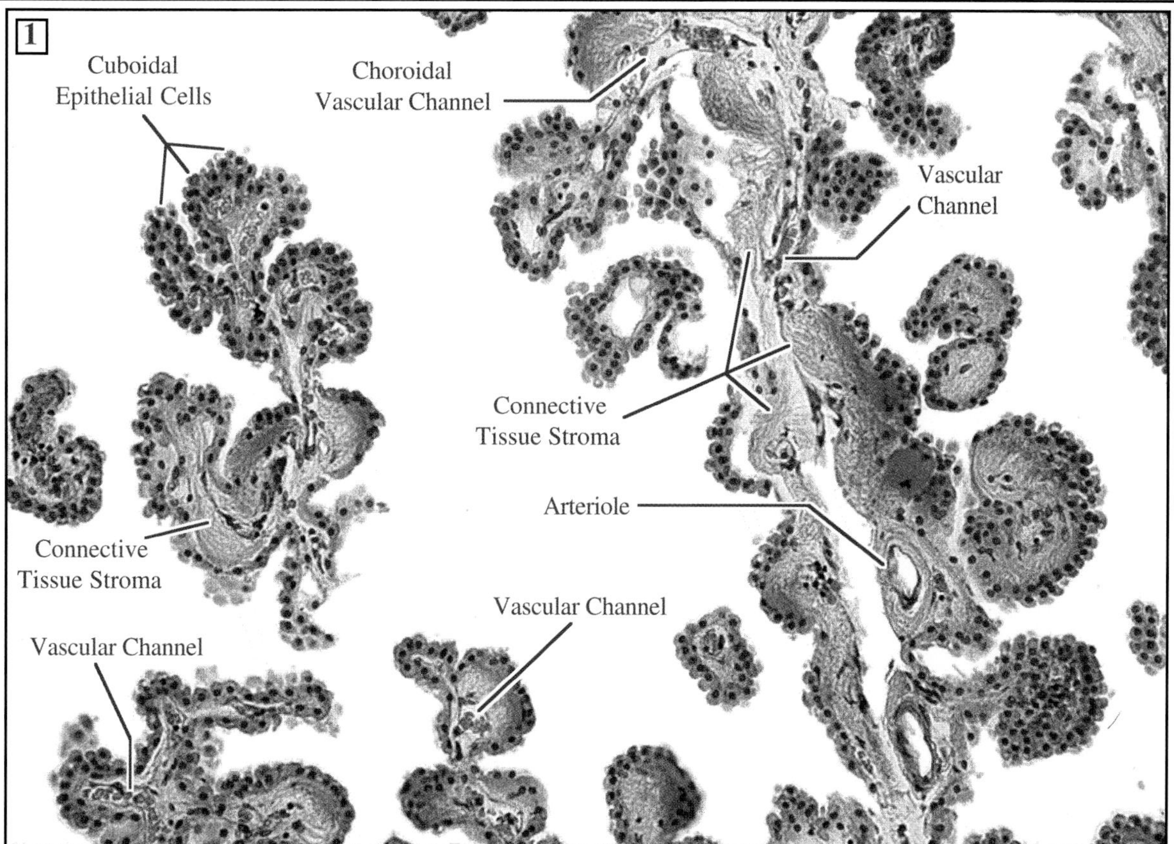

1: Choroid Plexus from the lateral ventricle, 100X original magnification
2: Subcortical white matter (frontoparietal), 250X original magnification

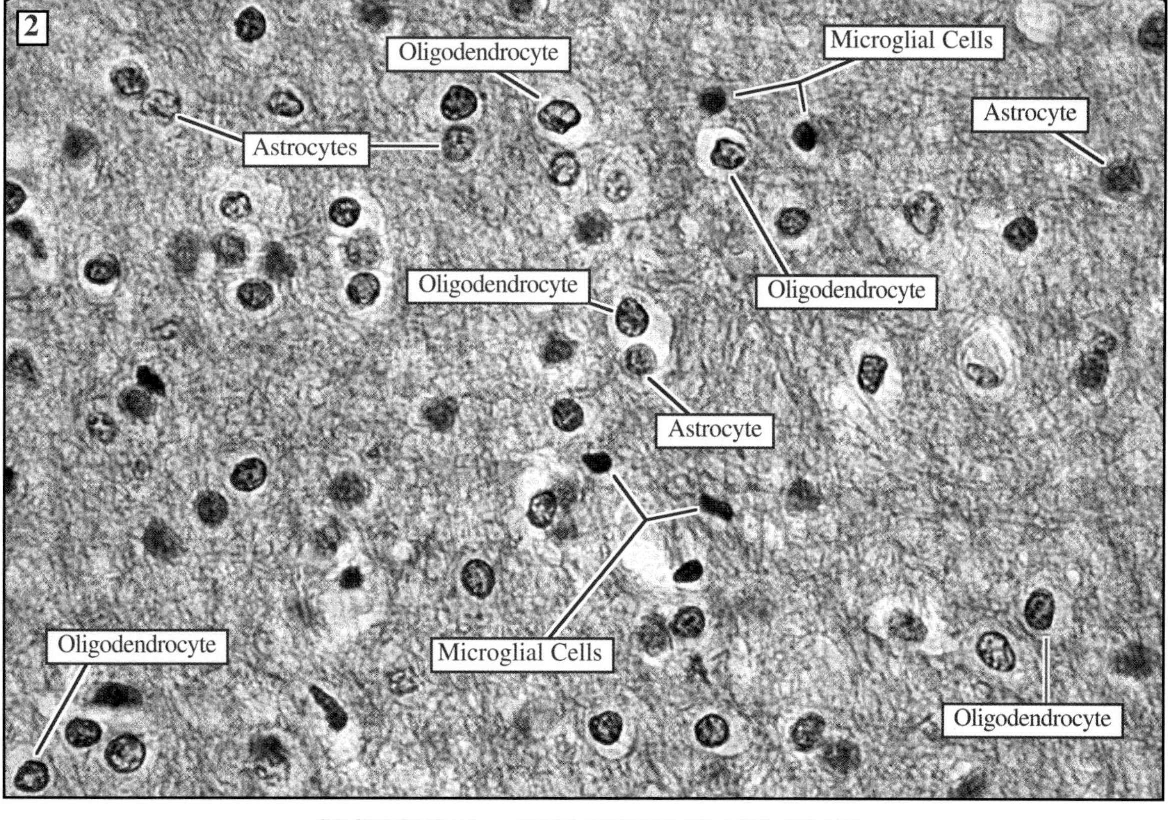

SECTIONS 12 μ, HEMATOXYLIN AND EOSIN

(A) MYELINATED FIBERS TRAVERSING THE DEEP LAYERS OF AREA 4 MOTOR CORTEX (100X)
(B) HISTOLOLOGY OF DEEP SUBCORTICAL WHITE MATTER (400X)

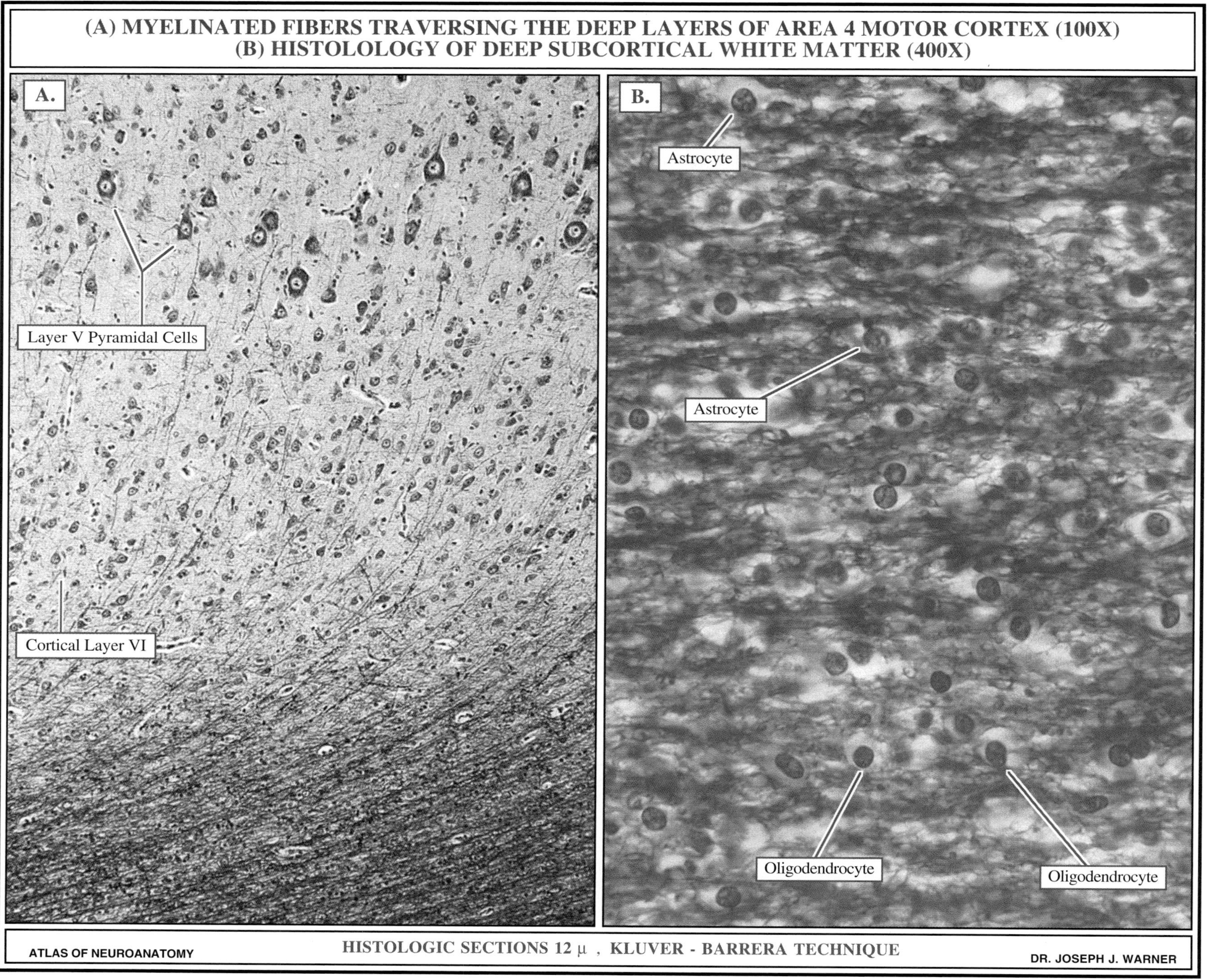

HISTOLOGIC SECTIONS 12 μ , KLUVER - BARRERA TECHNIQUE

ASTROCYTES AND THE CEREBROVASCULAR SYSTEM

The pia mater lines the small perivascular spaces (known as Virchow-Robin spaces) which accompany surface penetrating vessels for a limited depth into the cortex. This single epithelial cell layer lines the parenchymal surface of the central nervous system as the innermost of the meningeal layers, and surrounds microvascular structures (including arterioles) as they penetrate neural tissue.

Astrocytes are characterized by processes which extend (A) between neuronal cell bodies, (B) to the basal lamina surrounding blood vessels, and (C) to the surface of the central nervous system, subjacent to the pia mater. Astrocytic end feet and cell bodies thus form a continuous layer, referred to as the glia limitans, entirely enclosing the central nervous system. Astrocytic processes cover approximately 85% of cerebral capillary surface area, and along with cells of the pia, surround arterioles as well. The illustration below demonstrates the relationship of these astrocytic processes to a small arteriole.

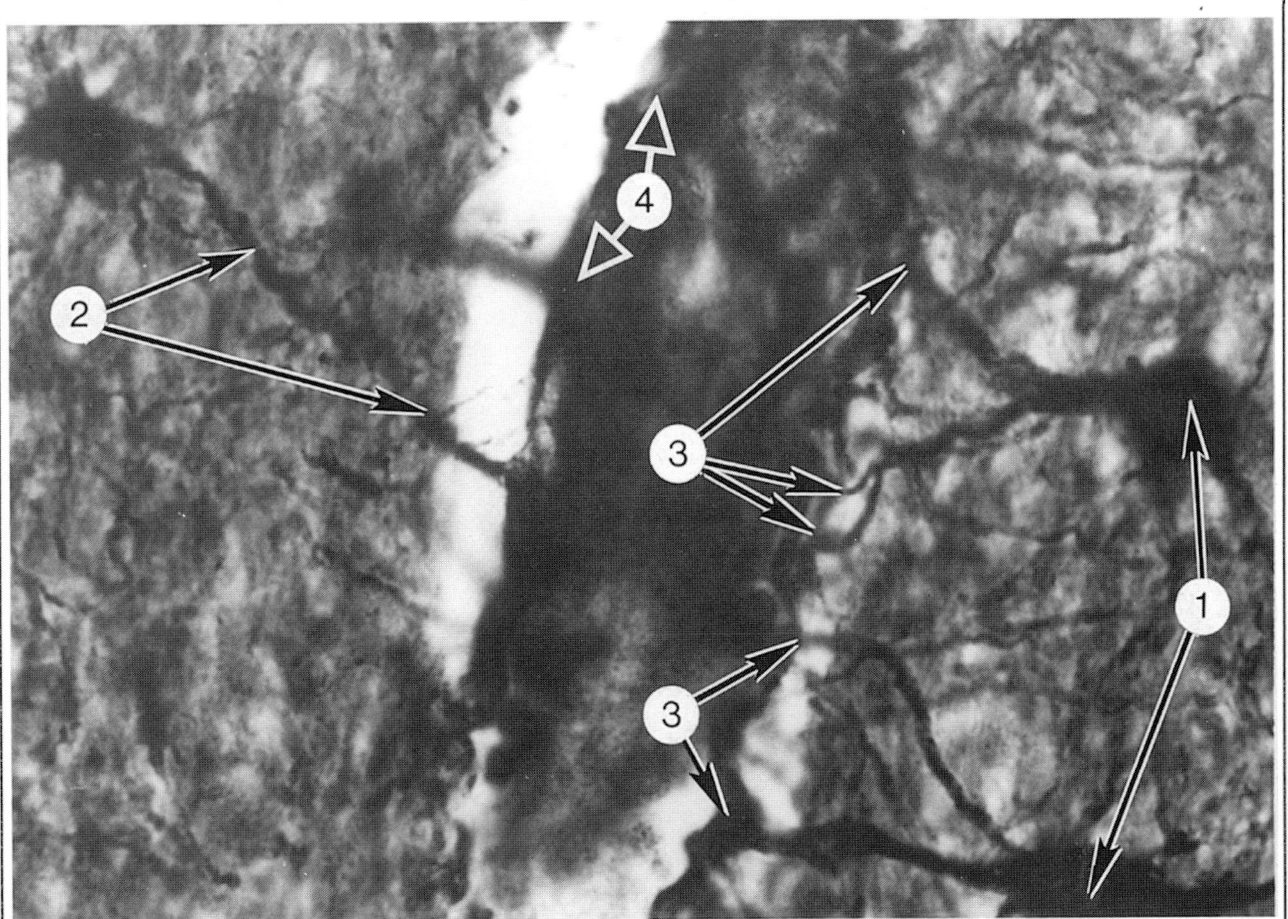

DESCRIPTION AND KEY TO NUMBERED STRUCTURES

Silver stained section of cerebral white matter, 25 μ, 400X. The perivascular space surrounding an arteriole is evident, (asymmetrically enlarged with histologic processing).

1. Astrocyte cell bodies, (fibrous or filamentous astrocytes are characterized by a smooth cellular contour, and are located primarily in white matter).
2. Astrocytic process, extending from the cell body to an arteriole.
3. Astrocytic end-feet contacting the basal lamina of the arteriole.
4. Arteriolar wall

CEREBELLUM, MORPHOLOGY OF THE FOLIA
LFB-PAS-HEMATOXYLIN, 12 μ SECTION, 40X ORIGINAL MAGNIFICATION

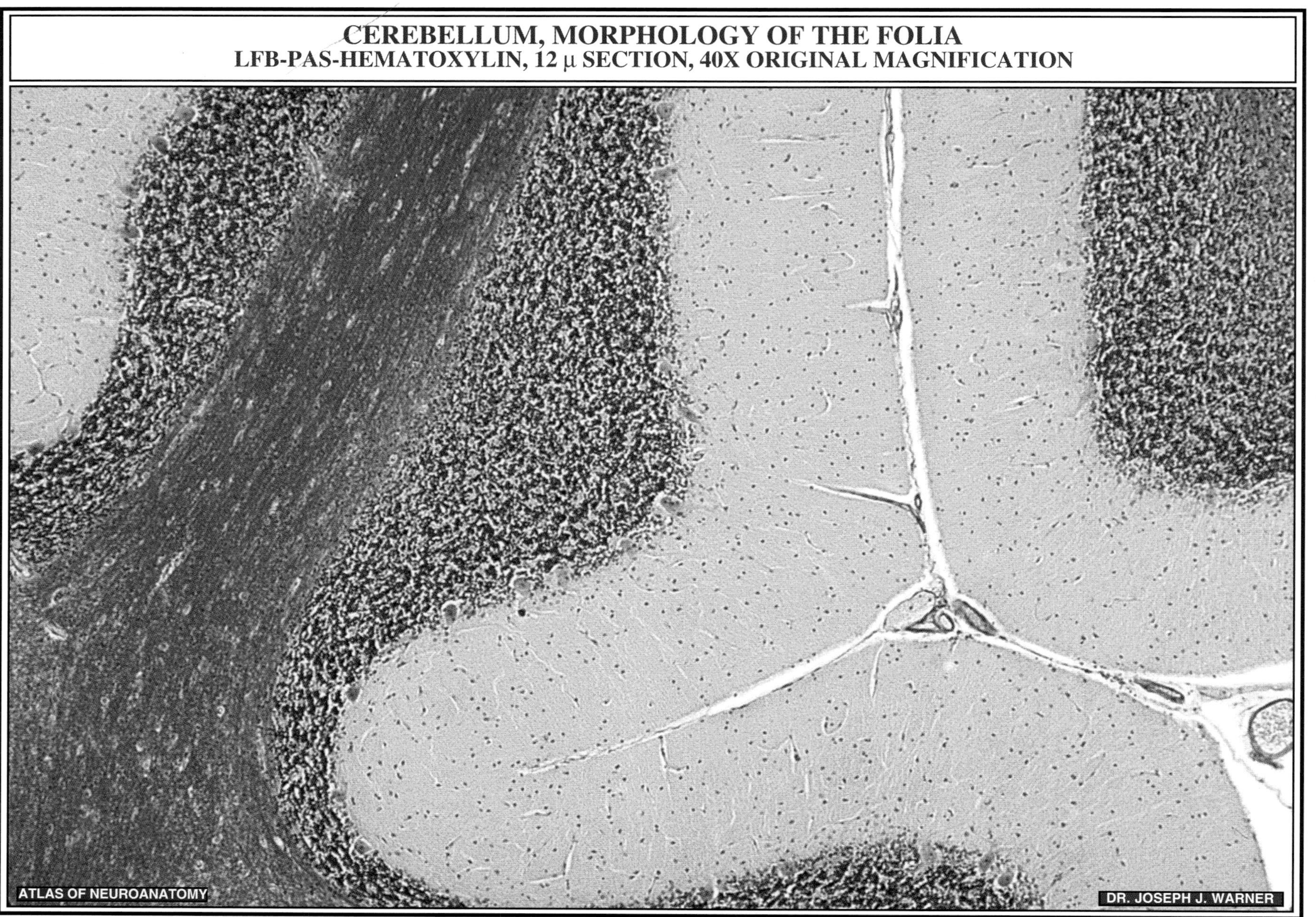

HISTOLOGY OF THE CEREBELLUM: BIELSCHOWSKY SILVER STAIN
SECTIONED PERPENDICULAR TO THE AXIS OF THE FOLIA, 12 μ, 40X

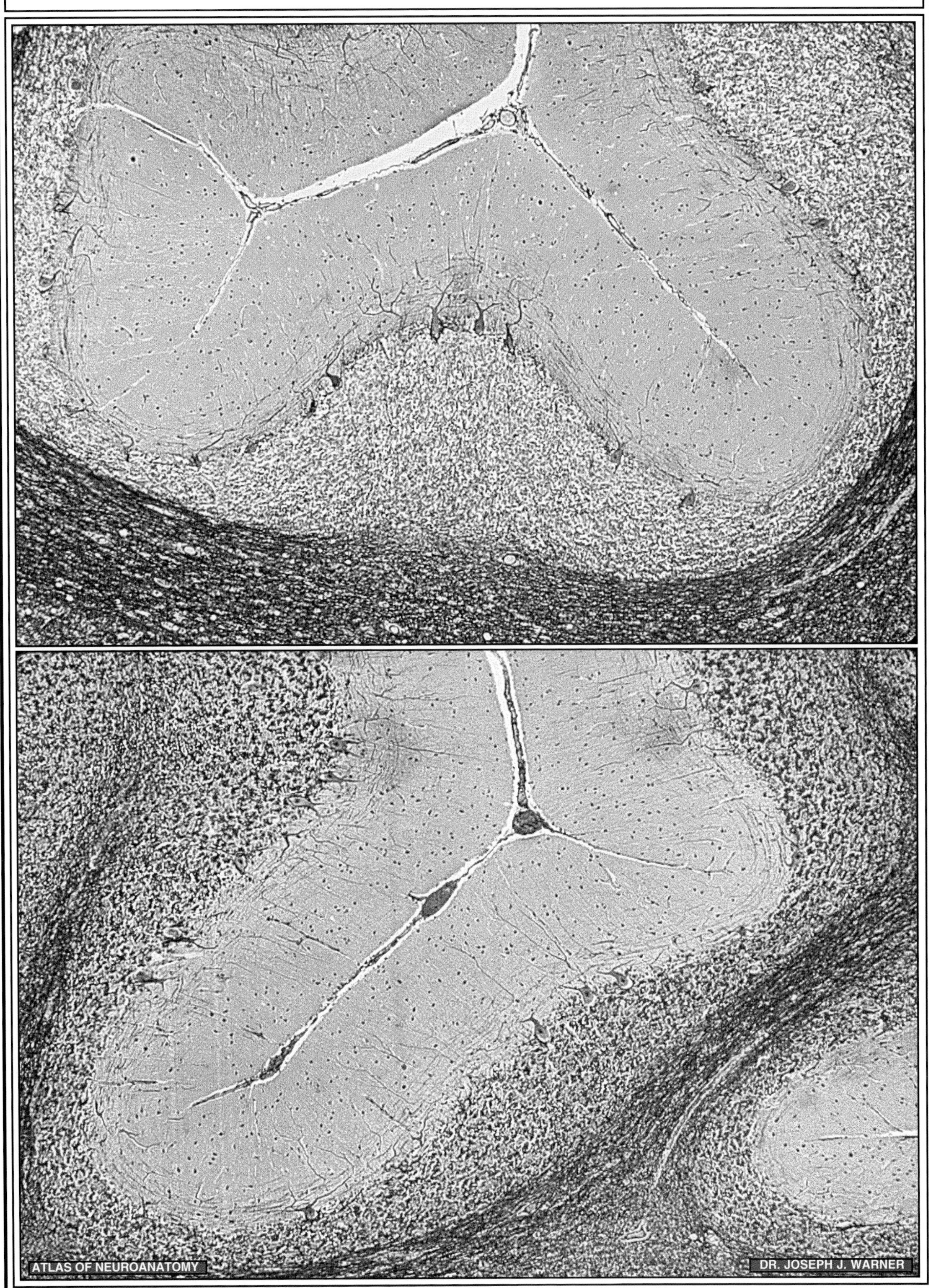

HISTOLOGY OF THE CEREBELLUM:
SECTIONED PERPENDICULAR TO THE AXIS OF THE FOLIA, 12 μ, 40X

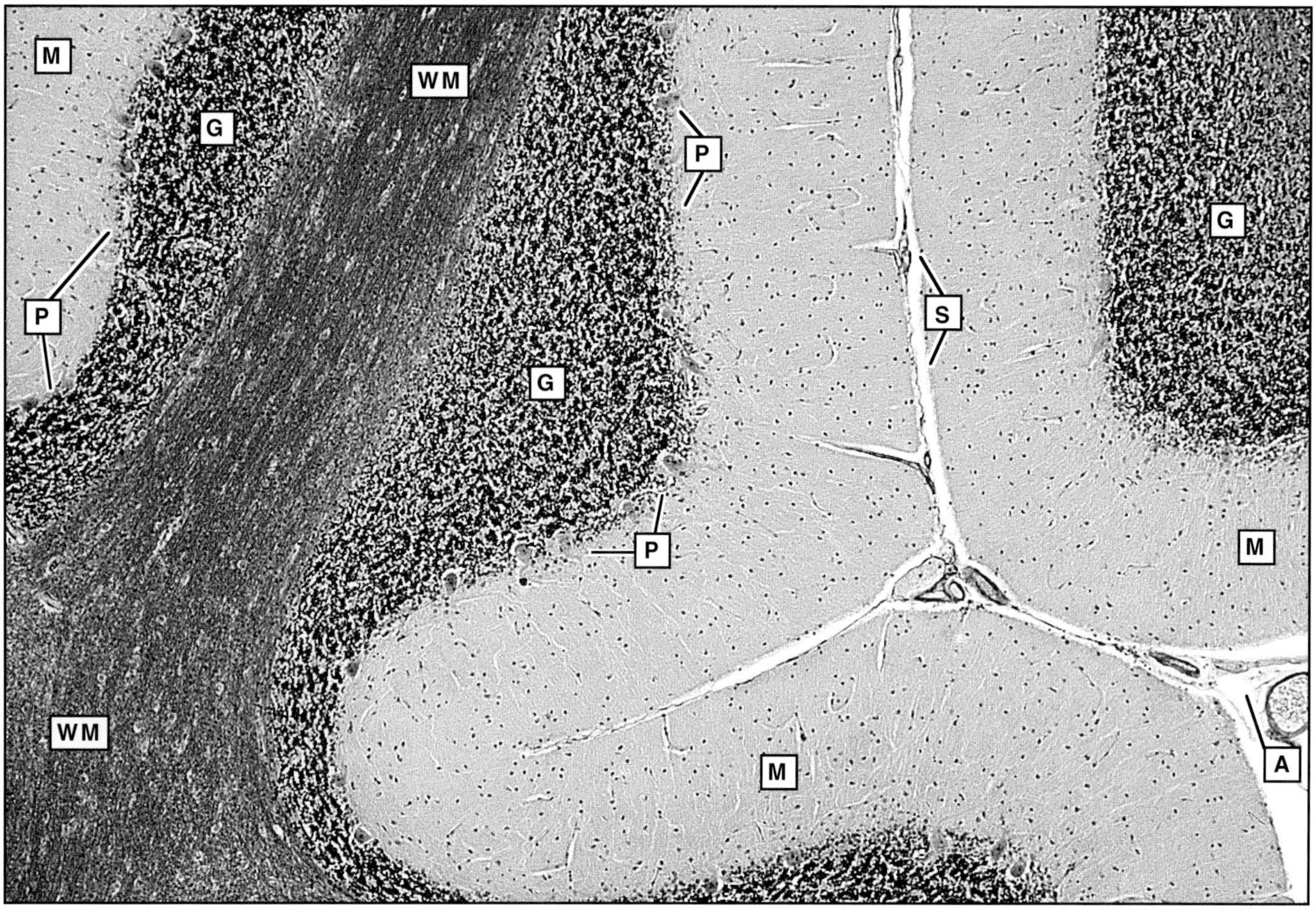

Above: Cerebellum sectioned transverse to the longitudinal axis of the folia (sagittal near midline or radial in the intermediate and lateral zones of the cerebellar hemisphere) stained with a combination myelin (Luxol Fast Blue) and Nissl stain demonstrates white matter and cortical layers. Dense cellularity is characteristic of the granular layer, in contrast to unmyelinated neuronal processes which comprise a major constituent of the molecular layer. *Below*: The Silver stain demonstrates neuronal processes, including Purkinje cell dendrites and parallel fibers in the molecular layer. A high density of axons in the white matter results in intense argyrophilia. These myelinated axons include Purkinje cell projections, recurrent collaterals, and afferent inputs (terminating as mossy or climbing fibers) to the cerebellar cortex.

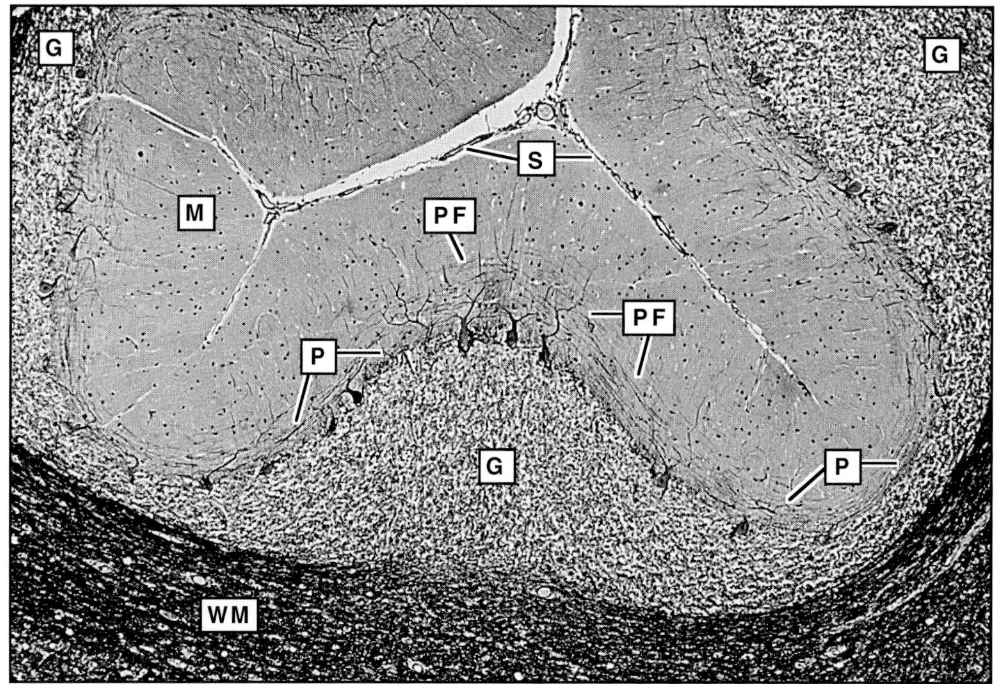

M: Molecular Layer
P: Purkinje Cell Layer
PF: Parallel Fibers
G: Granular Layer
WM: White Matter
S: Pial surface of Folium
A: Subarachnoid Space

ATLAS OF NEUROANATOMY
DR. JOSEPH J. WARNER

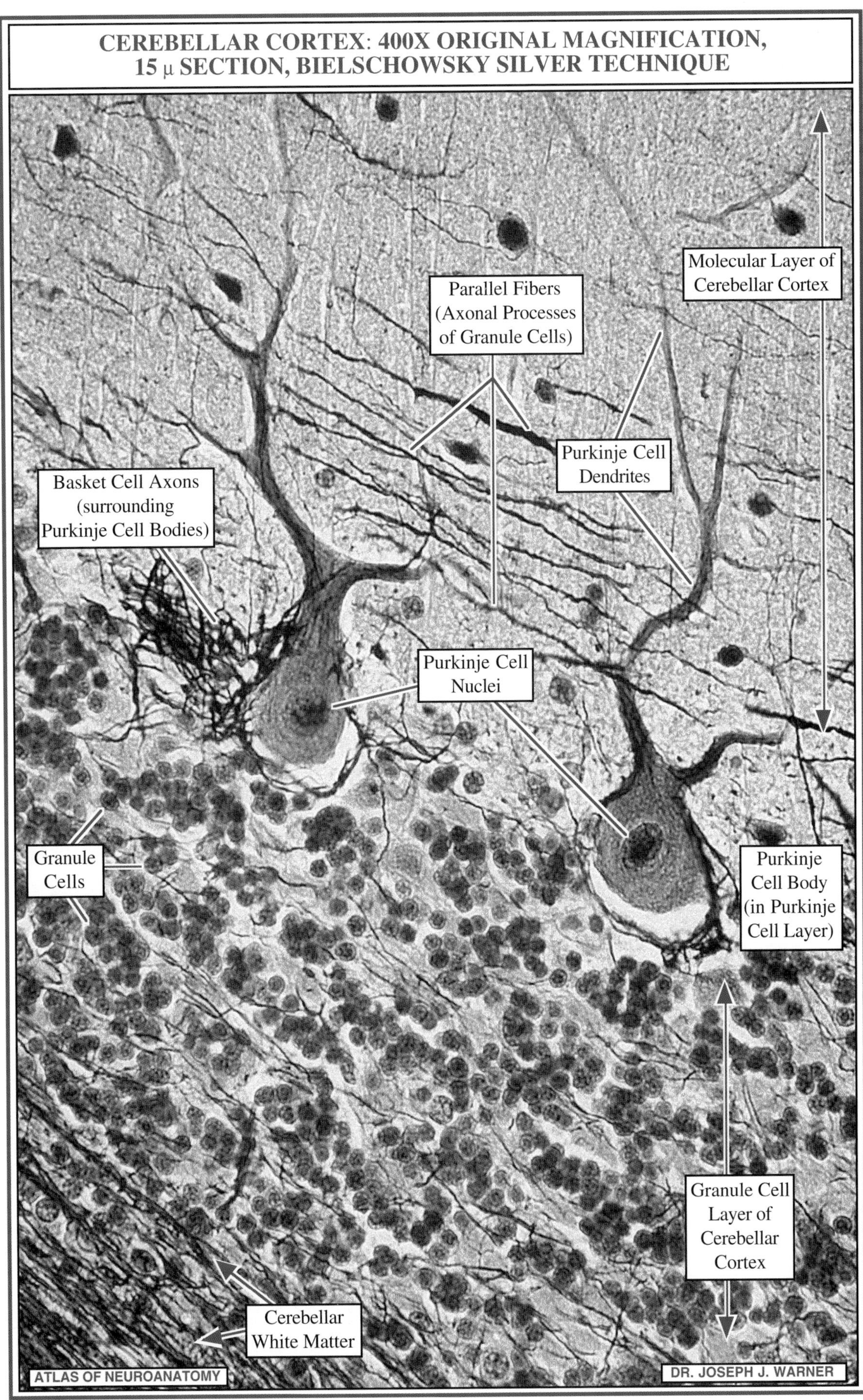
CEREBELLAR CORTEX: 400X ORIGINAL MAGNIFICATION,
15 μ SECTION, BIELSCHOWSKY SILVER TECHNIQUE
Molecular Layer of Cerebellar Cortex
Parallel Fibers (Axonal Processes of Granule Cells)
Purkinje Cell Dendrites
Basket Cell Axons (surrounding Purkinje Cell Bodies)
Purkinje Cell Nuclei
Granule Cells
Purkinje Cell Body (in Purkinje Cell Layer)
Granule Cell Layer of Cerebellar Cortex
Cerebellar White Matter
ATLAS OF NEUROANATOMY
DR. JOSEPH J. WARNER

CEREBELLAR CORTEX: PURKINJE CELLS AND PARALLEL FIBERS
BODIAN SILVER PROTEINATE PROCEDURE, 12 μ SECTION, 400X ORIGINAL MAGNIFICATION

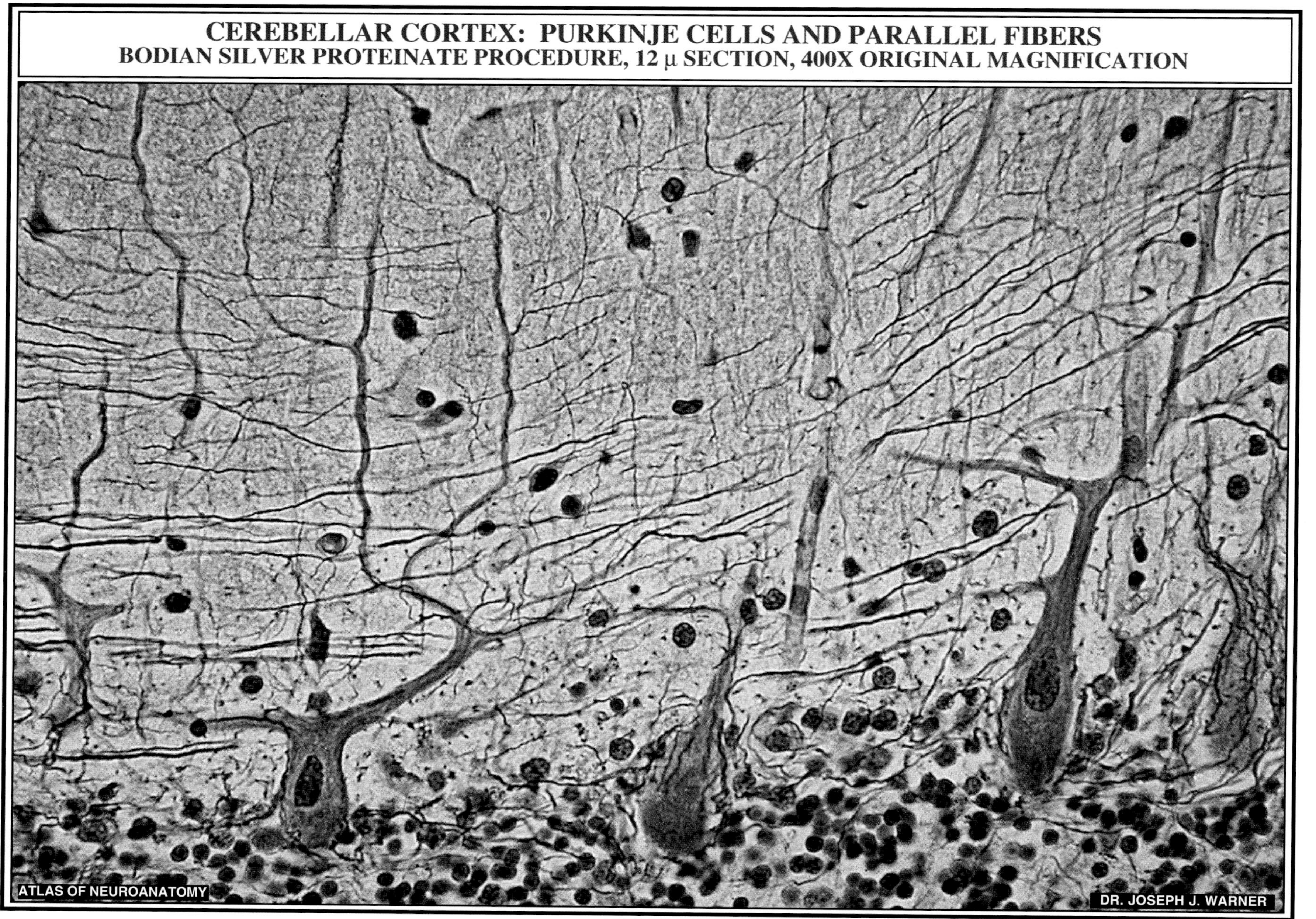

CEREBELLAR CORTEX: PURKINJE CELLS AND PARALLEL FIBERS
BODIAN SILVER PROTEINATE PROCEDURE, 12 μ SECTION
400X MAGNIFICATION

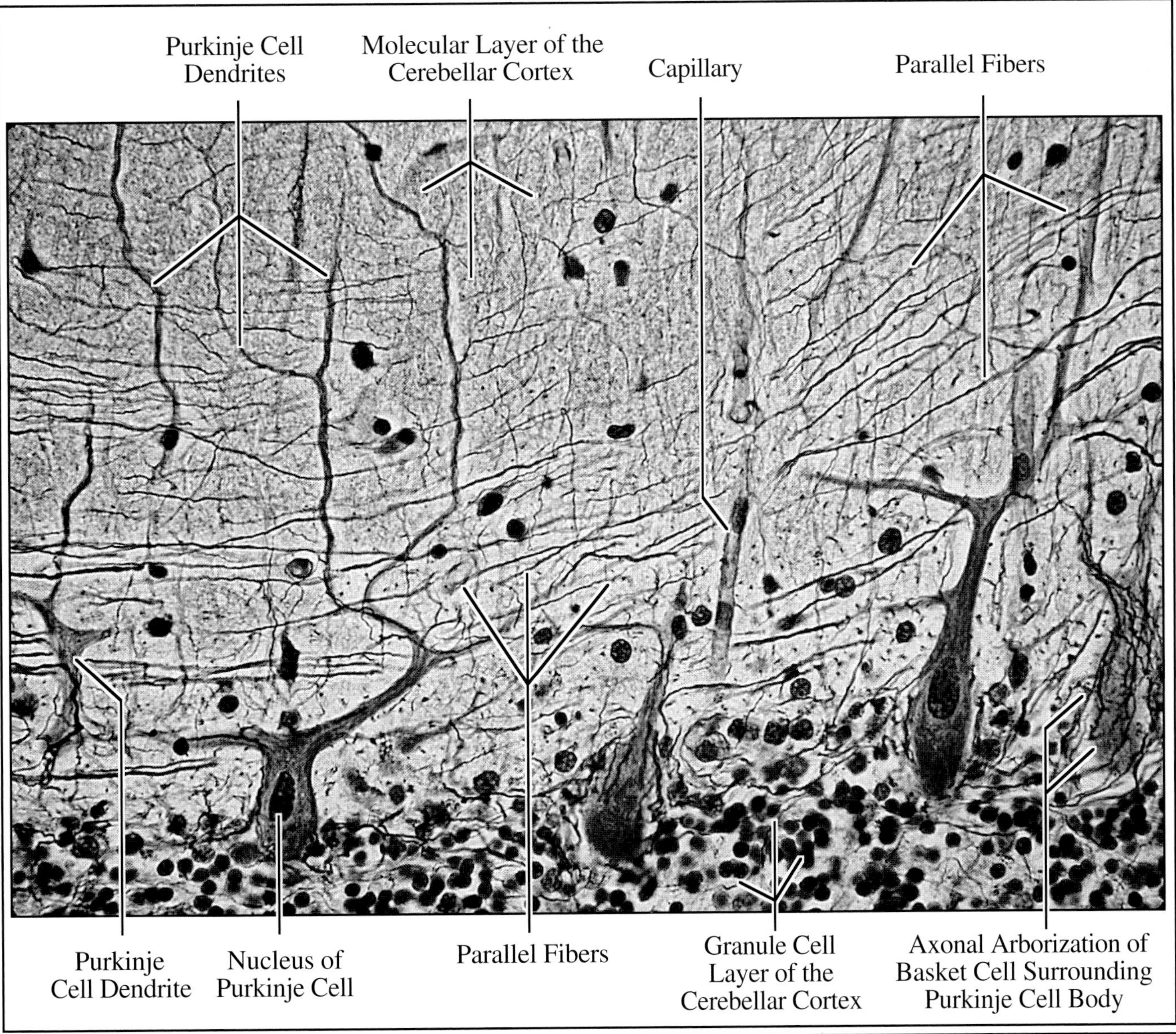

ORGANIZATION OF THE CEREBELLAR CORTEX

The cerebellar cortex is divided into three layers. Directly subjacent to the pial surface of the cerebellar folia is the *Molecular Layer*. Comprised chiefly of dendritic arborizations and axonal processes, this layer also includes two types of neurons. Outer stellate cells send unmyelinated axons (transverse to the longitudinal axis of the folia) that synapse on Purkinje cell dendrites. Basket cells, located adjacent to Purkinje cell bodies, are characterized by dendrites which ascend in the molecular layer, and unmyelinated axons which course perpendicular to the longitudinal axis of each folium. Descending collaterals of basket cell axons form an intricate plexus surrounding individual Each basket cell may form up to ten such axonal arborizations.

The *Purkinje Cell Layer* is comprised of large neurons with complex dendritic arborizations in the molecular layer. These dendritic structures are somewhat planar in morphology, with the plane of the Purkinje cell dendritic tree perpendicular to the longitudinal axis of each folium. Purkinje cell axons are myelinated, project to the deep cerebellar nuclei and give rise to recurrent collaterals which form axosomatic synapses on Golgi type II cells. Climbing fiber terminations, with cell bodies of origin within the inferior olivary nucleus, form complex axodendritic synapses with Purkinje cells.

ORGANIZATION OF THE CEREBELLAR CORTEX

Each climbing fiber branches into several fine terminations that form numerous contacts with one Purkinje cell. Collaterals of climbing fibers may form axosomatic synapses on the same cell as well as axodendritic synapses on adjacent Purkinje cells. In addition to their powerful synaptic influence on Purkinje cells, climbing fibers branch into collaterals that synapse with Golgi, stellate, and basket cells. (Fine collaterals also contact granule cell dendrites.)

The *Granular Layer* is comprised of granule cells, large Golgi type II cells, and smaller Golgi cells. Granule cells are characterized by 4 - 5 short dendritic processes and a long axon which projects into the molecular layer and bifurcates into parallel fibers. Parallel fibers, which form axodendritic synapses on Purkinje and Golgi cells, course parallel to the axis of each folium. One granule cell, by virtue of this arrangement of axonal terminations, synapses with several Purkinje cells. Granule cells receive excitatory input from mossy fiber terminations (in addition to climbing fiber collaterals) and inhibitory input from Golgi cells. Fibers of the dorsal and ventral spinocerebellar tracts, of the cuneocerebellar tract, and of pontocerebellar projections are among those which form mossy fiber terminations. Golgi cell dendrites extend through all layers of the cerebellar cortex. Their numerous axons form complex contacts with granule cell dendrites and mossy fiber terminations. Within the granular layer, several glomeruli are present. Each glomerulus is characterized histologically by a space between the granule cells occupied by a mossy fiber termination (rosette) in contact with numerous granule cell dendrites and with the axons and dendrites of Golgi cells.

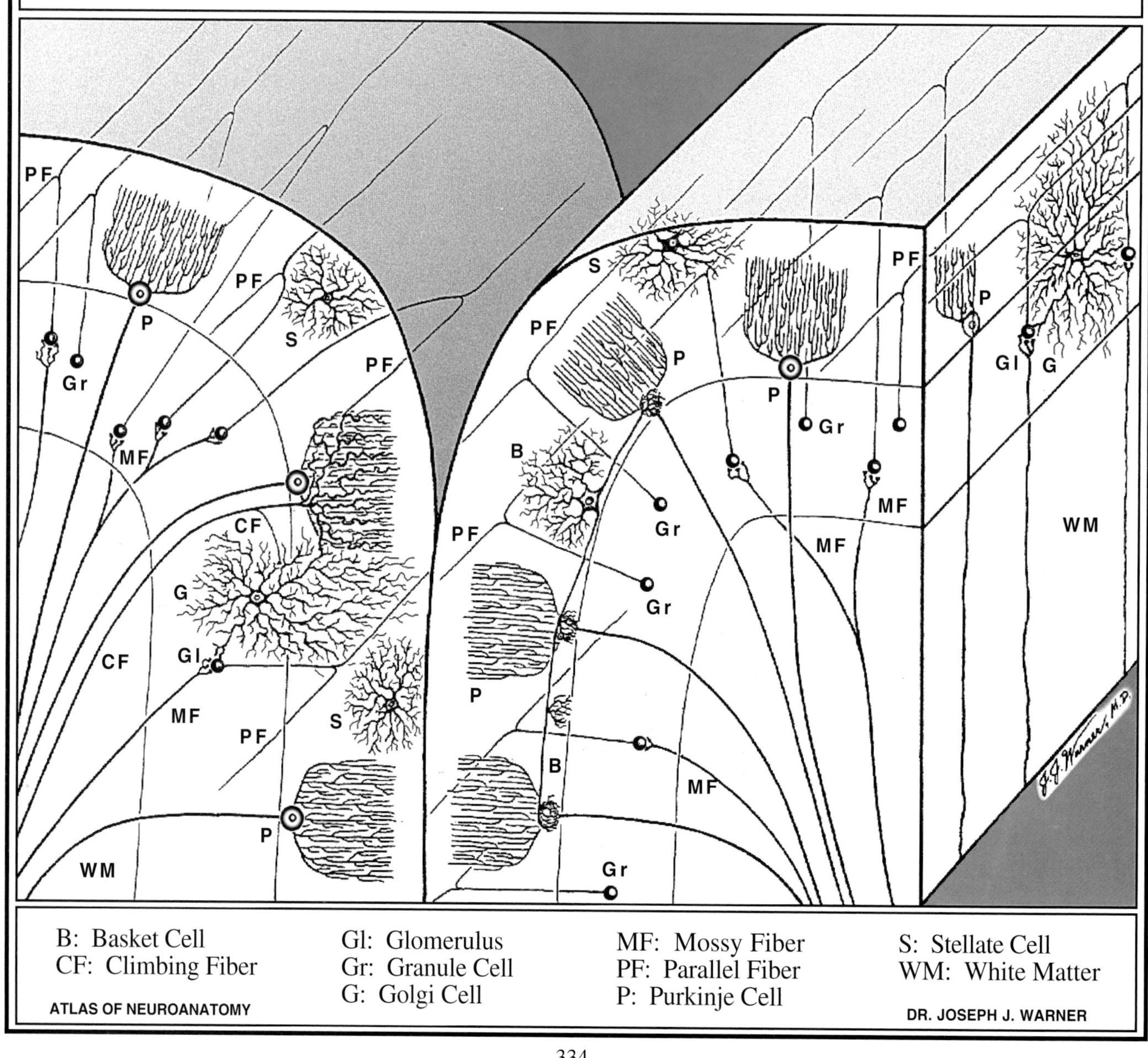

B: Basket Cell
CF: Climbing Fiber
Gl: Glomerulus
Gr: Granule Cell
G: Golgi Cell
MF: Mossy Fiber
PF: Parallel Fiber
P: Purkinje Cell
S: Stellate Cell
WM: White Matter

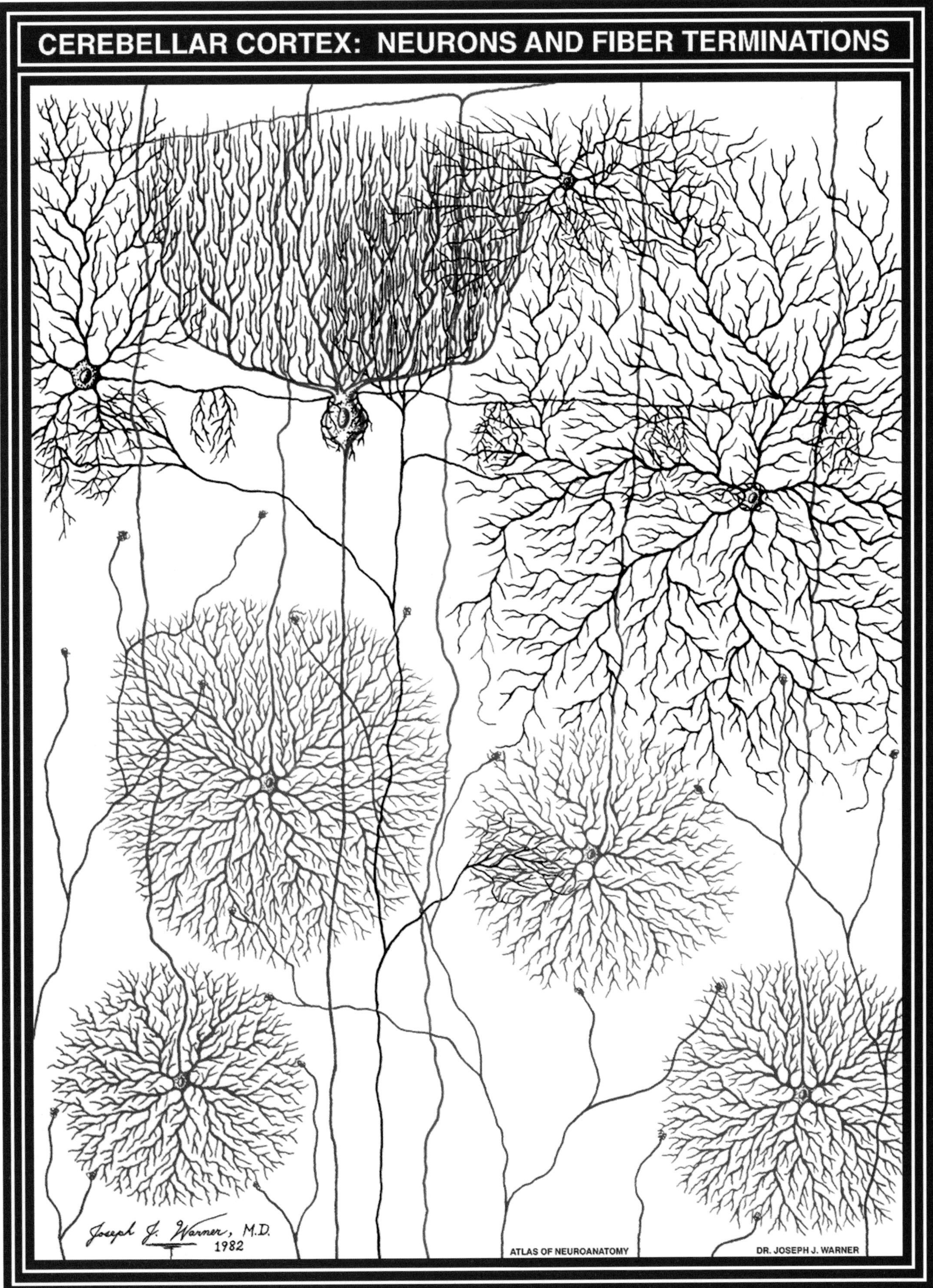
CEREBELLAR CORTEX: NEURONS AND FIBER TERMINATIONS
Joseph J. Warner, M.D.
1982
ATLAS OF NEUROANATOMY
DR. JOSEPH J. WARNER

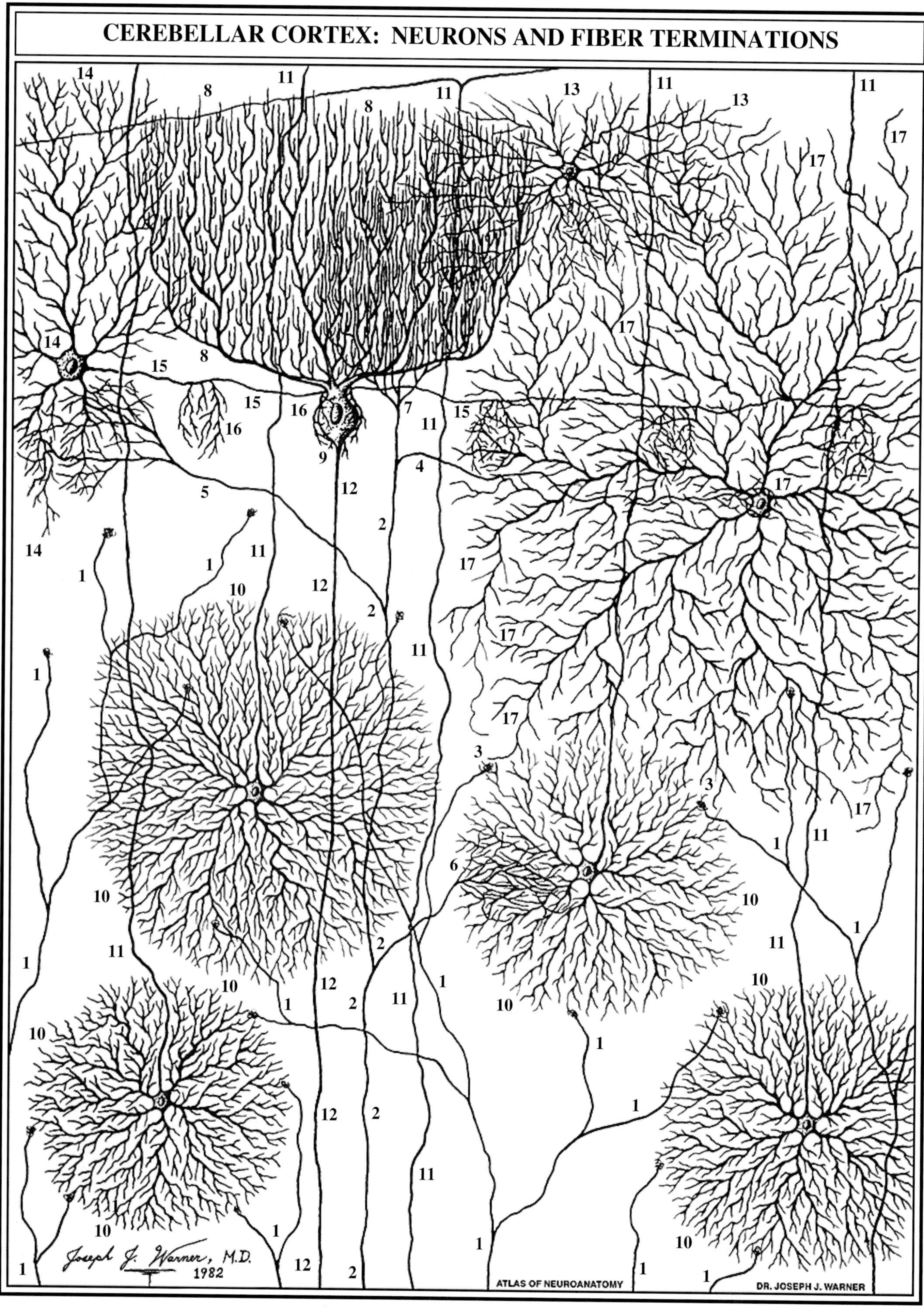
CEREBELLAR CORTEX: NEURONS AND FIBER TERMINATIONS
14
8
11
8
11
13
11
13
11
17
17
17
14
15
8
15
16
7
11
15
16
9
4
17
5
12
2
14
1
1
11
17
12
10
2
11
17
1
17
3
3
17
1
11
6
10
10
1
11
2
11
10
12
1
2
11
1
10
10
1
1
12
2
11
10
1
10
1
12
2
1
1
1
Joseph J. Warner, M.D.
1982
ATLAS OF NEUROANATOMY
DR. JOSEPH J. WARNER

CEREBELLAR CORTEX, NEURONS AND FIBER TERMINATIONS: KEY TO NUMBERED STRUCTURES

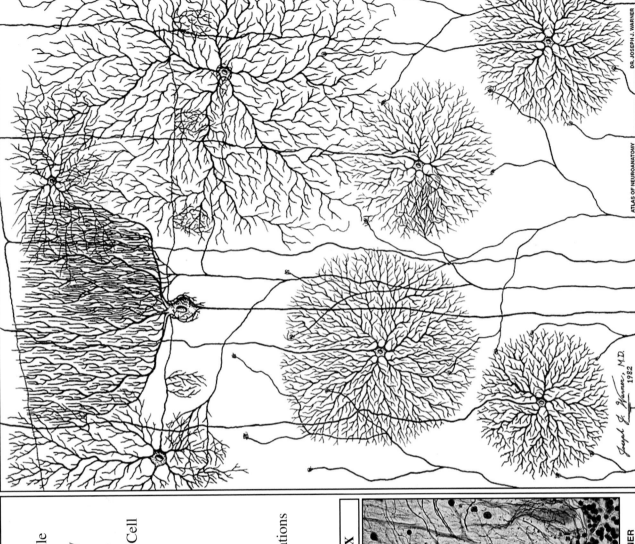

1. Mossy Fibers
2. Climbing Fibers
3. Glomerulus including Mossy Fiber Termination, Granule Cell Dendrites, and Golgi Cell Axons
4. Climbing Fiber Collateral projecting to Golgi Cell Body
5. Climbing Fiber Collateral projecting to Basket Cell
6. Climbing Fiber Collateral projecting to Granule Cell Dendrites
7. Climbing Fiber Terminations ascending along Purkinje Cell Dendritic Arborization
8. Dendritic Arborization of Purkinje Cell
9. Purkinje Cell
10. Granule Cell Dendrites
11. Granule Cell Axons (subsequently bifurcate to form Parallel Fibers)
12. Axon of Purkinje Cell
13. Stellate Cell Processes
14. Basket Cell Processes
15. Axon of Basket Cell with a series of terminal Arborizations
16. Axonal Arborization of Basket Cell (each of which surrounds a single Purkinje Cell)
17. Golgi Cell and its Processes

CEREBELLAR CORTEX: BODIAN SILVER, 12 μ, 400X

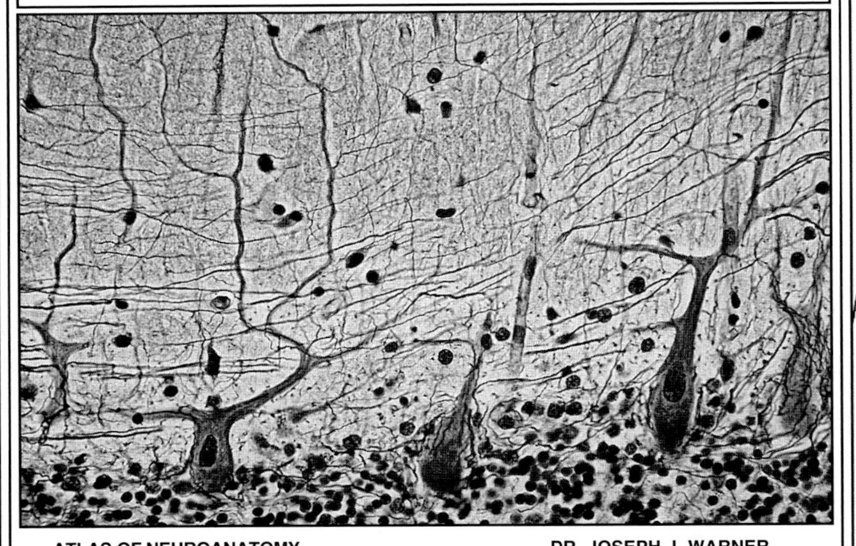

ATLAS OF NEUROANATOMY DR. JOSEPH J. WARNER

Joseph J. Warner, M.D. 1982

ATLAS OF NEUROANATOMY DR. JOSEPH J. WARNER

ANTERIOR HORN CELLS (MOTOR NEURONS) OF THE SPINAL CORD:
A. CERVICAL ANTERIOR HORN, BODIAN SILVER PROTEINATE TECHNIQUE
B. LUMBAR ANTERIOR HORN, BIELSCHOWSKY SILVER TECHNIQUE

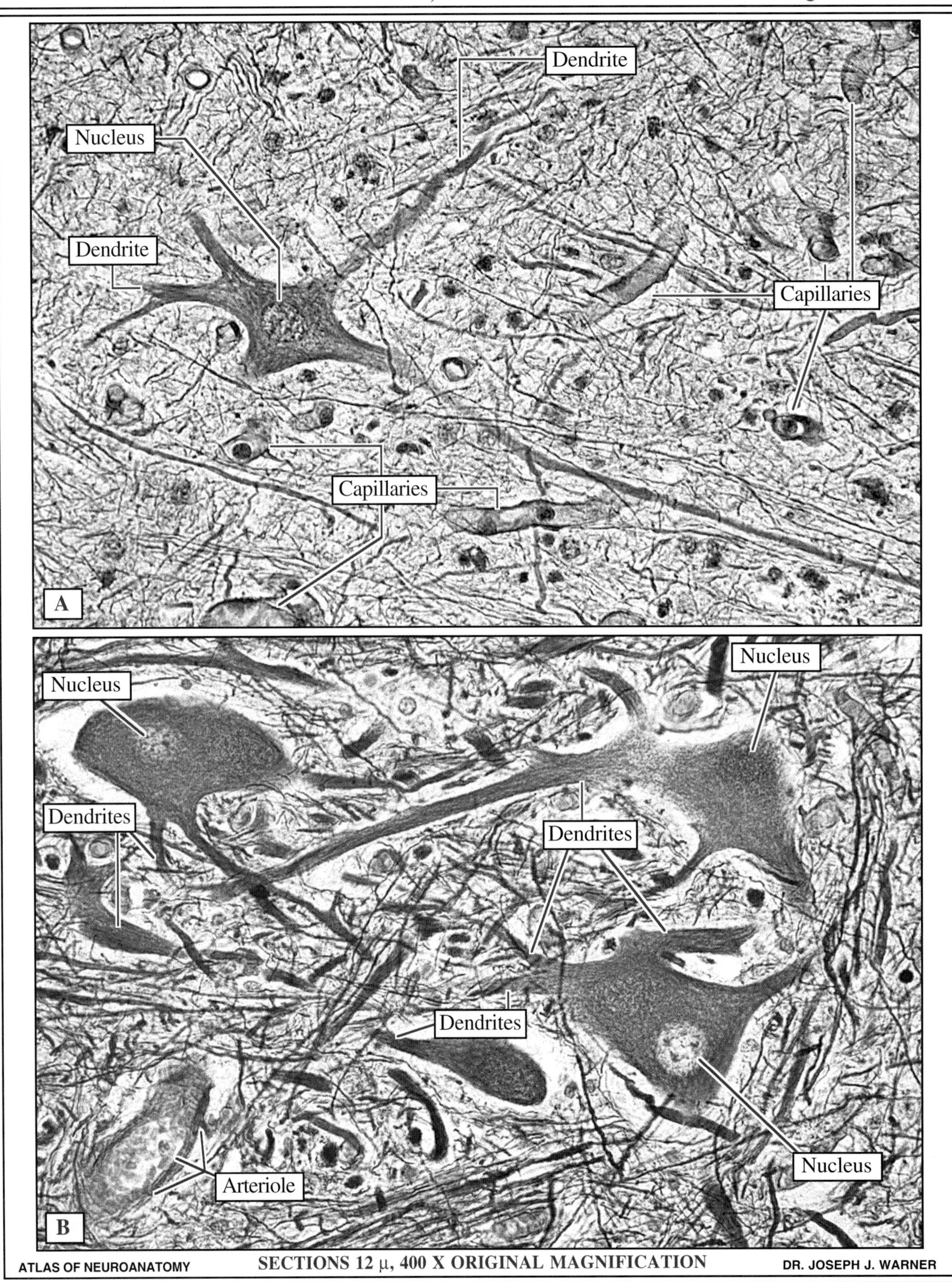

ATLAS OF NEUROANATOMY SECTIONS 12 μ, 400 X ORIGINAL MAGNIFICATION DR. JOSEPH J. WARNER

CERVICAL SPINAL CORD, CENTRAL REGION: 250X
12 μ SECTION, BODIAN SILVER PROTEINATE PROCEDURE

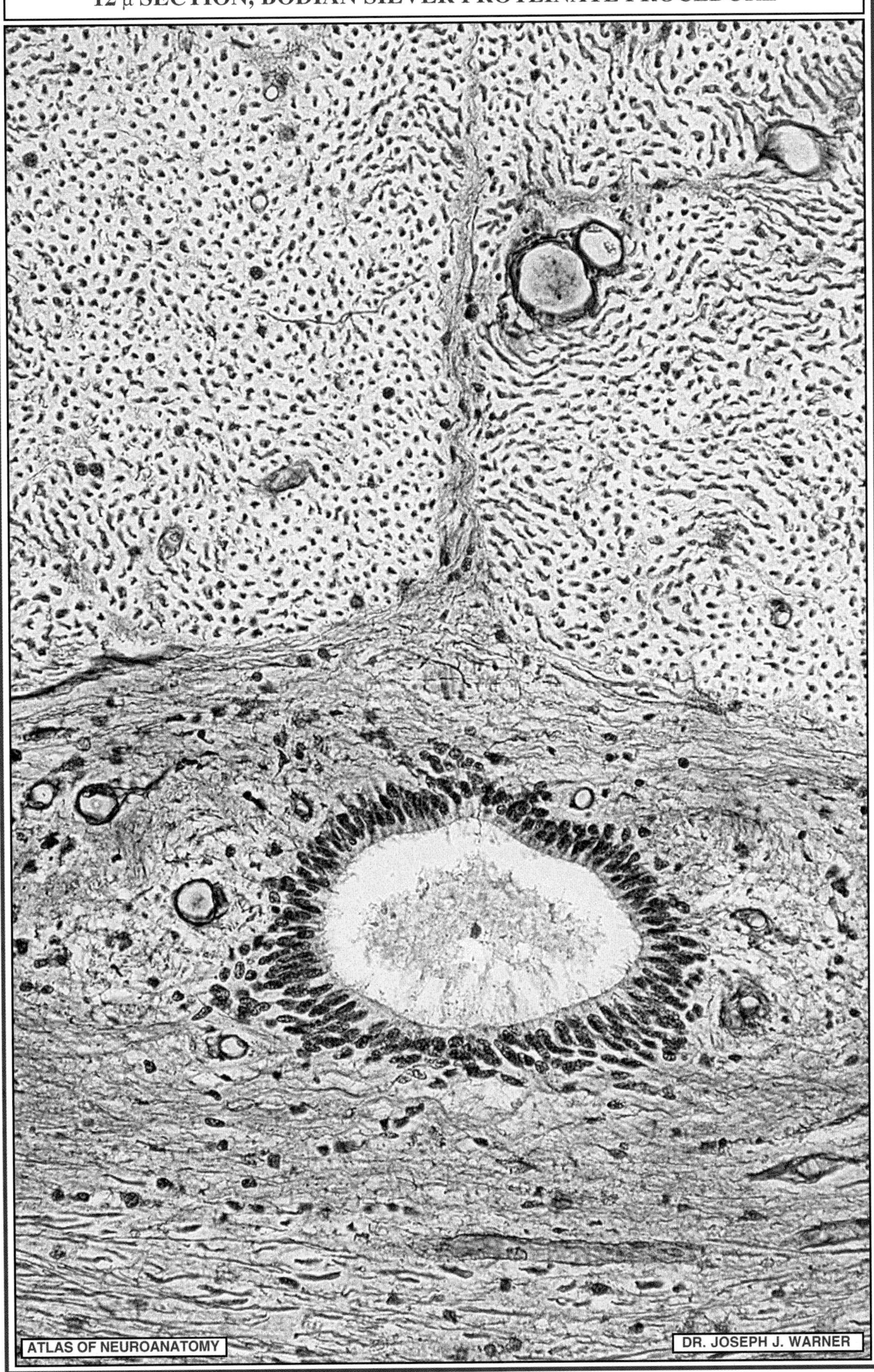

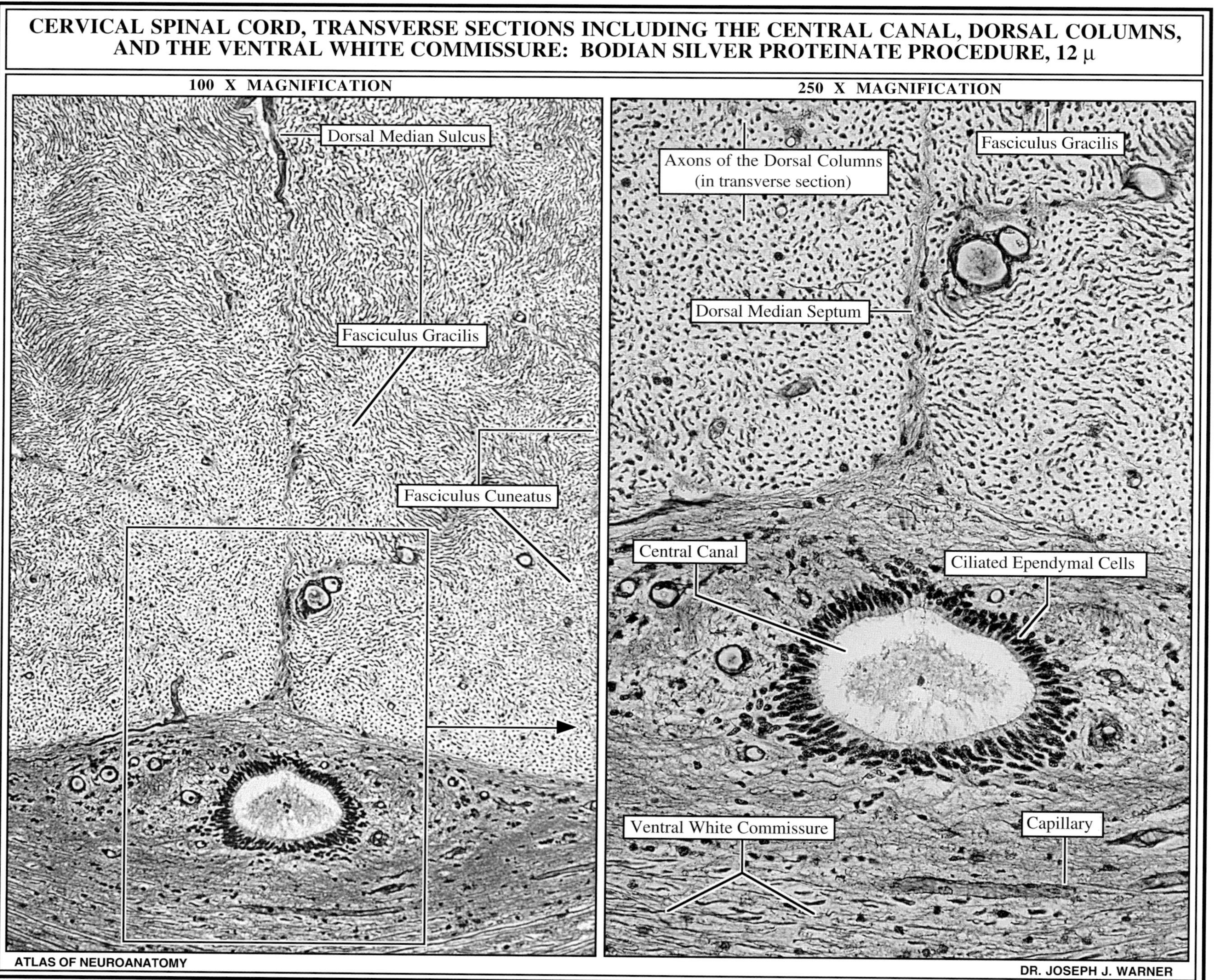
CERVICAL SPINAL CORD, TRANSVERSE SECTIONS INCLUDING THE CENTRAL CANAL, DORSAL COLUMNS, AND THE VENTRAL WHITE COMMISSURE: BODIAN SILVER PROTEINATE PROCEDURE, 12 μ
100 X MAGNIFICATION
Dorsal Median Sulcus
Fasciculus Gracilis
Fasciculus Cuneatus
250 X MAGNIFICATION
Axons of the Dorsal Columns
(in transverse section)
Fasciculus Gracilis
Dorsal Median Septum
Central Canal
Ciliated Ependymal Cells
Ventral White Commissure
Capillary
ATLAS OF NEUROANATOMY
DR. JOSEPH J. WARNER

HISTOLOGY OF PERIPHERAL GANGLIA: A COMPARISON OF (1) HEMATOXYLIN AND EOSIN AND (2) CRESYL ECHT VIOLET NISSL STAINED SECTIONS OF HUMAN LUMBAR DORSAL ROOT GANGLIA

1.

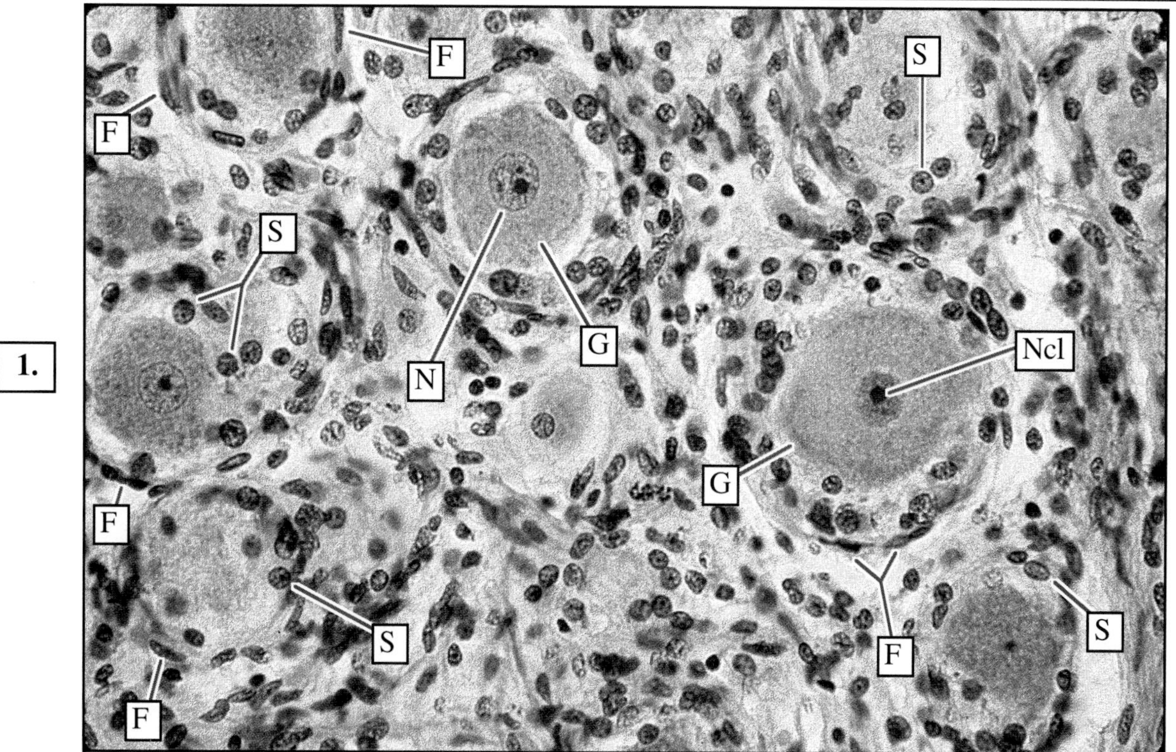

1. Hematoxylin and eosin stained section demonstrates neurons (G) characterized by spheroidal cell bodies and nuclei (N) with well-defined nucleoli (Ncl). Satellite cells (S) are situated circumferentially around the neurons. Fibroblasts are evident as spindle-shaped cells with elongated nuclei (F).

2.

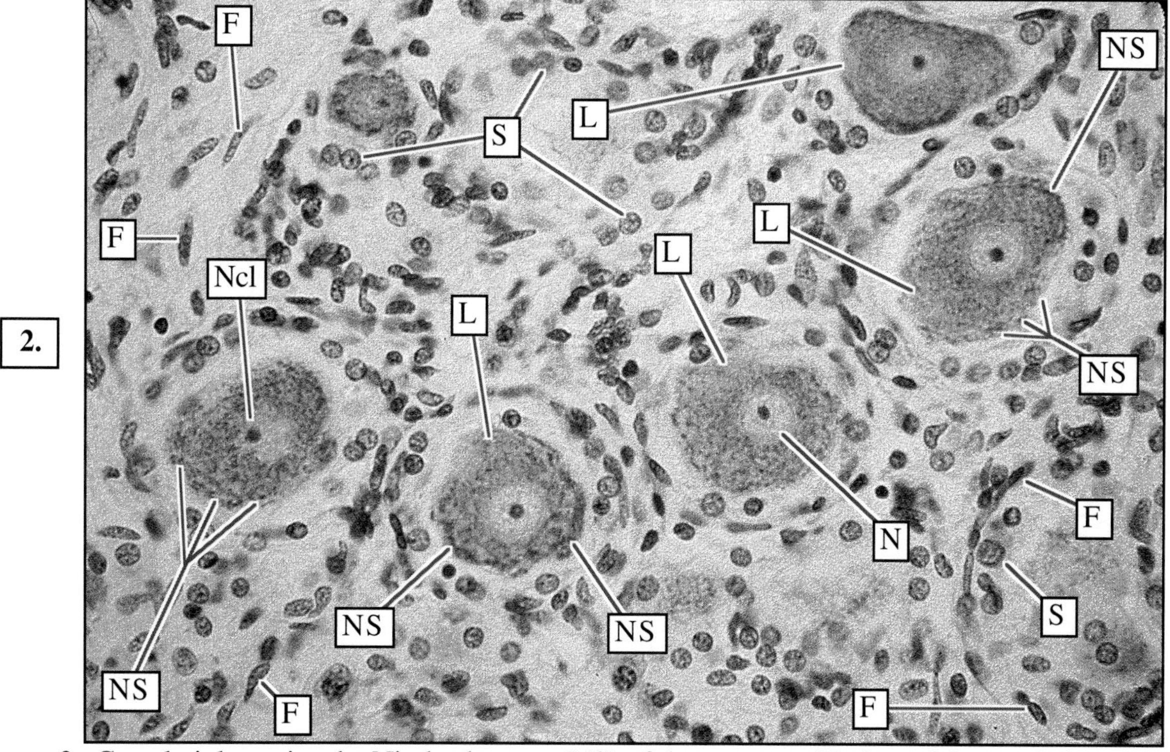

2. Cresyl violet stains the Nissl substance (NS) of the neurons. Their nuclei are pale in comparison to the cytoplasm, and contain a darkly stained nucleolus. Lipofuscin pigment (L) appears as golden-brown granular accumulations eccentrically located in the neuronal cytoplasm.

Sections: 250X original magnification

THE TRIGEMINAL GANGLION: 12 μ SECTION, BIELSCHOWSKY SILVER TECHNIQUE

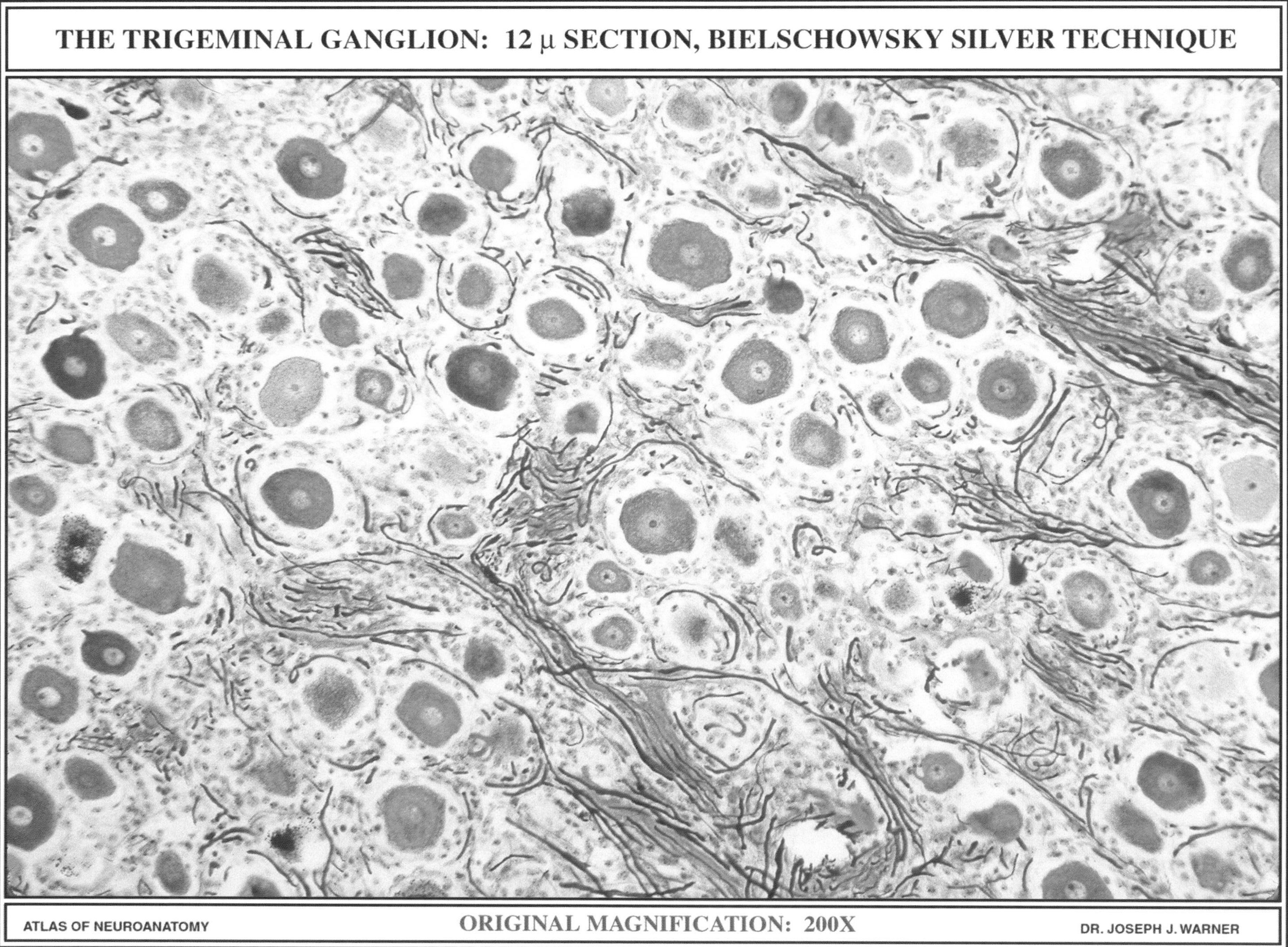

ORIGINAL MAGNIFICATION: 200X

HISTOLOGY OF PERIPHERAL NERVE: A COMPARISON OF (1) HEMATOXYLIN AND EOSIN AND (2) ANILINE BLUE TRICHROME STAINED LONGITUDINAL SECTIONS OF HUMAN FEMORAL NERVE

1.

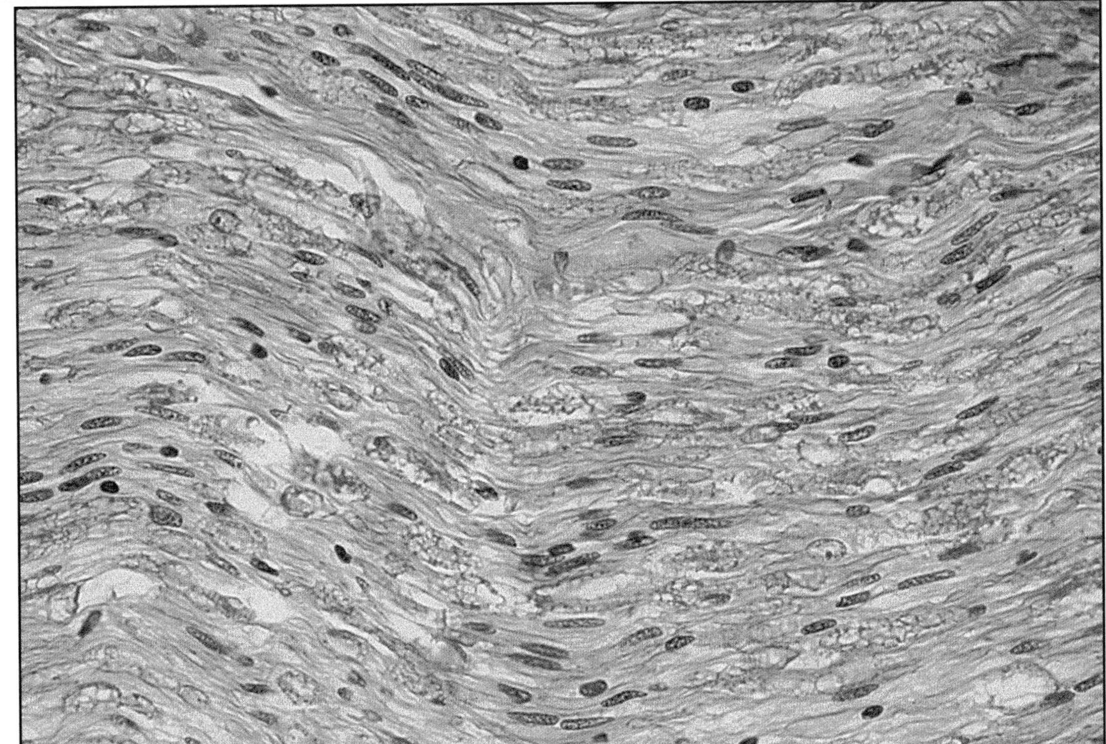

1. Longitudinal section of femoral nerve, 10 μ, hematoxylin and eosin stained, demonstrates nuclei of Schwann cells as well as of fibroblasts. Peripheral myelin (formed by Schwann cells) and collagen (comprising endoneurium, perineurium, and epineurium) are eosinophilic.

2.

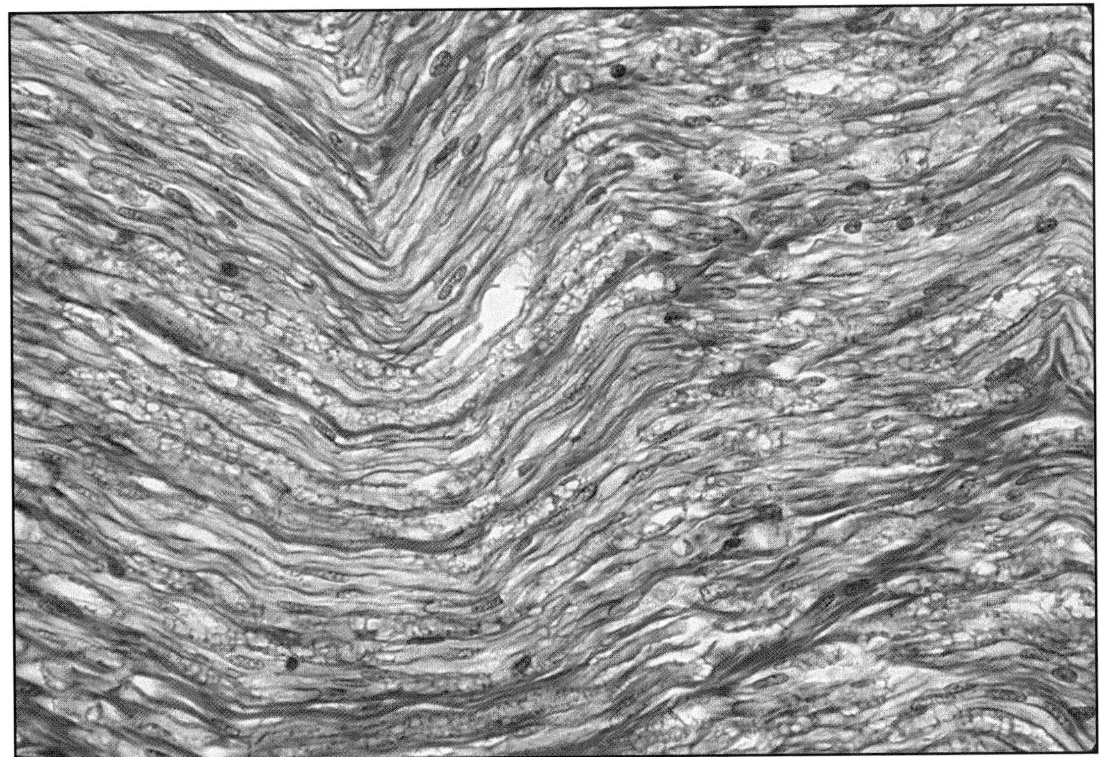

2. Longitudinal section of femoral nerve, 10 μ, aniline blue trichrome stained, distinguishes myelin (scarlet) from endoneurial, perineurial, and epineurial collagen (stained with aniline blue).

Sections: 100X original magnification

LONGITUDINAL SECTION OF HUMAN FEMORAL NERVE DEMONSTRATING MULTIPLE FIBER DIAMETERS: SECTION 10 µ , BODIAN SILVER TECHNIQUE, 400X ORIGINAL MAGNIFICATION

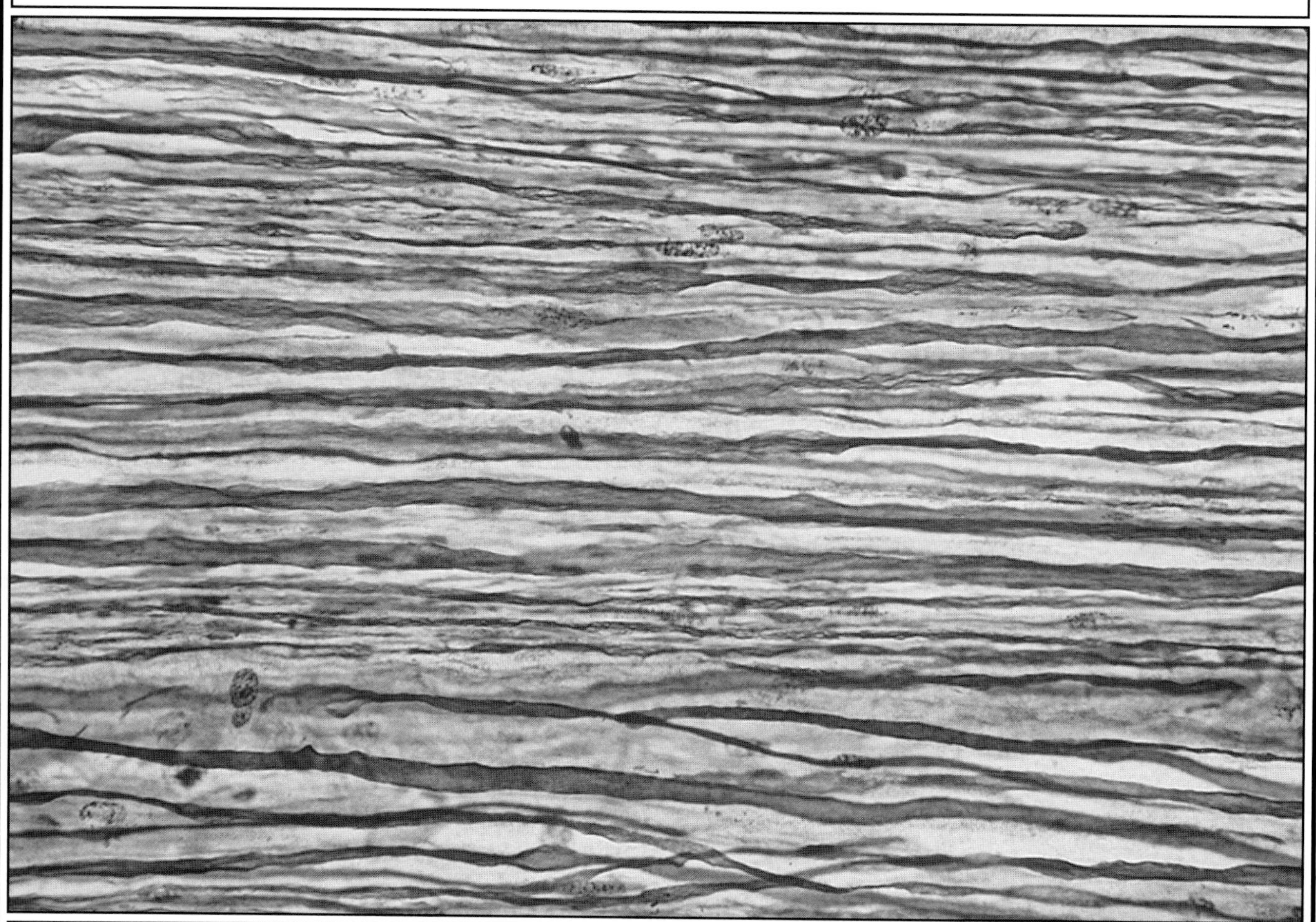

CLASSIFICATION OF AFFERENT FIBERS BASED UPON DIAMETER

FIBER TYPE	CONDUCTION VELOCITY		AFFERENT MODALITY OR RECEPTOR
Group I A alpha	70 - 120 meters / sec.	Ia	Primary muscle spindle afferents
		Ib	Golgi tendon organs
Group II A beta	25 - 70 meters / sec.	II	Secondary muscle spindle afferents Joint Receptors
		A beta	Cutaneous touch receptors
Group III A delta	10 - 30 meters / sec.	III	Muscle and visceral receptors (pressure and pain)
		A delta	Protopathic touch, pain, and temperature (cutaneous receptors)
Group IV Type C	0.5 - 2 meters / sec.	IV	Deep pain sensation
		C	Cutaneous pain and temperature sensation

Afferent fiber diameters fall into distinct categories that correlate with conduction velocity and general functional characteristics. Large fiber modalities include discriminative aspects of tactile sensation and afferent input from receptors involved in proprioception, detection of muscle length and mechanical tension. These are primarily represented by larger, myelinated fibers, which include Group I and II afferents. Group IV or Type C fibers are unmyelinated, characterized by a small diameter and slow conduction velocities. The histologic section of the femoral nerve contains both afferent and efferent (motor) fibers. The distinct fiber sizes are clearly demonstrated by the Bodian silver technique. Large-diameter fibers have the lowest threshold for activation by electrical stimulation. This property is demonstrable in transcutaneous electrical nerve stimulation (T.E.N.S.) in which large-fiber activation produces sensations similating vibration or touch, not perceived as painful. T.E.N.S.-induced afferent activation is used to modulate pain transmission.

PART IV: SECTIONAL NEUROANATOMY OF THE THALAMUS AND BASAL GANGLIA

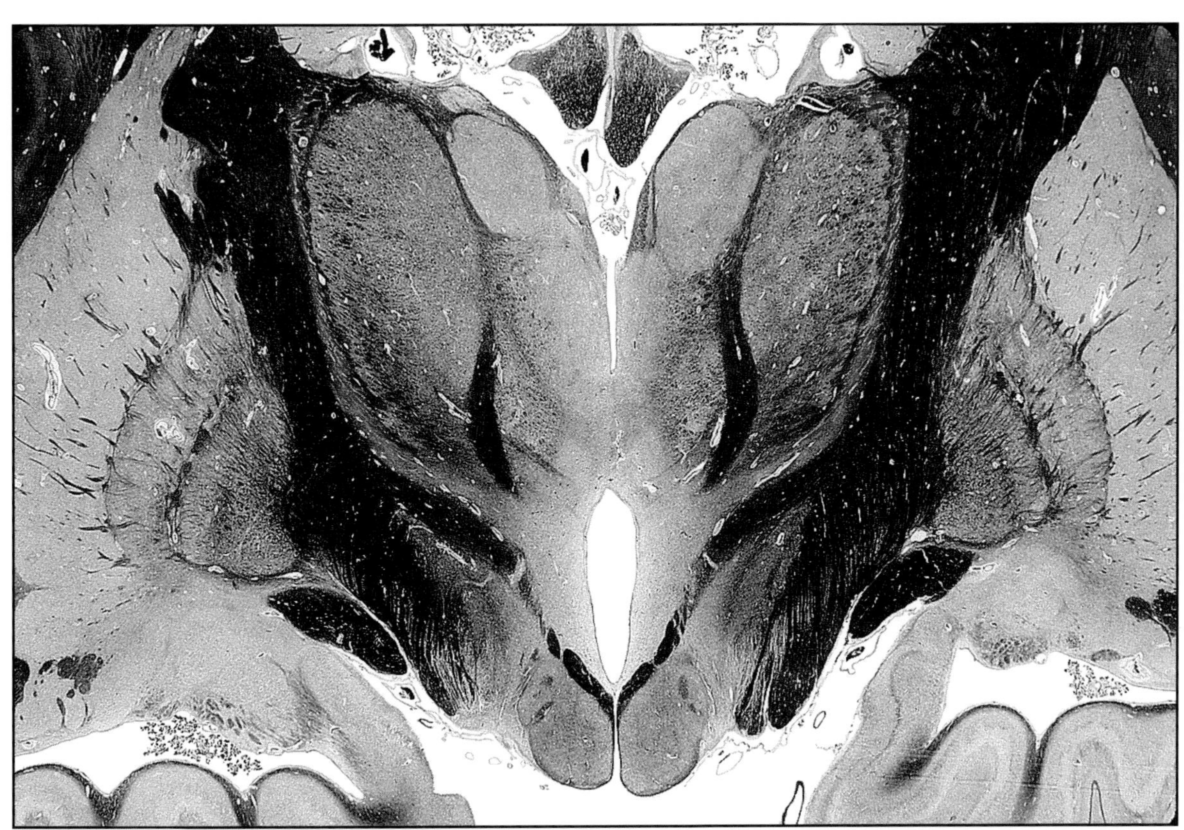

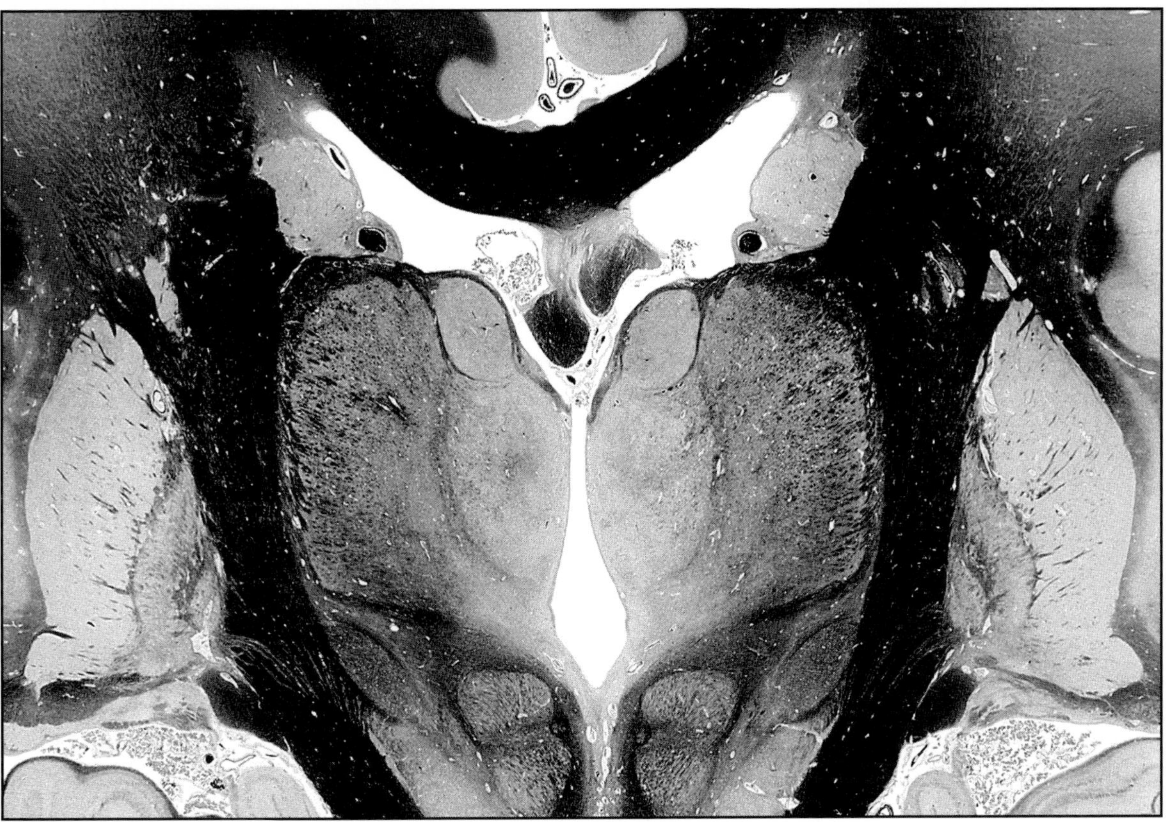

CORONAL SECTION OF THE BRAIN: LEVEL OF THE ANTERIOR COMMISSURE, OPTIC CHIASM, AND THE ANTERIOR PERFORATED SUBSTANCE

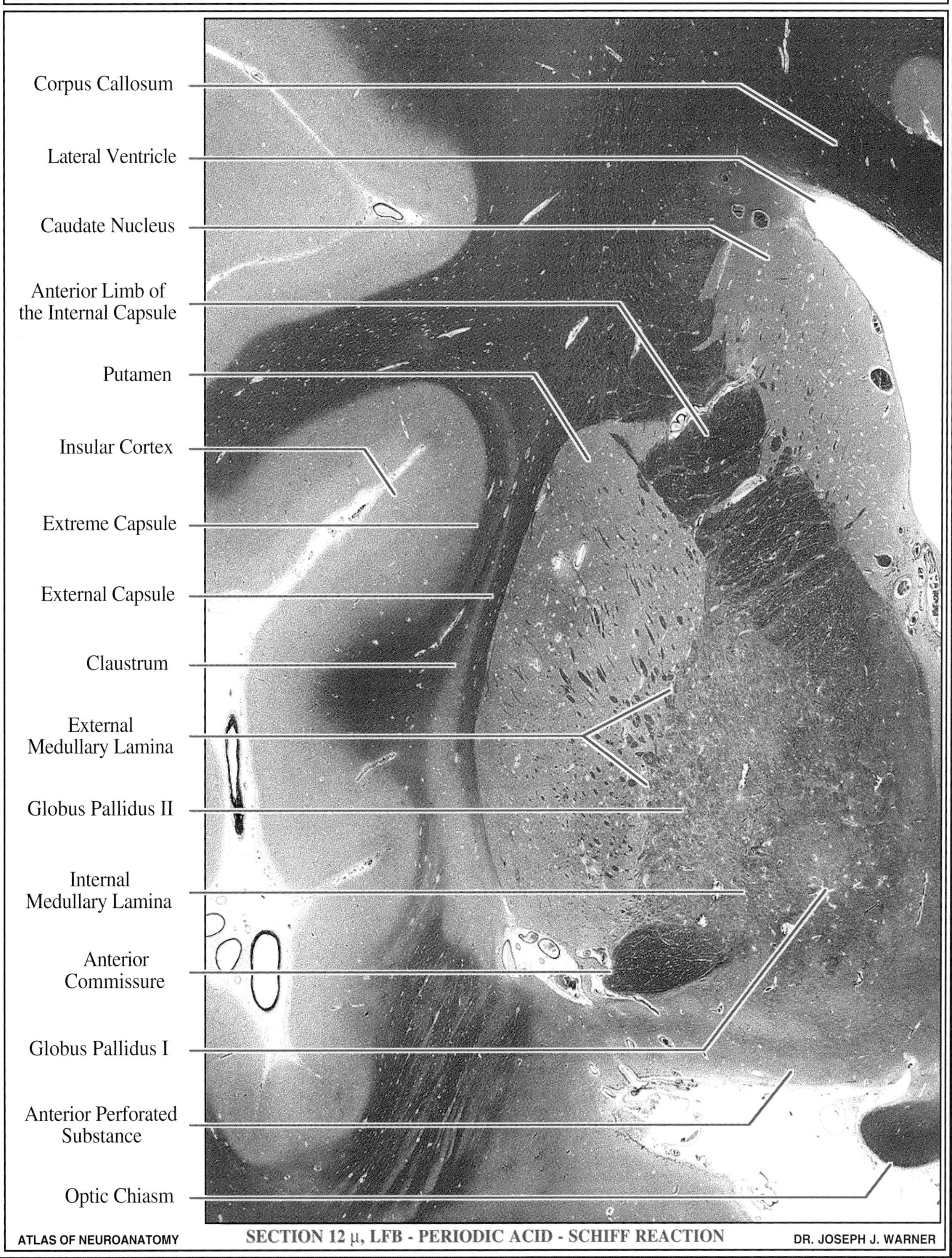

SECTION 12 μ, LFB - PERIODIC ACID - SCHIFF REACTION

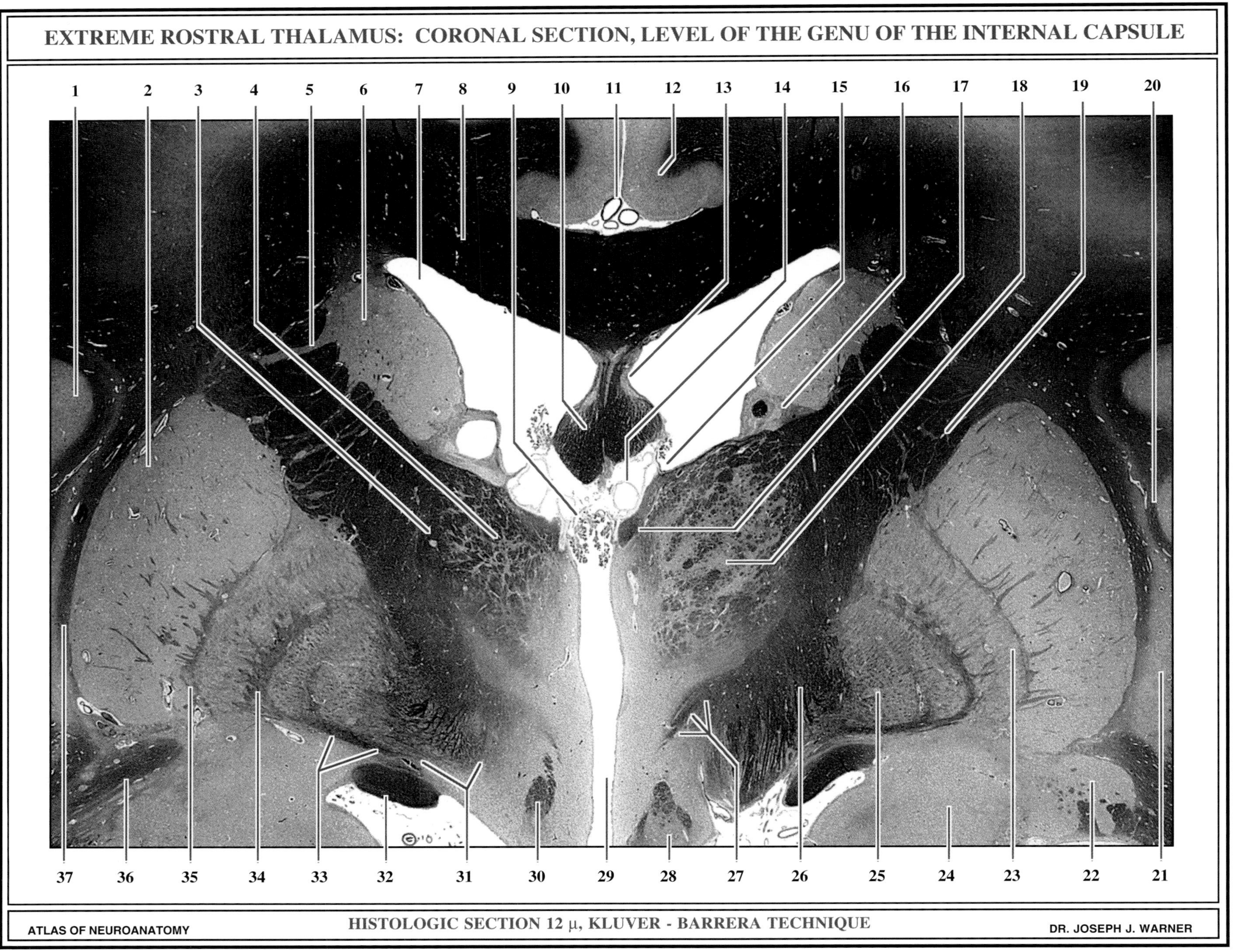

EXTREME ROSTRAL THALAMUS: CORONAL SECTION, LEVEL OF THE GENU OF THE INTERNAL CAPSULE
1 2 3 4 5 6 7 8 9 10 11 12 13 14 15 16 17 18 19 20
37 36 35 34 33 32 31 30 29 28 27 26 25 24 23 22 21
ATLAS OF NEUROANATOMY
HISTOLOGIC SECTION 12 μ, KLUVER - BARRERA TECHNIQUE
DR. JOSEPH J. WARNER

CORONAL SECTION OF THE BRAIN; LEVEL OF THE EXTREME ROSTRAL THALAMUS AND GENU OF THE INTERNAL CAPSULE: SECTION ORIENTATION AND KEY TO NUMBERED STRUCTURES

KEY TO NUMBERED STRUCTURES

1. Insula
2. Putamen
3. Genu of the Internal Capsule
4. Reticular Nucleus of the Thalamus and the Anterior Thalamic Radiations
5. Transcapsular Caudatolenticular Gray Stria
6. Caudate Nucleus
7. Body of the Lateral Ventricle
8. Corpus Callosum
9. Taenia Thalami
10. Fornix
11. Anterior Cerebral Arteries
12. Cingulate Cortex
13. Septum Pellucidum
14. Internal Cerebral Vein
15. Tela Choroidea*
16. Stria Terminalis and the Thalamostriate Vein
17. Stria Medullaris
18. Anterior Nuclear Group of the Thalamus
19. Anterior Limb of the Internal Capsule
20. Extreme Capsule
21. Claustrum
22. Tail of the Caudate Nucleus
23. Globus Pallidus II
24. Amygdala
25. Globus Pallidus I
26. Posterior Limb of the Internal Capsule
27. Lenticular Fasciculus
28. Mammillary Body (rostral aspect)
29. Third Ventricle
30. Fornix
31. Ansa Lenticularis
32. Optic Tract
33. Ansa Lenticularis
34. Internal Medullary Lamina
35. External Medullary Lamina
36. Anterior Commissure
37. External Capsule

*The taenia thalami forms the epithelial roof of the third ventricle. The tela choroidea separate the ventricles from the subarachnoid compartments.

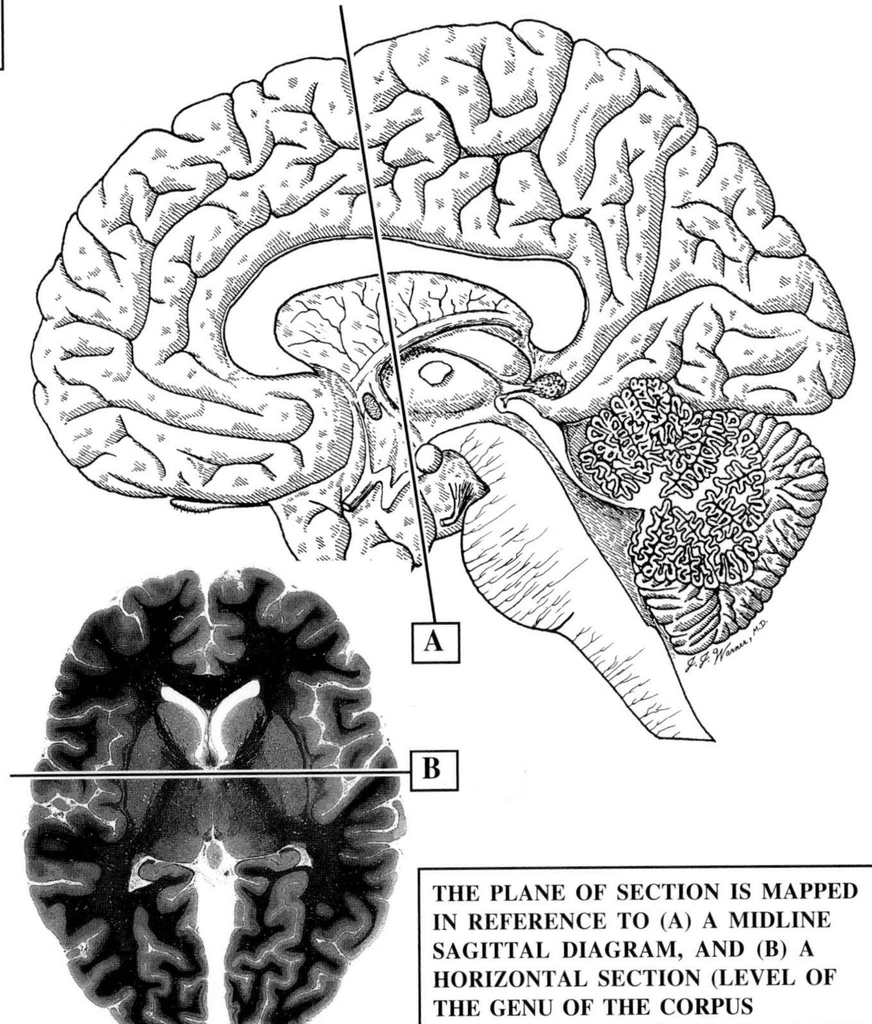

THE PLANE OF SECTION IS MAPPED IN REFERENCE TO (A) A MIDLINE SAGITTAL DIAGRAM, AND (B) A HORIZONTAL SECTION (LEVEL OF THE GENU OF THE CORPUS CALLOSUM AND THE PINEAL BODY)

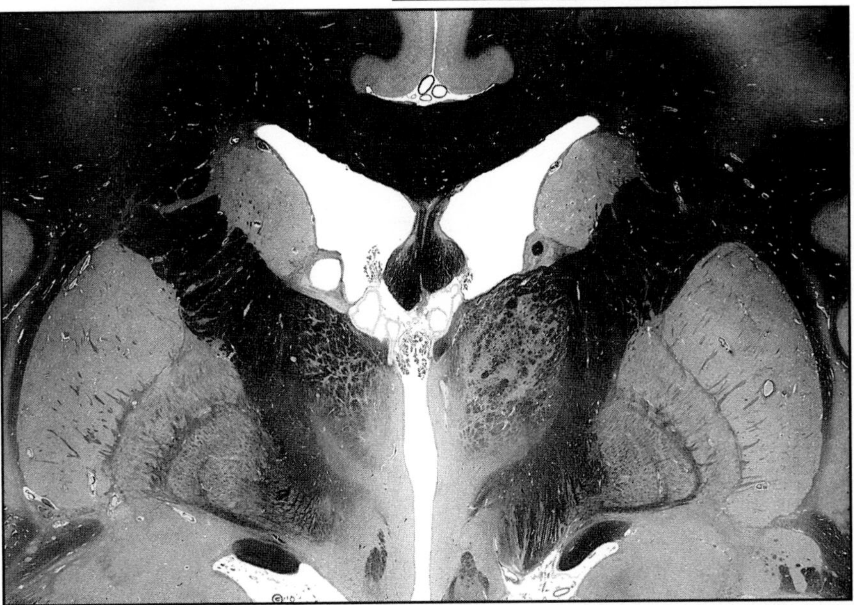

HISTOLOGICAL SECTION: 12 μ, KLUVER - BARRERA TECHNIQUE

CORONAL SECTION OF THE BRAIN; LEVEL OF THE EXTREME ROSTRAL THALAMUS AND GENU OF THE INTERNAL CAPSULE: PLANE MAPPED ON A HORIZONTAL REFERENCE SECTION

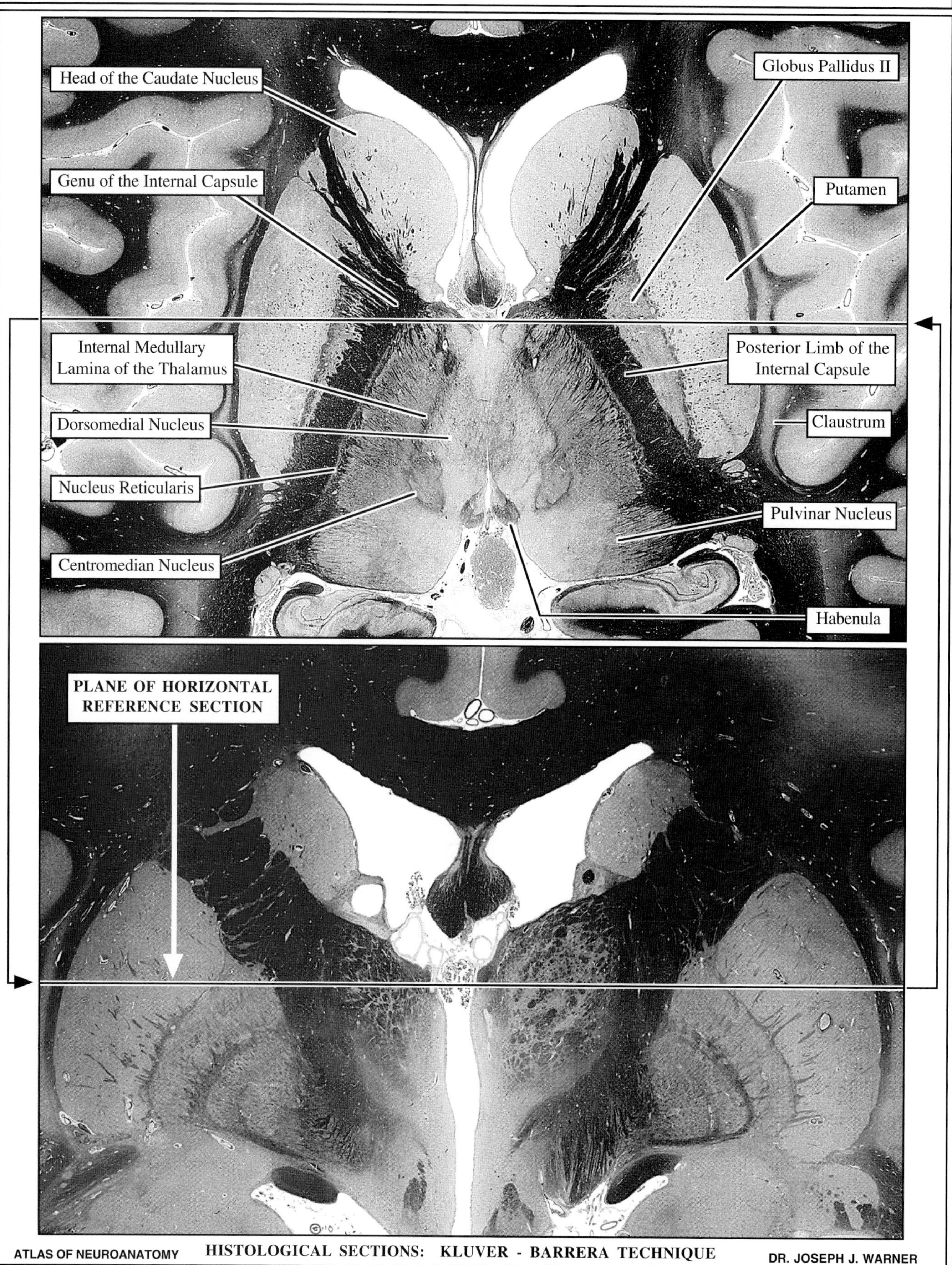

CORONAL SECTION OF THE BRAIN; LEVEL OF THE ANTERIOR NUCLEUS OF THE THALAMUS, THE MAMMILLOTHALAMIC TRACT, AND THE MAMMILLARY BODIES

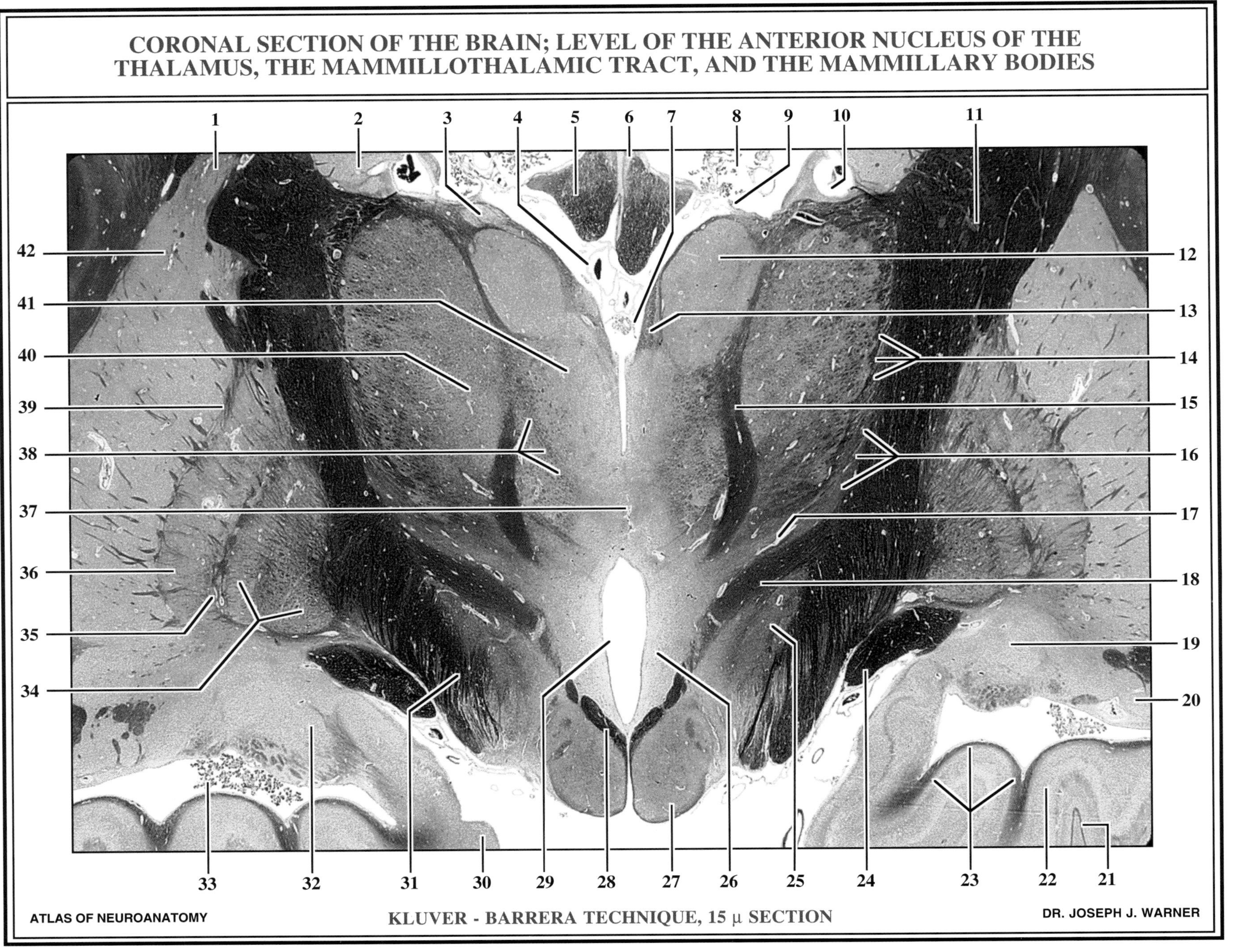

KLUVER - BARRERA TECHNIQUE, 15 μ SECTION

CORONAL SECTION OF THE BRAIN; LEVEL OF THE ANTERIOR NUCLEUS OF THE THALAMUS, THE MAMMILLOTHALAMIC TRACT, AND THE MAMMILLARY BODIES (MAGNIFIED VIEW): SECTION ORIENTATION AND KEY TO NUMBERED STRUCTURES

1. Transcapsular Caudatolenticular Gray Stria
2. Caudate Nucleus
3. Lateral Dorsal Nucleus of the Thalamus
4. Internal Cerebral Vein
5. Fornix
6. Septum Pellucidum
7. Taenia Thalami
8. Choroid Plexus in the Lateral Ventricle
9. Tela Choroidea
10. Thalamostriate Vein and Stria Terminalis
11. Posterior Limb of the Internal Capsule
12. Anterior Nucleus of the Thalamus
13. Stria Medullaris
14. External Medullary Lamina of the Thalamus
15. Mammillothalamic Tract
16. Nucleus Reticularis of the Thalamus
17. Zona Incerta
18. Lenticular Fasciculus (Field H2 of Forel)
19. Amygdala
20. Tail of the Caudate Nucleus (terminates in juxtaposition to the Amygdala)
21. Dentate Gyrus of the Hippocampus
22. Hippocampal Formation
23. Alveus
24. Optic Tract
25. Subthalamic Nucleus (rostral aspect)
26. Posterior Hypothalamus
27. Mammillary Body
28. Principal Mammillary Fasciculus
29. Third Ventricle
30. Uncus
31. Cerebral Peduncle
32. Amygdala
33. Choroid Plexus in the Temporal Horn of the Lateral Ventricle
34. Globus Pallidus I
35. Internal Medullary Lamina
36. Globus Pallidus II
37. Massa Intermedia
38. Internal Medullary Lamina of the Thalamus
39. External Medullary Lamina
40. Ventroanterior Nucleus of the Thalamus
41. Dorsomedial Nucleus of the Thalamus
42. Putamen

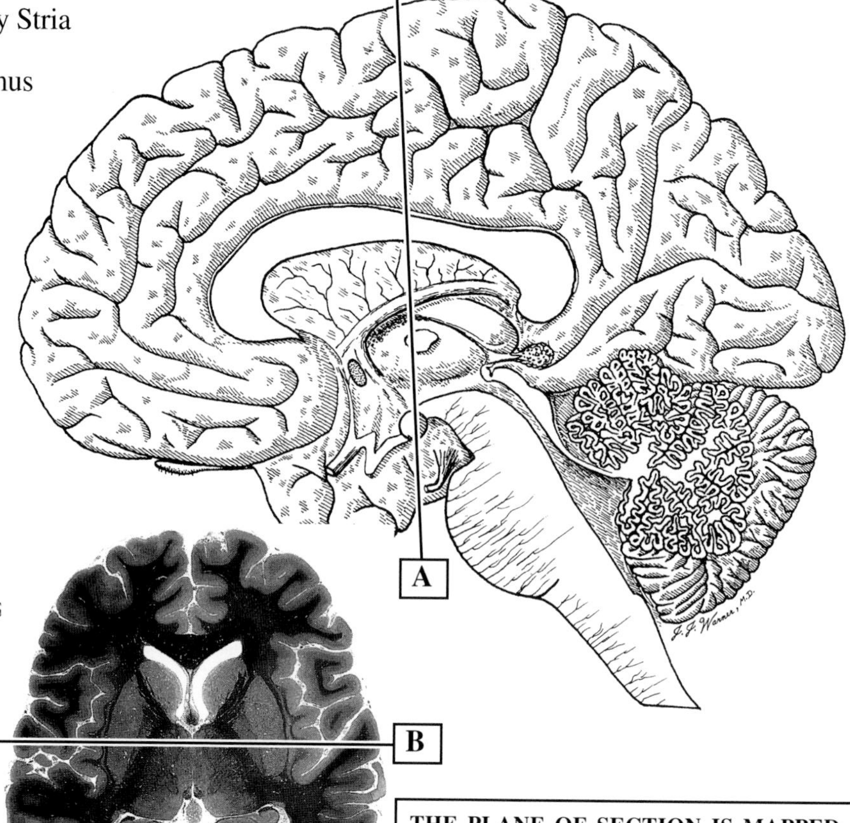

THE PLANE OF SECTION IS MAPPED IN REFERENCE TO (A) A MIDLINE SAGITTAL DIAGRAM, AND (B) A HORIZONTAL SECTION (LEVEL OF THE GENU OF THE CORPUS CALLOSUM AND THE PINEAL BODY)

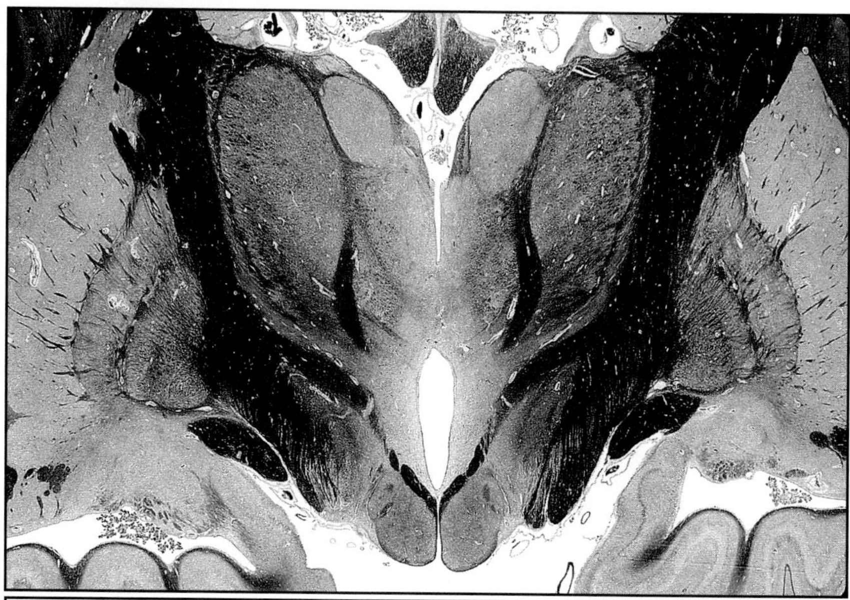

HISTOLOGICAL SECTION: 15 μ, KLUVER - BARRERA TECHNIQUE

CORONAL SECTION OF THE BRAIN; LEVEL OF THE ANTERIOR NUCLEUS OF THE THALAMUS AND OF THE MAMMILLARY BODIES (MAGNIFIED VIEW): CROSS-REFERENCES TO HORIZONTAL SECTIONS

A

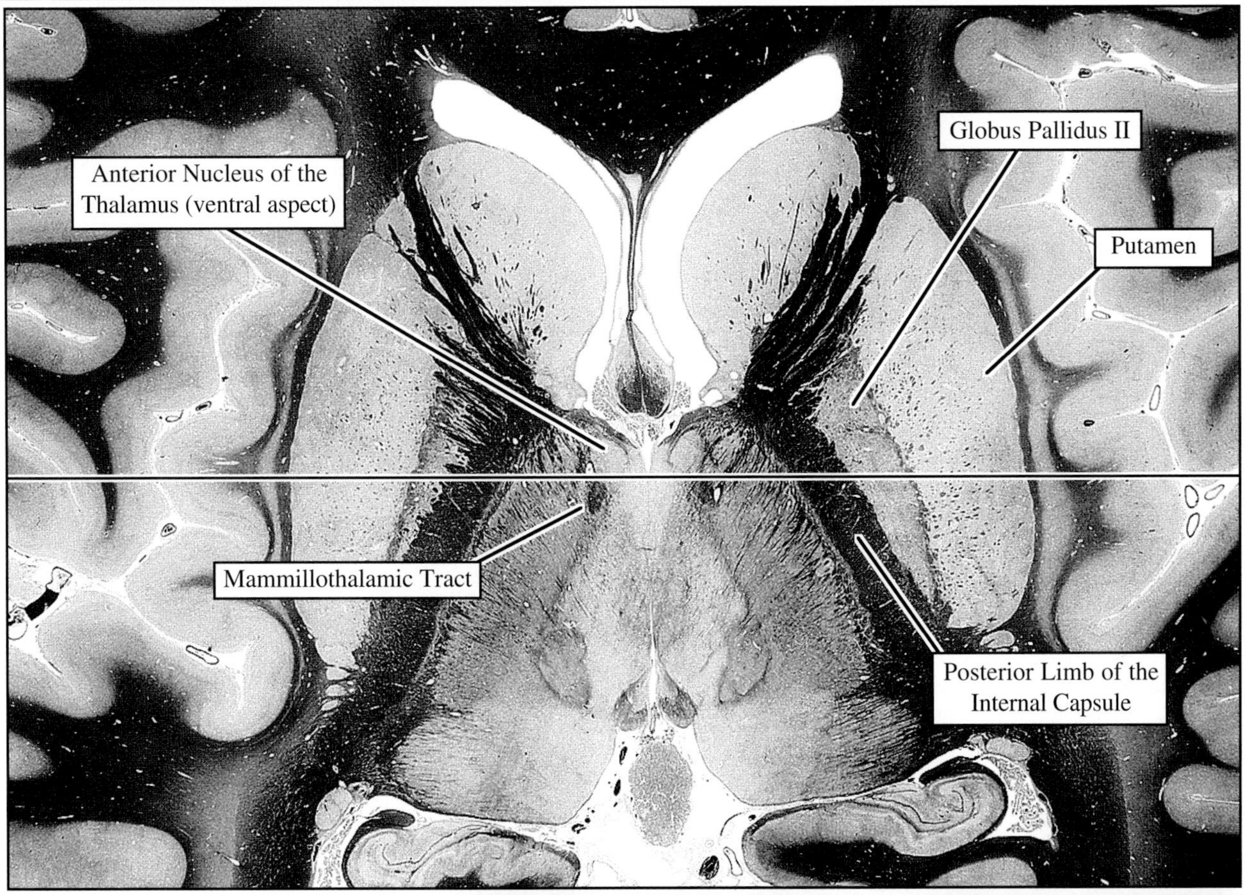

Anterior Nucleus of the Thalamus (ventral aspect)

Globus Pallidus II

Putamen

Mammillothalamic Tract

Posterior Limb of the Internal Capsule

HISTOLOGICAL SECTIONS: 15 μ, KLUVER-BARRERA TECHNIQUE

These reference sections emphasize the three-dimensional relationships between structures identified in the coronal plane. The intersection of the coronal plane with each horizontal section is indicated by a line. In section A, the position of the coronal plane with respect to the internal capsule, thalamus, and basal ganglia is demonstrated. In section B (through the mesencephalic-diencephalic transition), the position of the coronal plane relative to the cerebral peduncles, third ventricle, basal ganglia, and amygdala is shown. Note the bipartite or divided appearance that characterizes globus pallidus I on the coronal section and on the reference horizontal section (B). The more dorsal horizontal section (A) does not include globus pallidus I. The mammillothalamic tract, characterized by a slightly curved trajectory, courses in and out of the coronal plane of section. The rostral aspect of the subthalamic nucleus appears in this coronal plane.

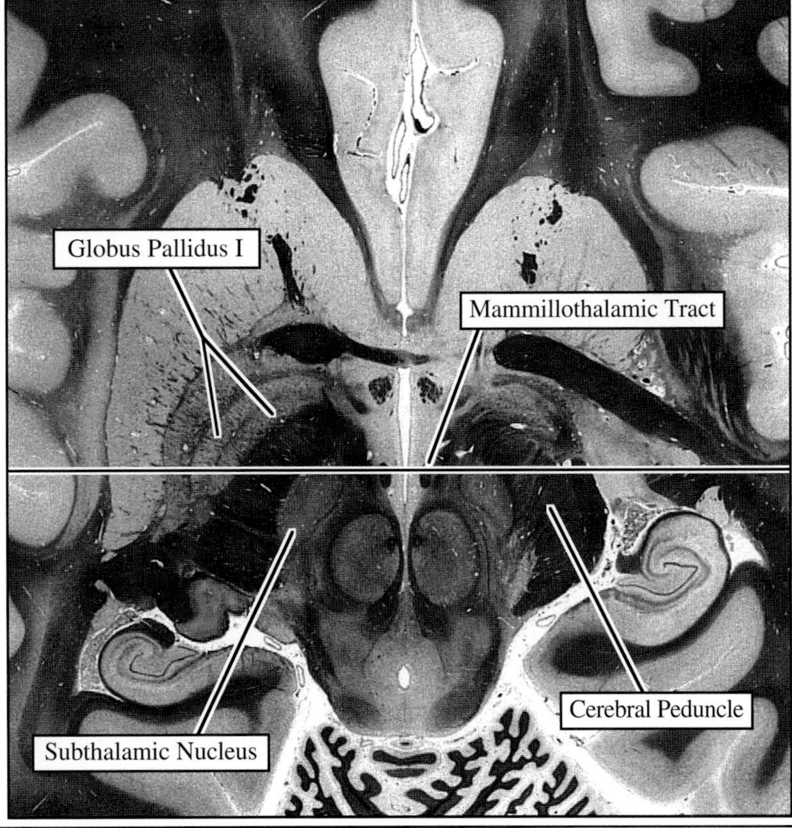

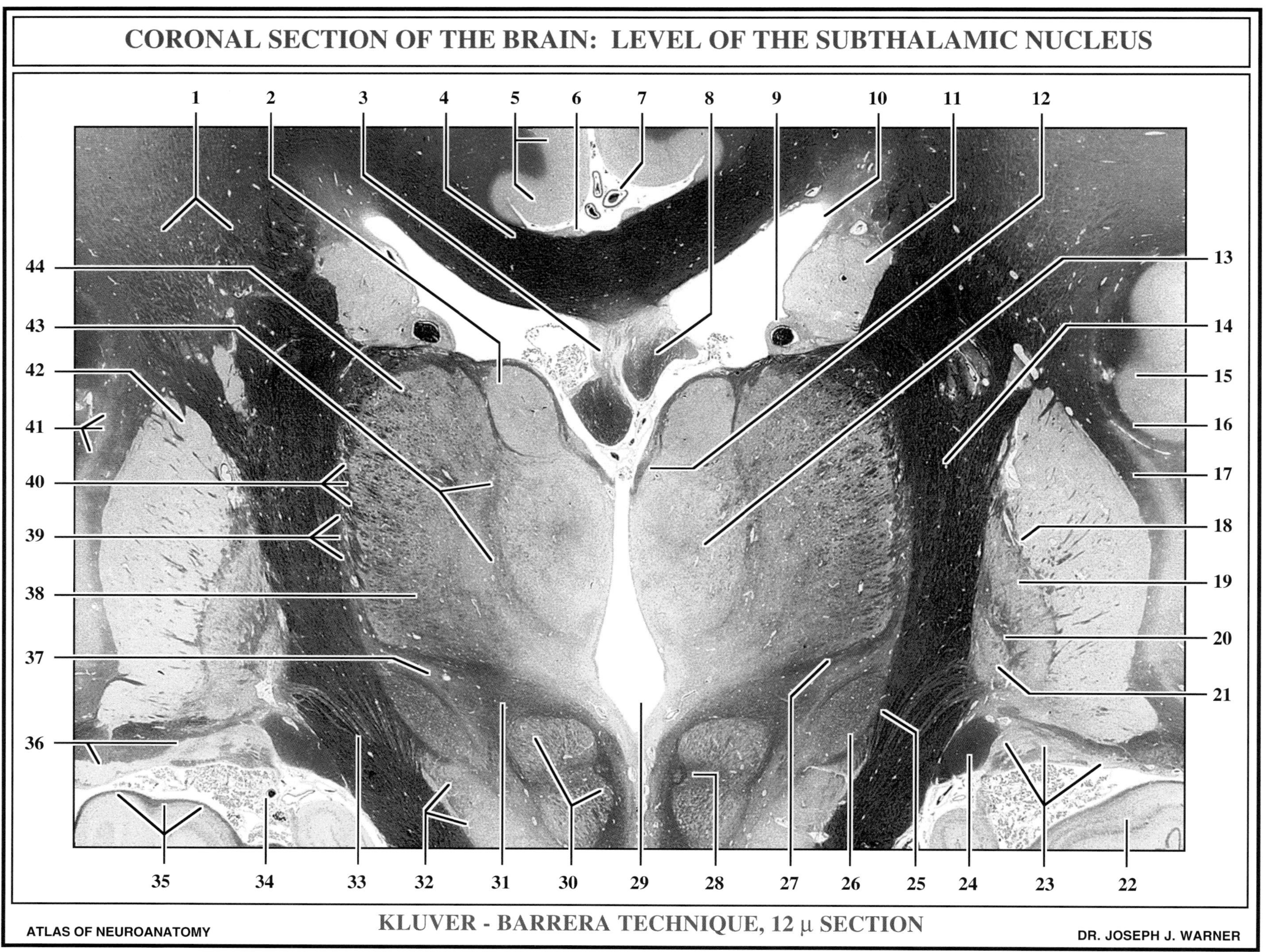

CORONAL SECTION OF THE BRAIN: LEVEL OF THE SUBTHALAMIC NUCLEUS
1
2
3
4
5
6
7
8
9
10
11
12
13
14
15
16
17
18
19
20
21
22
23
24
25
26
27
28
29
30
31
32
33
34
35
36
37
38
39
40
41
42
43
44
KLUVER - BARRERA TECHNIQUE, 12 μ SECTION
ATLAS OF NEUROANATOMY
DR. JOSEPH J. WARNER

CORONAL SECTION OF THE BRAIN; LEVEL OF THE SUBTHALAMIC NUCLEUS (MAGNIFIED): SECTION ORIENTATION AND KEY TO NUMBERED STRUCTURES

KEY TO NUMBERED STRUCTURES

1. Corona Radiata
2. Lateral Dorsal Nucleus of the Thalamus
3. Septum Pellucidum
4. Corpus Callosum
5. Cingulate Cortex
6. Induseum Griseum
7. Anterior Cerebral Artery
8. Fornix
9. Thalamostriate Vein and the Stria Terminalis
10. Lateral Ventricle
11. Caudate Nucleus
12. Stria Medullaris of the Thalamus
13. Dorsomedial Nucleus of the Thalamus
14. Posterior Limb of the Internal Capsule
15. Insular Cortex
16. Extreme Capsule
17. External Capsule
18. External Medullary Lamina
19. Globus Pallidus II
20. Internal Medullary Lamina
21. Globus Pallidus I
22. Hippocampus
23. Termination of the Tail of the Caudate at the caudal extent of the Amygdala
24. Optic Tract
25. Subthalamic Fasciculus (fibers comprise a part of the Capsule of the Subthalamic Nucleus)
26. Subthalamic Nucleus
27. Thalamic Fasciculus (Field H1 of Forel)
28. Fasciculus Retroflexus of Meynert (Habenulointerpeduncular Tract)
29. Third Ventricle
30. Red Nucleus
31. Dentatorubrothalamic Fibers
32. Substantia Nigra
33. Cerebral Peduncle
34. Choroid Plexus in the Temporal Horn of the Lateral Ventricle
35. Alveus
36. Tail of the Caudate Nucleus
37. Zona Incerta
38. Ventrolateral Nucleus of the Thalamus
39. Nucleus Reticularis of the Thalamus
40. External Medullary Lamina of the Thalamus
41. Claustrum
42. Putamen
43. Internal Medullary Lamina of the Thalamus
44. Lateral Posterior Nucleus of the Thalamus

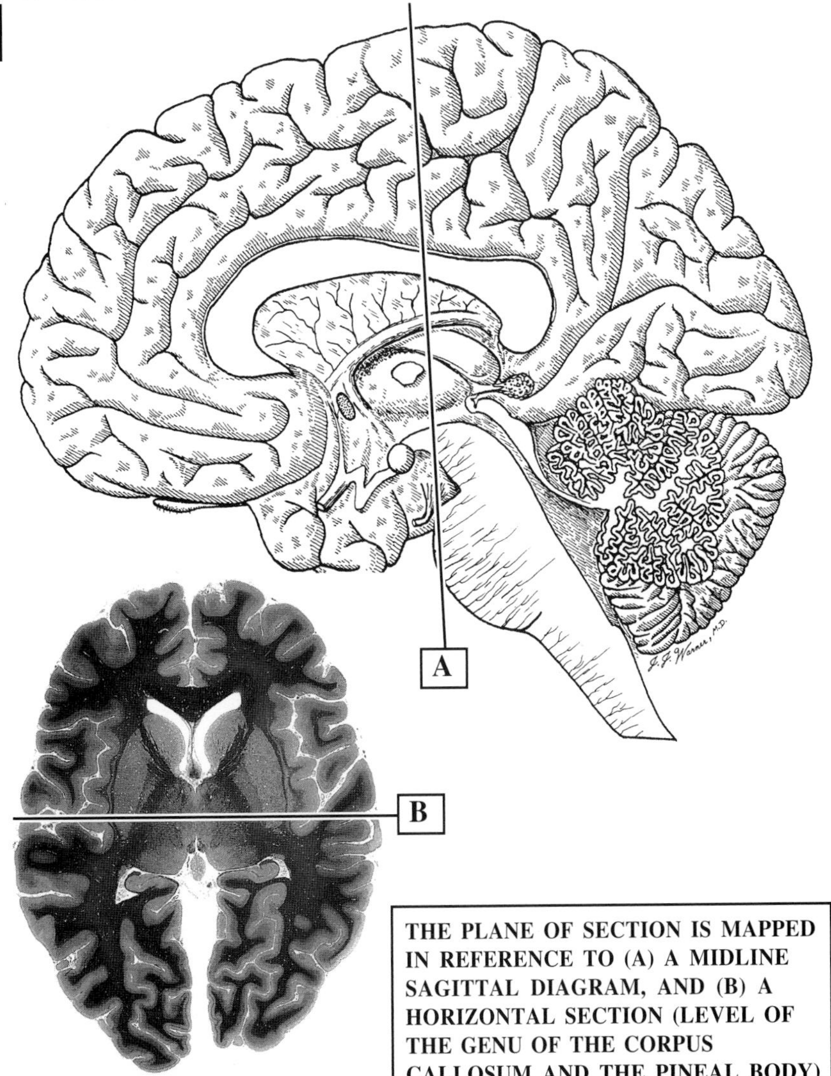

THE PLANE OF SECTION IS MAPPED IN REFERENCE TO (A) A MIDLINE SAGITTAL DIAGRAM, AND (B) A HORIZONTAL SECTION (LEVEL OF THE GENU OF THE CORPUS CALLOSUM AND THE PINEAL BODY)

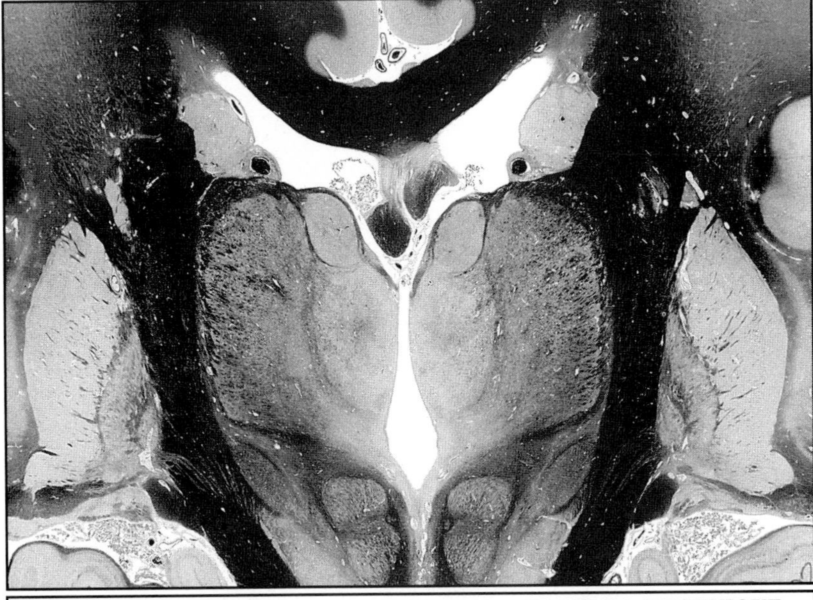

HISTOLOGICAL SECTION: 12 μ, KLUVER - BARRERA TECHNIQUE

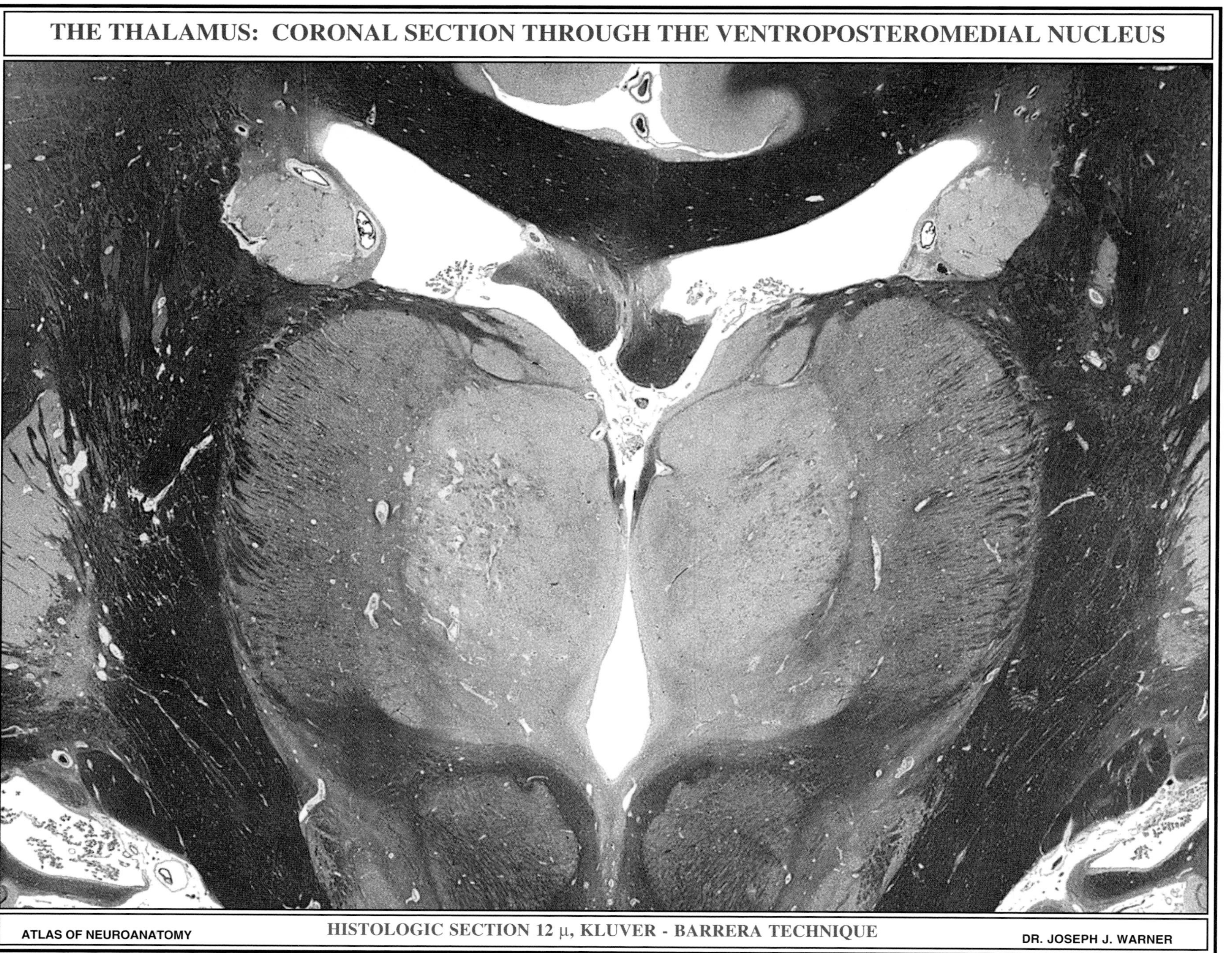
THE THALAMUS: CORONAL SECTION THROUGH THE VENTROPOSTEROMEDIAL NUCLEUS
ATLAS OF NEUROANATOMY
HISTOLOGIC SECTION 12 μ, KLUVER - BARRERA TECHNIQUE
DR. JOSEPH J. WARNER

THALAMUS, LEVEL OF VENTROPOSTEROMEDIAL AND ROSTRAL CENTROMEDIAN NUCLEI, RED NUCLEUS, SUBSTANTIA NIGRA

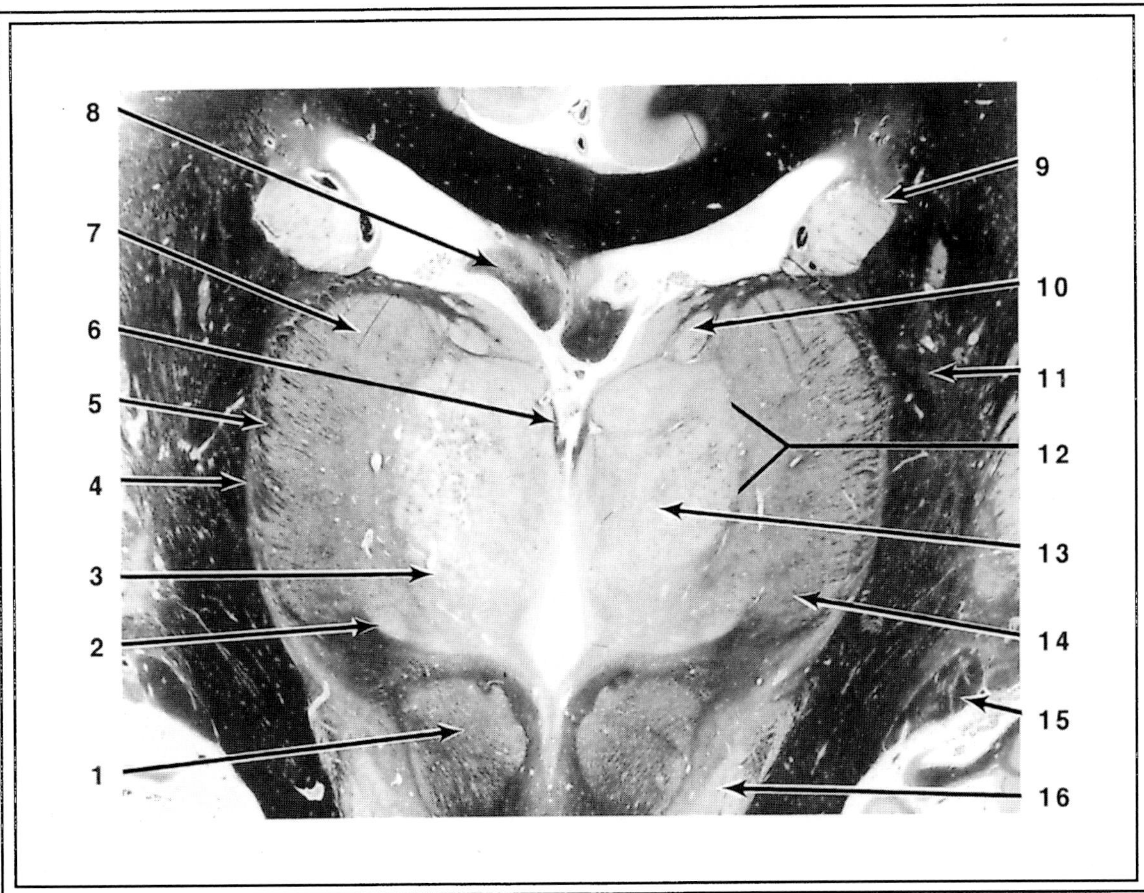

KEY TO NUMBERED STRUCTURES

1. Red Nucleus
2. Ventroposteromedial Nucleus
3. Centromedian Nucleus
4. Reticular Nucleus
5. External Medullary Lamina of the Thalamus
6. Stria Medullaris
7. Lateral Posterior Nucleus
8. Fornix
9. Caudate Nucleus
10. Lateral Dorsal Nucleus
11. Internal Capsule, Posterior Limb
12. Internal Medullary Lamina of the Thalamus
13. Dorsomedial Nucleus
14. Ventroposterolateral Nucleus
15. Optic Tract and rostral Lateral Geniculate Nucleus
16. Substantia Nigra

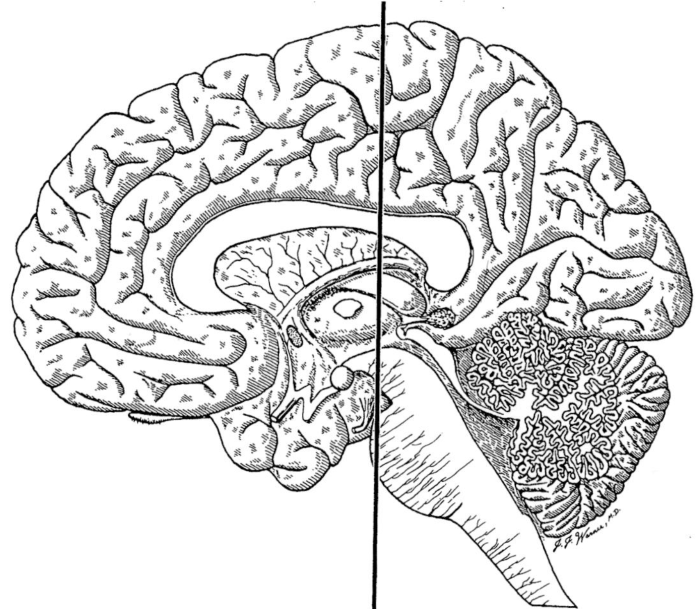

The internal medullary lamina of each thalamus extends ventrally from the anterior and lateral dorsal nuclei, then curves toward the third ventricle. In coronal sections through the mid-thalamus, this thin layer of white matter divides and passes on either side of the centromedian nucleus in each hemisphere, demarcating this structure from the other thalamic nuclei. (Nuclei thus enclosed by the internal medullary lamina are termed intralaminar nuclei). This relationship is clearly demonstrated by examination of stained horizontal sections through the centromedian nucleus. (Refer to subsequent figure).

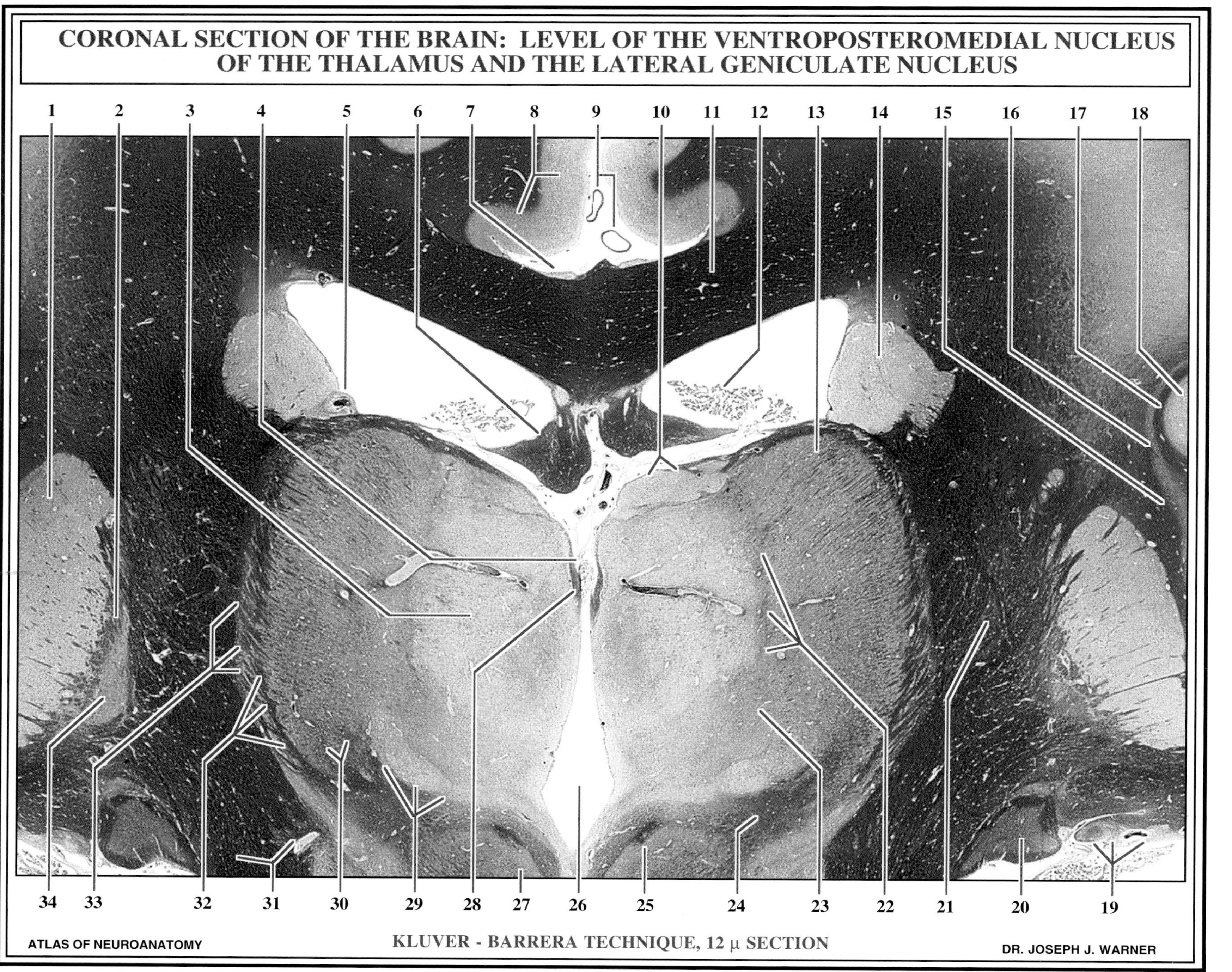
CORONAL SECTION OF THE BRAIN: LEVEL OF THE VENTROPOSTEROMEDIAL NUCLEUS OF THE THALAMUS AND THE LATERAL GENICULATE NUCLEUS
1
2
3
4
5
6
7
8
9
10
11
12
13
14
15
16
17
18
34
33
32
31
30
29
28
27
26
25
24
23
22
21
20
19
ATLAS OF NEUROANATOMY
KLUVER - BARRERA TECHNIQUE, 12 μ SECTION
DR. JOSEPH J. WARNER

CORONAL SECTION OF THE BRAIN; LEVEL OF THE LATERAL GENICULATE NUCLEUS AND THE VENTROPOSTEROMEDIAL NUCLEUS OF THE THALAMUS: SECTION ORIENTATION AND KEY TO NUMBERED STRUCTURES

KEY TO NUMBERED STRUCTURES

1. Putamen
2. Internal Medullary Lamina
3. Dorsomedial Nucleus of the Thalamus
4. Taenia Thalami*
5. Stria Terminalis and Thalamostriate Vein
6. Fornix
7. Induseum Griseum
8. Cingulate Cortex
9. Anterior Cerebral Arteries
10. Lateral Dorsal Nucleus of the Thalamus
11. Corpus Callosum
12. Choroid Plexus in the Body of the Lateral Ventricle
13. Lateral Posterior Nucleus of the Thalamus
14. Caudate Nucleus
15. External Capsule
16. Claustrum
17. Extreme Capsule
18. Insular Cortex
19. Tail of the Caudate Nucleus
20. Lateral Geniculate Nucleus
21. Posterior Limb of the Internal Capsule
22. Internal Medullary Lamina of the Thalamus
23. Centromedian Nucleus of the Thalamus
24. Dentatorubrothalamic Projections
25. Fasciculus Retroflexus of Meynert (Habenulointerpeduncular Tract)
26. Third Ventricle
27. Red Nucleus
28. Stria Medullaris
29. Ventroposteromedial Nucleus of the Thalamus
30. Ventroposterolateral Nucleus of the Thalamus
31. Cerebral Peduncle
32. External Medullary Lamina of the Thalamus
33. Nucleus Reticularis of the Thalamus
34. Globus Pallidus II

* The Taenia Thalami (a component of the epithalamus) forms the epithelial roof of the Third Ventricle adjacent to the Stria Medullaris.

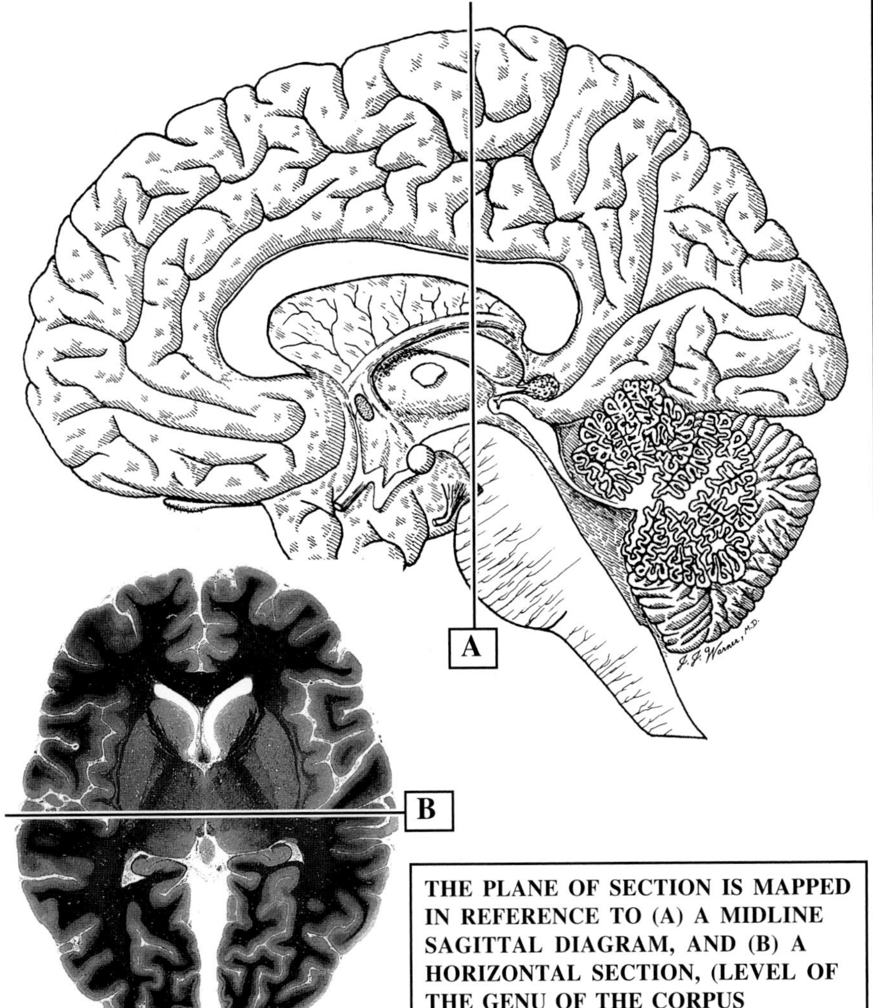

THE PLANE OF SECTION IS MAPPED IN REFERENCE TO (A) A MIDLINE SAGITTAL DIAGRAM, AND (B) A HORIZONTAL SECTION, (LEVEL OF THE GENU OF THE CORPUS CALLOSUM AND THE PINEAL BODY)

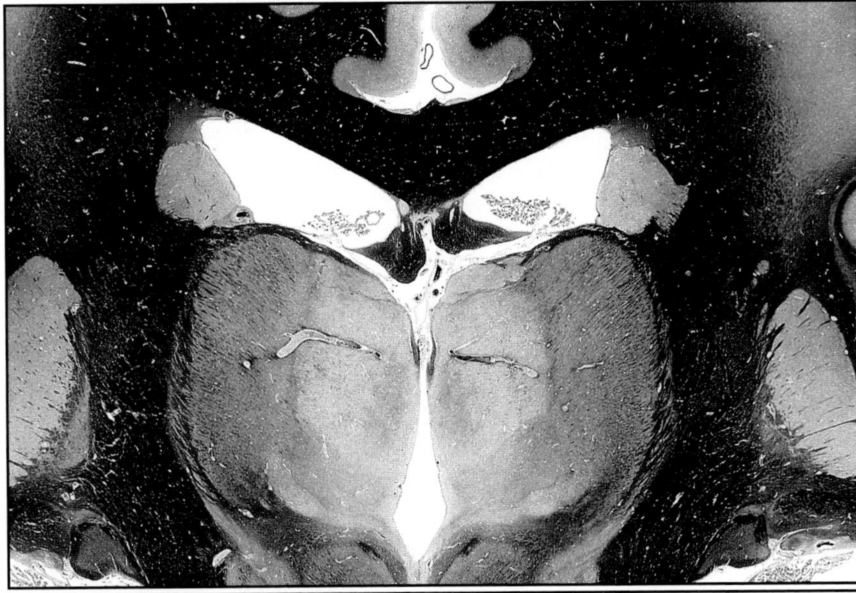

HISTOLOGICAL SECTION: 12 μ, KLUVER - BARRERA TECHNIQUE

CORONAL SECTION OF THE BRAIN; LEVEL OF THE LATERAL GENICULATE NUCLEUS AND THE VENTROPOSTEROMEDIAL NUCLEUS OF THE THALAMUS: PLANE MAPPED ON A HORIZONTAL REFERENCE SECTION

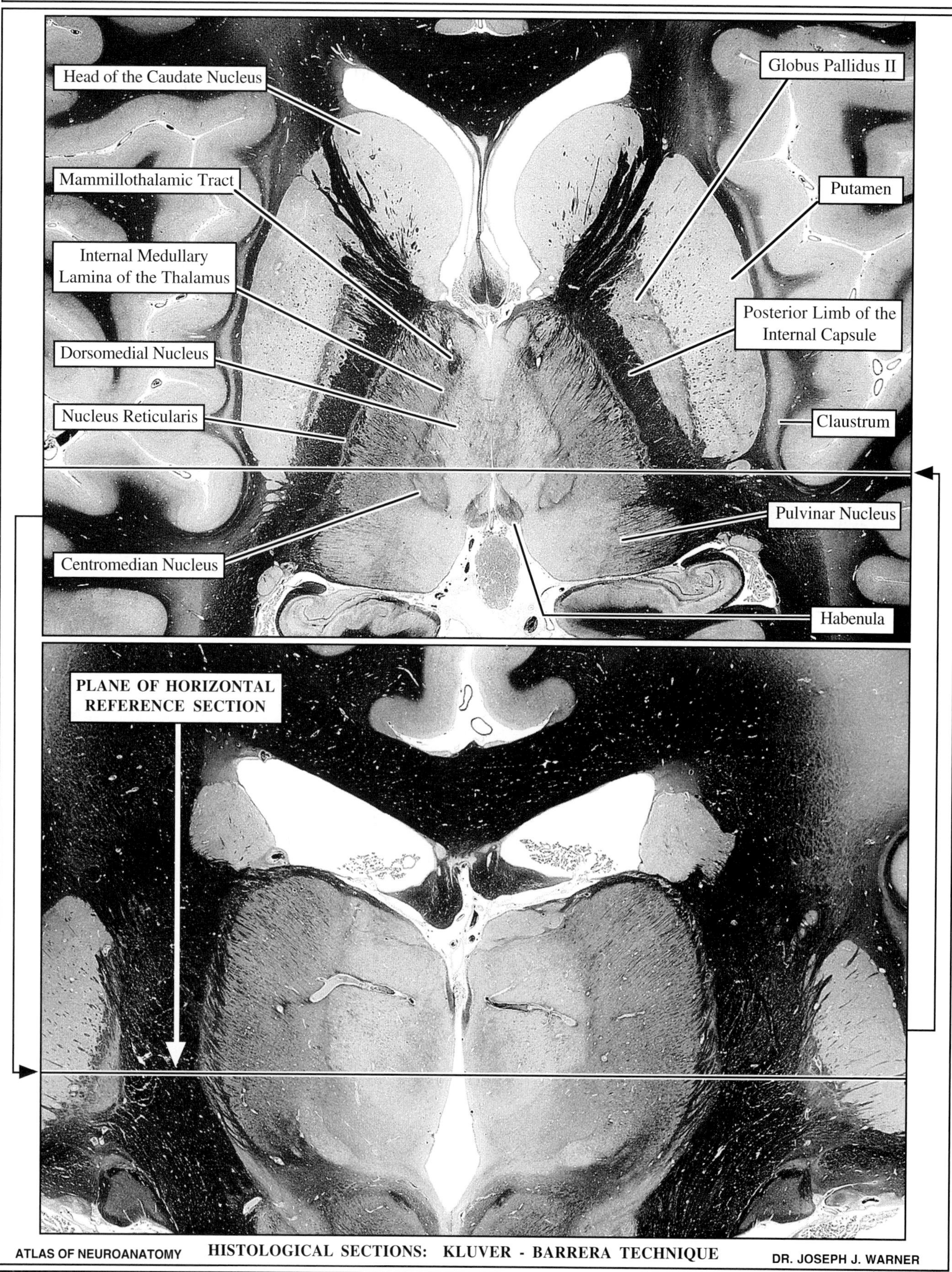

 HISTOLOGICAL SECTIONS: KLUVER - BARRERA TECHNIQUE

THE THALAMUS AND BASAL GANGLIA: HORIZONTAL SECTION AT THE LEVEL OF THE CENTROMEDIAN NUCLEUS OF THE THALAMUS

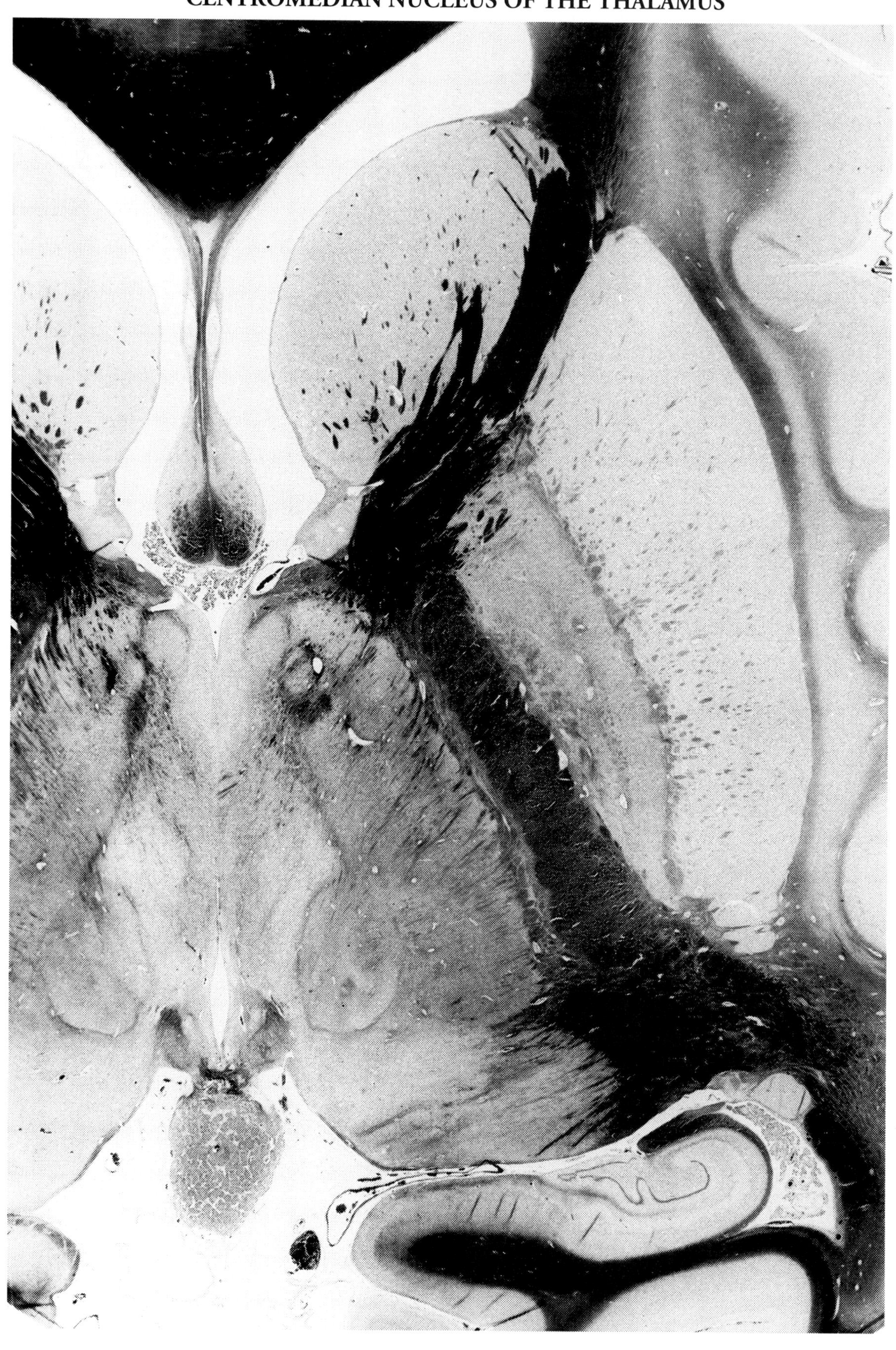

THALAMUS, LEVEL OF CENTROMEDIAN NUCLEI, HABENULAR COMMISSURE, PINEAL BODY, HORIZONTAL SECTION

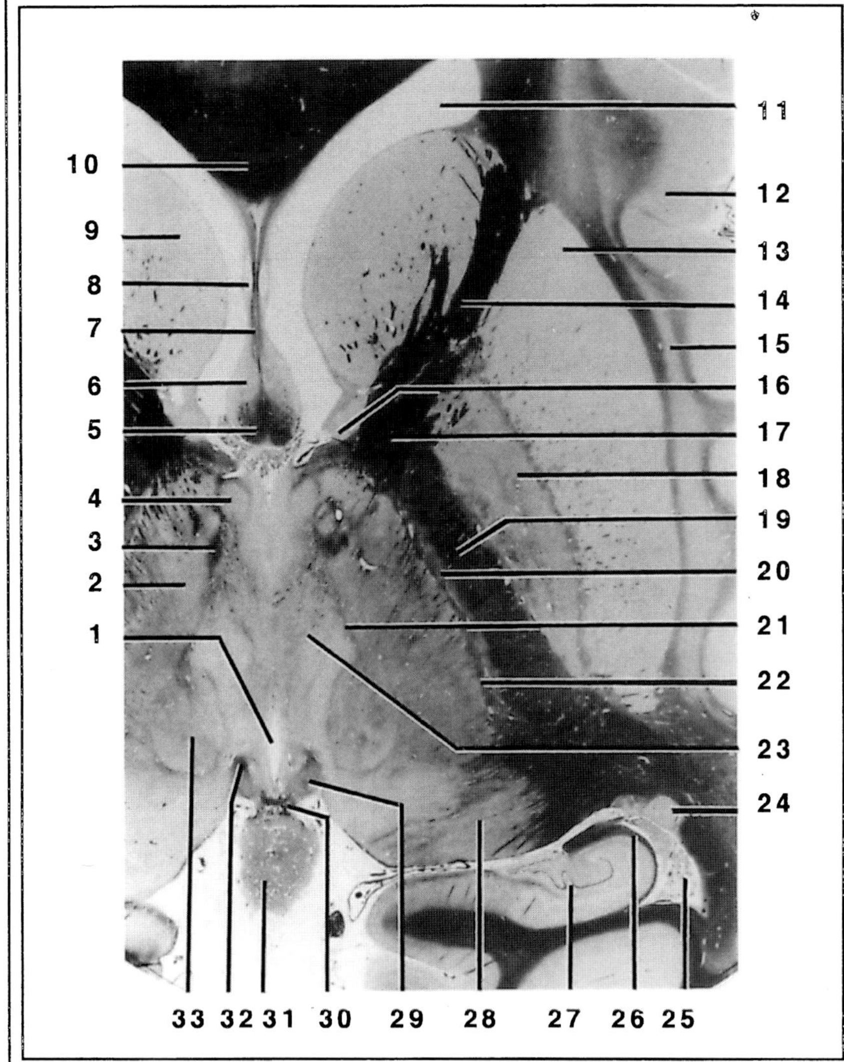

KEY TO NUMBERED STRUCTURES

1. Third Ventricle
2. Ventroanterior, Ventrolateral Nuclei
3. Mammillothalamic Tract
4. Anterior Nucleus of Thalamus
5. Fornix
6. Septal Nuclei
7. Septum Pellucidum
8. Septal Vein
9. Head of the Caudate Nucleus
10. Genu, Corpus Callosum
11. Anterior Horn, Lateral Ventricle
12. Insula
13. Putamen
14. Anterior Limb, Internal Capsule
15. Claustrum
16. Stria Terminalis and Thalamostriate Vein
17. Genu, Internal Capsule
18. Globus Pallidus II
19. Posterior Limb, Internal Capsule
20. Nucleus Reticularis, Thalamus
21. Internal Medullary Lamina of the Thalamus
22. External Medullary Lamina of the Thalamus
23. Dorsomedial Nucleus
24. Tail of the Caudate Nucleus
25. Temporal Horn, Lateral Ventricle
26. Fimbria of the Fornix
27. Hippocampus
28. Pulvinar Nucleus, Thalamus
29. Habenula
30. Habenular Commissure
31. Pineal body
32. Stria Medullaris
33. Centromedian Nucleus

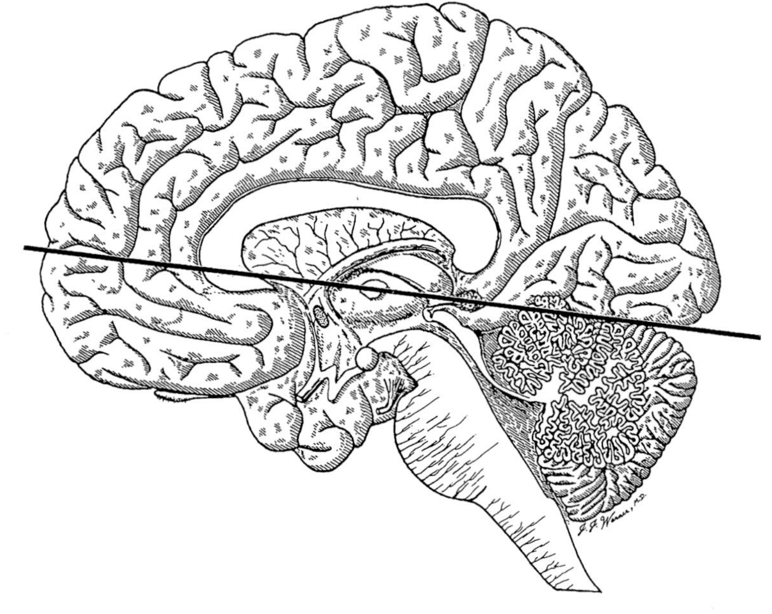

The internal medullary lamina divides and passes on either side of the centromedian nucleus in each hemisphere, demarcating this structure from the other thalamic nuclei. This relationship is clearly demonstrated by this horizontal section through the centromedian nucleus (15 μ, Kluver-Barrera technique). Plane of section is indicated on the midline sagittal diagram. Note the position of the habenula, the habenular commissure, and the pineal. This plane passes through the ventral aspect of the anterior nucleus of the thalamus. The superior extent of the mammillothalamic tract is visible, with its fibers sectioned transversely in this plane.

THALAMUS, CORONAL SECTION, LEVEL OF POSTERIOR COMMISSURE, MEDIAL AND LATERAL GENICULATE NUCLEI

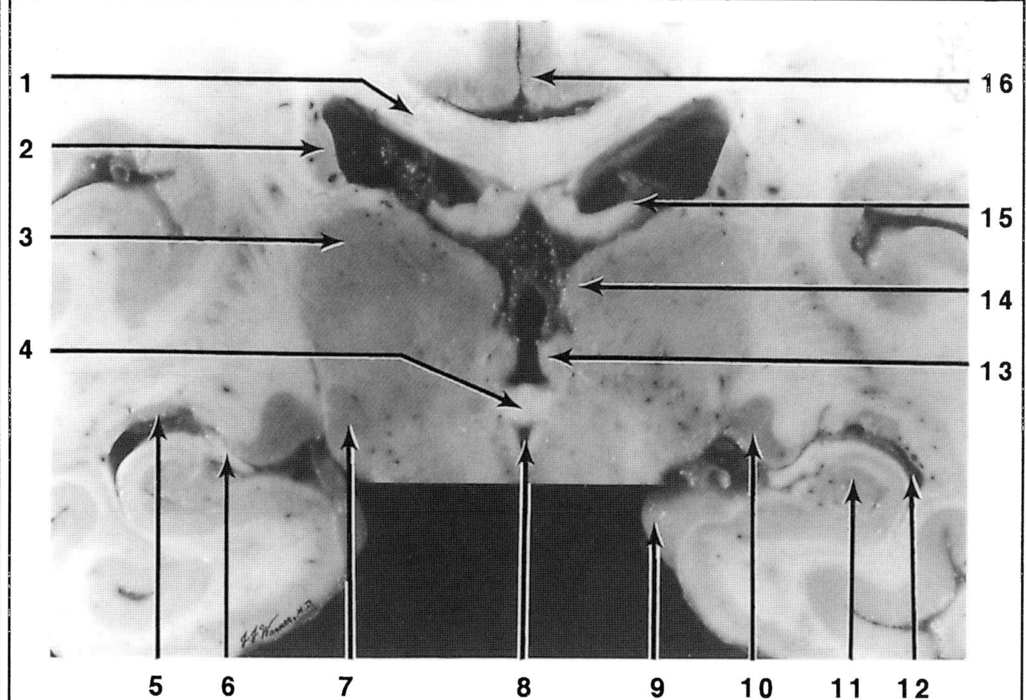

KEY TO NUMBERED STRUCTURES

1. Corpus Callosum
2. Caudate Nucleus
3. Lateral Posterior Nucleus, Thalamus
4. Posterior Commissure
5. Tail of Caudate N.
6. Fimbria of Fornix
7. Medial Geniculate Nucleus
8. Aqueduct of Sylvius
9. Parahippocampal Gyrus
10. Lateral Geniculate Nucleus
11. Hippocampus
12. Temporal horn of Lateral Ventricle
13. Habenula
14. Dorsomedial Nucleus, Thalamus
15. Fornix
16. Cingulate Gyrus

This section is viewed from a rostral to a caudal direction. The rostral aspect of the posterior commissure is broadly cylindrical, however when viewed in sagittal section, the posterior concavity of this structure is evident. The lateral geniculate nucleus is adjacent to the fimbria of the fornix, and may be seen dorsal to the hippocampus in the same sagittal plane. The medial geniculate nucleus is contiguous with the dorsolateral mesencephalon, and thus seen dorsal to the cerebral peduncle in sagittal sections. Both may be seen in the same horizontal plane in sections which pass through the mesencephalic-diencephalic transition.

PLANE OF SECTION MAPPED ON VENTRAL ASPECT OF THE BRAIN

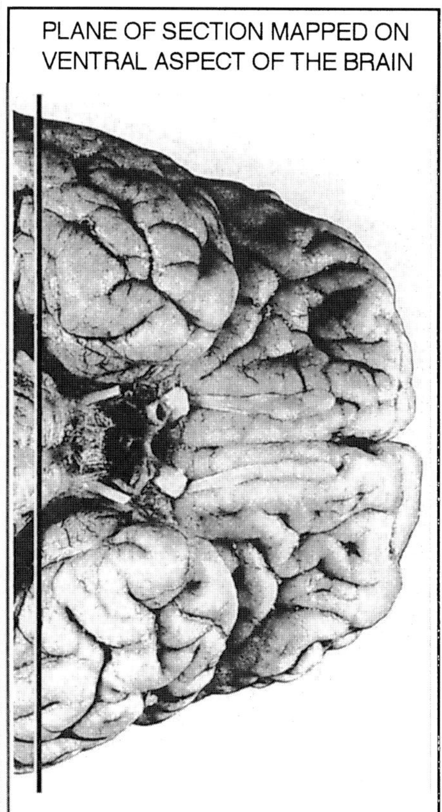

PLANE OF SECTION MAPPED ON MIDLINE SAGITTAL DIAGRAM OF THE BRAIN. (The brainstem has been removed by intercollicular transection).

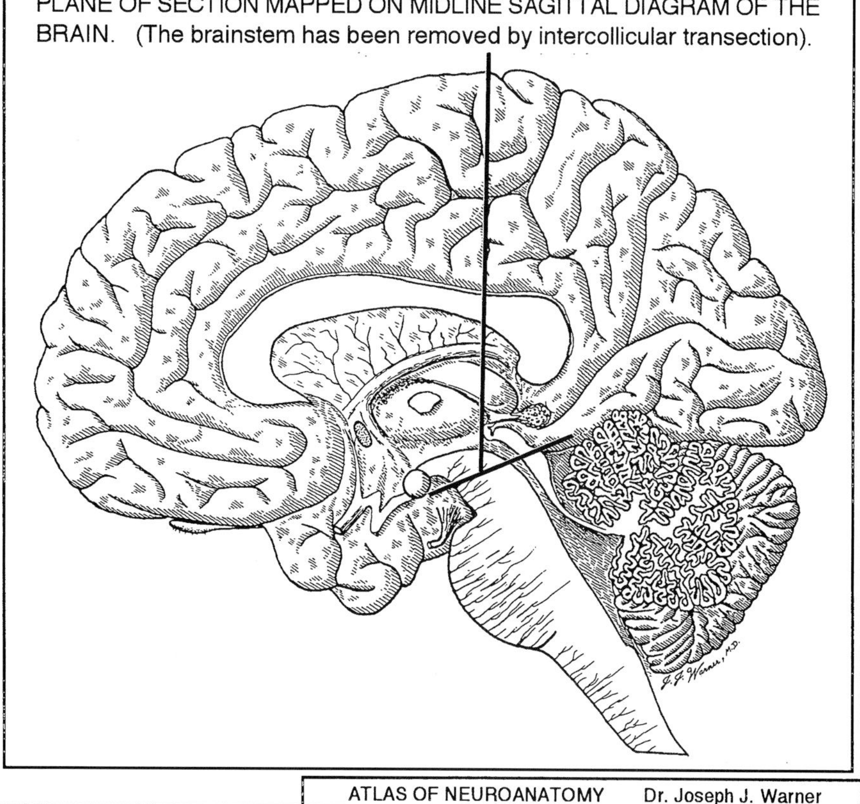

PART V: NEUROANATOMIC ORGANIZATION OF THE MESENCEPHALIC-DIENCEPHALIC TRANSITION

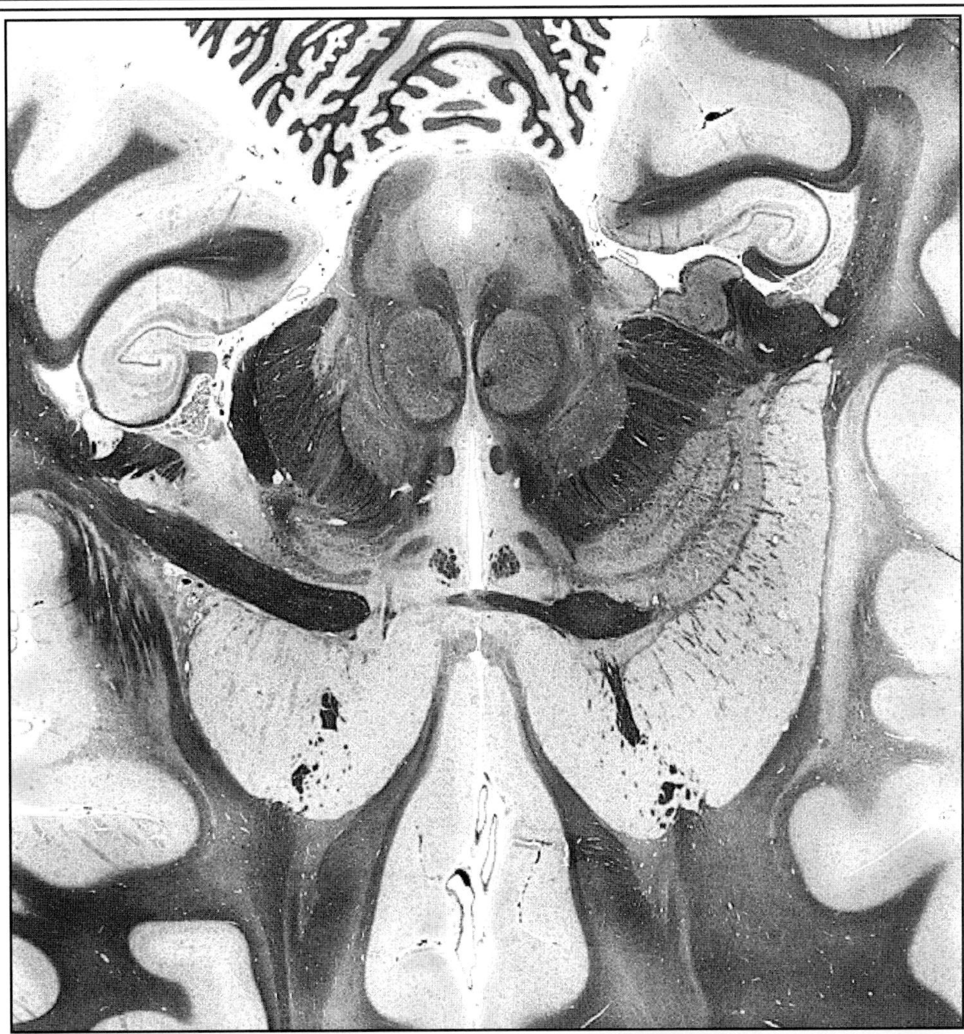

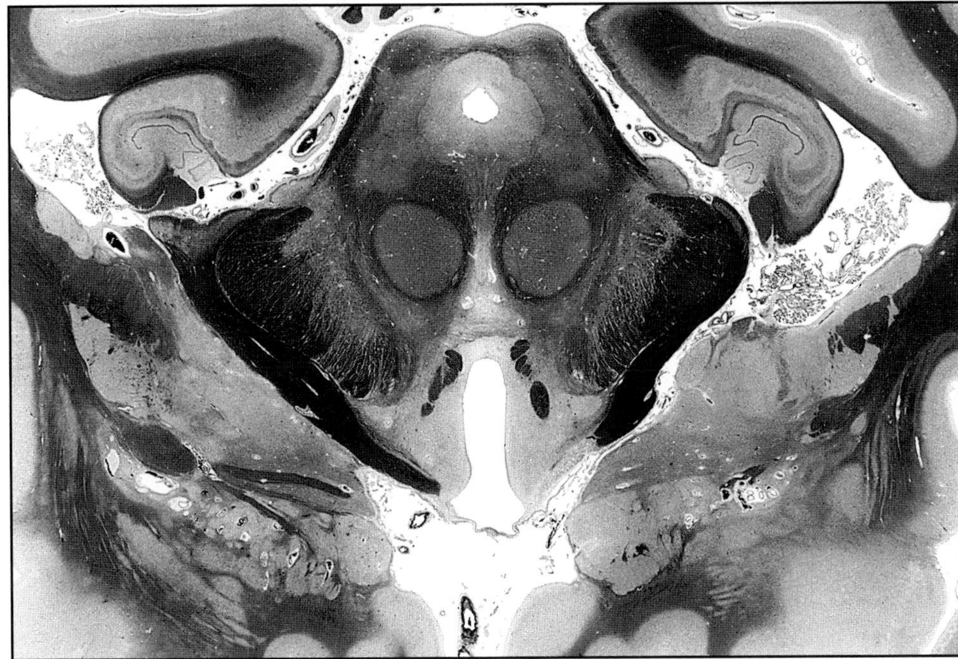

THE MESENCEPHALIC-DIENCEPHALIC TRANSITION: HORIZONTAL SECTION; LEVEL INCLUDING THE INFERIOR COLLICULUS, MEDIAL AND LATERAL GENICULATE NUCLEI, AND VENTRAL ASPECT OF THE ANTERIOR COMMISSURE

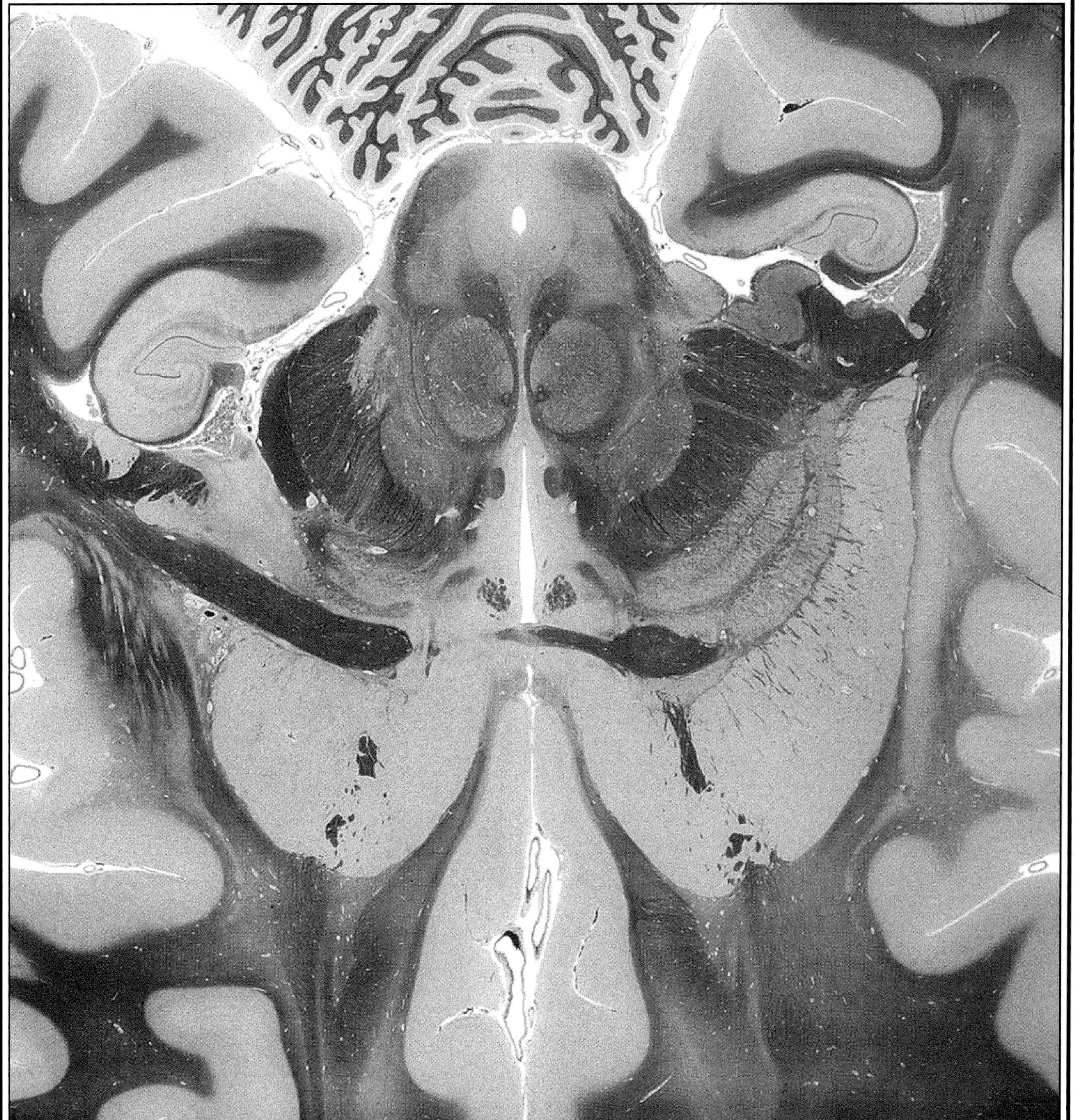

SECTION 15 μ, KLUVER-BARRERA TECHNIQUE

Major components of the mesencephalon and its relationship to diencephalic structures are demonstrated in this section. A transverse section through the mesencephalon at the level of the inferior colliculus would pass caudal to the red nuclei and include decussating fibers of the superior cerebellar peduncles. Although the inferior colliculus is included at this level, the orientation of this section is such that the red nuclei, the subthalamic nuclei, and the substantia nigra appear in the same plane. The brachium of the inferior colliculus is discernible from its origin to its termination in the medial geniculate nucleus.

THE MESENCEPHALIC-DIENCEPHALIC TRANSITION: HORIZONTAL SECTION; LEVEL INCLUDING THE INFERIOR COLLICULUS, MEDIAL AND LATERAL GENICULATE NUCLEI, AND VENTRAL ASPECT OF THE ANTERIOR COMMISSURE

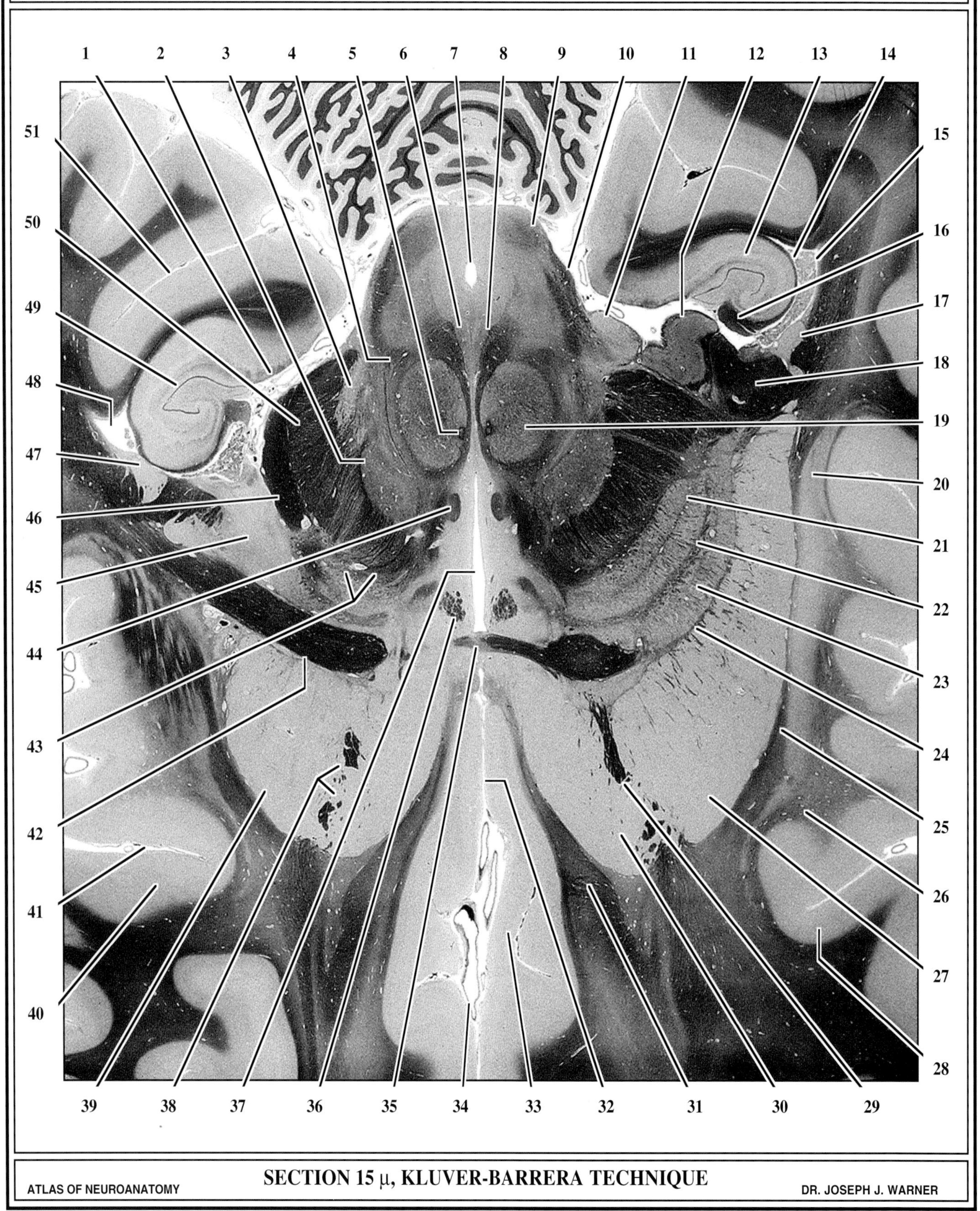

SECTION 15 μ, KLUVER-BARRERA TECHNIQUE

ATLAS OF NEUROANATOMY

DR. JOSEPH J. WARNER

THE MESENCEPHALIC-DIENCEPHALIC TRANSITION: HORIZONTAL SECTION; LEVEL INCLUDING THE INFERIOR COLLICULUS, MEDIAL AND LATERAL GENICULATE NUCLEI, AND VENTRAL ASPECT OF THE ANTERIOR COMMISSURE

KEY TO NUMBERED STRUCTURES

1. Superficial Medullary Stratum of the Subiculum
2. Subthalamic Nucleus
3. Substantia Nigra
4. Medial Lemniscus
5. Fasciculus Retroflexus of Meynert (Habenulo-interpeduncular Tract)
6. Oculomotor Nuclear Complex
7. Aqueduct of Sylvius
8. Medial Longitudinal Fasciculus
9. Inferior Colliculus
10. Brachium of the Inferior Colliculus
11. Medial Geniculate Nucleus
12. Lateral Geniculate Nucleus
13. Hippocampal Formation
14. Alveus
15. Choroid Plexus
16. Fimbria of the Fornix
17. Tail of the Caudate Nucleus
18. Meyer's Loop (Geniculocalcarine Radiations)
19. Red Nucleus
20. Claustrum
21. Globus Pallidus I (note bipartite appearance)
22. Internal Medullary Lamina
23. Globus Pallidus II
24. External Medullary Lamina
25. External Capsule
26. Extreme Capsule
27. Putamen
28. Insular Cortex
29. Anterior Limb of the Internal Capsule
30. Head of the Caudate Nucleus
31. Rostrum of the Corpus Callosum
32. Interhemispheric Fissure
33. Subcallosal Gyrus
34. Anterior Cerebral Artery
35. Anterior Commissure
36. Fornix (postcommissural component)
37. Third Ventricle
38. Nucleus Accumbens
39. Putamen
40. Insular Cortex
41. Circular Sulcus
42. Anterior Commissure
43. Subthalamic Fasciculus
44. Mammillothalamic Tract
45. Amygdala
46. Optic Tract
47. Tail of the Caudate Nucleus
48. Temporal Horn of the Lateral Ventricle
49. Dentate Gyrus of the Hippocampus
50. Cerebral Peduncle
51. Collateral Sulcus

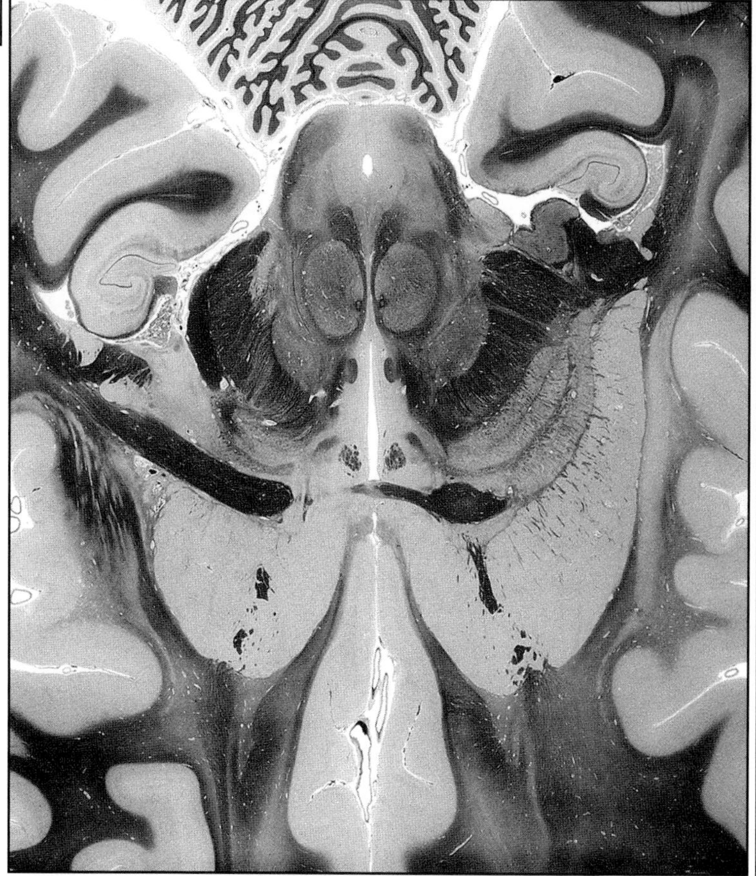

SECTION 15 μ, KLUVER - BARRERA TECHNIQUE

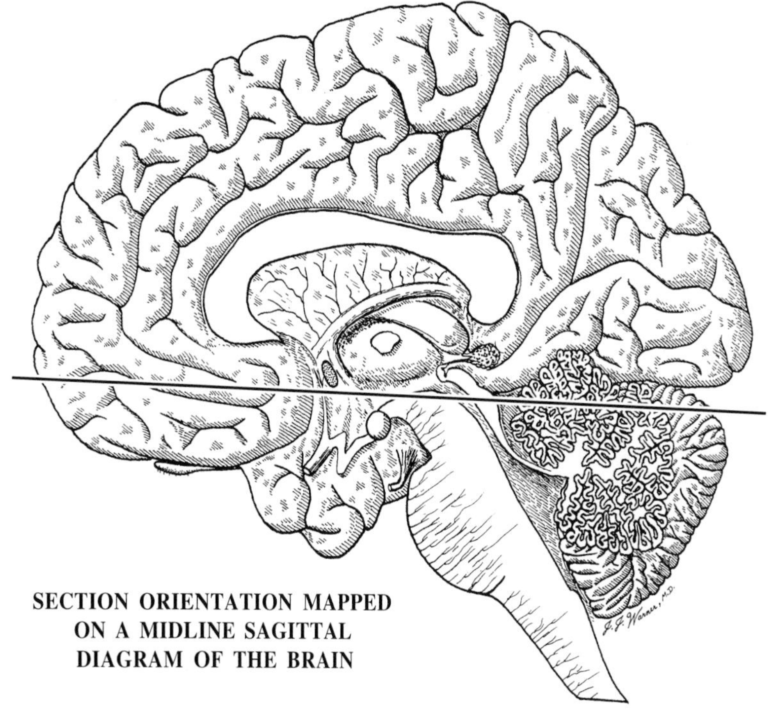

SECTION ORIENTATION MAPPED ON A MIDLINE SAGITTAL DIAGRAM OF THE BRAIN

MESENCEPHALON AND LATERAL GENICULATE NUCLEUS: HORIZONTAL SECTION

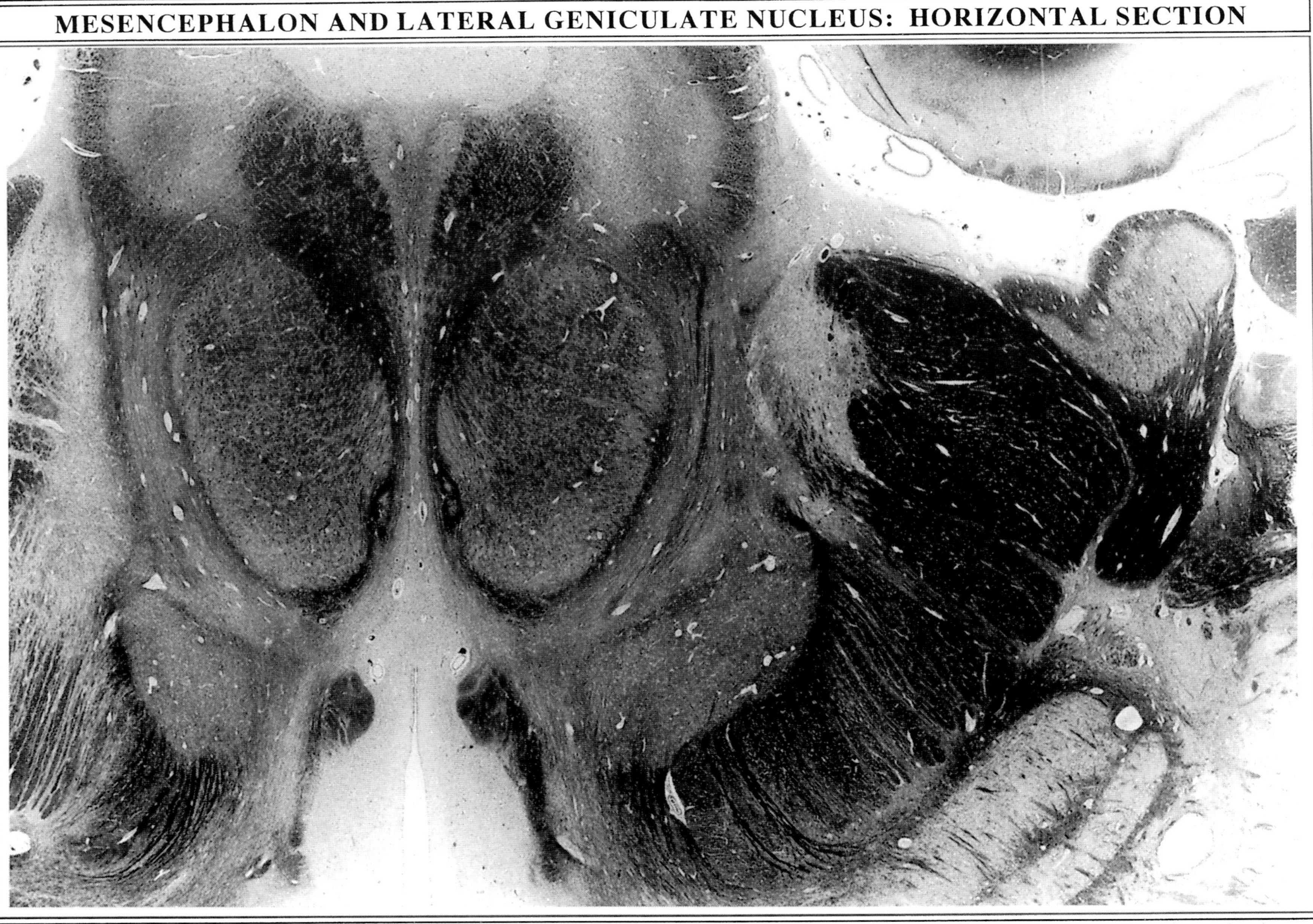

This horizontal section passes through the inferior colliculus, red nucleus, cerebral peduncles, and subthalamic region. The substantia nigra is located caudal to the subthalamic nucleus, however, this plane of section includes both pairs of structures. The globus pallidus is situated rostral and lateral to the cerebral peduncles. The optic tract is clearly shown as it courses circumferentially around the cerebral peduncle and terminates in the lateral geniculate nucleus..

THE MESENCEPHALIC-DIENCEPHALIC TRANSITION: SECTION PARALLEL TO THE SYLVIAN FISSURE; LEVEL INCLUDING THE OPTIC TRACTS AND THE HYPOTHALAMUS

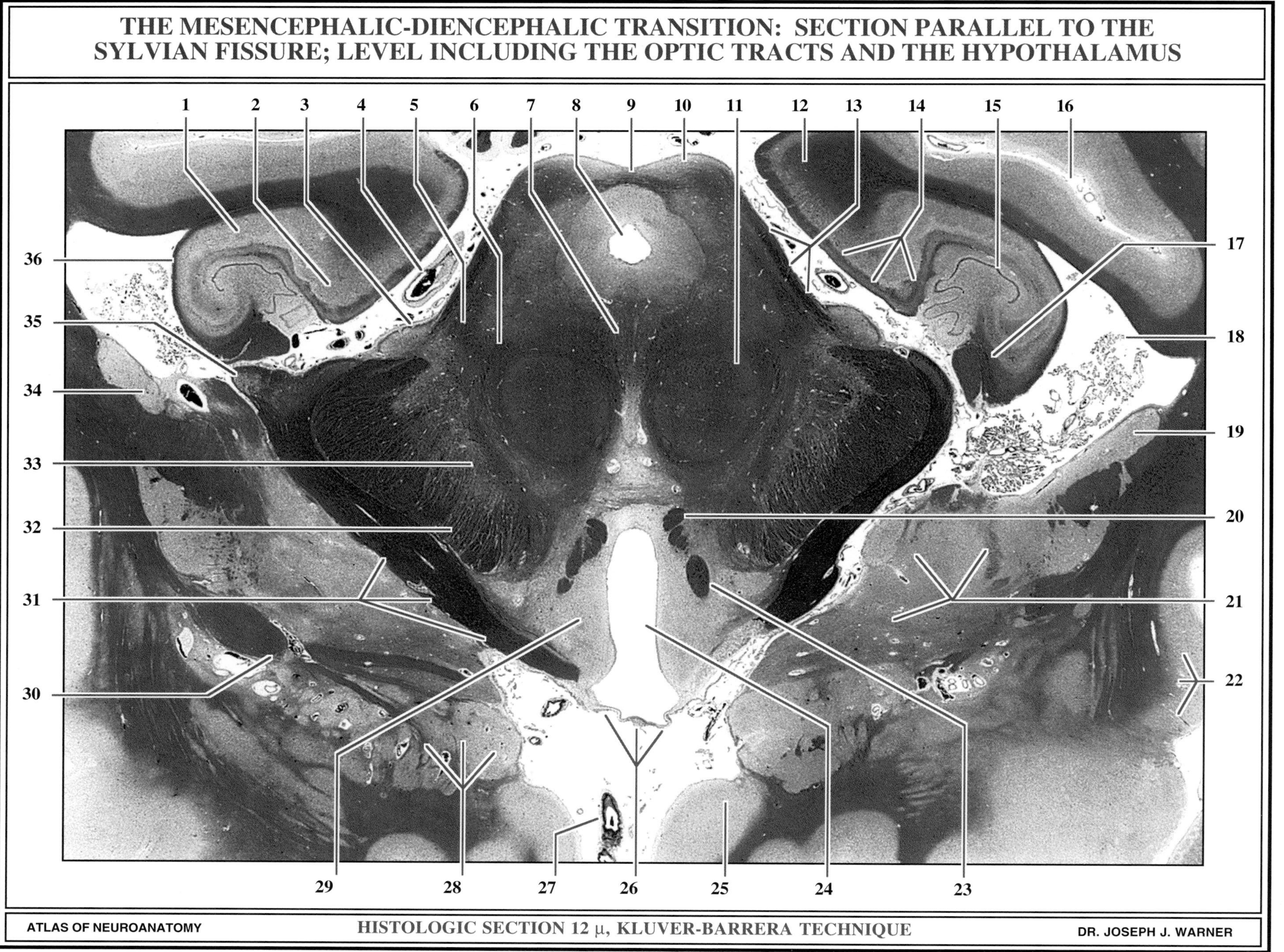

HISTOLOGIC SECTION 12 μ, KLUVER-BARRERA TECHNIQUE

THE MESENCEPHALIC-DIENCEPHALIC TRANSITION; SECTION PARALLEL TO THE SYLVIAN FISSURE, LEVEL INCLUDING THE OPTIC TRACTS AND THE HYPOTHALAMUS: SECTION ORIENTATION AND KEY TO NUMBERED STRUCTURES

KEY TO NUMBERED STRUCTURES

1. Hippocampal Formation
2. Subiculum
3. Medial Geniculate Nucleus
4. Posterior Cerebral Artery
5. Spinothalamic and Ventral Trigeminothalamic Tracts
6. Medial Lemniscus
7. Oculomotor Nuclear Complex
8. Aqueduct of Sylvius
9. Commissure of the Inferior Colliculus
10. Inferior Colliculus (rostral aspect)
11. Red Nucleus
12. Parahippocampal Gyrus
13. Brachium of the Inferior Colliculus
14. Superficial Medullary Stratum of the Subiculum
15. Dentate Gyrus of the Hippocampus
16. Collateral Sulcus
17. Fimbria of the Fornix
18. Choroid Plexus in the Temporal Horn of the Lateral Ventricle
19. Tail of the Caudate Nucleus
20. Mammillothalamic Tract
21. Amygdala
22. Insula
23. Fornix
24. Third Ventricle
25. Paraolfactory Gyrus
26. Lamina Terminalis
27. Anterior Cerebral Artery
28. Anterior Perforated Substance
29. Hypothalamus
30. Anterior Commissure
31. Optic Tract
32. Cerebral Peduncle
33. Substantia Nigra
34. Tail of the Caudate Nucleus
35. Lateral Geniculate Nucleus
36. Alveus

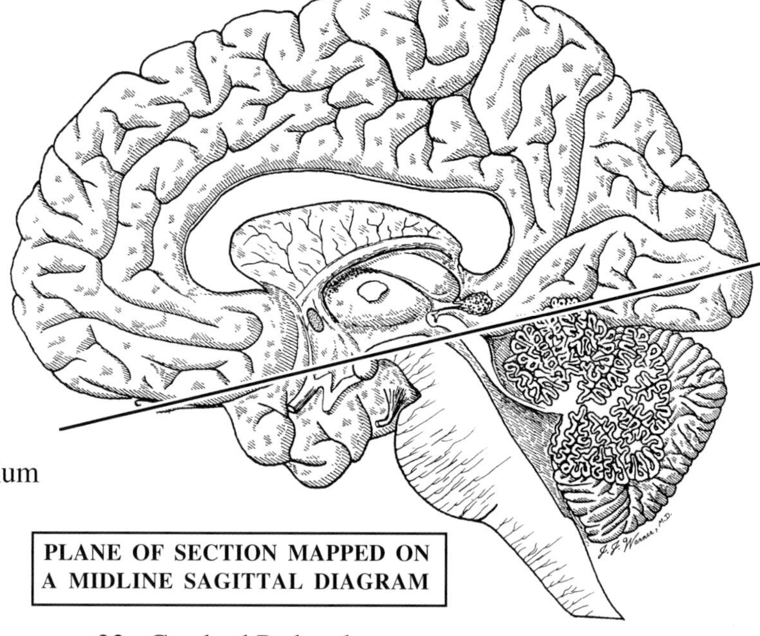

PLANE OF SECTION MAPPED ON A MIDLINE SAGITTAL DIAGRAM

This plane of section includes the rostral aspect of the inferior colliculi and the medial geniculate nuclei. In contrast to the horizontal section of the mesencephalic-diencephalic transition at the level of the inferior colliculus and medial geniculate nuclei (Figure A), the orientation of this section (parallel to the Sylvian fissure) demonstrates the course of the optic tract lateral to the hypothalamus and cerebral peduncles (Figure B).

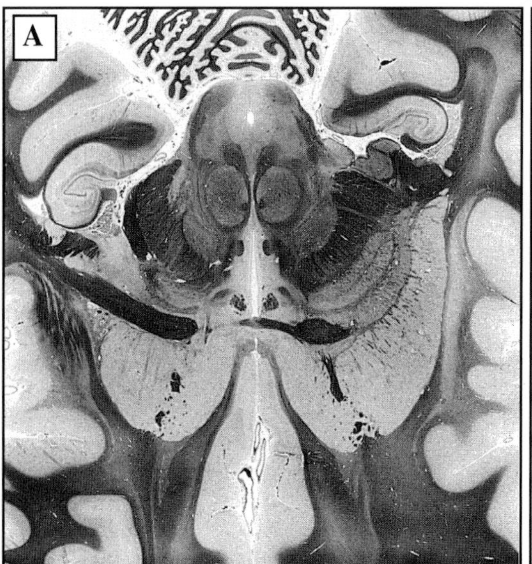

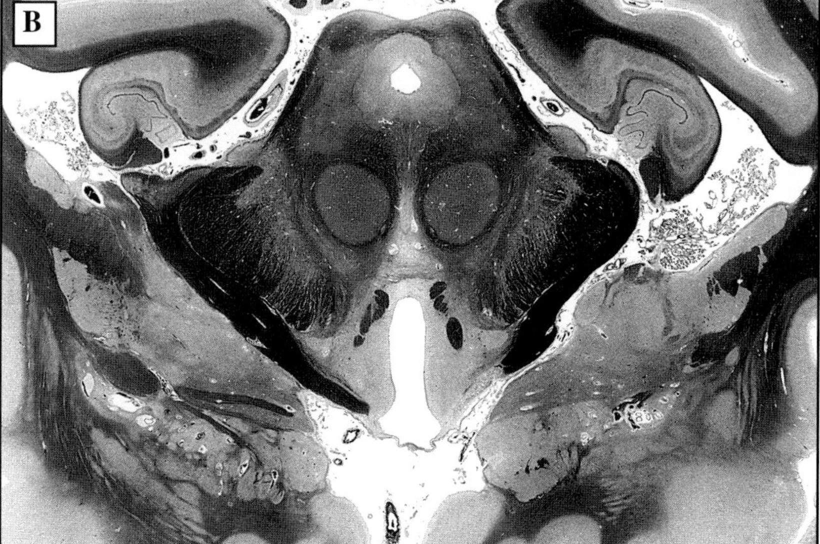

CEREBELLUM, BRAINSTEM, AND DIENCEPHALON: PARASAGITTAL SECTION

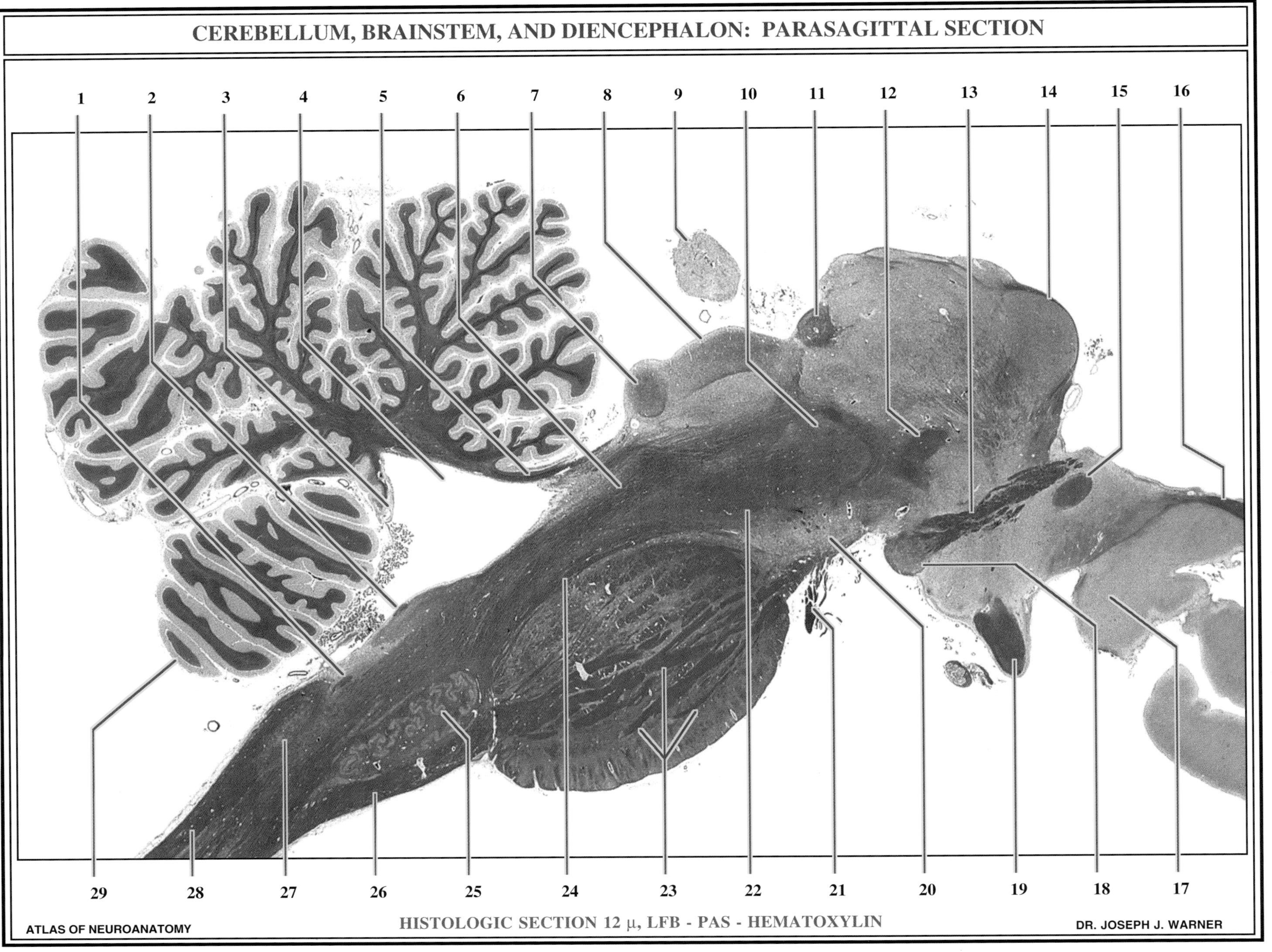

HISTOLOGIC SECTION 12 μ, LFB - PAS - HEMATOXYLIN

DR. JOSEPH J. WARNER

CEREBELLUM, BRAINSTEM, AND DIENCEPHALON: PARASAGITTAL SECTION

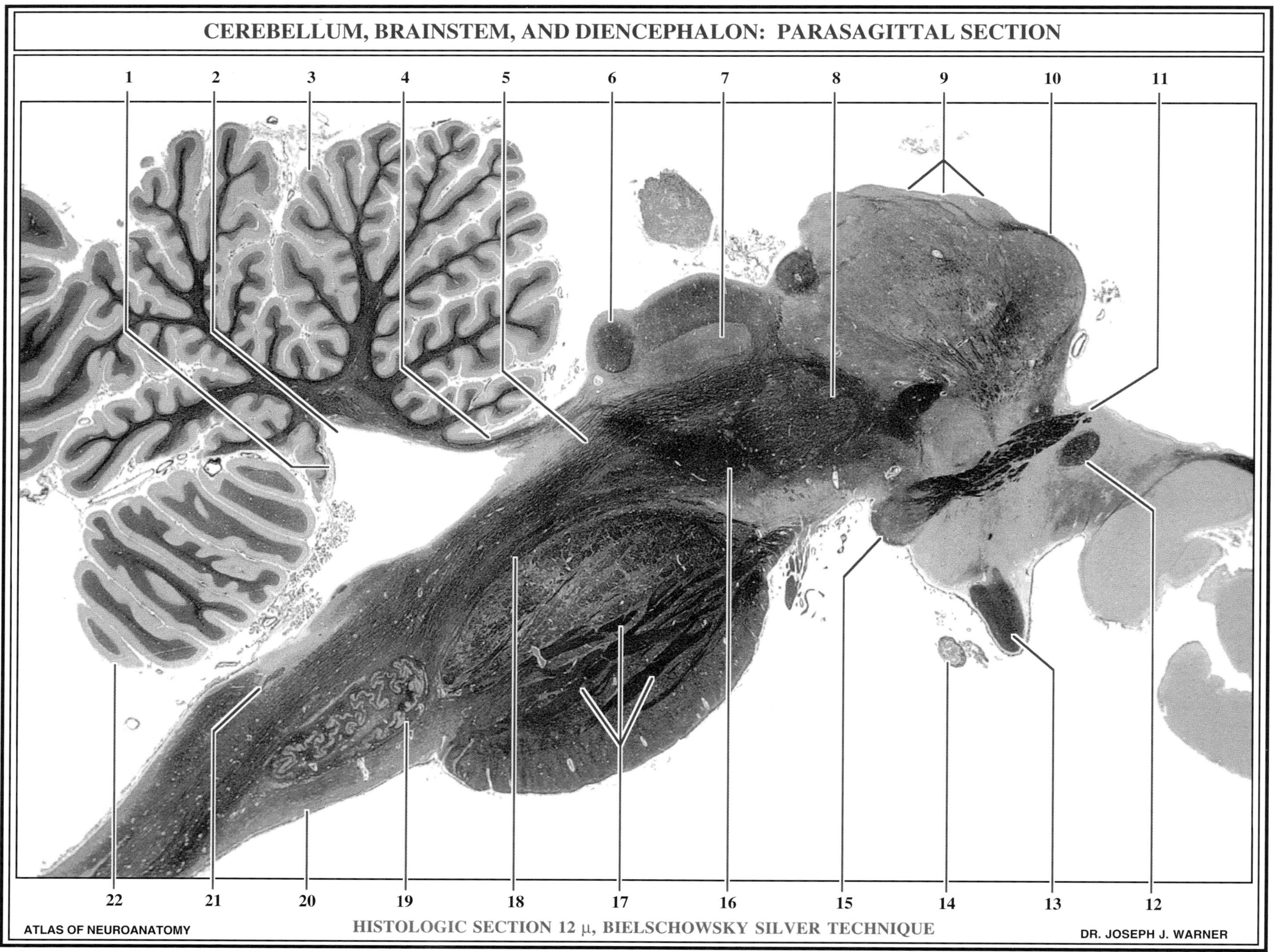

HISTOLOGIC SECTION 12 μ, BIELSCHOWSKY SILVER TECHNIQUE

ATLAS OF NEUROANATOMY

DR. JOSEPH J. WARNER

CEREBELLUM, BRAINSTEM, AND DIENCEPHALON; (A) LFB - PAS - HEMATOXYLIN AND (B) BIELSCHOWSKY SILVER STAINED 12 μ PARASAGITTAL SECTIONS: KEY TO NUMBERED STRUCTURES

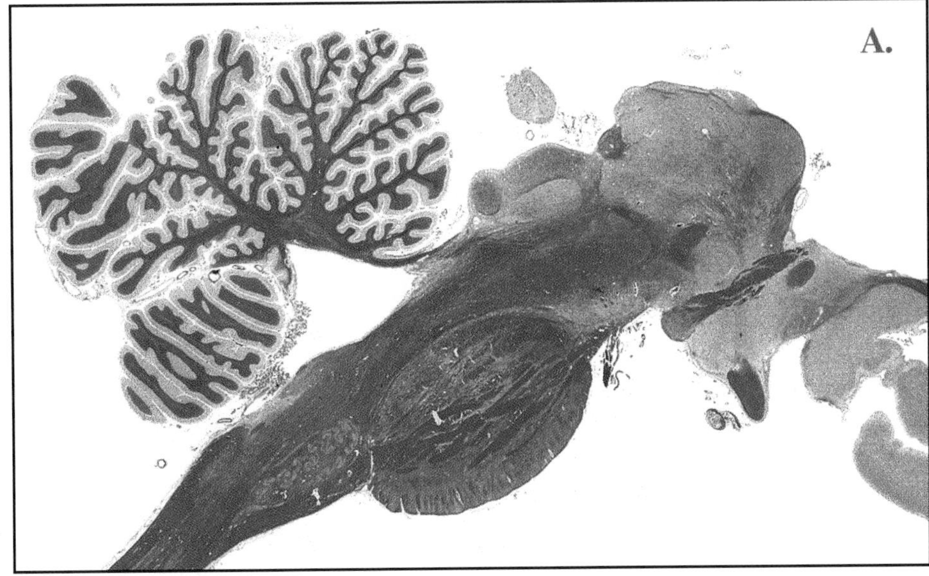

KEY FOR LFB - PAS - HEMATOXYLIN STAINED SECTION

1. Nucleus and Tractus Solitarius
2. Genu of the Facial (VII) Nerve
3. Inferior Medullary Velum
4. Fourth Ventricle
5. Superior Medullary Velum
6. Central Tegmental Tract
7. Inferior Colliculus
8. Superior Colliculus
9. Pineal Body
10. Red Nucleus
11. Brachium of the Superior Colliculus
12. Mammillothalamic Tract
13. Fornix (Post-commissural fibers)
14. Anterior Nucleus of the Thalamus
15. Anterior Commissure
16. Rostrum of the Corpus Callosum
17. Paraterminal Gyrus
18. Mammillary Body
19. Optic Chiasm
20. Substantia Nigra
21. Oculomotor (III) Nerve
22. Decussation of the Superior Cerebellar Peduncle
23. Corticobulbar and Corticospinal Fibers
24. Medial Lemniscus
25. Inferior Olivary Nucleus
27. Nucleus Gracilis
28. Fasciculus Gracilis
29. Cerebellar Tonsil

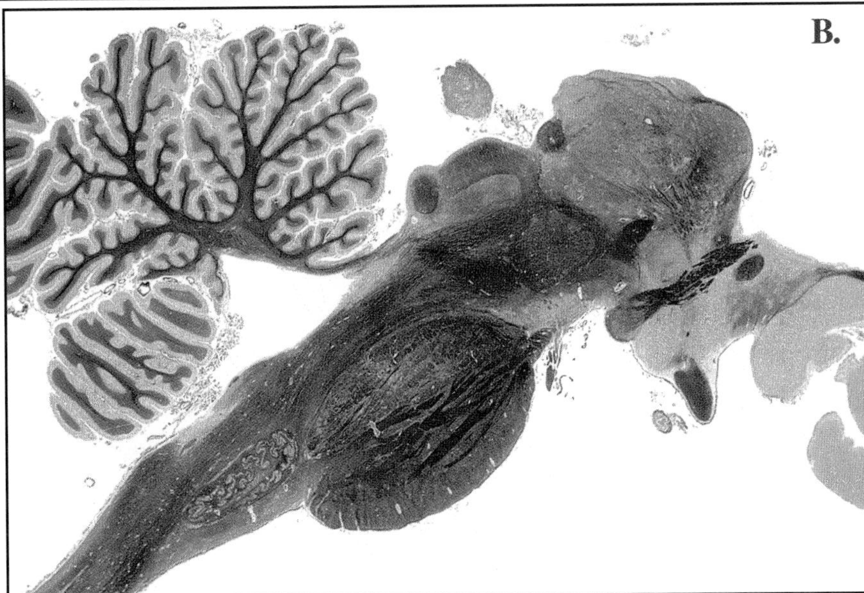

KEY FOR BIELSCHOWSKY SILVER STAINED SECTION

1. Inferior Medullary Velum
2. Fourth Ventricle
3. Superior Cerebellar Vermis
4. Superior (Anterior) Medullary Velum
5. Central Tegmental Tract
6. Inferior Colliculus
7. Periaqueductal Gray
8. Red Nucleus
9. Lateral Dorsal Nucleus of the Thalamus
10. Anterior Nucleus of the Thalamus
11. Fornix
12. Anterior Commissure
13. Optic Chiasm
14. Pituitary Stalk
15. Mammillary Body
16. Decussation of the Superior Cerebellar Peduncle
17. Corticobulbar and Corticospinal Fibers
18. Medial Lemniscus
19. Inferior Olivary Nucleus
20. Medullary Pyramid
21. Nucleus and Tractus Solitarius
22. Cerebellar Tonsil

ROSTRAL BRAINSTEM AND DIENCEPHALON: 15μ PARASAGITTAL SECTION, LFB-PAS STAIN

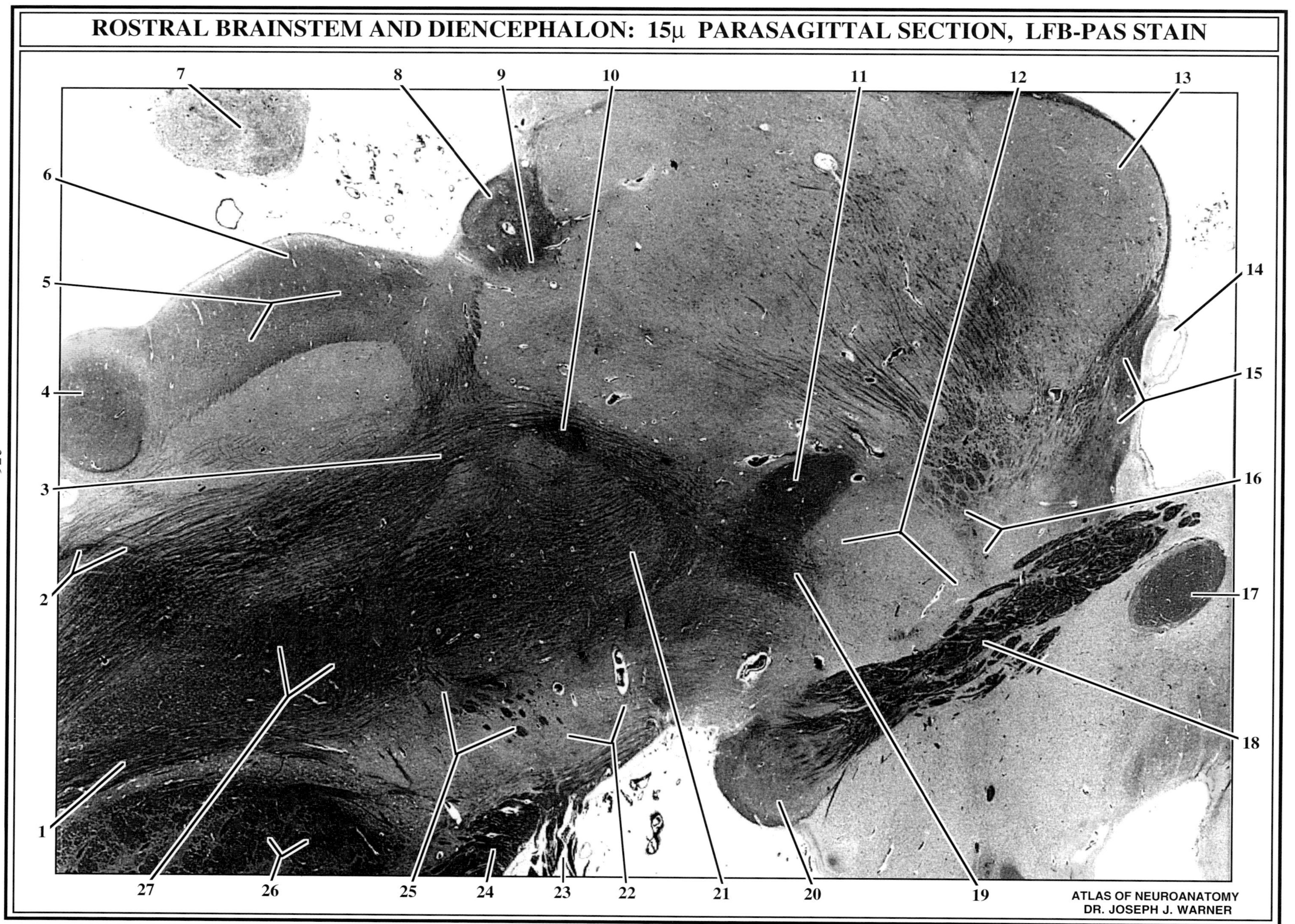

SAGITTAL SECTION MAP OF THE ROSTRAL BRAINSTEM AND DIENCEPHALON: REFERENCED TO A HORIZONTAL SECTION THROUGH THE MESENCEPHALIC-DIENCEPHALIC TRANSITION, 15μ, KLUVER-BARRERA TECHNIQUE

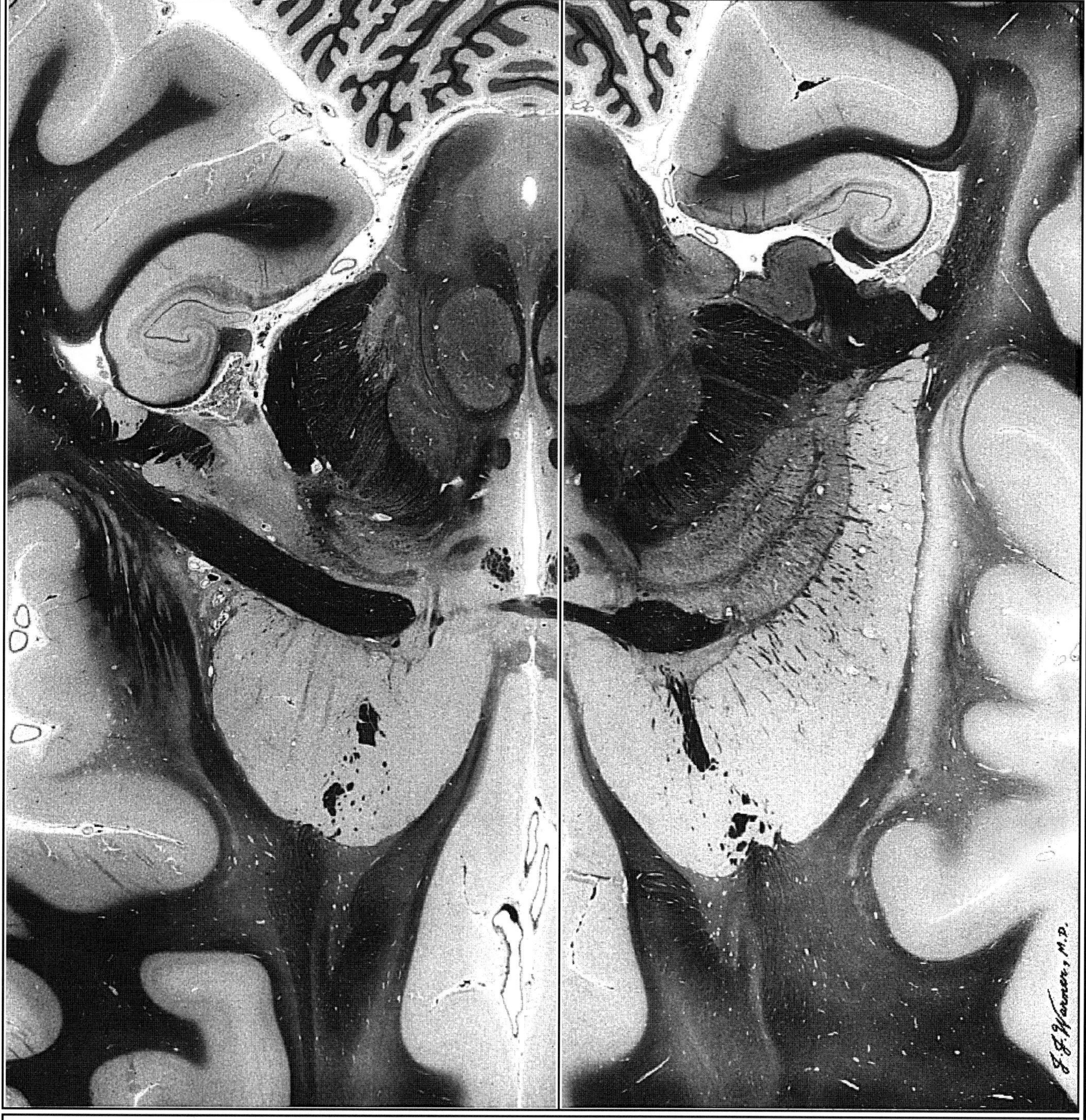

KEY TO NUMBERED STRUCTURES ON PARASAGITTAL SECTION THROUGH THE ROSTRAL BRAINSTEM AND DIENCEPHALON

1. Medial Lemniscus
2. Fibers of Superior Cerebellar Peduncle
3. Central Tegmental Tract
4. Inferior Colliculus
5. Stratum Opticum of Superior Colliculus
6. Superior Colliculus
7. Pineal Body
8. Brachium of the Superior Colliculus
9. Posterior Commissure
10. Habenulointerpeduncular Tract
11. Mammillothalamic Tract
12. Dorsomedial and Posterior Hypothalamic Nuclei
13. Anterior Nucleus (Thalamus)
14. Thalamostriate Vein
15. Stria Medullaris
16. Inferior Thalamic Peduncle
17. Anterior Commissure
18. Fornix
19. Lenticular Fasciculus, Field H2 of Forel
20. Mammillary Body
21. Red Nucleus
22. Substantia Nigra
23. Fascicles of Oculomotor Nerve
24. Cerebral Peduncle
25. Fascicles of Oculomotor Nerve
26. Transverse Pontocerebellar Fibers in Basis Pontis
27. Decussation of Superior Cerebellar Peduncle

ATLAS OF NEUROANATOMY
DR. JOSEPH J. WARNER

PARASAGITTAL SECTION, LEVEL OF THE MAMMILLARY BODY AND HABENULOINTERPEDUNCULAR TRACT, MAGNIFIED VIEW

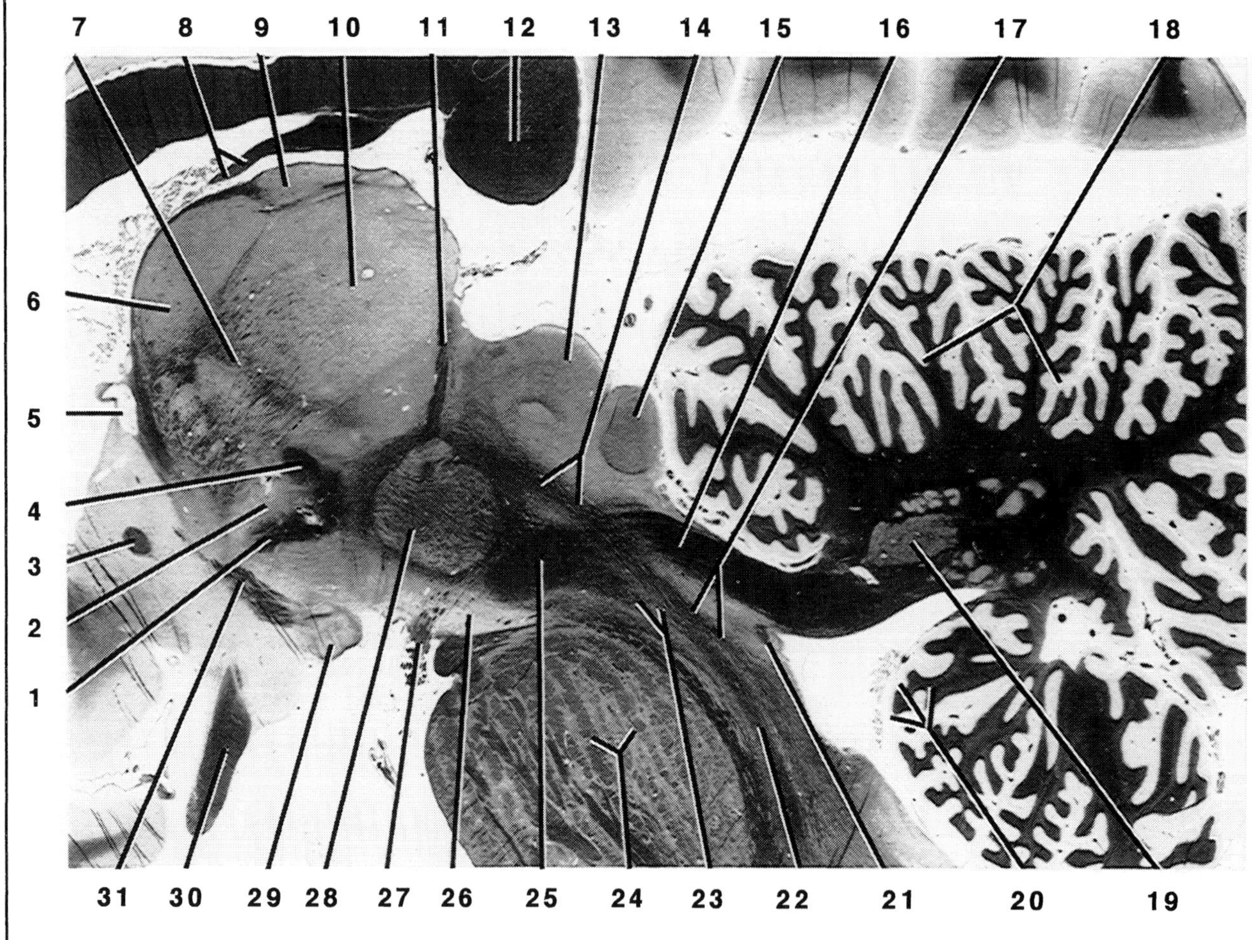

Sagittal Section, 15μ, Kluver-Barrera technique

KEY TO NUMBERED STRUCTURES

1. Field H2 of Forel (Lenticular Fasciculus)
2. Zona Incerta
3. Anterior Commissure
4. Mammillothalamic Tract
5. Thalamostriate Vein and Stria Terminalis
6. Anterior Nucleus of the Thalamus
7. Internal Medullary Lamina of the Thalamus
8. Fornix
9. Lateral Dorsal Nucleus of the Thalamus
10. Dorsomedial Nucleus of the Thalamus
11. Habenulointerpeduncular Tract
12. Splenium, Corpus Callosum
13. Superior Colliculus
14. Central Tegmental Tract (see #17)
15. Inferior Colliculus
16. Superior Cerebellar Peduncle
17. Central Tegmental Tract (see #14)
18. Anterior Lobe, Cerebellum
19. Emboliform Nucleus
20. Nodulus
21. Mesencephalic root of the Trigeminal Nerve
22. Medial Lemniscus
23. Medial Lemniscus and Ventral Trigeminothalamic fibers
24. Transverse Pontocerebellar Fibers
25. Decussation, Superior Cerebellar Peduncle
26. Substantia Nigra
27. Oculomotor Nerve
28. Red Nucleus
29. Mammillary Body
30. Optic Chiasm
31. Fornix

THE MESENCEPHALIC - DIENCEPHALIC TRANSITION: SAGITTAL SECTION THROUGH THE FASCICULUS RETROFLEXUS OF MEYNERT (HABENULOINTERPEDUNCULAR TRACT)

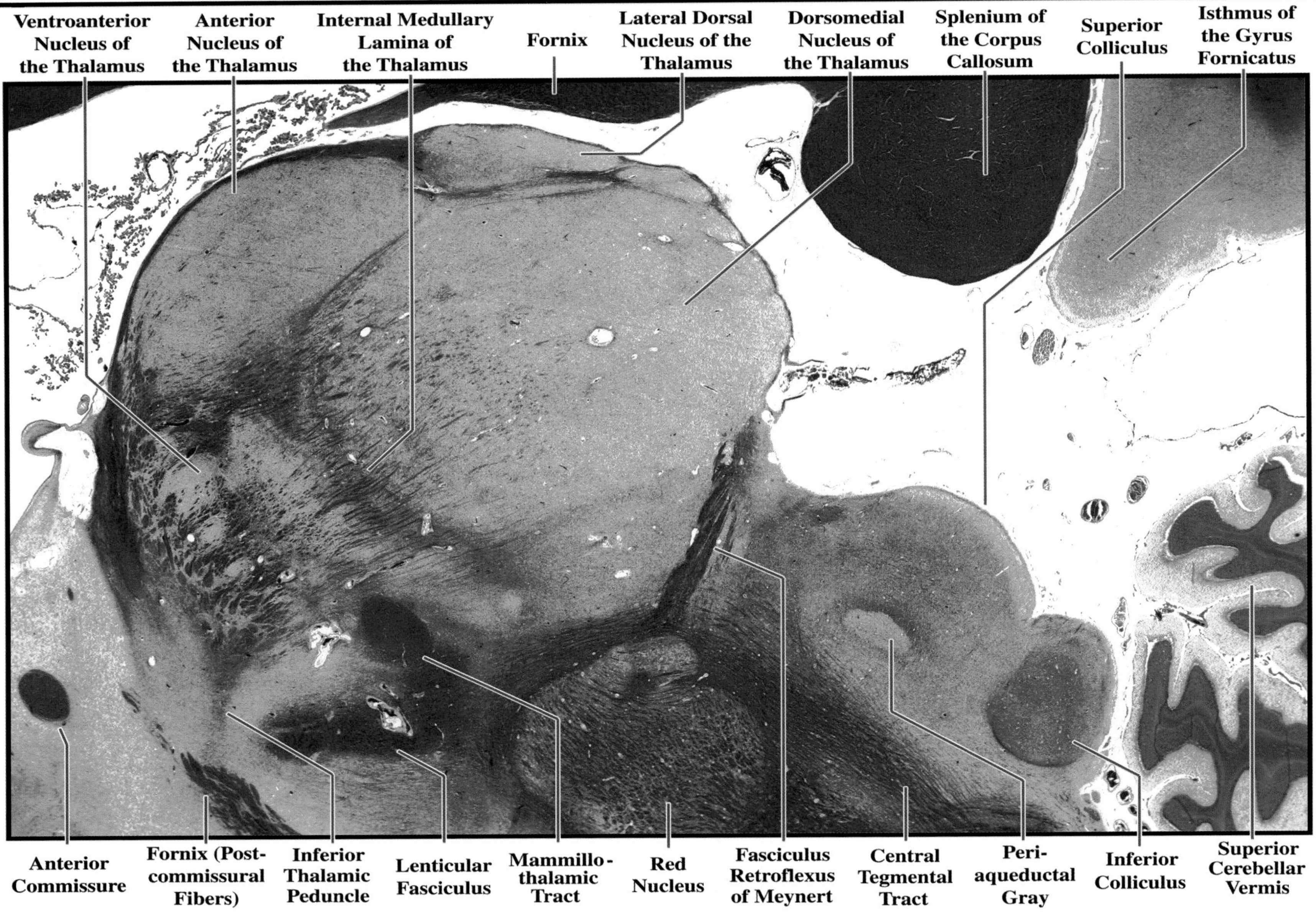

Ventroanterior Nucleus of the Thalamus
Anterior Nucleus of the Thalamus
Internal Medullary Lamina of the Thalamus
Fornix
Lateral Dorsal Nucleus of the Thalamus
Dorsomedial Nucleus of the Thalamus
Splenium of the Corpus Callosum
Superior Colliculus
Isthmus of the Gyrus Fornicatus

Anterior Commissure
Fornix (Post-commissural Fibers)
Inferior Thalamic Peduncle
Lenticular Fasciculus
Mammillo-thalamic Tract
Red Nucleus
Fasciculus Retroflexus of Meynert
Central Tegmental Tract
Peri-aqueductal Gray
Inferior Colliculus
Superior Cerebellar Vermis

Section 15 μ, Kluver - Barrera Technique

DR. JOSEPH J. WARNER

PARASAGITTAL SECTION, LEVEL INCLUDING THE CENTROMEDIAN NUCLEUS AND ROSTRAL COURSE OF THE LATERAL LEMNISCUS, MAGNIFIED VIEW

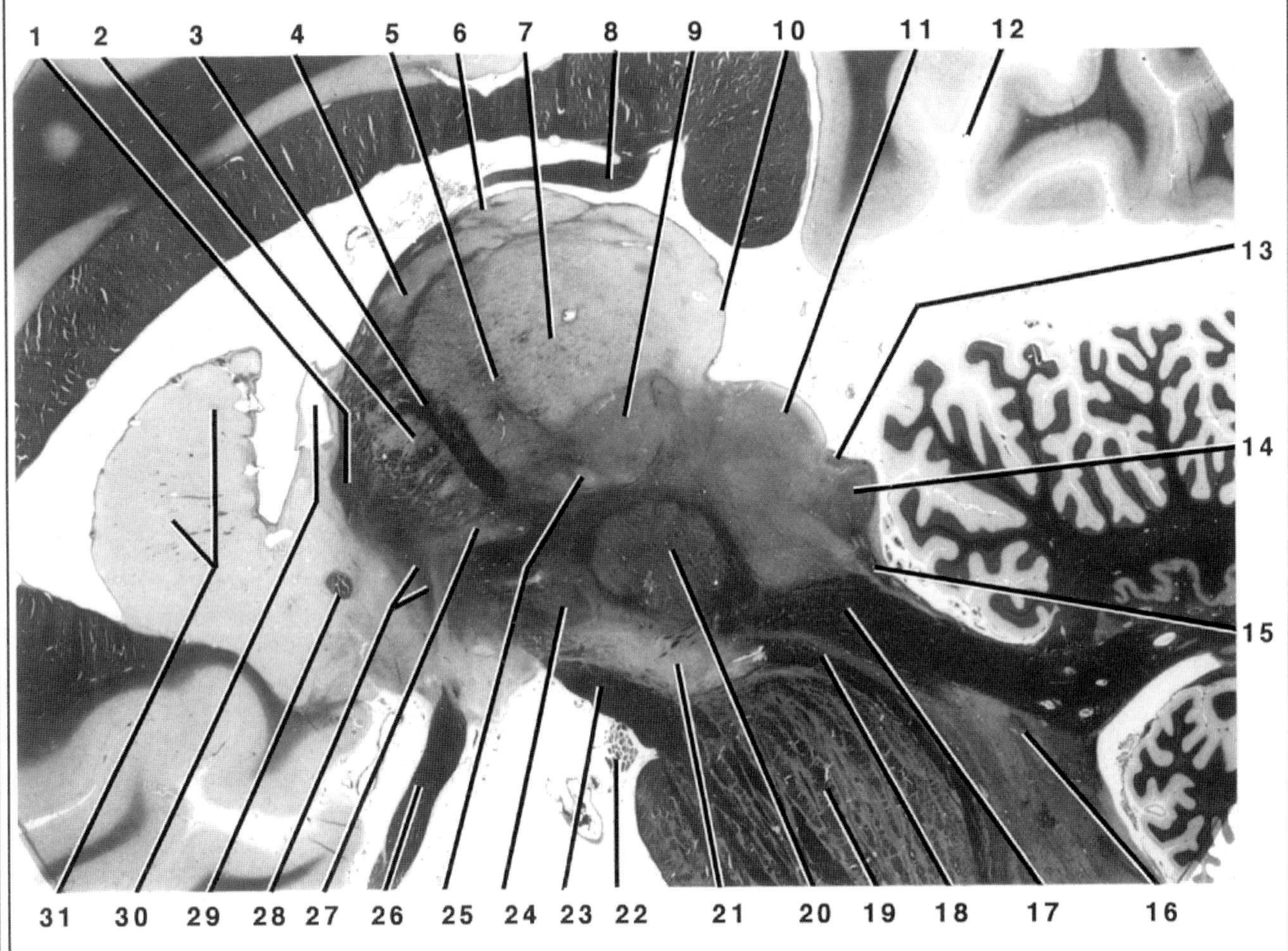

Sagittal Section, 15μ, Kluver-Barrera technique

KEY TO NUMBERED STRUCTURES

1. Anterior Thalamic Radiations (Peduncle)
2. Ventroanterior Nucleus of the Thalamus
3. Mammillothalamic Tract
4. Anterior Nucleus of the Thalamus
5. Internal Medullary Lamina of the Thalamus
6. Lateral Dorsal Nucleus of the Thalamus
7. Dorsomedial Nucleus of the Thalamus
8. Fornix
9. Centromedian Nucleus of the Thalamus
10. Pulvinar
11. Superior Colliculus
12. Parieto-occipital Sulcus
13. Brachium of Inferior Colliculus
14. Inferior Colliculus
15. Lateral Lemniscus
16. Mesencephalic root of the Trigeminal Nerve
17. Superior Cerebellar Peduncle
18. Medial Lemniscus
19. Transverse Pontocerebellar fibers
20. Red Nucleus
21. Substantia Nigra
22. Fascicles of Oculomotor Nerve
23. Cerebral Peduncle
24. Subthalamic Nucleus
25. Ventroposteromedial Nucleus of the Thalamus
26. Optic Chiasm
27. Zona Incerta
28. Inferior Thalamic Peduncle
29. Anterior Commissure
30. Thalamostriate Vein and adjacent Stria Terminalis
31. Head of the Caudate Nucleus

THE MESENCEPHALIC-DIENCEPHALIC TRANSITION: SECTION PARALLEL TO THE PARIETO-OCCIPITAL SULCUS, LEVEL INCLUDING THE MEDIAL AND LATERAL GENICULATE NUCLEI

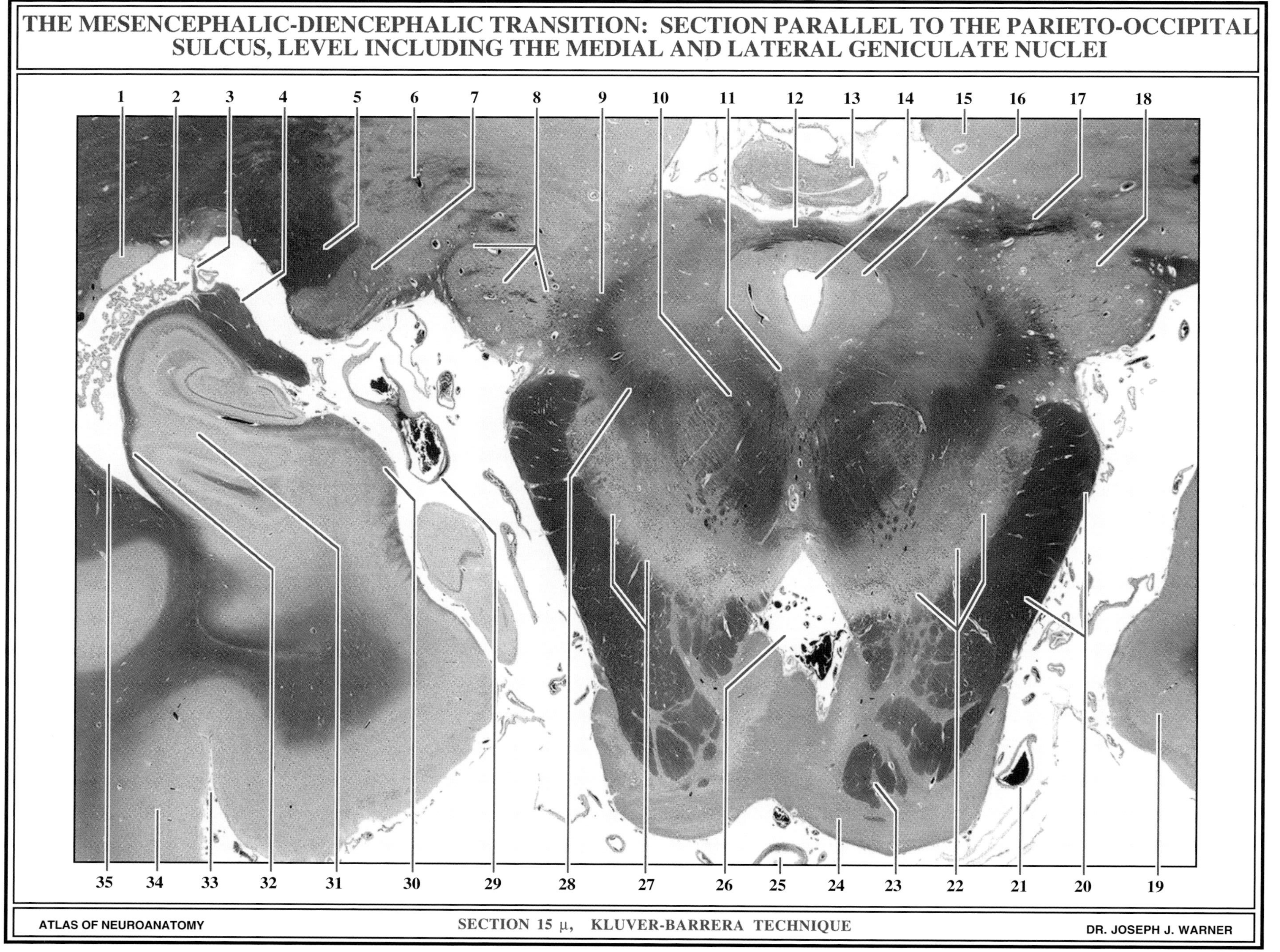

SECTION 15 μ, KLUVER-BARRERA TECHNIQUE

DR. JOSEPH J. WARNER

THE MESENCEPHALIC-DIENCEPHALIC TRANSITION: PLANE PARALLEL TO THE PARIETO-OCCIPITAL SULCUS, LEVEL INCLUDING THE LATERAL AND MEDIAL GENICULATE NUCLEI; MAGNIFIED VIEW SECTION ORIENTATION AND KEY TO NUMBERED STRUCTURES

KEY TO NUMBERED STRUCTURES

1. Tail of the Caudate Nucleus
2. Choroid Plexus
3. Tela Choroidea
4. Fimbria of the Fornix
5. Geniculocalcarine (Optic) Radiations
6. Lateral Pulvinar Nucleus of the Thalamus
7. Lateral Geniculate Nucleus
8. Medial Geniculate Nucleus
9. Spinothalamic Tract
10. Dentatorubrothalamic Fibers
11. Oculomotor (III) Nuclear Complex
12. Transition from the Posterior Commissure to the Commissure of the Superior Colliculus
13. Pineal Body
14. Aqueduct of Sylvius
15. Medial Pulvinar Nucleus of the Thalamus
16. Periaqueductal Gray
17. Brachium of the Superior Colliculus
18. Medial Geniculate Nucleus
19. Parahippocampal Gyrus
20. Cerebral Peduncle
21. Superior Cerebellar Artery
22. Substantia Nigra Pars Compacta
23. Frontopontine Fibers
24. Basis Pontis
25. Basilar Artery
26. Interpeduncular Fossa
27. Substantia Nigra Pars Reticulata
28. Medial Lemniscus
29. Posterior Cerebral Artery
30. Superficial Medullary Stratum of the Subiculum
31. Hippocampal Formation
32. Alveus
33. Collateral Sulcus
34. Fusiform Gyrus
35. Temporal Horn of the Lateral Ventricle

This plane of section through the mesencephalic-diencephalic junction includes the rostral basis pontis, interpeduncular fossa, and pretectal region of the dorsal mesencephalon. The brachium of the superior colliculus is clearly demonstrated as it courses ventral to the medial aspect of the pulvinar nucleus of the thalamus and dorsal to the medial geniculate nucleus.

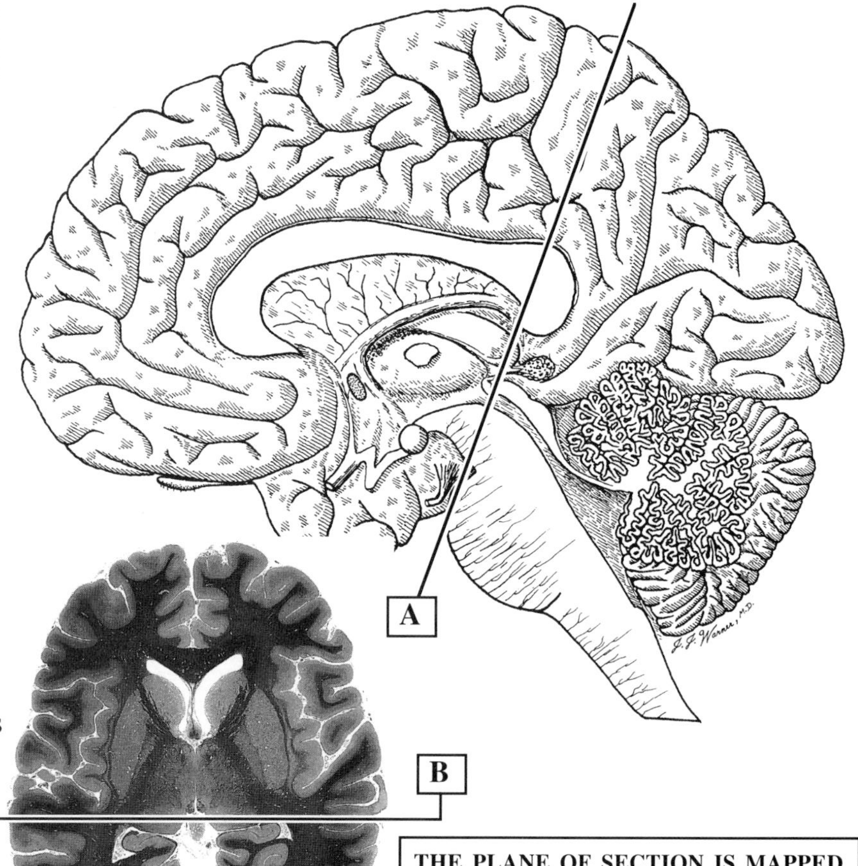

THE PLANE OF SECTION IS MAPPED IN REFERENCE TO (A) A MIDLINE SAGITTAL DIAGRAM, AND (B) A HORIZONTAL SECTION, (LEVEL OF THE GENU OF THE CORPUS CALLOSUM AND THE PINEAL BODY)

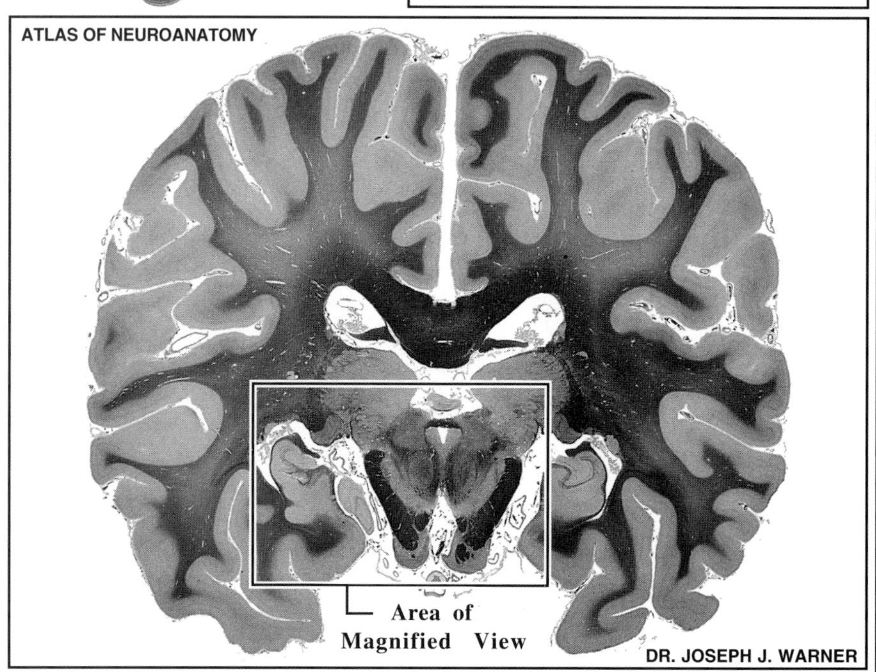

HORIZONTAL SECTION OF THE BRAIN (MAGNIFIED VIEW): LEVEL OF THE MAMMILLARY BODIES, THE OLFACTORY TRACT, AND THE INFUNDIBULAR RECESS OF THE THIRD VENTRICLE

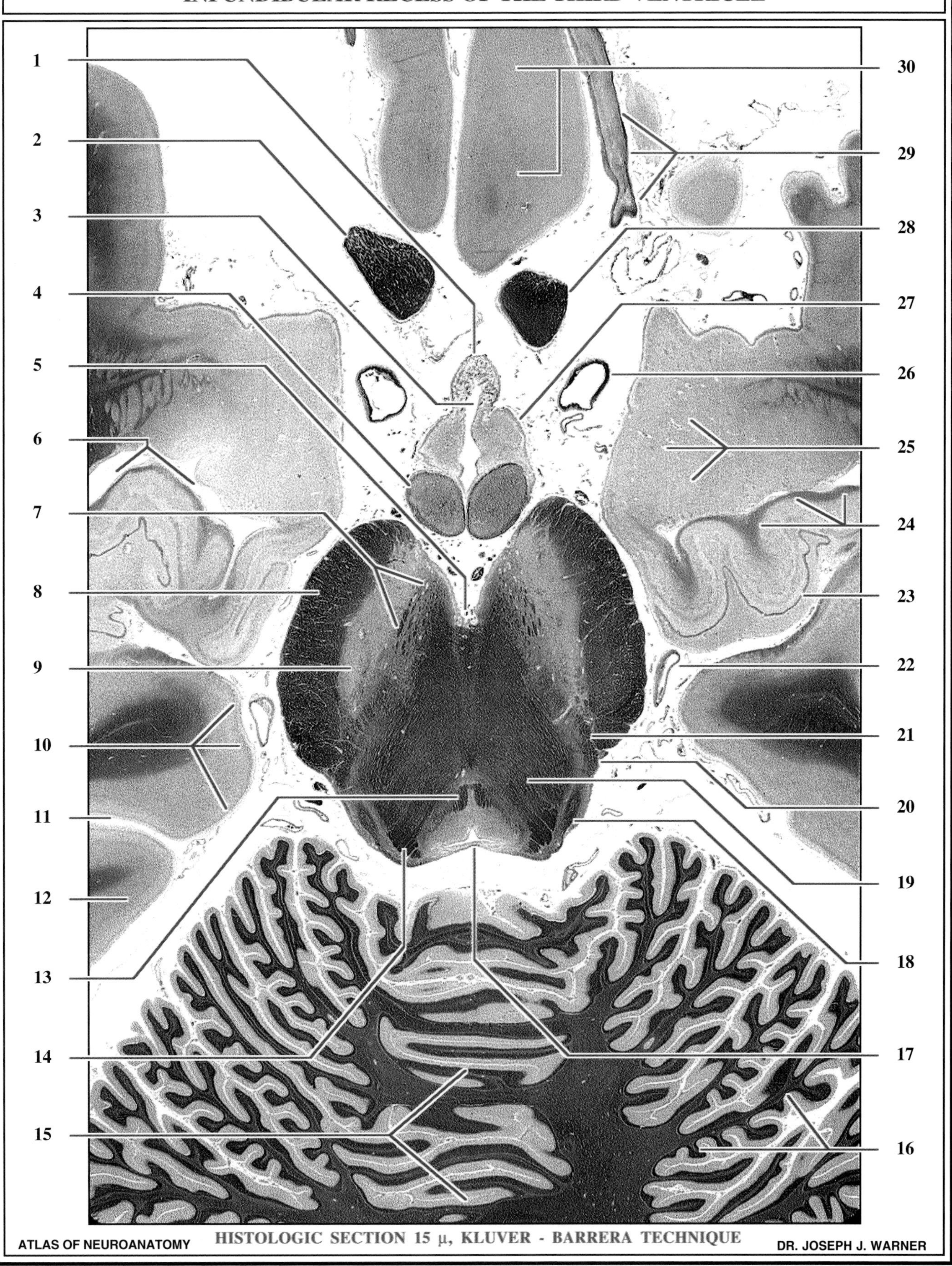

ATLAS OF NEUROANATOMY

HISTOLOGIC SECTION 15 µ, KLUVER - BARRERA TECHNIQUE

DR. JOSEPH J. WARNER

HORIZONTAL SECTION OF THE BRAIN (MAGNIFIED VIEW): LEVEL OF THE MAMMILLARY BODIES, THE OLFACTORY TRACT, AND THE INFUNDIBULAR RECESS OF THE THIRD VENTRICLE

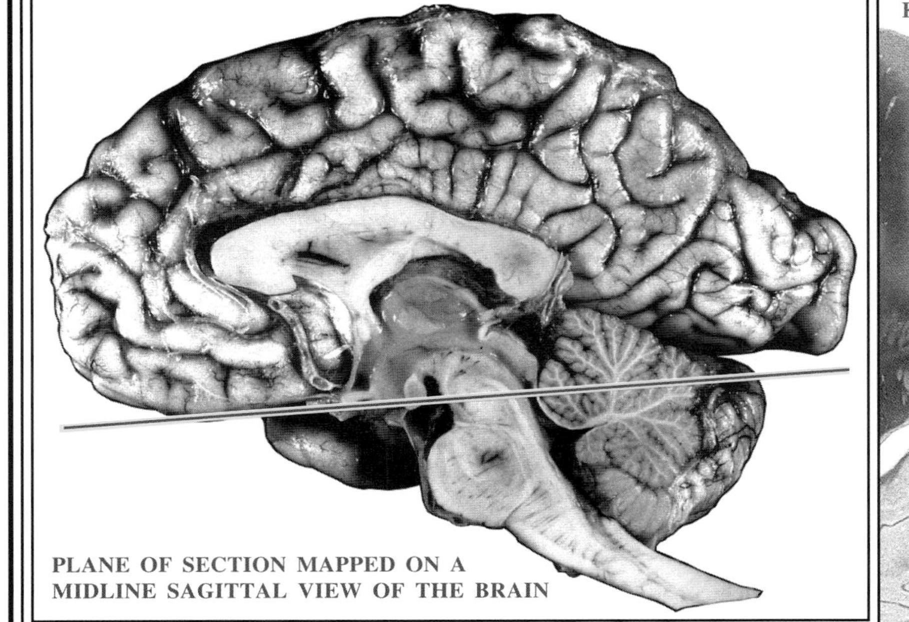

PLANE OF SECTION MAPPED ON A MIDLINE SAGITTAL VIEW OF THE BRAIN

KLUVER-BARRERA TECHNIQUE

SECTION 15 µ

KEY TO NUMBERED STRUCTURES

1. Pituitary Stalk
2. Optic Nerve
3. Infundibular Recess of the Third Ventricle
4. Mammillary Body
5. Interpeduncular Fossa
6. Temporal Horn of the Lateral Ventricle
7. Fascicles of the Oculomotor (III) Nerve
8. Cerebral Peduncle
9. Substantia Nigra
10. Parahippocampal Gyrus
11. Collateral Sulcus
12. Fusiform Gyrus
13. Medial Longitudinal Fasciculus
14. Superior Cerebellar Peduncle
15. Cerebellar Vermis
16. Anterior Lobe of the Cerebellum
17. Anterior Medullary Velum
18. Lateral Lemniscus
19. Decussation of the Superior Cerebellar Peduncle
20. Spinothalamic Tract
21. Medial Lemniscus
22. Posterior Cerebral Artery
23. Dentate Gyrus of the Hippocampus
24. Alveus
25. Amygdala
26. Internal Carotid Artery
27. Hypothalamus
28. Optic Nerve
29. Olfactory Tract
30. Gyrus Rectus

ATLAS OF NEUROANATOMY

DR. JOSEPH J. WARNER

HORIZONTAL SECTION OF THE BRAIN (MAGNIFIED): LEVEL INCLUDING THE SUPRAOPTIC RECESS OF THE THIRD VENTRICLE AND THE LAMINA TERMINALIS

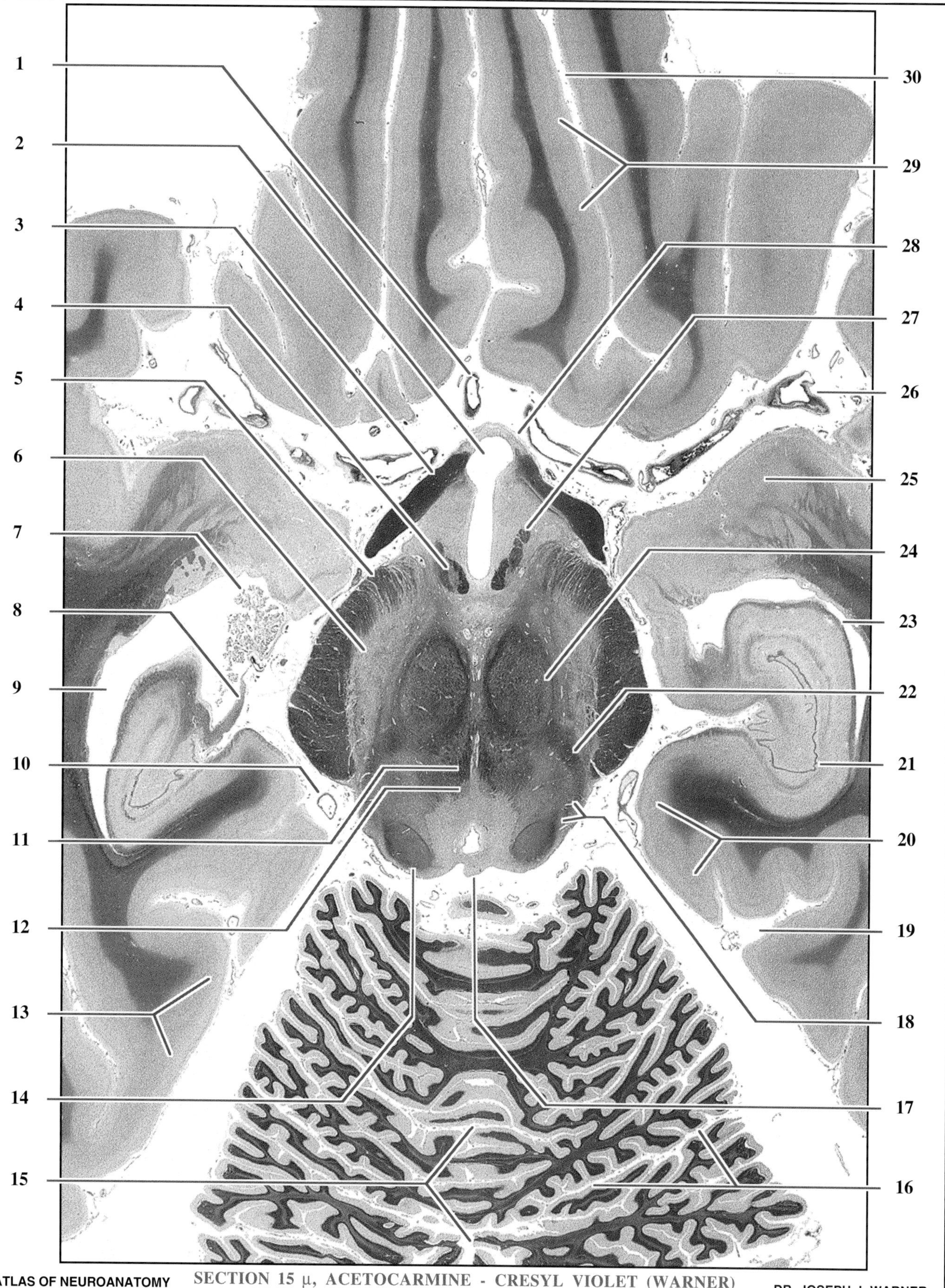

1
2
3
4
5
6
7
8
9
10
11
12
13
14
15

30
29
28
27
26
25
24
23
22
21
20
19
18
17
16

SECTION 15 μ, ACETOCARMINE - CRESYL VIOLET (WARNER)

HORIZONTAL SECTION OF THE BRAIN (MAGNIFIED VIEW): LEVEL INCLUDING THE SUPRAOPTIC RECESS OF THE THIRD VENTRICLE, THE LAMINA TERMINALIS, AND THE OPTIC TRACTS

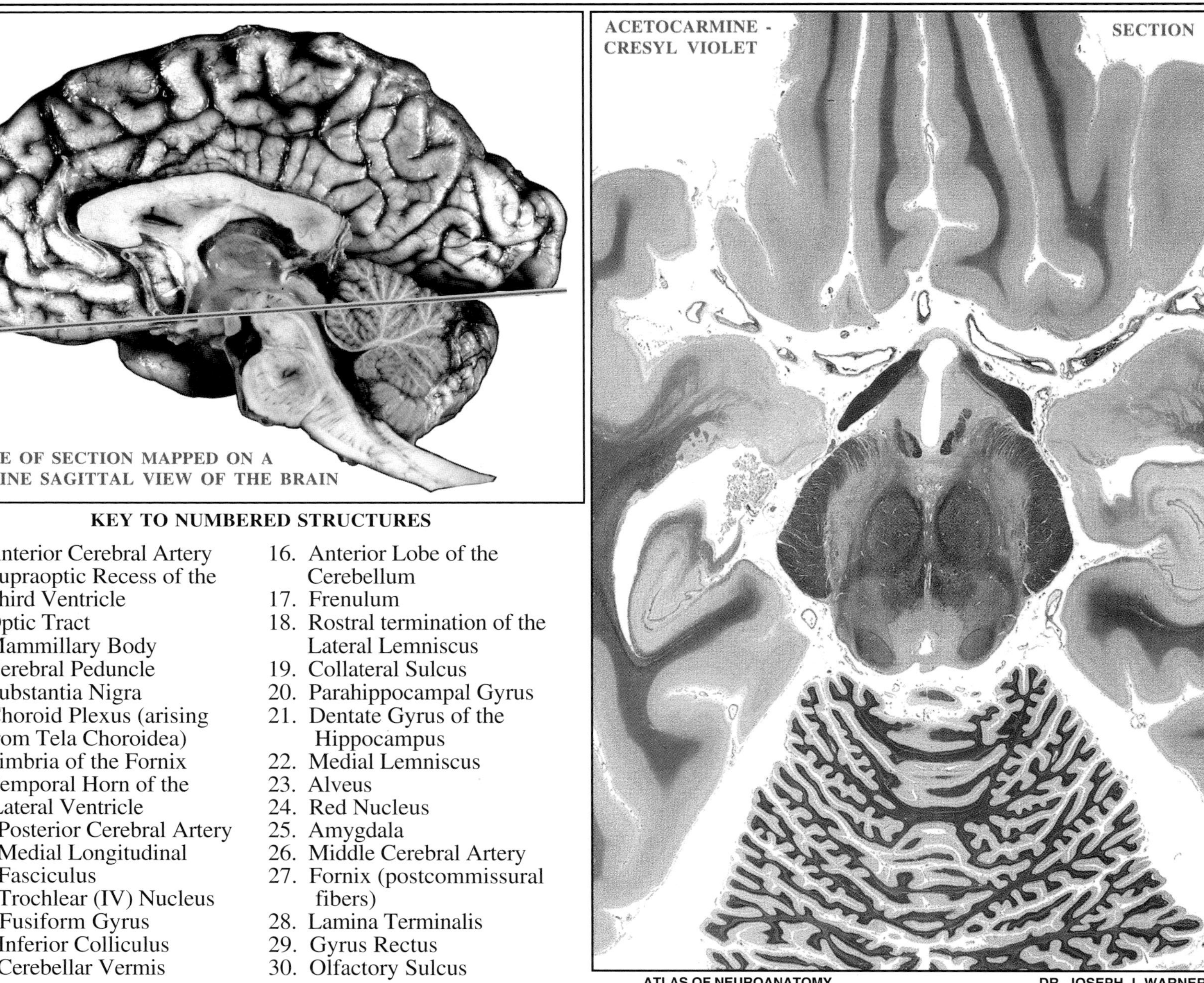

KEY TO NUMBERED STRUCTURES

1. Anterior Cerebral Artery
2. Supraoptic Recess of the Third Ventricle
3. Optic Tract
4. Mammillary Body
5. Cerebral Peduncle
6. Substantia Nigra
7. Choroid Plexus (arising from Tela Choroidea)
8. Fimbria of the Fornix
9. Temporal Horn of the Lateral Ventricle
10. Posterior Cerebral Artery
11. Medial Longitudinal Fasciculus
12. Trochlear (IV) Nucleus
13. Fusiform Gyrus
14. Inferior Colliculus
15. Cerebellar Vermis
16. Anterior Lobe of the Cerebellum
17. Frenulum
18. Rostral termination of the Lateral Lemniscus
19. Collateral Sulcus
20. Parahippocampal Gyrus
21. Dentate Gyrus of the Hippocampus
22. Medial Lemniscus
23. Alveus
24. Red Nucleus
25. Amygdala
26. Middle Cerebral Artery
27. Fornix (postcommissural fibers)
28. Lamina Terminalis
29. Gyrus Rectus
30. Olfactory Sulcus

PART VI: SECTIONAL NEUROANATOMY OF THE BRAINSTEM, CEREBELLUM, AND SPINAL CORD

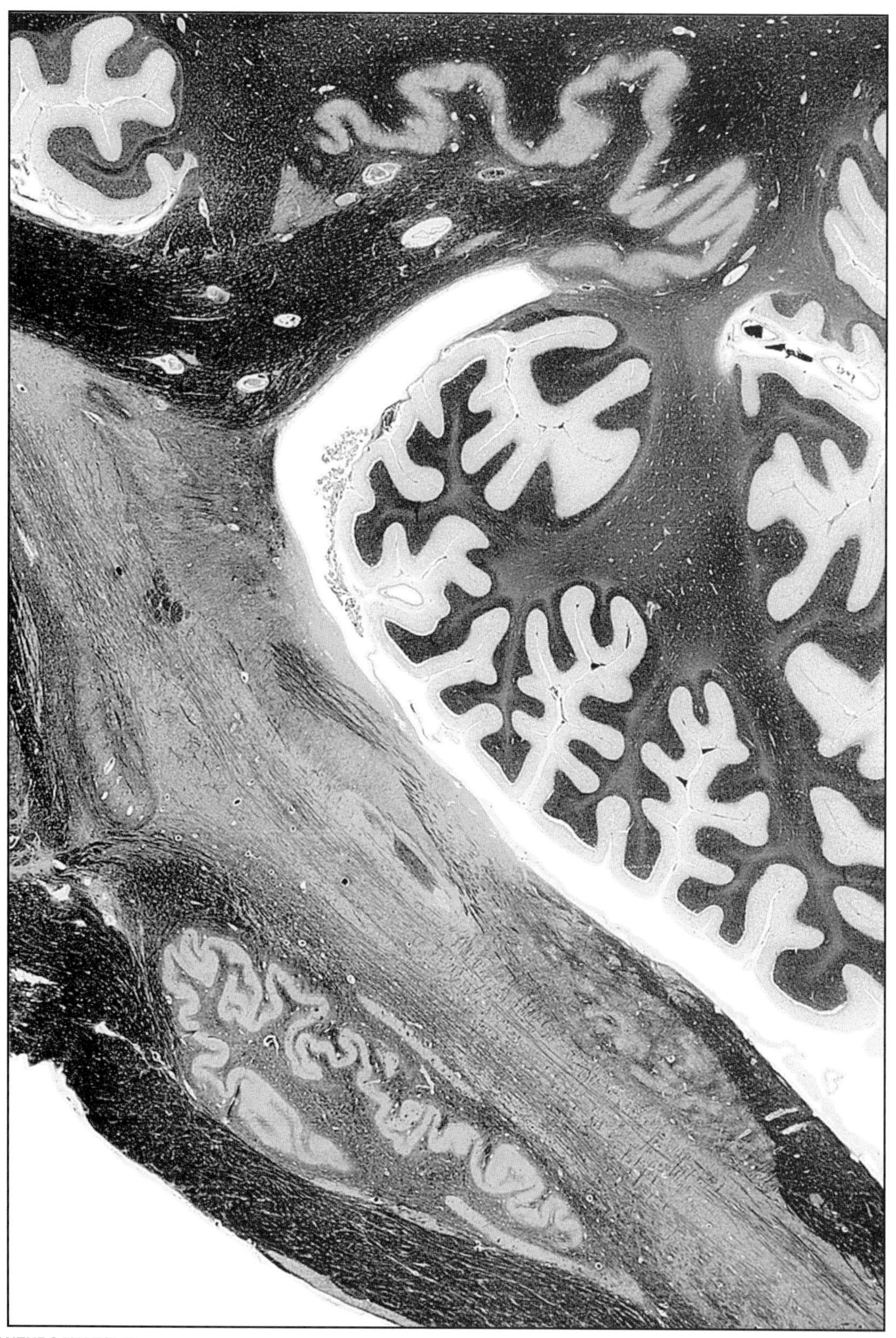

SAGITTAL SECTION: LEVEL OF THE MAMMILLOTHALAMIC TRACT, 15 μ, KLUVER-BARRERA TECHNIQUE

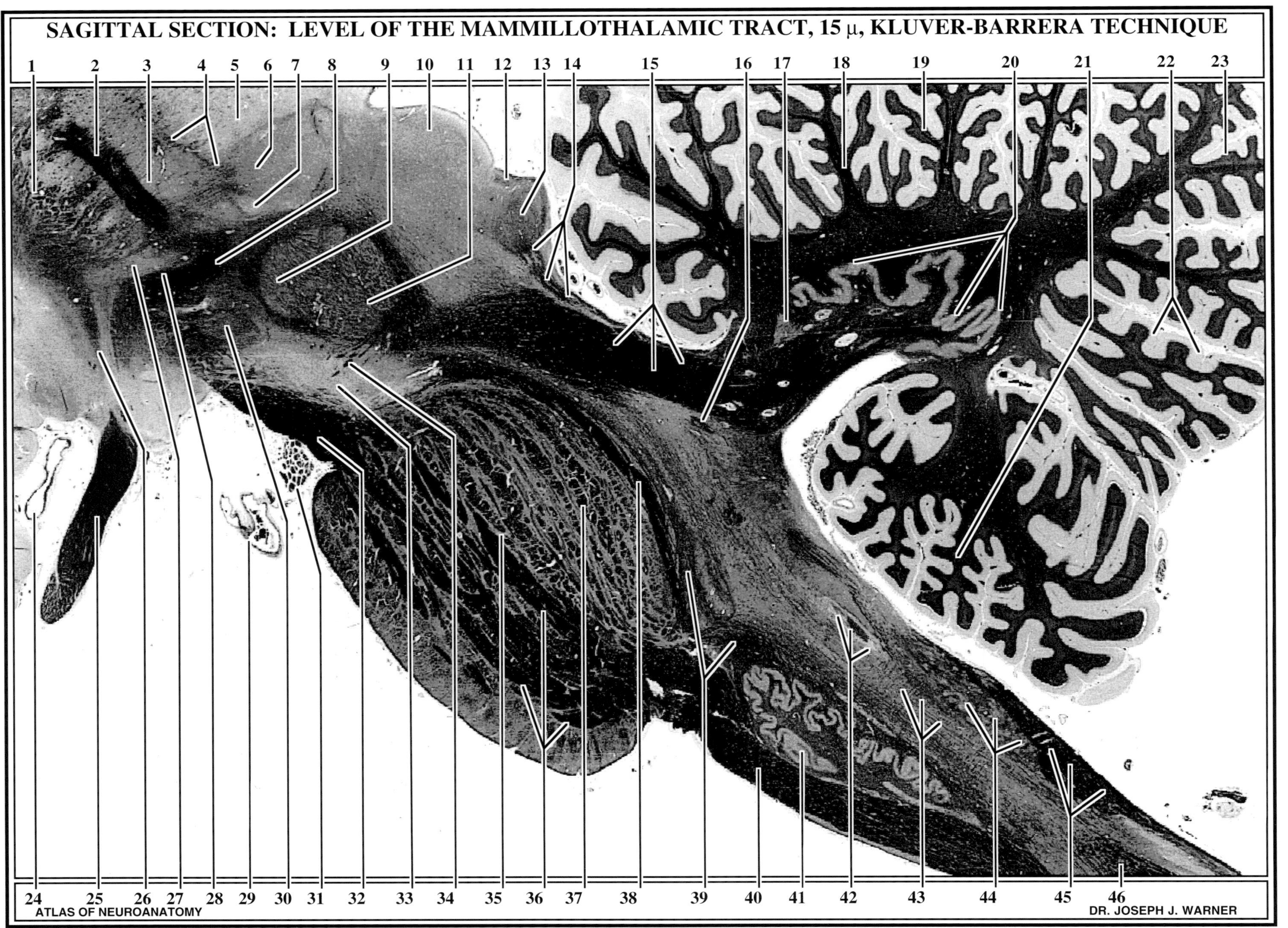

DR. JOSEPH J. WARNER

PARAMEDIAN SAGITTAL SECTION: LEVEL OF THE INTRATHALAMIC COURSE OF THE MAMMILLOTHALAMIC TRACT AND OF THE ROSTRAL TERMINATION OF THE LATERAL LEMNISCUS, 15 μ, KLUVER-BARRERA TECHNIQUE

SAGITTAL PLANE MAPPED ON A HORIZONTAL SECTION THROUGH THE MESENCEPHALIC-DIENCEPHALIC JUNCTION (REFERENCED INTERSECTION STRUCTURES LABELED)

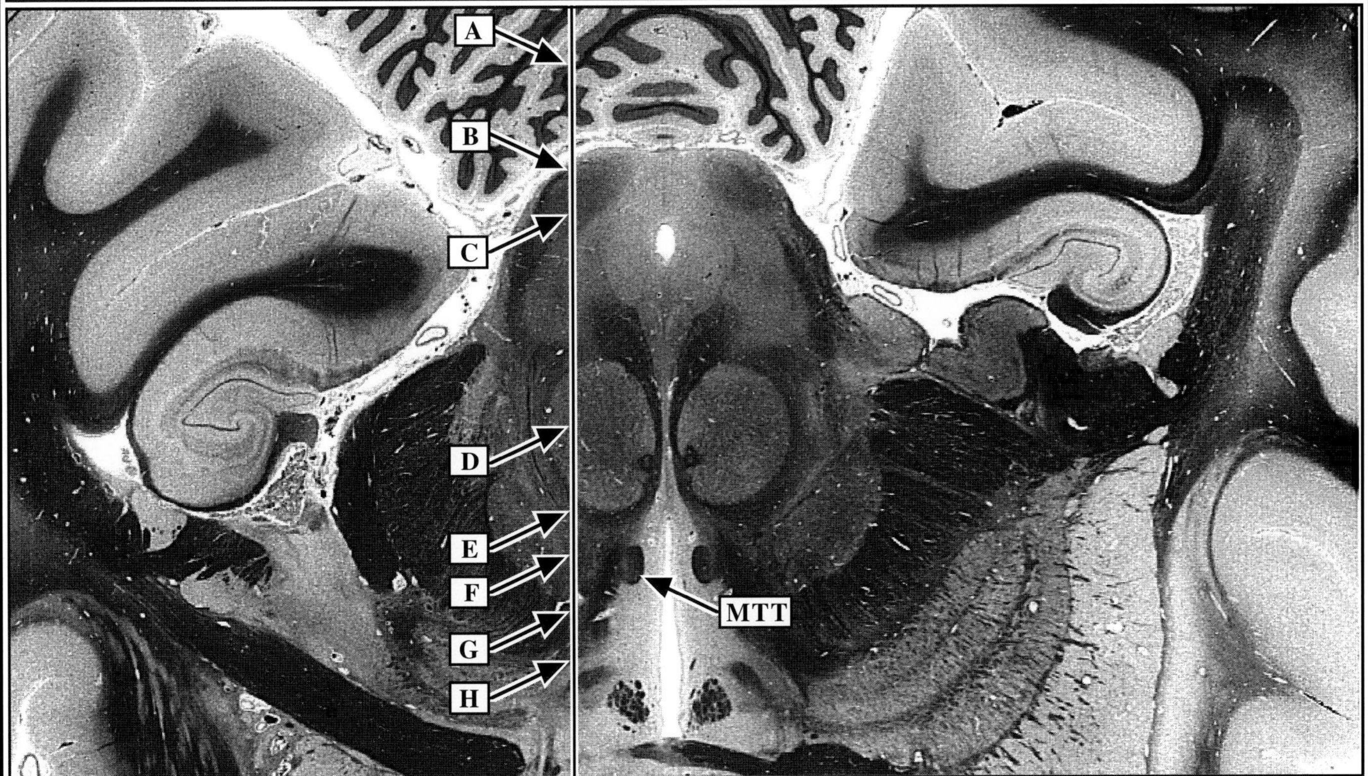

REFERENCED INTERSECTION STRUCTURES

At the level of this horizontal section, the mammillothalamic tract* (MTT) passes medial to the sagittal plane mapped above. As this tract courses dorsally from the mammillary body toward the anterior nucleus of the thalamus, it curves laterally on either side of the third ventricle. Thus, the intrathalamic segment of the mammillothalamic tract passes through the sagittal plane mapped in this figure, whereas the ventral aspect of the tract is distinctly medial to this plane. Note that the mammillothalamic tract courses medial to the Fields of Forel.

A. Anterior Lobe of Cerebellum
B. Rostral Fibers, Lateral Lemniscus
C. Red Nucleus
D. Substantia Nigra
E. Subthalamic Nucleus
F. Medial aspect, Cerebral Peduncle
G, H. Fields of Forel
MTT. Mammillothalamic Tract*

KEY TO NUMBERED STRUCTURES

1. Ventroanterior Nucleus
2. Mammillothalamic Tract
3. Ventrolateral Nucleus
4. Internal Medullary Lamina of the Thalamus
5. Dorsomedial Nucleus
6. Centromedian Nucleus
7. Ventroposteromedial Nucleus
8. Field H of Forel
9. Red Nucleus, rostral aspect
10. Superior Colliculus
11. Red Nucleus, caudal aspect (primary location of Magnocellular component)
12. Brachium of Inferior Colliculus
13. Inferior Colliculus
14. Lateral Lemniscus
15. Superior Cerebellar Peduncle
16. Mesencephalic Root of the Trigeminal Nerve
17. Emboliform Nucleus
18. White Matter of Folium
19. Granule Cell Layer, Cerebellar Cortex
20. Dentate Nucleus
21. Cerebellar Tonsil
22. Molecular layer, Cerebellar Cortex
23. Purkinje Cell Layer, Cerebellar Cortex
24. Anterior Cerebral Artery
25. Optic Chiasm, Tract
26. Inferior Thalamic Peduncle
27. Zona Incerta
28. Lenticular Fasciculus (Field H2)
29. Posterior Cerebral Artery
30. Subthalamic Nucleus
31. Oculomotor Nerve
32. Cerebral Peduncle
33. Substantia Nigra
34. Fascicles of Oculomotor Nerve
35. Pontine Nuclei (Gray)
36. Corticospinal, Corticobulbar Fibers
37. Transverse Pontocerebellar Fibers
38. Medial Lemniscus
39. Central Tegmental Tract
40. Medullary Pyramid
41. Inferior Olivary Nucleus
42. Nucleus and Tractus Solitarius
43. Internal Arcuate Fibers
44. Nucleus Cuneatus
45. Fasciculus Cuneatus
46. Pyramidal Decussation, Corticospinal Tract

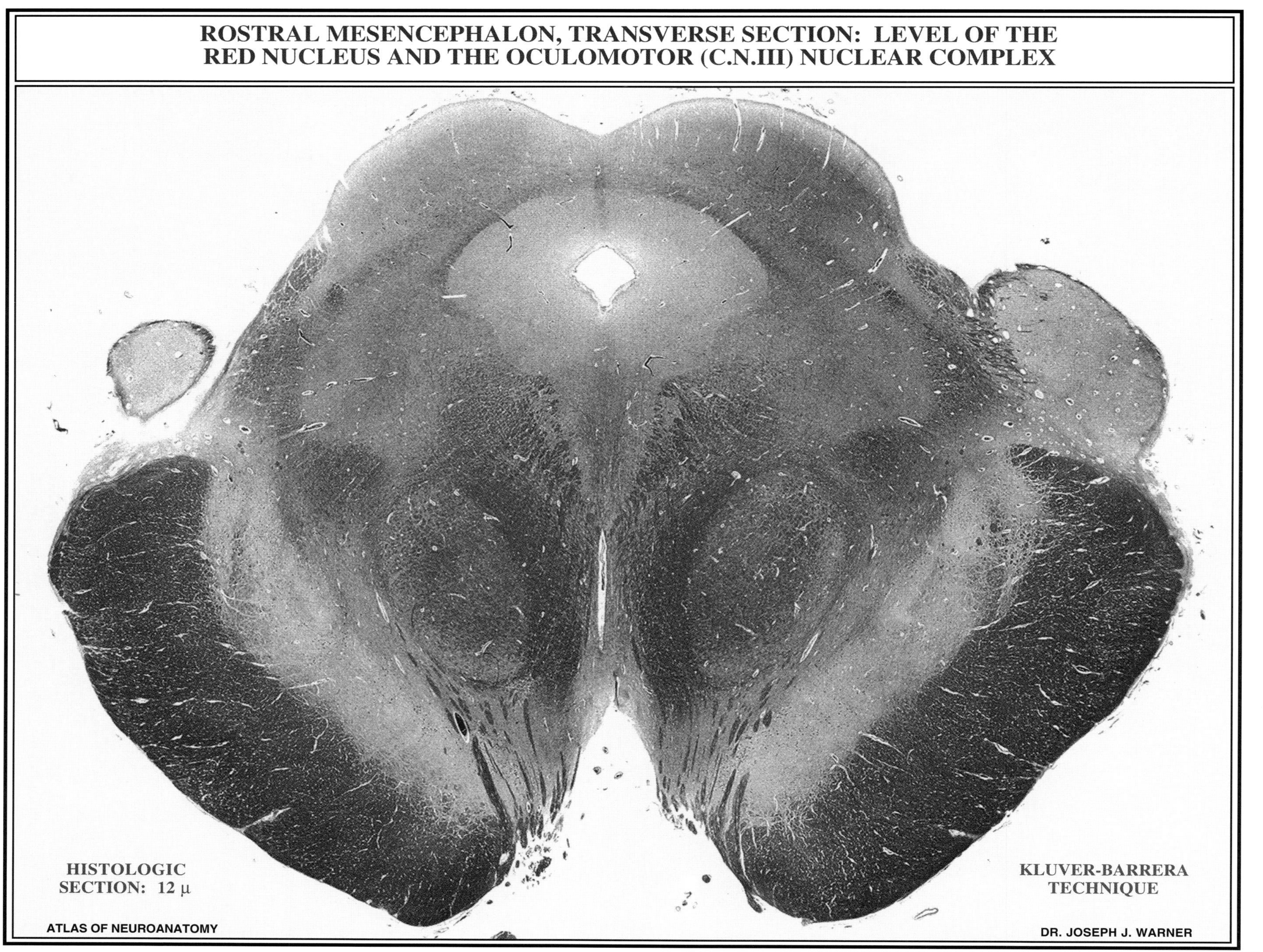
ROSTRAL MESENCEPHALON, TRANSVERSE SECTION: LEVEL OF THE
RED NUCLEUS AND THE OCULOMOTOR (C.N.III) NUCLEAR COMPLEX
HISTOLOGIC
SECTION: 12 μ
KLUVER-BARRERA
TECHNIQUE
ATLAS OF NEUROANATOMY
DR. JOSEPH J. WARNER

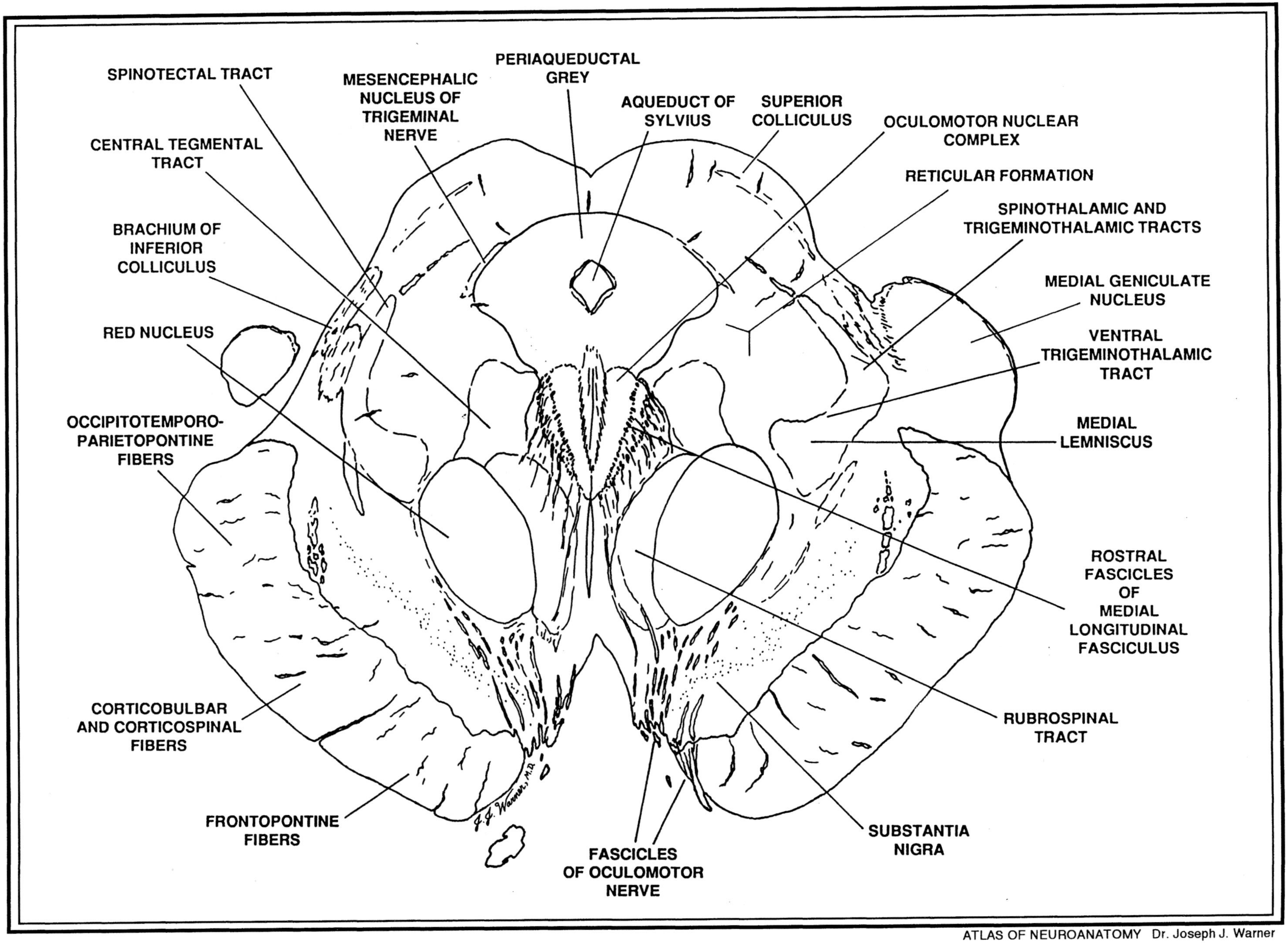

SPINOTECTAL TRACT

MESENCEPHALIC NUCLEUS OF TRIGEMINAL NERVE

PERIAQUEDUCTAL GREY

AQUEDUCT OF SYLVIUS

SUPERIOR COLLICULUS

OCULOMOTOR NUCLEAR COMPLEX

CENTRAL TEGMENTAL TRACT

RETICULAR FORMATION

SPINOTHALAMIC AND TRIGEMINOTHALAMIC TRACTS

BRACHIUM OF INFERIOR COLLICULUS

MEDIAL GENICULATE NUCLEUS

RED NUCLEUS

VENTRAL TRIGEMINOTHALAMIC TRACT

OCCIPITOTEMPORO-PARIETOPONTINE FIBERS

MEDIAL LEMNISCUS

ROSTRAL FASCICLES OF MEDIAL LONGITUDINAL FASCICULUS

CORTICOBULBAR AND CORTICOSPINAL FIBERS

RUBROSPINAL TRACT

FRONTOPONTINE FIBERS

J.J. Warner, M.D.

SUBSTANTIA NIGRA

FASCICLES OF OCULOMOTOR NERVE

CAUDAL MESENCEPHALON, TRANSVERSE SECTION: LEVEL OF THE INFERIOR COLLICULUS AND THE DECUSSATION OF THE SUPERIOR CEREBELLAR PEDUNCLES

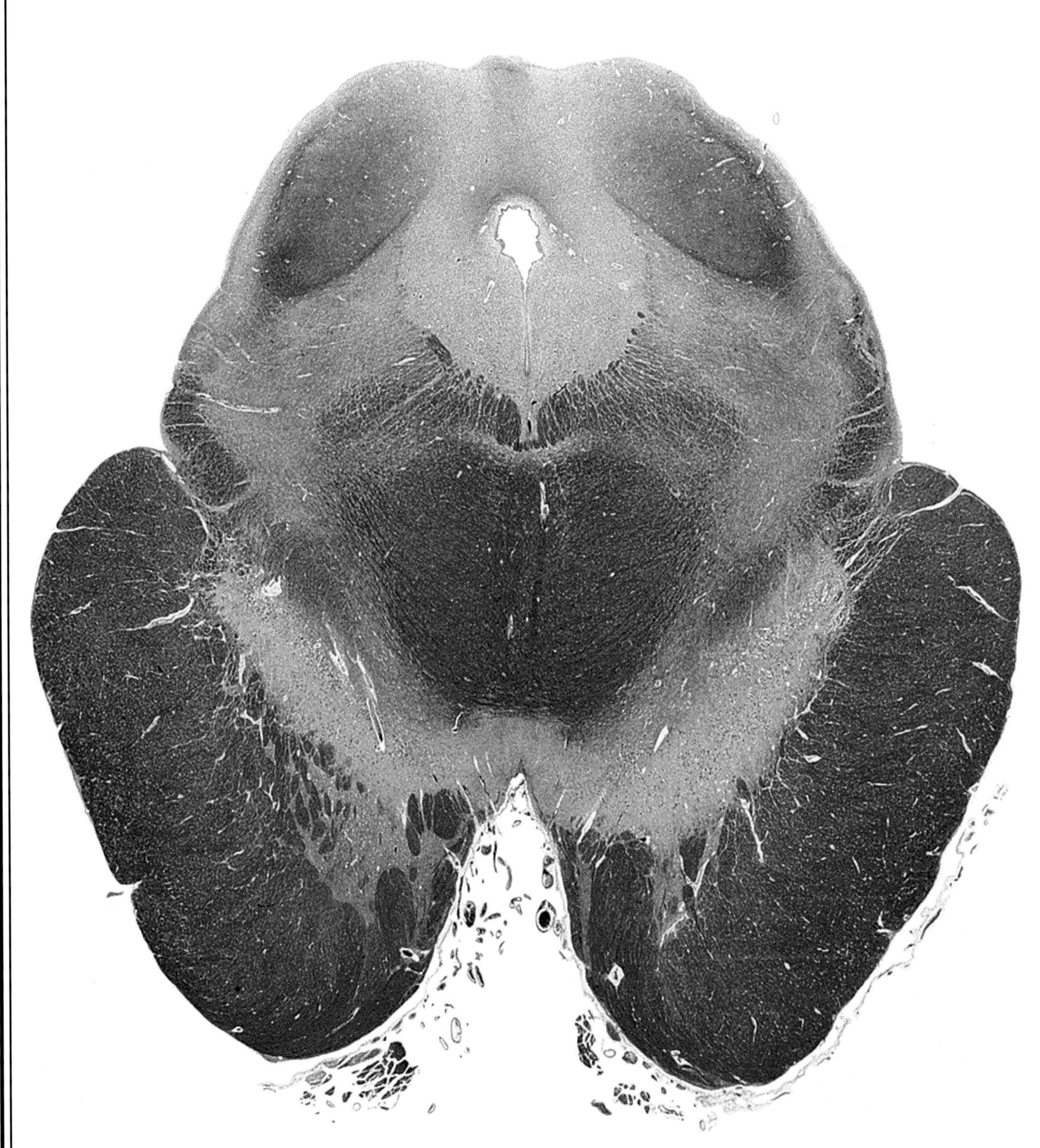

SECTION 12 μ, KLUVER-BARRERA TECHNIQUE

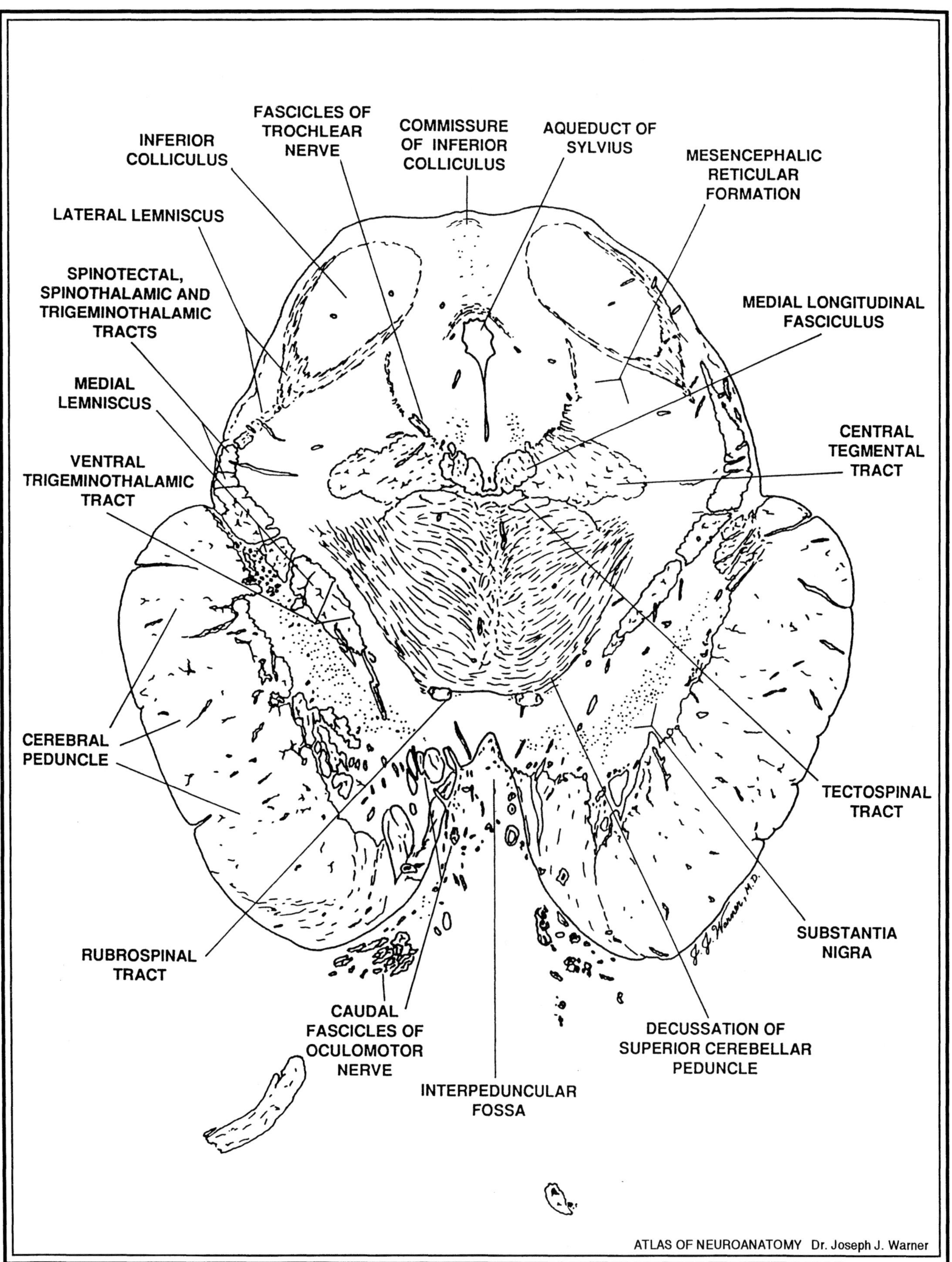

INFERIOR COLLICULUS
FASCICLES OF TROCHLEAR NERVE
COMMISSURE OF INFERIOR COLLICULUS
AQUEDUCT OF SYLVIUS
MESENCEPHALIC RETICULAR FORMATION
LATERAL LEMNISCUS
SPINOTECTAL, SPINOTHALAMIC AND TRIGEMINOTHALAMIC TRACTS
MEDIAL LONGITUDINAL FASCICULUS
MEDIAL LEMNISCUS
CENTRAL TEGMENTAL TRACT
VENTRAL TRIGEMINOTHALAMIC TRACT
CEREBRAL PEDUNCLE
TECTOSPINAL TRACT
SUBSTANTIA NIGRA
RUBROSPINAL TRACT
CAUDAL FASCICLES OF OCULOMOTOR NERVE
DECUSSATION OF SUPERIOR CEREBELLAR PEDUNCLE
INTERPEDUNCULAR FOSSA
J. J. Warner, M.D.

MESENCEPHALON, TRANSVERSE SECTION: LEVEL OF THE TROCHLEAR (IV) NUCLEUS AND THE DECUSSATION OF THE SUPERIOR CEREBELLAR PEDUNCLES

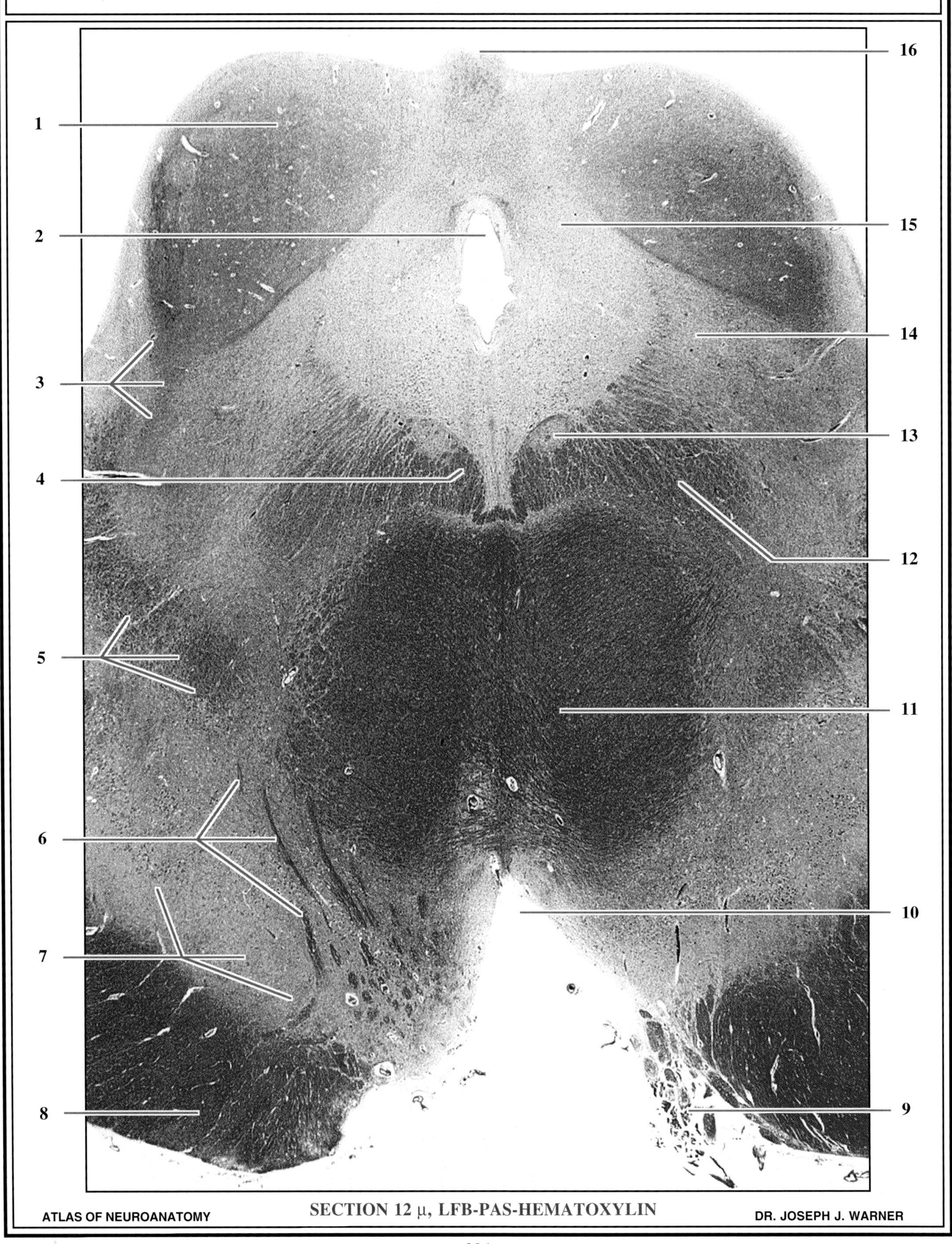

SECTION 12 μ, LFB-PAS-HEMATOXYLIN

MESENCEPHALON, TRANSVERSE SECTION: LEVEL OF THE TROCHLEAR (IV) NUCLEUS AND THE DECUSSATION OF THE SUPERIOR CEREBELLAR PEDUNCLES: SECTION ORIENTATION AND KEY TO NUMBERED STRUCTURES

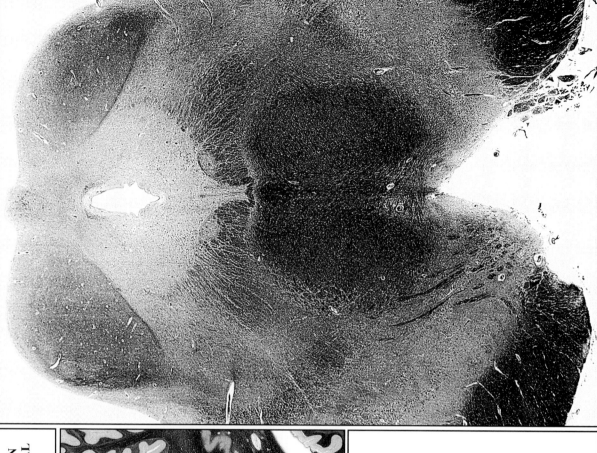

SECTION PLANE MAPPED ON A SAGITTAL HISTOLOGIC SECTION THROUGH THE SUPERIOR CEREBELLAR PEDUNCLE AND ROSTRAL TERMINATION OF THE LATERAL LEMNISCUS

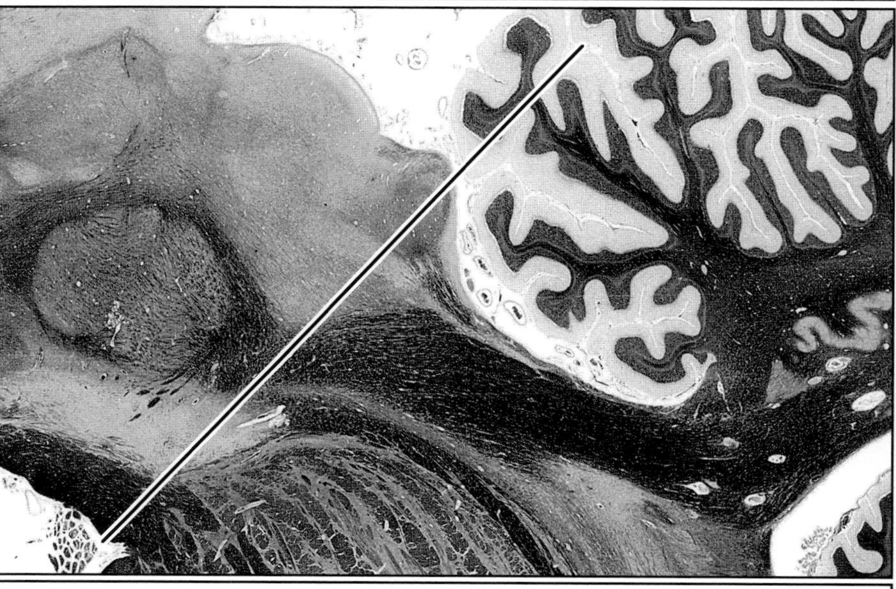

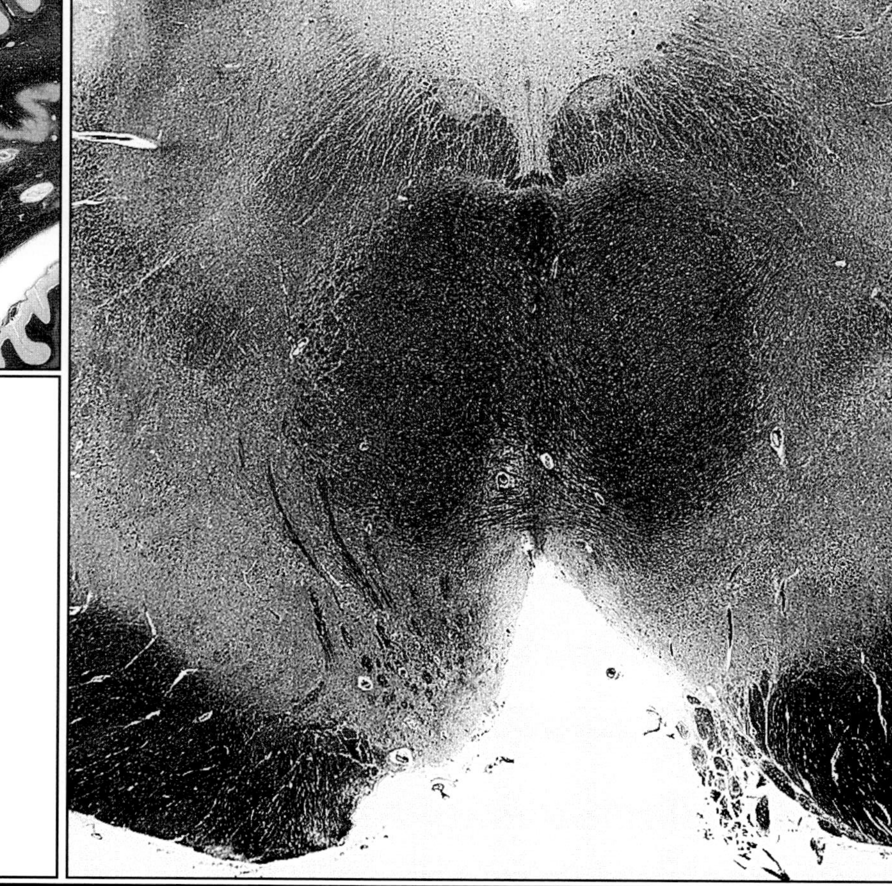

1. Inferior Colliculus
2. Aqueduct of Sylvius
3. Lateral Lemniscus (termination)
4. Medial Longitudinal Fasciculus
5. Medial Lemniscus
6. Fascicles of the Oculomotor (III) Nerve
7. Substantia Nigra
8. Cerebral Peduncle
9. Fascicles of the Oculomotor (III) Nerve
10. Interpeduncular Fossa
11. Decussation of the Superior Cerebellar Peduncle
12. Central Tegmental Tract
13. Trochlear (IV) Nucleus
14. Mesencephalic Trigeminal Nucleus
15. Periaqueductal Gray
16. Frenulum

CAUDAL MESENCEPHALON: GROSS TRANSVERSE SECTION DEMONSTRATING THE TROCHLEAR (IV) NERVES

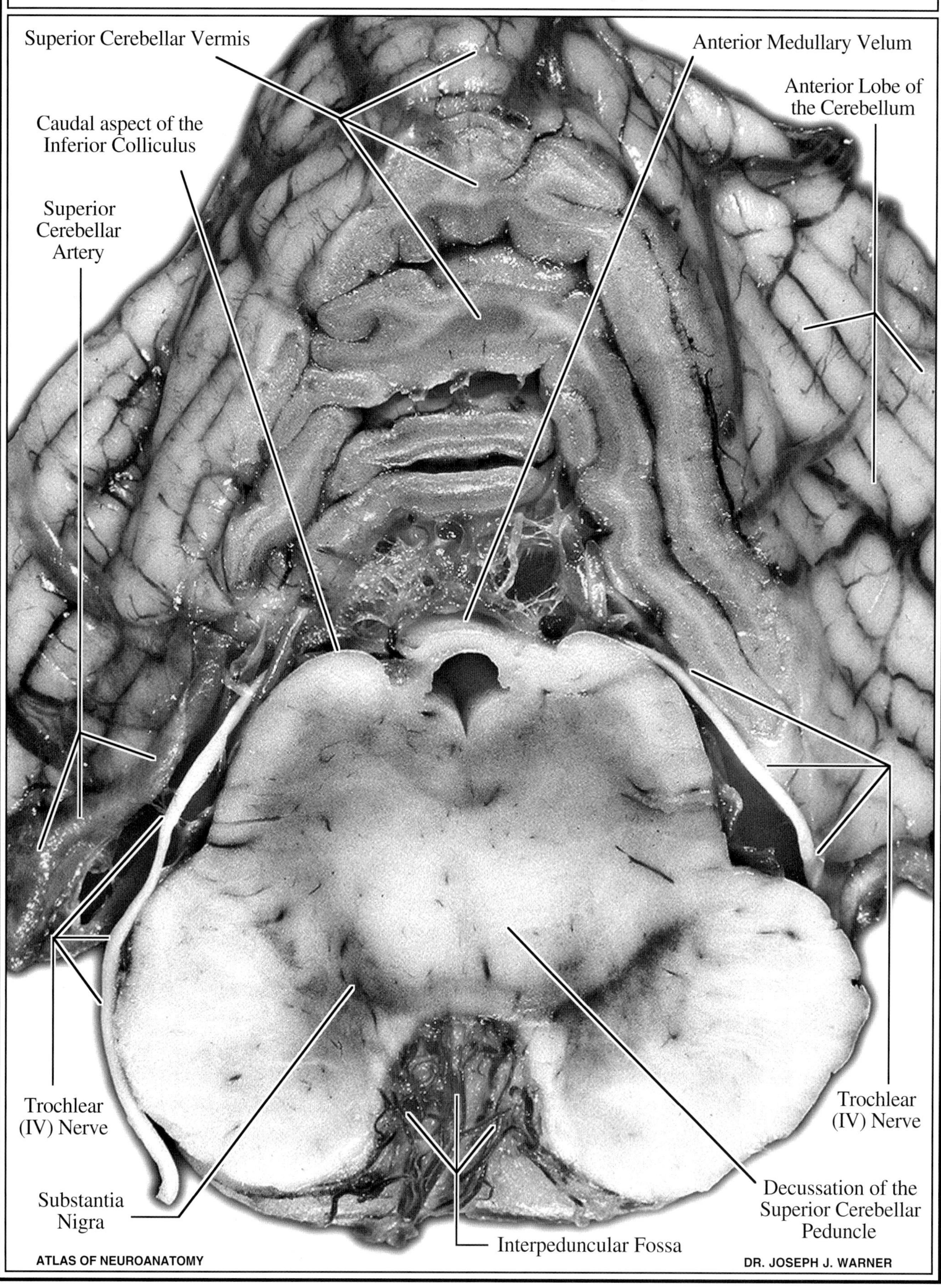

HORIZONTAL SECTION OF THE PONTOMESENCEPHALIC JUNCTION: COLOR INFRARED PHOTOGRAPH OF TISSUE PROCESSED WITH LONG TERM CUPRIC ACETATE - ACETIC ACID - FORMALIN PROTOCOL (WARNER)

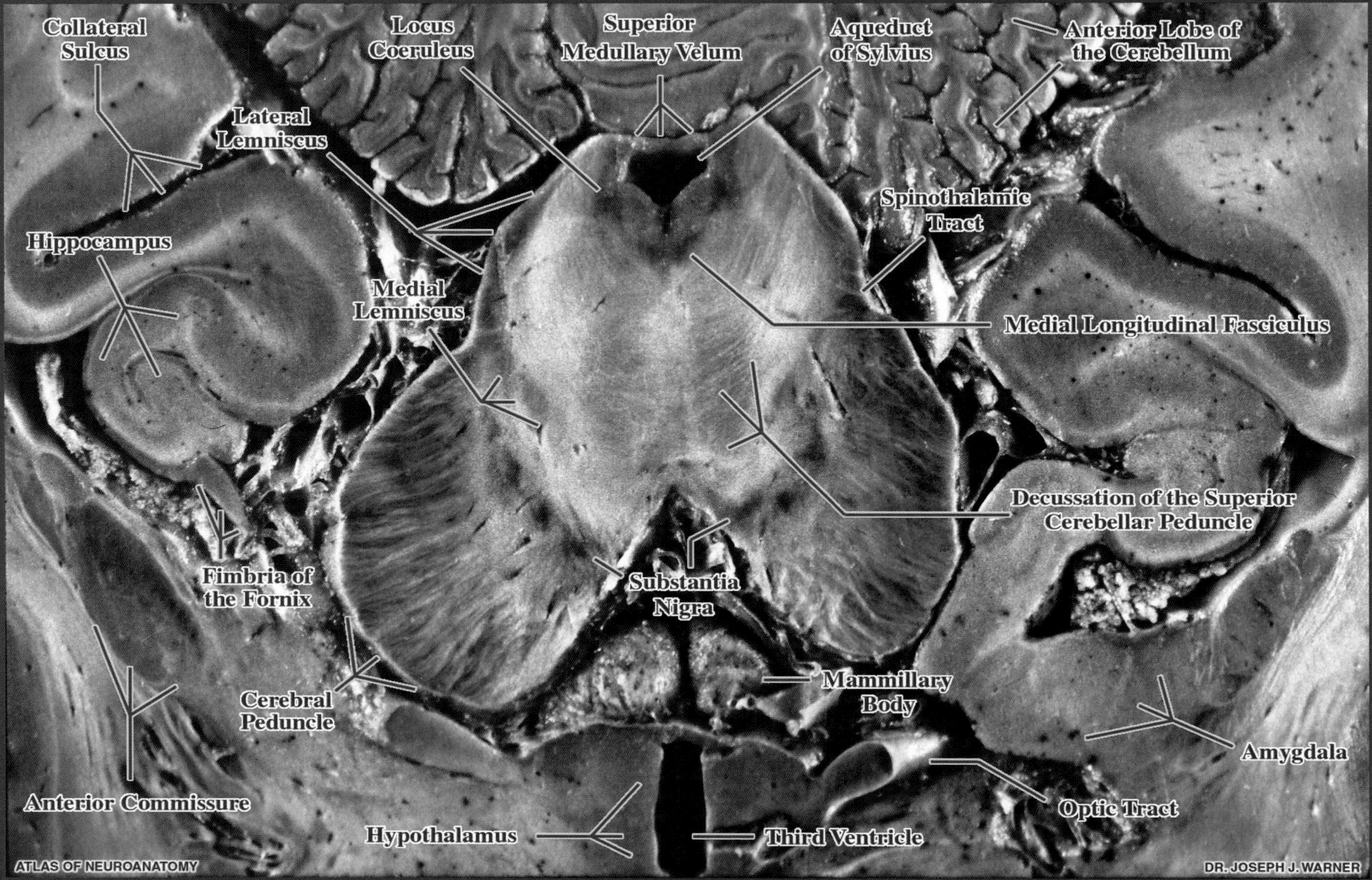

Collateral Sulcus
Locus Coeruleus
Superior Medullary Velum
Aqueduct of Sylvius
Anterior Lobe of the Cerebellum
Lateral Lemniscus
Spinothalamic Tract
Hippocampus
Medial Lemniscus
Medial Longitudinal Fasciculus
Decussation of the Superior Cerebellar Peduncle
Fimbria of the Fornix
Substantia Nigra
Cerebral Peduncle
Mammillary Body
Amygdala
Anterior Commissure
Optic Tract
Hypothalamus
Third Ventricle
ATLAS OF NEUROANATOMY
DR. JOSEPH J. WARNER

ROSTRAL PONS, TRANSVERSE SECTION: LEVEL OF THE CAUDAL ASPECT OF THE DECUSSATION OF THE SUPERIOR CEREBELLAR PEDUNCLES

HISTOLOGIC SECTION: 12 μ

LFB - PAS- HEMATOXYLIN

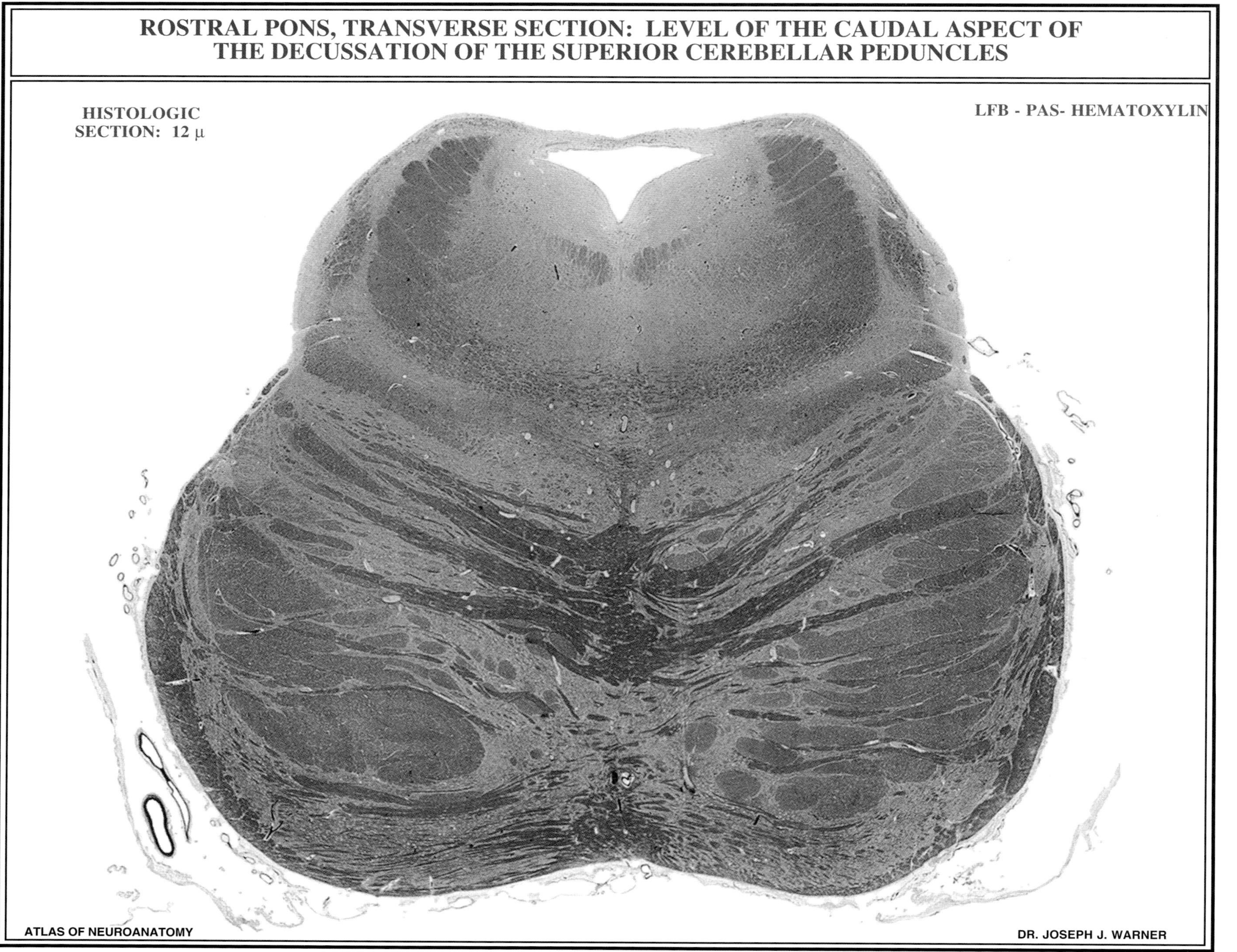

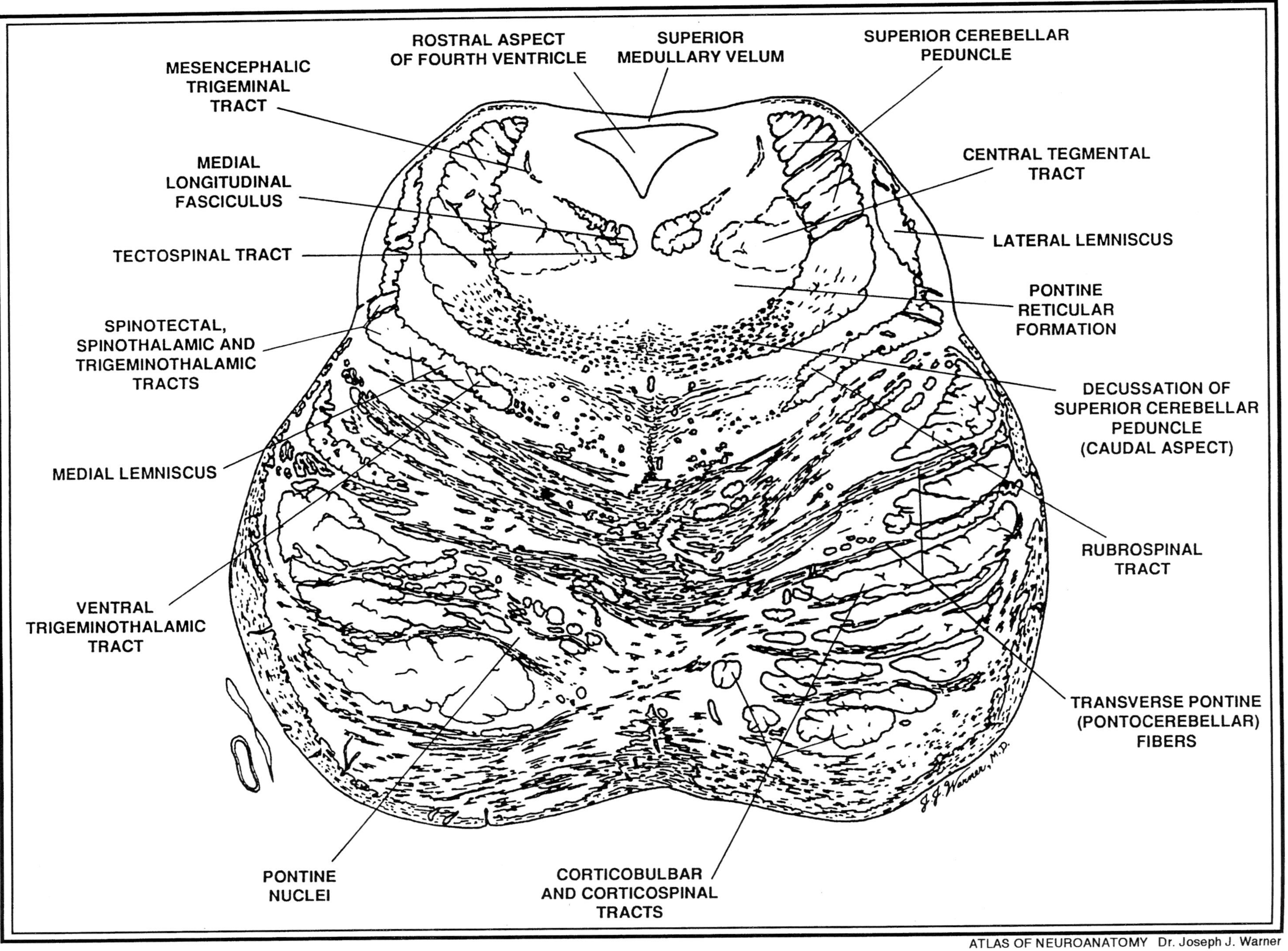
MESENCEPHALIC TRIGEMINAL TRACT
ROSTRAL ASPECT OF FOURTH VENTRICLE
SUPERIOR MEDULLARY VELUM
SUPERIOR CEREBELLAR PEDUNCLE
MEDIAL LONGITUDINAL FASCICULUS
CENTRAL TEGMENTAL TRACT
TECTOSPINAL TRACT
LATERAL LEMNISCUS
PONTINE RETICULAR FORMATION
SPINOTECTAL, SPINOTHALAMIC AND TRIGEMINOTHALAMIC TRACTS
DECUSSATION OF SUPERIOR CEREBELLAR PEDUNCLE (CAUDAL ASPECT)
MEDIAL LEMNISCUS
RUBROSPINAL TRACT
VENTRAL TRIGEMINOTHALAMIC TRACT
TRANSVERSE PONTINE (PONTOCEREBELLAR) FIBERS
PONTINE NUCLEI
CORTICOBULBAR AND CORTICOSPINAL TRACTS

ROSTRAL PONS, TRANSVERSE SECTION: LEVEL INCLUDING THE LOCUS COERULEUS

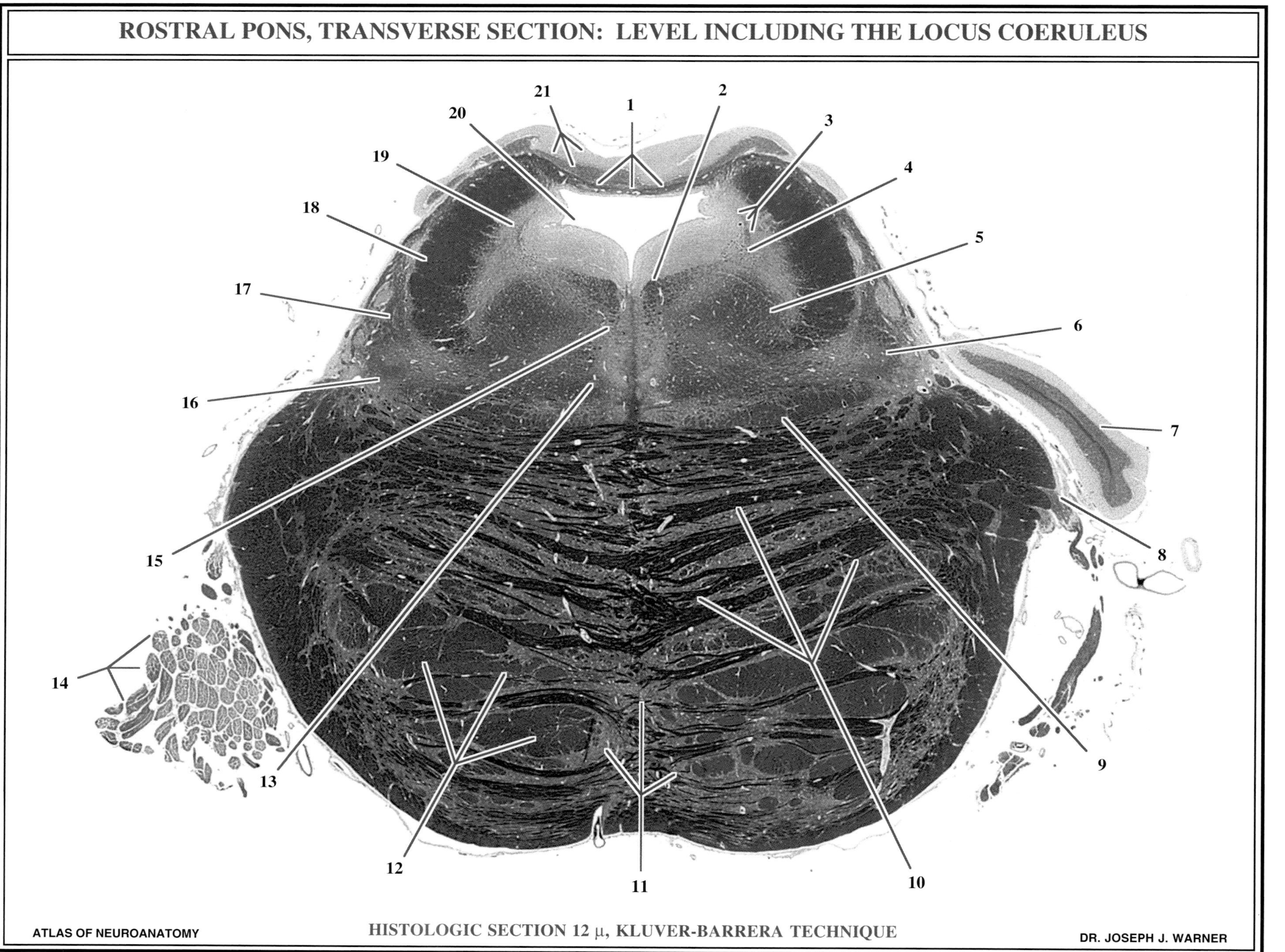

HISTOLOGIC SECTION 12 μ, KLUVER-BARRERA TECHNIQUE

DR. JOSEPH J. WARNER

ROSTRAL PONS, TRANSVERSE SECTION; LEVEL INCLUDING THE LOCUS COERULEUS: SECTION ORIENTATION AND KEY TO NUMBERED STRUCTURES

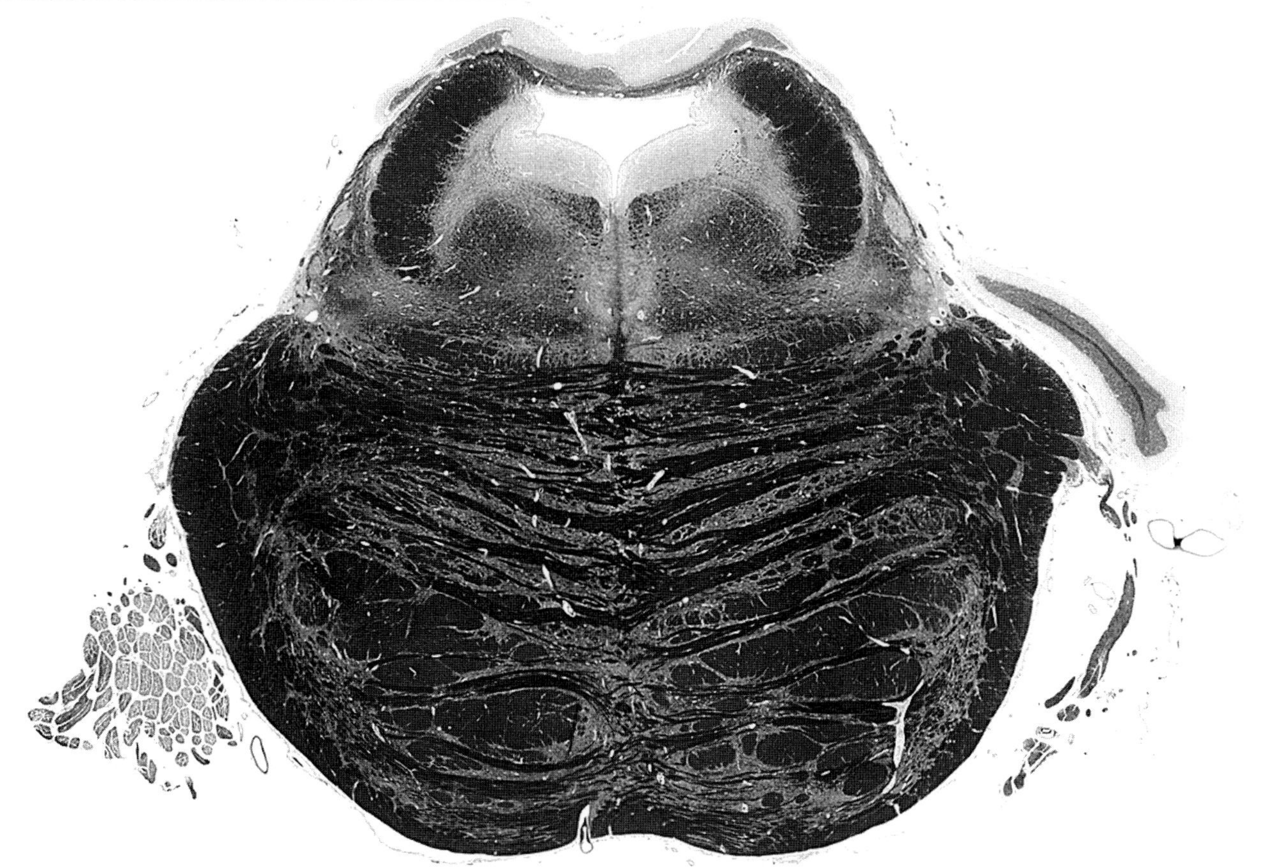

1. Superior (Anterior) Medullary Velum
2. Medial Longitudinal Fasciculus
3. Mesencephalic Tract of the Trigeminal Nerve
4. Locus Coeruleus
5. Central Tegmental Tract
6. Chief Sensory Nucleus of the Trigeminal Nerve (rostral extent)
7. Folium of Anterior Lobe of the Cerebellum
8. Fascicles of the Trigeminal Nerve (V)
9. Medial Lemniscus and the Ventral Trigeminothalamic Tract
10. Transverse Pontocerebellar Fibers
11. Pontine Nuclei
12. Corticobulbar and Corticospinal Fibers
13. Rubrospinal Tract
14. Trigeminal Nerve (V)
15. Tectospinal Tract
16. Spinothalamic and Ventral Trigeminothalamic Tracts
17. Lateral Lemniscus
18. Superior Cerebellar Peduncle
19. Mesencephalic Trigeminal Nucleus
20. Fourth Ventricle
21. Lingula of the Cerebellum

PLANE OF SECTION MAPPED IN REFERENCE TO A PARAMEDIAN SAGITTAL SECTION INCLUDING THE SUPERIOR CEREBELLAR PEDUNCLE

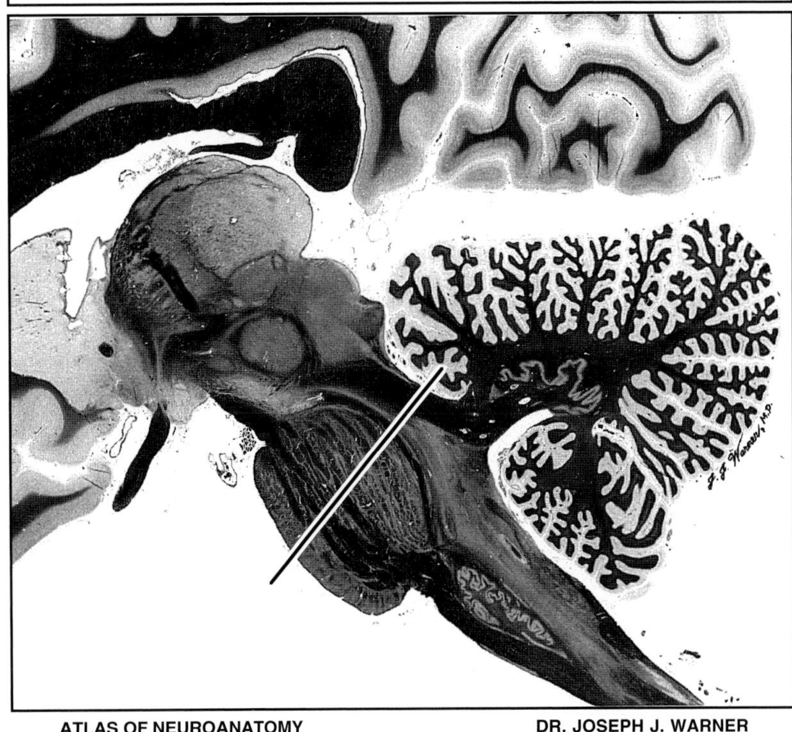

DORSOLATERAL PONS, TRANSVERSE SECTION: MAGNIFIED VIEW DEMONSTRATING THE LOCUS COERULEUS AND THE MESENCEPHALIC TRIGEMINAL TRACT AND NUCLEUS

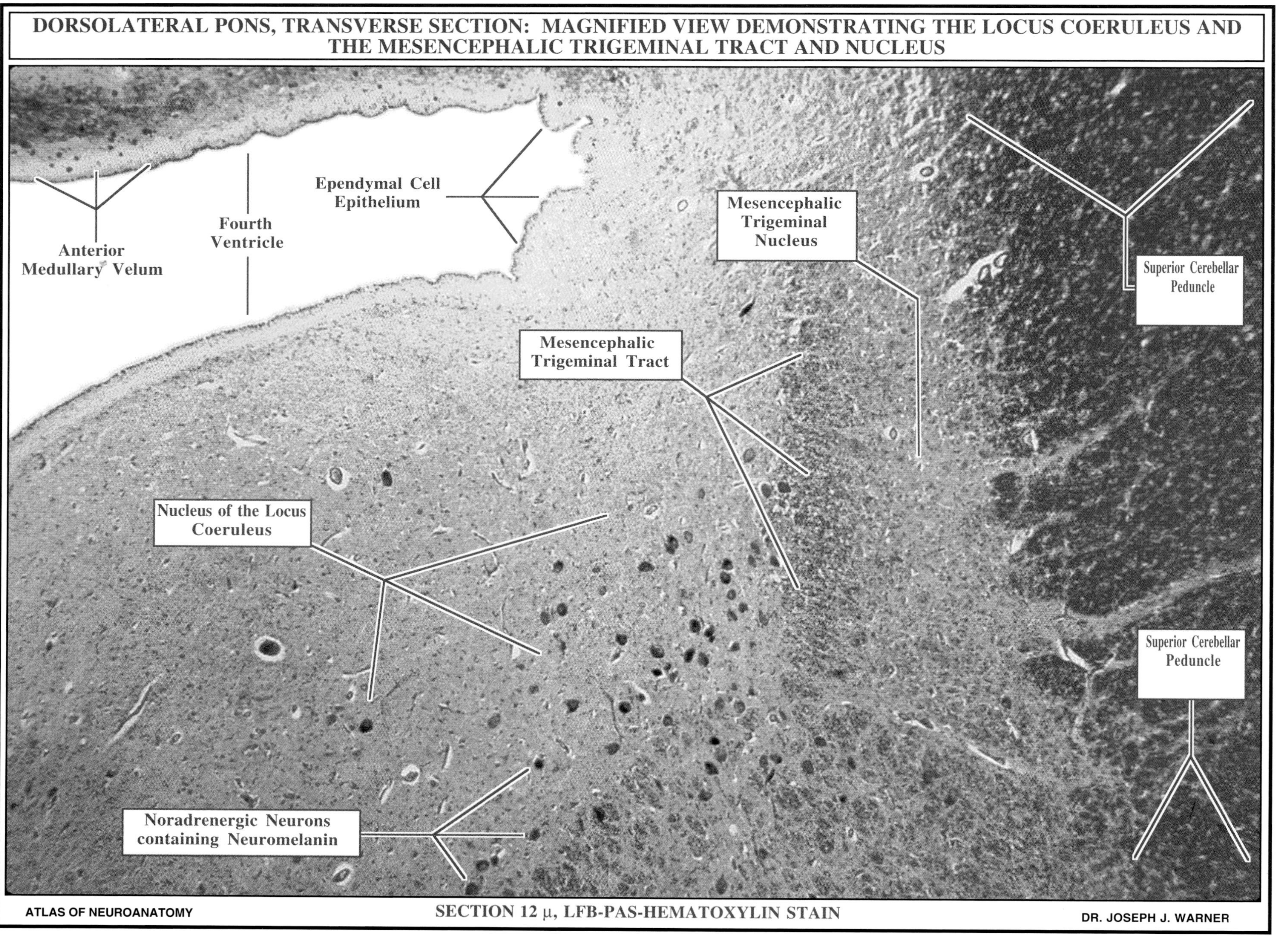

SECTION 12 μ, LFB-PAS-HEMATOXYLIN STAIN

TRANSVERSE SECTION OF THE PONS AND CEREBELLUM: LEVEL INCLUDING THE SUPERIOR AND MIDDLE CEREBELLAR PEDUNCLES AND THE TRIGEMINAL NERVES

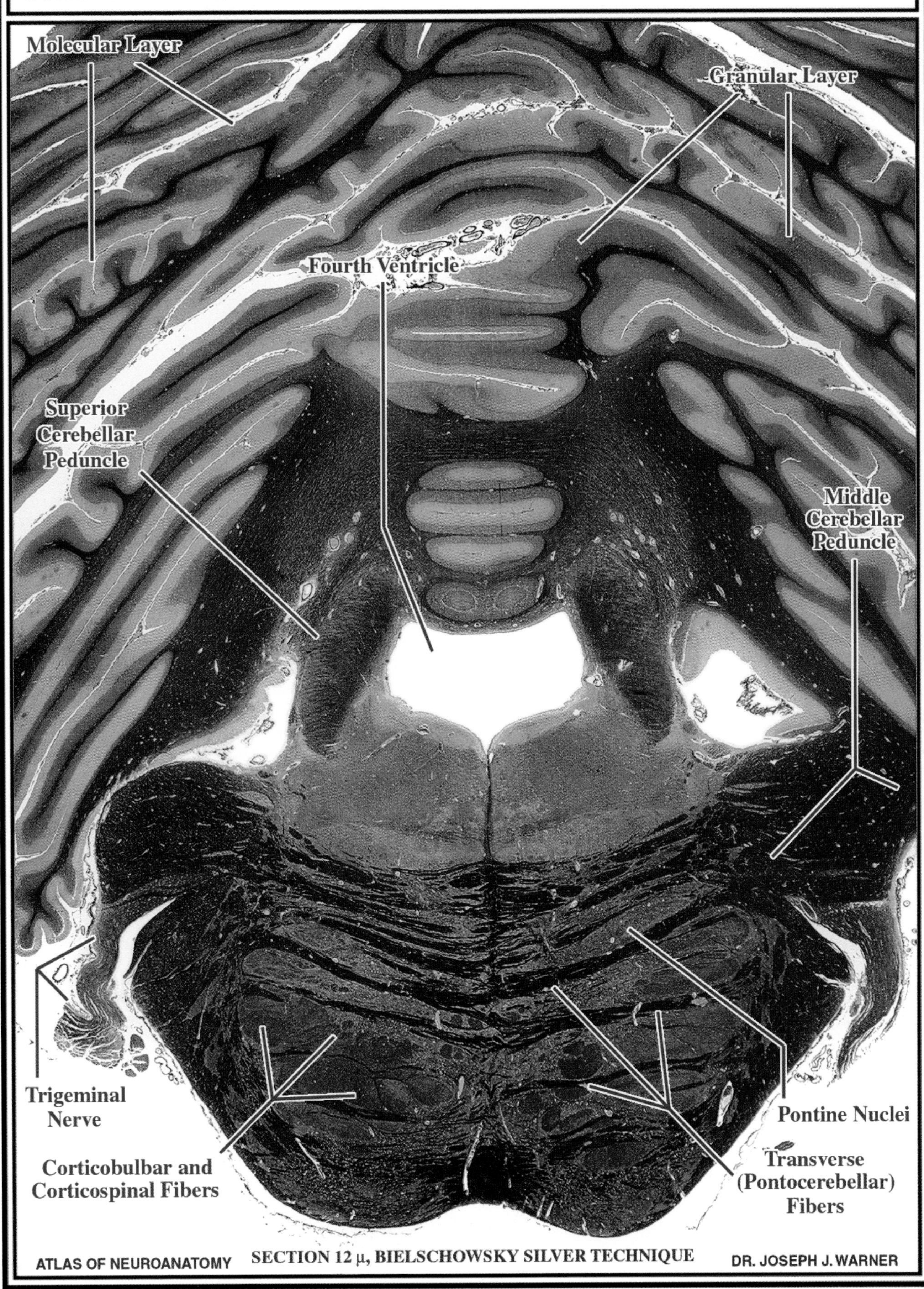

ATLAS OF NEUROANATOMY SECTION 12 μ, BIELSCHOWSKY SILVER TECHNIQUE DR. JOSEPH J. WARNER

SAGITTAL SECTION OF THE ROSTRAL PONS, CEREBELLUM, AND THE MESENCEPHALIC-DIENCEPHALIC JUNCTION: PARASAGITTAL PLANE INCLUDING THE SUPERIOR CEREBELLAR PEDUNCLE AND THE TERMINATION OF THE LATERAL LEMNISCUS AT THE INFERIOR COLLICULUS

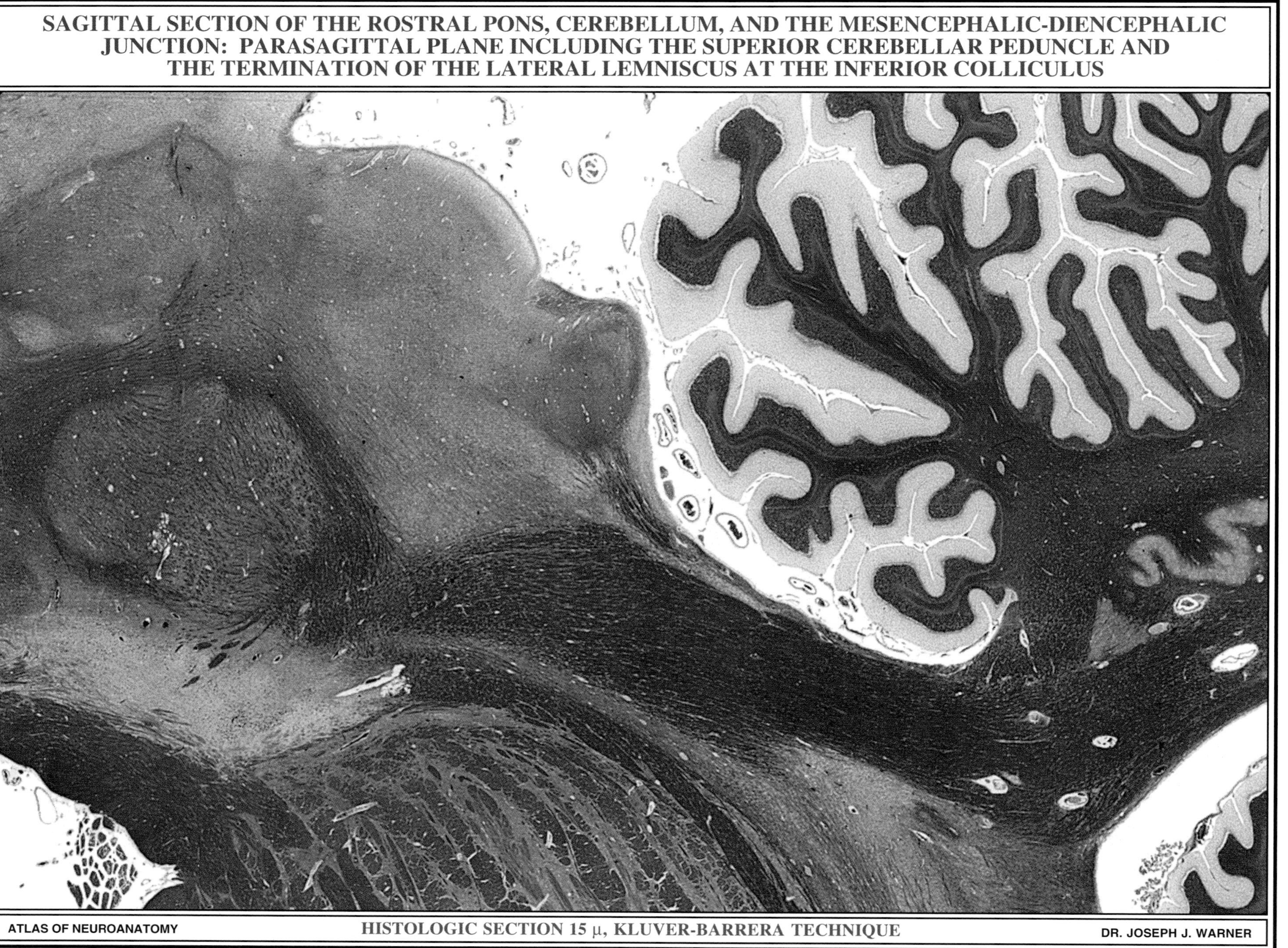

HISTOLOGIC SECTION 15 μ, KLUVER-BARRERA TECHNIQUE

DR. JOSEPH J. WARNER

SAGITTAL SECTION OF THE ROSTRAL PONS, CEREBELLUM, AND THE MESENCEPHALIC-DIENCEPHALIC JUNCTION: PARASAGITTAL PLANE INCLUDING THE SUPERIOR CEREBELLAR PEDUNCLE AND THE TERMINATION OF THE LATERAL LEMNISCUS AT THE INFERIOR COLLICULUS

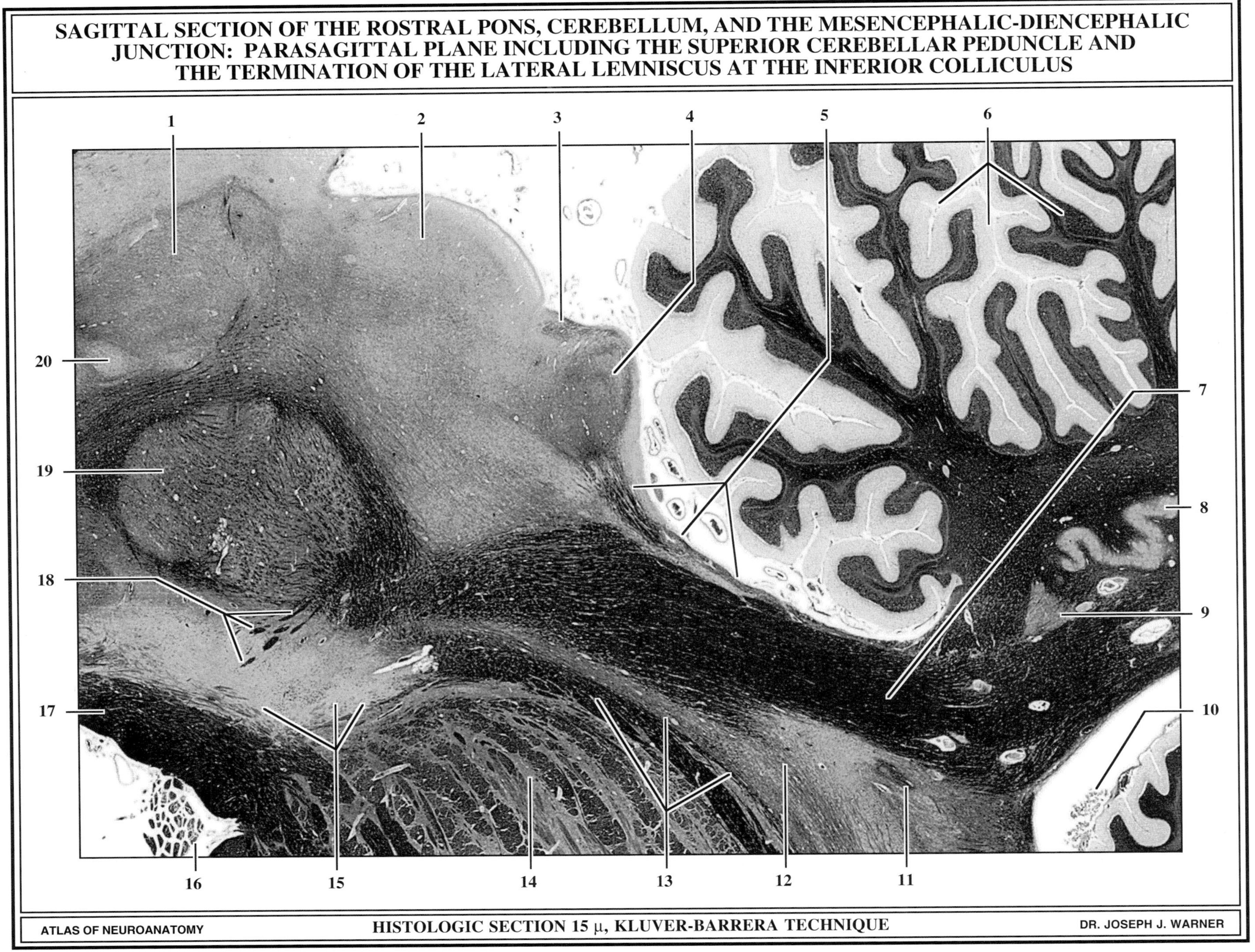

ATLAS OF NEUROANATOMY

HISTOLOGIC SECTION 15 μ, KLUVER-BARRERA TECHNIQUE

DR. JOSEPH J. WARNER

SAGITTAL SECTION OF THE ROSTRAL PONS, CEREBELLUM, AND THE MESENCEPHALIC-DIENCEPHALIC JUNCTION; MAGNIFIED VIEW INCLUDING THE SUPERIOR CEREBELLAR PEDUNCLE AND THE TERMINATION OF THE LATERAL LEMNISCUS AT THE INFERIOR COLLICULUS: SECTION ORIENTATION AND KEY TO NUMBERED STRUCTURES

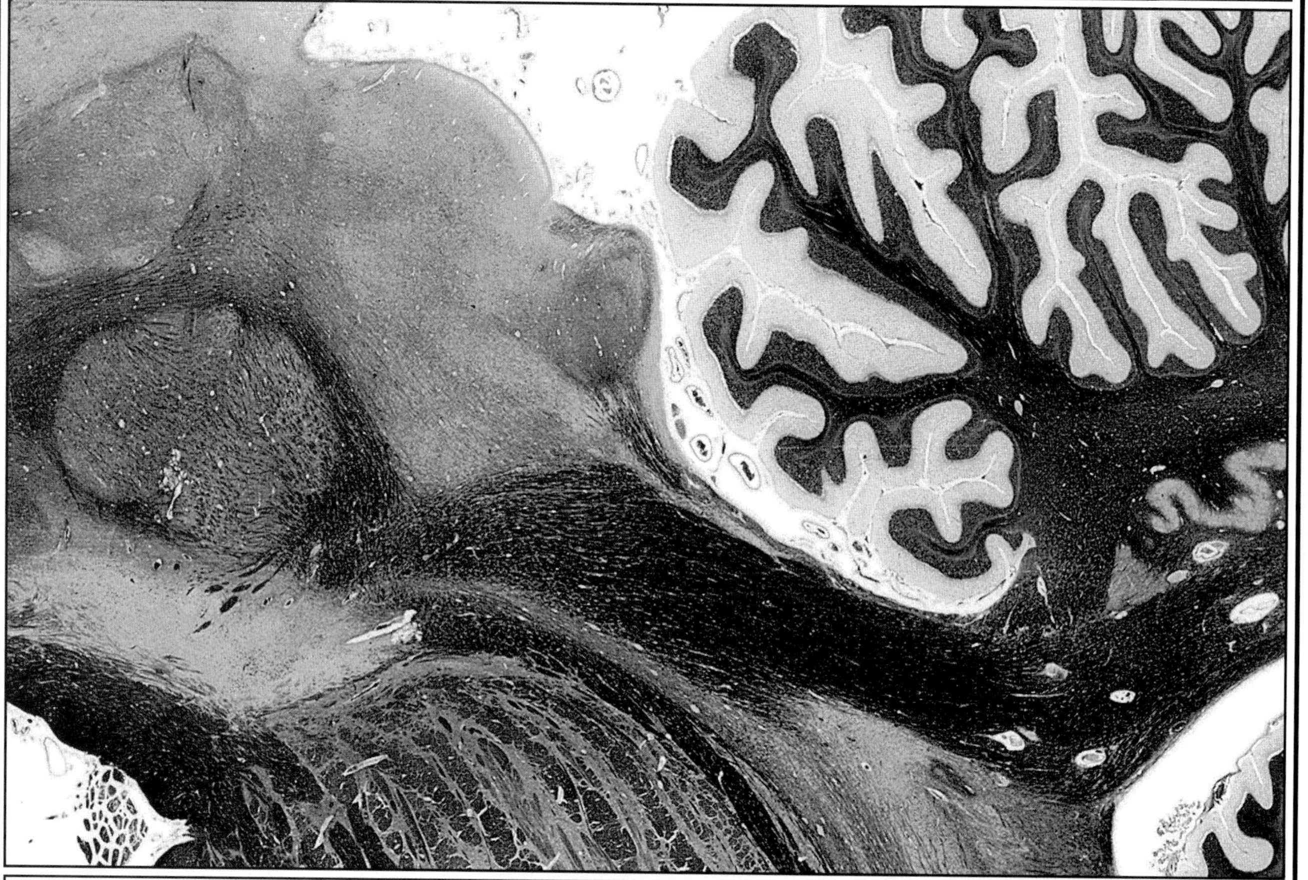

KEY TO NUMBERED STRUCTURES

1. Centromedian Nucleus of the Thalamus
2. Superior Colliculus
3. Brachium of the Inferior Colliculus
4. Inferior Colliculus
5. Lateral Lemniscus
6. Anterior Lobe of the Cerebellum
7. Superior Cerebellar Peduncle
8. Dentate Nucleus of the Cerebellum
9. Emboliform Nucleus of the Cerebellum
10. Choroid Plexus
11. Mesencephalic Tract of the Trigeminal Nerve
12. Central Tegmental Tract
13. Medial Lemniscus
14. Pontine Nuclei
15. Substantia Nigra
16. Oculomotor (III) Nerve
17. Cerebral Peduncle
18. Fascicles of the Oculomotor (III) Nerve
19. Red Nucleus
20. Ventroposteromedial Nucleus of the Thalamus

AREA OF MAGNIFIED VIEW OUTLINED ON THE COMPLETE PARAMEDIAN SAGITTAL SECTION

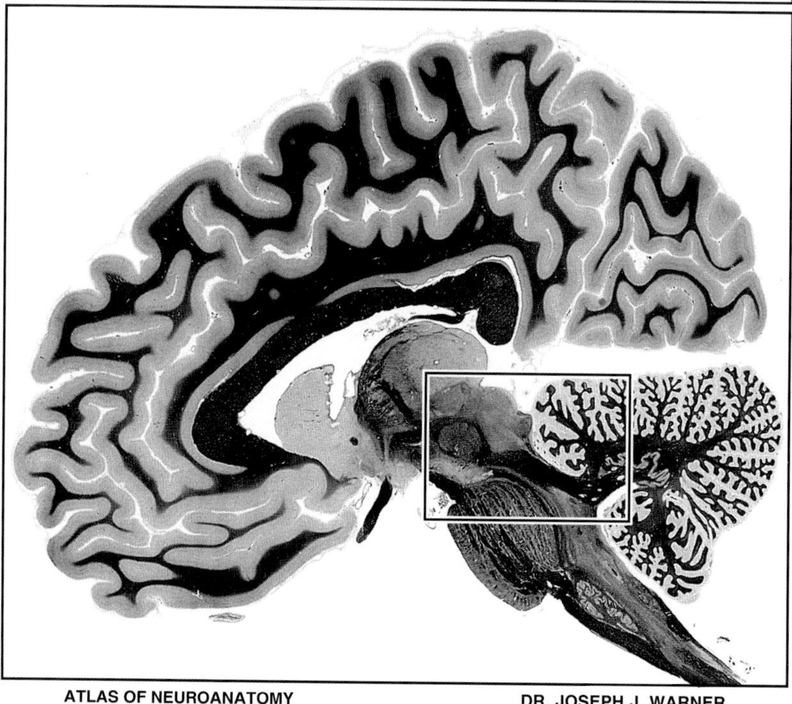

CEREBELLUM, TRANSVERSE PLANE OF SECTION THROUGH THE PONS, LEVEL OF THE MIDDLE CEREBELLAR PEDUNCLES; MAGNIFIED VIEW INCLUDING THE DENTATE NUCLEI, NODULUS, AND THE ROOF OF THE FOURTH VENTRICLE: SECTION 15 μ, KLUVER-BARRERA TECHNIQUE

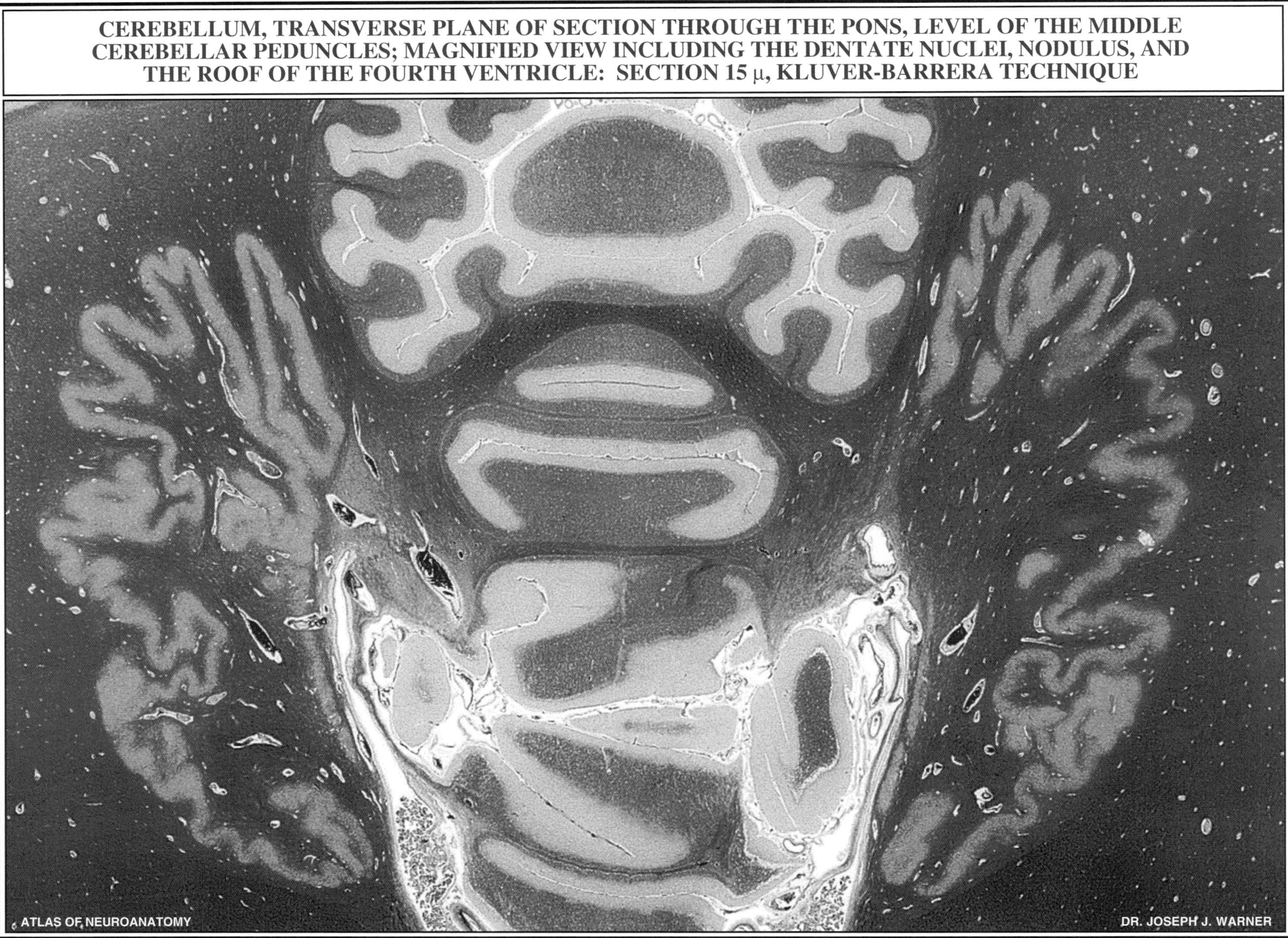

PONS AND CEREBELLUM: TRANSVERSE SECTION THROUGH THE DENTATE NUCLEI AND MIDDLE CEREBELLAR PEDUNCLES

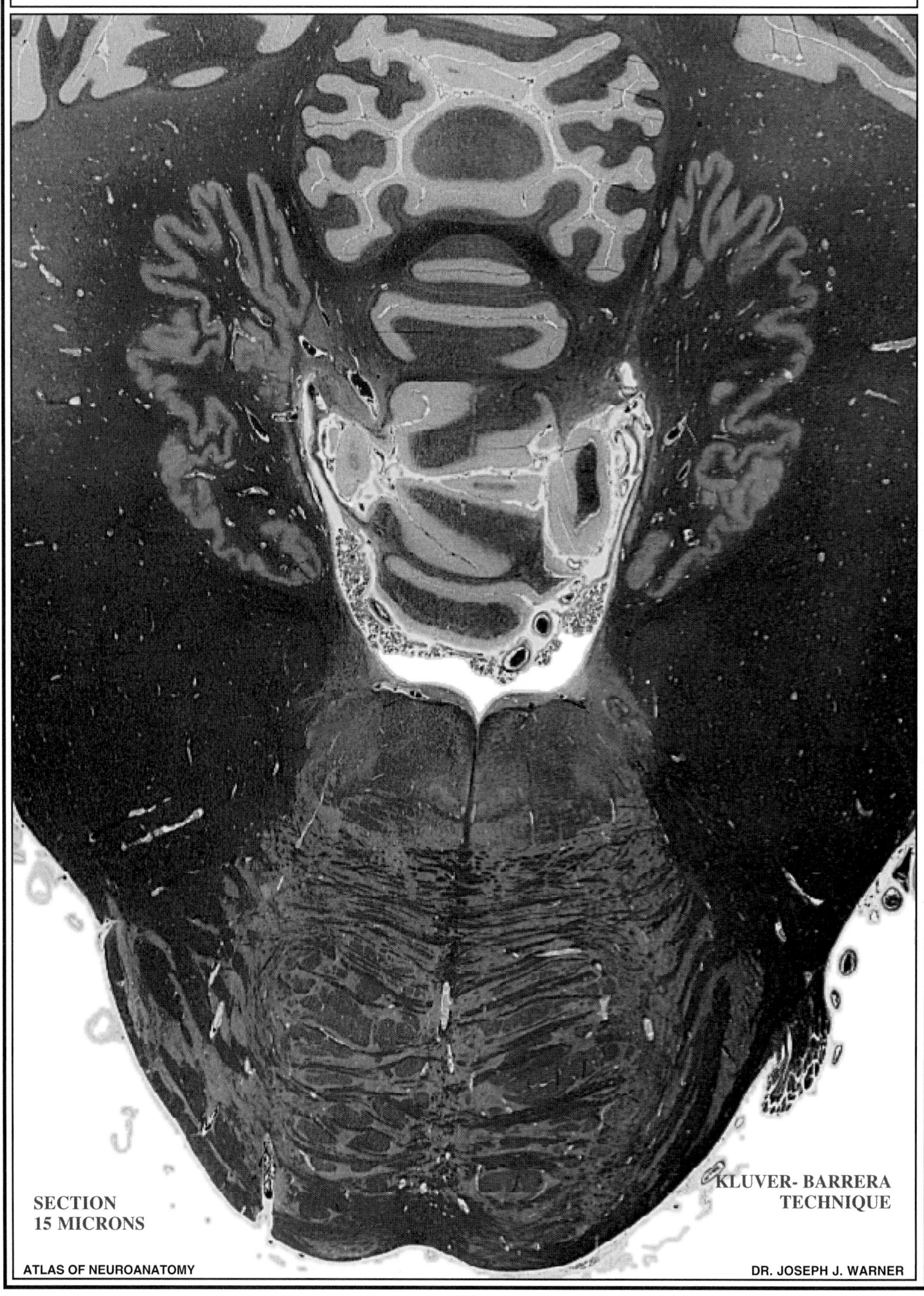

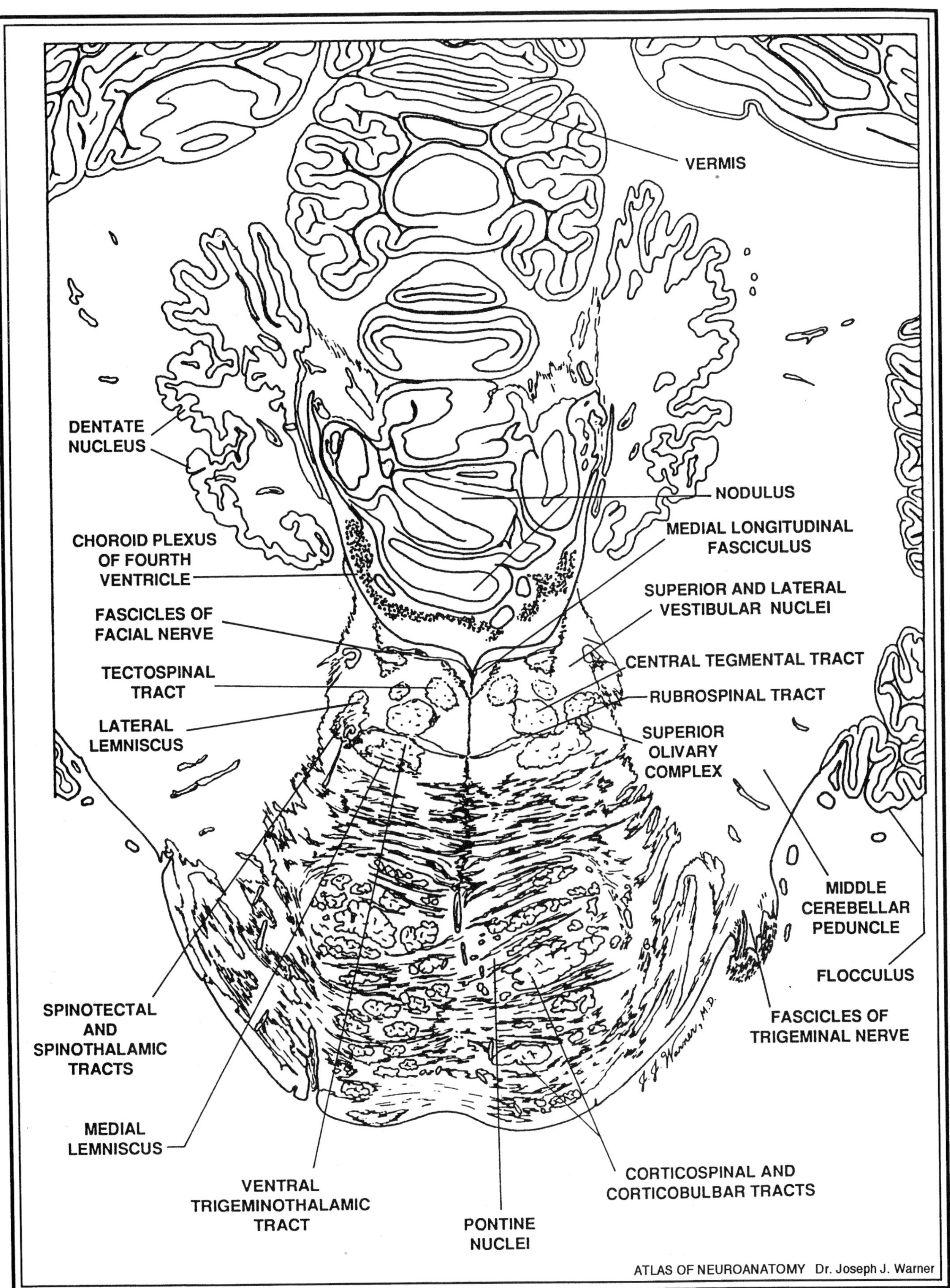
VERMIS
DENTATE NUCLEUS
NODULUS
MEDIAL LONGITUDINAL FASCICULUS
CHOROID PLEXUS OF FOURTH VENTRICLE
SUPERIOR AND LATERAL VESTIBULAR NUCLEI
FASCICLES OF FACIAL NERVE
CENTRAL TEGMENTAL TRACT
TECTOSPINAL TRACT
RUBROSPINAL TRACT
LATERAL LEMNISCUS
SUPERIOR OLIVARY COMPLEX
MIDDLE CEREBELLAR PEDUNCLE
FLOCCULUS
SPINOTECTAL AND SPINOTHALAMIC TRACTS
FASCICLES OF TRIGEMINAL NERVE
MEDIAL LEMNISCUS
VENTRAL TRIGEMINOTHALAMIC TRACT
PONTINE NUCLEI
CORTICOSPINAL AND CORTICOBULBAR TRACTS
J. J. Warner, M.D.
ATLAS OF NEUROANATOMY Dr. Joseph J. Warner

SECTION PARALLEL TO THE LONGITUDINAL AXIS OF THE BRAINSTEM: LEVEL INCLUDING THE LOCUS COERULEUS AND THE VENTROPOSTEROMEDIAL NUCLEUS OF THE THALAMUS

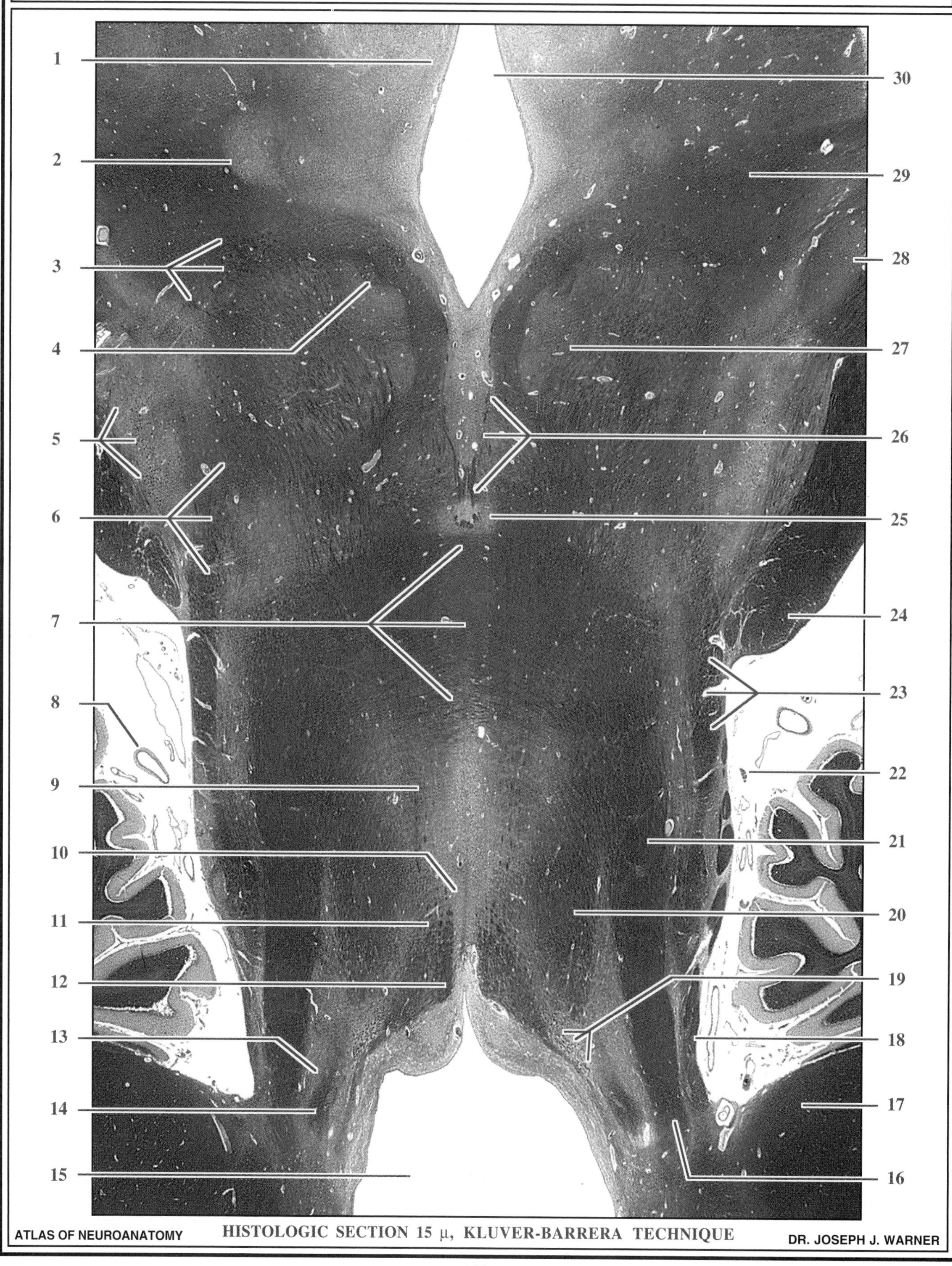

ATLAS OF NEUROANATOMY — HISTOLOGIC SECTION 15 μ, KLUVER-BARRERA TECHNIQUE — DR. JOSEPH J. WARNER

SECTION PARALLEL TO THE LONGITUDINAL AXIS OF THE BRAINSTEM: LEVEL INCLUDING THE LOCUS COERULEUS AND THE VENTROPOSTEROMEDIAL NUCLEUS OF THE THALAMUS

SECTION ORIENTATION AND KEY TO NUMBERED STRUCTURES

1. Dorsomedial Nucleus of the Thalamus
2. Ventroposteromedial Nucleus of the Thalamus*
3. Dentatorubrothalamic Fibers
4. Fasciculus Retroflexus of Meynert (Habenulointerpeduncular Tract)
5. Substantia Nigra
6. Ventral Trigeminothalamic and Spinothalamic Tracts and the Medial Lemniscus
7. Decussation of the Superior Cerebellar Peduncle*
8. Superior Cerebellar Artery
9. Rubrospinal Tract
10. Dorsal Raphe Nuclei
11. Tectospinal Tract
12. Medial Longitudinal Fasciculus
13. Mesencephalic Trigeminal Nucleus
14. Mesencephalic Trigeminal Tract
15. Fourth Ventricle
16. Superior Cerebellar Peduncle*
17. Middle Cerebellar Peduncle
18. Lateral Lemniscus
19. Locus Coeruleus
20. Central Tegmental Tract
21. Superior Cerebellar Peduncle*
22. Trochlear (IV) Nerve
23. Spinothalamic Tract
24. Cerebral Peduncle
25. Oculomotor Nuclear Complex
26. Fascicles of the Oculomotor (III) Nerve
27. Red Nucleus*
28. Subthalamic Nucleus
29. Thalamic Fasciculus (Field H1 of Forel)
30. Third Ventricle

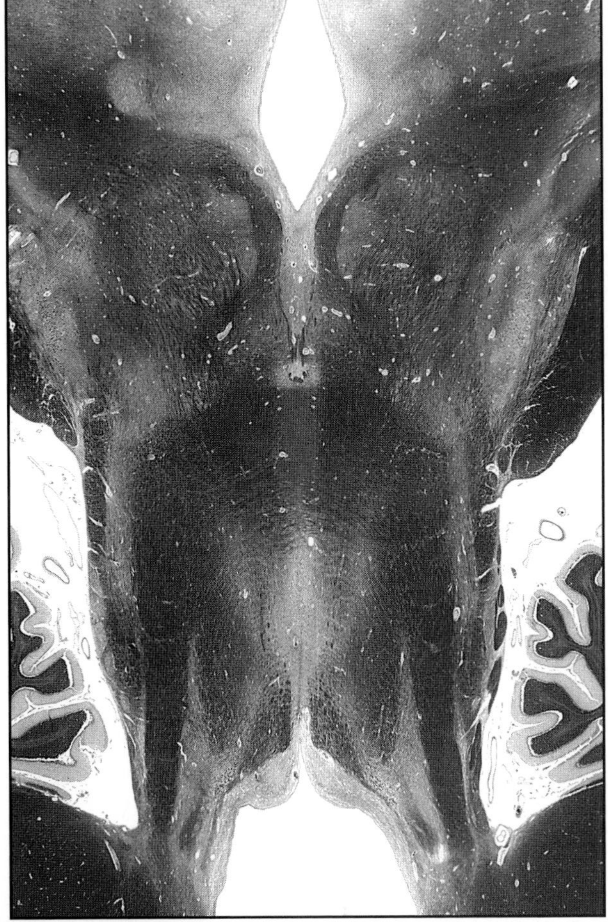

MAP OF SECTION PLANE REFERENCED TO A PARASAGITTAL HISTOLOGIC SECTION OF THE BRAIN

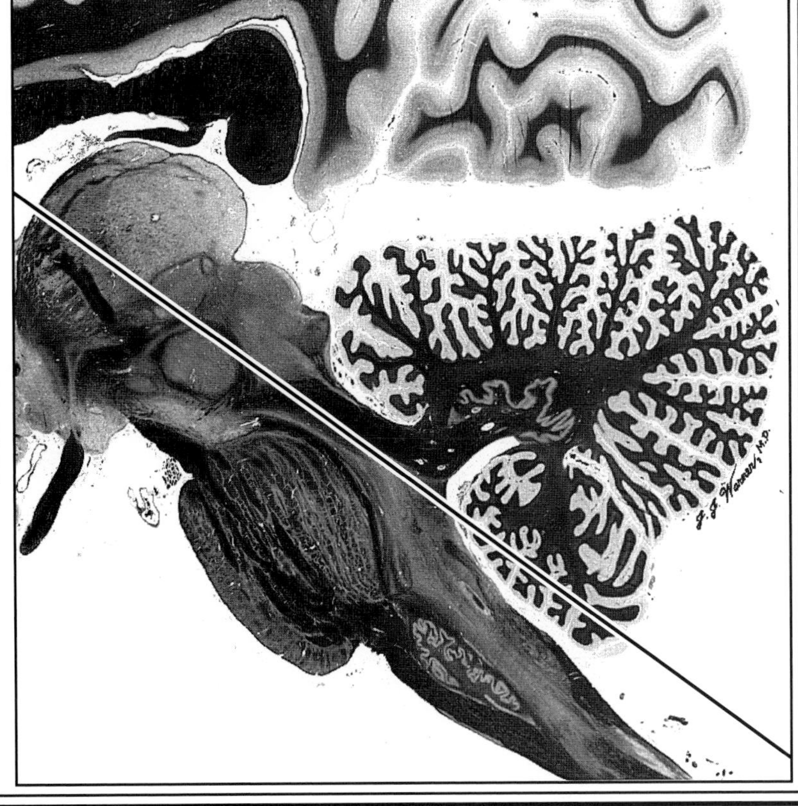

*Note intersection points, including the ventroposteromedial nucleus of the thalamus, the red nucleus, and the superior cerebellar peduncle.

HISTOLOGIC SECTIONS 15 μ, KLUVER-BARRERA TECHNIQUE

TRANSVERSE SECTION OF THE PONS: LEVEL OF INCLUDING THE ROSTRAL ASPECT OF THE SPINAL TRACT AND NUCLEUS OF THE TRIGEMINAL NERVE

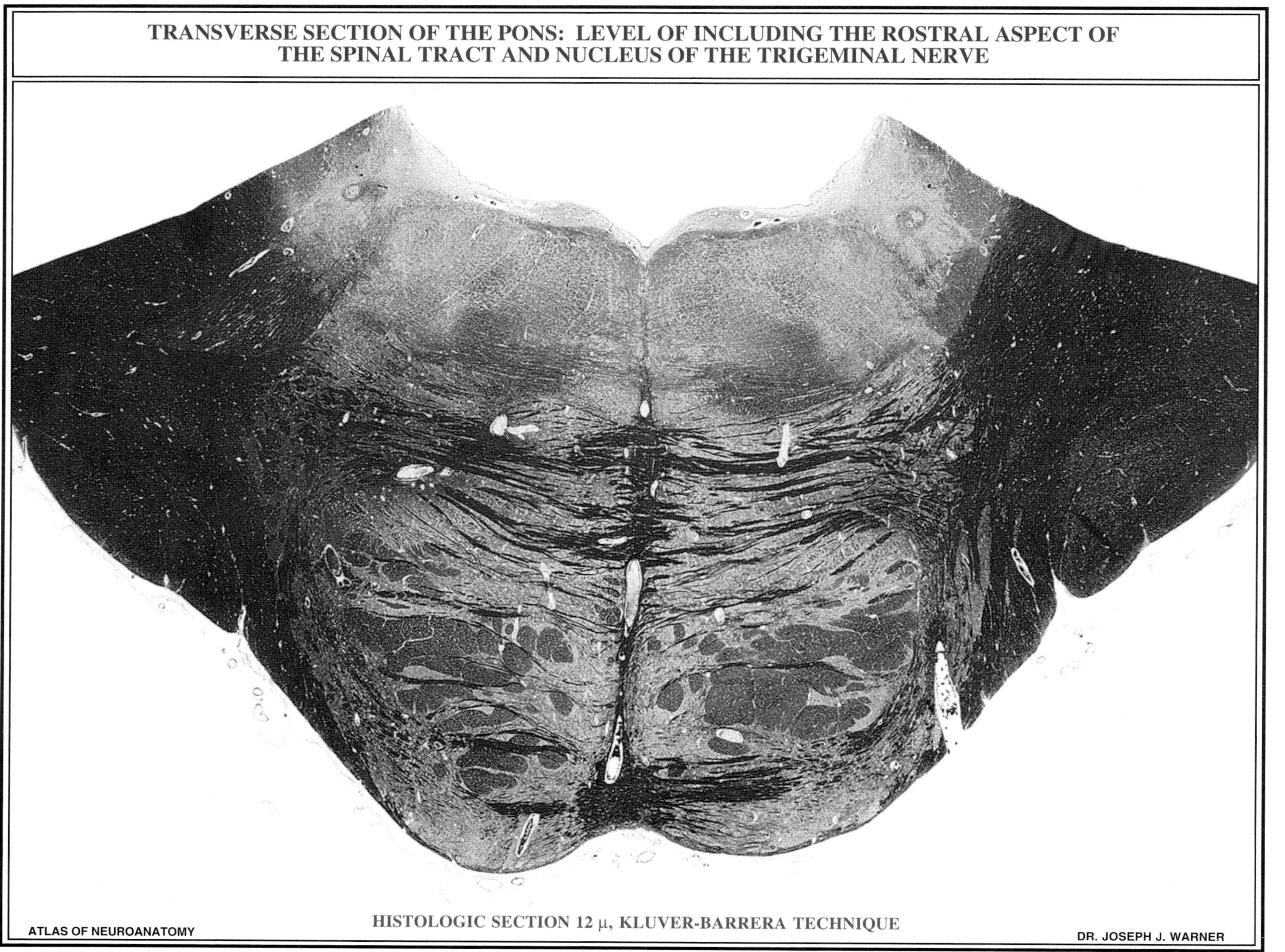

HISTOLOGIC SECTION 12 μ, KLUVER-BARRERA TECHNIQUE

DR. JOSEPH J. WARNER

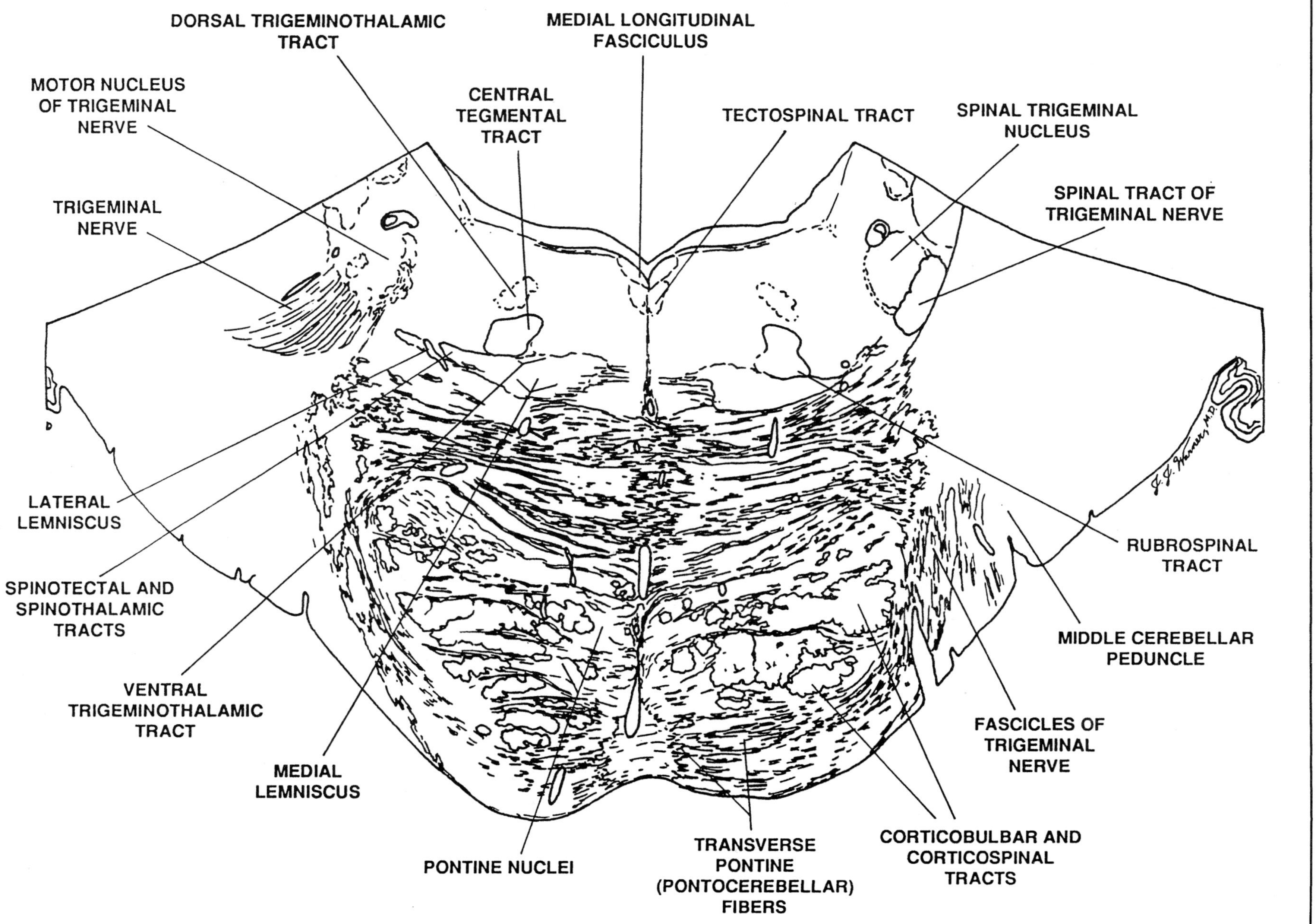

DORSAL TRIGEMINOTHALAMIC TRACT

MEDIAL LONGITUDINAL FASCICULUS

MOTOR NUCLEUS OF TRIGEMINAL NERVE

CENTRAL TEGMENTAL TRACT

TECTOSPINAL TRACT

SPINAL TRIGEMINAL NUCLEUS

SPINAL TRACT OF TRIGEMINAL NERVE

TRIGEMINAL NERVE

LATERAL LEMNISCUS

RUBROSPINAL TRACT

SPINOTECTAL AND SPINOTHALAMIC TRACTS

MIDDLE CEREBELLAR PEDUNCLE

VENTRAL TRIGEMINOTHALAMIC TRACT

FASCICLES OF TRIGEMINAL NERVE

MEDIAL LEMNISCUS

PONTINE NUCLEI

TRANSVERSE PONTINE (PONTOCEREBELLAR) FIBERS

CORTICOBULBAR AND CORTICOSPINAL TRACTS

CAUDAL PONS, TRANSVERSE SECTION: LEVEL OF THE NUCLEI AND FASCICLES OF THE ABDUCENS (VI) AND FACIAL (VII) NERVES

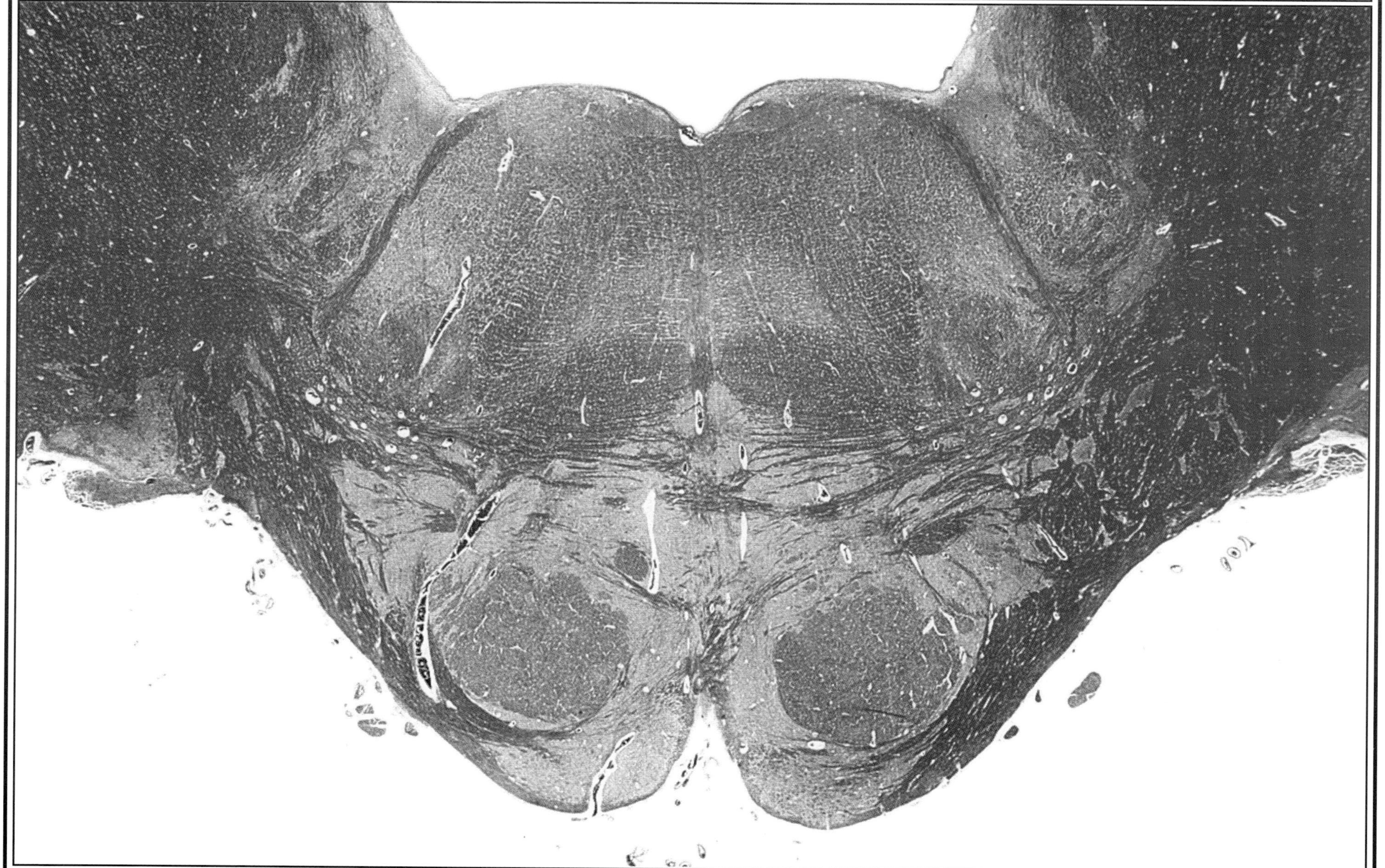

SECTION 12 μ, KLUVER-BARRERA TECHNIQUE

CAUDAL PONS, TRANSVERSE SECTION: LEVEL OF THE NUCLEI AND FASCICLES OF THE ABDUCENS (VI) AND FACIAL (VII) NERVES

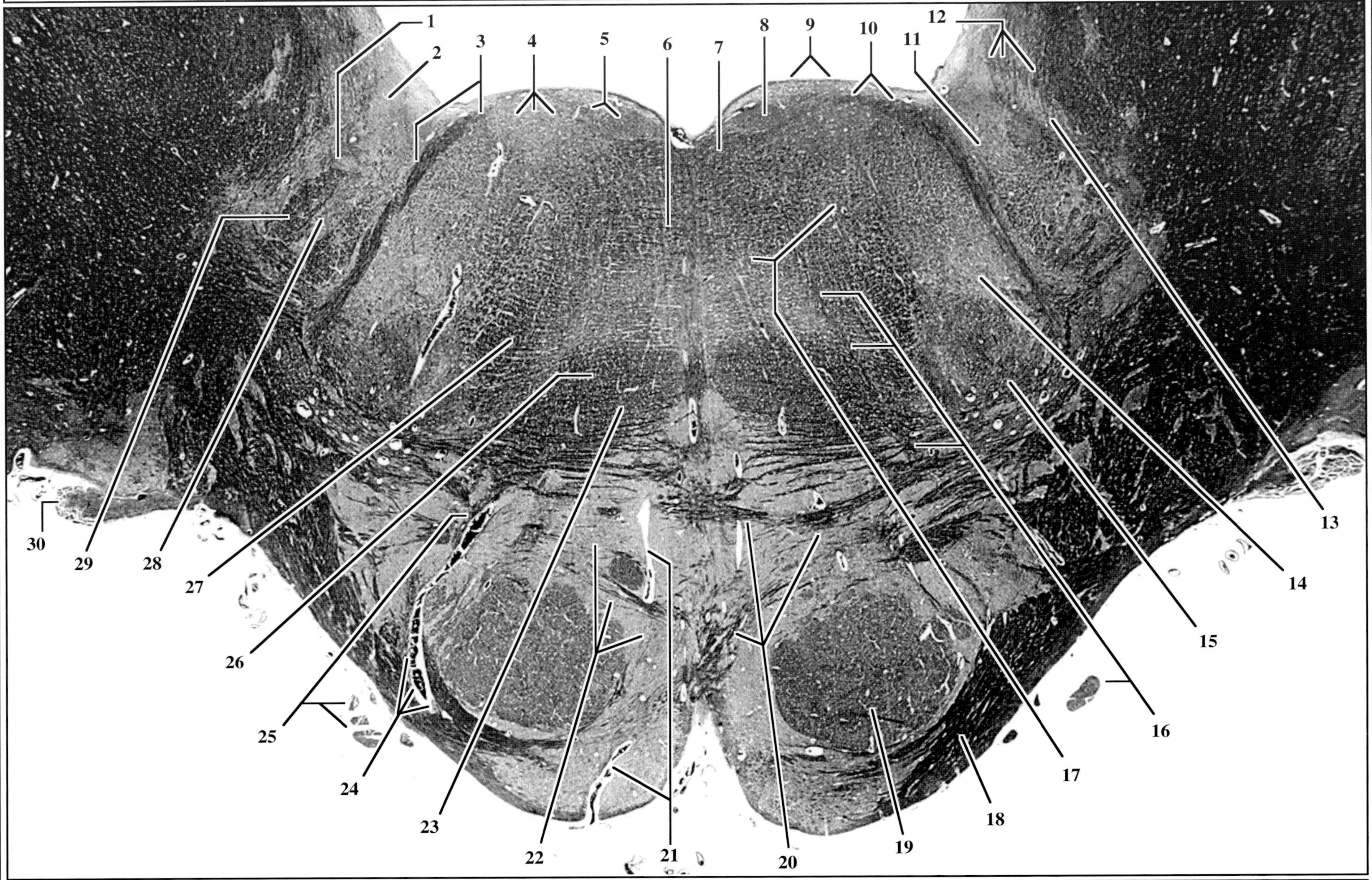
1
2
3
4
5
6
7
8
9
10
11
12
13
14
15
16
17
18
19
20
21
22
23
24
25
26
27
28
29
30

ATLAS OF NEUROANATOMY

SECTION 12 μ, KLUVER-BARRERA TECHNIQUE

DR. JOSEPH J. WARNER

CAUDAL PONS, TRANSVERSE SECTION: LEVEL OF THE NUCLEI AND FASCICLES OF THE ABDUCENS (VI) AND FACIAL (VII) NERVES: SECTION MAP AND KEY TO NUMBERED STRUCTURES

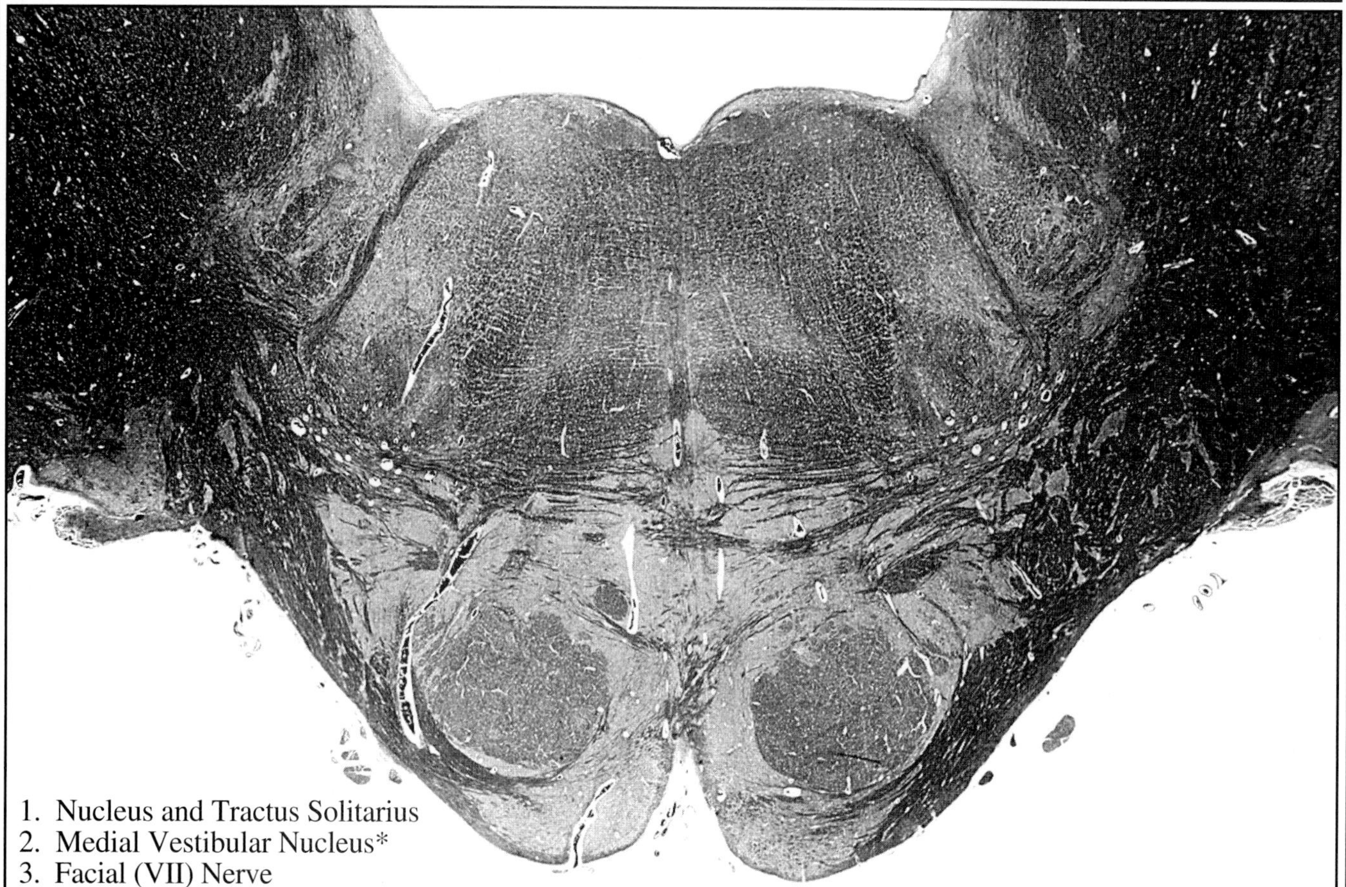

1. Nucleus and Tractus Solitarius
2. Medial Vestibular Nucleus*
3. Facial (VII) Nerve
4. Abducens (VI) Nucleus
5. Genu of the Facial Nerve
6. Tectospinal Tract
7. Medial Longitudinal Fasciculus
8. Genu of the Facial Nerve
9. Facial Colliculus
10. Facial (VII) Nerve
11. Superior Salivatory Nucleus
12. Juxtarestiform Body*
13. Lateral Vestibular Nucleus*
14. Facial (VII) Nucleus
15. Anterolateral Tract System
16. Fascicles of the Abducens (VI) Nerve
17. Pontine Reticular Formation
18. Pontocerebellar Fibers
19. Corticobulbar and Corticospinal Tracts
20. Transverse Pontocerebellar Fibers
21. Paramedian Pontine Arteries
22. Pontine Nuclei
23. Medial Lemniscus
24. Short Circumferential Artery
25. Fascicles of the Abducens (VI) Nerve
26. Ventral Trigeminothalamic Tract
27. Central Tegmental Tract
28. Spinal Trigeminal Nucleus
29. Spinal Trigeminal Tract
30. Facial (VII) Nerve

TRANSVERSE PLANE MAPPED ON A SAGITTAL SECTION OF THE CAUDAL PONS AND MEDULLA

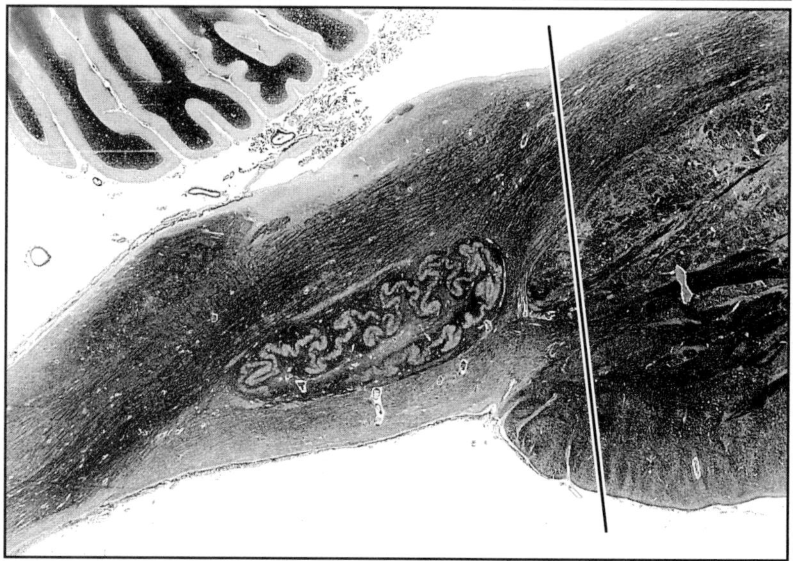

* The Juxtarestiform Body, with the Hook Fibers of Russell, include tracts interconnecting the vestibular nuclei with the cerebellum. These fibers join cerebellar afferents from more caudal levels to enter the inferior cerebellar peduncle.

PONTOMEDULLARY JUNCTION AND CEREBELLUM: OBLIQUE SECTION (PARALLEL TO THE PARIETO-OCCIPITAL SULCUS) DEMONSTRATING THE DEEP CEREBELLAR NUCLEI

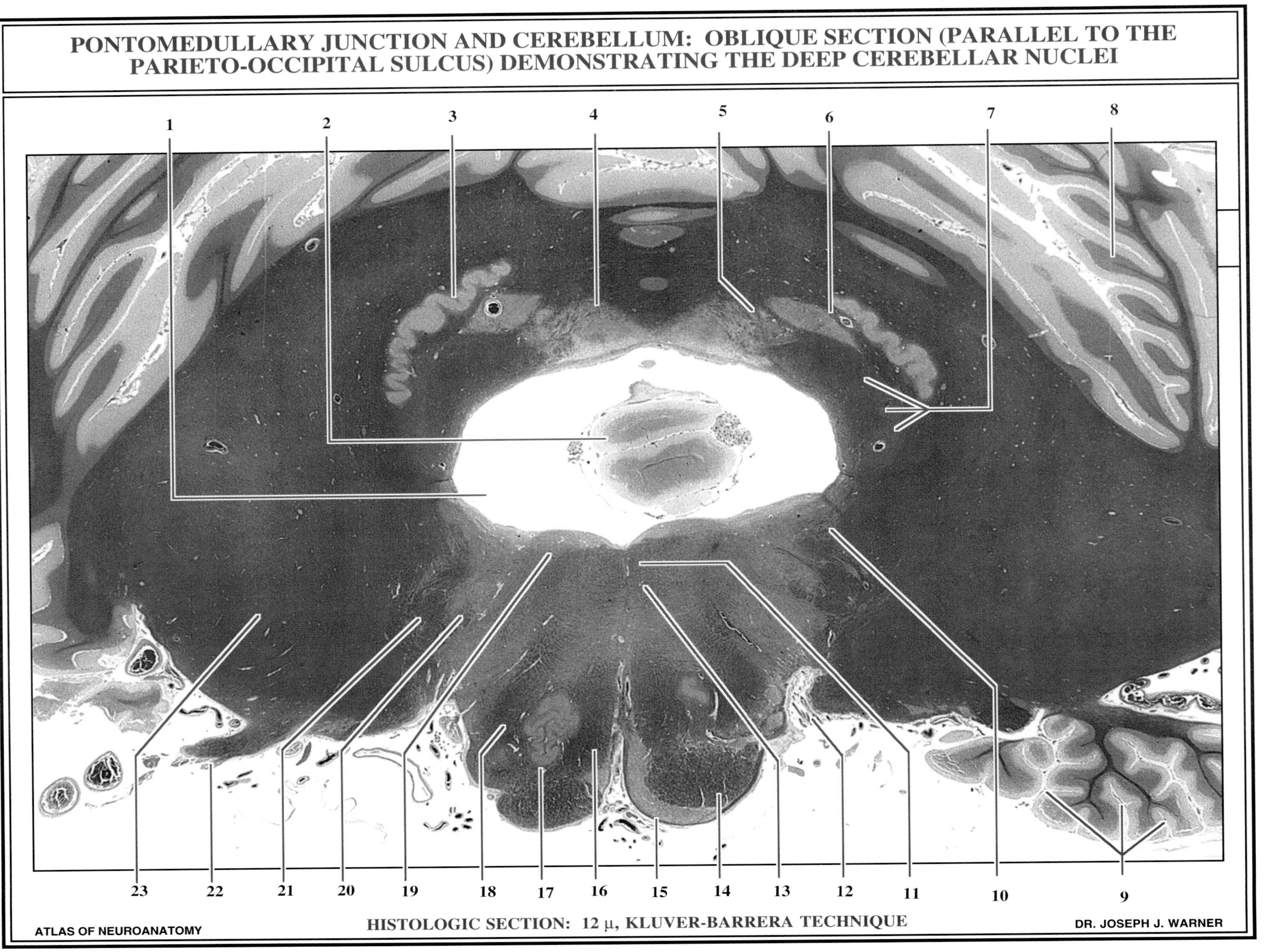

HISTOLOGIC SECTION: 12 μ, KLUVER-BARRERA TECHNIQUE

DR. JOSEPH J. WARNER

PONTOMEDULLARY JUNCTION AND CEREBELLUM; OBLIQUE SECTION (PARALLEL TO THE PARIETO-OCCIPITAL SULCUS) DEMONSTRATING THE DEEP CEREBELLAR NUCLEI: SECTION ORIENTATION AND KEY TO NUMBERED STRUCTURES

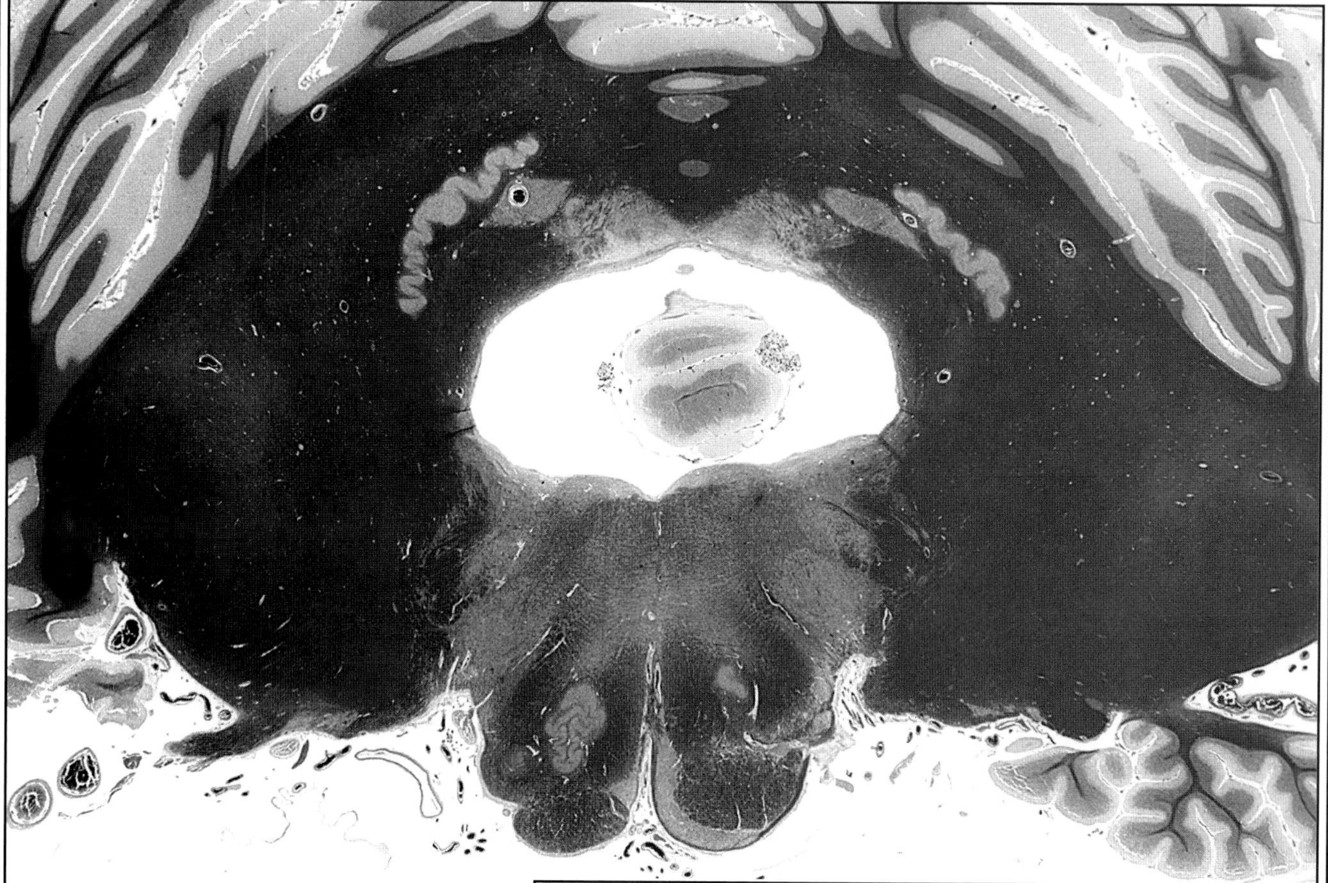

1. Fourth Ventricle
2. Nodulus
3. Dentate Nucleus
4. Fastigial Nucleus
5. Globose Nucleus
6. Emboliform Nucleus
7. Superior Cerebellar Peduncle
8. Granular Layer of the Cerebellar Cortex
9. Flocculus
10. Lateral Vestibular Nucleus
11. Medial Longitudinal Fasciculus
12. Pontomedullary Sulcus
13. Tectospinal Tract
14. Medullary Pyramid
15. Arcuate Nucleus
16. Medial Lemniscus
17. Inferior Olivary Nucleus
18. Central Tegmental Tract
19. Abducens (VI) Nucleus
20. Spinal Nucleus of the Trigeminal Nerve
21. Spinal Tract of the Trigeminal Nerve
22. Facial (VII) Nerve
23. Middle Cerebellar Peduncle

OBLIQUE PLANE MAPPED ON A PARAMEDIAN SAGITTAL SECTION INCLUDING THE SUPERIOR CEREBELLAR PEDUNCLE

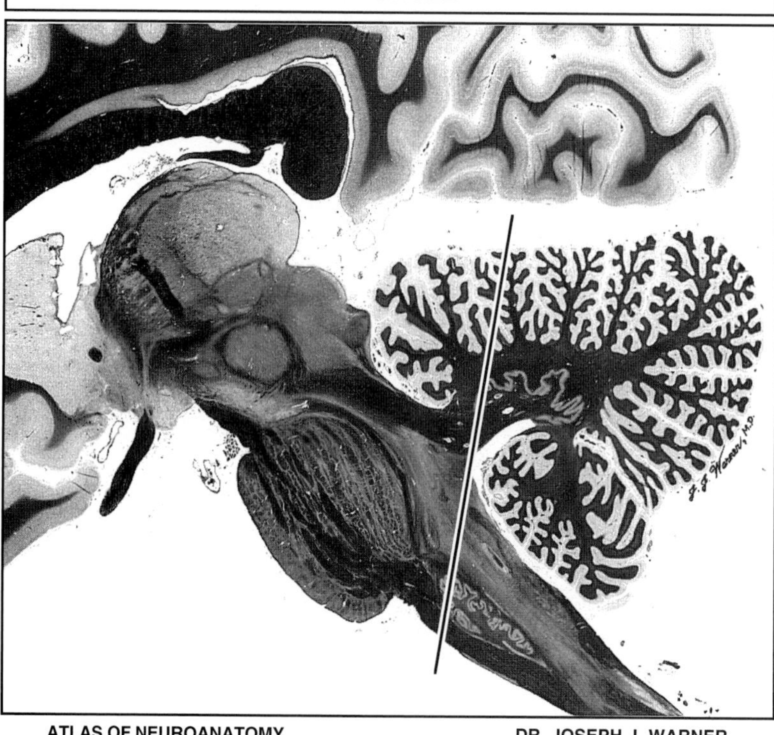

ROSTRAL MEDULLA, TRANSVERSE SECTION: LEVEL OF THE VESTIBULOCOCHLEAR (VIII) AND GLOSSOPHARYNGEAL (IX) NERVES

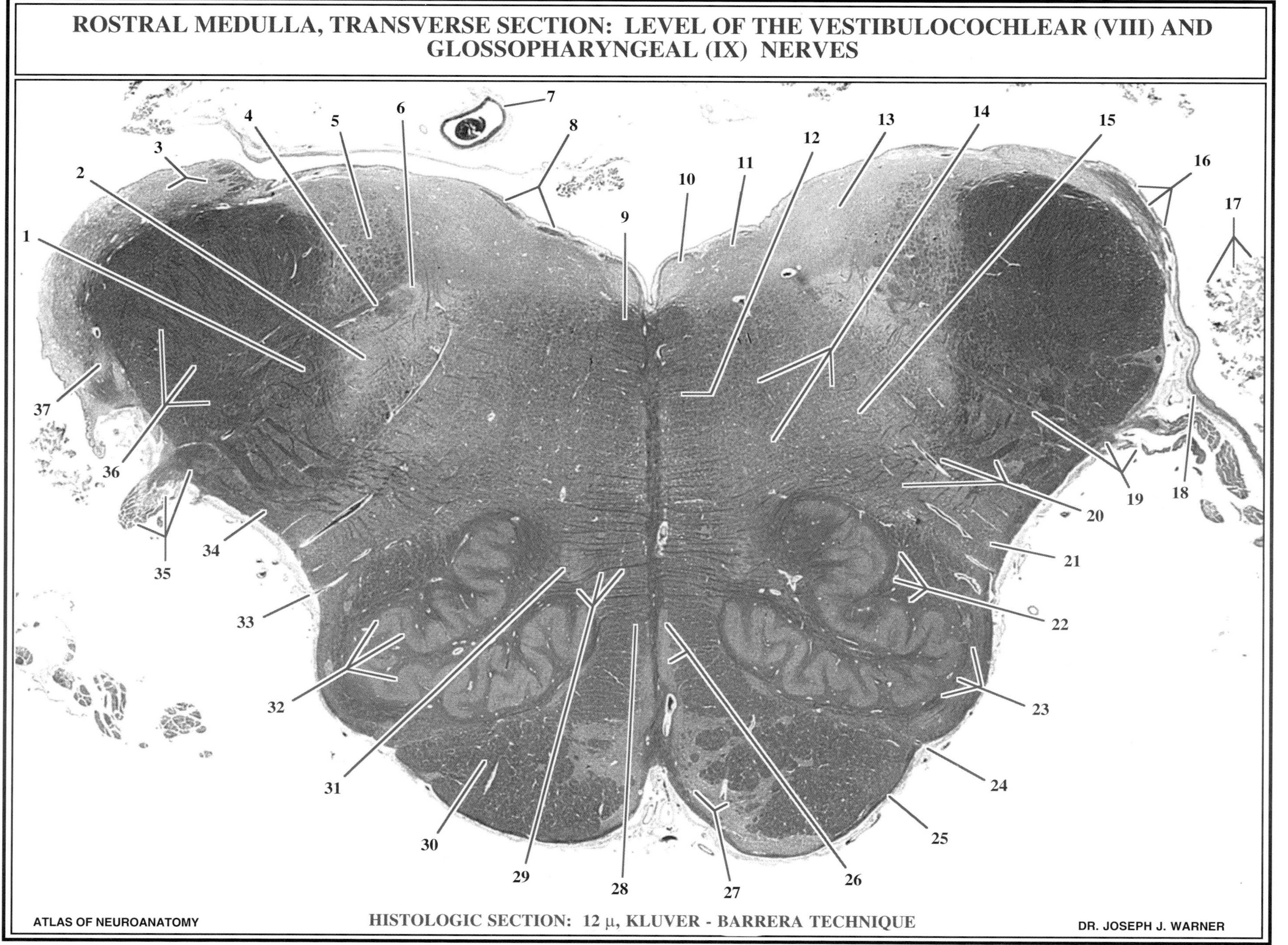

HISTOLOGIC SECTION: 12 μ, KLUVER - BARRERA TECHNIQUE

DR. JOSEPH J. WARNER

ROSTRAL MEDULLA, TRANSVERSE SECTION; LEVEL OF THE VESTIBULOCOCHLEAR (VIII) AND GLOSSOPHARYNGEAL (IX) NERVES SECTION MAP AND KEY TO NUMBERED STRUCTURES

1. Spinal Tract of the Trigeminal Nerve
2. Spinal Nucleus of the Trigeminal Nerve
3. Dorsal Cochlear Nucleus
4. Tractus Solitarius
5. Inferior Vestibular Nucleus
6. Nucleus Solitarius
7. Posterior Inferior Cerebellar Artery
8. Stria Medullares of the Fourth Ventricle
9. Medial Longitudinal Fasciculus
10. Nucleus Prepositus
11. Dorsal Efferent Nucleus of the Vagus (rostral aspect)
12. Tectospinal Tract
13. Medial Vestibular Nucleus
14. Reticular Formation
15. Nucleus Ambiguus
16. Fascicles of the Vestibulocochlear (VIII) Nerve
17. Choroid Plexus adjacent to the Foramen of Luschka
18. Fascicles of the Vestibulocochlear (VIII) Nerve
19. Fascicles of the Glossopharyngeal (IX) Nerve
20. Olivocerebellar Fibers
21. Spinothalamic Tract

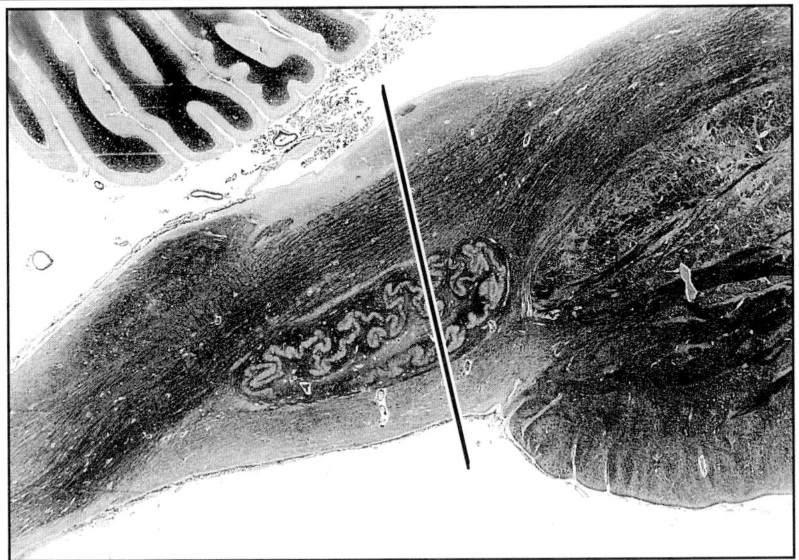

22, 23. Central Tegmental Tract (termination surrounds the Inferior Olivary Nucleus)
24. Post-olivary Fissure
25. External Arcuate Fibers
26. Median Raphe Nucleus
27. Arcuate Nucleus
28. Medial Lemniscus
29. Olivocerebellar Fibers
30. Pyramidal Tract
31. Medial Accessory Olivary Nucleus
32. Inferior Olivary Nucleus
33. Post-olivary Fissure
34. Ventral Spinocerebellar Tract
35. Glossopharyngeal (IX) Nerve
36. Inferior Cerebellar Peduncle
37. Inferior Cochlear Nucleus

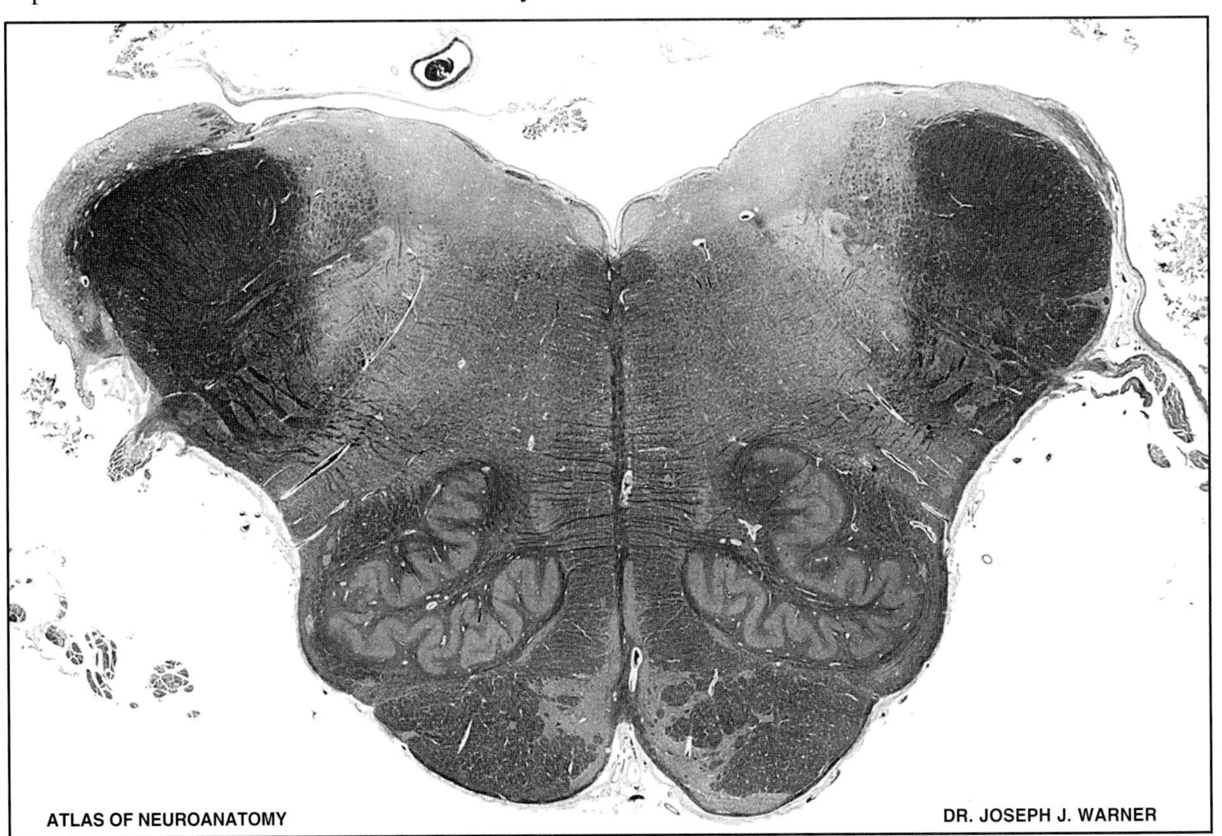

ROSTRAL MEDULLA, TRANSVERSE SECTION: LEVEL OF THE VESTIBULOCOCHLEAR (VIII) AND GLOSSOPHARYNGEAL (IX) NERVES

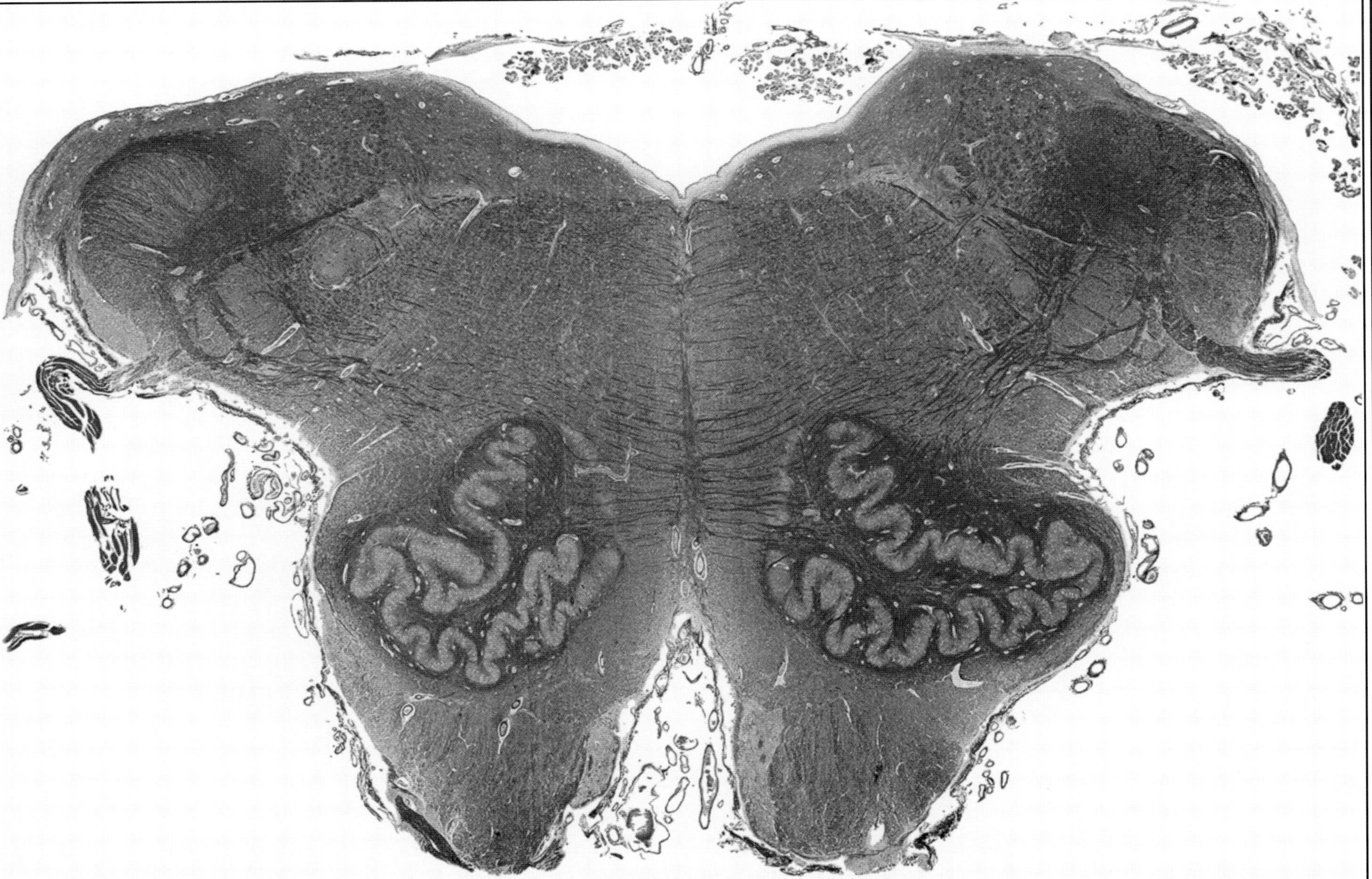

ATLAS OF NEUROANATOMY

SECTION 12 μ, BIELSCHOWSKY SILVER TECHNIQUE

DR. JOSEPH J. WARNER

ROSTRAL MEDULLA, TRANSVERSE SECTION: LEVEL OF THE VESTIBULOCOCHLEAR (VIII) AND GLOSSOPHARYNGEAL (IX) NERVES

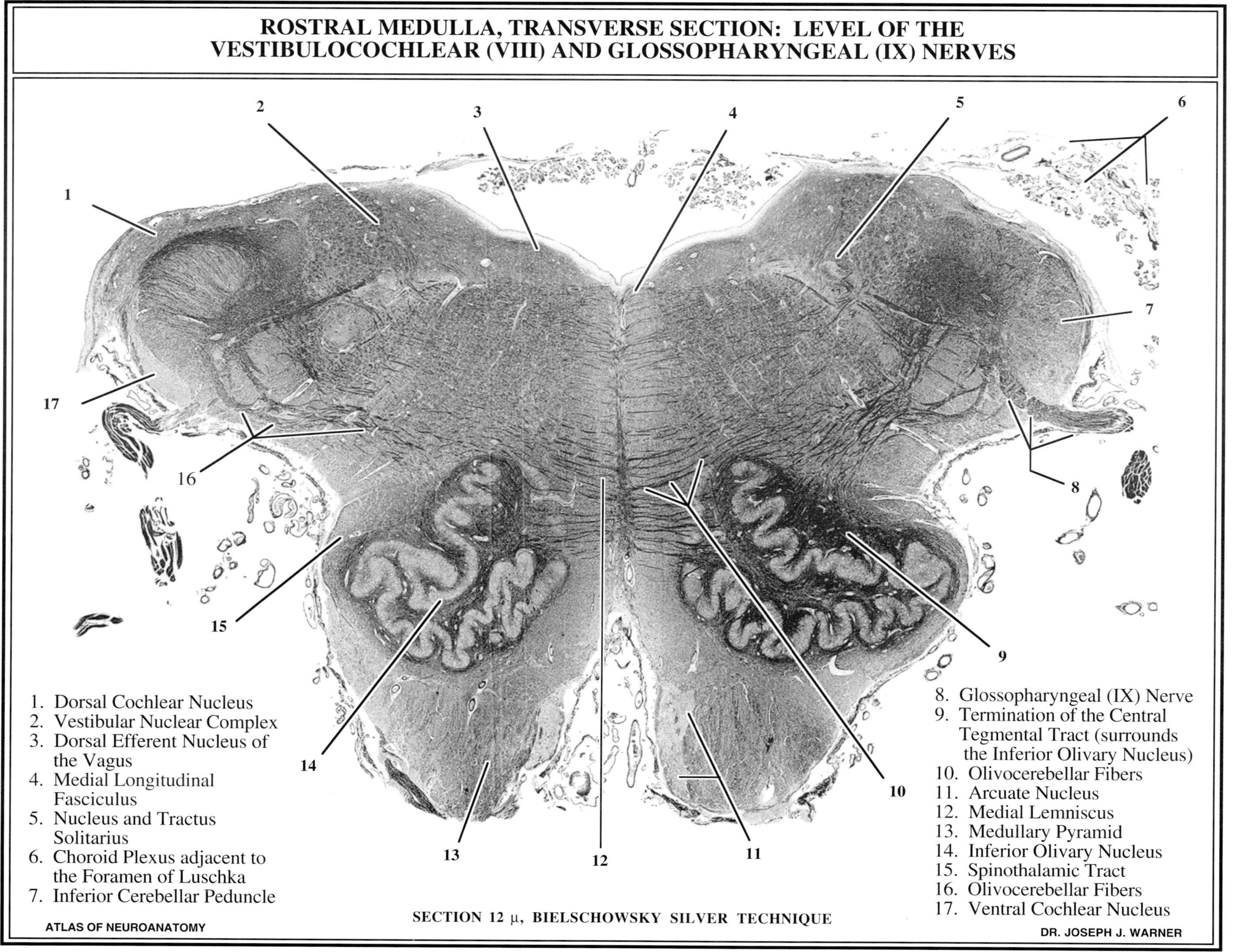

1. Dorsal Cochlear Nucleus
2. Vestibular Nuclear Complex
3. Dorsal Efferent Nucleus of the Vagus
4. Medial Longitudinal Fasciculus
5. Nucleus and Tractus Solitarius
6. Choroid Plexus adjacent to the Foramen of Luschka
7. Inferior Cerebellar Peduncle
8. Glossopharyngeal (IX) Nerve
9. Termination of the Central Tegmental Tract (surrounds the Inferior Olivary Nucleus)
10. Olivocerebellar Fibers
11. Arcuate Nucleus
12. Medial Lemniscus
13. Medullary Pyramid
14. Inferior Olivary Nucleus
15. Spinothalamic Tract
16. Olivocerebellar Fibers
17. Ventral Cochlear Nucleus

SECTION 12 μ, BIELSCHOWSKY SILVER TECHNIQUE

MEDULLA, HORIZONTAL SECTION INTERSECTING THE PONTOMEDULLARY SULCUS: LEVEL INCLUDING THE BASIS PONTIS, THE HYPOGLOSSAL NUCLEUS, AND THE DORSAL EFFERENT NUCLEUS OF THE VAGUS

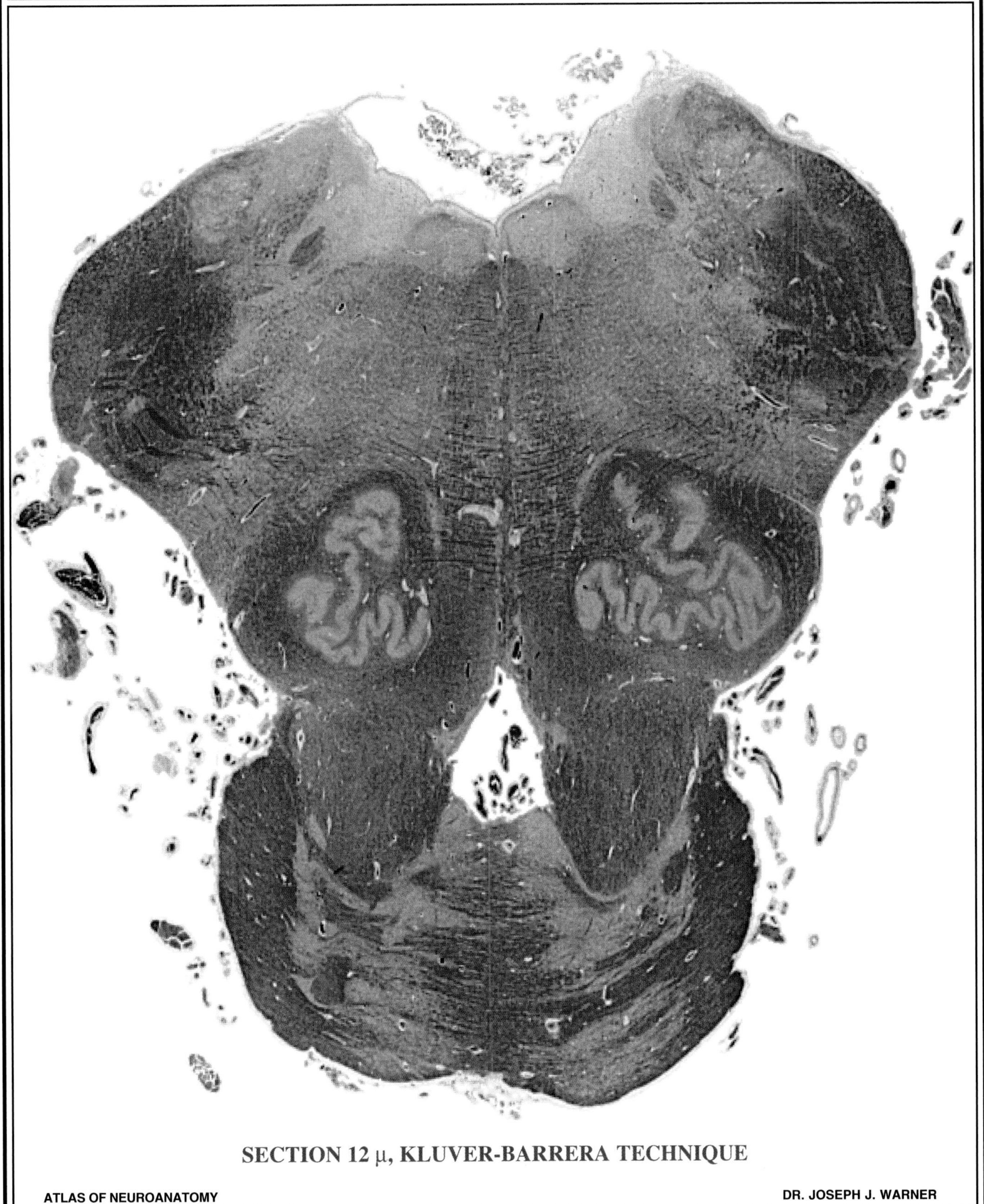

SECTION 12 μ, KLUVER-BARRERA TECHNIQUE

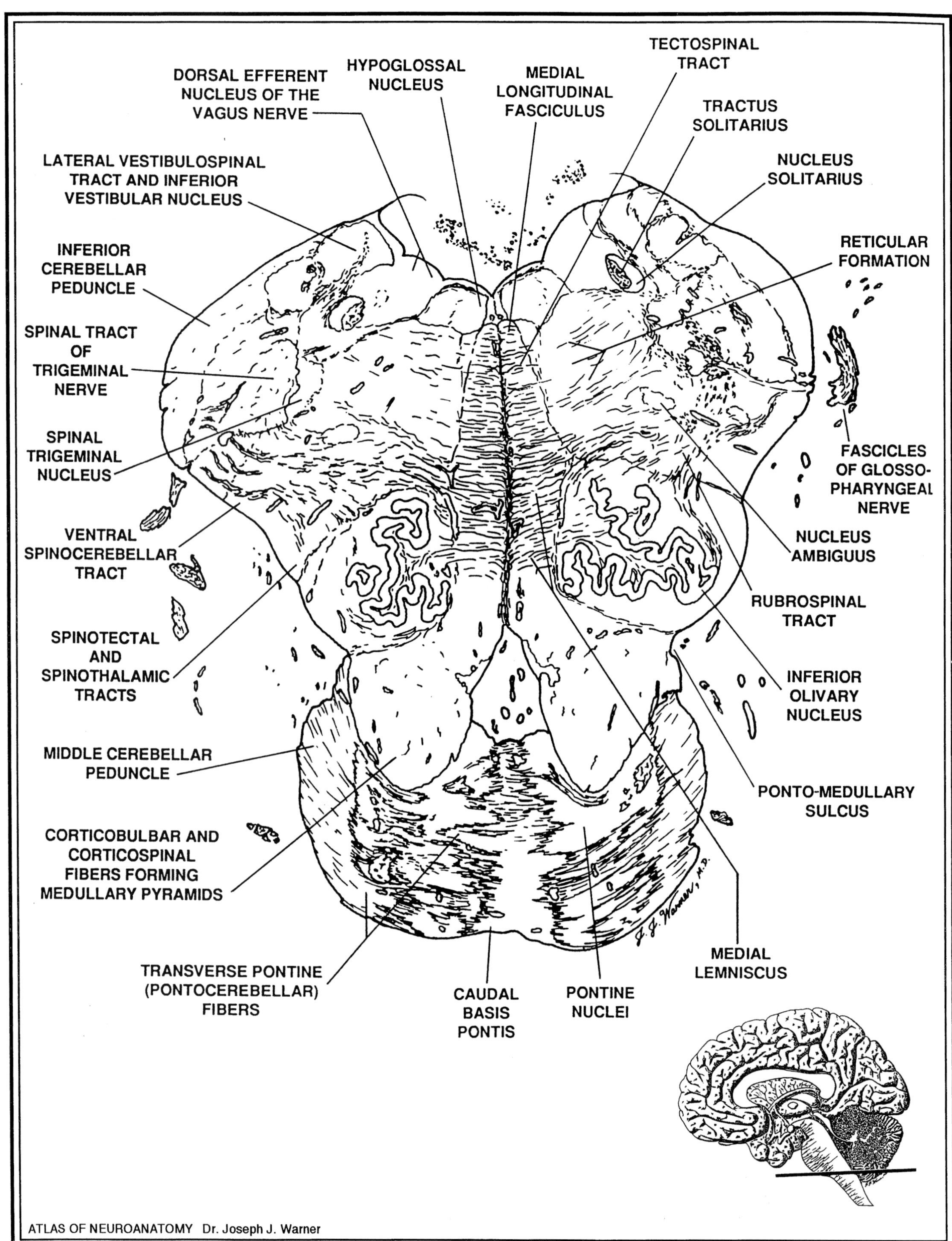

TECTOSPINAL TRACT
DORSAL EFFERENT NUCLEUS OF THE VAGUS NERVE
HYPOGLOSSAL NUCLEUS
MEDIAL LONGITUDINAL FASCICULUS
TRACTUS SOLITARIUS
LATERAL VESTIBULOSPINAL TRACT AND INFERIOR VESTIBULAR NUCLEUS
NUCLEUS SOLITARIUS
INFERIOR CEREBELLAR PEDUNCLE
RETICULAR FORMATION
SPINAL TRACT OF TRIGEMINAL NERVE
SPINAL TRIGEMINAL NUCLEUS
FASCICLES OF GLOSSO-PHARYNGEAL NERVE
VENTRAL SPINOCEREBELLAR TRACT
NUCLEUS AMBIGUUS
RUBROSPINAL TRACT
SPINOTECTAL AND SPINOTHALAMIC TRACTS
INFERIOR OLIVARY NUCLEUS
MIDDLE CEREBELLAR PEDUNCLE
PONTO-MEDULLARY SULCUS
CORTICOBULBAR AND CORTICOSPINAL FIBERS FORMING MEDULLARY PYRAMIDS
J. J. Warner, M.D.
MEDIAL LEMNISCUS
TRANSVERSE PONTINE (PONTOCEREBELLAR) FIBERS
CAUDAL BASIS PONTIS
PONTINE NUCLEI
ATLAS OF NEUROANATOMY Dr. Joseph J. Warner

MEDULLA, TRANSVERSE SECTION: LEVEL OF THE ROSTRAL ASPECT OF THE HYPOGLOSSAL NUCLEUS

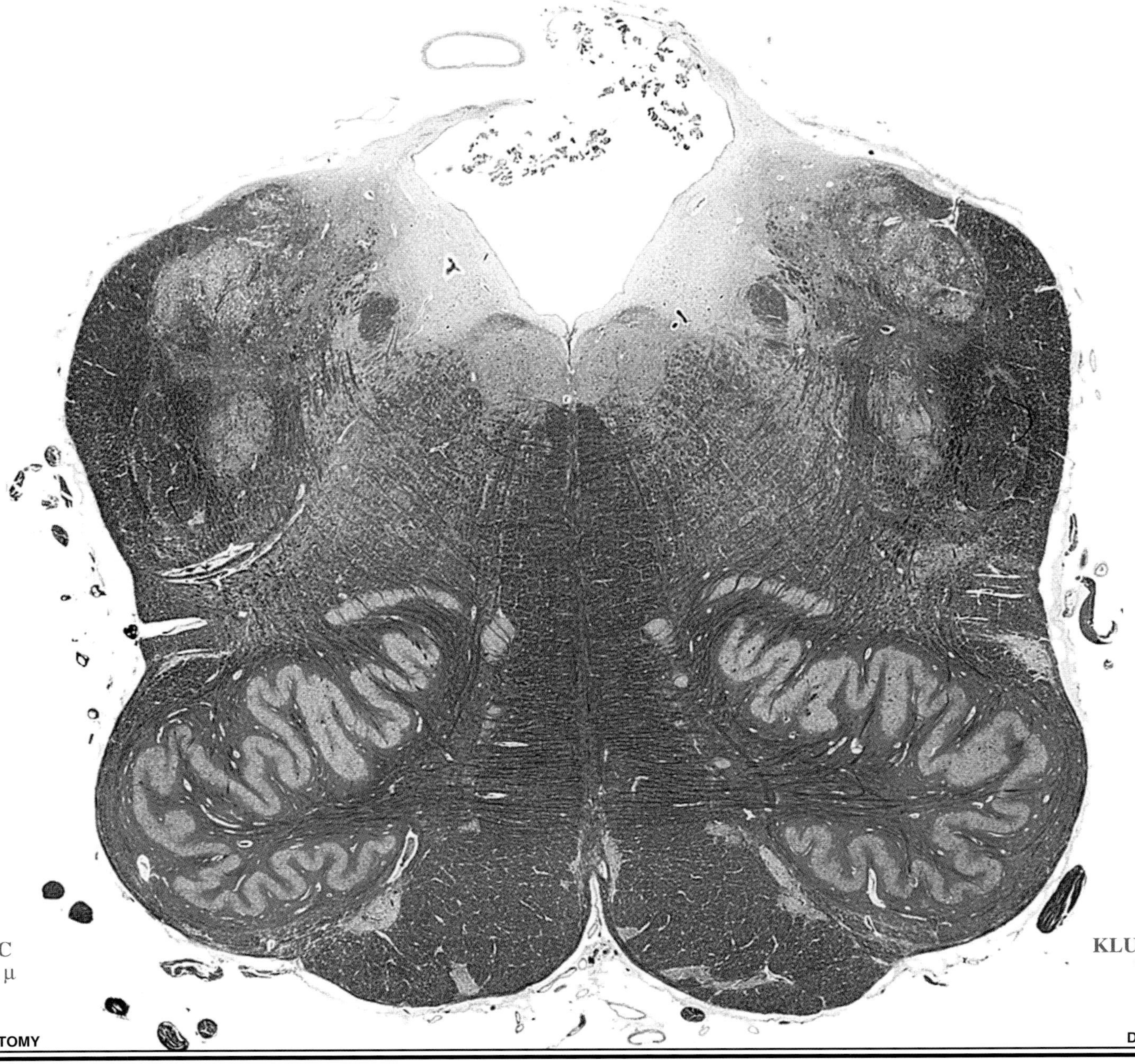

HISTOLOGIC
SECTION: 12 μ

KLUVER - BARRERA
TECHNIQUE

ATLAS OF NEUROANATOMY

DR. JOSEPH J. WARNER

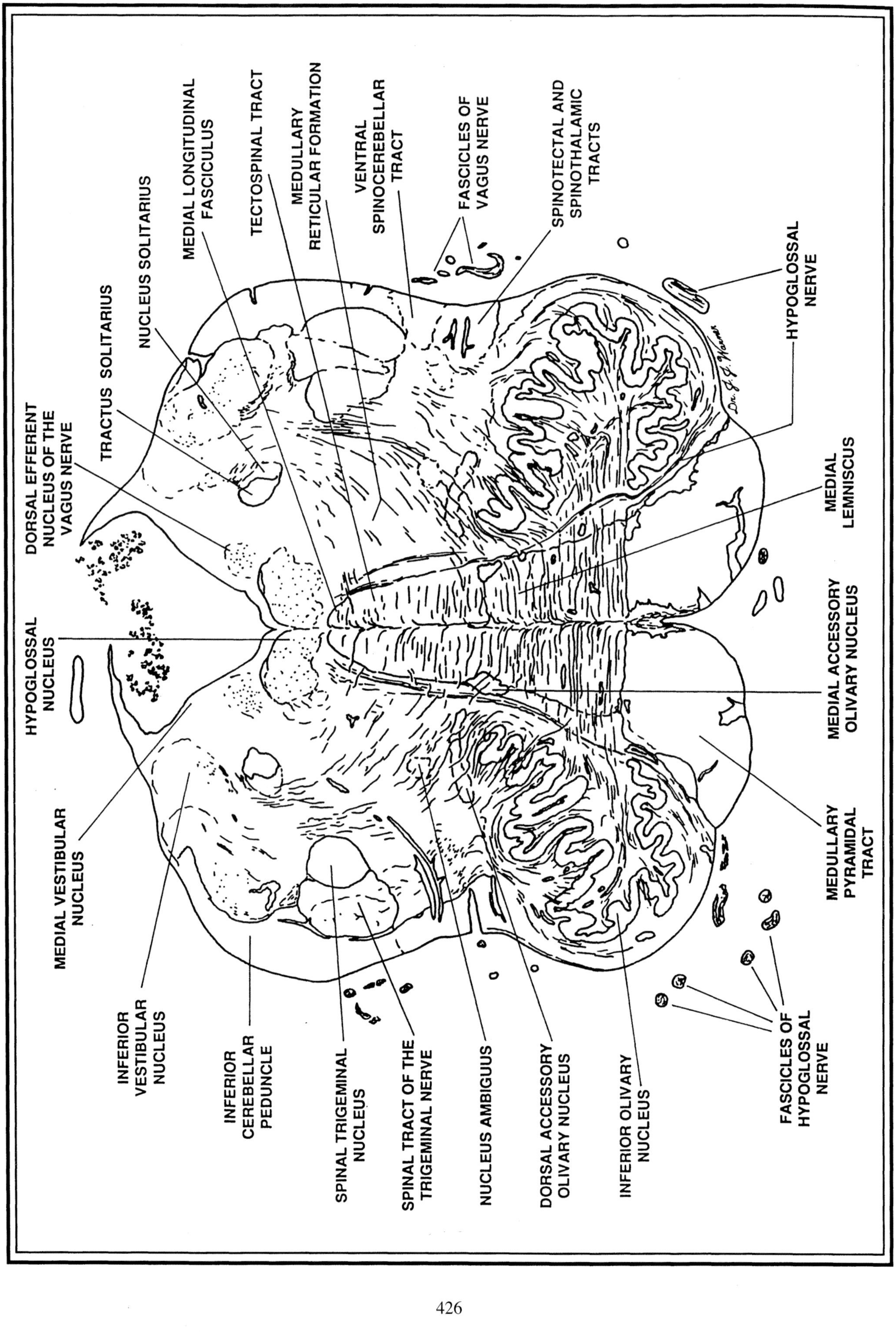

HYPOGLOSSAL NUCLEUS
DORSAL EFFERENT NUCLEUS OF THE VAGUS NERVE
MEDIAL VESTIBULAR NUCLEUS
TRACTUS SOLITARIUS
NUCLEUS SOLITARIUS
INFERIOR VESTIBULAR NUCLEUS
MEDIAL LONGITUDINAL FASCICULUS
INFERIOR CEREBELLAR PEDUNCLE
TECTOSPINAL TRACT
MEDULLARY RETICULAR FORMATION
SPINAL TRIGEMINAL NUCLEUS
VENTRAL SPINOCEREBELLAR TRACT
SPINAL TRACT OF THE TRIGEMINAL NERVE
FASCICLES OF VAGUS NERVE
NUCLEUS AMBIGUUS
DORSAL ACCESSORY OLIVARY NUCLEUS
SPINOTECTAL AND SPINOTHALAMIC TRACTS
INFERIOR OLIVARY NUCLEUS
Dr. J. J. Warner
FASCICLES OF HYPOGLOSSAL NERVE
HYPOGLOSSAL NERVE
MEDULLARY PYRAMIDAL TRACT
MEDIAL ACCESSORY OLIVARY NUCLEUS
MEDIAL LEMNISCUS

MEDULLA, TRANSVERSE SECTION: MAGNIFIED VIEW INCLUDING THE NUCLEUS AND FASCICLES OF THE HYPOGLOSSAL NERVE (XII), DORSAL EFFERENT NUCLEUS OF THE VAGUS, TRACTUS SOLITARIUS, AND THE DORSAL ACCESSORY OLIVARY NUCLEUS

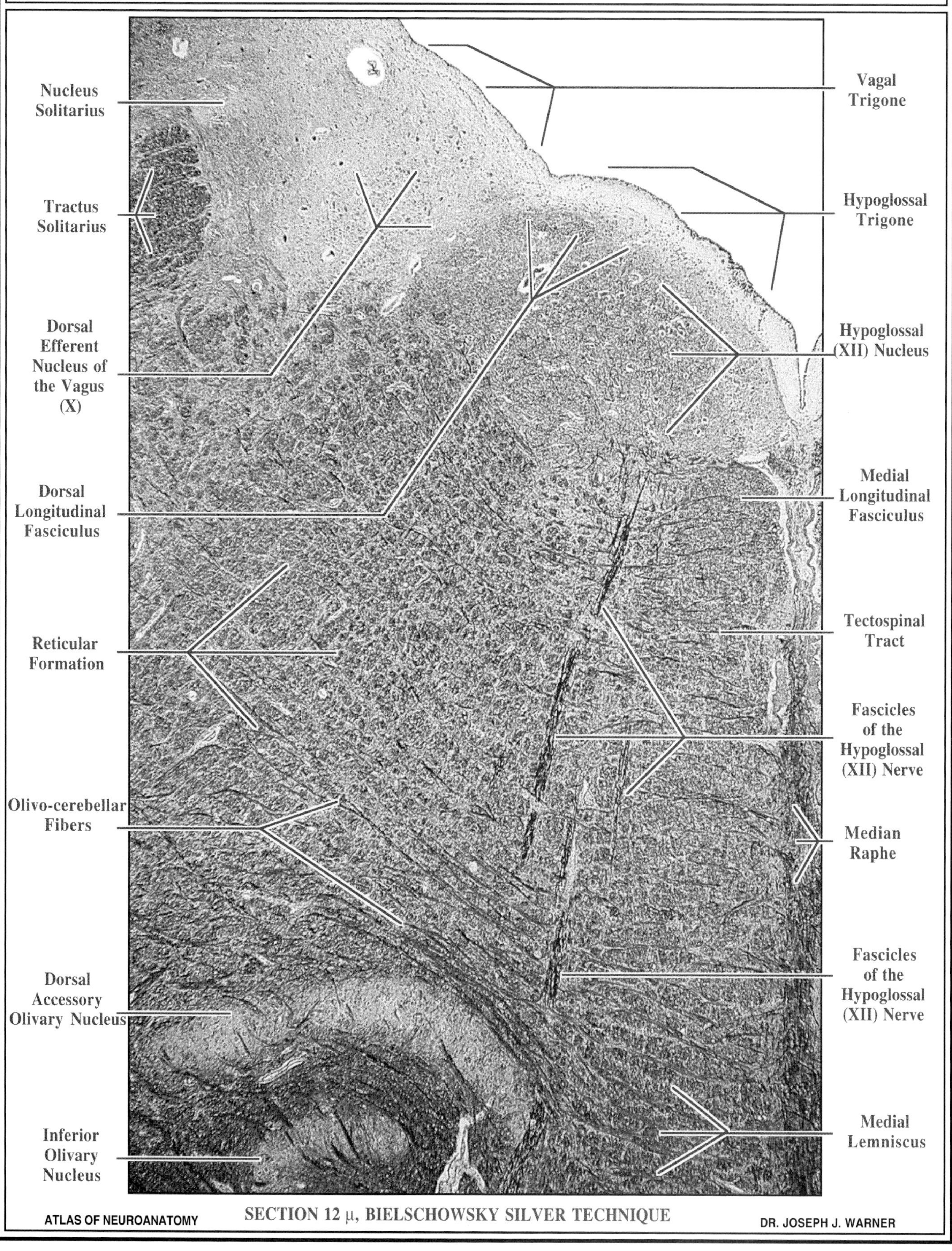

SECTION 12 μ, BIELSCHOWSKY SILVER TECHNIQUE

MEDULLA, MID-CAUDAL LEVEL, SECTION ORIENTATION APPROXIMATING THE HORIZONTAL PLANE: 12 μ, KLUVER-BARRERA TECHNIQUE

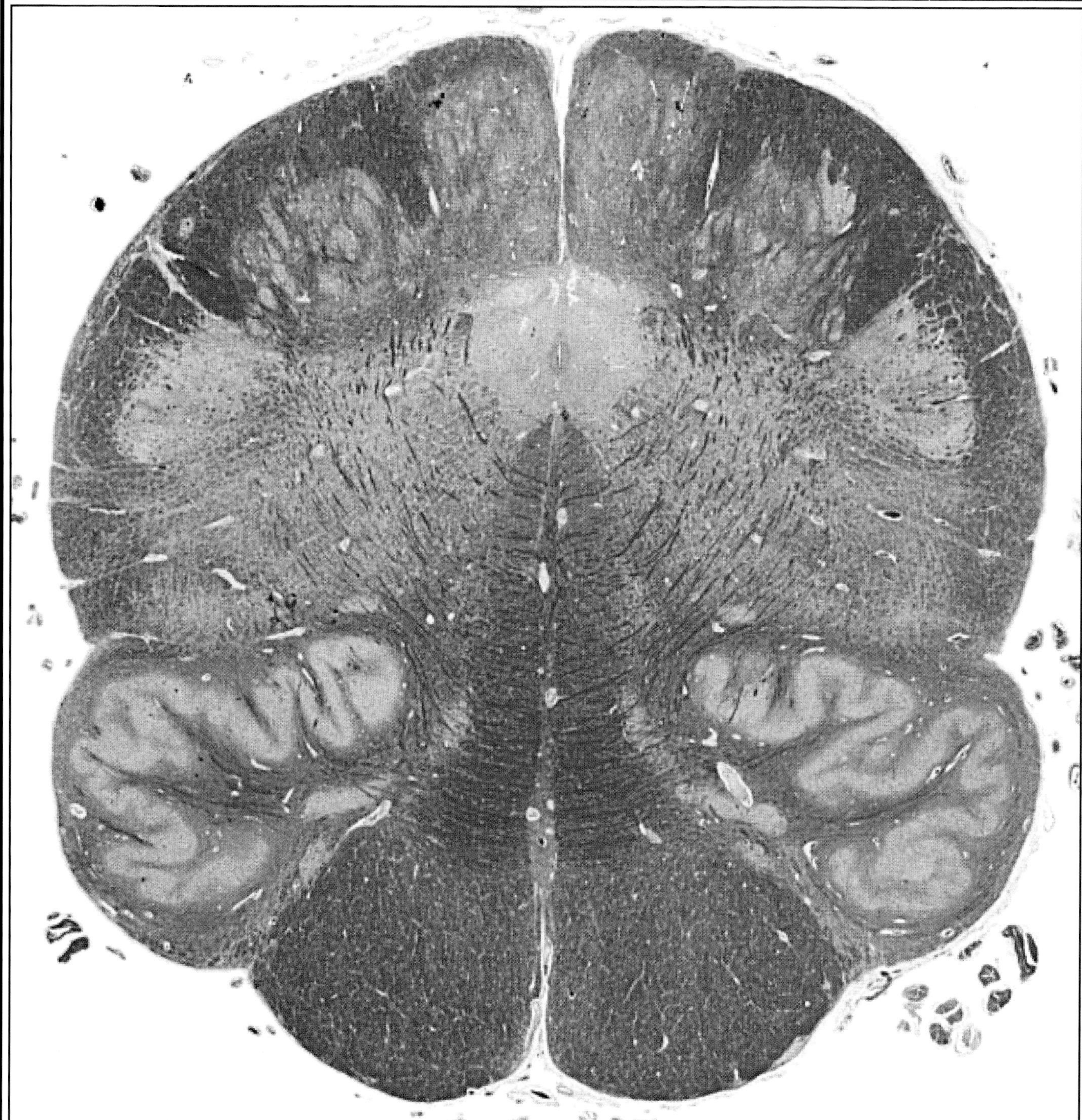

This plane of section is distinct from the conventional transverse orientation, which is characterized by the appearance of the hypoglossal and dorsal efferent nucleus of the vagus in the same level as the central region of the inferior olivary nucleus (refer to transverse sections at the level of cranial nerves X and XII). This section, by virtue of its orientation, demonstrates more caudal structures on the dorsal aspect (nucleus gracilis and cuneatus) in comparison with the configuration of the inferior olivary nucleus which is characteristic of more rostral levels of the medulla. Note the clearly discernible course of the internal arcuate fibers, as they pass ventromedially from their origin in nucleus gracilis and nucleus cuneatus. These fibers cross the midline, and ascend in the medial lemniscus (contralateral to their cell bodies of origin) to terminate in the ventroposterolateral nucleus of the thalamus.

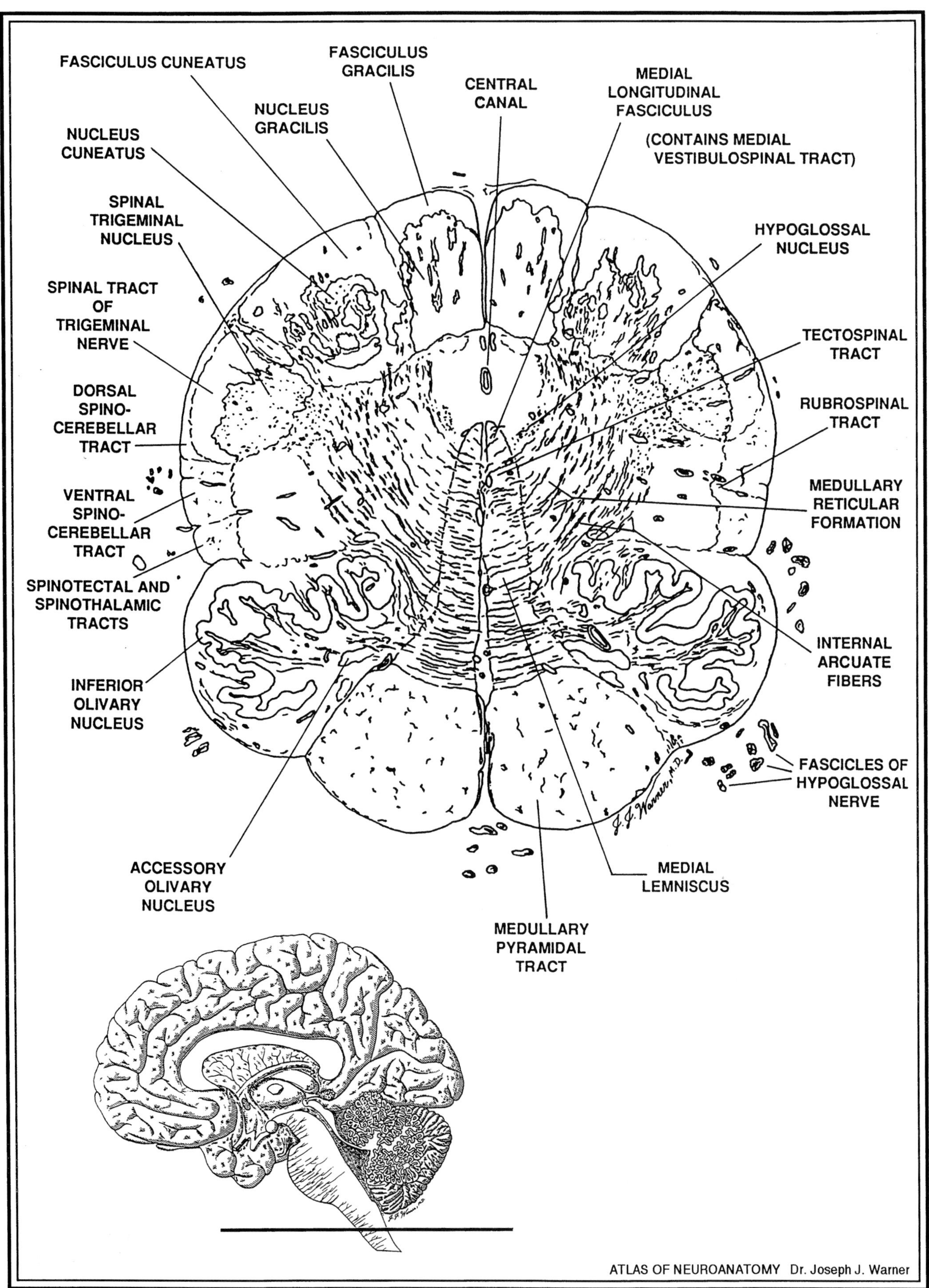
FASCICULUS CUNEATUS
FASCICULUS GRACILIS
CENTRAL CANAL
MEDIAL LONGITUDINAL FASCICULUS
(CONTAINS MEDIAL VESTIBULOSPINAL TRACT)
NUCLEUS GRACILIS
NUCLEUS CUNEATUS
SPINAL TRIGEMINAL NUCLEUS
HYPOGLOSSAL NUCLEUS
SPINAL TRACT OF TRIGEMINAL NERVE
TECTOSPINAL TRACT
DORSAL SPINO-CEREBELLAR TRACT
RUBROSPINAL TRACT
VENTRAL SPINO-CEREBELLAR TRACT
MEDULLARY RETICULAR FORMATION
SPINOTECTAL AND SPINOTHALAMIC TRACTS
INTERNAL ARCUATE FIBERS
INFERIOR OLIVARY NUCLEUS
FASCICLES OF HYPOGLOSSAL NERVE
ACCESSORY OLIVARY NUCLEUS
MEDIAL LEMNISCUS
MEDULLARY PYRAMIDAL TRACT

ATLAS OF NEUROANATOMY Dr. Joseph J. Warner

SAGITTAL SECTION OF THE MEDULLA, CAUDAL PONS, AND CEREBELLUM; LEVEL OF NUCLEUS CUNEATUS, FASCICULUS CUNEATUS, AND THE INTERNAL ARCUATE FIBERS: 15 μ SECTION, KLUVER-BARRERA TECHNIQUE

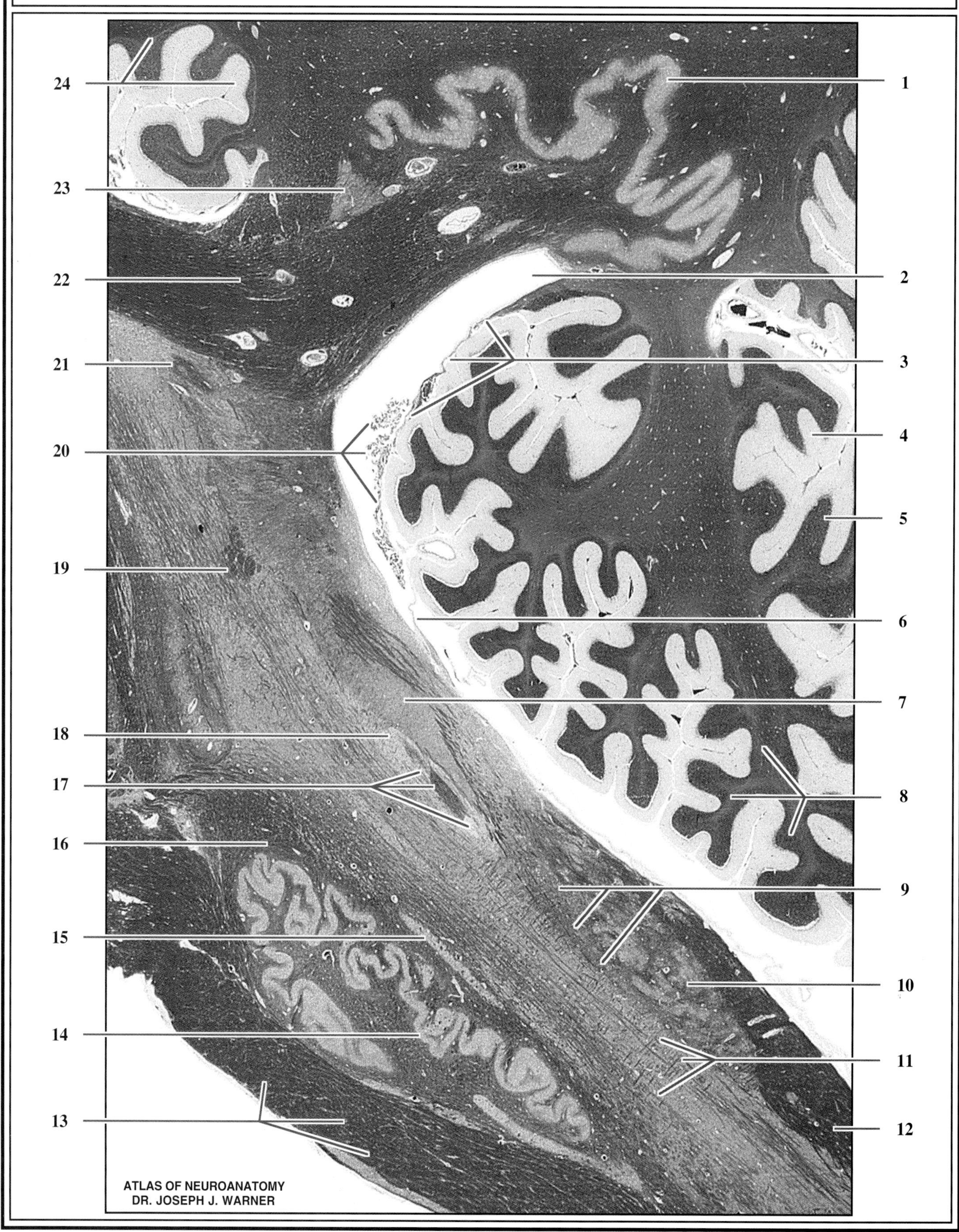

SAGITTAL SECTION OF THE MEDULLA, CAUDAL PONS, AND CEREBELLUM; LEVEL OF NUCLEUS CUNEATUS, FASCICULUS CUNEATUS, AND THE INTERNAL ARCUATE FIBERS: 15 μ SECTION, KLUVER-BARRERA TECHNIQUE

KEY TO NUMBERED STRUCTURES

1. Dentate Nucleus of the Cerebellum
2. Fourth Ventricle
3. Inferior (Posterior) Medullary Velum
4. Molecular Layer, Cerebellar Cortex
5. Granular Layer, Cerebellar Cortex
6. Tela Choroidea (interposed between ventricle and subarachnoid space)
7. Medial Vestibular Nucleus
8. Cerebellar Tonsil
9. Internal Arcuate Fibers
10. Nucleus Cuneatus
11. Internal Arcuate Fibers
12. Fasciculus Cuneatus
13. Medullary Pyramid
14. Inferior Olivary Nucleus
15. Dorsal Accessory Olivary Nucleus
16. Central Tegmental Tract
17. Nucleus and Tractus Solitarius
18. Dorsal Efferent Nucleus of the Vagus (X) Nerve
19. Facial (VII) Nerve
20. Choroid Plexus
21. Mesencephalic Root of the Trigeminal (V) Nerve
22. Superior Cerebellar Peduncle
23. Nucleus Interpositus
24. Anterior Lobe of the Cerebellum

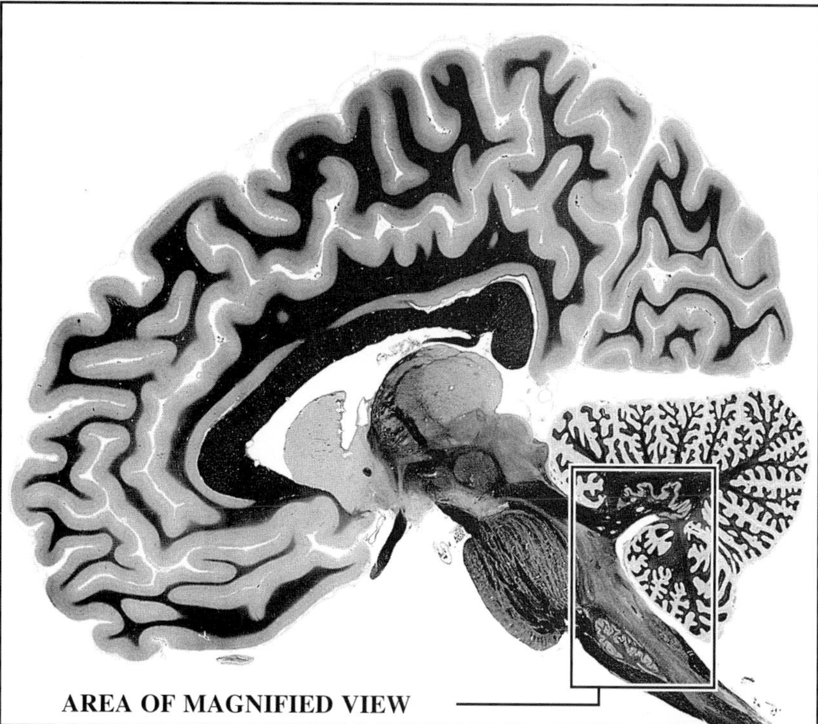

AREA OF MAGNIFIED VIEW

SAGITTAL PLANE REFERENCED TO A HORIZONTAL SECTION OF THE MEDULLA

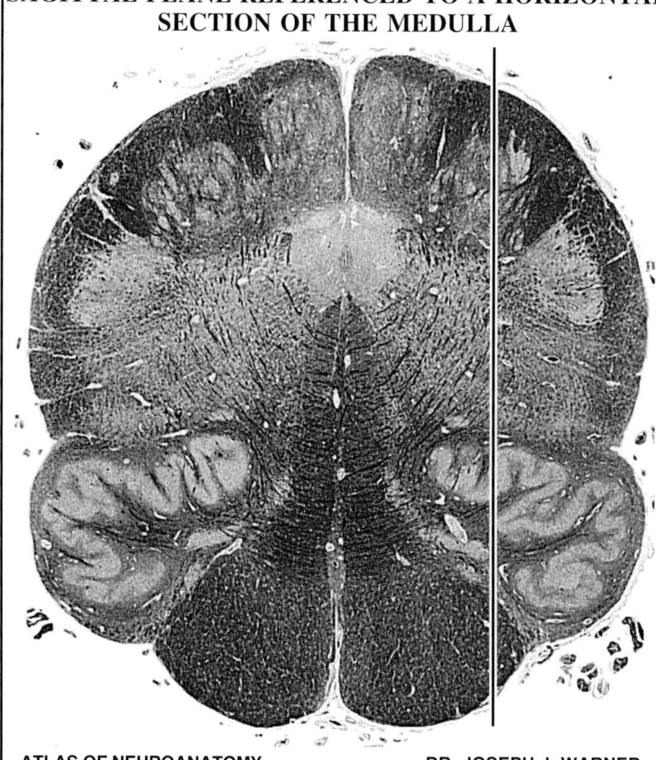

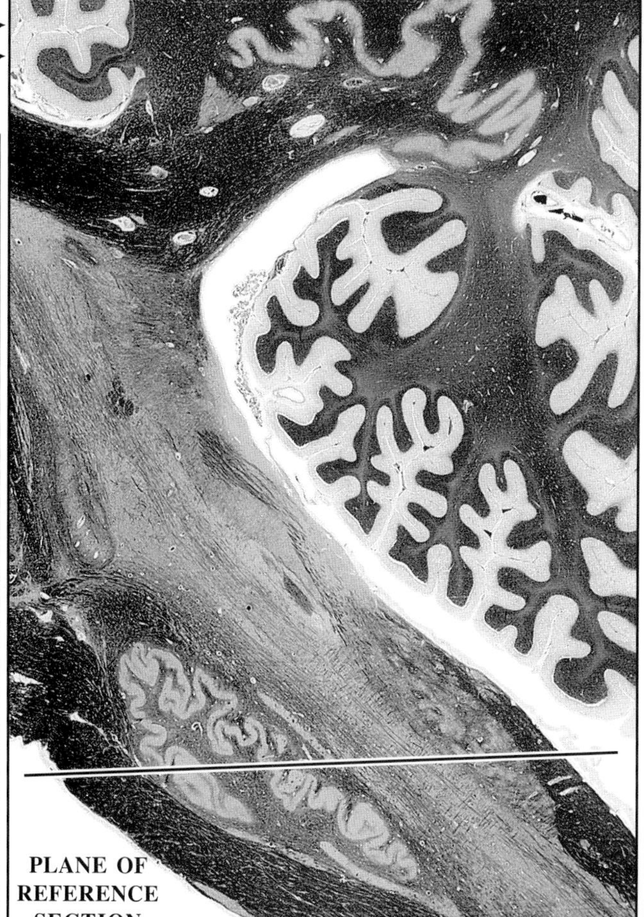

PLANE OF REFERENCE SECTION

OBLIQUE SECTION (APPROXIMATING THE CORONAL PLANE) OF THE BRAINSTEM: LEVEL INCLUDING THE SUPERIOR AND INFERIOR COLLICULI, THE LATERAL AND MEDIAL LEMNISCI, THE MIDDLE CEREBELLAR PEDUNCLES, THE INFERIOR OLIVARY NUCLEI, AND THE MEDULLARY PYRAMIDS

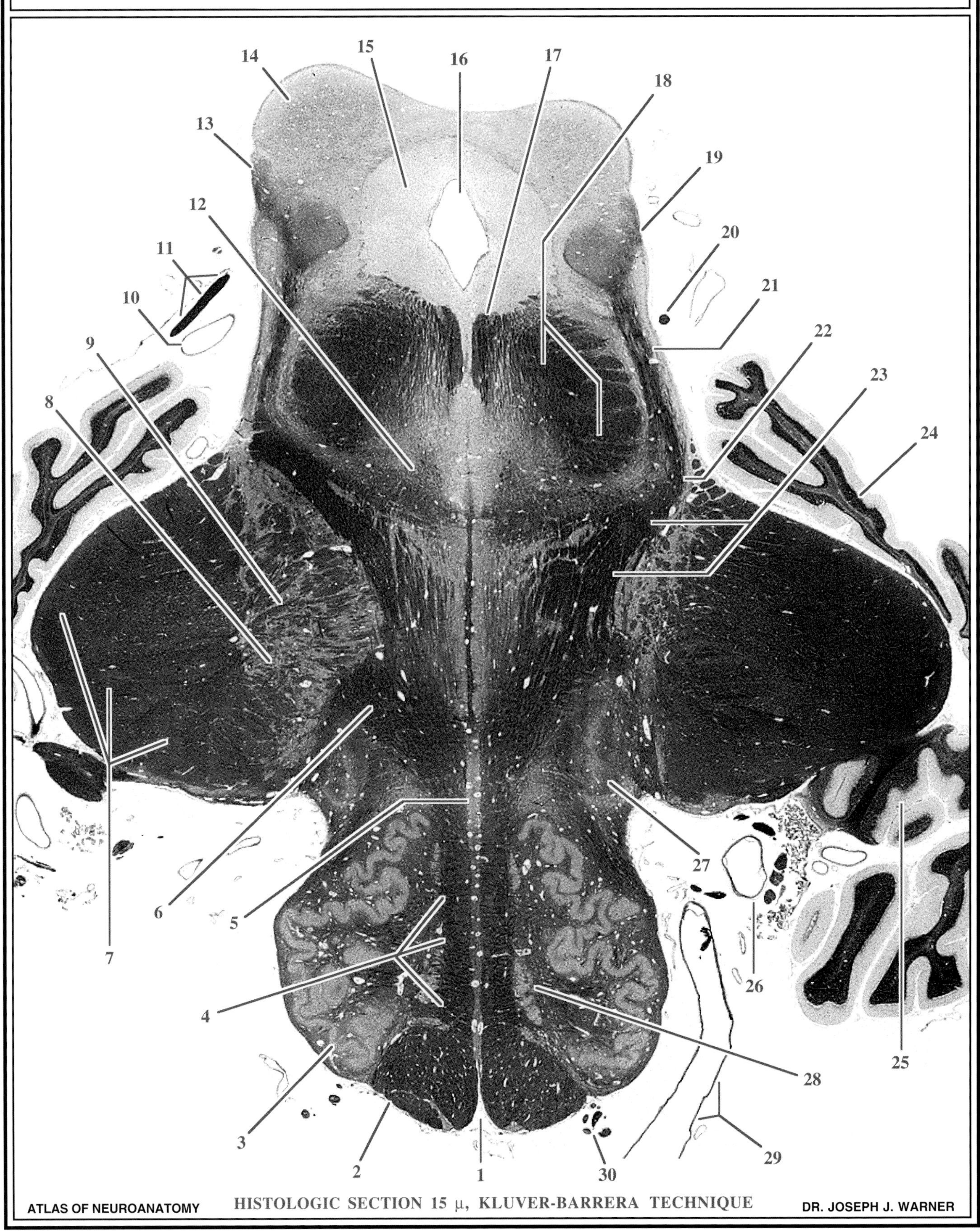

ATLAS OF NEUROANATOMY — HISTOLOGIC SECTION 15 μ, KLUVER-BARRERA TECHNIQUE — DR. JOSEPH J. WARNER

OBLIQUE SECTION (APPROXIMATING THE CORONAL PLANE) OF THE BRAINSTEM: LEVEL INCLUDING THE SUPERIOR AND INFERIOR COLLICULI, THE LATERAL AND MEDIAL LEMNISCI, THE MIDDLE CEREBELLAR PEDUNCLES, THE INFERIOR OLIVARY NUCLEI, AND THE MEDULLARY PYRAMIDS

KEY TO NUMBERED STRUCTURES

1. Ventral Median Fissure
2. Medullary Pyramid
3. Inferior Olivary Nucleus
4. Medial Lemniscus*
5. Median Raphe Nuclei
6. Central Tegmental Tract*
7. Middle Cerebellar Peduncle
8. Pontine Nuclei
9. Transverse (Pontocerebellar) Fibers
10. Superior Cerebellar Artery
11. Trochlear (IV) Nerve
12. Central Tegmental Tract*
13. Brachium of the Inferior Colliculus
14. Superior Colliculus
15. Periaqueductal Gray
16. Aqueduct of Sylvius
17. Medial Longitudinal Fasciculus
18. Superior Cerebellar Peduncle
19. Inferior Colliculus
20. Trochlear (IV) Nerve
21. Lateral Lemniscus
22. Spinothalamic Tract
23. Medial Lemniscus*
24. Folium of the Anterior Lobe of the Cerebellum
25. Flocculus
26. Posterior Inferior Cerebellar Artery
27. Spinal Tract of the Trigeminal Nerve
28. Medial Accessory Olivary Nucleus
29. Vertebral Artery
30. Fascicles of the Hypoglossal (XII) Nerve

* The arcuate course of the central tegmental tract and of the medial lemniscus is evident on sagittal sections, as these tracts pass dorsal to the basis pontis. Each of these tracts passes through this plane of section twice (see section orientation map). The central tegmental tract originates in the red nucleus, passes through the pontine tegmentum, then curves ventrally to terminate in the inferior olivary nucleus. Each medial lemniscus shifts dorsolaterally as it courses rostrally from the medulla through the pons and mesencephalon, and terminates in the thalamus.

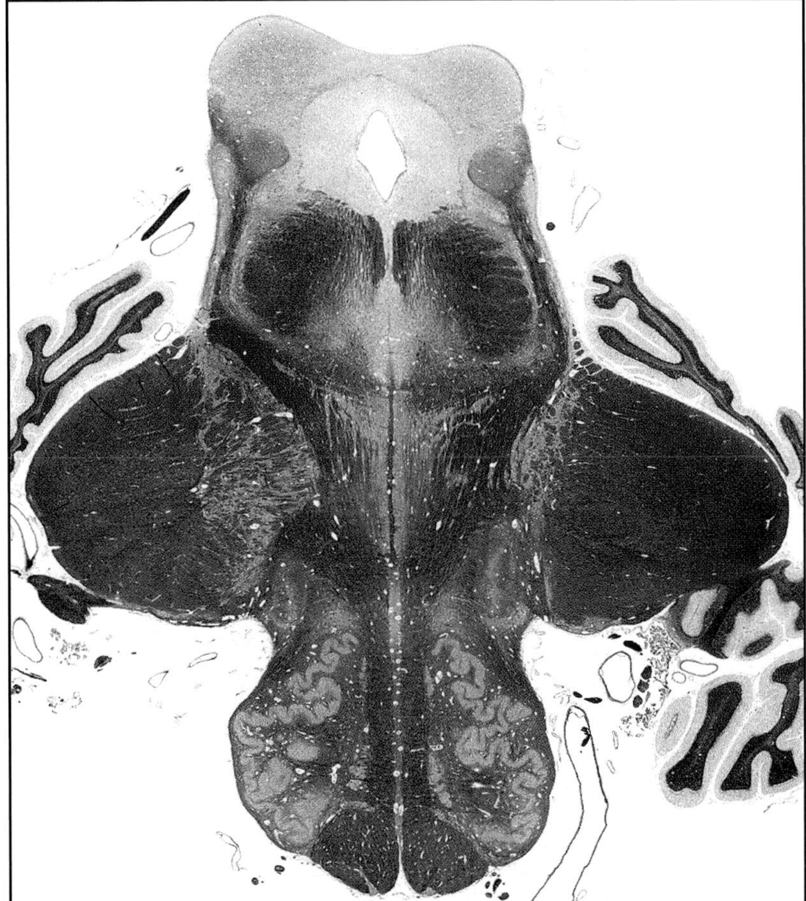

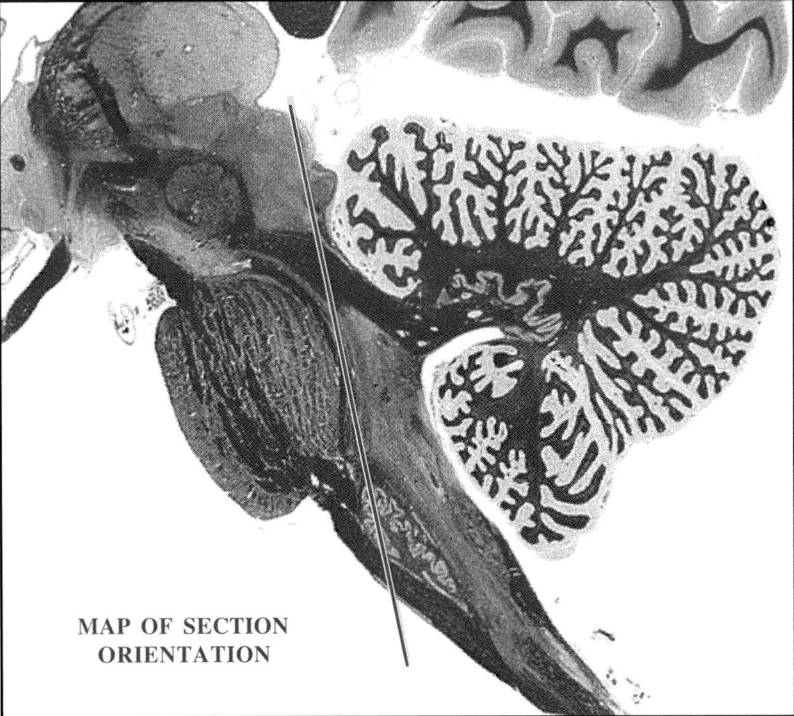

MAP OF SECTION ORIENTATION

HISTOLOGIC SECTIONS 15 μ, KLUVER-BARRERA TECHNIQUE

MEDULLA, TRANSVERSE SECTION: LEVEL OF THE CONVERGENCE OF THE VAGAL TRIGONE DORSAL TO THE HYPOGLOSSAL NUCLEI (CAUDAL OBEX)

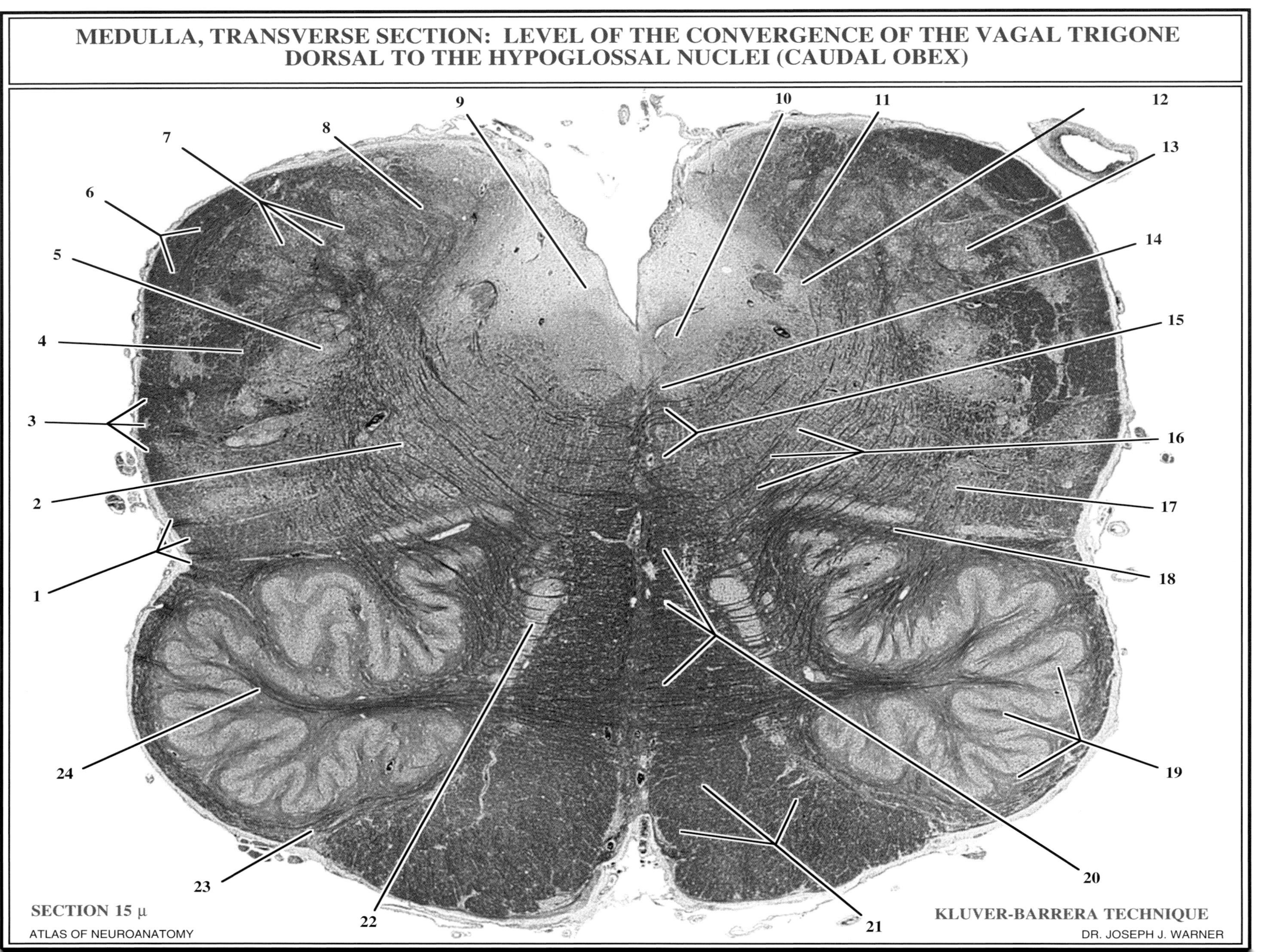

MEDULLA, TRANSVERSE SECTION, 15 μ, KLUVER-BARRERA TECHNIQUE
KEY TO NUMBERED STRUCTURES AND SECTION ORIENTATION MAP

1. Lateral Spinothalamic Tract
2. Nucleus Ambiguus
3. Ventral Spinocerebellar Tract
4. Spinal Tract of the Trigeminal Nerve
5. Spinal Trigeminal Nucleus
6. Dorsal Spinocerebellar Tract
7. Nucleus Cuneatus
8. Nucleus Gracilis
9. Dorsal Efferent Nucleus of the Vagus (X)
10. Hypoglossal Nucleus (XII)
11. Tractus Solitarius
12. Nucleus Solitarius
13. Lateral (Accessory) Cuneate Nucleus
14. Medial Longitudinal Fasciculus
15. Tectospinal Tract
16. Internal Arcuate Fibers
17. Lateral Reticular Nucleus
18. Dorsal Accessory Olivary Nucleus
19. Inferior Olivary Nucleus
20. Medial Lemniscus
21. Medullary Pyramid
22. Medial Accessory Olivary Nucleus
23. Fascicles of the Hypoglossal (XII) Nerve
24. Olivocerebellar Fibers

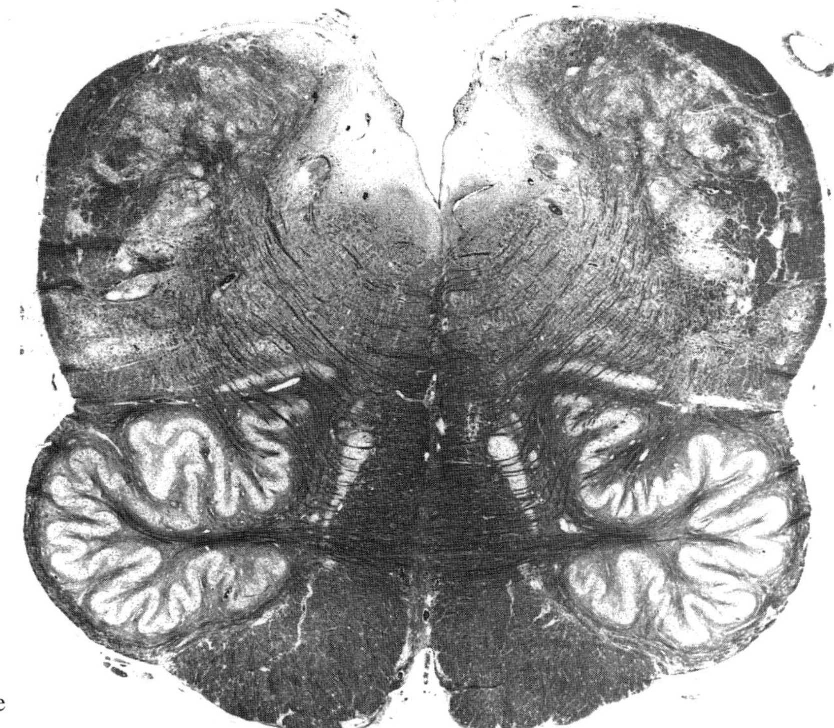

The plane of section includes the nucleus gracilis and nucleus cuneatus. This level is rostral to the majority of the fibers of the fasciculi gracilis and cuneatus. The internal arcuate fibers (lemniscal sensory decussation) are clearly discernible at this level.

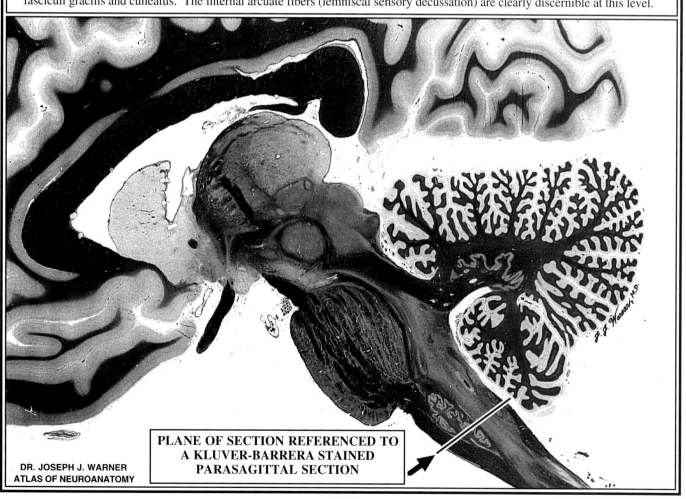

PLANE OF SECTION REFERENCED TO A KLUVER-BARRERA STAINED PARASAGITTAL SECTION

MEDULLA , CAUDAL PONS AND CEREBELLUM: SAGITTAL SECTION, 15 μ, BIELSCHOWSKY SILVER STAIN
LEVEL OF THE INFERIOR OLIVARY NUCLEUS, MEDIAL VESTIBULAR NUCLEUS, NUCLEUS AND TRACTUS SOLITARIUS, AND THE CENTRAL TEGMENTAL TRACT

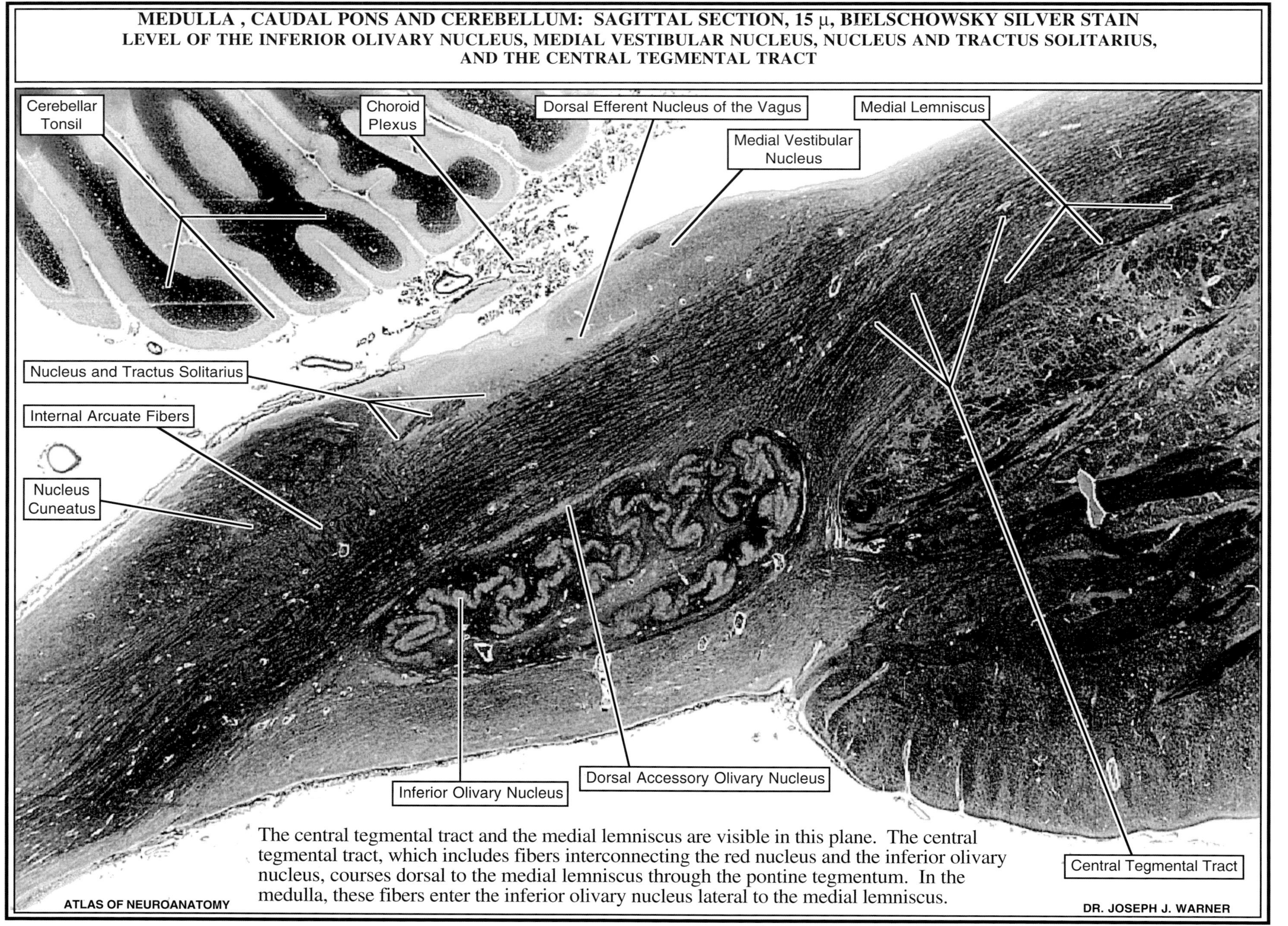

The central tegmental tract and the medial lemniscus are visible in this plane. The central tegmental tract, which includes fibers interconnecting the red nucleus and the inferior olivary nucleus, courses dorsal to the medial lemniscus through the pontine tegmentum. In the medulla, these fibers enter the inferior olivary nucleus lateral to the medial lemniscus.

MEDULLA, CAUDAL, TRANSVERSE SECTION: LEVEL OF THE NUCLEUS GRACILIS, NUCLEUS AND FASCICULUS CUNEATUS, AND OF THE ACCESSORY CUNEATE NUCLEUS

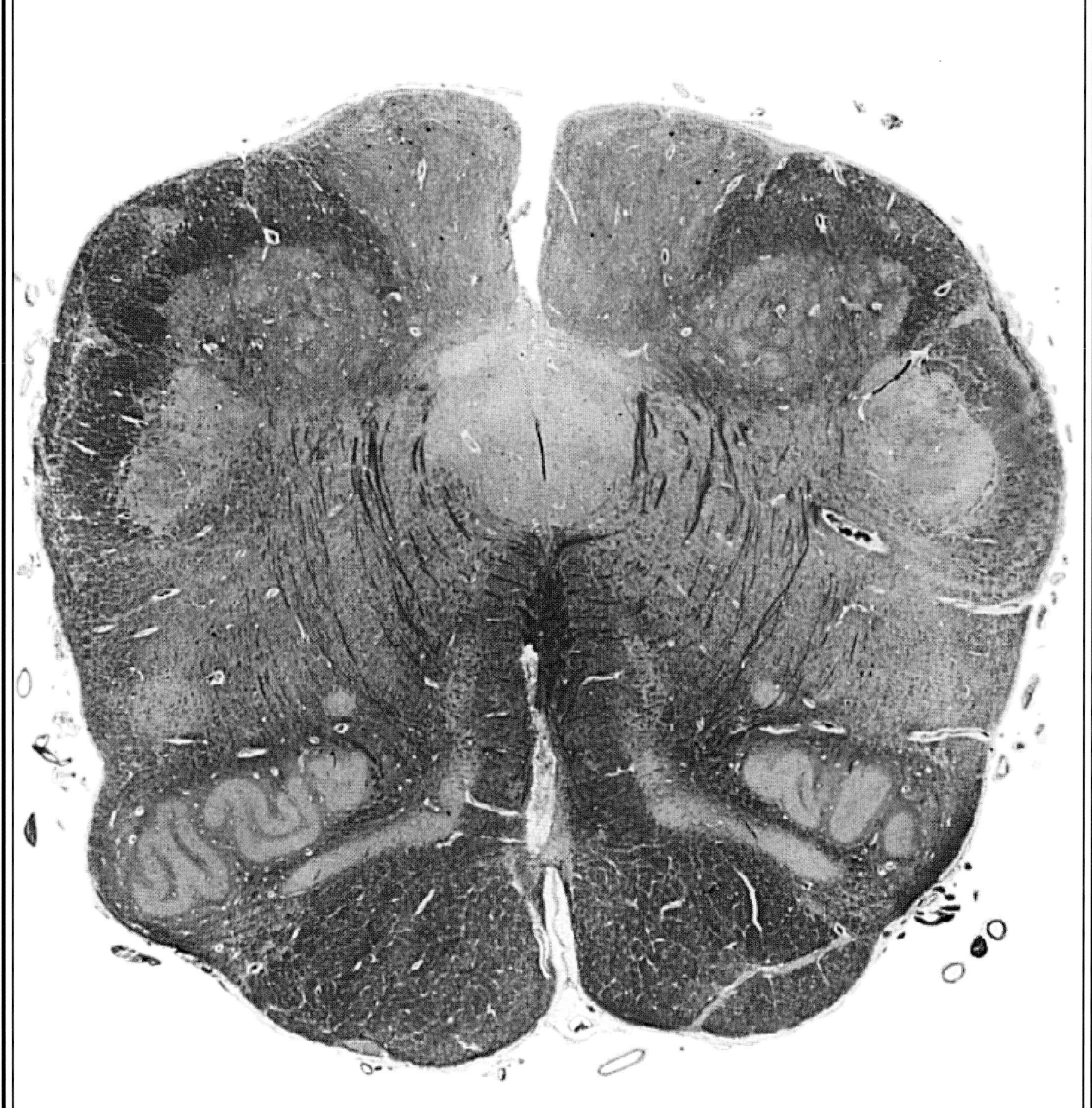

12 μ SECTION, KLUVER-BARRERA TECHNIQUE

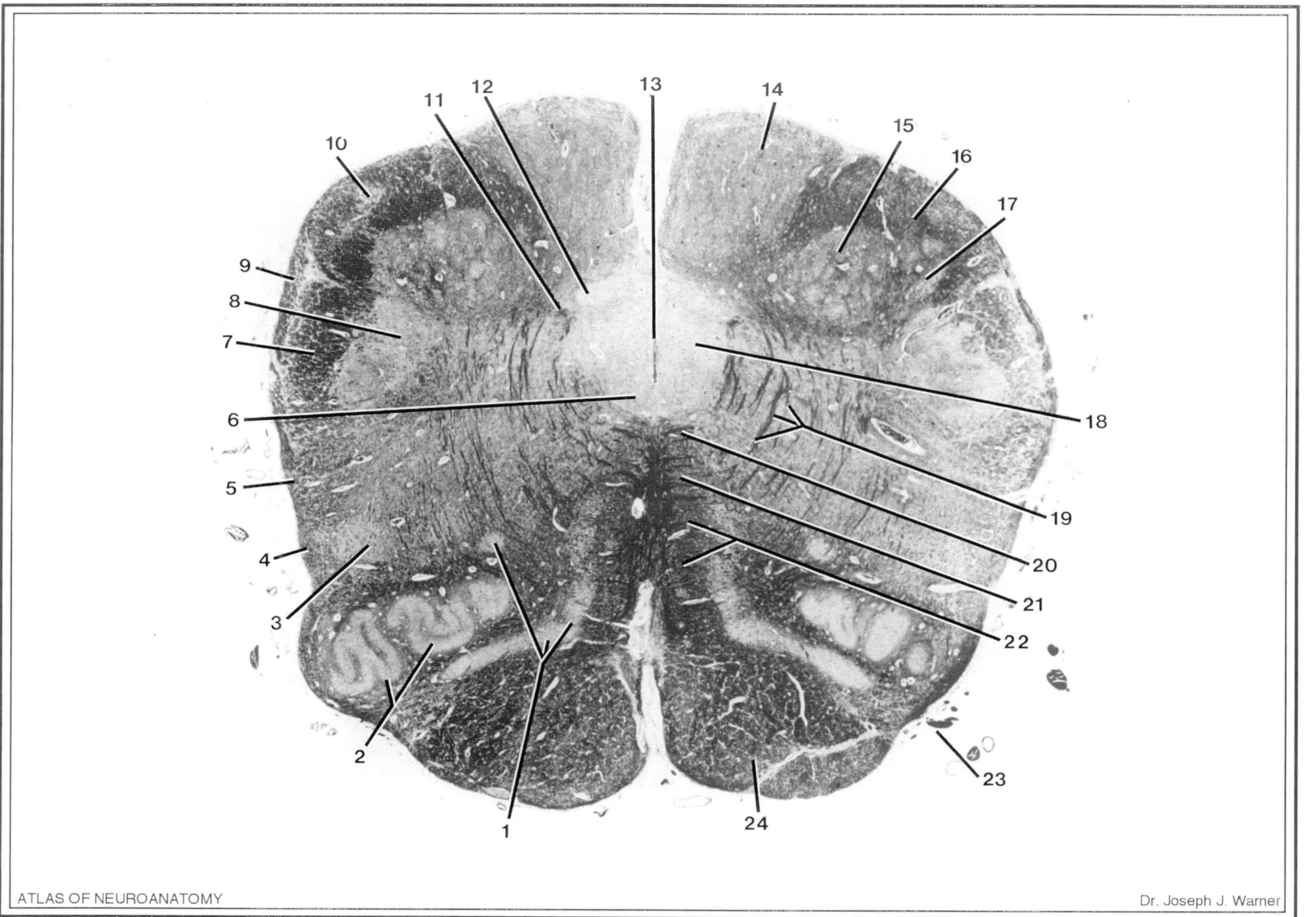

13
12
11
14
15
16
10
17
9
8
7
6
18
5
19
4
20
3
21
22
2
23
24
1
ATLAS OF NEUROANATOMY
Dr. Joseph J. Warner

CAUDAL MEDULLA, TRANSVERSE 15 μ SECTION, KLUVER-BARRERA TECHNIQUE
KEY TO NUMBERED STRUCTURES AND SECTION ORIENTATION MAP

1. Dorsal and Medial Accessory Olivary Nuclei
2. Inferior Olivary Nucleus
3. Lateral Reticular Nucleus
4. Lateral Spinothalamic Tract
5. Ventral Spinocerebellar Tract
6. Hypoglossal Nucleus (XII)
7. Spinal Tract of the Trigeminal Nerve
8. Spinal Trigeminal Nucleus
9. Dorsal Spinocerebellar Tract
10. Lateral (Accessory) Cuneate Nucleus
11. Tractus Solitarius
12. Nucleus Solitarius
13. Central Canal
14. Nucleus Gracilis
15. Nucleus Cuneatus
16. Fasciculus Cuneatus
17. Lateral (Accessory) Cuneate Nucleus
18. Dorsal Efferent Nucleus of the Vagus
19. Internal Arcuate Fibers (sensory decussation forming the Medial Lemniscus)
20. Medial Longitudinal Fasciculus
21. Tectospinal Tract
22. Medial Lemniscus
23. Fascicles of the Hypoglossal (XII) Nerve
24. Medullary Pyramid

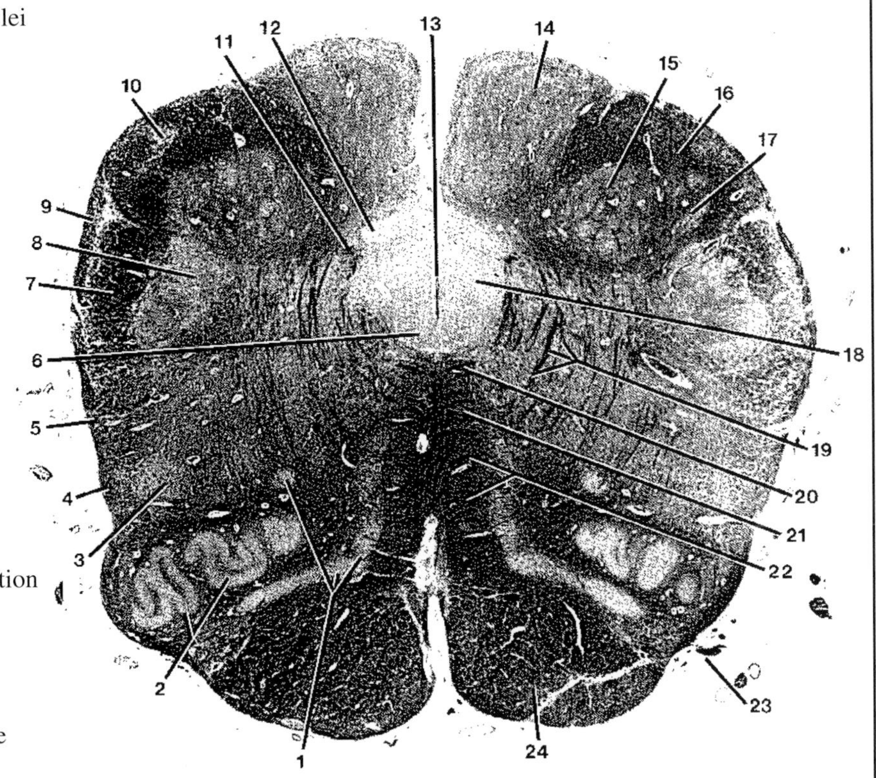

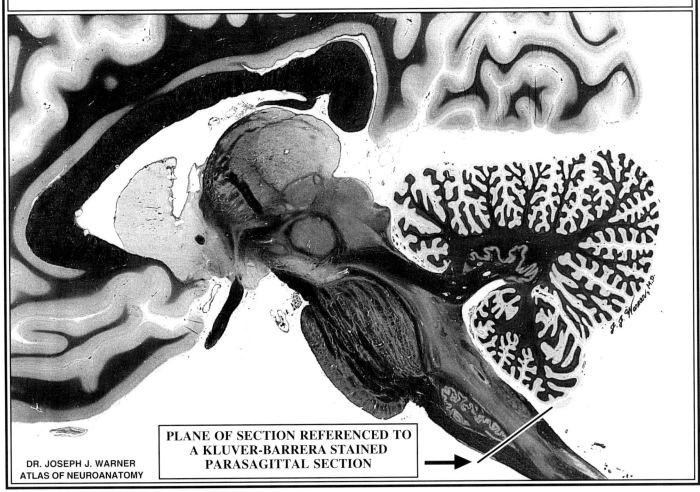

PLANE OF SECTION REFERENCED TO A KLUVER-BARRERA STAINED PARASAGITTAL SECTION

DR. JOSEPH J. WARNER
ATLAS OF NEUROANATOMY

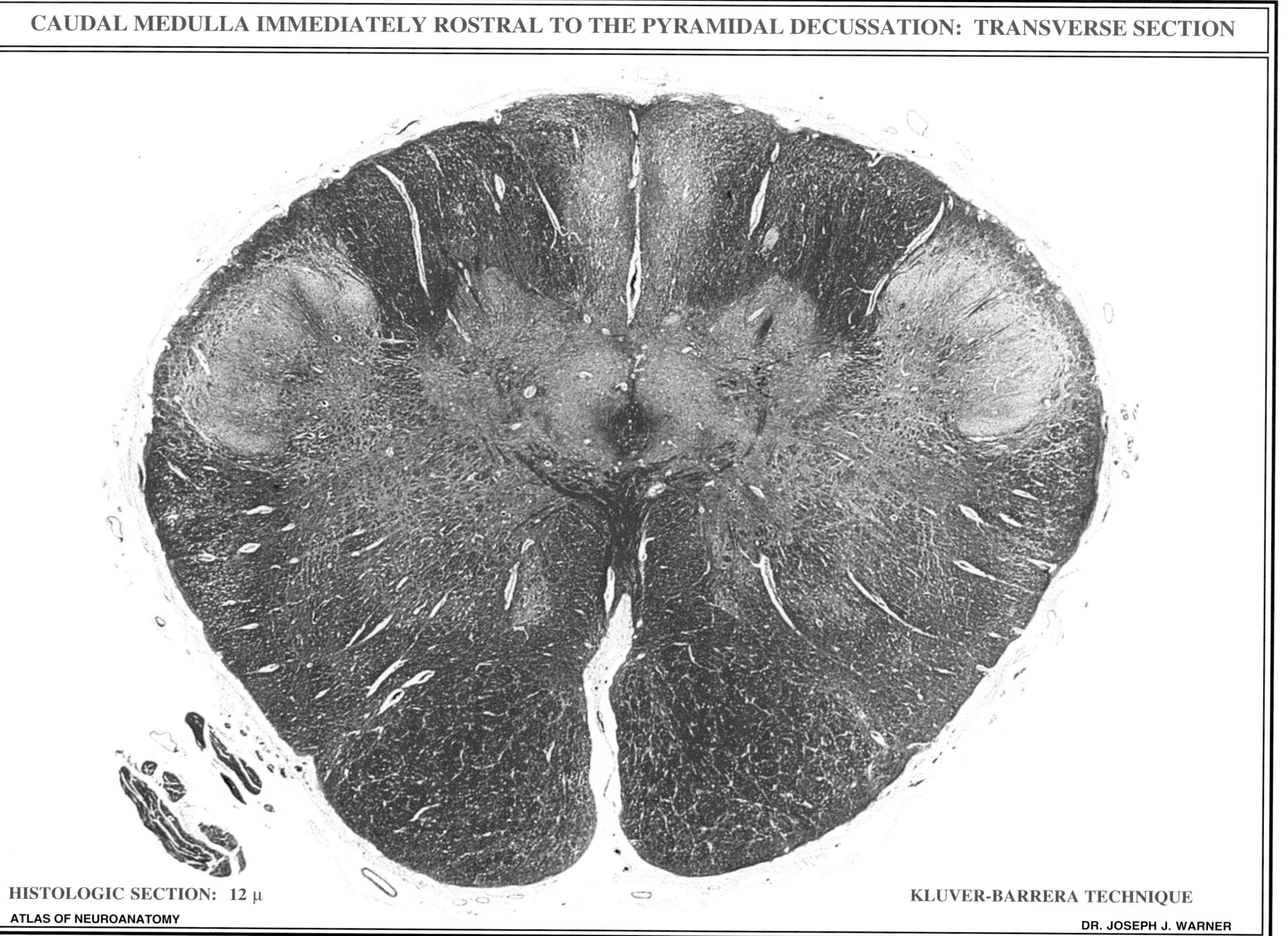
CAUDAL MEDULLA IMMEDIATELY ROSTRAL TO THE PYRAMIDAL DECUSSATION: TRANSVERSE SECTION
HISTOLOGIC SECTION: 12 μ
KLUVER-BARRERA TECHNIQUE
ATLAS OF NEUROANATOMY
DR. JOSEPH J. WARNER

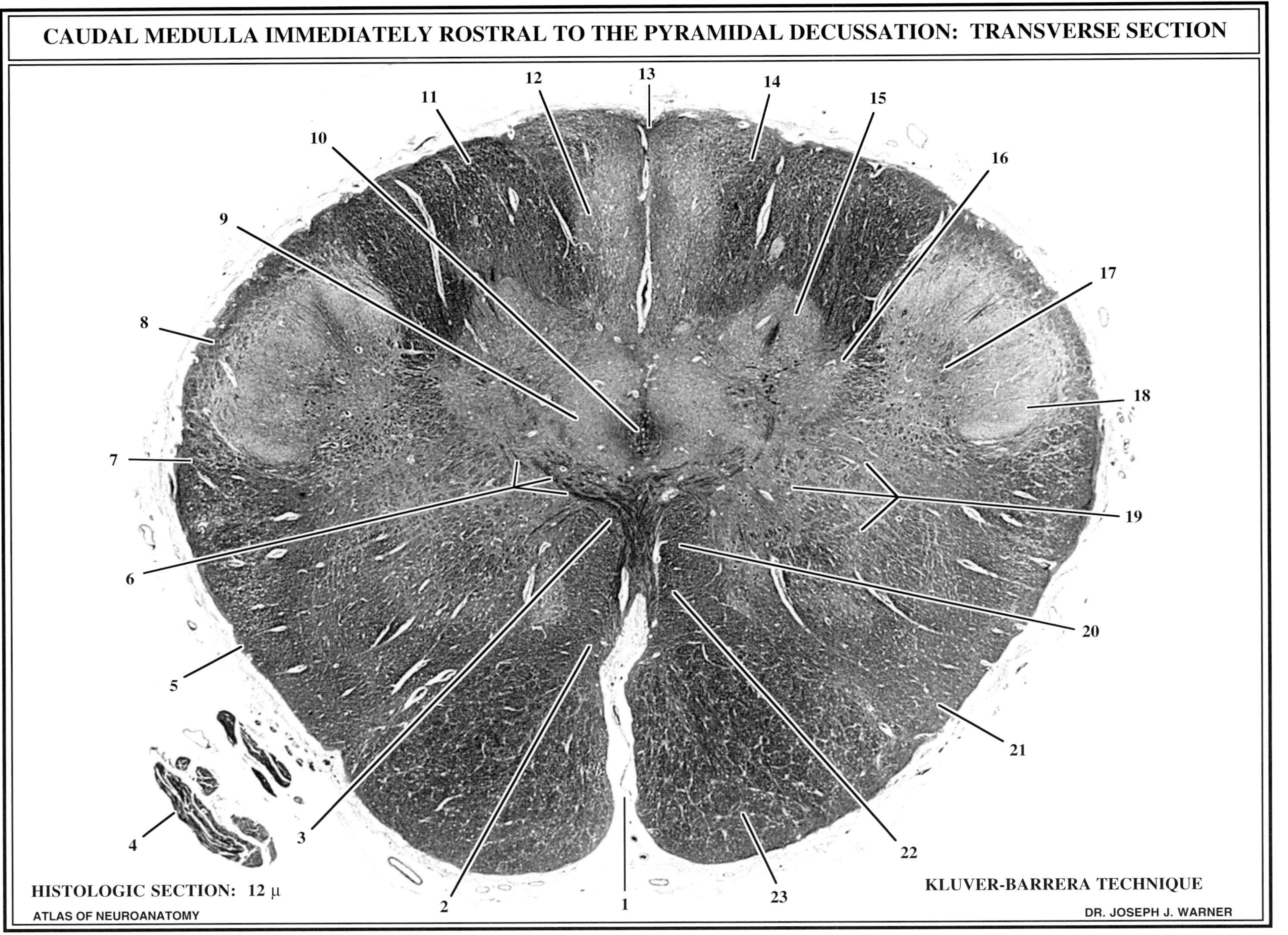
CAUDAL MEDULLA IMMEDIATELY ROSTRAL TO THE PYRAMIDAL DECUSSATION: TRANSVERSE SECTION
1
2
3
4
5
6
7
8
9
10
11
12
13
14
15
16
17
18
19
20
21
22
23
HISTOLOGIC SECTION: 12 μ
ATLAS OF NEUROANATOMY
KLUVER-BARRERA TECHNIQUE
DR. JOSEPH J. WARNER

CAUDAL MEDULLA, TRANSVERSE SECTION: LEVEL IMMEDIATELY ROSTRAL TO THE PYRAMIDAL DECUSSATION: SECTION MAP AND KEY TO NUMBERED STRUCTURES

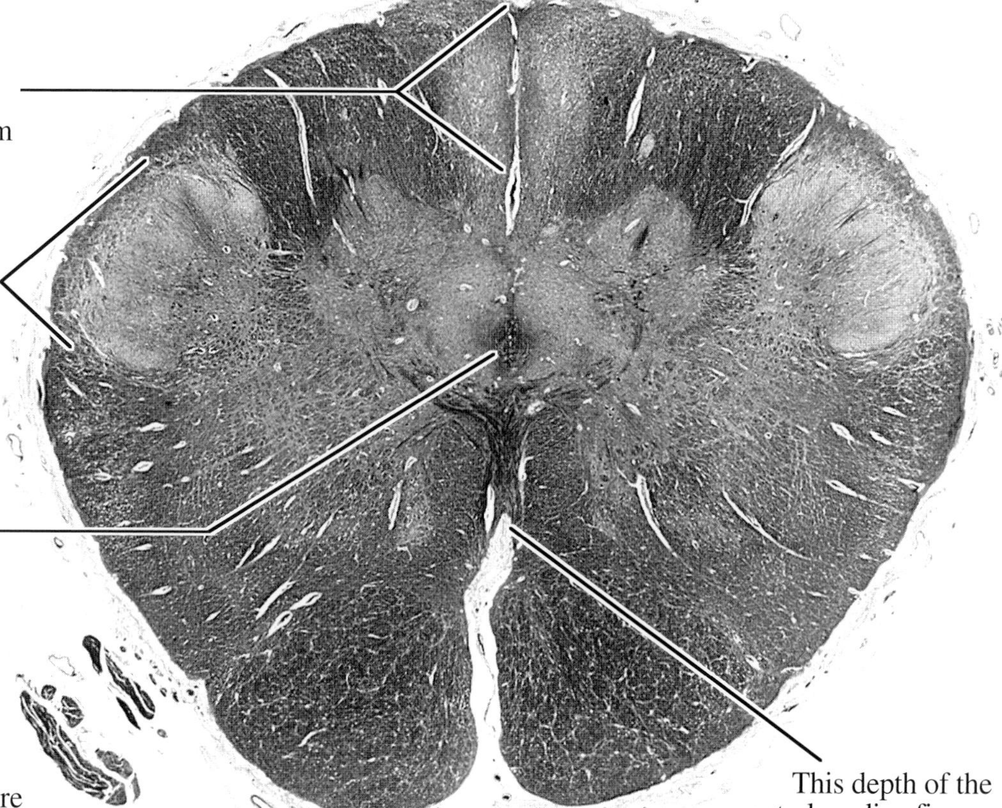

The floor of the fourth ventricle and the obex is replaced by the dorsal median sulcus and septum
The spinal tract and nucleus of the trigeminal nerve continues into rostral segments of the cervical spinal cord
The central canal appears caudal to the obex, and continues through the spinal cord dorsal to the ventral white commissure.
This depth of the ventral median fissure characterizes spinal levels.

1. Ventral Median Fissure
2. Rostral extent of the Pyramidal Decussation
3. Medial Longitudinal Fasciculus (contains the Medial Vestibulospinal Tract)
4. Fascicles of the Hypoglossal (XII) Nerve
5. Ventral Spinocerebellar Tract
6. Internal Arcuate Fibers
7. Dorsal Spinocerebellar Tract
8. Spinal Trigeminal Tract
9. Central Gray
10. Central Canal
11. Fasciculus Cuneatus
12. Nucleus Gracilis
13. Dorsal Median Sulcus
14. Fasciculus Gracilis
15. Nucleus Cuneatus
16. Accessory Cuneate Nucleus
17. Spinal Nucleus of the Trigeminal Nerve, Magnocellular Division
18. Spinal Nucleus of the Trigeminal Nerve, Division Gelatinosa
19. Reticular Formation
20. Tectospinal Tract
21. Spinothalamic and Spinotectal Tracts
22. Medial Lemniscus
23. Medullary Pyramid

Sections adjacent to the pyramidal decussation demonstrate characteristics of both the cervical spinal cord and the medulla. The central canal, the dorsal median sulcus, and the ventral median fissure are anatomic landmarks of the spinal cord.

TRANSVERSE PLANE MAPPED ON A SAGITTAL SECTION OF THE CAUDAL PONS AND MEDULLA

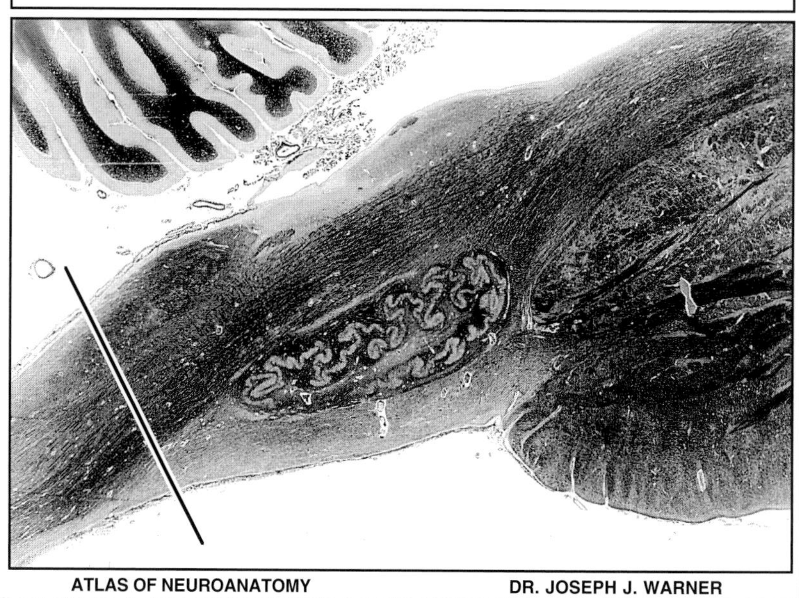

CERVICAL SPINAL CORD: TRANSVERSE SECTION THROUGH THE CERVICAL ENLARGEMENT

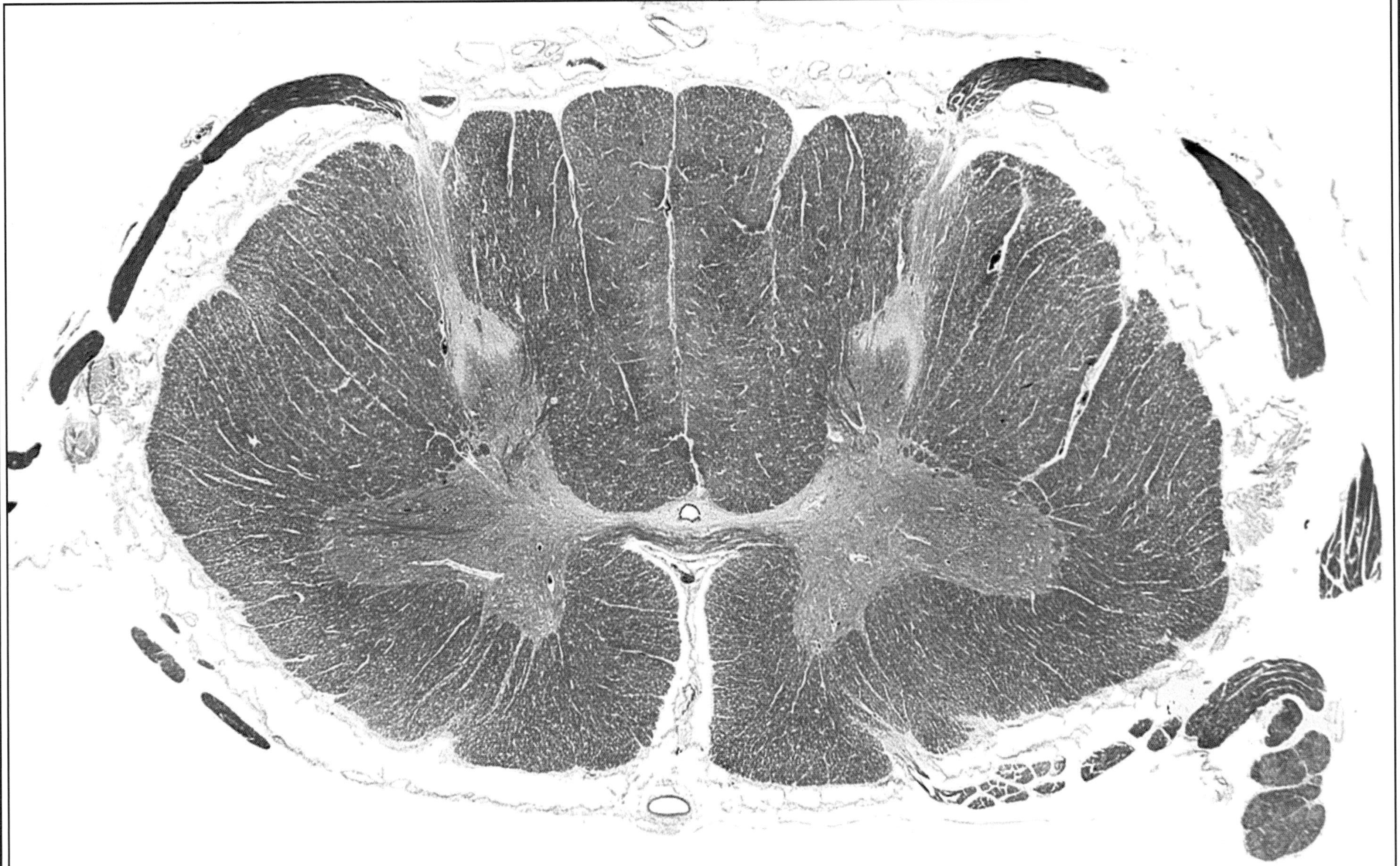

HISTOLOGIC SECTION 12 μ, LFB-PAS TECHNIQUE

DR. JOSEPH J. WARNER

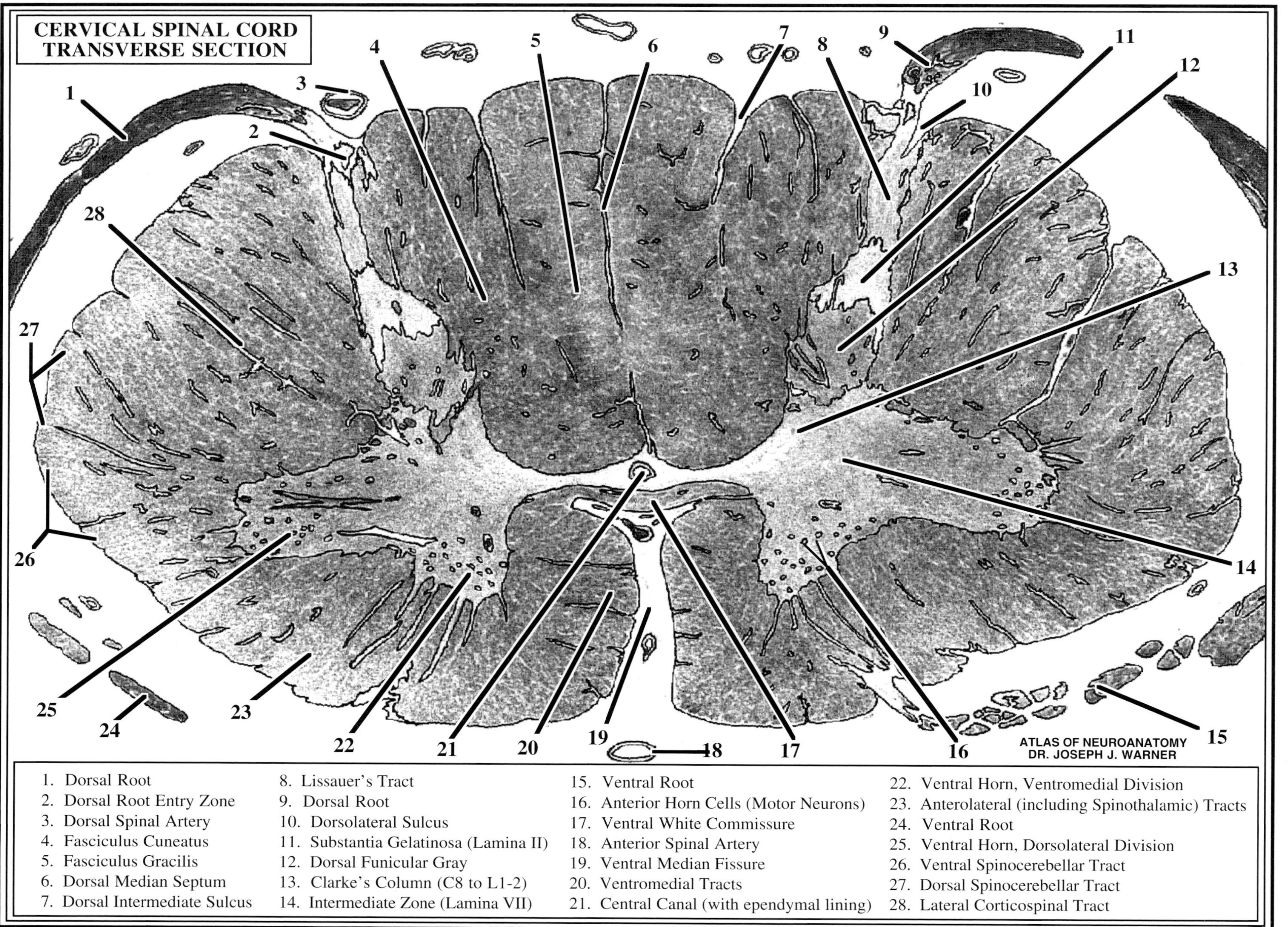
CERVICAL SPINAL CORD TRANSVERSE SECTION
1
2
3
4
5
6
7
8
9
10
11
12
13
14
15
16
17
18
19
20
21
22
23
24
25
26
27
28
ATLAS OF NEUROANATOMY
DR. JOSEPH J. WARNER
1. Dorsal Root
2. Dorsal Root Entry Zone
3. Dorsal Spinal Artery
4. Fasciculus Cuneatus
5. Fasciculus Gracilis
6. Dorsal Median Septum
7. Dorsal Intermediate Sulcus
8. Lissauer's Tract
9. Dorsal Root
10. Dorsolateral Sulcus
11. Substantia Gelatinosa (Lamina II)
12. Dorsal Funicular Gray
13. Clarke's Column (C8 to L1-2)
14. Intermediate Zone (Lamina VII)
15. Ventral Root
16. Anterior Horn Cells (Motor Neurons)
17. Ventral White Commissure
18. Anterior Spinal Artery
19. Ventral Median Fissure
20. Ventromedial Tracts
21. Central Canal (with ependymal lining)
22. Ventral Horn, Ventromedial Division
23. Anterolateral (including Spinothalamic) Tracts
24. Ventral Root
25. Ventral Horn, Dorsolateral Division
26. Ventral Spinocerebellar Tract
27. Dorsal Spinocerebellar Tract
28. Lateral Corticospinal Tract

TRANSVERSE SECTIONS OF THE CERVICAL SPINAL CORD: (A) LFB-PAS MYELIN STAIN, AND (B) BODIAN SILVER PROTEINATE TECHNIQUE

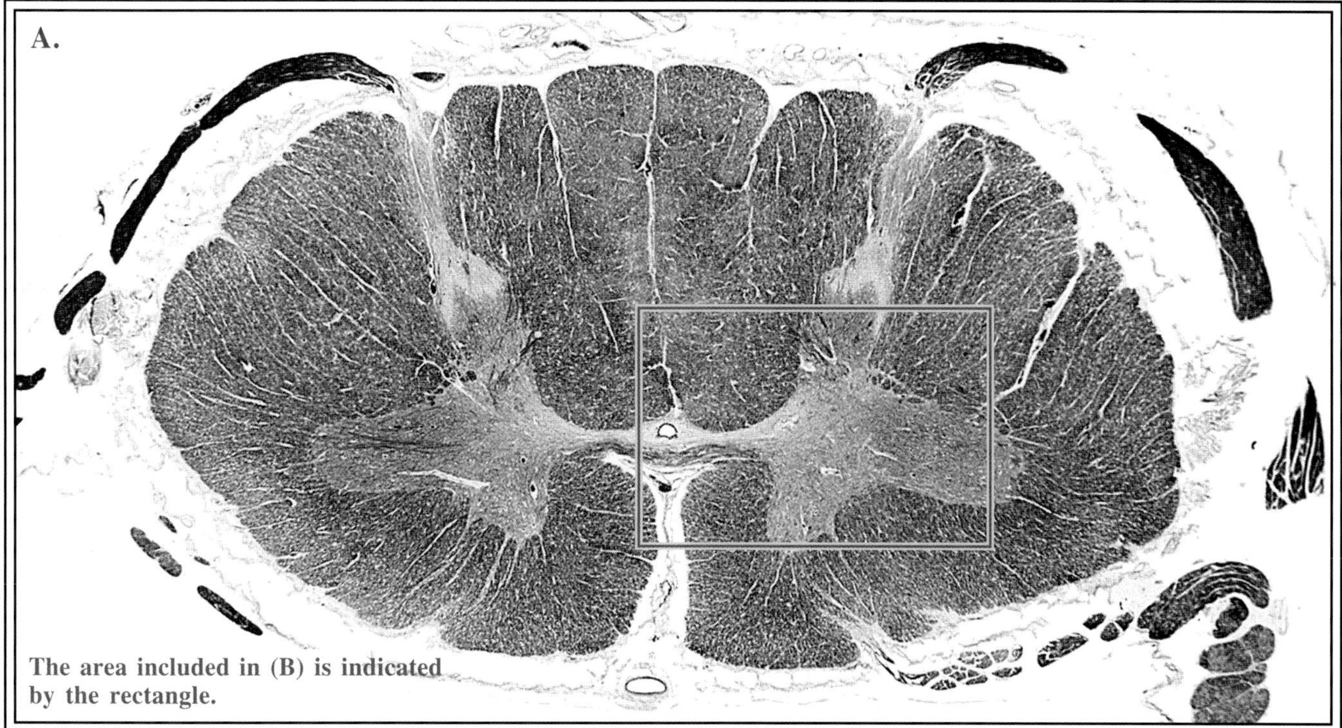

The area included in (B) is indicated by the rectangle.

The organization of myelinated fibers is shown on the LFB-PAS stained histologic section (A). In contrast, the section stained with the Bodian Silver Proteinate technique demonstrates neurons and their processes (B).

B.

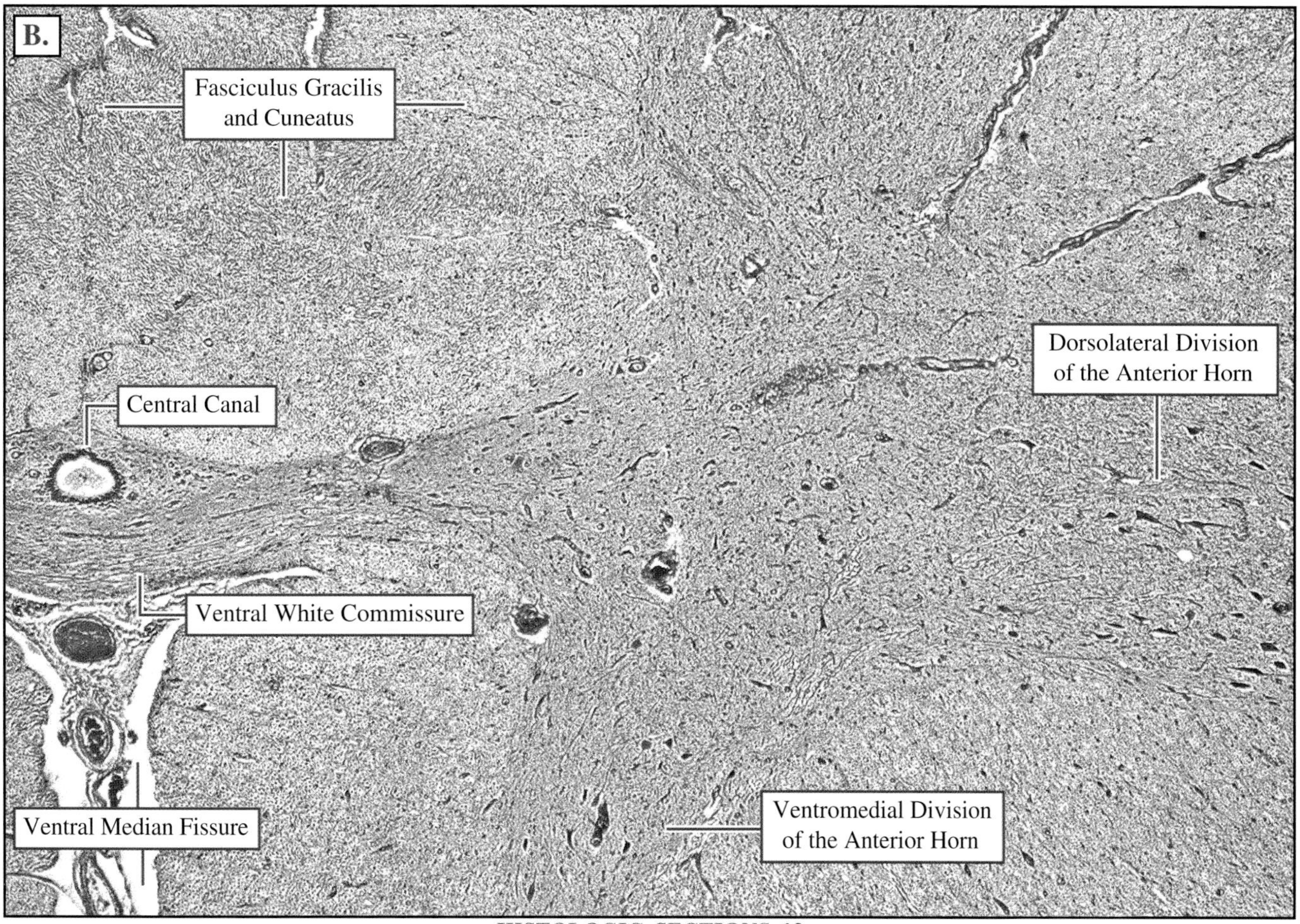

Fasciculus Gracilis and Cuneatus

Dorsolateral Division of the Anterior Horn

Central Canal

Ventral White Commissure

Ventral Median Fissure

Ventromedial Division of the Anterior Horn

THORACIC SPINAL CORD: TRANSVERSE SECTION THROUGH THE T6 LEVEL

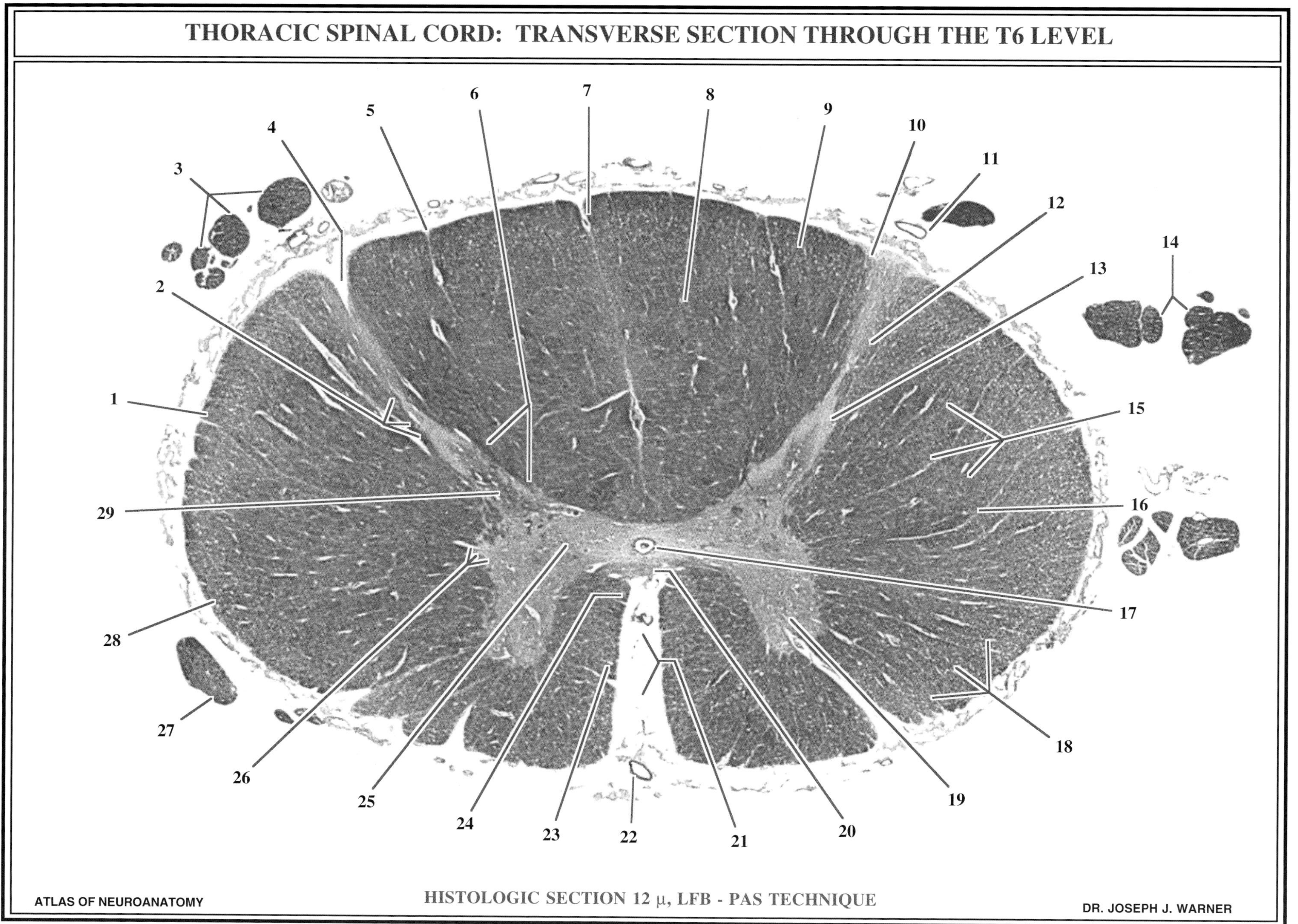

HISTOLOGIC SECTION 12 μ, LFB - PAS TECHNIQUE

DR. JOSEPH J. WARNER

THORACIC SPINAL CORD; TRANSVERSE SECTION THROUGH T6: KEY TO NUMBERED STRUCTURES

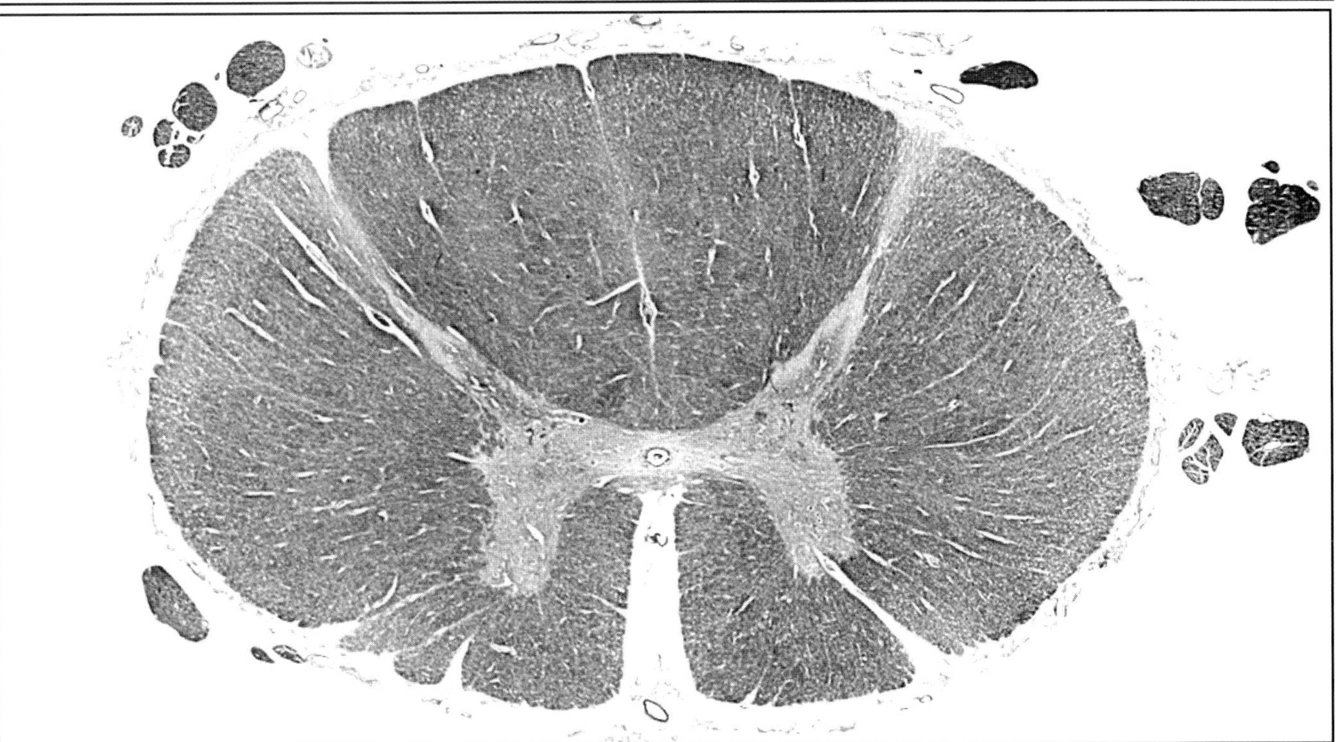

1. Dorsal Spinocerebellar Tract
2. Propriospinal System
3. Dorsal Roots
4. Dorsolateral Sulcus
5. Dorsal Intermediate Sulcus
6. Propriospinal System
7. Dorsal Median Sulcus
8. Fasciculus Gracilis
9. Fasciculus Cuneatus
10. Medial Division Fibers (of the dorsal root)
11. Dorsal Spinal Artery (bilateral)
12. Lissauer's Tract
13. Substantia Gelatinosa (Lamina II)
14. Dorsal Roots
15. Corticospinal Tract
16. Rubrospinal Tract (overlaps with the corticospinal fibers)
17. Central Canal
18. Spinothalamic Tract (component of the anterolateral system)
19. Ventral or Anterior Horn
20. Ventral White Commissure
21. Ventral Median Fissure
22. Anterior Spinal Artery
23. Ventral Corticospinal Tract
24. Medial Vestibulospinal Tract
25. Nucleus Dorsalis of Clark
26. Intermediolateral Cell Column
27. Ventral Root
28. Ventral Spinocerebellar Tract
29. Nucleus Proprius

Comparison of the thoracic spinal cord with the cervical or lumbar levels reveals a relatively diminutive size of the anterior or ventral horns. In contrast to the motor neuron pools innervating either the upper or lower extremities, the thoracic somatic motor innervation involves primarily axial musculature, including the intercostal muscles. The large ventromedial and dorsolateral divisions of the anterior horn of the cervical cord (refer to figure) are replaced by a smaller ventromedial anterior horn in the thoracic cord. The high white to gray matter ratio of the thoracic spinal cord is attributable to massive ascending and descending tracts communicating with lumbosacral levels. The intermediolateral cell column of the thoracic cord contains preganglionic sympathetic neurons modulated by ipsilateral descending projections from the hypothalamus.

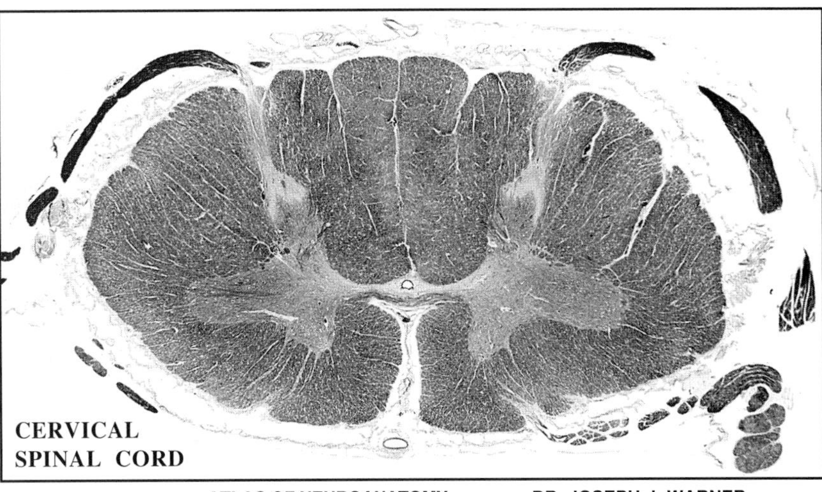

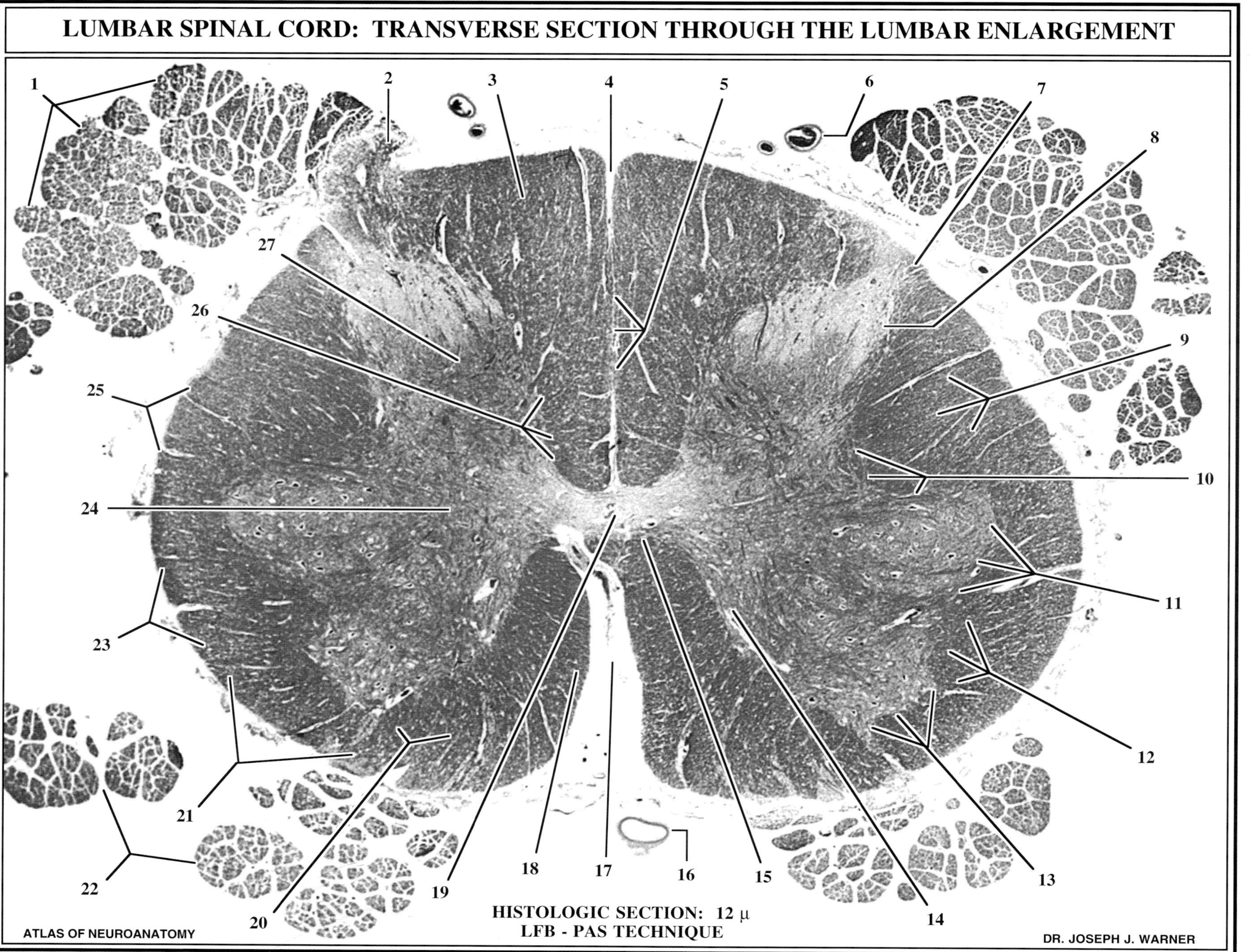
LUMBAR SPINAL CORD: TRANSVERSE SECTION THROUGH THE LUMBAR ENLARGEMENT
1
2
3
4
5
6
7
8
9
10
11
12
13
14
15
16
17
18
19
20
21
22
23
24
25
26
27
HISTOLOGIC SECTION: 12 μ
LFB - PAS TECHNIQUE
ATLAS OF NEUROANATOMY
DR. JOSEPH J. WARNER

LUMBAR SPINAL CORD; TRANSVERSE SECTION THROUGH THE LUMBAR ENLARGEMENT: KEY TO NUMBERED STRUCTURES

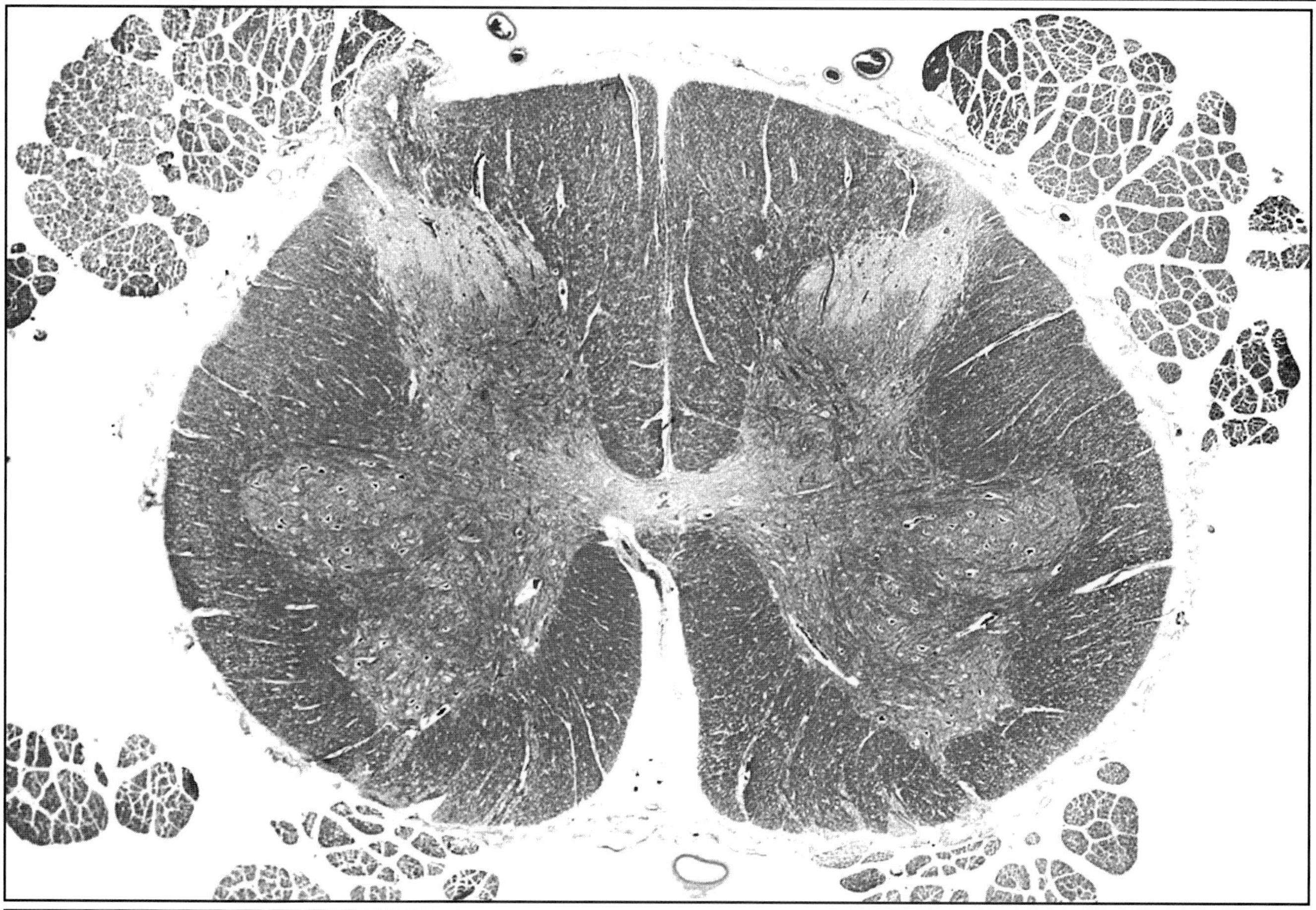

KEY TO NUMBERED STRUCTURES

1. Dorsal Roots
2. Medial Division Fibers (of the dorsal root)
3. Fasciculus Gracilis
4. Dorsal Median Sulcus
5. Dorsal Median Septum
6. Dorsal Spinal Artery (bilateral)
7. Lissauer's Tract
8. Substantia Gelatinosa (Lamina II)
9. Corticospinal Tract
10. Propriospinal System
11. Anterior Horn, Dorsolateral Division
12. Medullary Reticulospinal Tract
13. Anterior Horn, Ventromedial Division
14. Medial Motor Nuclei
15. Ventral White Commissure
16. Anterior Spinal Artery
17. Ventral Median Fissure
18. Ventral Corticospinal Tract
19. Central Canal
20. Lateral Vestibulospinal and Pontine Reticulospinal Tracts
21. Spinothalamic Tract
22. Ventral Roots
23. Ventral Spinocerebellar Tract
24. Intermediate Zone (Lamina VII)
25. Dorsal Spinocerebellar Tract
26. Propriospinal System
27. Nucleus Proprius

The high gray to white matter volume ratio of the lumbar spinal cord is segmentally related to the lumbosacral plexus. As in the cervical spinal cord, motor neuron pools are grouped into ventromedial and dorsolateral divisions. (Refer to figure below).

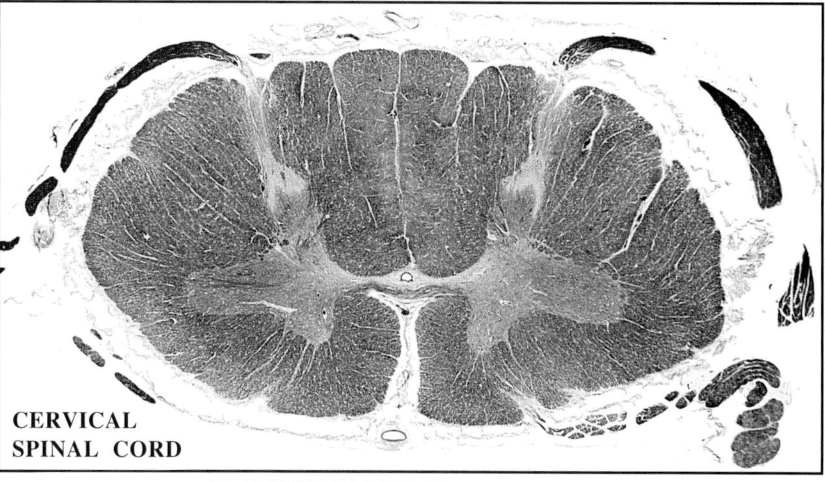

LUMBAR SPINAL CORD, TRANSVERSE SECTION THROUGH THE LUMBAR ENLARGEMENT: (A) LFB-PAS AND (B) BIELSCHOWSKY SILVER TECHNIQUE

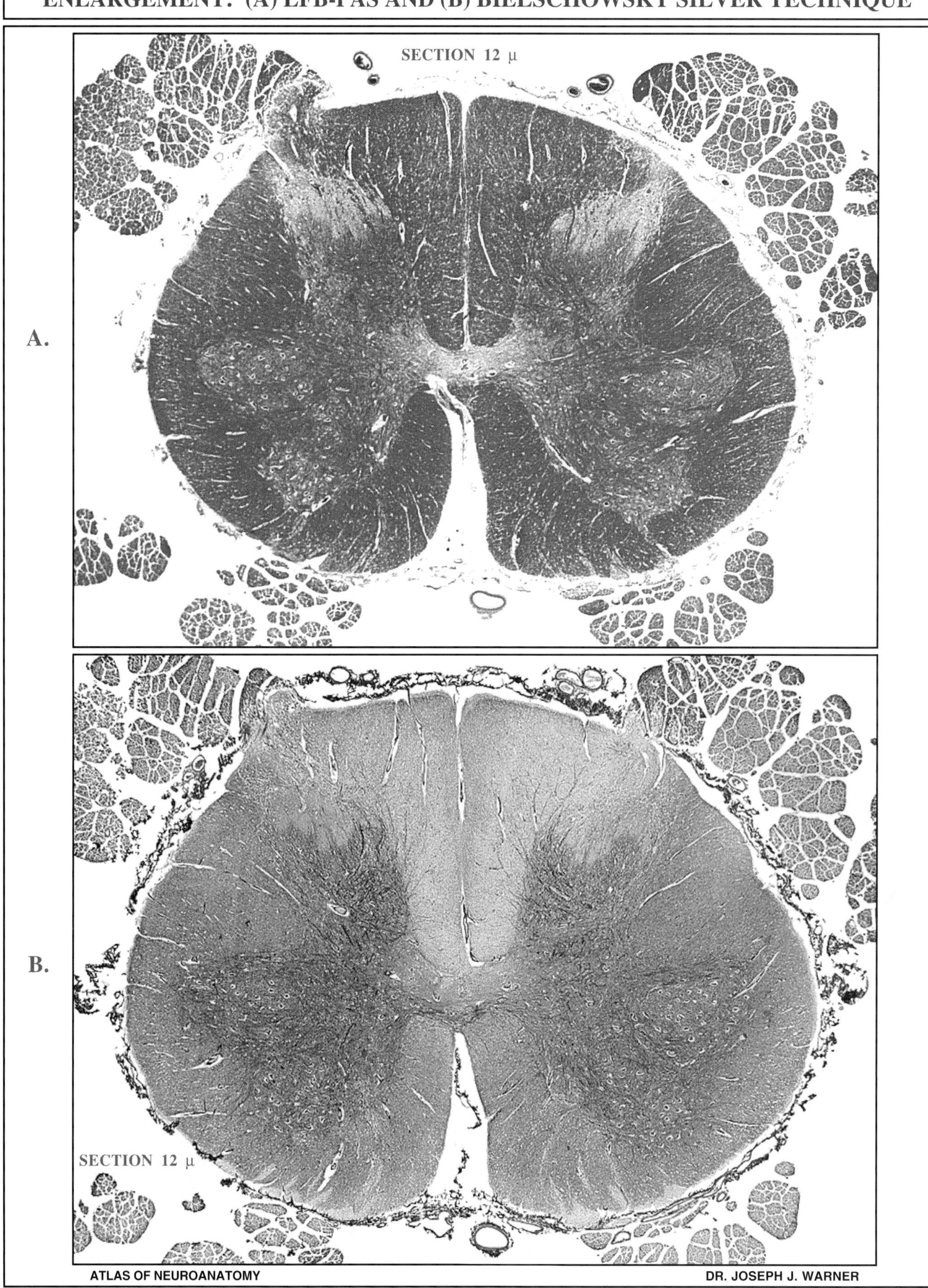

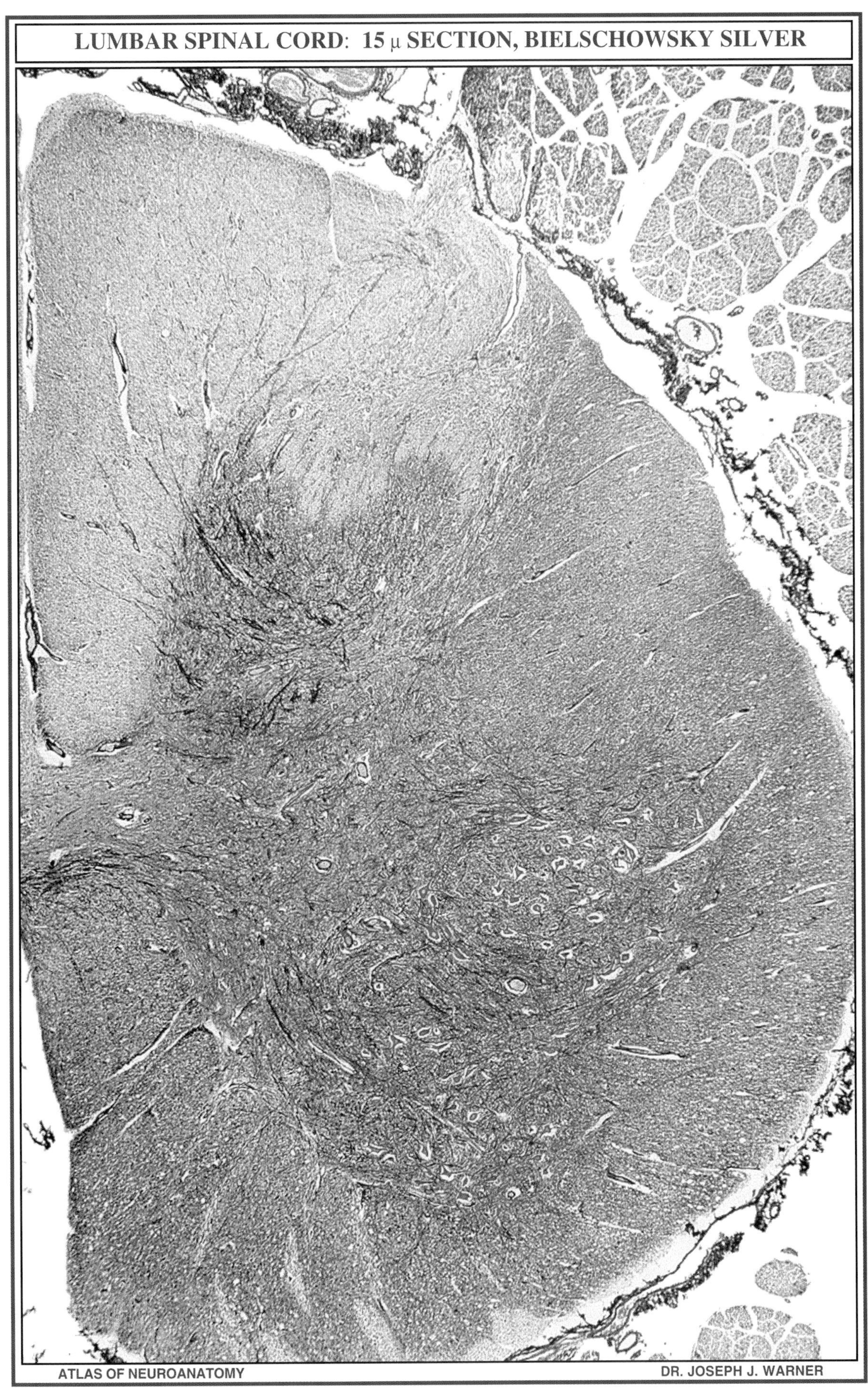
LUMBAR SPINAL CORD: 15 μ SECTION, BIELSCHOWSKY SILVER
ATLAS OF NEUROANATOMY
DR. JOSEPH J. WARNER

LUMBAR SPINAL CORD, TRANSVERSE SECTION: BIELSCHOWSKY SILVER TECHNIQUE, 15 μ

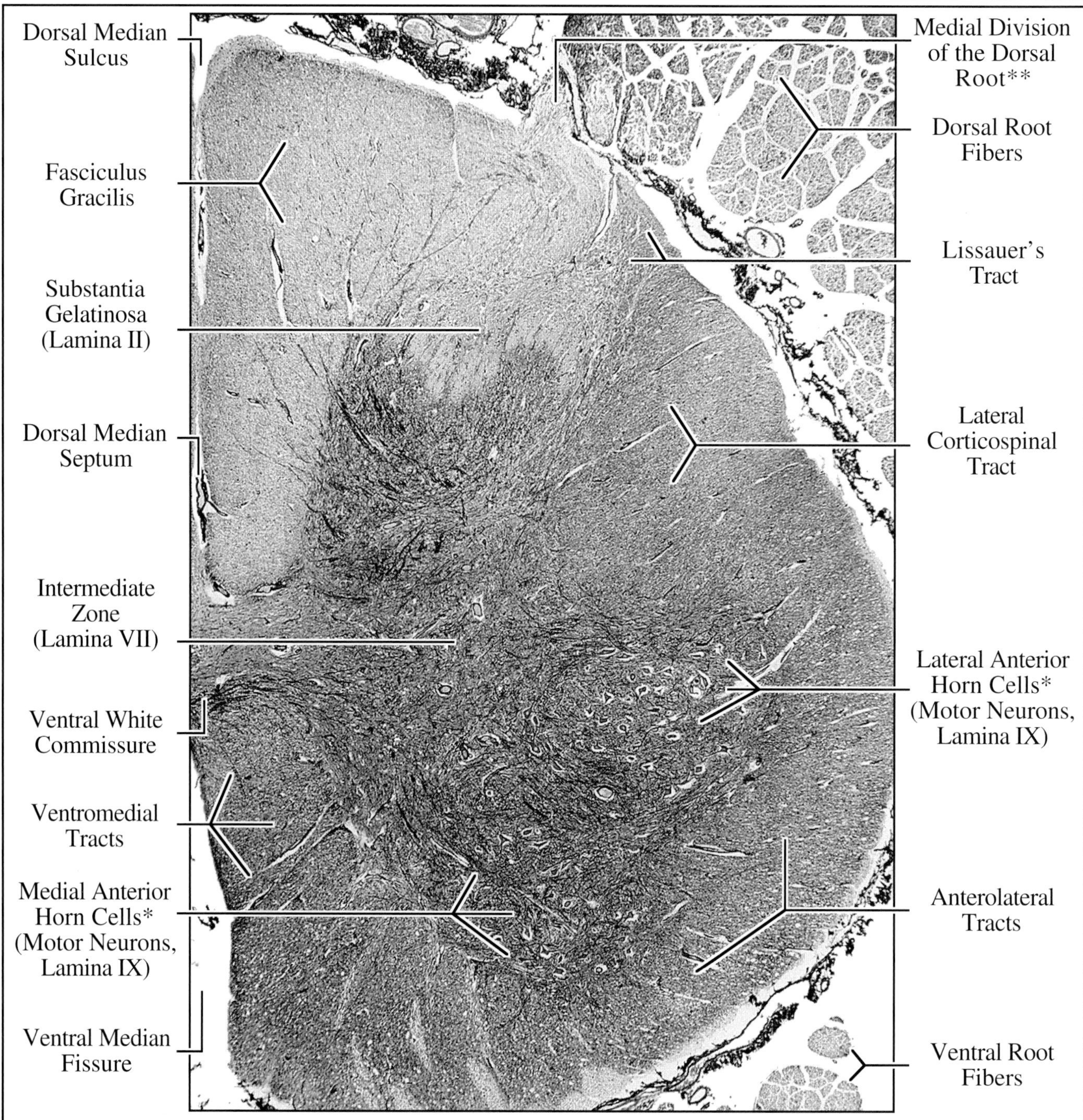

This transverse section includes one half of the spinal cord. The midline is defined by the ventral median fissure and the dorsal median sulcus. The dorsal median septum, a connective tissue layer extending ventrally from the dorsal median sulcus, passes between the left and the right fasciculus gracilis. The central canal is a midline structure just dorsal to the ventral white commissure. The Bielschowsky silver stain demonstrates neuronal processes and stains neurofibrillar elements of the neuronal cell bodies. Thus, even at this low magnification, large motor neurons are clearly discernible in the anterior horn. The nuclei of several neurons in this section are demarcated by a lucency in the center of the cell body.

*Motor neurons are not uniformly distributed throughout the anterior horn. Rather, they are segregated into groups or motor neuron pools, characterized by a somatotopic organization. Division of the anterior horn into ventromedial and dorsolateral divisions is quite prominent in the lumbar and cervical enlargements. **Fibers of the medial division of the dorsal root pass directly into the fasciculus gracilis.

A COMPARISON OF TRANSVERSE SECTIONS OF THE SPINAL CORD AT LUMBAR, THORACIC, AND CERVICAL LEVELS

A direct comparison of transverse sections of the lumbar, thoracic, and cervical spinal cord levels emphasizes the clear morphologic differences between these levels. On the basis of tract organization, gray to white matter ratio, and the specific components of the spinal gray, the general level of a given section may be readily identified. The dorsal columns of the lumbar spinal cord contain only the fasciculus gracilis bilaterally. Proceeding in a rostral direction, the fasciculus cuneatus appears as ascending fibers enter the dorsal columns lateral to fasciculus gracilis. In the lumbosacral cord, the lateral corticospinal tract is diminished in size in contrast to more rostral levels. Division of the anterior or ventral horn into ventromedial and dorsolateral divisions is discernible in the lumbar spinal cord, as it is in cervical levels. (This division of the ventral horn is not a characteristic of the thoracic spinal cord.)

An important aspect of the thoracic spinal cord is the presence of the intermediolateral cell column, containing preganglionic sympathetic neurons. The orientation of root fibers differs between lumbosacral and cervical levels. At cervical levels, roots course at an angle that is either perpendicular or oblique to the longitudinal axis of the spinal cord. At lumbar and sacral levels, roots are almost parallel to this axis. Thus, dorsal and ventral root fibers appear in oblique or longitudinal orientation in transverse histologic sections at cervical levels, in contrast to the transverse sectional appearance of root fibers at lumbar and sacral levels.

The external contour of transverse sections at the cervical and lumbar levels is also distinct. At the cervical enlargement, the cord has a smaller anteroposterior to mediolateral dimensional ratio than that of the lumbar spinal cord. These differences are clearly evident on studies such as computerized tomography and magnetic resonance imaging.

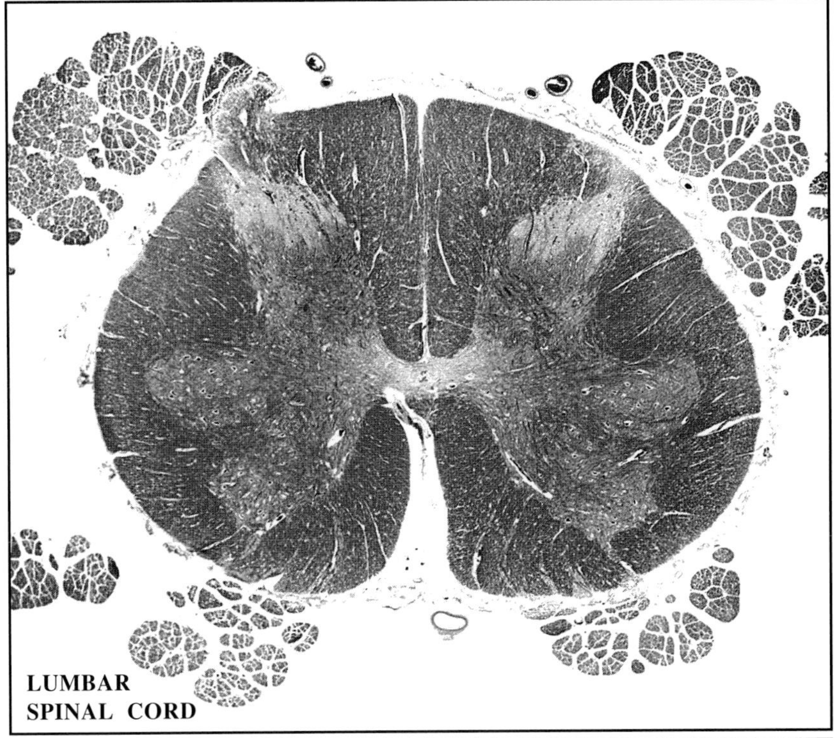

LUMBAR SPINAL CORD

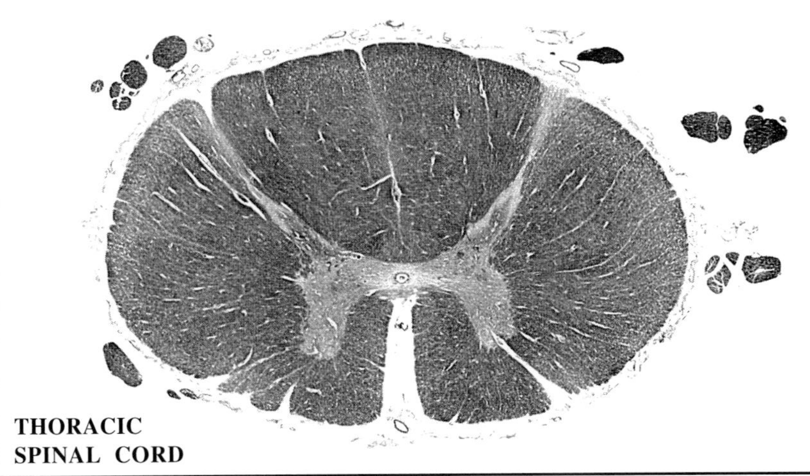

THORACIC SPINAL CORD

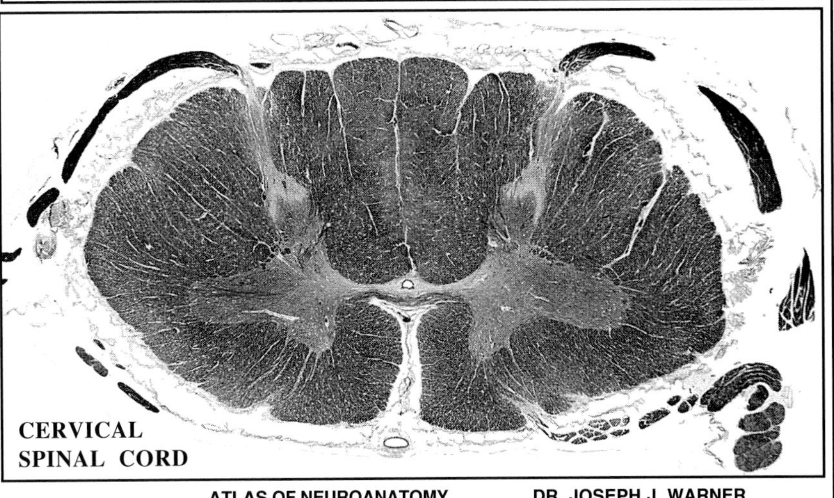

CERVICAL SPINAL CORD

PART VII: SCHEMATIC DIAGRAMS OF SYSTEMS ORGANIZATION AND CONNECTIVITY

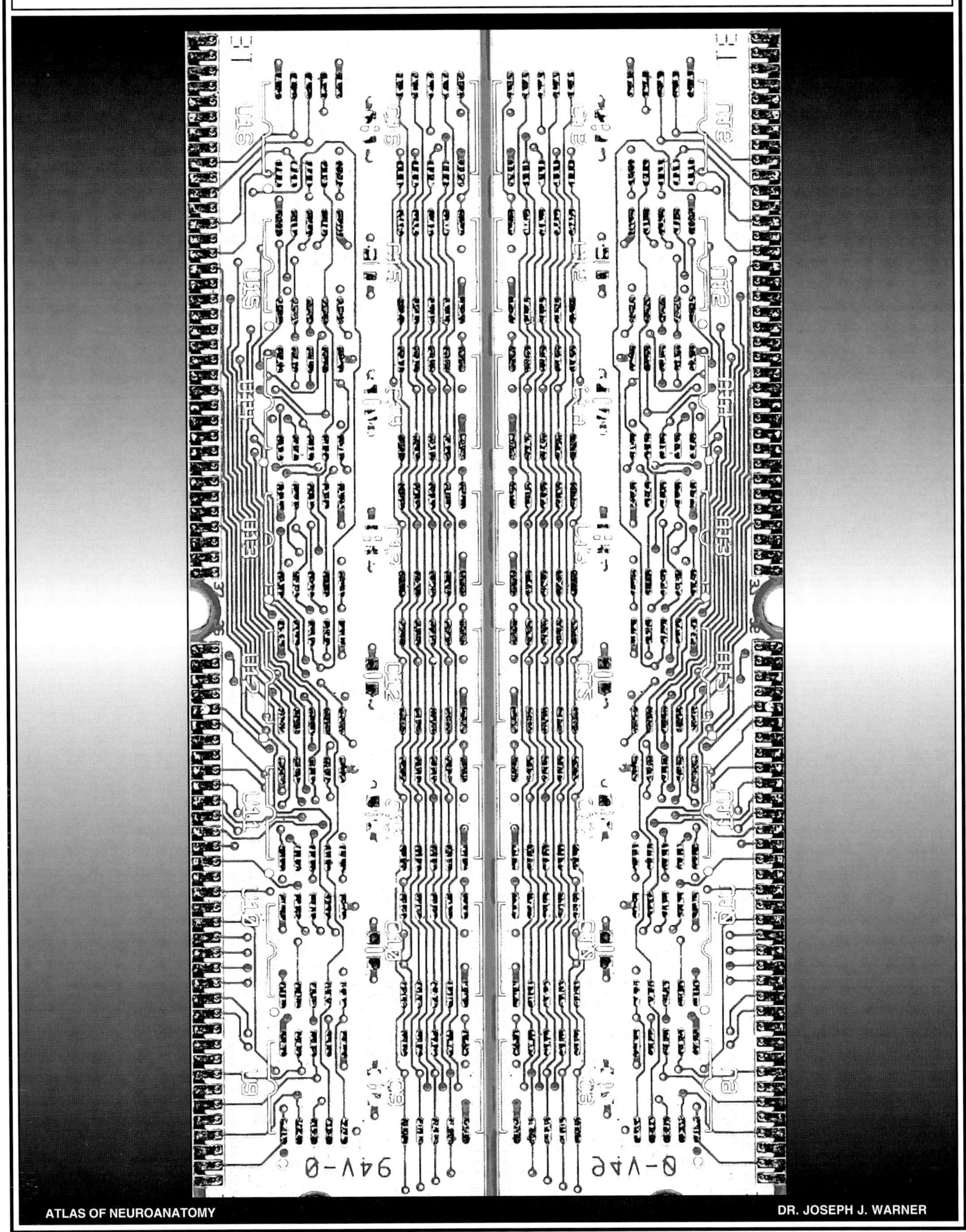

ATLAS OF NEUROANATOMY

DR. JOSEPH J. WARNER

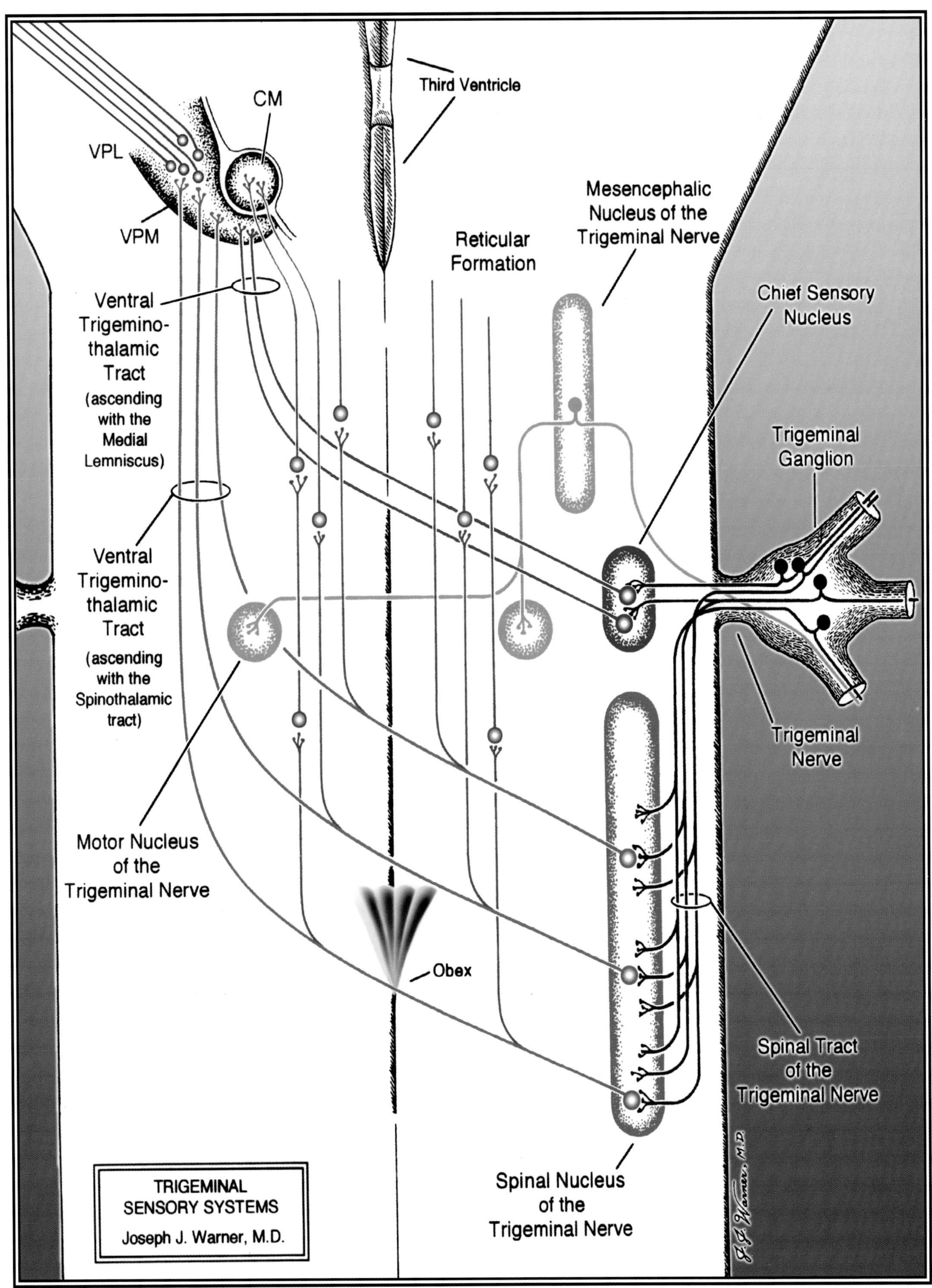

Third Ventricle
CM
VPL
VPM
Mesencephalic Nucleus of the Trigeminal Nerve
Reticular Formation
Ventral Trigemino-thalamic Tract (ascending with the Medial Lemniscus)
Chief Sensory Nucleus
Trigeminal Ganglion
Ventral Trigemino-thalamic Tract (ascending with the Spinothalamic tract)
Trigeminal Nerve
Motor Nucleus of the Trigeminal Nerve
Obex
Spinal Tract of the Trigeminal Nerve
Spinal Nucleus of the Trigeminal Nerve
TRIGEMINAL SENSORY SYSTEMS
Joseph J. Warner, M.D.
J.J. Warner, M.D.

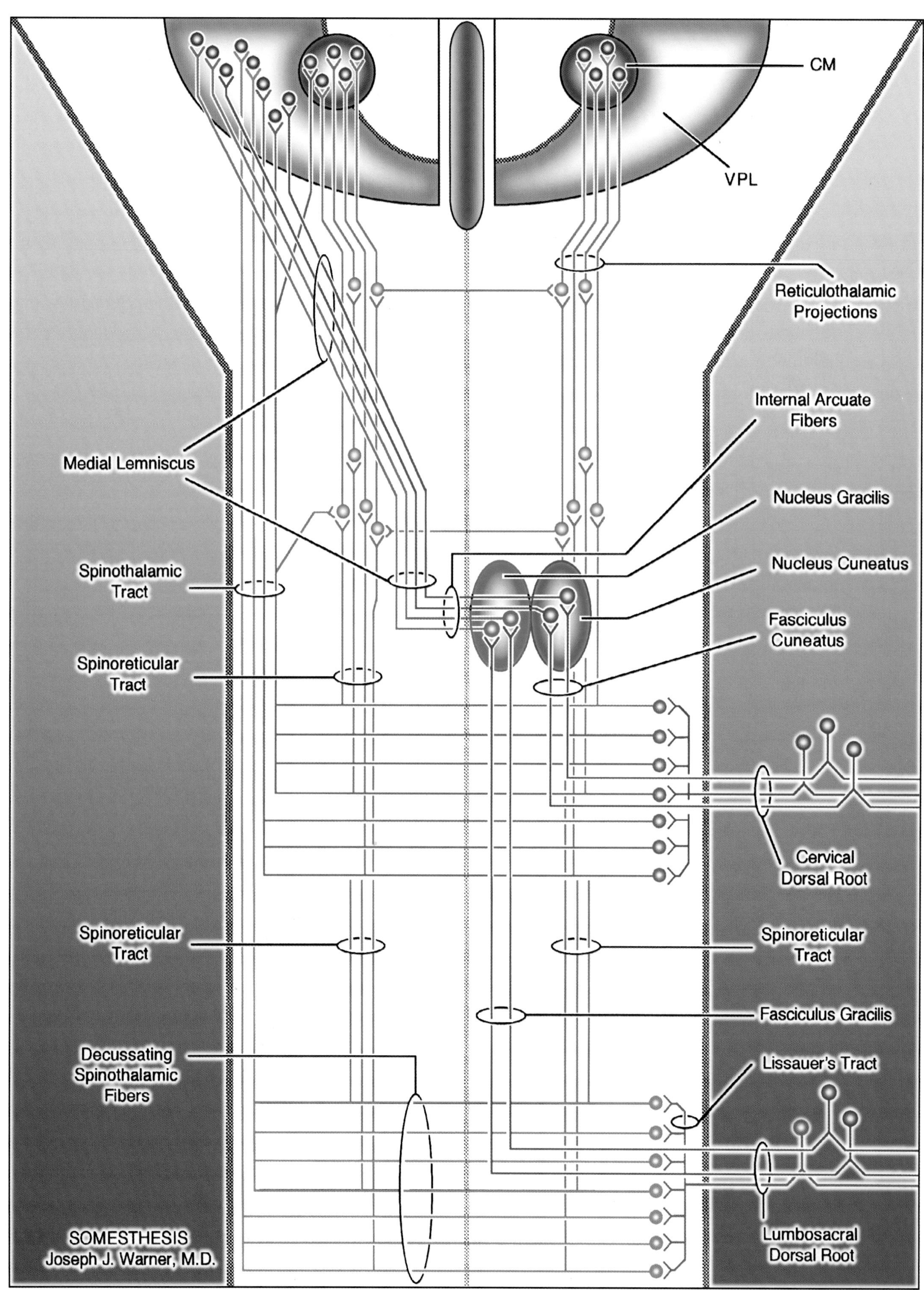
CM
VPL
Reticulothalamic Projections
Internal Arcuate Fibers
Medial Lemniscus
Nucleus Gracilis
Nucleus Cuneatus
Spinothalamic Tract
Fasciculus Cuneatus
Spinoreticular Tract
Cervical Dorsal Root
Spinoreticular Tract
Spinoreticular Tract
Fasciculus Gracilis
Decussating Spinothalamic Fibers
Lissauer's Tract
SOMESTHESIS
Joseph J. Warner, M.D.
Lumbosacral Dorsal Root

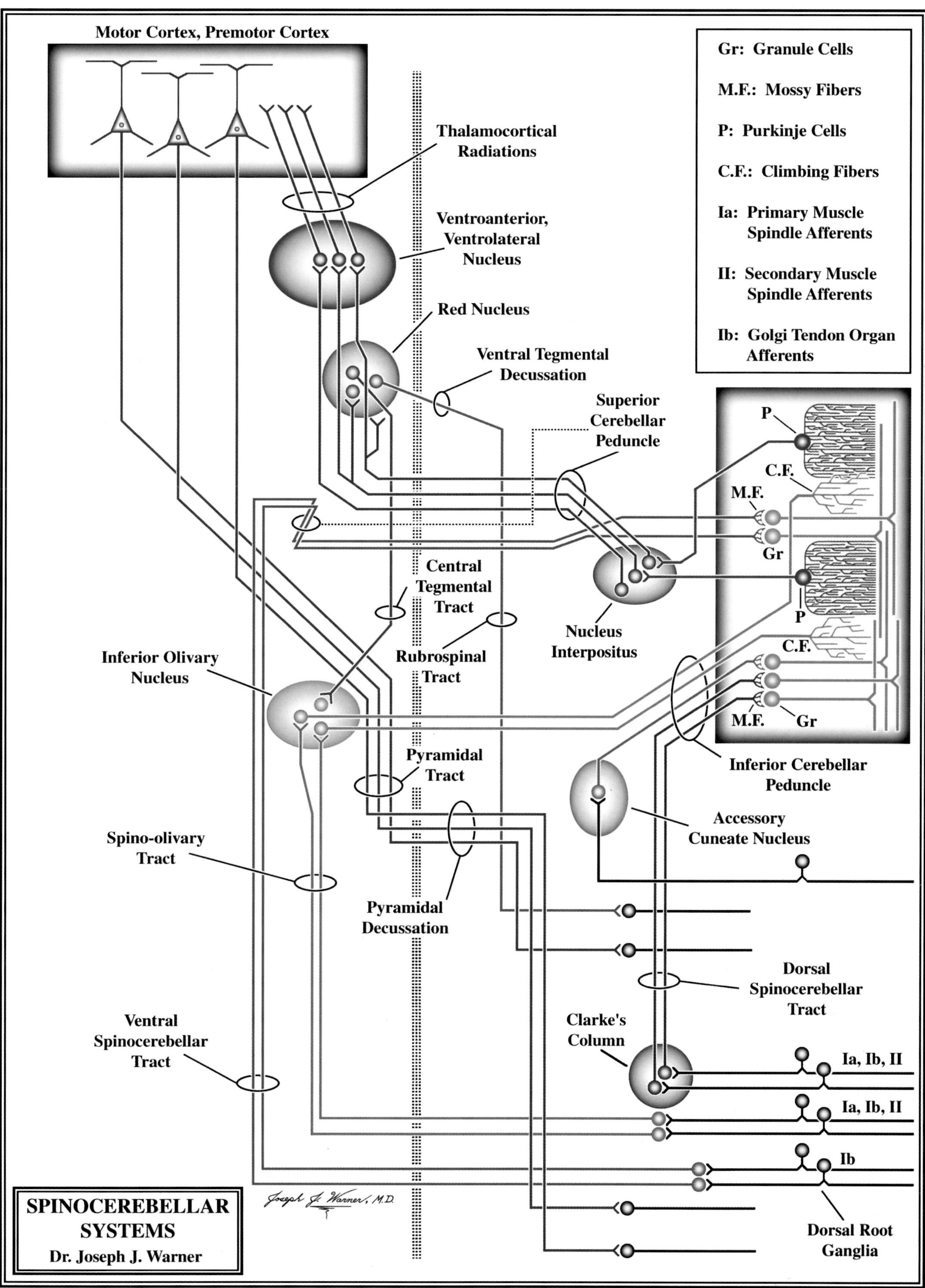
Motor Cortex, Premotor Cortex
Thalamocortical Radiations
Ventroanterior, Ventrolateral Nucleus
Red Nucleus
Ventral Tegmental Decussation
Superior Cerebellar Peduncle
Gr: Granule Cells
M.F.: Mossy Fibers
P: Purkinje Cells
C.F.: Climbing Fibers
Ia: Primary Muscle Spindle Afferents
II: Secondary Muscle Spindle Afferents
Ib: Golgi Tendon Organ Afferents
P
C.F.
M.F.
Gr
P
C.F.
M.F.
Gr
Central Tegmental Tract
Rubrospinal Tract
Nucleus Interpositus
Inferior Olivary Nucleus
Inferior Cerebellar Peduncle
Pyramidal Tract
Accessory Cuneate Nucleus
Spino-olivary Tract
Pyramidal Decussation
Dorsal Spinocerebellar Tract
Clarke's Column
Ventral Spinocerebellar Tract
Ia, Ib, II
Ia, Ib, II
Ib
Dorsal Root Ganglia
SPINOCEREBELLAR SYSTEMS
Dr. Joseph J. Warner
Joseph J. Warner, M.D.

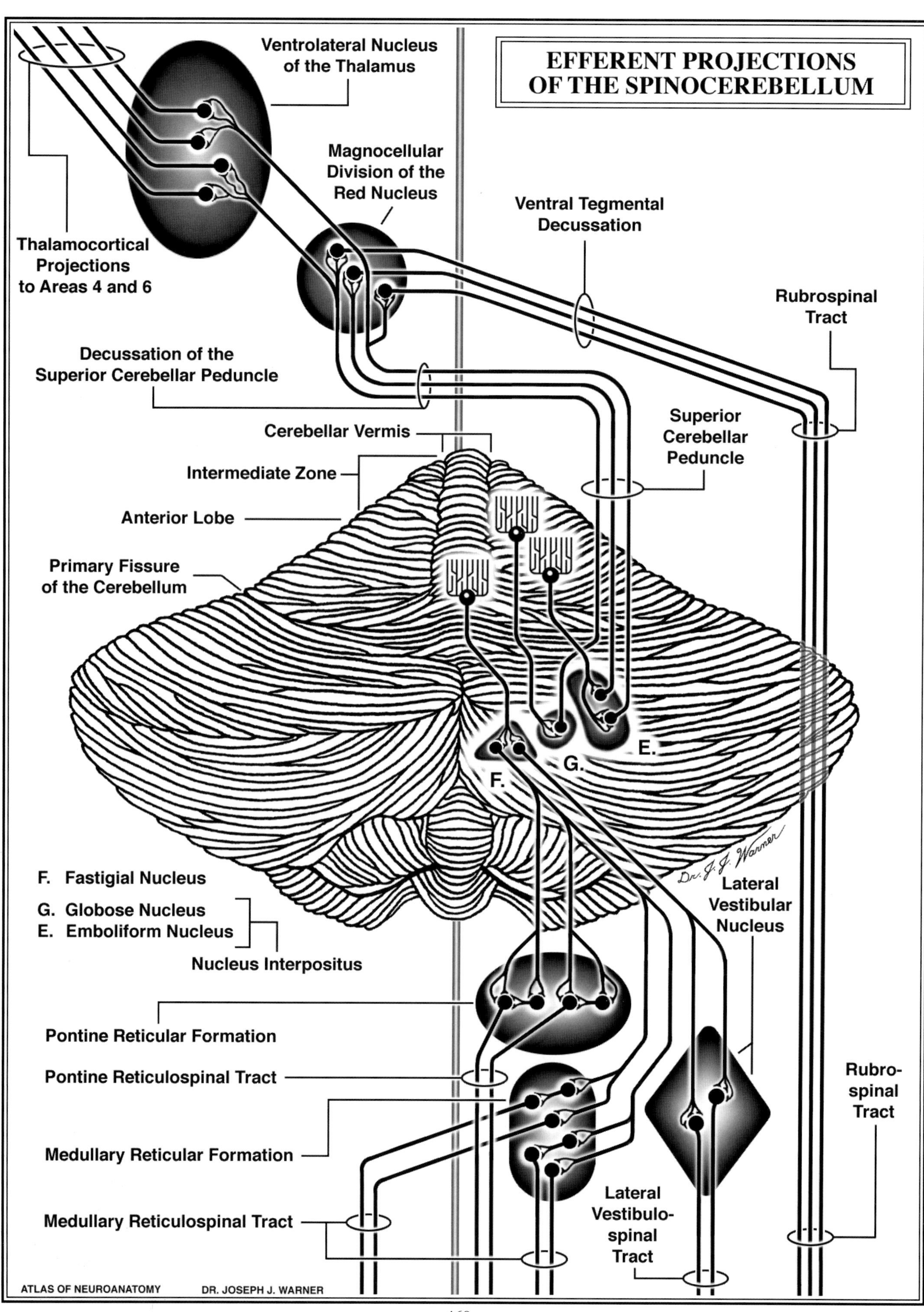
EFFERENT PROJECTIONS OF THE SPINOCEREBELLUM
Ventrolateral Nucleus of the Thalamus
Magnocellular Division of the Red Nucleus
Thalamocortical Projections to Areas 4 and 6
Ventral Tegmental Decussation
Rubrospinal Tract
Decussation of the Superior Cerebellar Peduncle
Cerebellar Vermis
Superior Cerebellar Peduncle
Intermediate Zone
Anterior Lobe
Primary Fissure of the Cerebellum
E.
G.
F.
Dr. J. J. Warner
F. Fastigial Nucleus
G. Globose Nucleus
E. Emboliform Nucleus
Nucleus Interpositus
Lateral Vestibular Nucleus
Pontine Reticular Formation
Pontine Reticulospinal Tract
Medullary Reticular Formation
Rubro-spinal Tract
Medullary Reticulospinal Tract
Lateral Vestibulo-spinal Tract
ATLAS OF NEUROANATOMY
DR. JOSEPH J. WARNER

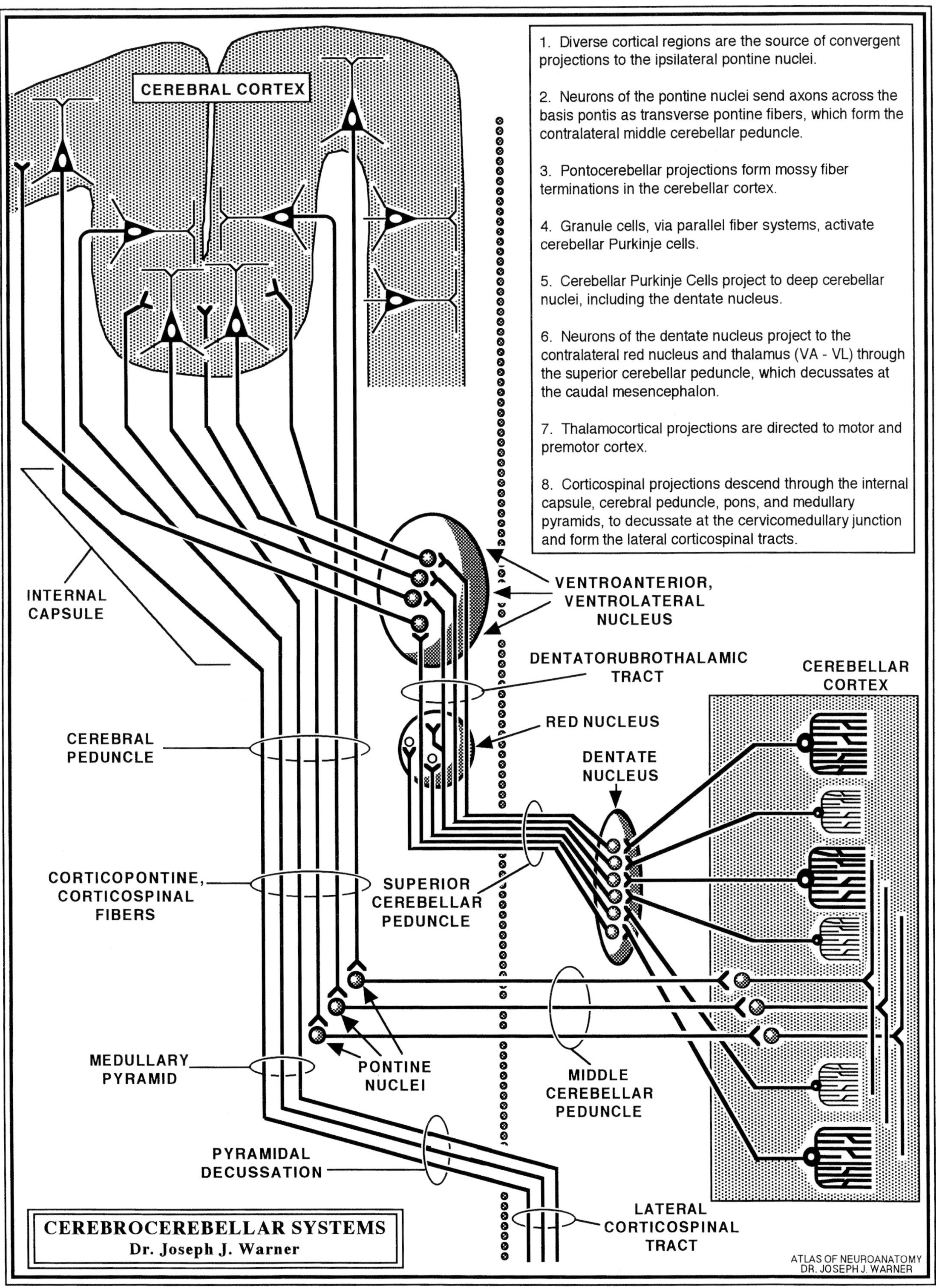
CEREBRAL CORTEX
1. Diverse cortical regions are the source of convergent projections to the ipsilateral pontine nuclei.
2. Neurons of the pontine nuclei send axons across the basis pontis as transverse pontine fibers, which form the contralateral middle cerebellar peduncle.
3. Pontocerebellar projections form mossy fiber terminations in the cerebellar cortex.
4. Granule cells, via parallel fiber systems, activate cerebellar Purkinje cells.
5. Cerebellar Purkinje Cells project to deep cerebellar nuclei, including the dentate nucleus.
6. Neurons of the dentate nucleus project to the contralateral red nucleus and thalamus (VA - VL) through the superior cerebellar peduncle, which decussates at the caudal mesencephalon.
7. Thalamocortical projections are directed to motor and premotor cortex.
8. Corticospinal projections descend through the internal capsule, cerebral peduncle, pons, and medullary pyramids, to decussate at the cervicomedullary junction and form the lateral corticospinal tracts.
INTERNAL CAPSULE
VENTROANTERIOR, VENTROLATERAL NUCLEUS
DENTATORUBROTHALAMIC TRACT
CEREBELLAR CORTEX
CEREBRAL PEDUNCLE
RED NUCLEUS
DENTATE NUCLEUS
CORTICOPONTINE, CORTICOSPINAL FIBERS
SUPERIOR CEREBELLAR PEDUNCLE
MEDULLARY PYRAMID
PONTINE NUCLEI
MIDDLE CEREBELLAR PEDUNCLE
PYRAMIDAL DECUSSATION
LATERAL CORTICOSPINAL TRACT
CEREBROCEREBELLAR SYSTEMS
Dr. Joseph J. Warner
ATLAS OF NEUROANATOMY
DR. JOSEPH J. WARNER

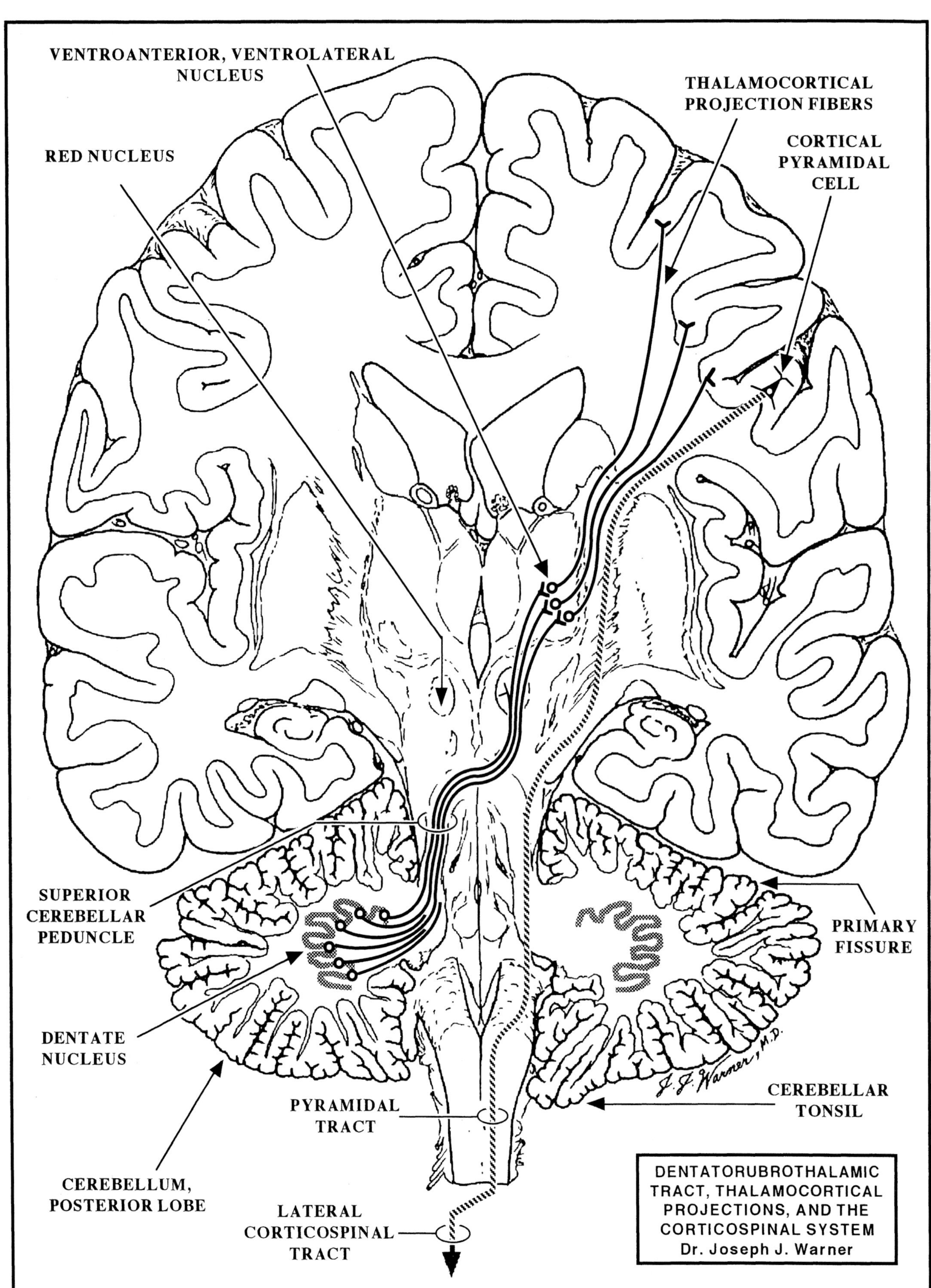

DENTATORUBROTHALAMIC TRACT, THALAMOCORTICAL PROJECTIONS, AND THE CORTICOSPINAL SYSTEM
Dr. Joseph J. Warner

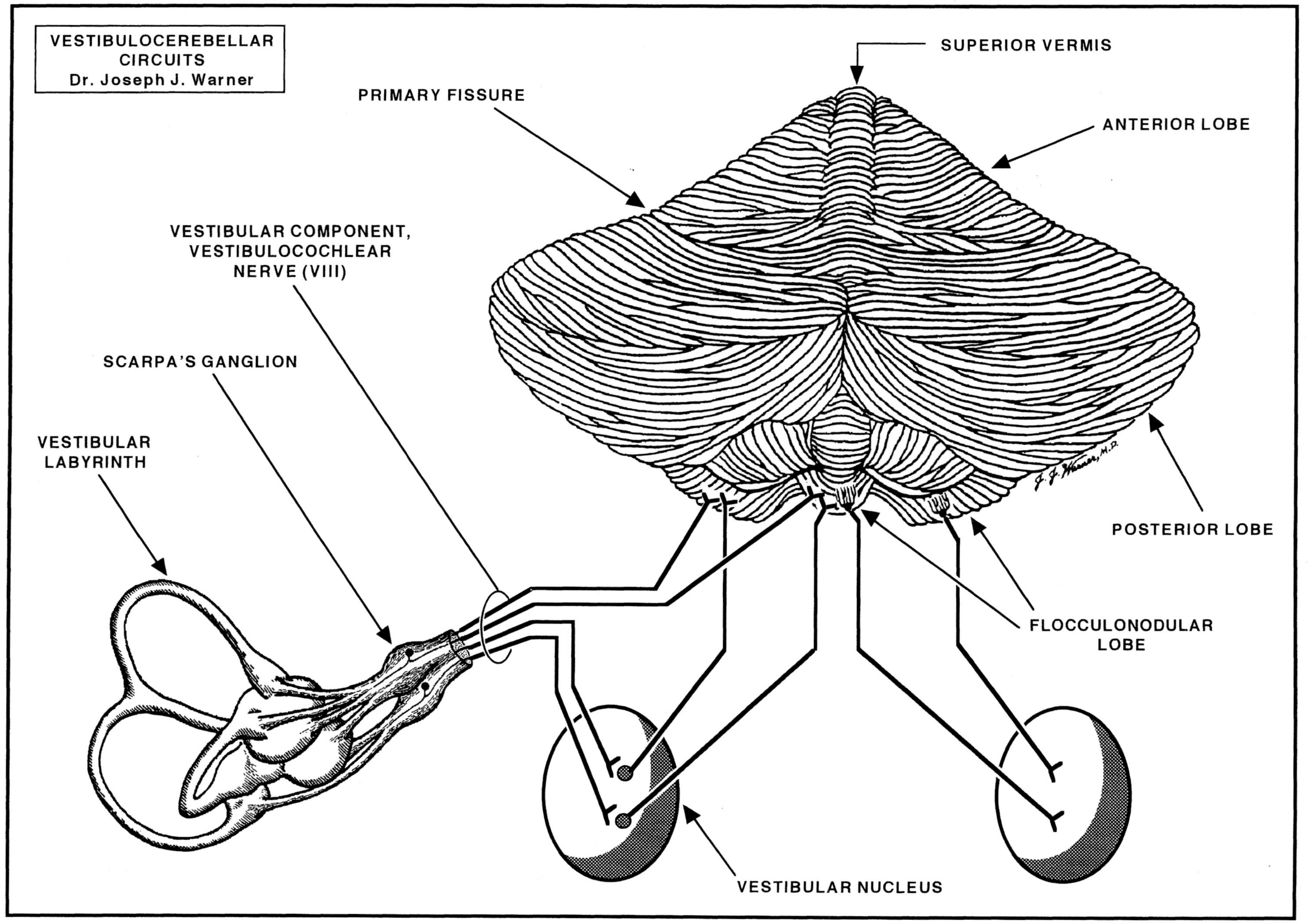
VESTIBULOCEREBELLAR
CIRCUITS
Dr. Joseph J. Warner
SUPERIOR VERMIS
PRIMARY FISSURE
ANTERIOR LOBE
VESTIBULAR COMPONENT,
VESTIBULOCOCHLEAR
NERVE (VIII)
SCARPA'S GANGLION
VESTIBULAR
LABYRINTH
POSTERIOR LOBE
FLOCCULONODULAR
LOBE
VESTIBULAR NUCLEUS

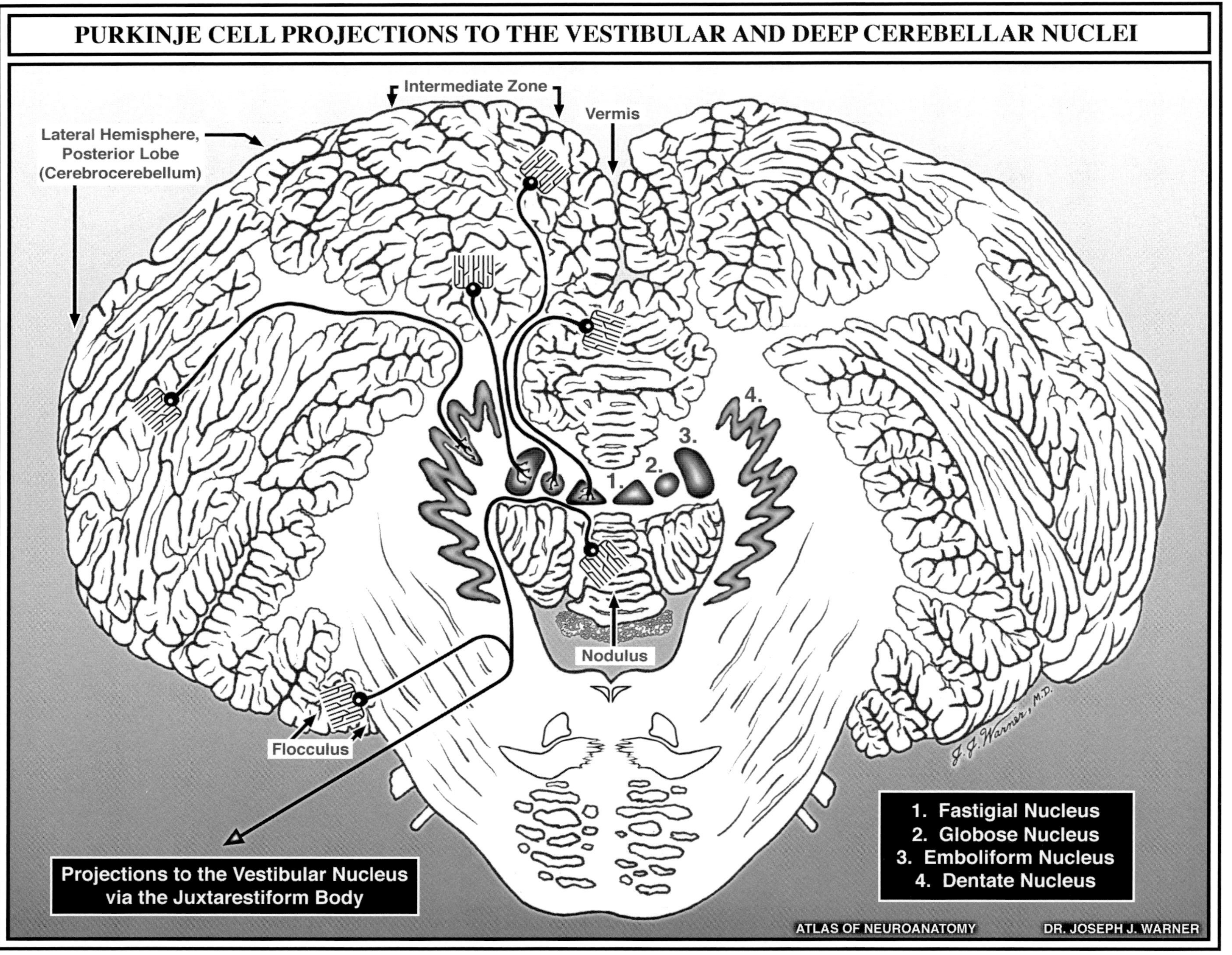
PURKINJE CELL PROJECTIONS TO THE VESTIBULAR AND DEEP CEREBELLAR NUCLEI
Intermediate Zone
Vermis
Lateral Hemisphere,
Posterior Lobe
(Cerebrocerebellum)
4.
3.
2.
1.
Nodulus
Flocculus
J. J. Warner, M.D.
Projections to the Vestibular Nucleus
via the Juxtarestiform Body
1. Fastigial Nucleus
2. Globose Nucleus
3. Emboliform Nucleus
4. Dentate Nucleus
ATLAS OF NEUROANATOMY
DR. JOSEPH J. WARNER

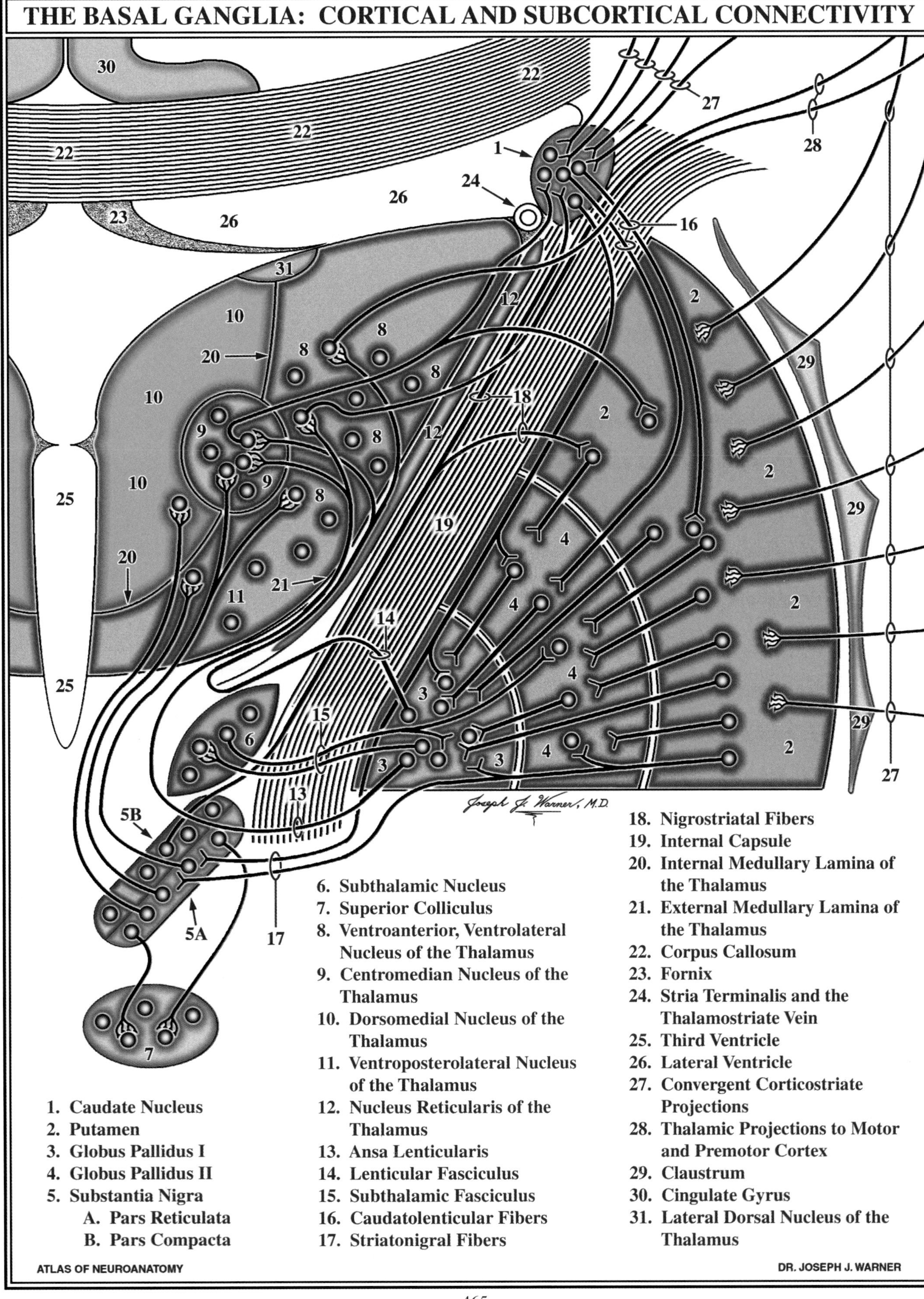
THE BASAL GANGLIA: CORTICAL AND SUBCORTICAL CONNECTIVITY
Joseph J. Warner, M.D.
1. Caudate Nucleus
2. Putamen
3. Globus Pallidus I
4. Globus Pallidus II
5. Substantia Nigra
A. Pars Reticulata
B. Pars Compacta
6. Subthalamic Nucleus
7. Superior Colliculus
8. Ventroanterior, Ventrolateral Nucleus of the Thalamus
9. Centromedian Nucleus of the Thalamus
10. Dorsomedial Nucleus of the Thalamus
11. Ventroposterolateral Nucleus of the Thalamus
12. Nucleus Reticularis of the Thalamus
13. Ansa Lenticularis
14. Lenticular Fasciculus
15. Subthalamic Fasciculus
16. Caudatolenticular Fibers
17. Striatonigral Fibers
18. Nigrostriatal Fibers
19. Internal Capsule
20. Internal Medullary Lamina of the Thalamus
21. External Medullary Lamina of the Thalamus
22. Corpus Callosum
23. Fornix
24. Stria Terminalis and the Thalamostriate Vein
25. Third Ventricle
26. Lateral Ventricle
27. Convergent Corticostriate Projections
28. Thalamic Projections to Motor and Premotor Cortex
29. Claustrum
30. Cingulate Gyrus
31. Lateral Dorsal Nucleus of the Thalamus
ATLAS OF NEUROANATOMY
DR. JOSEPH J. WARNER

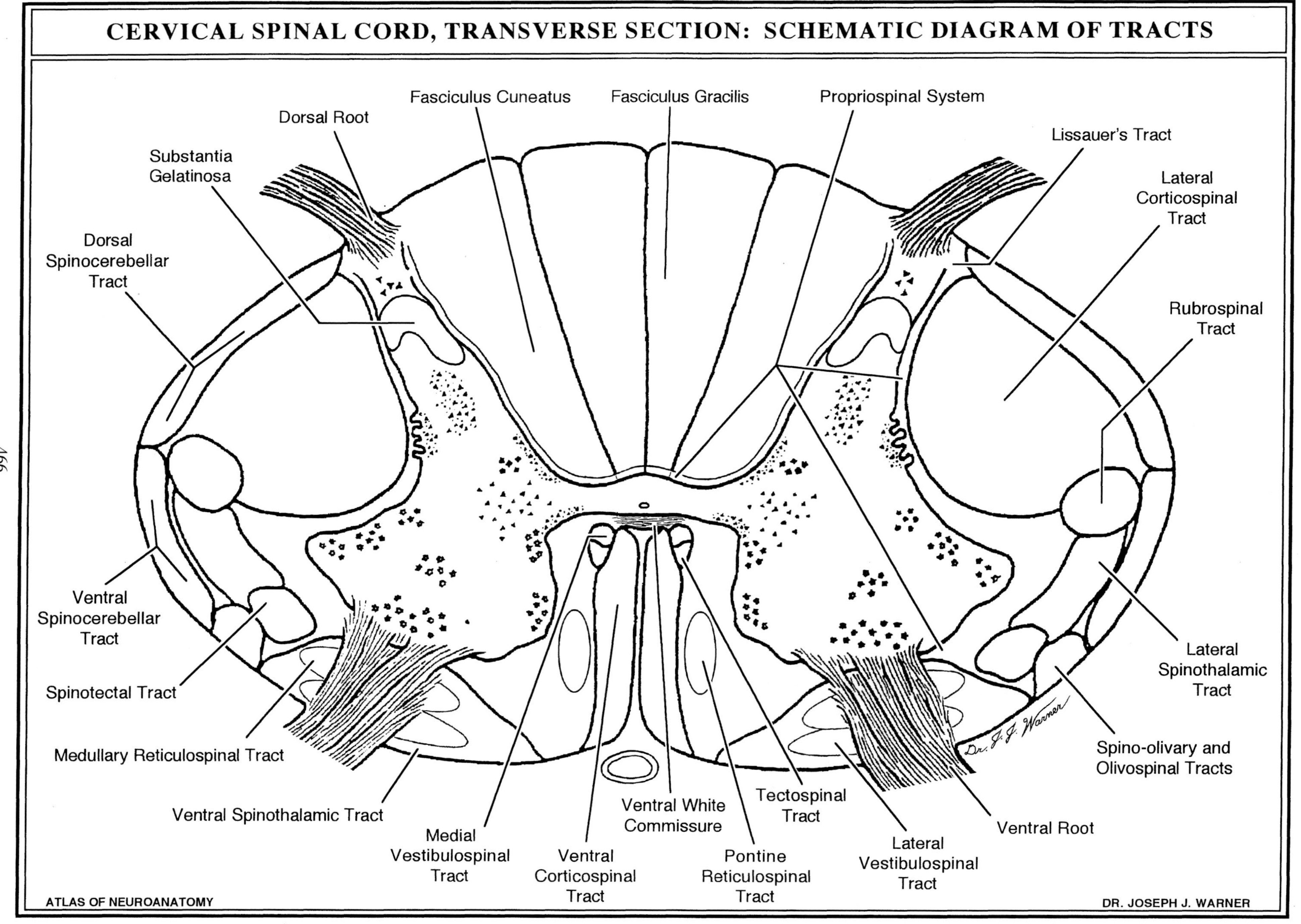
CERVICAL SPINAL CORD, TRANSVERSE SECTION: SCHEMATIC DIAGRAM OF TRACTS
Fasciculus Cuneatus
Fasciculus Gracilis
Propriospinal System
Dorsal Root
Lissauer's Tract
Substantia Gelatinosa
Lateral Corticospinal Tract
Dorsal Spinocerebellar Tract
Rubrospinal Tract
Ventral Spinocerebellar Tract
Lateral Spinothalamic Tract
Spinotectal Tract
Medullary Reticulospinal Tract
Spino-olivary and Olivospinal Tracts
Ventral Spinothalamic Tract
Tectospinal Tract
Ventral White Commissure
Ventral Root
Medial Vestibulospinal Tract
Lateral Vestibulospinal Tract
Ventral Corticospinal Tract
Pontine Reticulospinal Tract
ATLAS OF NEUROANATOMY
DR. JOSEPH J. WARNER

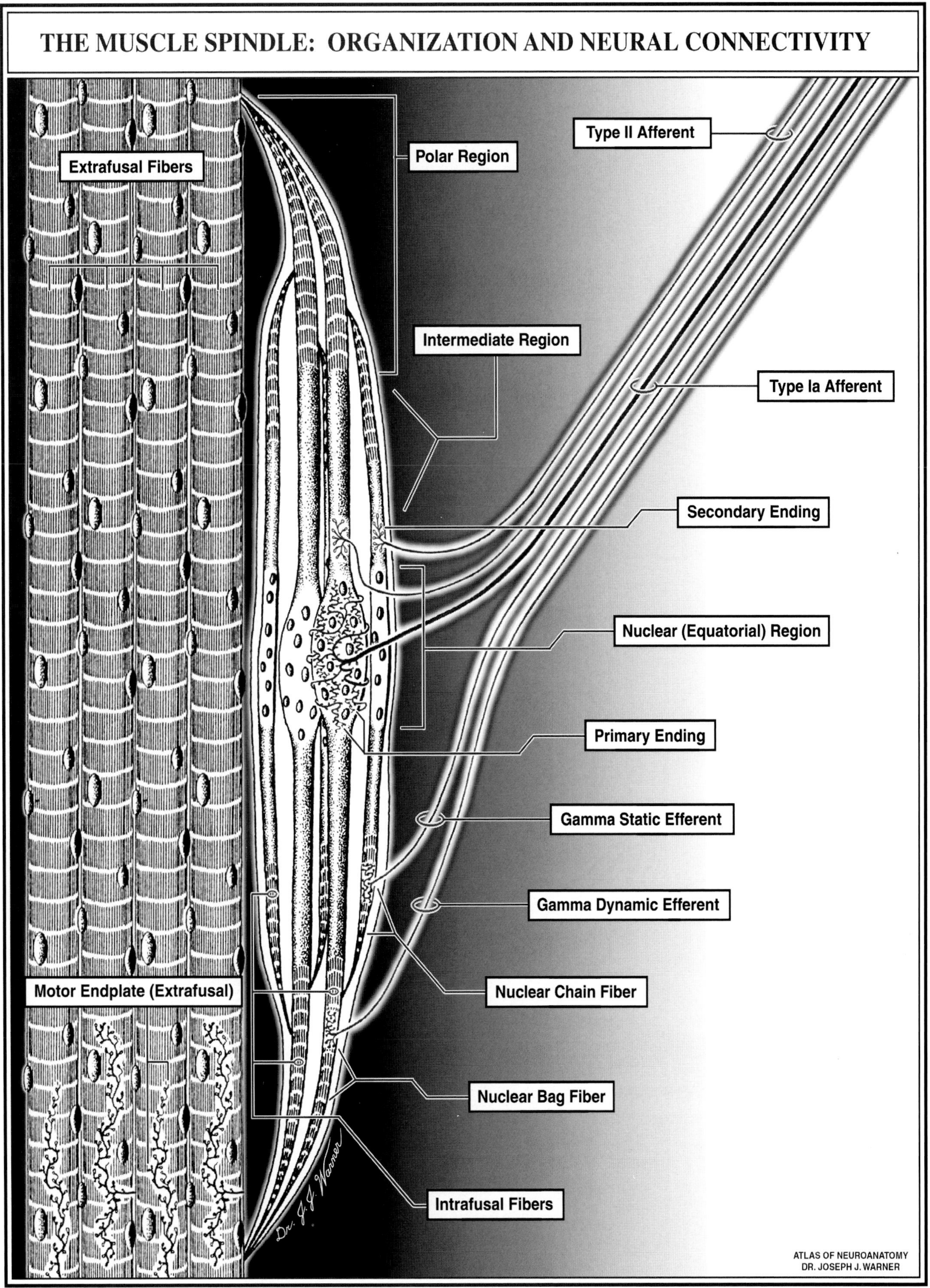
THE MUSCLE SPINDLE: ORGANIZATION AND NEURAL CONNECTIVITY
Extrafusal Fibers
Polar Region
Type II Afferent
Intermediate Region
Type Ia Afferent
Secondary Ending
Nuclear (Equatorial) Region
Primary Ending
Gamma Static Efferent
Gamma Dynamic Efferent
Motor Endplate (Extrafusal)
Nuclear Chain Fiber
Nuclear Bag Fiber
Intrafusal Fibers
Dr. J. J. Warner
ATLAS OF NEUROANATOMY
DR. JOSEPH J. WARNER

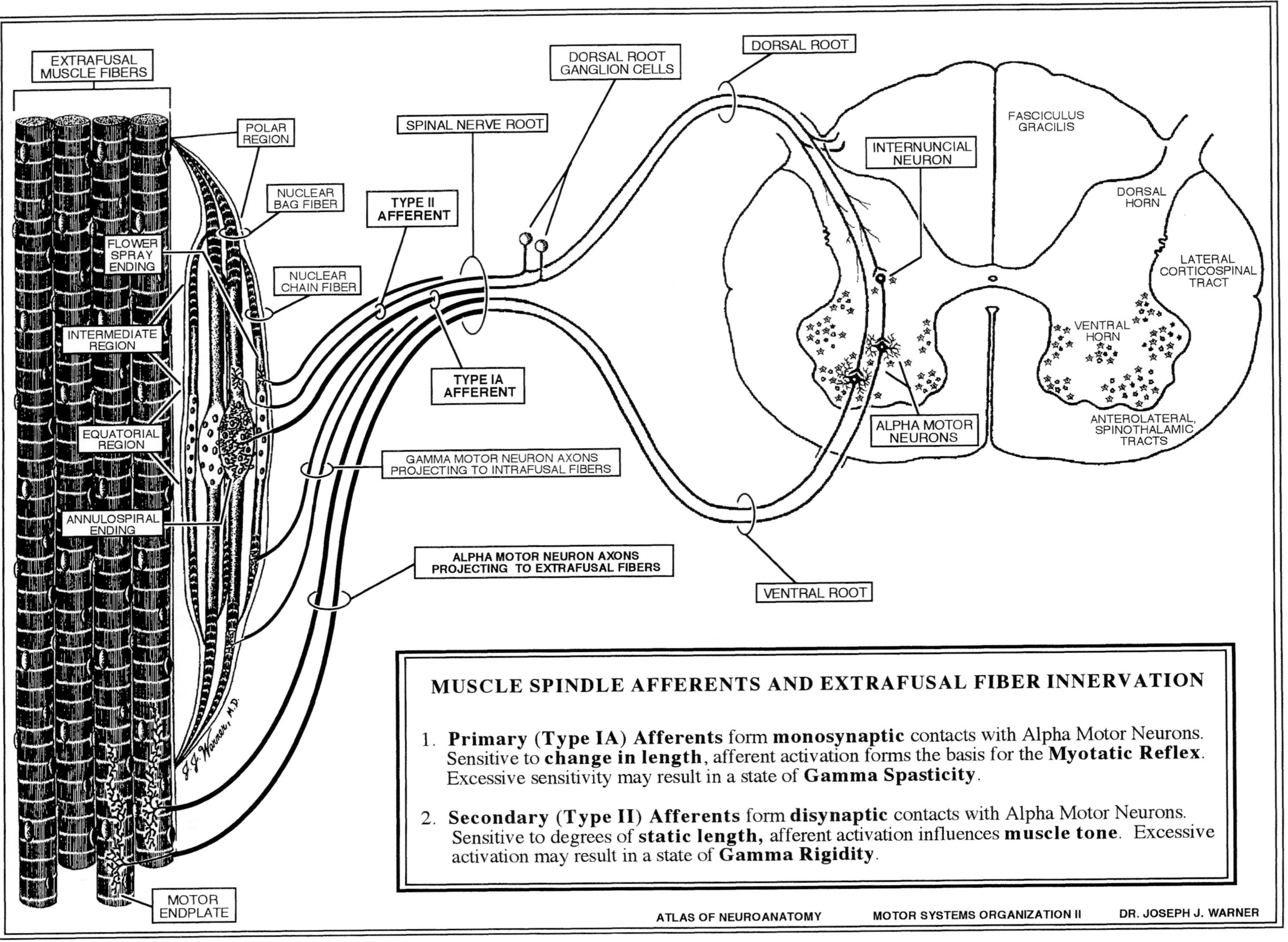

MUSCLE SPINDLE AFFERENTS AND EXTRAFUSAL FIBER INNERVATION

1. **Primary (Type IA) Afferents** form **monosynaptic** contacts with Alpha Motor Neurons. Sensitive to **change in length**, afferent activation forms the basis for the **Myotatic Reflex**. Excessive sensitivity may result in a state of **Gamma Spasticity**.

2. **Secondary (Type II) Afferents** form **disynaptic** contacts with Alpha Motor Neurons. Sensitive to degrees of **static length,** afferent activation influences **muscle tone**. Excessive activation may result in a state of **Gamma Rigidity**.

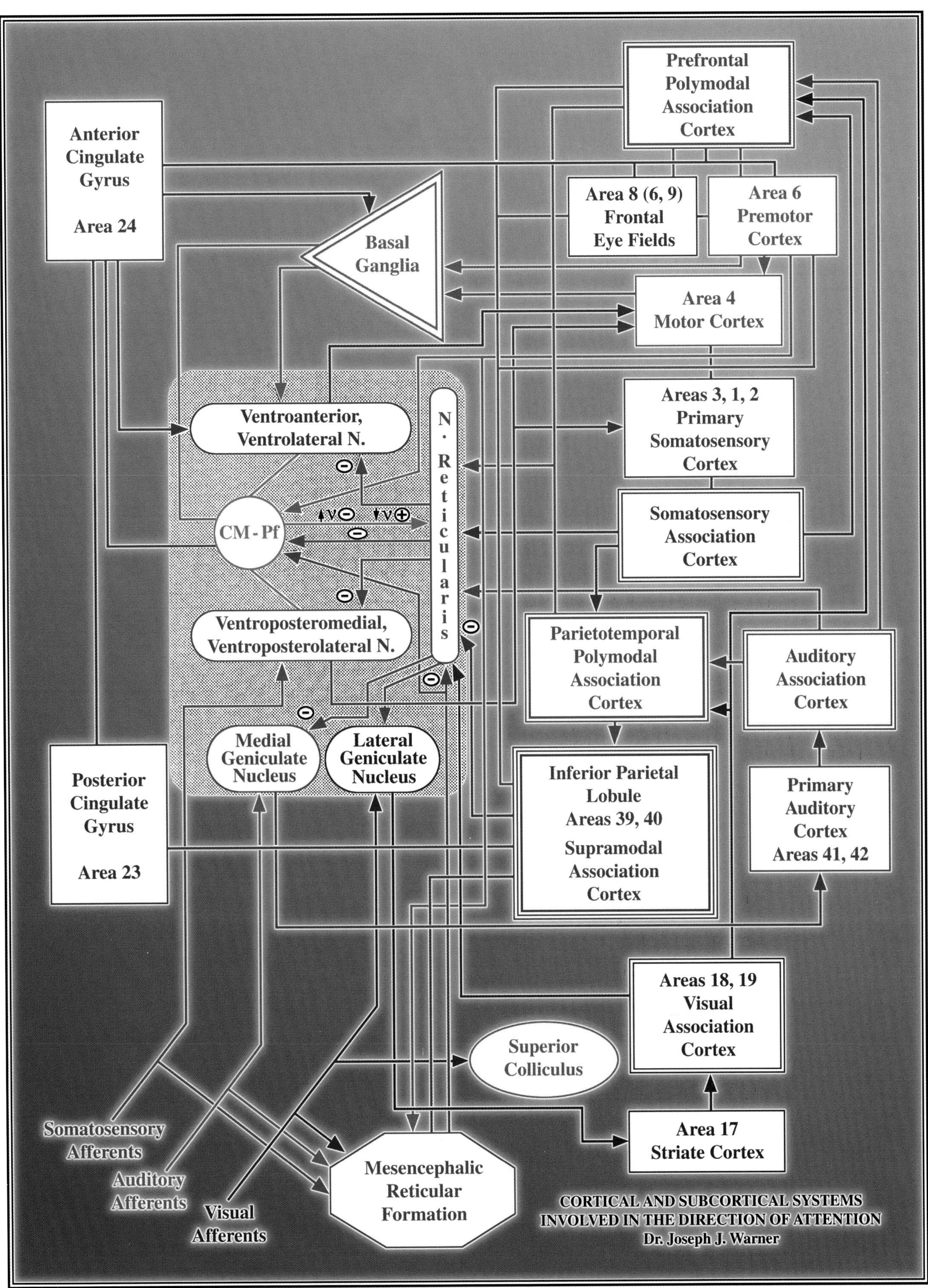

Prefrontal Polymodal Association Cortex
Anterior Cingulate Gyrus
Area 24
Area 8 (6, 9) Frontal Eye Fields
Area 6 Premotor Cortex
Basal Ganglia
Area 4 Motor Cortex
Areas 3, 1, 2 Primary Somatosensory Cortex
Ventroanterior, Ventrolateral N.
N. Reticularis
CM - Pf
Somatosensory Association Cortex
Ventroposteromedial, Ventroposterolateral N.
Parietotemporal Polymodal Association Cortex
Auditory Association Cortex
Medial Geniculate Nucleus
Lateral Geniculate Nucleus
Posterior Cingulate Gyrus
Area 23
Inferior Parietal Lobule
Areas 39, 40
Supramodal Association Cortex
Primary Auditory Cortex
Areas 41, 42
Areas 18, 19 Visual Association Cortex
Superior Colliculus
Area 17 Striate Cortex
Somatosensory Afferents
Auditory Afferents
Visual Afferents
Mesencephalic Reticular Formation
CORTICAL AND SUBCORTICAL SYSTEMS INVOLVED IN THE DIRECTION OF ATTENTION
Dr. Joseph J. Warner

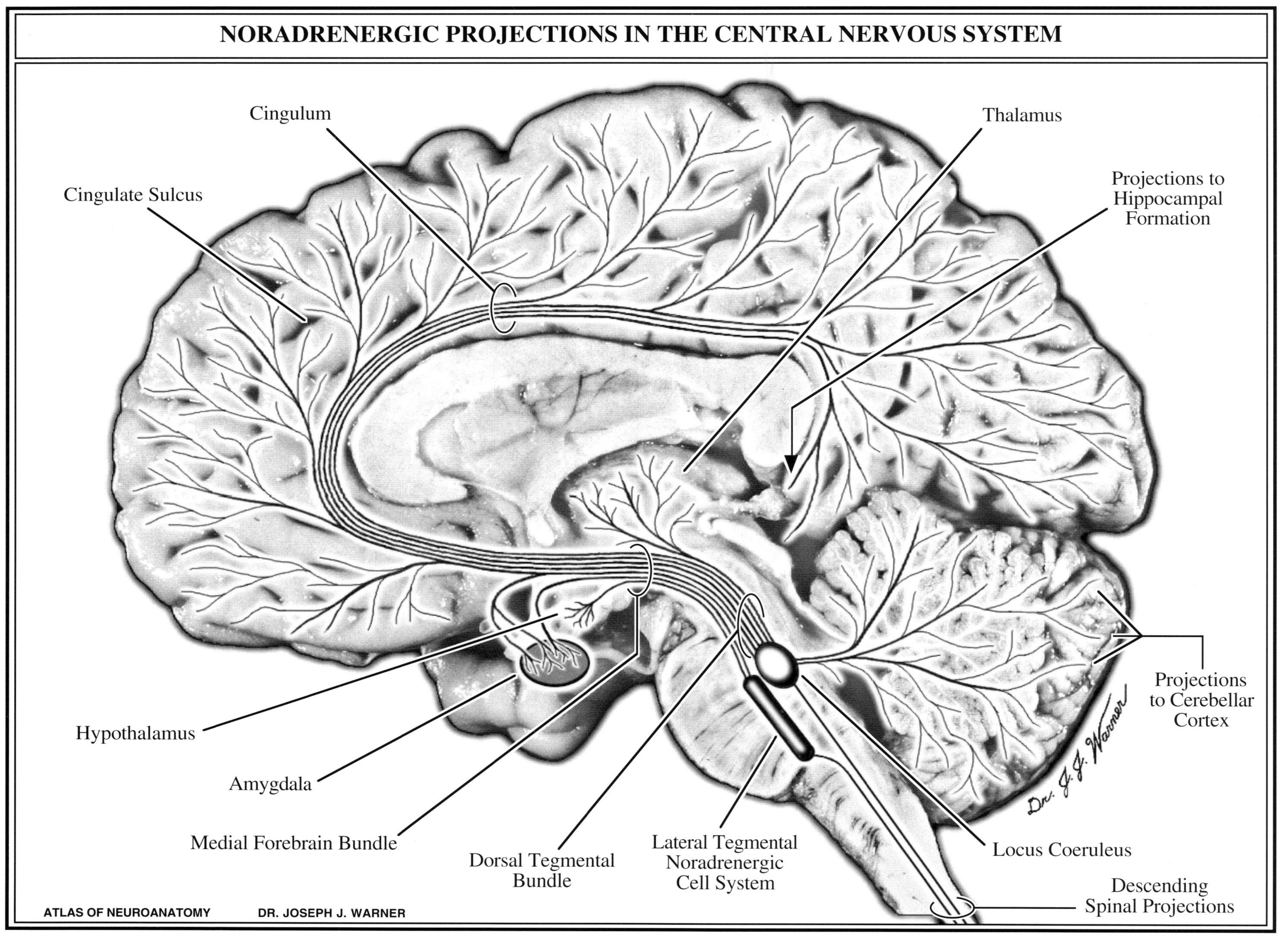
NORADRENERGIC PROJECTIONS IN THE CENTRAL NERVOUS SYSTEM
Cingulum
Thalamus
Cingulate Sulcus
Projections to Hippocampal Formation
Projections to Cerebellar Cortex
Hypothalamus
Amygdala
Medial Forebrain Bundle
Dorsal Tegmental Bundle
Lateral Tegmental Noradrenergic Cell System
Locus Coeruleus
Descending Spinal Projections
Dr. J. J. Warner
ATLAS OF NEUROANATOMY
DR. JOSEPH J. WARNER

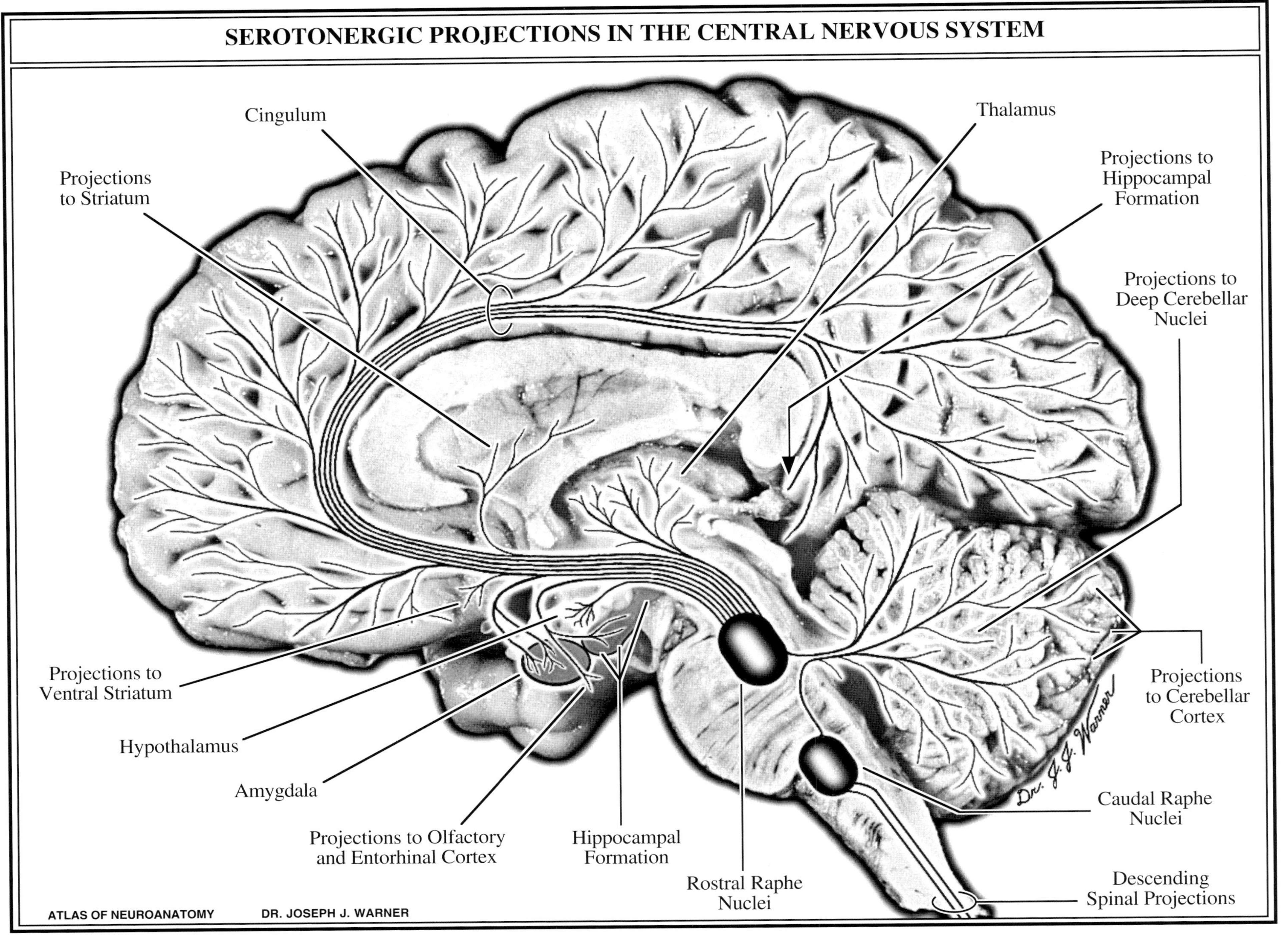
SEROTONERGIC PROJECTIONS IN THE CENTRAL NERVOUS SYSTEM
Cingulum
Thalamus
Projections to Striatum
Projections to Hippocampal Formation
Projections to Deep Cerebellar Nuclei
Projections to Ventral Striatum
Hypothalamus
Amygdala
Projections to Olfactory and Entorhinal Cortex
Hippocampal Formation
Rostral Raphe Nuclei
Projections to Cerebellar Cortex
Caudal Raphe Nuclei
Descending Spinal Projections
Dr. J. J. Warner
ATLAS OF NEUROANATOMY
DR. JOSEPH J. WARNER

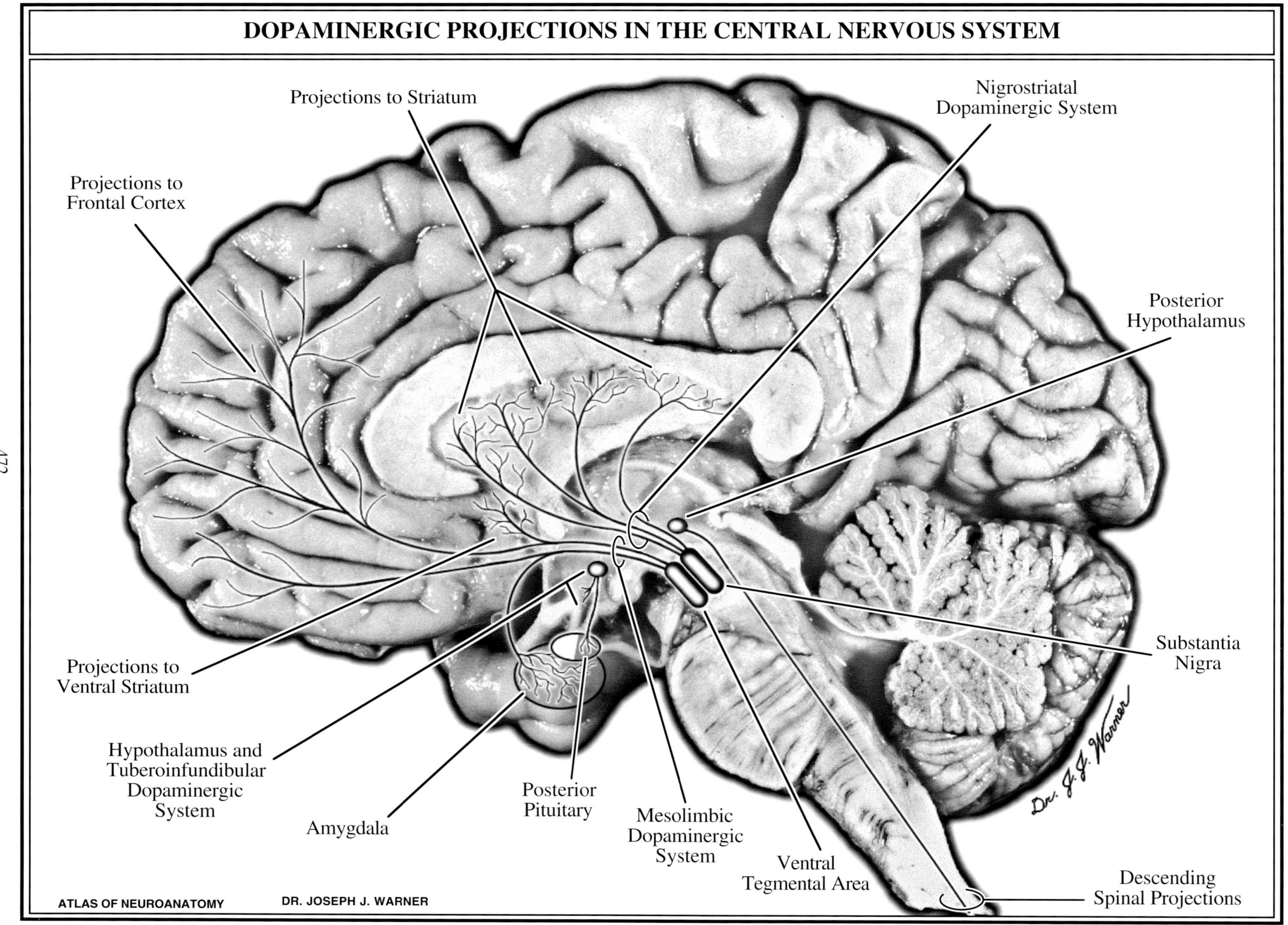

DOPAMINERGIC PROJECTIONS IN THE CENTRAL NERVOUS SYSTEM
Projections to Striatum
Nigrostriatal Dopaminergic System
Projections to Frontal Cortex
Posterior Hypothalamus
Substantia Nigra
Projections to Ventral Striatum
Hypothalamus and Tuberoinfundibular Dopaminergic System
Amygdala
Posterior Pituitary
Mesolimbic Dopaminergic System
Ventral Tegmental Area
Descending Spinal Projections
Dr. J. J. Warner
ATLAS OF NEUROANATOMY
DR. JOSEPH J. WARNER

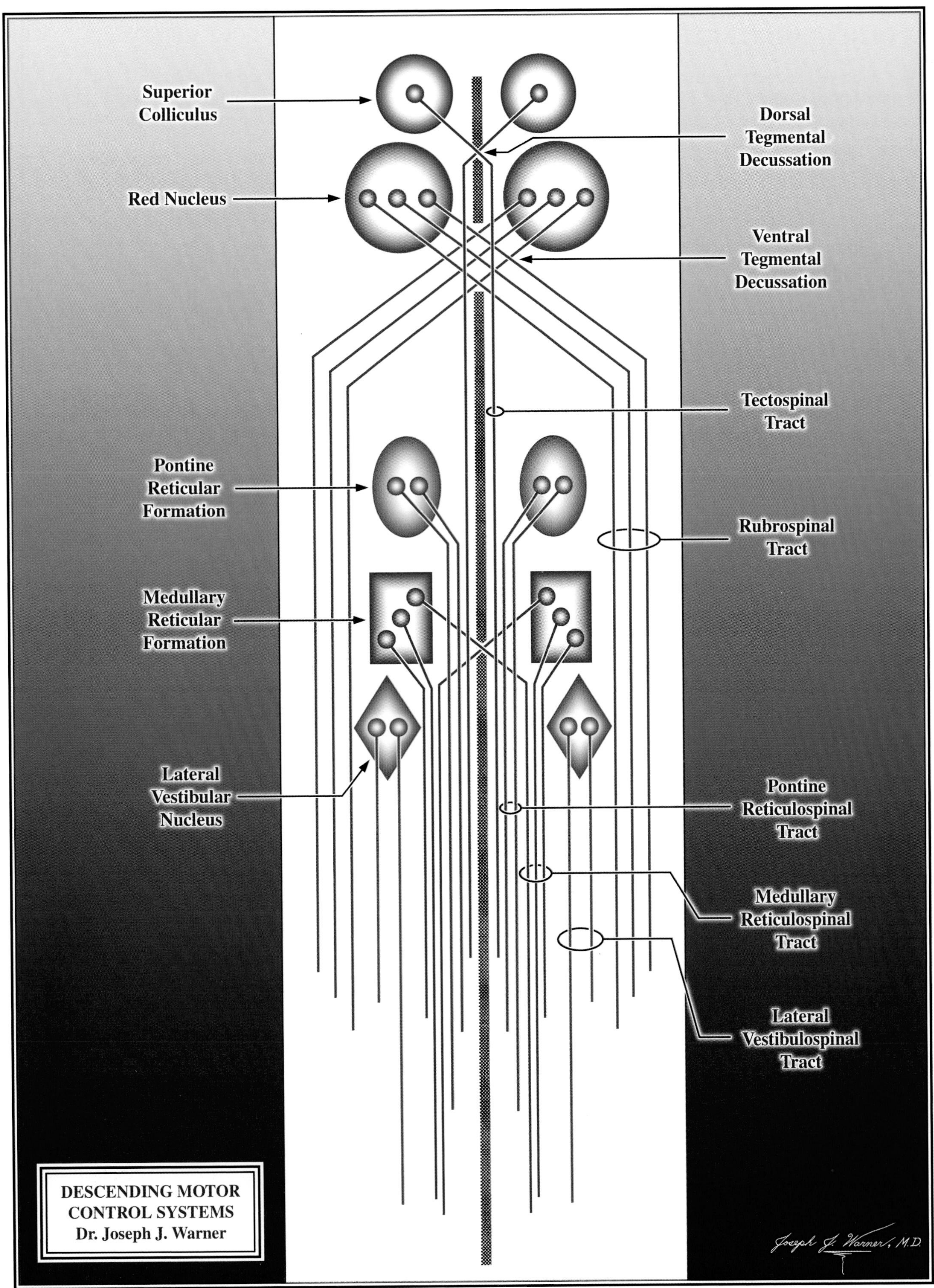

Superior Colliculus
Dorsal Tegmental Decussation
Red Nucleus
Ventral Tegmental Decussation
Tectospinal Tract
Pontine Reticular Formation
Rubrospinal Tract
Medullary Reticular Formation
Lateral Vestibular Nucleus
Pontine Reticulospinal Tract
Medullary Reticulospinal Tract
Lateral Vestibulospinal Tract
DESCENDING MOTOR CONTROL SYSTEMS
Dr. Joseph J. Warner
Joseph J. Warner, M.D.

DESCENDING MOTOR CONTROL SYSTEMS: CASE PRESENTATION

A 67-year-old right-handed male was brought to the emergency room, having been found unresponsive on the floor by a family member. The past medical history included significant hypertension and atherosclerotic cardiovascular disease with angina pectoris. He had no prior history of stroke or other neurologic symptomatology. The patient smoked one to two packs of cigarettes per day. Medications included antihypertensives and nitroglycerin p.r.n. chest pain. His compliance with his medications was often questionable, and on many physician visits, his blood pressure was in the range of 170 to 200 (systolic) and 100 to 120 (diastolic).

Neurologic findings included the following: The patient was unresponsive to verbal stimulation. Infrequent semipurposeful spontaneous movements of the left arm and leg were noted, however the patient did not move his right arm or leg. A left gaze preference was noted along with head deviation to the left. Tactile stimulation increased the left arm and leg movements, however no movement of the right side could be elicited. Noxious stimulation produced an asymmetric grimace, with evidence of a right upper motor neuron facial paresis. At the time of initial examination by emergency room staff, both pupils were equal (3 mm in diameter) and sluggishly reactive to light. Preparations were made for emergent computerized tomography, which was performed after the initial examination. (Refer to figure A).

Repeat examination was performed approximately one hour after his arrival to the emergency room. His blood pressure was 190/120 in both arms with a pulse of 60 per minute. A Cheyne-Stokes respiratory pattern was noted. Tactile stimulation evoked no discernible response, and noxious stimulation resulted in posturing of the right arm characterized by adduction at the shoulder, and flexion across the elbow, wrist, and of the digits. Examination of the pupils revealed the left to be 5 mm in diameter and minimally reactive to direct or consensual light stimulation. The right pupil was 3 mm in diameter and reactive to light in either eye. The left gaze preference persisted, with both eyes conjugately deviated to the left.

Treatment was initiated for increased intracranial pressure, including intravenous dexamethasone and mannitol (a hyperosmolar agent). Despite this intervention, a further change in his neurologic status ensued over the next two to three hours. Spontaneous posturing, which increased with noxious stimulation, was observed. This posturing was characterized by extension and internal rotation of both upper extremities. The movements previously observed in the left arm and leg ceased, and the flexor posturing was no longer elicitable. A decision for endotracheal intubation and controlled hyperventilation was made in order to attempt to alleviate the increased intracranial pressure associated with the diagnosis of hypertensive intracerebral hemorrhage.

Despite this intervention, the patient developed ventricular arrhythmias refractory to medical therapy. It was decided that cardiopulmonary resuscitation would not be attempted in the event of cardiac arrest. The patient expired within 24 hours of presentation, and neuropathologic examination was performed.

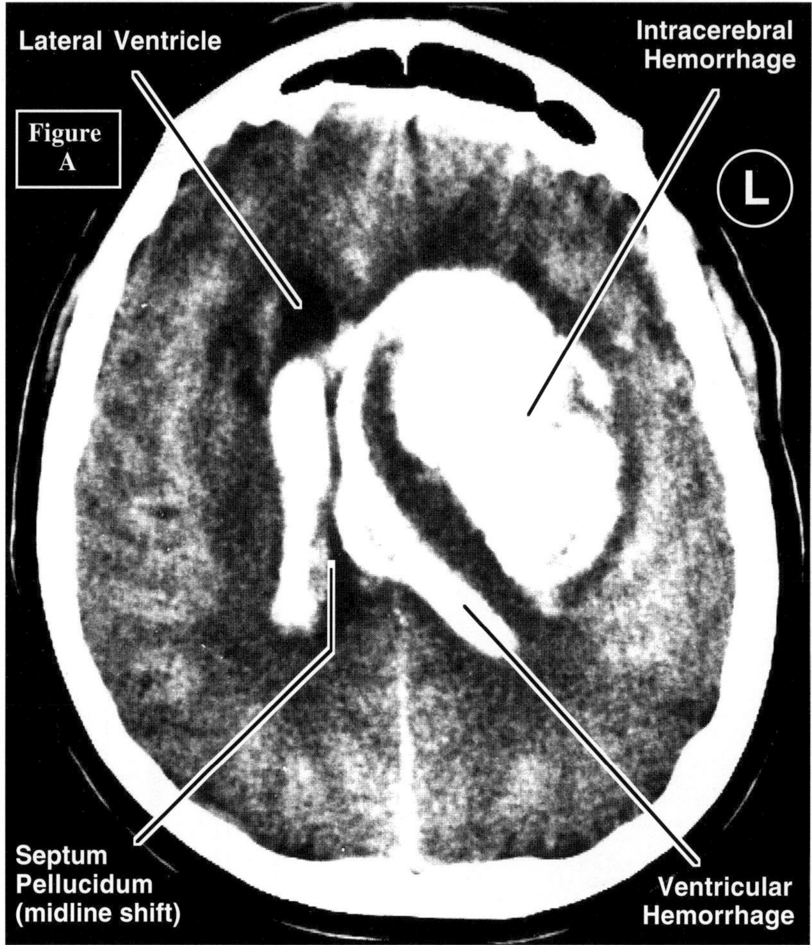

Computerized tomography demonstrated a left hemispheric intracerebral hemorrhage, likely of hypertensive etiology, with rupture into the ventricles (V) and mass effect with midline shift The hemorrhage most likely originated in the putamen.

HYPERTENSIVE INTRACEREBRAL HEMORRHAGE OF PUTAMENAL ORIGIN WITH MASS EFFECT AND RUPTURE INTO THE VENTRICULAR SYSTEM

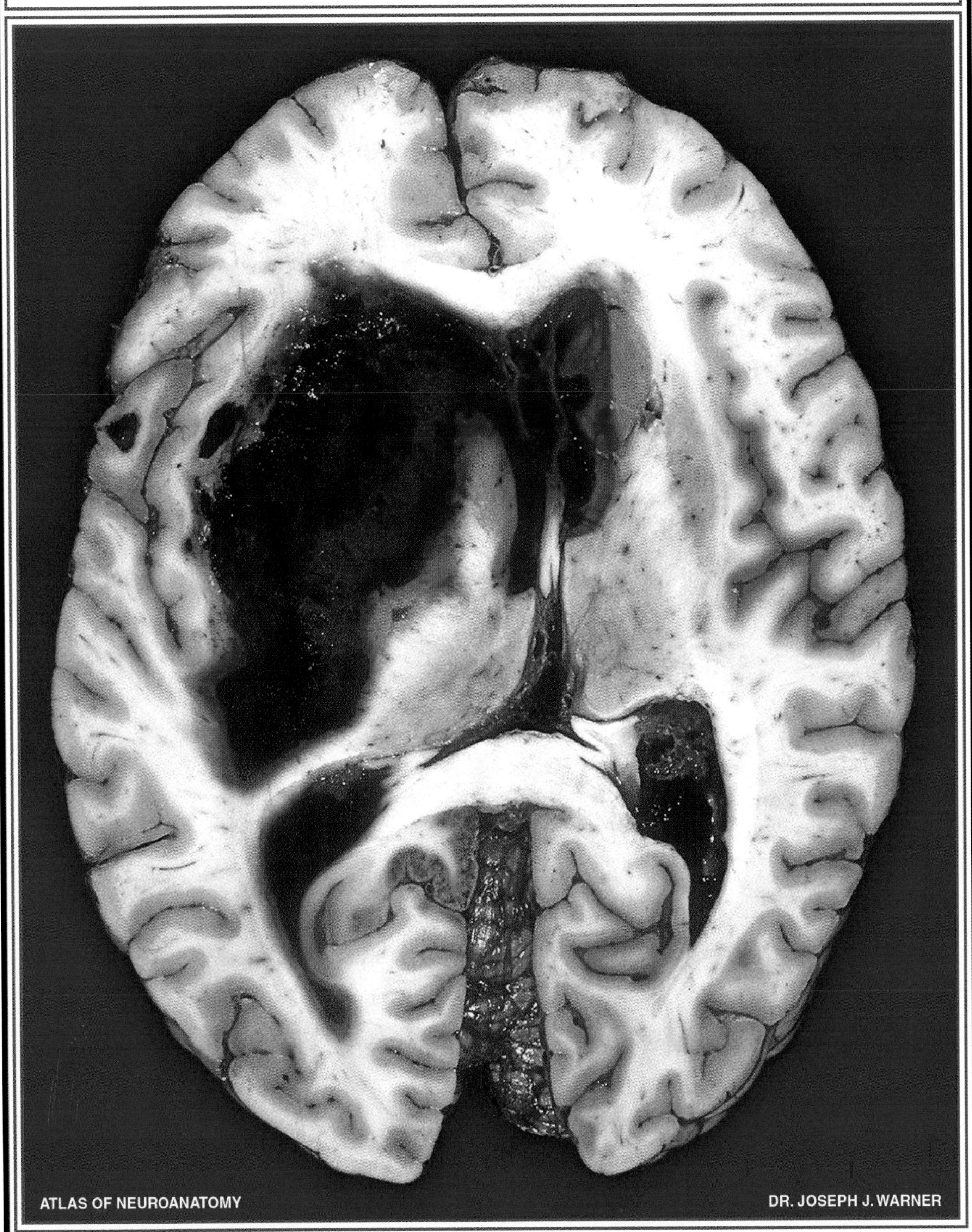

ATLAS OF NEUROANATOMY

DR. JOSEPH J. WARNER

HYPERTENSIVE INTRACEREBRAL HEMORRHAGE WITH MASS EFFECT, RUPTURE INTO THE VENTRICULAR SYSTEM, AND SUBARACHNOID EXTENSION

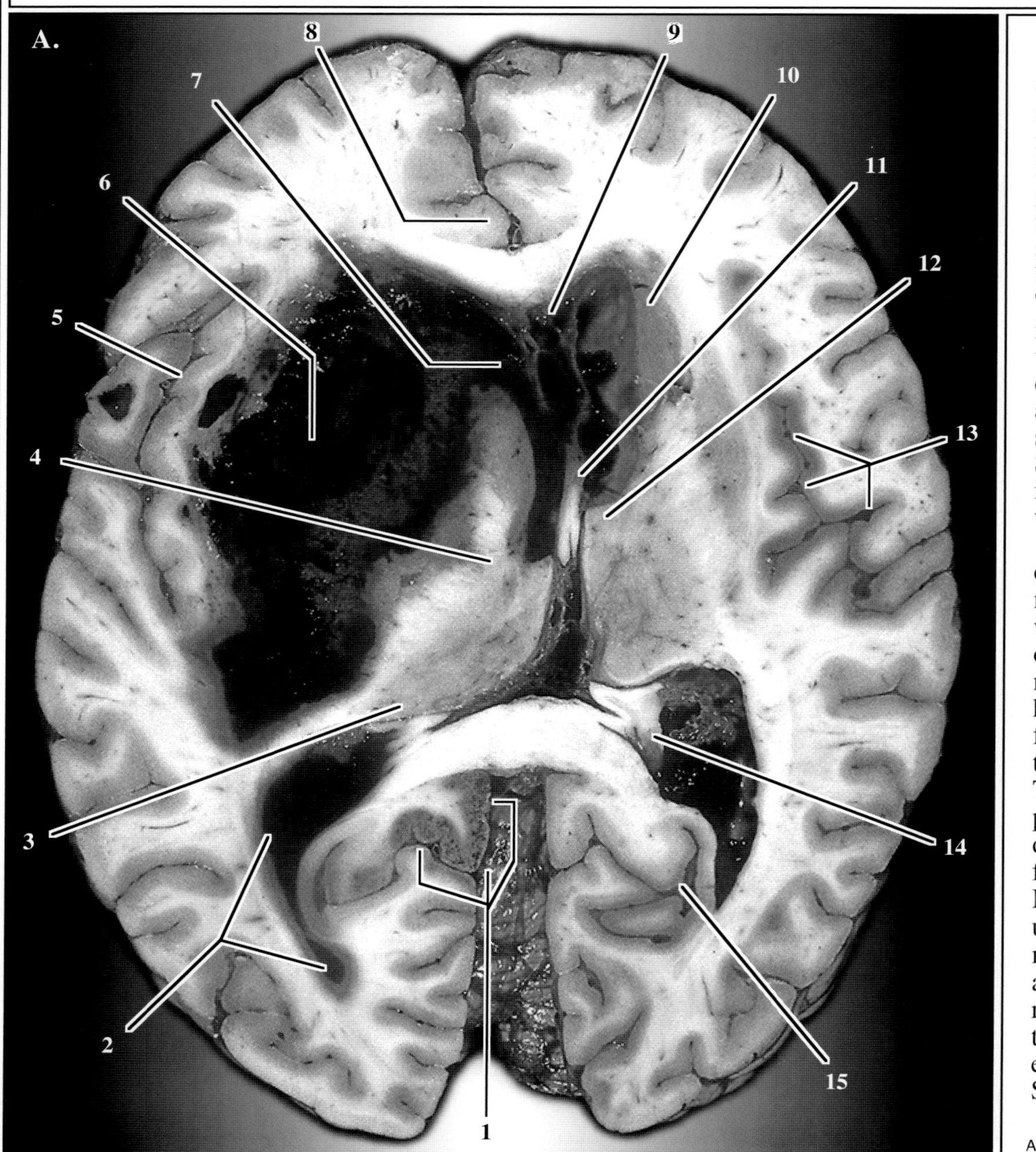

The pathophysiology of this case includes direct effects of increased intracranial pressure as well as secondary changes associated with intraventricular rupture and subarachnoid extension. Massive intracerebral hemorrhage originating within the basal ganglia is often associated with dissection of blood through adjacent white matter. Subcortical "U" fibers act as a mechanical barrier that resists dissection of blood to the surface of the cerebral hemisphere. Therefore, the "path of least resistance" frequently involves centripetal dissection and rupture into the ventricular system. Once this occurs, additional complications include acute obstructive hydrocephalus and extension of the hemorrhage into the subarachnoid space via the foramena of Luschka and Magendie. Subarachnoid blood acts as a chemical irritant, resulting in meningeal inflammation and secondary cerebral vasospasm.

As a result of supratentorial mass effect, direct compression of one or both posterior cerebral arteries may occur, with infarction within all or part of that vascular distribution. In this case, ipsilateral infarction of retrosplenial cortex is grossly visible. Contralateral midline shift is demonstrated, including subfalcine herniation of the cingulate gyrus. (The anatomy of the falx cerebri is characterized by incomplete extension into the interhemispheric fissure between the frontal lobes. Therefore, subfalcine herniation may be more pronounced rostrally.) In this case, the hemorrhage has dissected into the rostral temporal lobe and into the frontal white matter adjacent to the nucleus accumbens. Mass effect involving the temporal lobe has resulted in uncal herniation and contralateral shift of the mesencephalon. The insular cortex is laterally displaced and distorted ipsilateral to the hemorrhage. The site of rupture into the ventricular system is shown adjacent to the head of the caudate nucleus. Bilateral subarachnoid extension of the hemorrhage is evident, especially in the Sylvian and interhemispheric fissures.

HYPERTENSIVE INTRACEREBRAL HEMORRHAGE WITH MASS EFFECT, RUPTURE INTO THE VENTRICULAR SYSTEM, AND SUBARACHNOID EXTENSION

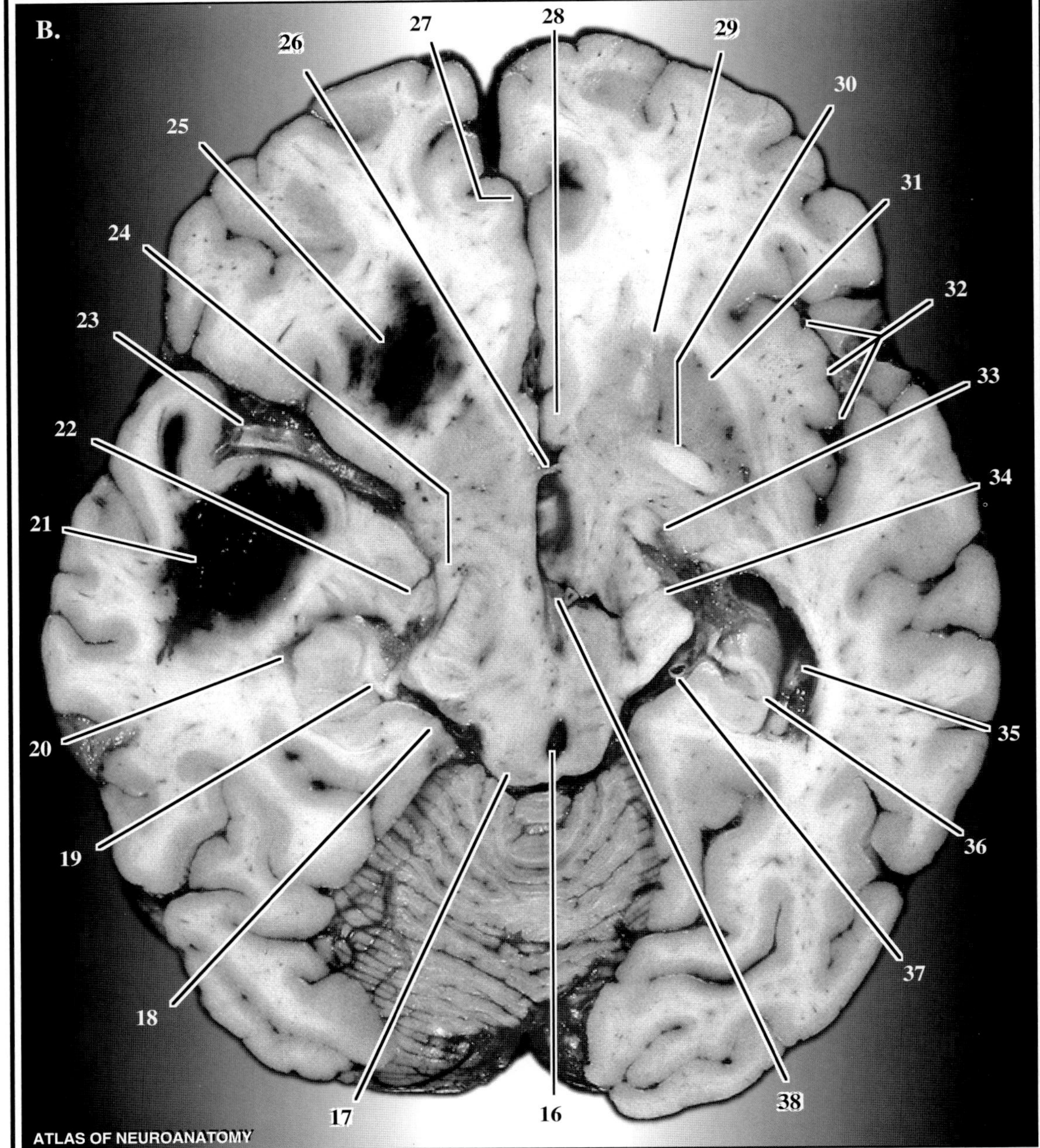

HORIZONTAL SECTIONS: (A.) LEVEL OF THE ANTERIOR NUCLEUS OF THE THALAMUS, AND (B.) LEVEL OF THE MESENCEPHALON

KEY TO NUMBERED STRUCTURES

1. Infarction involving Retrosplenial Cortex
2. Blood in the Occipital Horn of the Lateral Ventricle
3. Pulvinar Nucleus of the Thalamus
4. Genu of the Internal Capsule
5. Insula (laterally displaced)
6. Intracerebral Hemorrhage (origin in the Putamen)
7. Site of Rupture into the Lateral Ventricle
8. Subfalcine Herniation of the Cingulate Gyrus
9. Blood within Cavum Septum Pellucidum
10. Head of the Caudate Nucleus
11. Septal Nuclei
12. Anterior Nucleus of the Thalamus
13. Subarachnoid blood within the Sylvian Fissure
14. Crus of the Fornix
15. Calcarine Fissure
16. Blood within the Aqueduct of Sylvius
17. Inferior Colliculus
18. Parahippocampal Gyrus
19. Fimbria of the Fornix
20. Temporal Horn of the Lateral Ventricle
21. Extension of Hemorrhage into the Temporal Lobe
22. Medial Shift of the Uncus
23. Middle Cerebral Artery
24. Optic Tract
25. Extension of Hemorrhage into the Frontal Lobe
26. Lamina Terminalis
27. Subfalcine Herniation of the Subcallosal Gyrus
28. Paraterminal Gyrus
29. Anterior Limb of the Internal Capsule
30. Anterior Commissure
31. Putamen
32. Subarachnoid Blood over the Insular Cortex
33. Optic Tract
34. Cerebral Peduncle
35. Temporal Horn of the Lateral Ventricle
36. Hippocampal Formation
37. Posterior Cerebral Artery
38. Third Ventricle

DR. JOSEPH J. WARNER

DESCENDING MOTOR CONTROL SYSTEMS: PATHOPHYSIOLOGY

An analysis of this case must include an understanding of the pathophysiologic significance of the flexor followed by extensor posturing observed during this patient's clinical course. Initially, the patient presented with findings which included a right hemiparesis of the face, arm, and leg. Together with the left gaze preference, these findings indicate a left hemisphere lesion. The history of hypertension raises the question of infarction secondary to atherosclerotic cerebrovascular disease. With the sudden onset of coma, however, an acute increase in intracranial pressure secondary to intracranial hemorrhage must be considered. Hypertensive intracerebral hemorrhage is a likely possibility in this patient's differential diagnosis. Common sites for hypertensive hemorrhage include the basal ganglia, thalamus, cerebellum, and base of the pons. As previously indicated, the combined left gaze preference and right hemiparesis suggest a lesion within the left cerebral hemisphere.

Subsequent changes, however, include flexor posturing of the right upper extremity. The apparent facilitation of flexor muscle groups as described in this case is known as *decorticate posturing*. To analyze the significance of this finding, a review of subcortical centers which influence motor function is necessary. Referring to the first diagram, several subcortical centers are delineated. The first of these is an area of the brain which includes the subthalamic region (as distinguished from the subthalamic nucleus), the Fields of Forel, and the rostral mesencephalic tegmentum. The second center is the red nucleus. Caudally, the pontine reticular formation has a major influence on patterns of muscle activation. The lateral vestibular nucleus is included in this analysis, although its role in the posturing observed in this case is limited by the influence of direct cerebellar projections into the nucleus. Finally, the medullary reticular formation is diagrammatically represented. This structure exerts a major influence on the activation or facilitation of specific muscle groups.

Referring to the second diagram, the hierarchical organization of the cerebral cortex and subcortical motor centers is shown. In the intact brain, these subcortical centers are directly influenced by cortical activity. The cerebral cortex, via projection fibers from pyramidal cells, has a complex modulatory effect on subcortical motor systems. An important influence, as represented schematically, is the inhibitory effect the cortex exerts upon the subthalamic region, Fields of Forel, and rostral mesencephalic tegmentum, which will be considered as a functional unit. In addition, the cerebral cortex modulates activity within the pontine reticular formation, and directly facilitates the medullary reticular formation. Thus, in addition to the corticospinal and corticobulbar projection systems, the cerebral cortex controls motor activity through the modulation of several subcortical structures.

The hierarchy is not limited to the cortex. As delineated in the schematic diagram, the subthalamic region, Fields of Forel, and rostral mesencephalic tegmentum collectively inhibit the pontine reticular formation and facilitate the medullary reticular formation. The vestibular labyrinth, via Scarpa's ganglion and the vestibular afferent fibers in the Vestibulocochlear (VIII) nerve, has a direct excitatory effect on the pontine reticular formation and on the lateral vestibular nucleus. In the pontine reticular formation, this excitatory influence is "balanced" via projections from the cerebral cortex and from the subthalamic region. In the lateral vestibular nucleus, direct projections from the vestibulocerebellum exert an inhibitory influence, thus controlling the response of this structure to vestibular input.

In order to consider how this complex modulatory system of excitation and inhibition influences muscle activation, descending tracts from these structures are represented in the third diagram. Predominant effects of these projections on gamma and alpha motor neurons in the spinal cord are outlined for each system. Functional correlations of pathophysiologic abnormalities may thus be analyzed. As delineated, the subthalamic region, Fields of Forel, and the rostral mesencephalic tegmentum collectively influence motor activity of the upper extremities. The rubrospinal tract is known to facilitate activation of flexor alpha and gamma motor neurons for the upper extremities. The significance of this effect in the human nervous system is questionable (in contrast to the powerful effects which have been demonstrated through neurophysiologic studies in feline and other animal models). The pontine reticulospinal tract facilitates extensor gamma motor neurons (and is thus dependent upon the integrity of the gamma loop). The medullary reticulospinal tract transmits activity which facilitates flexor alpha and gamma motor neurons, and inhibits extensor motor neurons. Finally, the vestibulospinal tract transmits activity which exerts a powerful excitatory effect on extensor alpha motor neurons, although it has some effect on gamma motor neurons as well.

DECORTICATE AND DECEREBRATE POSTURING

Pathologic states may affect cortical control of the subthalamic region, Fields of Forel, and the rostral mesencephalic tegmentum. Unilateral lesions which have this effect are generally accompanied by contralateral decorticate posturing. In the case presented, the progressive mass effect of an acute intracerebral hemorrhage interrupted the normal cortical influence on subcortical motor control systems. As shown in the diagram of the decorticate state, disinhibition or "release" of the subthalamic region results in inhibition of the pontine reticulospinal system, and increased excitatory input to the medullary reticulospinal system. Through these projections, the predominant descending motor influence of the subthalamic region, Fields of Forel, and rostral mesencephalic tegmentum is exerted upon flexor gamma and alpha motor neurons of the upper extremity. The concomitant influence of the red nucleus and the rubrospinal system may contribute to increased flexor tone. These combined effects manifest themselves in the decorticate state.

As the mass effect expands, dysfunction descends to the intercollicular level of the mesencephalon. Interference with the descending influence of the subthalamic region, the Fields of Forel, and the rostral mesencephalic tegmentum (and of the red nucleus) results in disinhibition of the pontine reticulospinal system. This disinhibition, along with tonic driving of the pontine reticular formation by vestibular afferent activity, results in unopposed facilitation of extensor gamma motor neurons. Together with disfacilitation of the medullary reticulospinal system, excitation of pontine reticulospinal projections produces a state of extensor rigidity. This appears clinically as extension and internal rotation of the upper extremities as described in this case. Such posturing is termed *decerebrate rigidity.* (Refer to the figure delineating the pathophysiology of the decerebrate state).

Although the lateral vestibulospinal system facilitates extensor alpha motor neurons, this descending influence does not directly contribute to the state of decerebrate rigidity. Activation of the lateral vestibular nucleus by afferents from the vestibular labyrinth (via Scarpa's ganglion and the vestibulocochlear nerve) is "balanced" by direct inhibitory projections from the vestibulocerebellum. Thus, it is unlikely that the lateral vestibulospinal system is directly involved in decerebrate posturing.

Neurophysiologic studies in felines and other animal models have demonstrated that dorsal rhizotomy (section of the dorsal roots) abolishes decerebrate rigidity. Reviewing the gamma system (refer to figure), muscle spindle afferents (Type IA and Type II) enter the spinal cord via the dorsal roots. Gamma motor neurons influence the sensitivity and afferent activity of the spindle itself. Through monosynaptic and disynaptic reflex pathways respectively, type IA and type II afferents control alpha motor neuron activation. Thus, dorsal rhizotomy disables the gamma system. The abolition of decerebrate rigidity by dorsal rhizotomy indicates that this state is dependent upon the integrity of gamma systems. Thus, *decerebration* is associated with a state of *gamma rigidity.* Further lesion studies have elucidated mechanisms by which the vestibulospinal system controls motor activity. If cerebellar ablation is performed on a dorsal rhizotomized specimen (in which decerebrate rigidity has been abolished), a state of extensor rigidity reappears. Given the disabled status of the gamma system in such preparations, this rigidity must represent a direct effect on alpha motor neurons. Cerebellar ablation removes the inhibitory vestibulocerebellar influence on the lateral vestibular nucleus. Unopposed tonic driving of the *lateral vestibulospinal system* by vestibular afferents follows such an ablation, and results in a state of *alpha rigidity.*

Mass effect in this case presents as a rostrocaudal progression of neural dysfunction, with hemiparesis followed by decorticate posturing, then bilateral decerebration. The laterality of the lesion in a bilaterally decerebrate patient may not be immediately evident from the clinical presentation. If mass effect displaces the mesencephalon contralaterally (e.g. during transtentorial herniation), the cerebral peduncle contralateral to the mass lesion may be compressed against the adjacent tentorial incisura (Kernohan's notch phenomenon), and motor signs will appear ipsilateral to the lesion. In such a case, important clues to lesion laterality include the history of progression of motor signs and the sequential appearance of any pupillary asymmetry. Parasympathetic pupillary fibers traverse the surface of the oculomotor (III) nerve. Intercalated between the posterior cerebral and superior cerebellar arteries with movement restricted by the tentorial edge, the oculomotor nerve is susceptible to compression ipsilateral to the side of an expanding supratentorial mass. Parasympathetic fibers are compromised early. Thus, the side of initial pupillary dilatation generally indicates the laterality of the lesion.

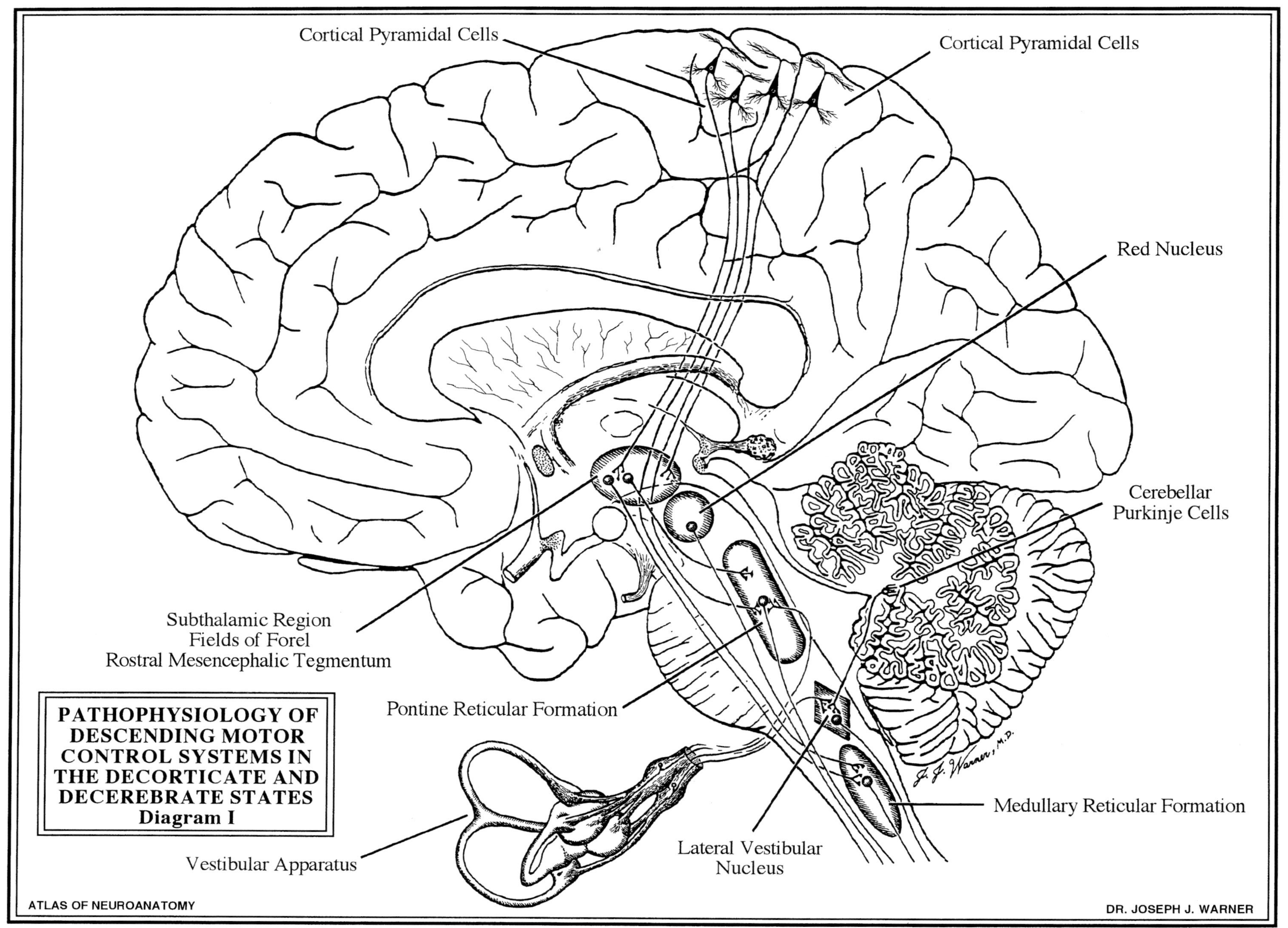
Cortical Pyramidal Cells
Cortical Pyramidal Cells
Red Nucleus
Cerebellar
Purkinje Cells
Subthalamic Region
Fields of Forel
Rostral Mesencephalic Tegmentum
PATHOPHYSIOLOGY OF
DESCENDING MOTOR
CONTROL SYSTEMS IN
THE DECORTICATE AND
DECEREBRATE STATES
Diagram I
Pontine Reticular Formation
Medullary Reticular Formation
Vestibular Apparatus
Lateral Vestibular
Nucleus
ATLAS OF NEUROANATOMY
DR. JOSEPH J. WARNER

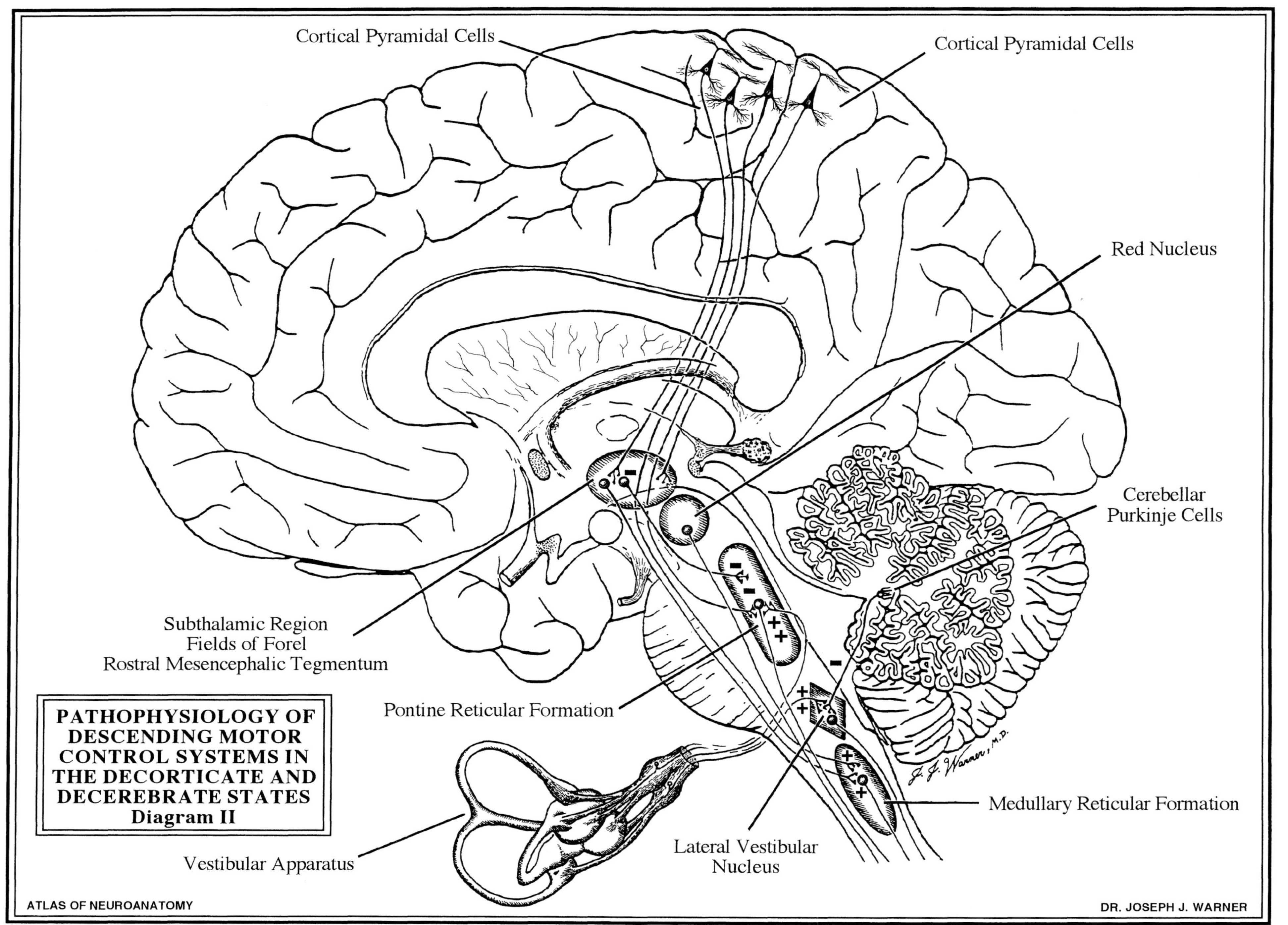

PATHOPHYSIOLOGY OF DESCENDING MOTOR CONTROL SYSTEMS IN THE DECORTICATE AND DECEREBRATE STATES
Diagram II

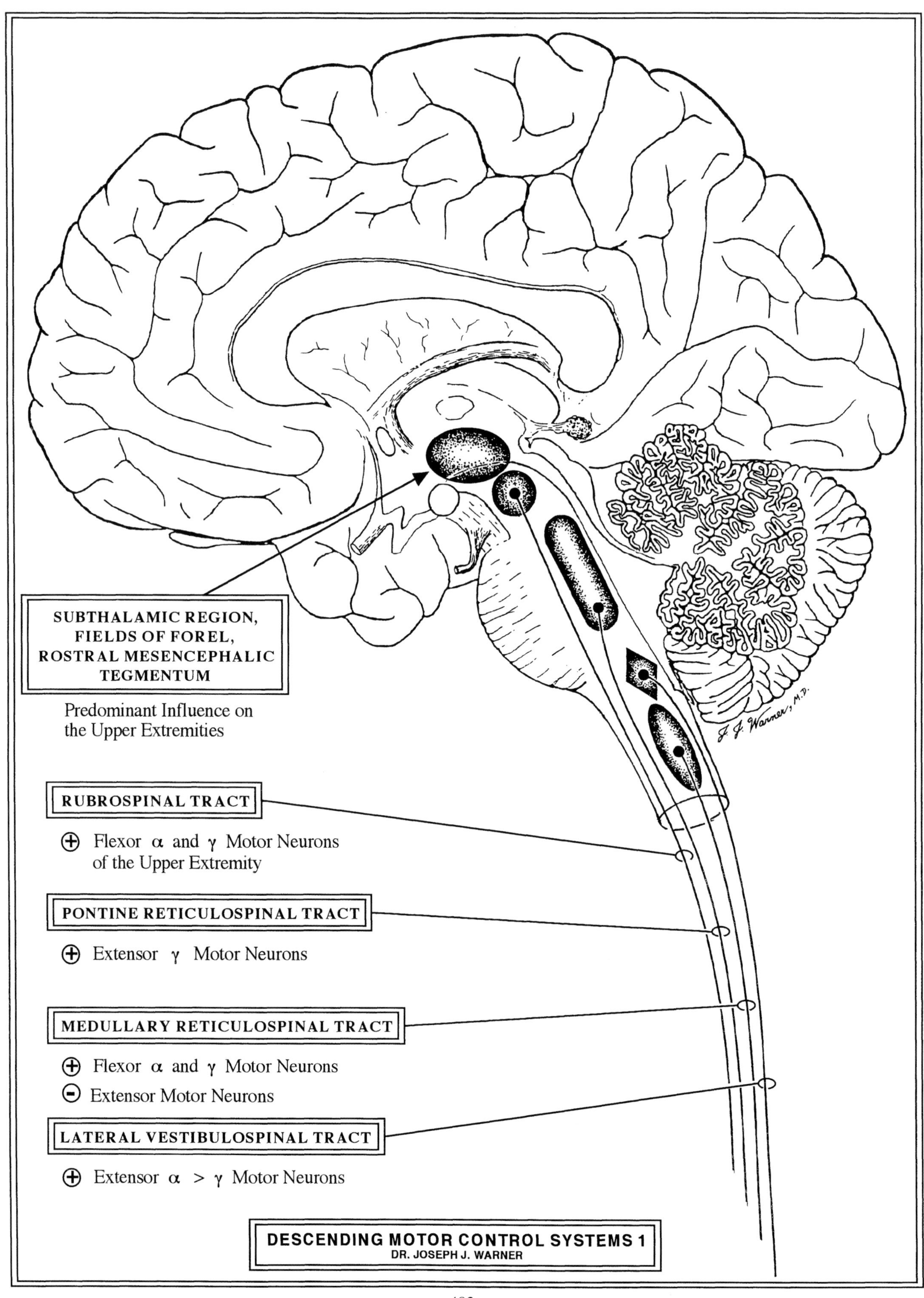
SUBTHALAMIC REGION, FIELDS OF FOREL, ROSTRAL MESENCEPHALIC TEGMENTUM
Predominant Influence on the Upper Extremities
RUBROSPINAL TRACT
⊕ Flexor α and γ Motor Neurons of the Upper Extremity
PONTINE RETICULOSPINAL TRACT
⊕ Extensor γ Motor Neurons
MEDULLARY RETICULOSPINAL TRACT
⊕ Flexor α and γ Motor Neurons
⊖ Extensor Motor Neurons
LATERAL VESTIBULOSPINAL TRACT
⊕ Extensor α > γ Motor Neurons
J. J. Warner, M.D.
DESCENDING MOTOR CONTROL SYSTEMS 1
DR. JOSEPH J. WARNER

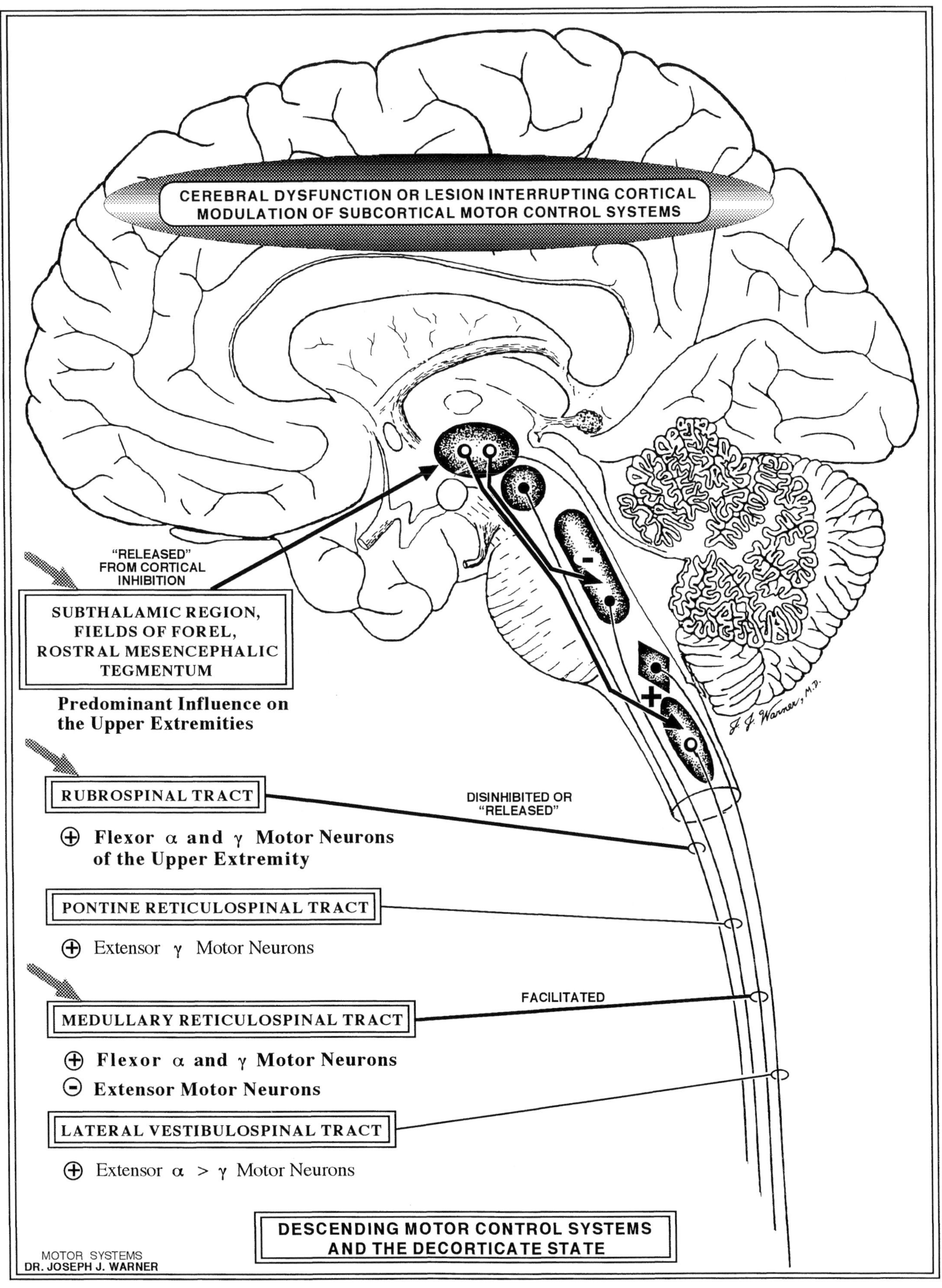
CEREBRAL DYSFUNCTION OR LESION INTERRUPTING CORTICAL MODULATION OF SUBCORTICAL MOTOR CONTROL SYSTEMS
"RELEASED" FROM CORTICAL INHIBITION
SUBTHALAMIC REGION, FIELDS OF FOREL, ROSTRAL MESENCEPHALIC TEGMENTUM
Predominant Influence on the Upper Extremities
RUBROSPINAL TRACT
⊕ Flexor α and γ Motor Neurons of the Upper Extremity
DISINHIBITED OR "RELEASED"
PONTINE RETICULOSPINAL TRACT
⊕ Extensor γ Motor Neurons
FACILITATED
MEDULLARY RETICULOSPINAL TRACT
⊕ Flexor α and γ Motor Neurons
⊖ Extensor Motor Neurons
LATERAL VESTIBULOSPINAL TRACT
⊕ Extensor α > γ Motor Neurons
F. J. Warner, M.D.
DESCENDING MOTOR CONTROL SYSTEMS AND THE DECORTICATE STATE
MOTOR SYSTEMS
DR. JOSEPH J. WARNER

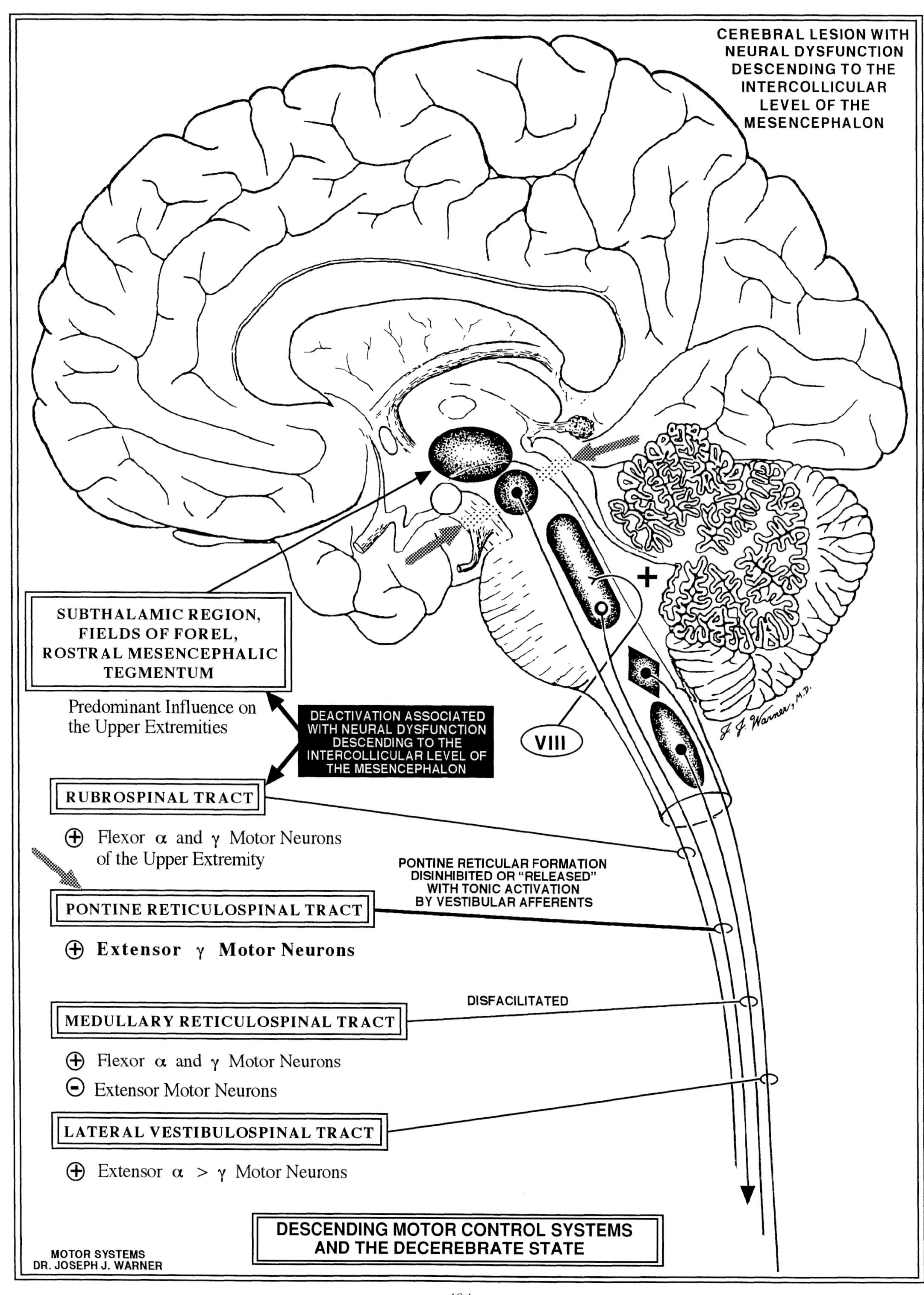
CEREBRAL LESION WITH NEURAL DYSFUNCTION DESCENDING TO THE INTERCOLLICULAR LEVEL OF THE MESENCEPHALON
SUBTHALAMIC REGION, FIELDS OF FOREL, ROSTRAL MESENCEPHALIC TEGMENTUM
Predominant Influence on the Upper Extremities
DEACTIVATION ASSOCIATED WITH NEURAL DYSFUNCTION DESCENDING TO THE INTERCOLLICULAR LEVEL OF THE MESENCEPHALON
VIII
+
J. J. Warner, M.D.
RUBROSPINAL TRACT
⊕ Flexor α and γ Motor Neurons of the Upper Extremity
PONTINE RETICULAR FORMATION DISINHIBITED OR "RELEASED" WITH TONIC ACTIVATION BY VESTIBULAR AFFERENTS
PONTINE RETICULOSPINAL TRACT
⊕ Extensor γ Motor Neurons
DISFACILITATED
MEDULLARY RETICULOSPINAL TRACT
⊕ Flexor α and γ Motor Neurons
⊖ Extensor Motor Neurons
LATERAL VESTIBULOSPINAL TRACT
⊕ Extensor α > γ Motor Neurons
DESCENDING MOTOR CONTROL SYSTEMS AND THE DECEREBRATE STATE
MOTOR SYSTEMS
DR. JOSEPH J. WARNER

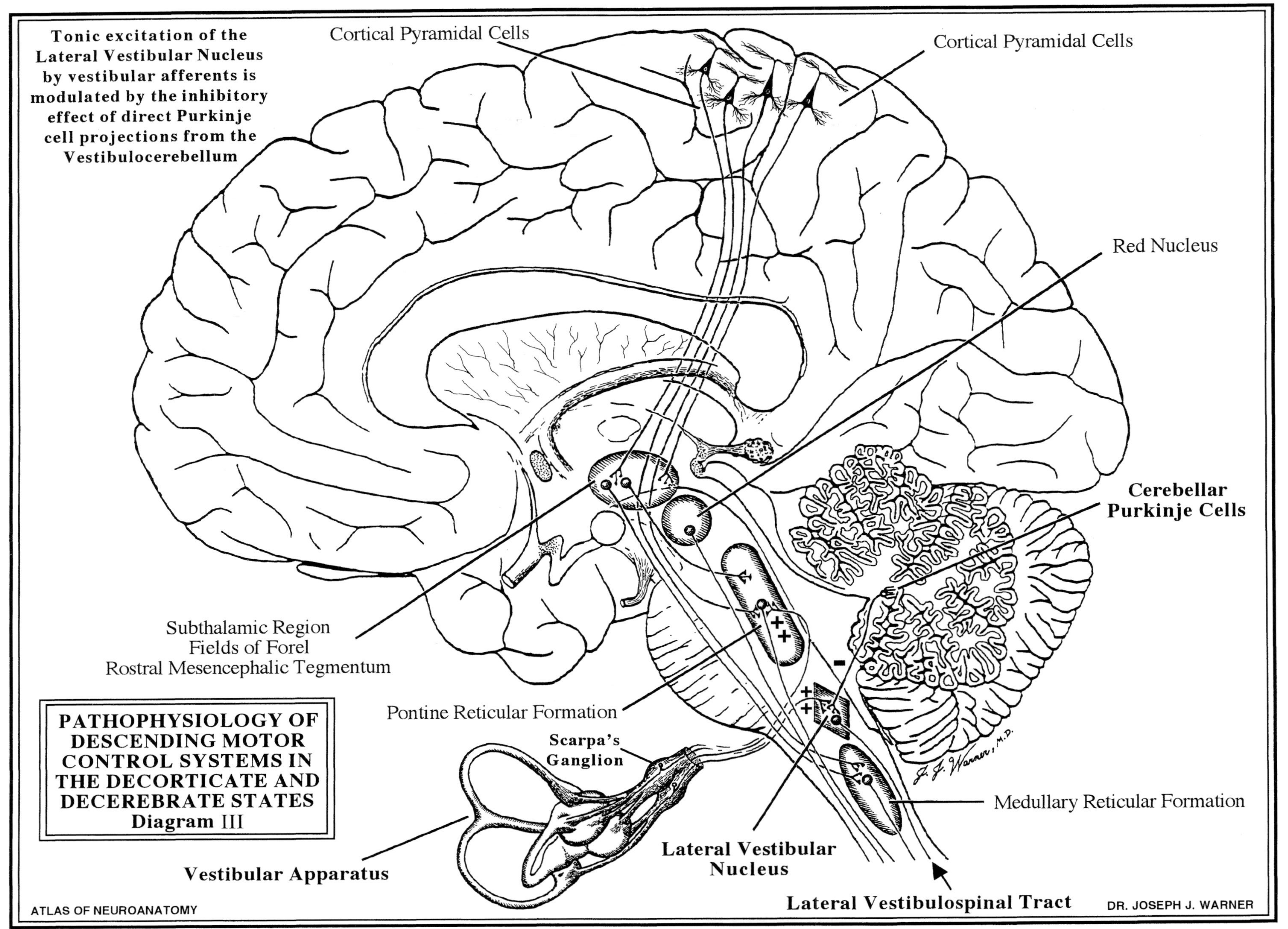
Tonic excitation of the Lateral Vestibular Nucleus by vestibular afferents is modulated by the inhibitory effect of direct Purkinje cell projections from the Vestibulocerebellum
Cortical Pyramidal Cells
Cortical Pyramidal Cells
Red Nucleus
Cerebellar Purkinje Cells
Subthalamic Region
Fields of Forel
Rostral Mesencephalic Tegmentum
Pontine Reticular Formation
Scarpa's Ganglion
Medullary Reticular Formation
Lateral Vestibular Nucleus
Vestibular Apparatus
Lateral Vestibulospinal Tract
PATHOPHYSIOLOGY OF DESCENDING MOTOR CONTROL SYSTEMS IN THE DECORTICATE AND DECEREBRATE STATES Diagram III
ATLAS OF NEUROANATOMY
DR. JOSEPH J. WARNER

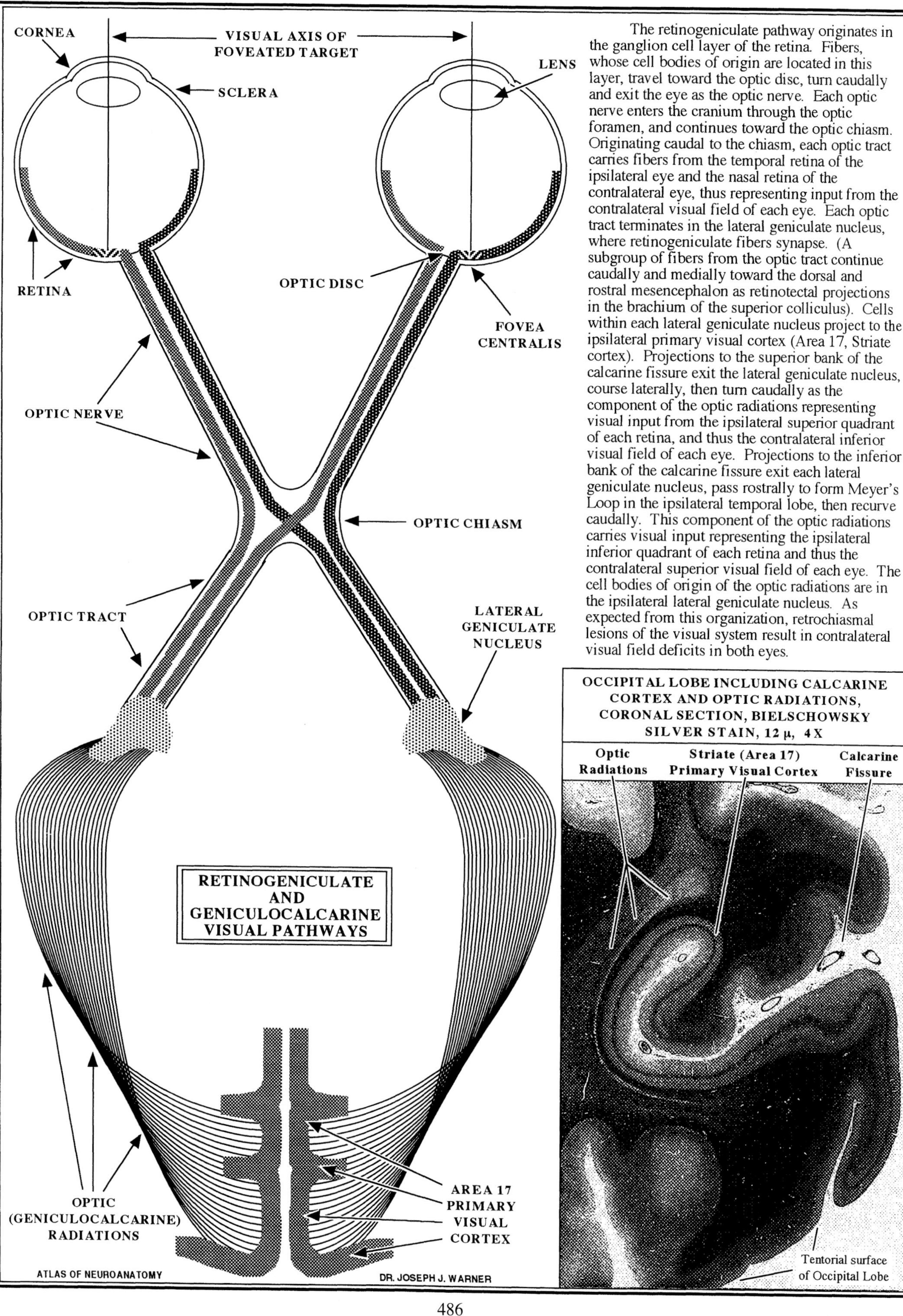

The retinogeniculate pathway originates in the ganglion cell layer of the retina. Fibers, whose cell bodies of origin are located in this layer, travel toward the optic disc, turn caudally and exit the eye as the optic nerve. Each optic nerve enters the cranium through the optic foramen, and continues toward the optic chiasm. Originating caudal to the chiasm, each optic tract carries fibers from the temporal retina of the ipsilateral eye and the nasal retina of the contralateral eye, thus representing input from the contralateral visual field of each eye. Each optic tract terminates in the lateral geniculate nucleus, where retinogeniculate fibers synapse. (A subgroup of fibers from the optic tract continue caudally and medially toward the dorsal and rostral mesencephalon as retinotectal projections in the brachium of the superior colliculus). Cells within each lateral geniculate nucleus project to the ipsilateral primary visual cortex (Area 17, Striate cortex). Projections to the superior bank of the calcarine fissure exit the lateral geniculate nucleus, course laterally, then turn caudally as the component of the optic radiations representing visual input from the ipsilateral superior quadrant of each retina, and thus the contralateral inferior visual field of each eye. Projections to the inferior bank of the calcarine fissure exit each lateral geniculate nucleus, pass rostrally to form Meyer's Loop in the ipsilateral temporal lobe, then recurve caudally. This component of the optic radiations carries visual input representing the ipsilateral inferior quadrant of each retina and thus the contralateral superior visual field of each eye. The cell bodies of origin of the optic radiations are in the ipsilateral lateral geniculate nucleus. As expected from this organization, retrochiasmal lesions of the visual system result in contralateral visual field deficits in both eyes.

OCCIPITAL LOBE INCLUDING CALCARINE CORTEX AND OPTIC RADIATIONS, CORONAL SECTION, BIELSCHOWSKY SILVER STAIN, 12 μ, 4X

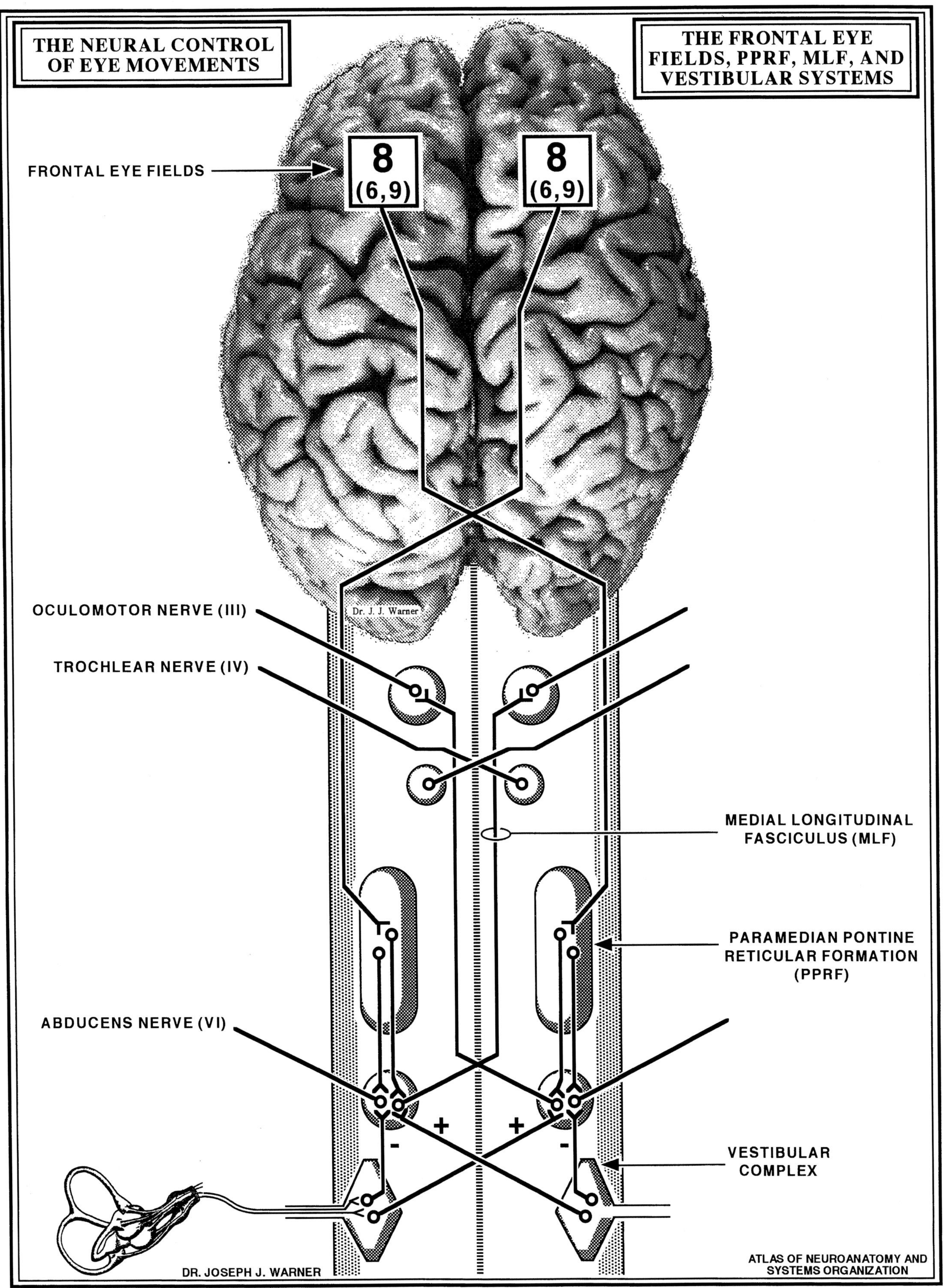
THE NEURAL CONTROL OF EYE MOVEMENTS
THE FRONTAL EYE FIELDS, PPRF, MLF, AND VESTIBULAR SYSTEMS
FRONTAL EYE FIELDS
8 (6,9)
8 (6,9)
Dr. J. J. Warner
OCULOMOTOR NERVE (III)
TROCHLEAR NERVE (IV)
MEDIAL LONGITUDINAL FASCICULUS (MLF)
PARAMEDIAN PONTINE RETICULAR FORMATION (PPRF)
ABDUCENS NERVE (VI)
+
+
-
-
VESTIBULAR COMPLEX
DR. JOSEPH J. WARNER
ATLAS OF NEUROANATOMY AND SYSTEMS ORGANIZATION

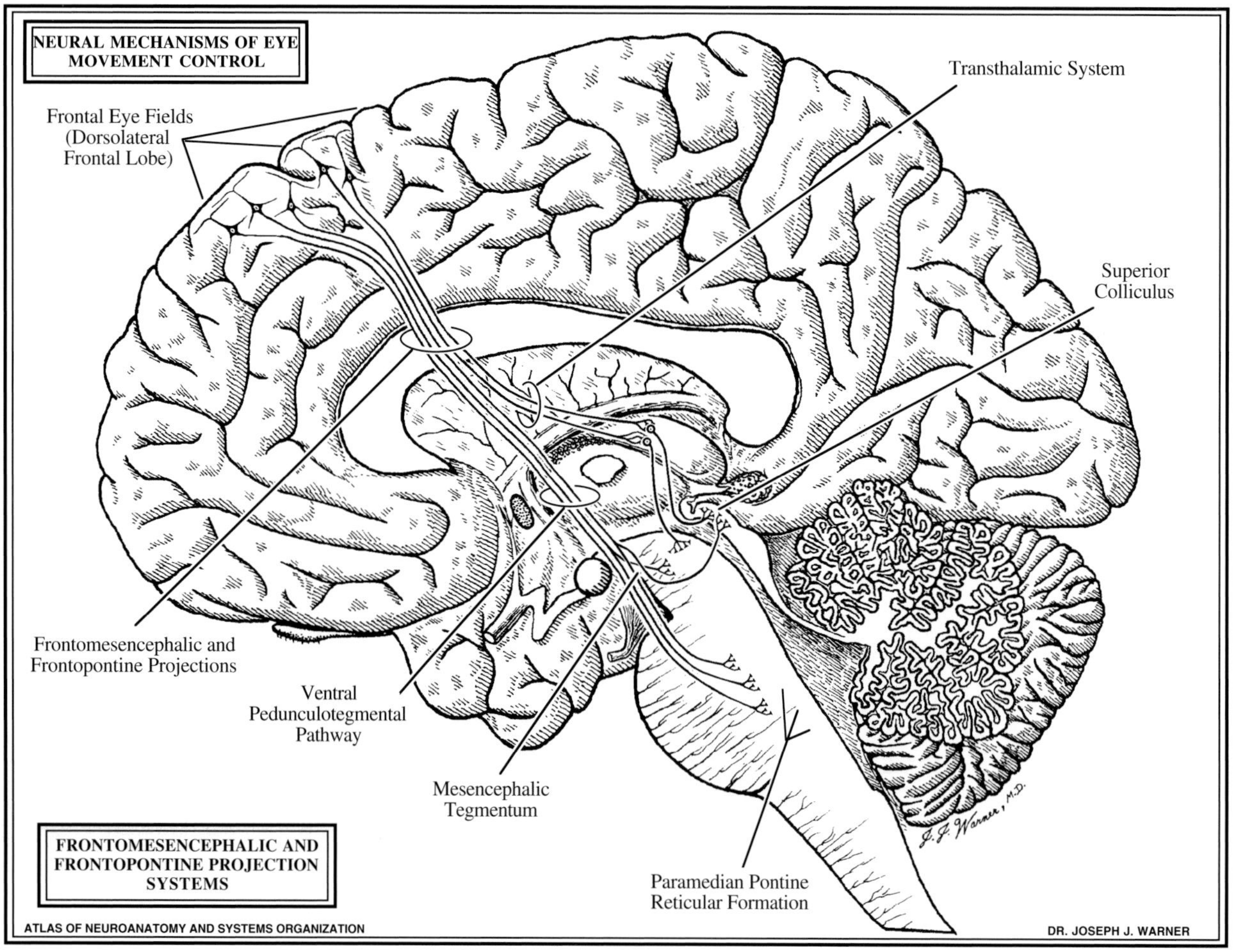

NEURAL MECHANISMS OF EYE MOVEMENT CONTROL

FRONTOMESENCEPHALIC AND FRONTOPONTINE PROJECTION SYSTEMS

ATLAS OF NEUROANATOMY AND SYSTEMS ORGANIZATION

DR. JOSEPH J. WARNER

NEURAL MECHANISMS OF EYE MOVEMENT CONTROL

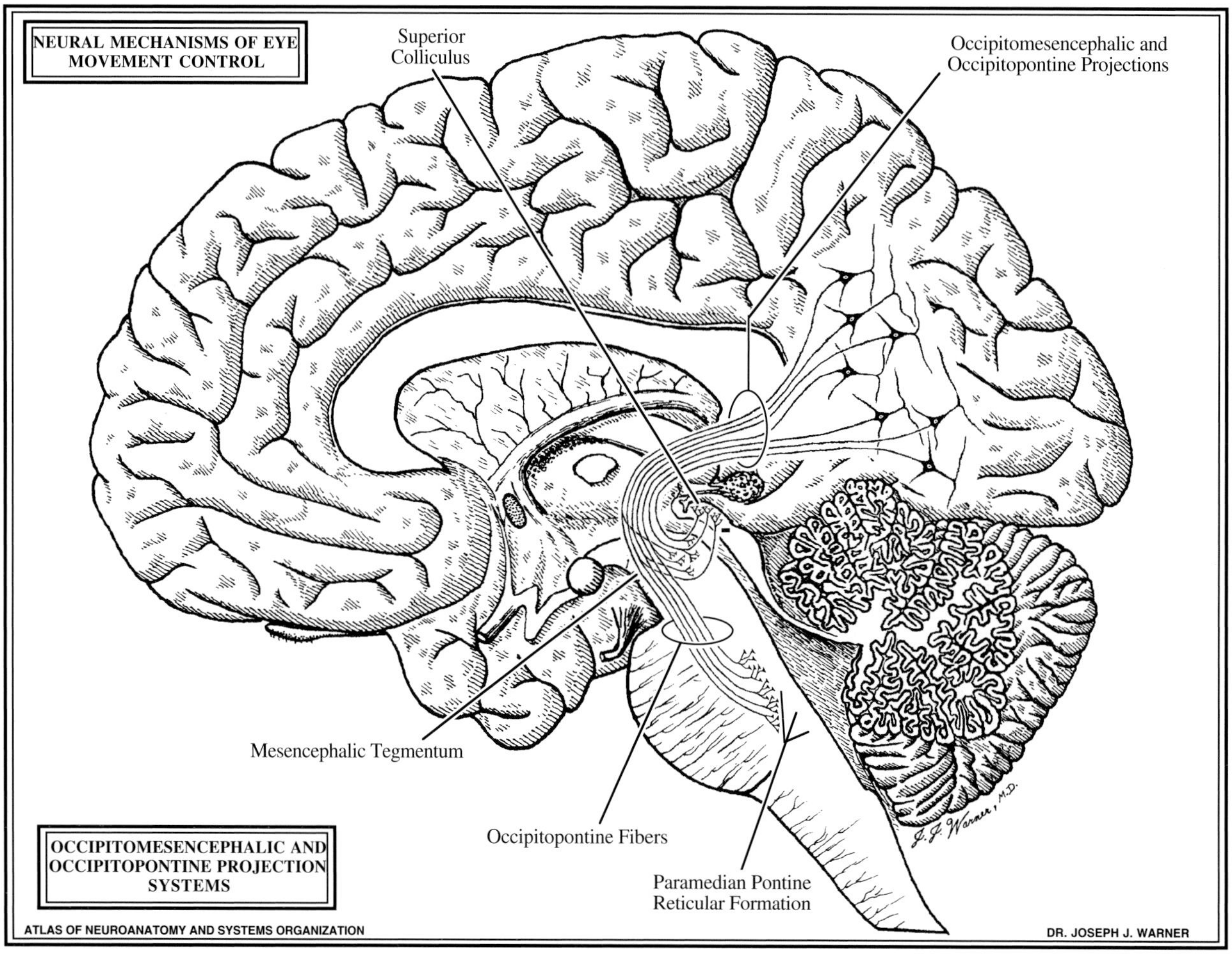

OCCIPITOMESENCEPHALIC AND OCCIPITOPONTINE PROJECTION SYSTEMS

ATLAS OF NEUROANATOMY AND SYSTEMS ORGANIZATION

DR. JOSEPH J. WARNER

NEURAL CONTROL OF EYE MOVEMENTS: THE FRONTAL EYE FIELDS AND OCCIPITOPARIETAL PURSUIT CENTERS

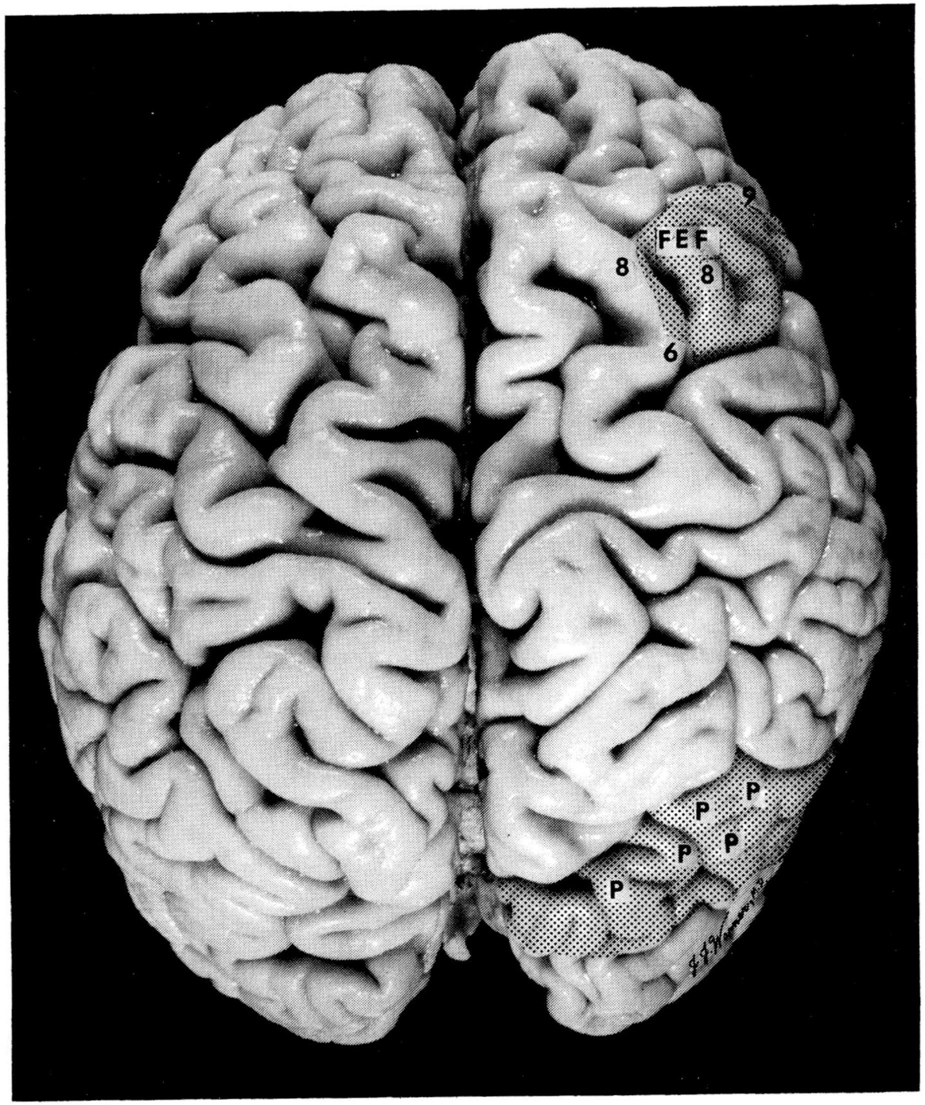

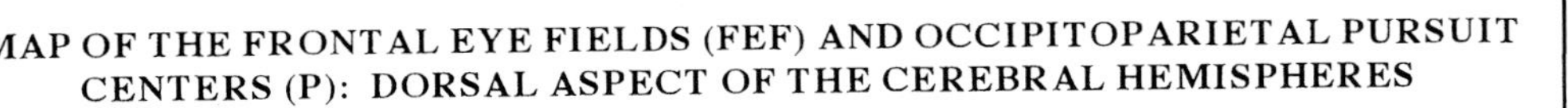

MAP OF THE FRONTAL EYE FIELDS (FEF) AND OCCIPITOPARIETAL PURSUIT CENTERS (P): DORSAL ASPECT OF THE CEREBRAL HEMISPHERES

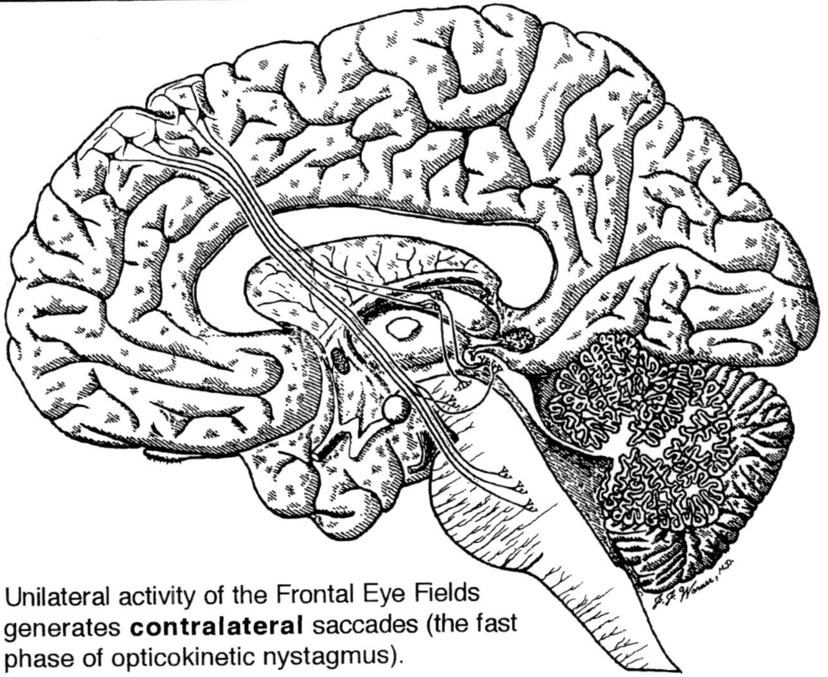

Unilateral activity of the Frontal Eye Fields generates **contralateral** saccades (the fast phase of opticokinetic nystagmus).

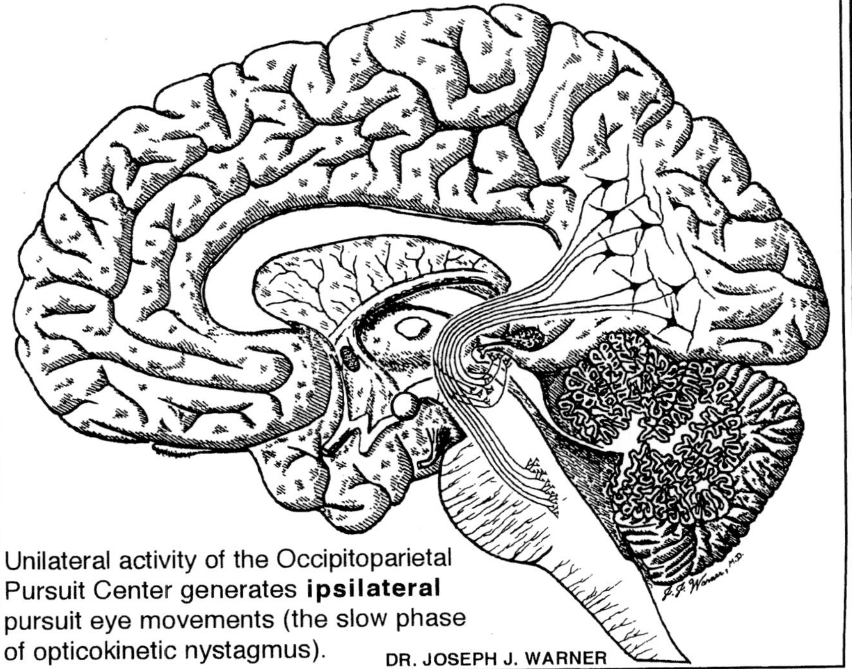

Unilateral activity of the Occipitoparietal Pursuit Center generates **ipsilateral** pursuit eye movements (the slow phase of opticokinetic nystagmus).

DR. JOSEPH J. WARNER

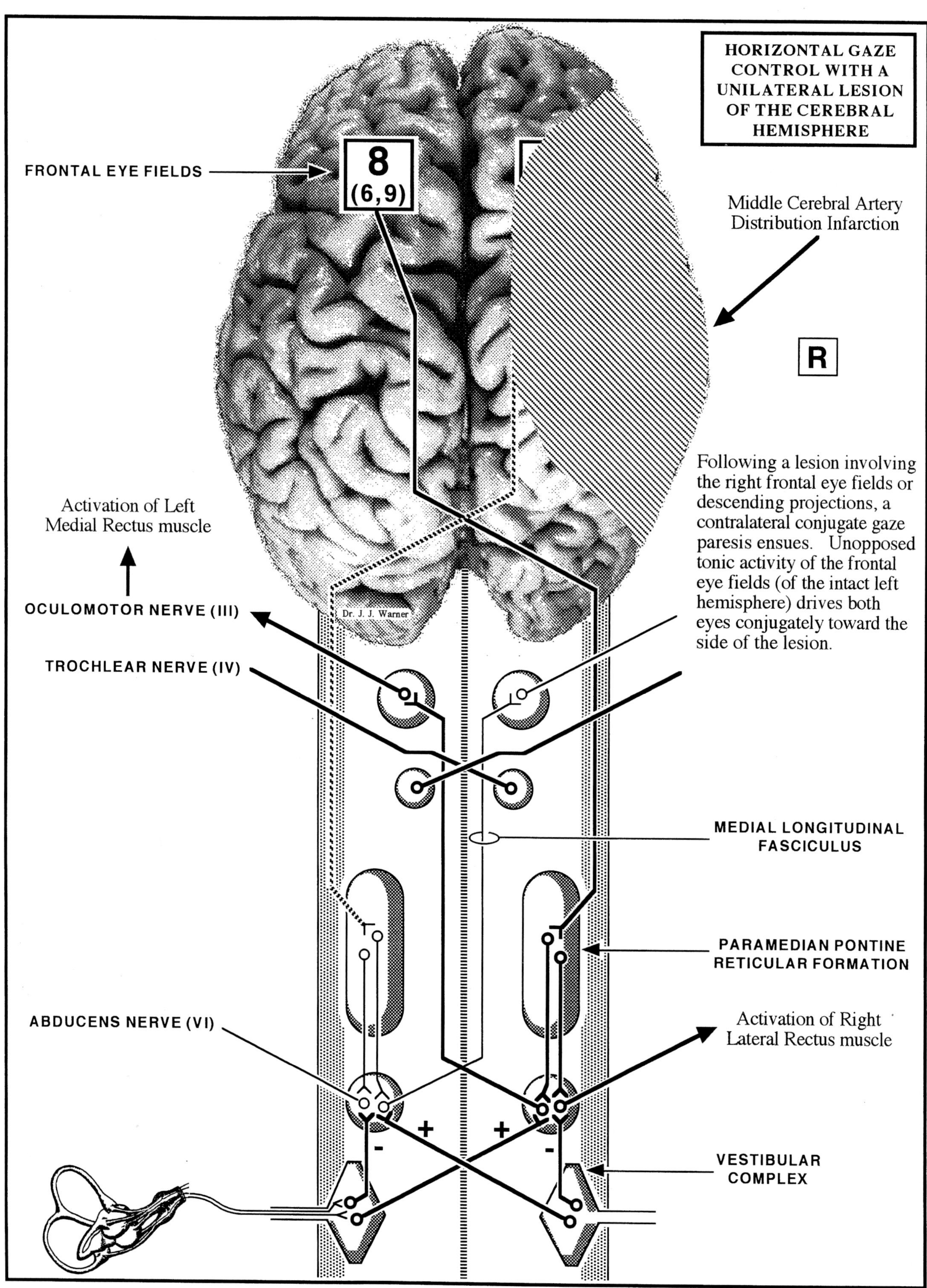
HORIZONTAL GAZE CONTROL WITH A UNILATERAL LESION OF THE CEREBRAL HEMISPHERE
FRONTAL EYE FIELDS
8
(6,9)
Middle Cerebral Artery Distribution Infarction
R
Following a lesion involving the right frontal eye fields or descending projections, a contralateral conjugate gaze paresis ensues. Unopposed tonic activity of the frontal eye fields (of the intact left hemisphere) drives both eyes conjugately toward the side of the lesion.
Activation of Left Medial Rectus muscle
OCULOMOTOR NERVE (III)
Dr. J. J. Warner
TROCHLEAR NERVE (IV)
MEDIAL LONGITUDINAL FASCICULUS
PARAMEDIAN PONTINE RETICULAR FORMATION
ABDUCENS NERVE (VI)
Activation of Right Lateral Rectus muscle
+
+
-
-
VESTIBULAR COMPLEX

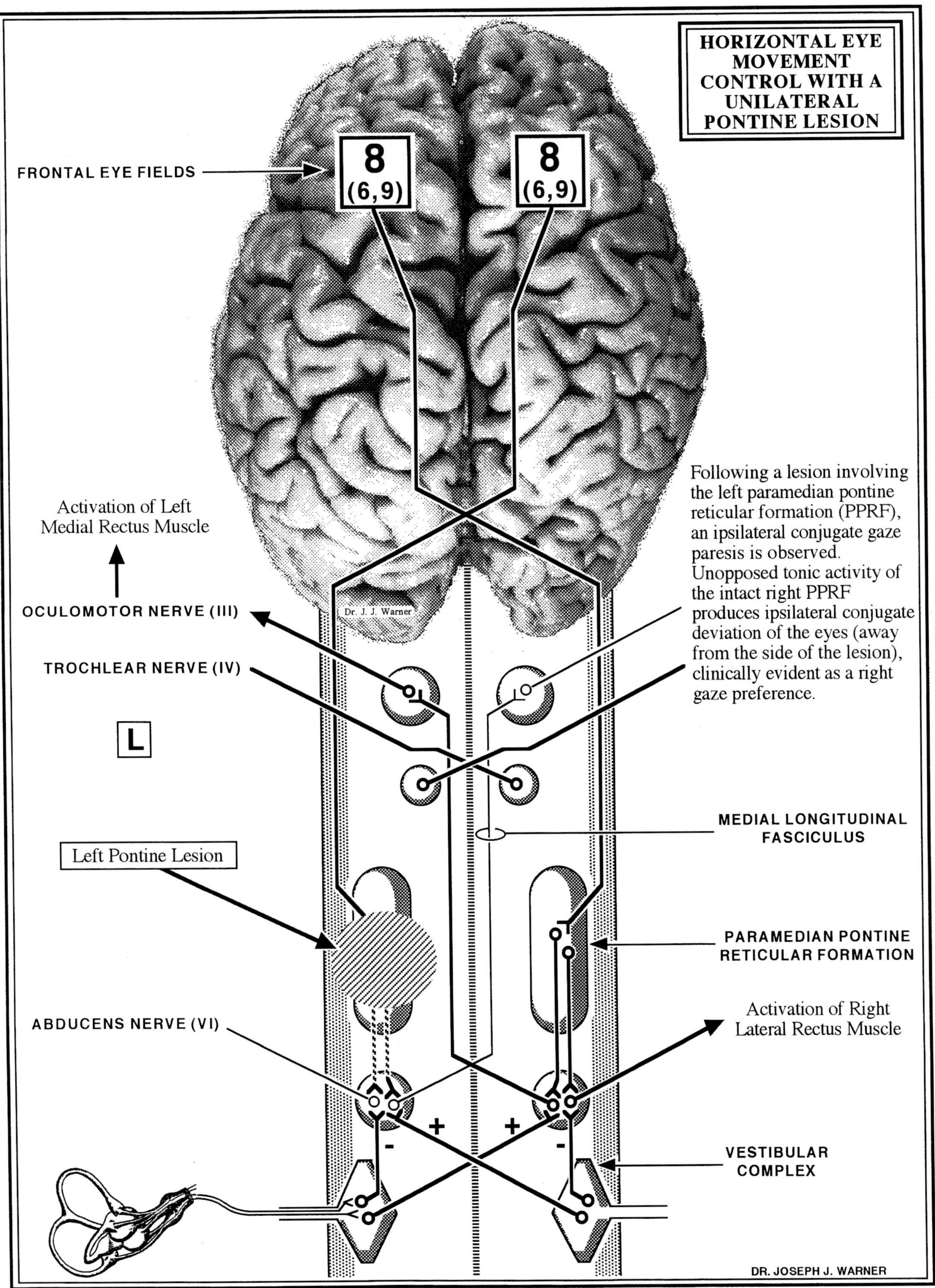
HORIZONTAL EYE MOVEMENT CONTROL WITH A UNILATERAL PONTINE LESION
FRONTAL EYE FIELDS
8
(6,9)
8
(6,9)
Activation of Left Medial Rectus Muscle
OCULOMOTOR NERVE (III)
Dr. J. J. Warner
TROCHLEAR NERVE (IV)
L
Following a lesion involving the left paramedian pontine reticular formation (PPRF), an ipsilateral conjugate gaze paresis is observed. Unopposed tonic activity of the intact right PPRF produces ipsilateral conjugate deviation of the eyes (away from the side of the lesion), clinically evident as a right gaze preference.
MEDIAL LONGITUDINAL FASCICULUS
Left Pontine Lesion
PARAMEDIAN PONTINE RETICULAR FORMATION
ABDUCENS NERVE (VI)
Activation of Right Lateral Rectus Muscle
+
+
-
-
VESTIBULAR COMPLEX
DR. JOSEPH J. WARNER

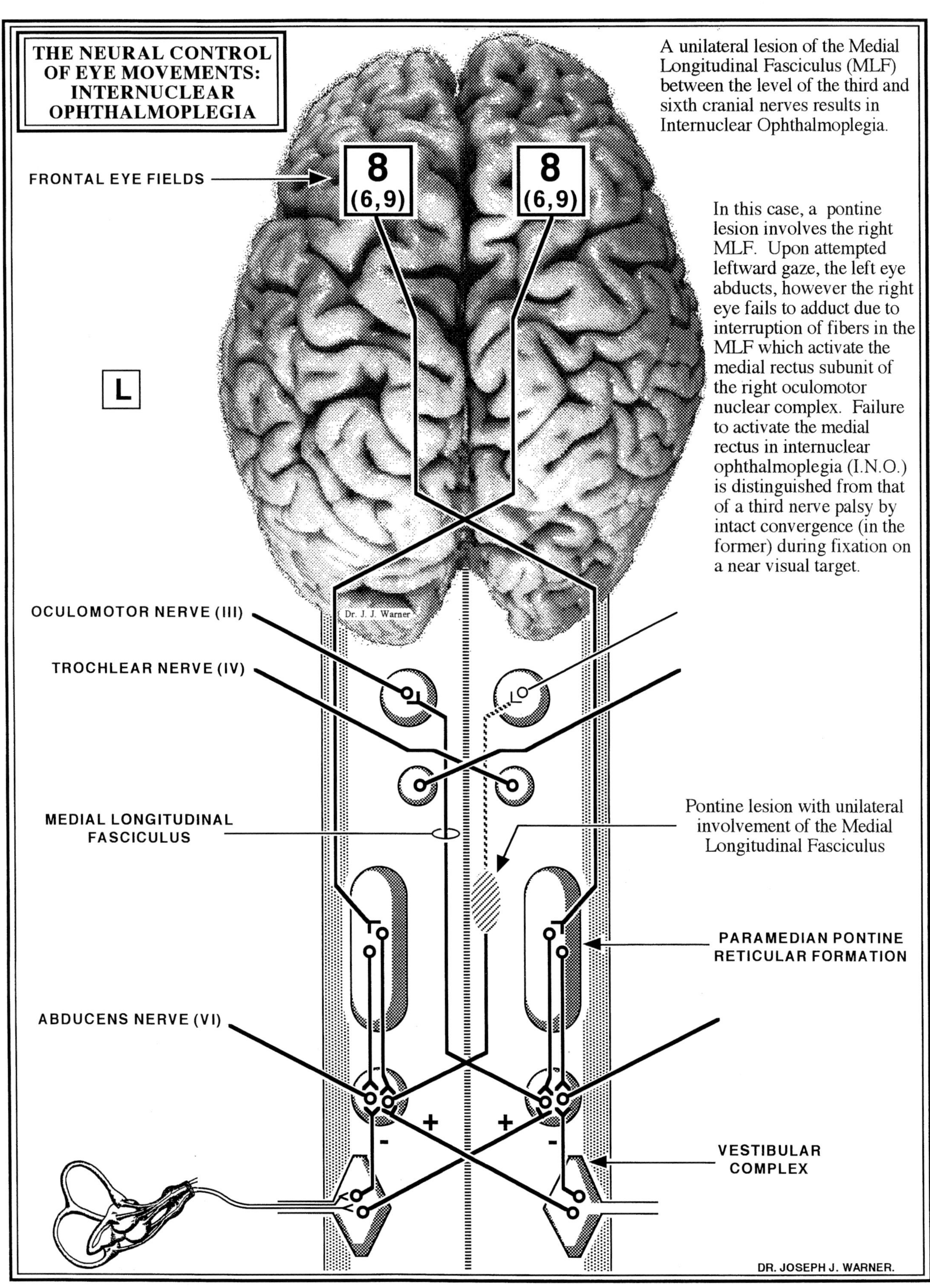
THE NEURAL CONTROL OF EYE MOVEMENTS: INTERNUCLEAR OPHTHALMOPLEGIA
A unilateral lesion of the Medial Longitudinal Fasciculus (MLF) between the level of the third and sixth cranial nerves results in Internuclear Ophthalmoplegia.
FRONTAL EYE FIELDS
8
(6,9)
8
(6,9)
In this case, a pontine lesion involves the right MLF. Upon attempted leftward gaze, the left eye abducts, however the right eye fails to adduct due to interruption of fibers in the MLF which activate the medial rectus subunit of the right oculomotor nuclear complex. Failure to activate the medial rectus in internuclear ophthalmoplegia (I.N.O.) is distinguished from that of a third nerve palsy by intact convergence (in the former) during fixation on a near visual target.
L
Dr. J. J. Warner
OCULOMOTOR NERVE (III)
TROCHLEAR NERVE (IV)
MEDIAL LONGITUDINAL FASCICULUS
Pontine lesion with unilateral involvement of the Medial Longitudinal Fasciculus
PARAMEDIAN PONTINE RETICULAR FORMATION
ABDUCENS NERVE (VI)
+
+
-
-
VESTIBULAR COMPLEX
DR. JOSEPH J. WARNER.

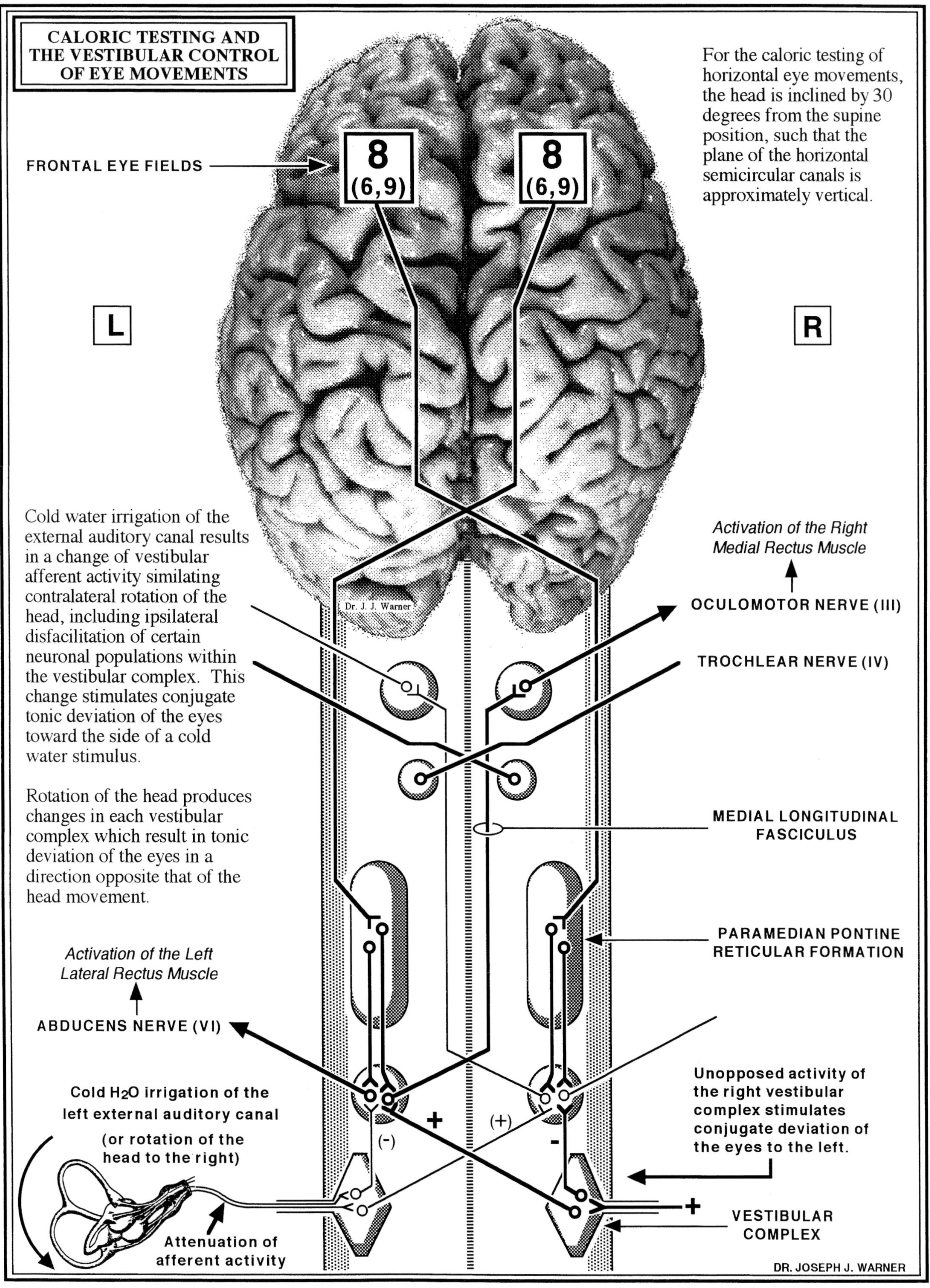

CALORIC TESTING AND THE VESTIBULAR CONTROL OF EYE MOVEMENTS
For the caloric testing of horizontal eye movements, the head is inclined by 30 degrees from the supine position, such that the plane of the horizontal semicircular canals is approximately vertical.
FRONTAL EYE FIELDS
8 (6,9)
8 (6,9)
L
R
Cold water irrigation of the external auditory canal results in a change of vestibular afferent activity similating contralateral rotation of the head, including ipsilateral disfacilitation of certain neuronal populations within the vestibular complex. This change stimulates conjugate tonic deviation of the eyes toward the side of a cold water stimulus.
Rotation of the head produces changes in each vestibular complex which result in tonic deviation of the eyes in a direction opposite that of the head movement.
Activation of the Right Medial Rectus Muscle
OCULOMOTOR NERVE (III)
TROCHLEAR NERVE (IV)
Dr. J. J. Warner
MEDIAL LONGITUDINAL FASCICULUS
PARAMEDIAN PONTINE RETICULAR FORMATION
Activation of the Left Lateral Rectus Muscle
ABDUCENS NERVE (VI)
Cold H_2O irrigation of the left external auditory canal
(or rotation of the head to the right)
+
(+)
(-)
-
Unopposed activity of the right vestibular complex stimulates conjugate deviation of the eyes to the left.
+
VESTIBULAR COMPLEX
Attenuation of afferent activity
DR. JOSEPH J. WARNER

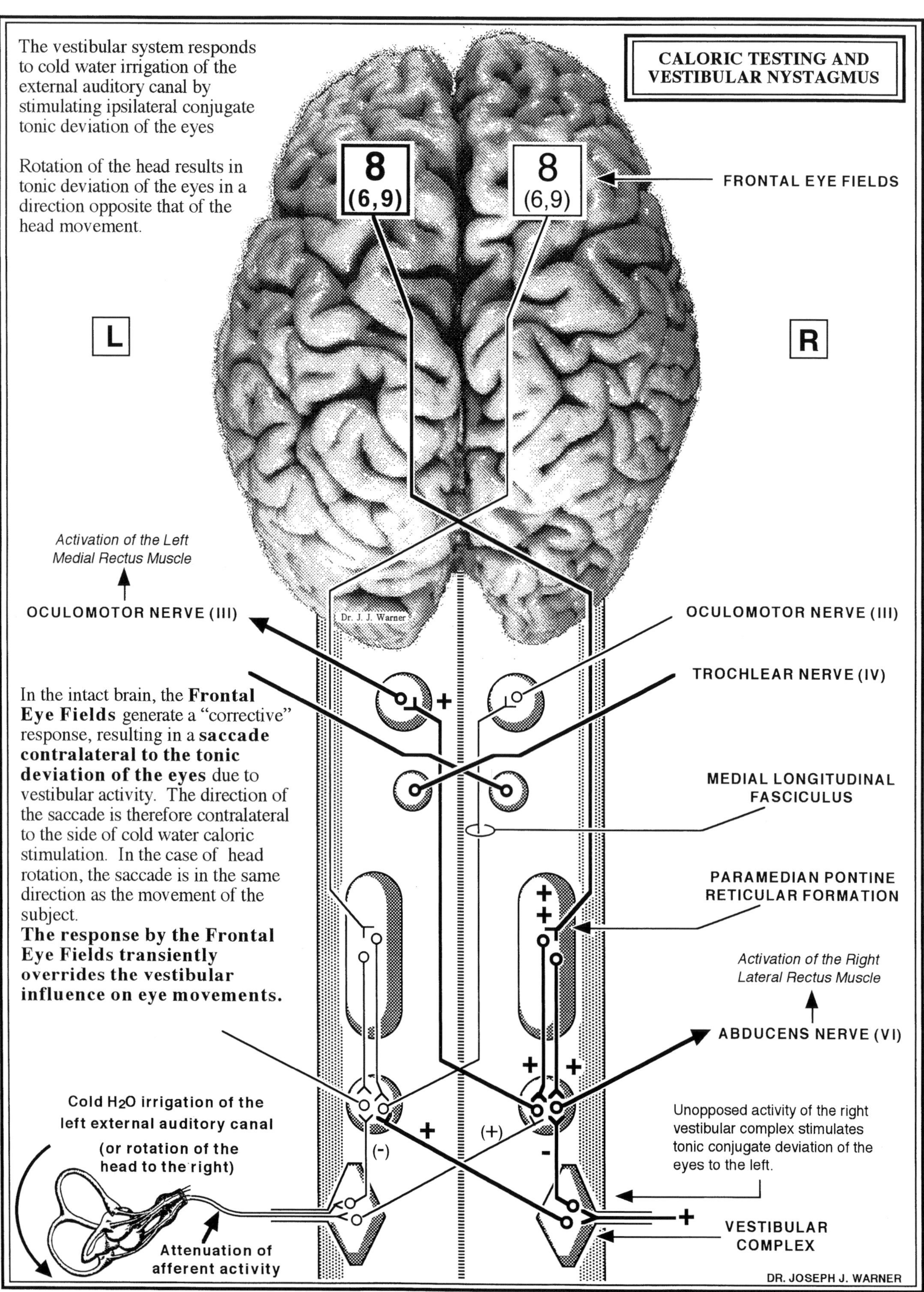
CALORIC TESTING AND VESTIBULAR NYSTAGMUS
The vestibular system responds to cold water irrigation of the external auditory canal by stimulating ipsilateral conjugate tonic deviation of the eyes
Rotation of the head results in tonic deviation of the eyes in a direction opposite that of the head movement.
8
(6,9)
8
(6,9)
FRONTAL EYE FIELDS
L
R
Activation of the Left Medial Rectus Muscle
OCULOMOTOR NERVE (III)
Dr. J. J. Warner
OCULOMOTOR NERVE (III)
TROCHLEAR NERVE (IV)
In the intact brain, the **Frontal Eye Fields** generate a "corrective" response, resulting in a **saccade contralateral to the tonic deviation of the eyes** due to vestibular activity. The direction of the saccade is therefore contralateral to the side of cold water caloric stimulation. In the case of head rotation, the saccade is in the same direction as the movement of the subject.
The response by the Frontal Eye Fields transiently overrides the vestibular influence on eye movements.
MEDIAL LONGITUDINAL FASCICULUS
PARAMEDIAN PONTINE RETICULAR FORMATION
Activation of the Right Lateral Rectus Muscle
ABDUCENS NERVE (VI)
Cold H_2O irrigation of the left external auditory canal
(or rotation of the head to the right)
Unopposed activity of the right vestibular complex stimulates tonic conjugate deviation of the eyes to the left.
Attenuation of afferent activity
VESTIBULAR COMPLEX
DR. JOSEPH J. WARNER

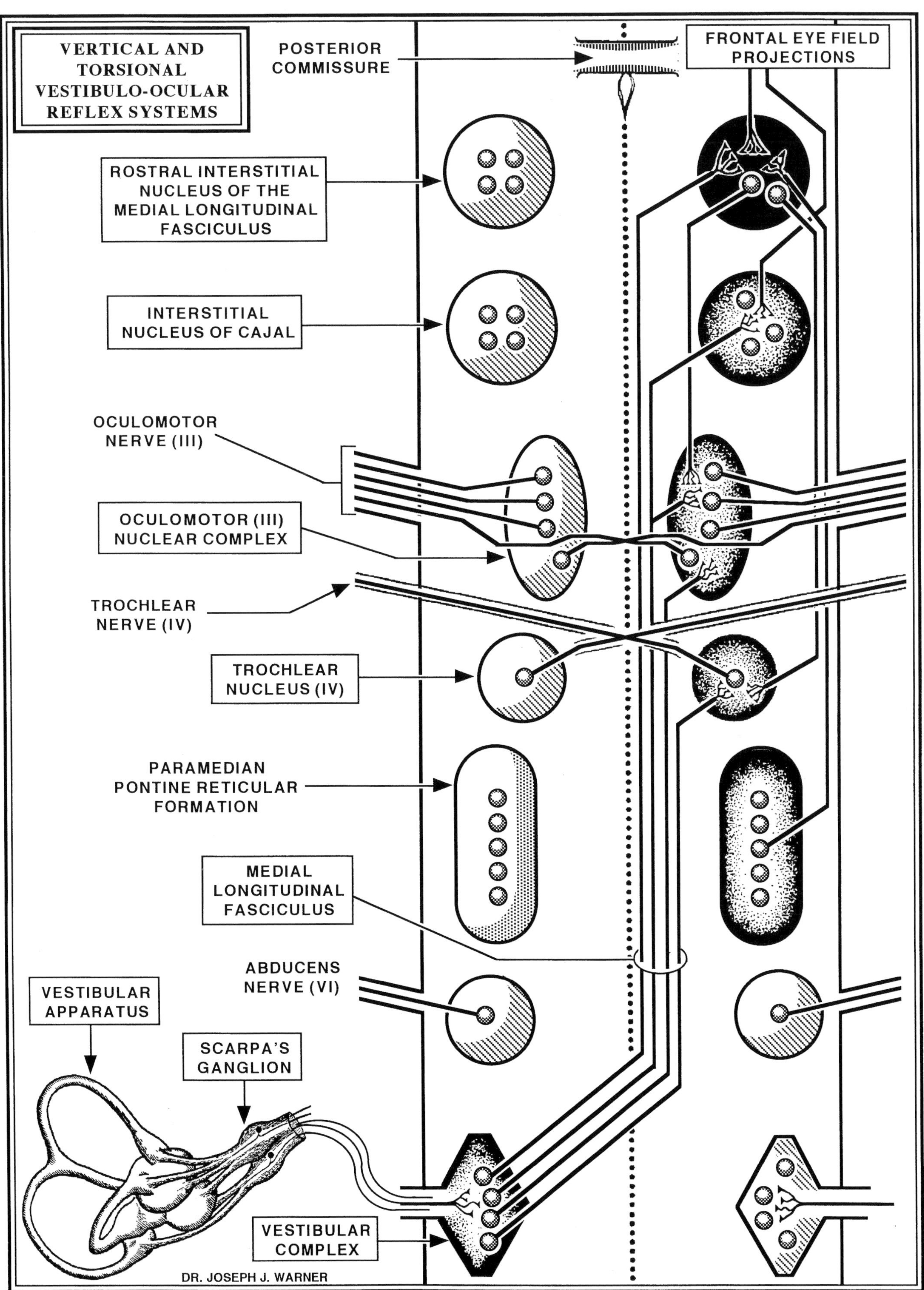

VERTICAL AND TORSIONAL VESTIBULO-OCULAR REFLEX SYSTEMS
POSTERIOR COMMISSURE
FRONTAL EYE FIELD PROJECTIONS
ROSTRAL INTERSTITIAL NUCLEUS OF THE MEDIAL LONGITUDINAL FASCICULUS
INTERSTITIAL NUCLEUS OF CAJAL
OCULOMOTOR NERVE (III)
OCULOMOTOR (III) NUCLEAR COMPLEX
TROCHLEAR NERVE (IV)
TROCHLEAR NUCLEUS (IV)
PARAMEDIAN PONTINE RETICULAR FORMATION
MEDIAL LONGITUDINAL FASCICULUS
ABDUCENS NERVE (VI)
VESTIBULAR APPARATUS
SCARPA'S GANGLION
VESTIBULAR COMPLEX
DR. JOSEPH J. WARNER

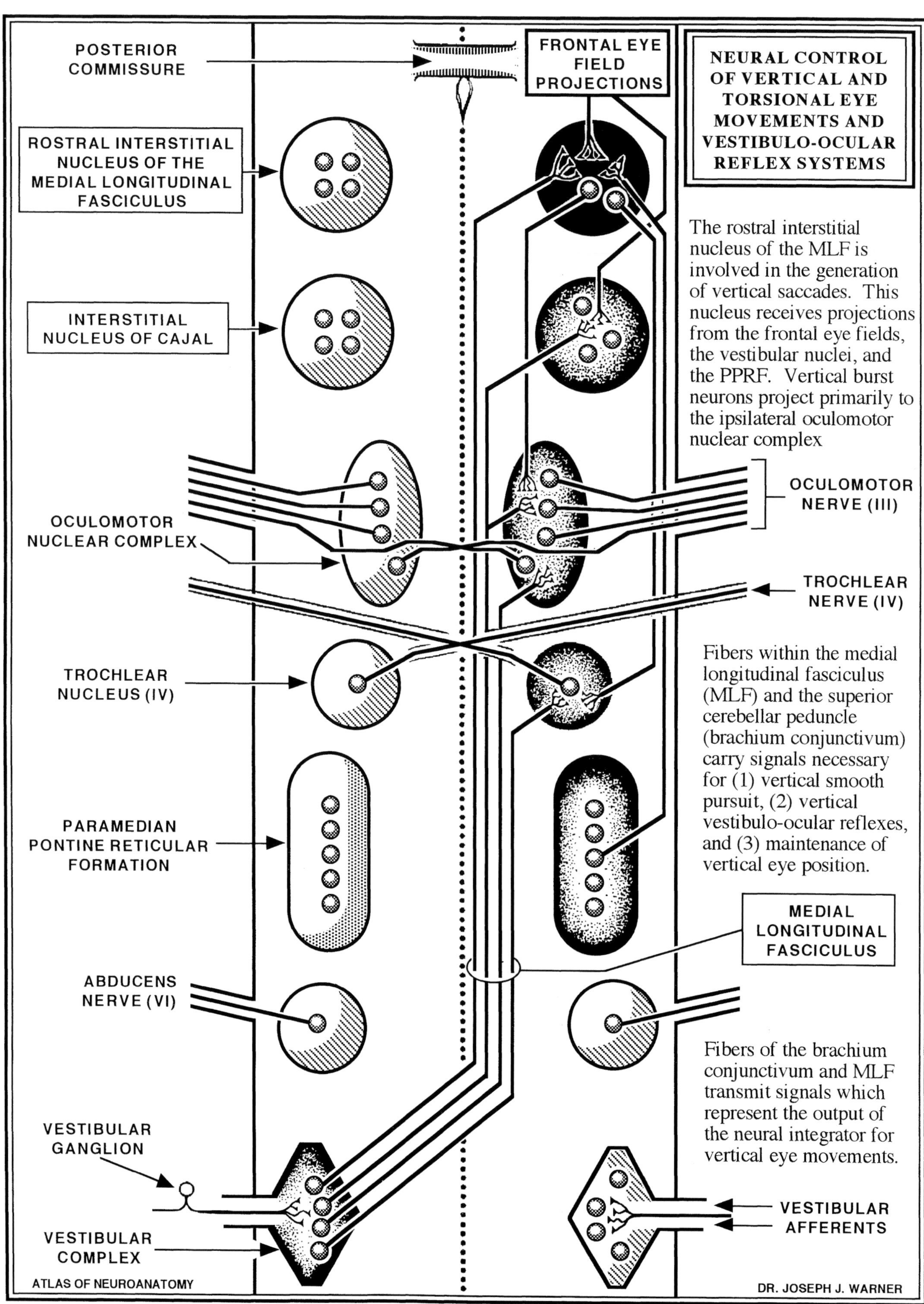
POSTERIOR COMMISSURE
FRONTAL EYE FIELD PROJECTIONS
NEURAL CONTROL OF VERTICAL AND TORSIONAL EYE MOVEMENTS AND VESTIBULO-OCULAR REFLEX SYSTEMS
ROSTRAL INTERSTITIAL NUCLEUS OF THE MEDIAL LONGITUDINAL FASCICULUS
The rostral interstitial nucleus of the MLF is involved in the generation of vertical saccades. This nucleus receives projections from the frontal eye fields, the vestibular nuclei, and the PPRF. Vertical burst neurons project primarily to the ipsilateral oculomotor nuclear complex
INTERSTITIAL NUCLEUS OF CAJAL
OCULOMOTOR NERVE (III)
OCULOMOTOR NUCLEAR COMPLEX
TROCHLEAR NERVE (IV)
TROCHLEAR NUCLEUS (IV)
Fibers within the medial longitudinal fasciculus (MLF) and the superior cerebellar peduncle (brachium conjunctivum) carry signals necessary for (1) vertical smooth pursuit, (2) vertical vestibulo-ocular reflexes, and (3) maintenance of vertical eye position.
PARAMEDIAN PONTINE RETICULAR FORMATION
MEDIAL LONGITUDINAL FASCICULUS
ABDUCENS NERVE (VI)
Fibers of the brachium conjunctivum and MLF transmit signals which represent the output of the neural integrator for vertical eye movements.
VESTIBULAR GANGLION
VESTIBULAR AFFERENTS
VESTIBULAR COMPLEX
ATLAS OF NEUROANATOMY
DR. JOSEPH J. WARNER

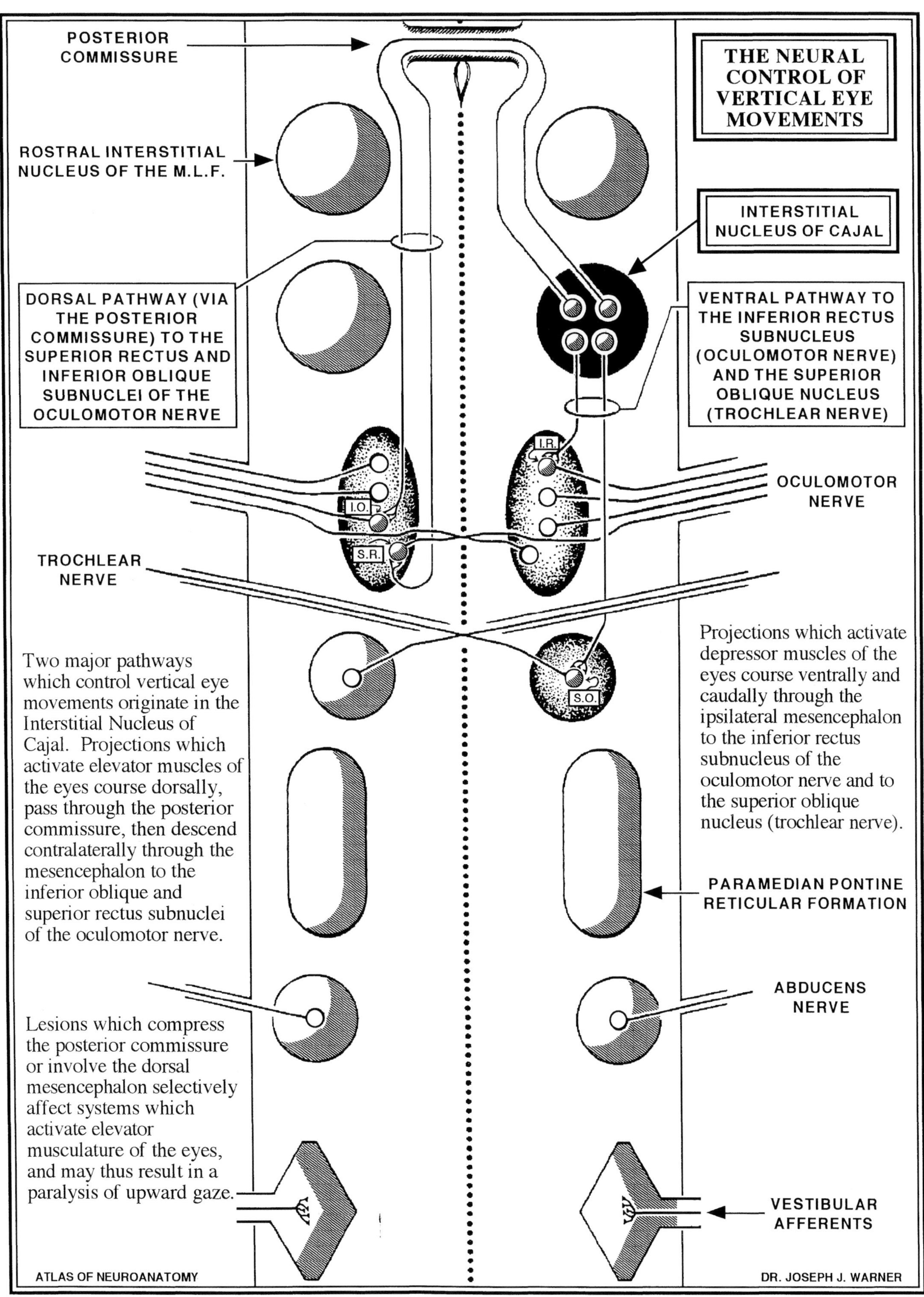
THE NEURAL CONTROL OF VERTICAL EYE MOVEMENTS
POSTERIOR COMMISSURE
ROSTRAL INTERSTITIAL NUCLEUS OF THE M.L.F.
INTERSTITIAL NUCLEUS OF CAJAL
DORSAL PATHWAY (VIA THE POSTERIOR COMMISSURE) TO THE SUPERIOR RECTUS AND INFERIOR OBLIQUE SUBNUCLEI OF THE OCULOMOTOR NERVE
VENTRAL PATHWAY TO THE INFERIOR RECTUS SUBNUCLEUS (OCULOMOTOR NERVE) AND THE SUPERIOR OBLIQUE NUCLEUS (TROCHLEAR NERVE)
I.R.
I.O.
S.R.
OCULOMOTOR NERVE
TROCHLEAR NERVE
S.O.
Two major pathways which control vertical eye movements originate in the Interstitial Nucleus of Cajal. Projections which activate elevator muscles of the eyes course dorsally, pass through the posterior commissure, then descend contralaterally through the mesencephalon to the inferior oblique and superior rectus subnuclei of the oculomotor nerve.
Projections which activate depressor muscles of the eyes course ventrally and caudally through the ipsilateral mesencephalon to the inferior rectus subnucleus of the oculomotor nerve and to the superior oblique nucleus (trochlear nerve).
PARAMEDIAN PONTINE RETICULAR FORMATION
ABDUCENS NERVE
Lesions which compress the posterior commissure or involve the dorsal mesencephalon selectively affect systems which activate elevator musculature of the eyes, and may thus result in a paralysis of upward gaze.
VESTIBULAR AFFERENTS
ATLAS OF NEUROANATOMY
DR. JOSEPH J. WARNER

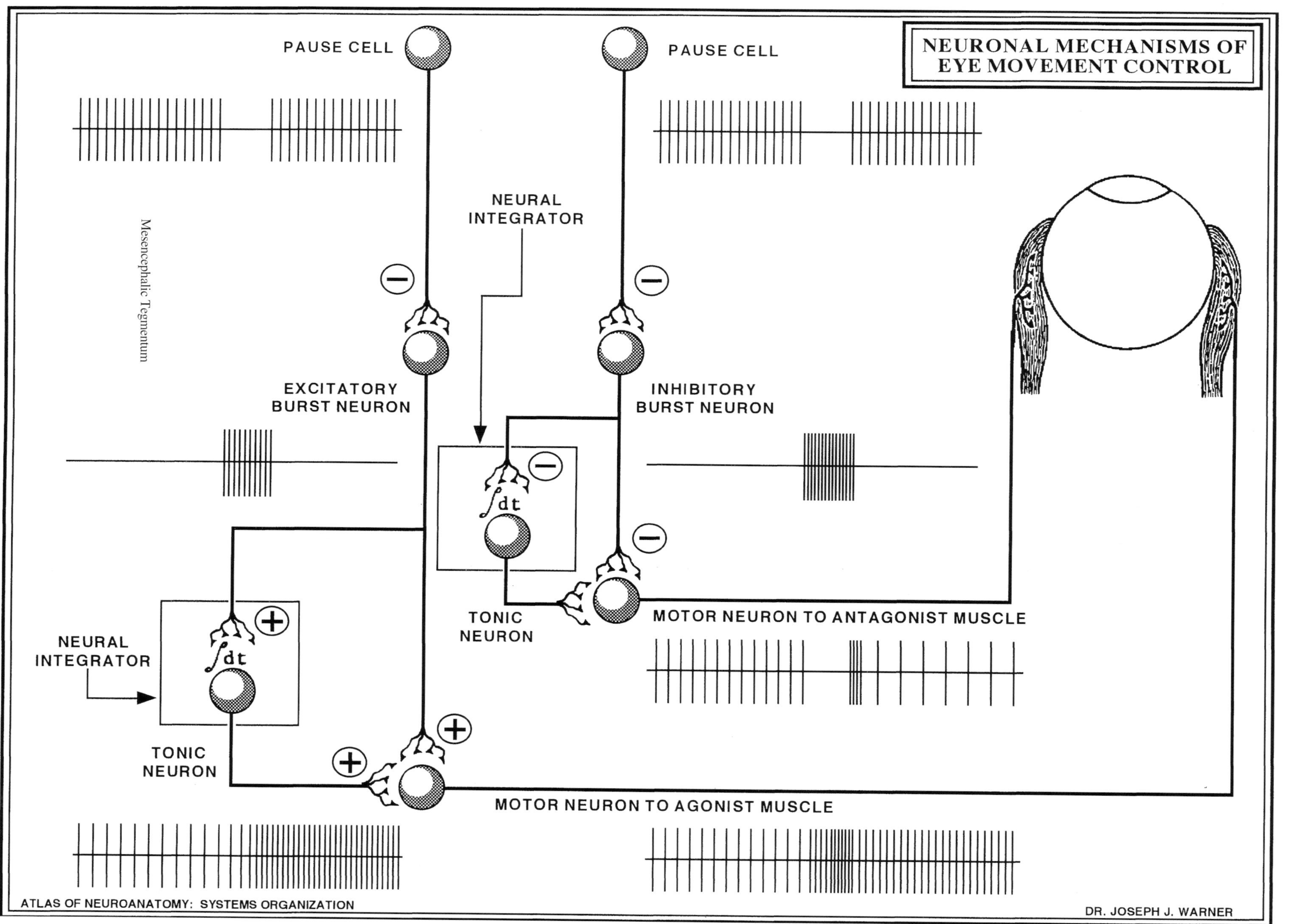
NEURONAL MECHANISMS OF
EYE MOVEMENT CONTROL
PAUSE CELL
PAUSE CELL
NEURAL
INTEGRATOR
EXCITATORY
BURST NEURON
INHIBITORY
BURST NEURON
∫dt
∫dt
TONIC
NEURON
MOTOR NEURON TO ANTAGONIST MUSCLE
NEURAL
INTEGRATOR
TONIC
NEURON
MOTOR NEURON TO AGONIST MUSCLE
ATLAS OF NEUROANATOMY: SYSTEMS ORGANIZATION
DR. JOSEPH J. WARNER

Mesencephalic Tegmentum

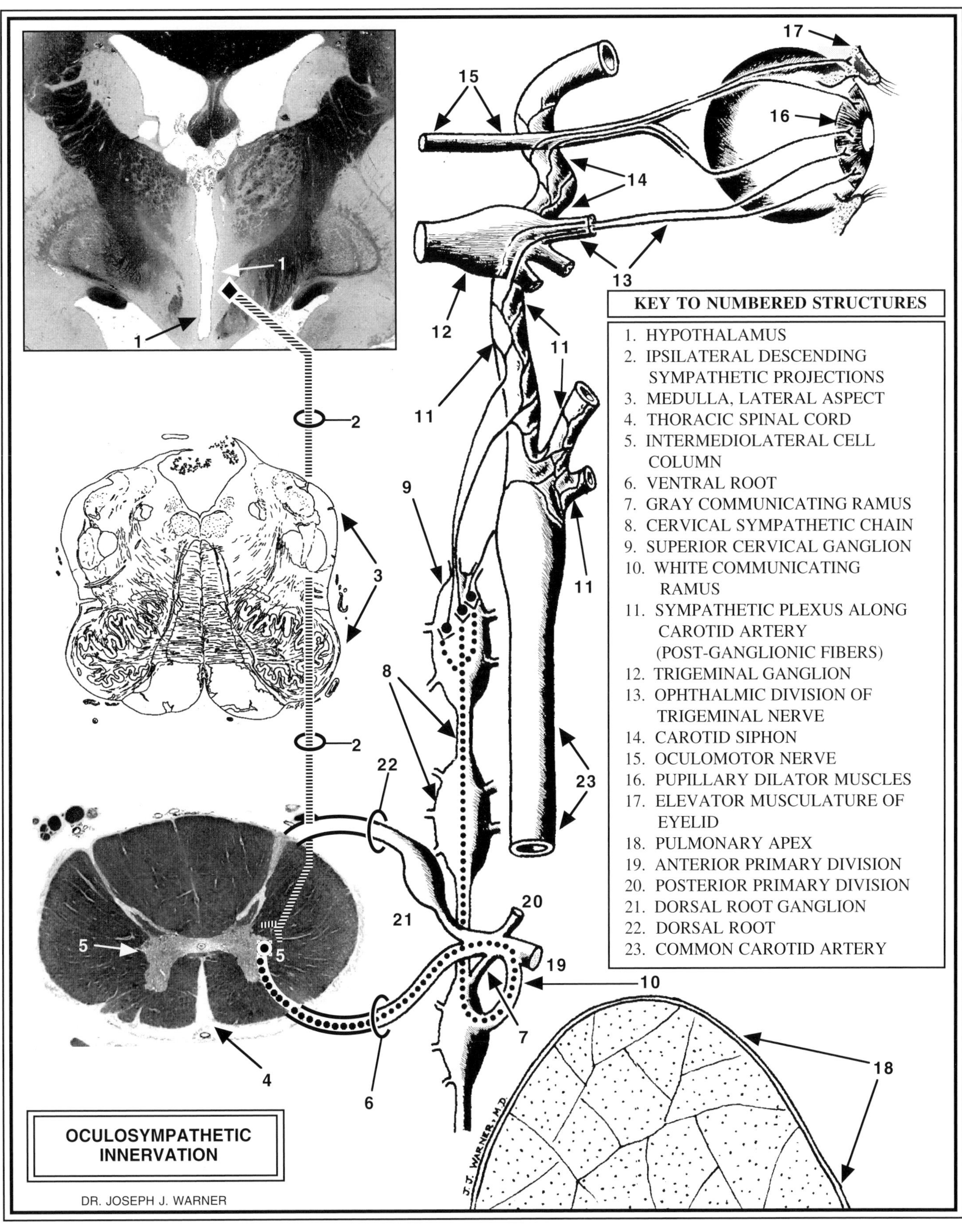

1
1
2
2
3
4
5
5
6
7
8
9
10
11
11
11
11
12
13
14
15
16
17
18
19
20
21
22
23
KEY TO NUMBERED STRUCTURES
1. HYPOTHALAMUS
2. IPSILATERAL DESCENDING SYMPATHETIC PROJECTIONS
3. MEDULLA, LATERAL ASPECT
4. THORACIC SPINAL CORD
5. INTERMEDIOLATERAL CELL COLUMN
6. VENTRAL ROOT
7. GRAY COMMUNICATING RAMUS
8. CERVICAL SYMPATHETIC CHAIN
9. SUPERIOR CERVICAL GANGLION
10. WHITE COMMUNICATING RAMUS
11. SYMPATHETIC PLEXUS ALONG CAROTID ARTERY (POST-GANGLIONIC FIBERS)
12. TRIGEMINAL GANGLION
13. OPHTHALMIC DIVISION OF TRIGEMINAL NERVE
14. CAROTID SIPHON
15. OCULOMOTOR NERVE
16. PUPILLARY DILATOR MUSCLES
17. ELEVATOR MUSCULATURE OF EYELID
18. PULMONARY APEX
19. ANTERIOR PRIMARY DIVISION
20. POSTERIOR PRIMARY DIVISION
21. DORSAL ROOT GANGLION
22. DORSAL ROOT
23. COMMON CAROTID ARTERY
J. J. WARNER, M.D.
OCULOSYMPATHETIC INNERVATION
DR. JOSEPH J. WARNER

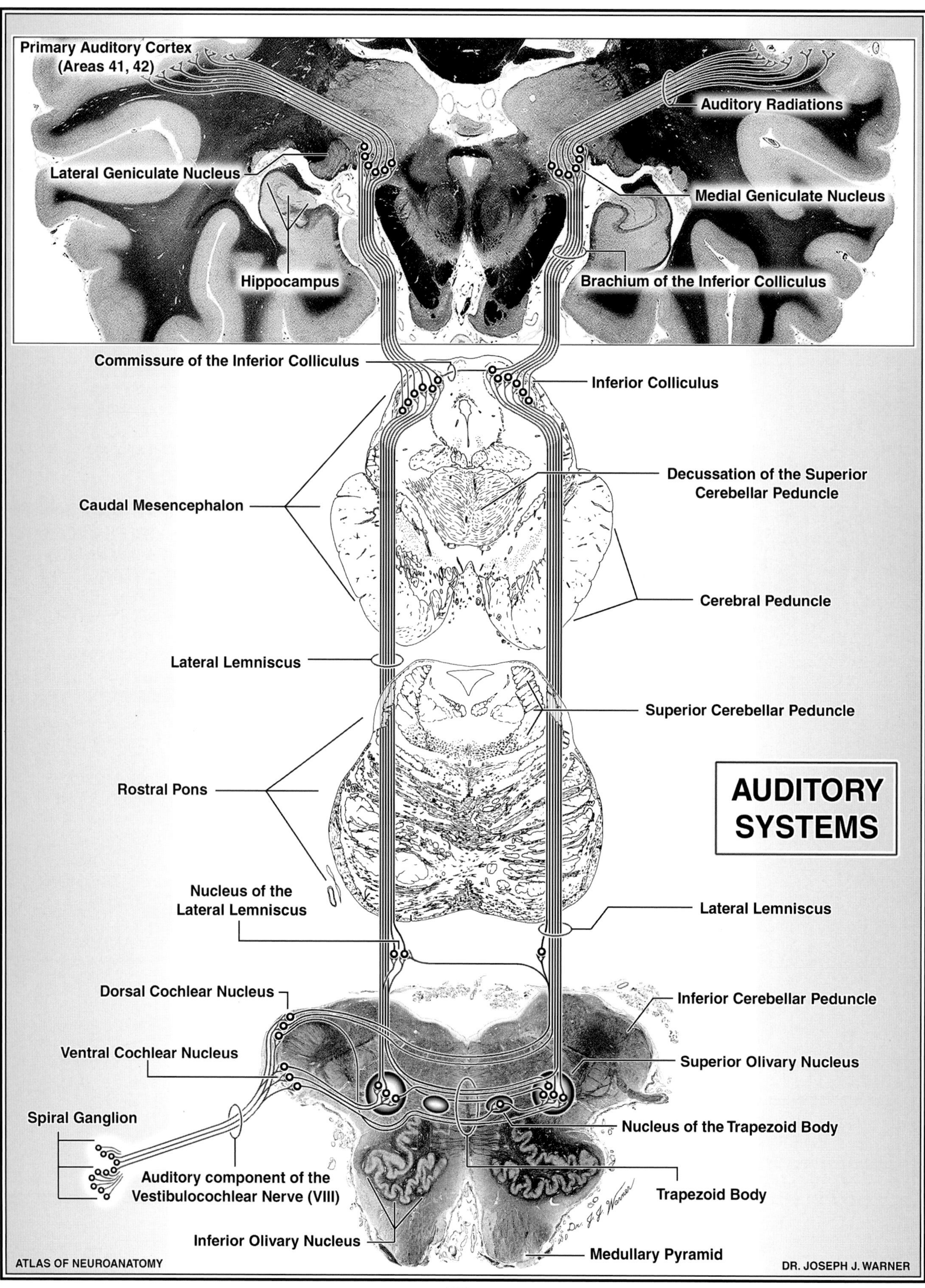
Primary Auditory Cortex
(Areas 41, 42)
Auditory Radiations
Lateral Geniculate Nucleus
Medial Geniculate Nucleus
Hippocampus
Brachium of the Inferior Colliculus
Commissure of the Inferior Colliculus
Inferior Colliculus
Decussation of the Superior
Cerebellar Peduncle
Caudal Mesencephalon
Cerebral Peduncle
Lateral Lemniscus
Superior Cerebellar Peduncle
Rostral Pons
AUDITORY
SYSTEMS
Nucleus of the
Lateral Lemniscus
Lateral Lemniscus
Dorsal Cochlear Nucleus
Inferior Cerebellar Peduncle
Ventral Cochlear Nucleus
Superior Olivary Nucleus
Spiral Ganglion
Nucleus of the Trapezoid Body
Auditory component of the
Vestibulocochlear Nerve (VIII)
Trapezoid Body
Inferior Olivary Nucleus
Medullary Pyramid
ATLAS OF NEUROANATOMY
DR. JOSEPH J. WARNER

PART VIII: FUNCTIONAL NEUROANATOMY AND PATHOPHYSIOLOGY: CLINICAL CASE CORRELATIONS

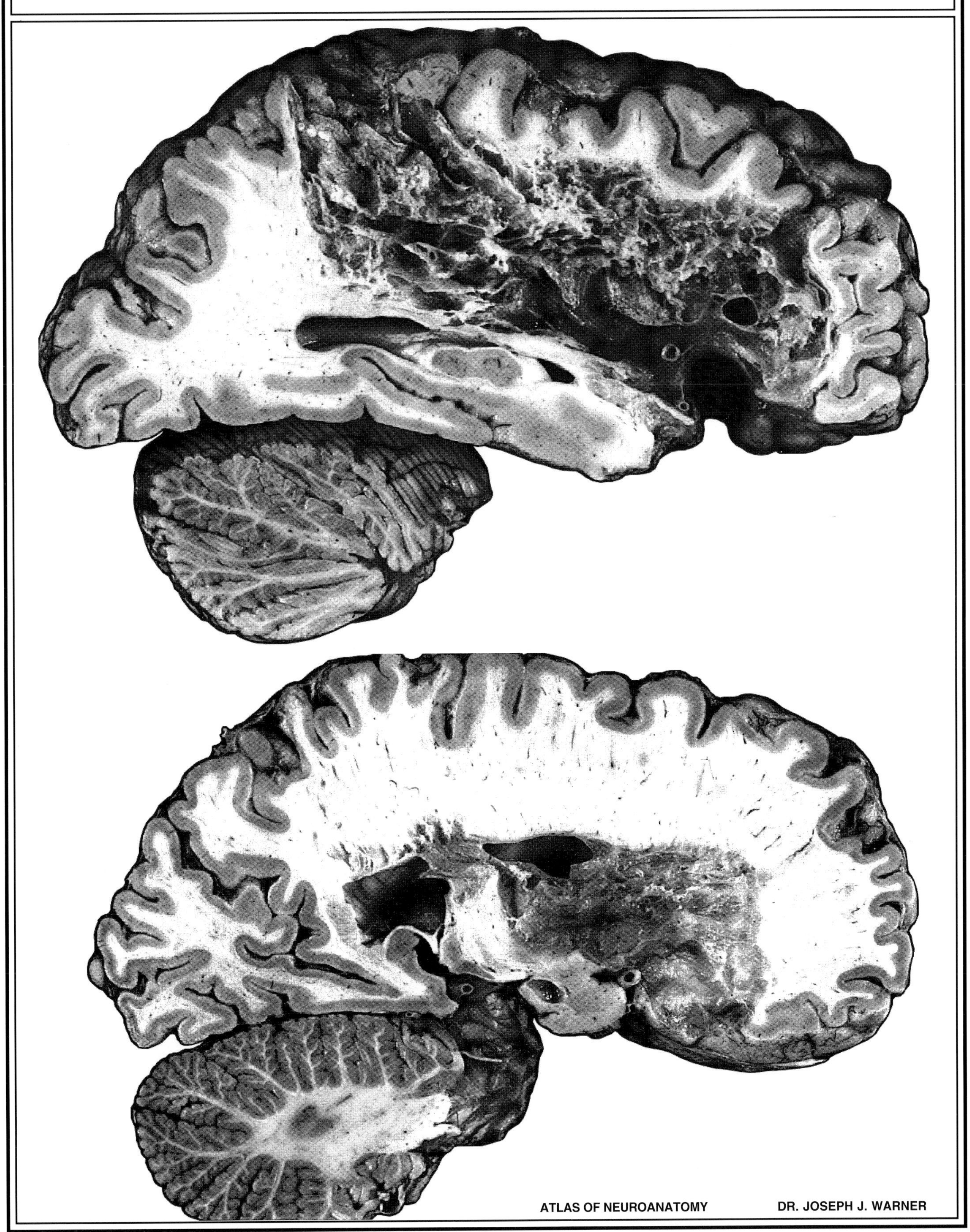

CASE PRESENTATION

This 65-year-old female presented to the hospital with a complaint of her right leg "giving way" accompanied by a feeling of "heaviness" of her right leg "like there's no circulation to it." The patient noticed these deficits upon arising from her bed in the morning. She denied any similar symptoms prior to that night. The patient did give a history of a "light stroke" affecting her left arm three years prior to this admission. She indicated that those deficits had resolved over a two-month period.

Neurologic findings included a somewhat flat affect. The patient acknowledged feeling "a little depressed about all this." She was somewhat slow to respond to questions or tasks during the examination. Her speech was hesitant, characterized by mild word-finding difficulty with occasional circumlocution. Comprehension and repetition were normal. She had difficulty with the performance of skilled motor movements on command, including the mimicking of correct movements and gestures. She frequently used "body part as object" when attempting to demonstrate the use of tools or household utensils. This problem was recognized by the patient, and was observed in both hands.
The elemental neurologic examination revealed a mild left gaze preference, and a moderate contralateral paresis of the right leg, especially noticeable in the flexor musculature. Sensation to pinprick, temperature, light touch and vibration was mildly diminished over the right leg. Right-sided hyperreflexia and a right Babinski sign were present.

CASE ANALYSIS

The history of the acute onset of deficits suggests a thromboembolic or other occlusive cerebrovascular process. An overview of the signs and symptoms indicates a cerebral lesion (as opposed to brainstem or more caudal localization). An important clue is the combination of right-sided sensorimotor findings with a left gaze preference.

Neurobehavioural changes include elements of depression and prolonged response latency which may be associated with frontal lobe dysfunction. The word-finding difficulty with circumlocution indicates the presence of anomia (assigning names to objects) rather than agnosia (failure to recognize or identify familiar objects). The inability to perform skilled motor tasks on command, (including inappropriate or inaccurate movements) is termed apraxia. The diagnosis of apraxia depends upon the determination that such deficits are not explicable on the basis of sensorimotor or cerebellar dysfunction. The left hemisphere appears to be dominant for the programming and control of skilled motor movements, with specific types of apraxia often arising from lesions involving certain cortical regions. Such lesions generally affect the motor performance bilaterally. Lesions of the anterior corpus callosum may produce unilateral apraxia by disconnecting left hemispheric premotor (Area 6) cortical projections to homologous regions of the right hemisphere.

The neurologic signs and symptoms indicate unilateral deficits of corticospinal, spinothalamic, and dorsal column - medial lemniscal systems. Since involvement of these systems affects the same side of the body, a spinal cord localization is essentially eliminated. The relationship between the laterality of the gaze preference and of the sensorimotor findings indicates a cerebral localization. Comparison of the distribution of the sensorimotor findings to the cortical somatotopic representation indicates involvement of medial or parasagittal sensorimotor cortex. The left gaze preference is consistent with a lesion of the left frontal eye fields, which includes certain regions of Brodmann's Areas 8, 6, and 9 in the superior and middle frontal convolutions.

Returning to the hypothesized cerebrovascular pathogenesis, this medial and parasagittal frontal localization suggests involvement of the left Anterior Cerebral Artery distribution.

CLINICAL COURSE

A Computerized Tomographic scan was performed approximately 24 hours after the onset of the patient's symptomatology. (Refer to Figure). This neuroimaging study revealed an area of decreased attenuation involving the medial and parasagittal aspect of the frontal lobe consistent with infarction in the distribution of the Anterior Cerebral Artery. Another lucency (approx. 1 cm in diameter) was discerned in the left parietal cortex raising the question of an embolic source affecting two vascular distributions. A third lesion, somewhat linear in contour, was demonstrated in the dorsolateral aspect of the right frontal lobe, extending anterolaterally from the periventricular white matter to the cortical surface. Given the history consistent with previous stroke in the right hemisphere, this lesion was presumed to be related to that earlier clinical event.

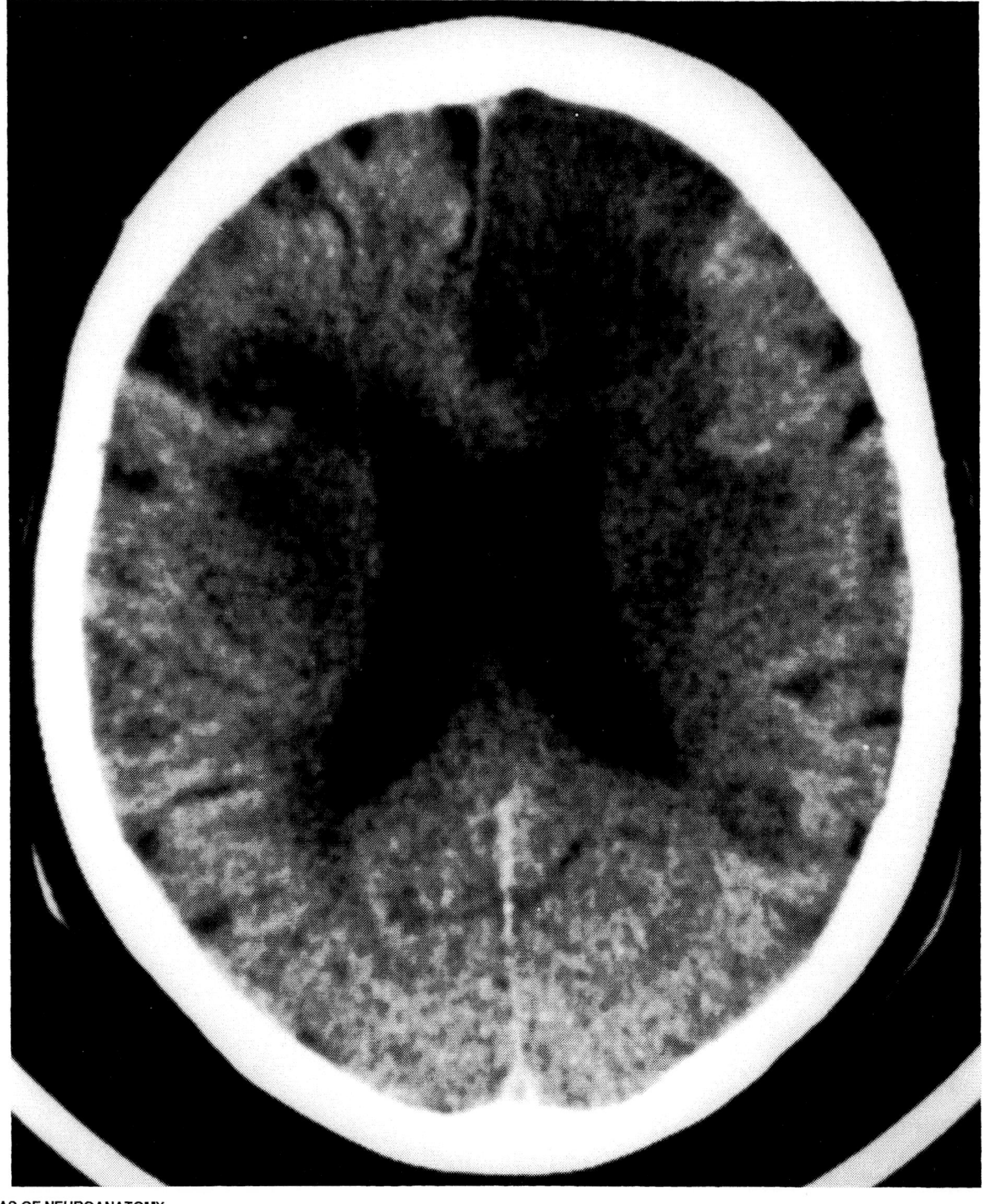

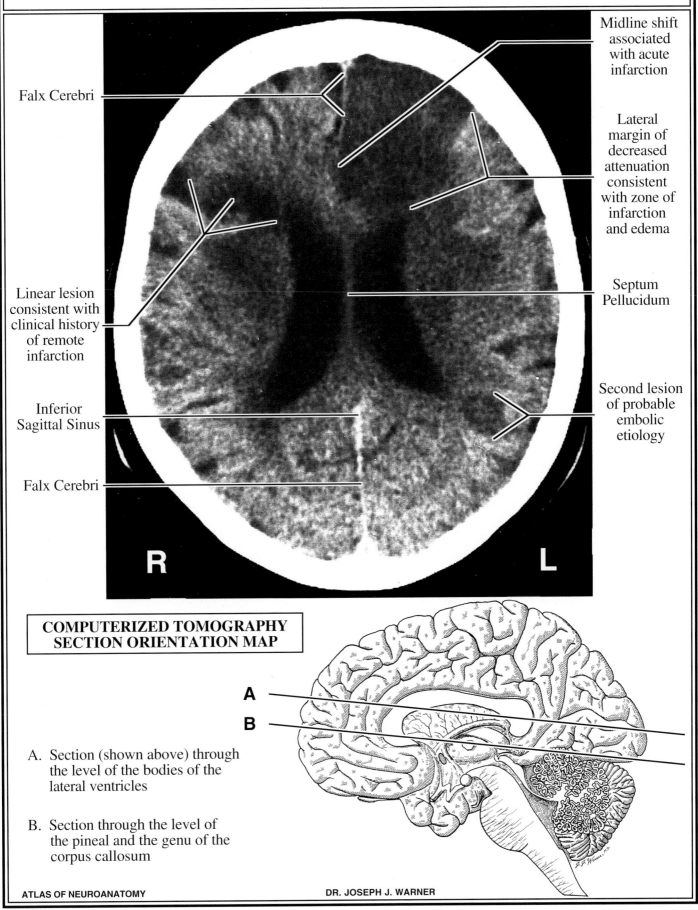

ANTERIOR CEREBRAL ARTERY DISTRIBUTION INFARCTION: COMPUTERIZED TOMOGRAPHY

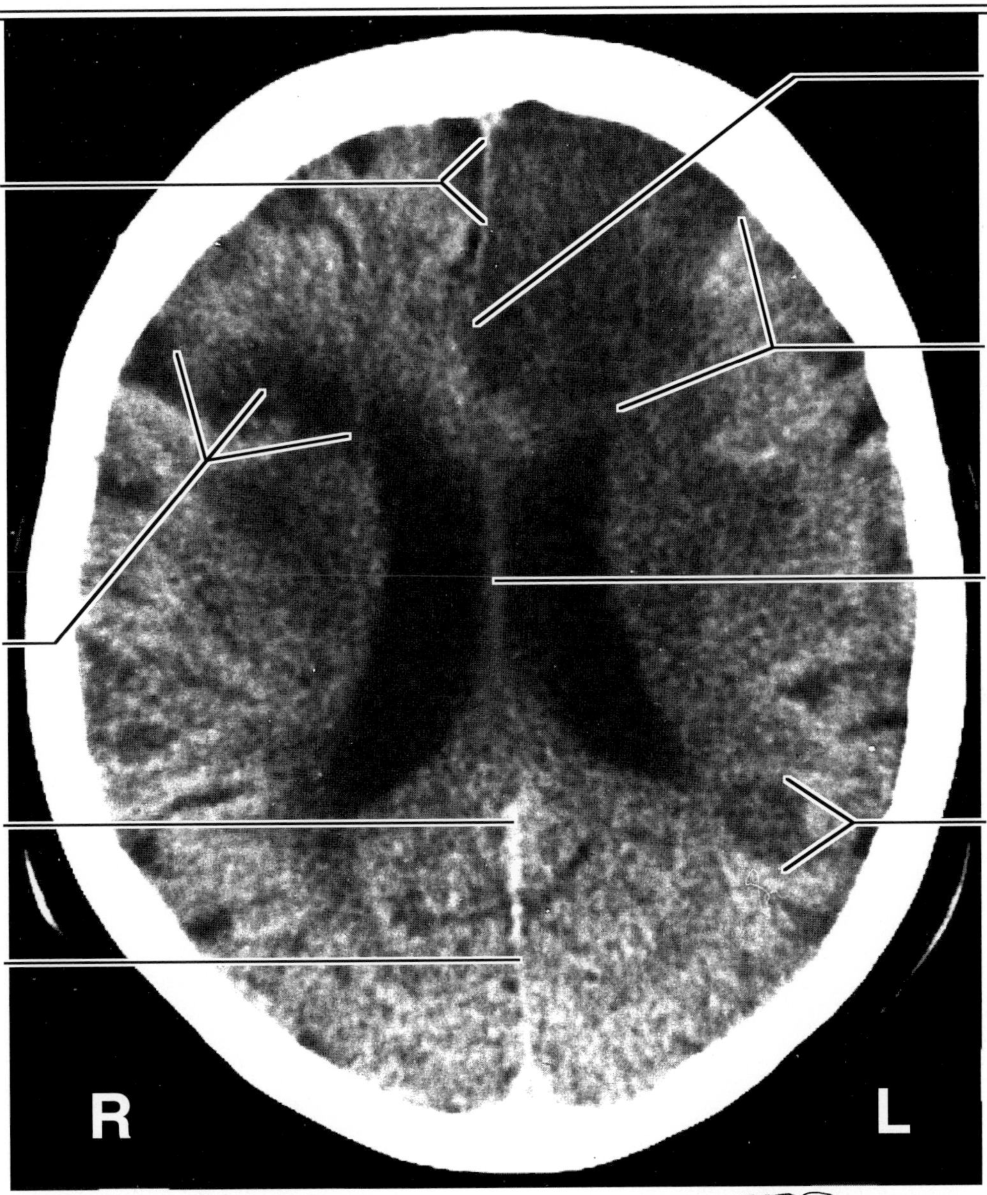

Midline shift associated with acute infarction

Falx Cerebri

Lateral margin of decreased attenuation consistent with zone of infarction and edema

Linear lesion consistent with clinical history of remote infarction

Septum Pellucidum

Second lesion of probable embolic etiology

Inferior Sagittal Sinus

Falx Cerebri

R

L

COMPUTERIZED TOMOGRAPHY SECTION ORIENTATION MAP

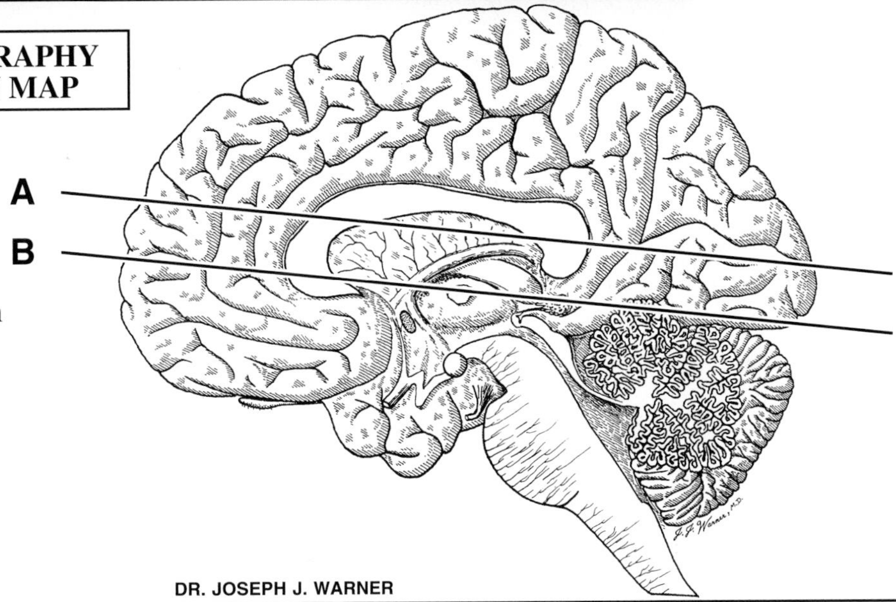

A

B

A. Section (shown above) through the level of the bodies of the lateral ventricles

B. Section through the level of the pineal and the genu of the corpus callosum

ANTERIOR CEREBRAL ARTERY DISTRIBUTION INFARCTION: COMPUTERIZED TOMOGRAPHY AND SUBSEQUENT CLINICAL COURSE

Computerized Tomography through the level of the pineal and the genu of the corpus callosum demonstrated lucency in the distribution of the anterior cerebral artery. (Refer to figure).

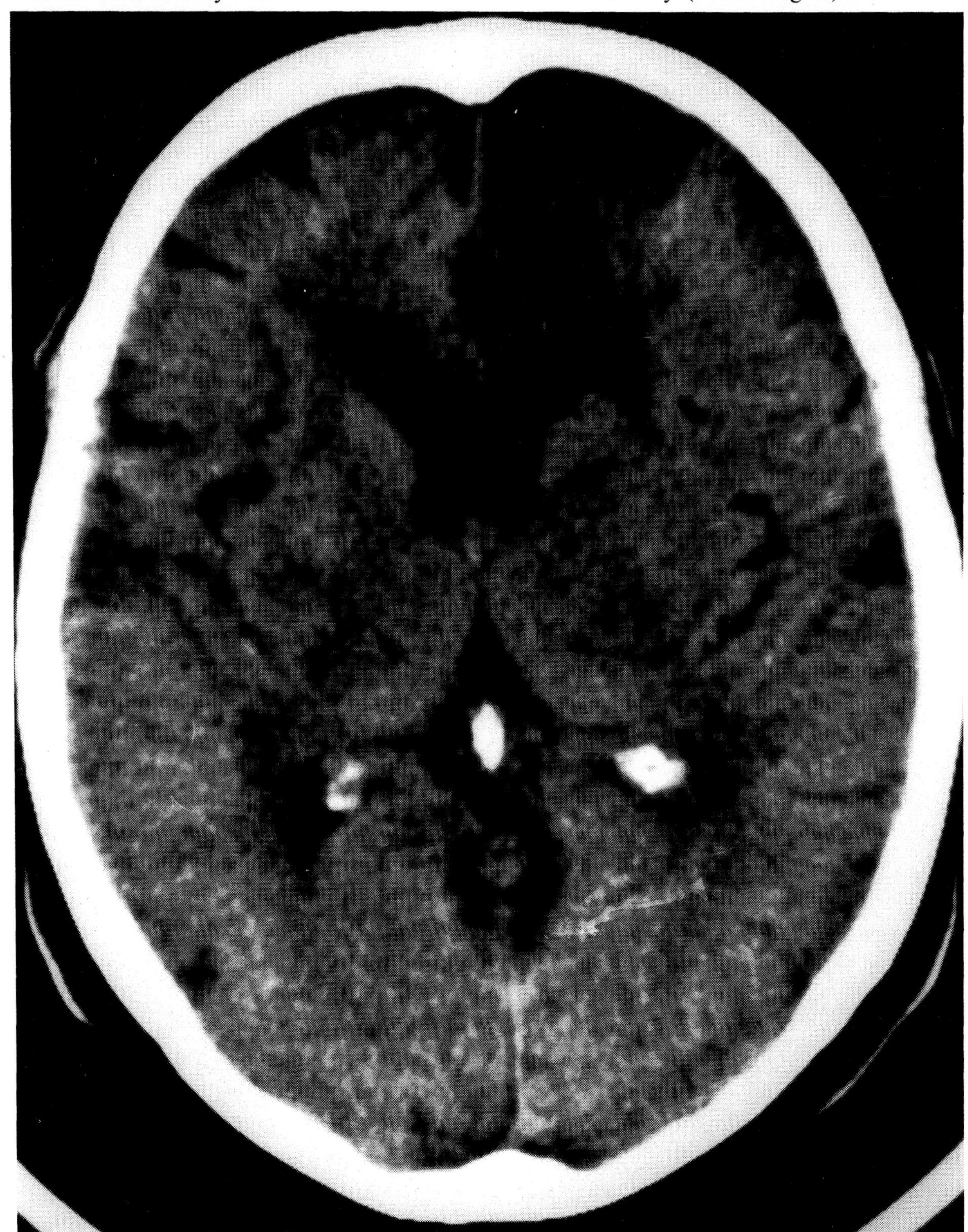

The subsequent clinical course included a progression of neurologic deficits accompanied by a mild degree of somnolence. These changes were attributed to edema and/or hemorrhage into the zone of infarction. The patient expired following an acute massive anterolateral myocardial infarction with cardiogenic shock. Pathologic examination of the brain was performed.

HEMORRHAGIC INFARCTION IN THE DISTRIBUTION OF THE LEFT ANTERIOR CEREBRAL ARTERY: EXTERNAL ROSTROCAUDAL VIEW OF THE BRAIN

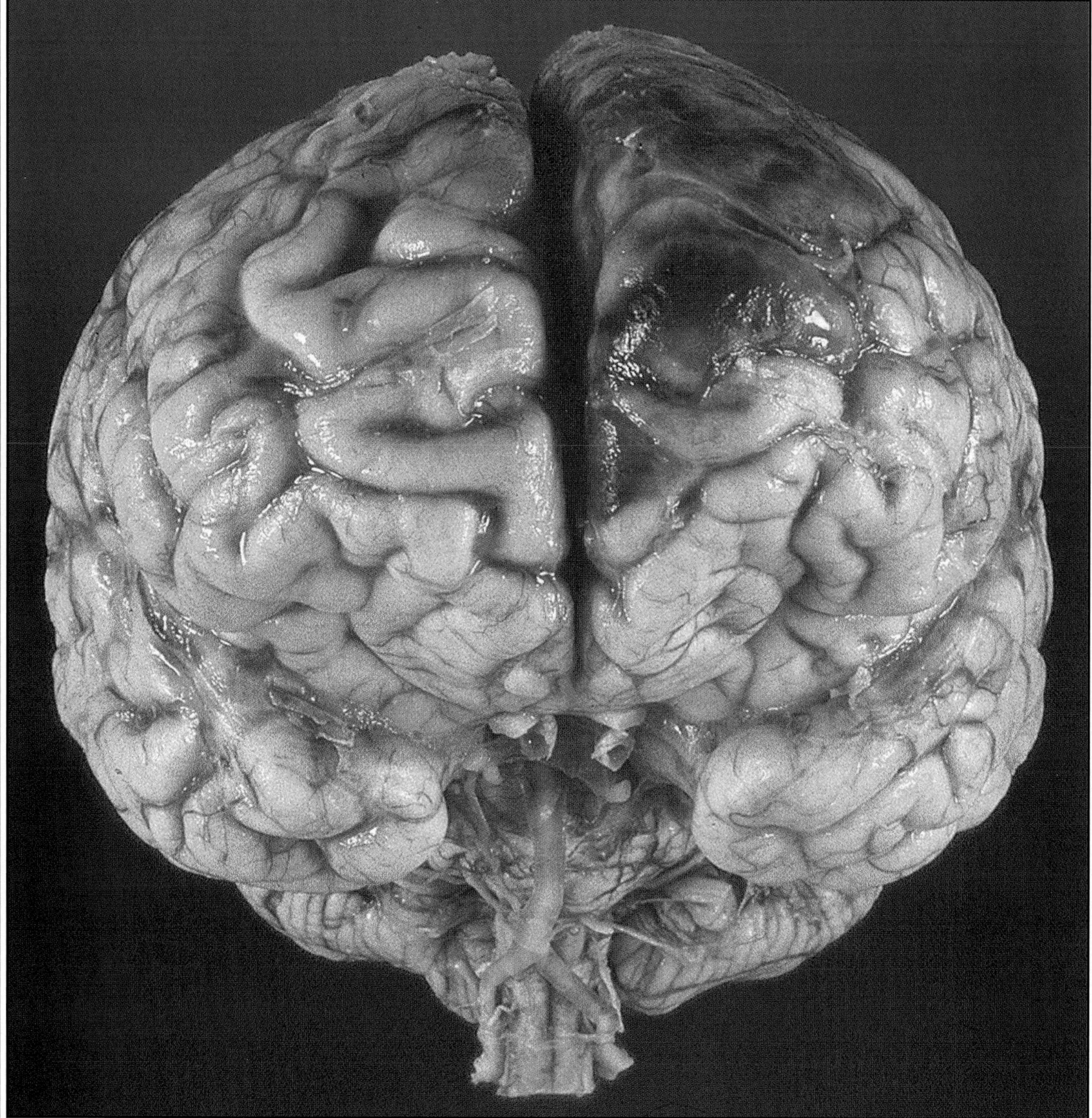

This rostrocaudal view of the frontal lobes demonstrates an area of surface discoloration and flattening of the gyri consistent with hemorrhage and mass effect. On pathologic examination, the distribution of these changes extended laterally from the midline to include the superior frontal convolution of the left cerebral hemisphere. Neither the lateral aspect of the frontal lobe nor the temporal lobe appeared to be involved on gross examination. The region of surface discoloration was accompanied by palpable subjacent softening of the brain. The remainder of the left hemisphere appeared externally normal. In this case, the lesion involving the medial and parasagittal frontal lobe was characteristic of an infarction within the distribution of the left anterior cerebral artery. Infarction in this vascular territory might involve the left frontal eye fields resulting in an ipsilateral gaze preference. Involvement of the paramedian sensorimotor cortex would be associated with contralateral hemiparesis and altered sensory perception, particularly evident in the lower extremity.

ANTERIOR CEREBRAL ARTERY DISTRIBUTION INFARCTION: HORIZONTAL SECTION FOR CT - PATHOLOGIC CASE CORRELATION

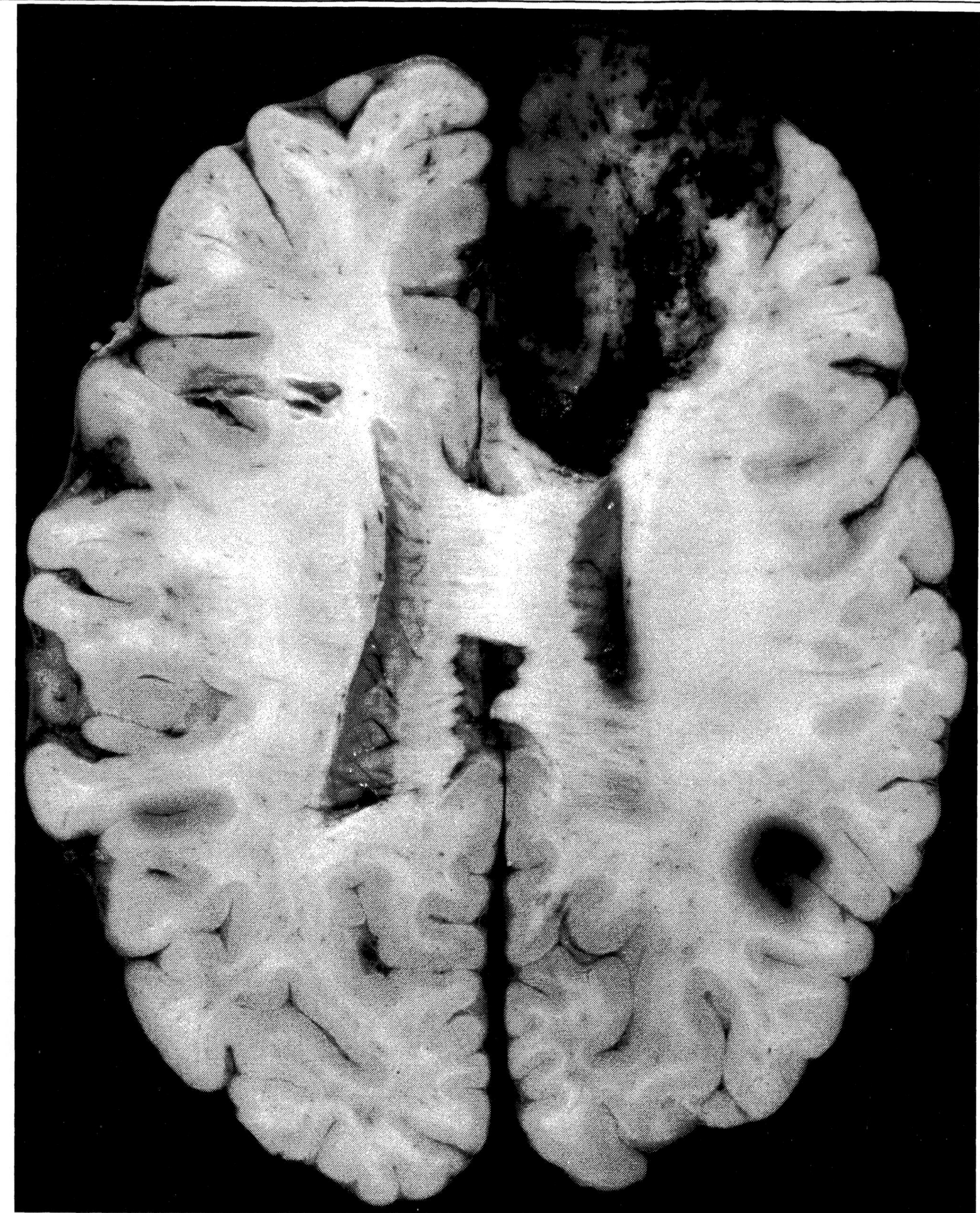

This pathologic specimen has been sectioned to correlate with the computerized tomographic scan through the level of the bodies of the lateral ventricles (Section map level A). Pathologic examination revealed diffuse multifocal hemorrhagic change with extension into the subarachnoid space.

ANTERIOR CEREBRAL ARTERY DISTRIBUTION INFARCTION: HORIZONTAL SECTION FOR CT - PATHOLOGIC CASE CORRELATION

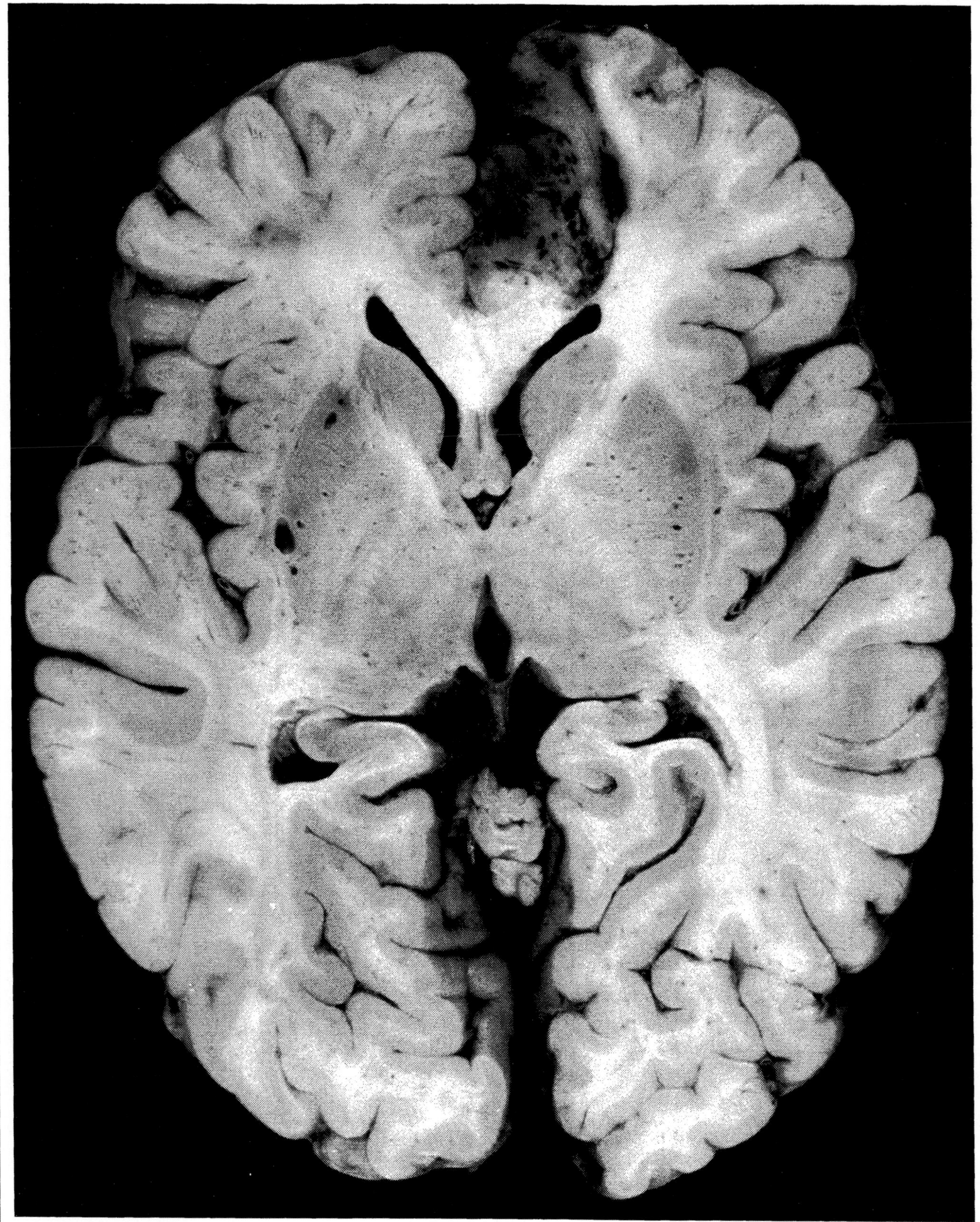

This pathologic specimen has been sectioned to correlate with the computerized tomographic scan through the level of the pineal and the genu of the corpus callosum. (Section map level B).

LEFT ANTERIOR CEREBRAL ARTERY DISTRIBUTION HEMORRHAGIC INFARCTION: HORIZONTAL SECTION

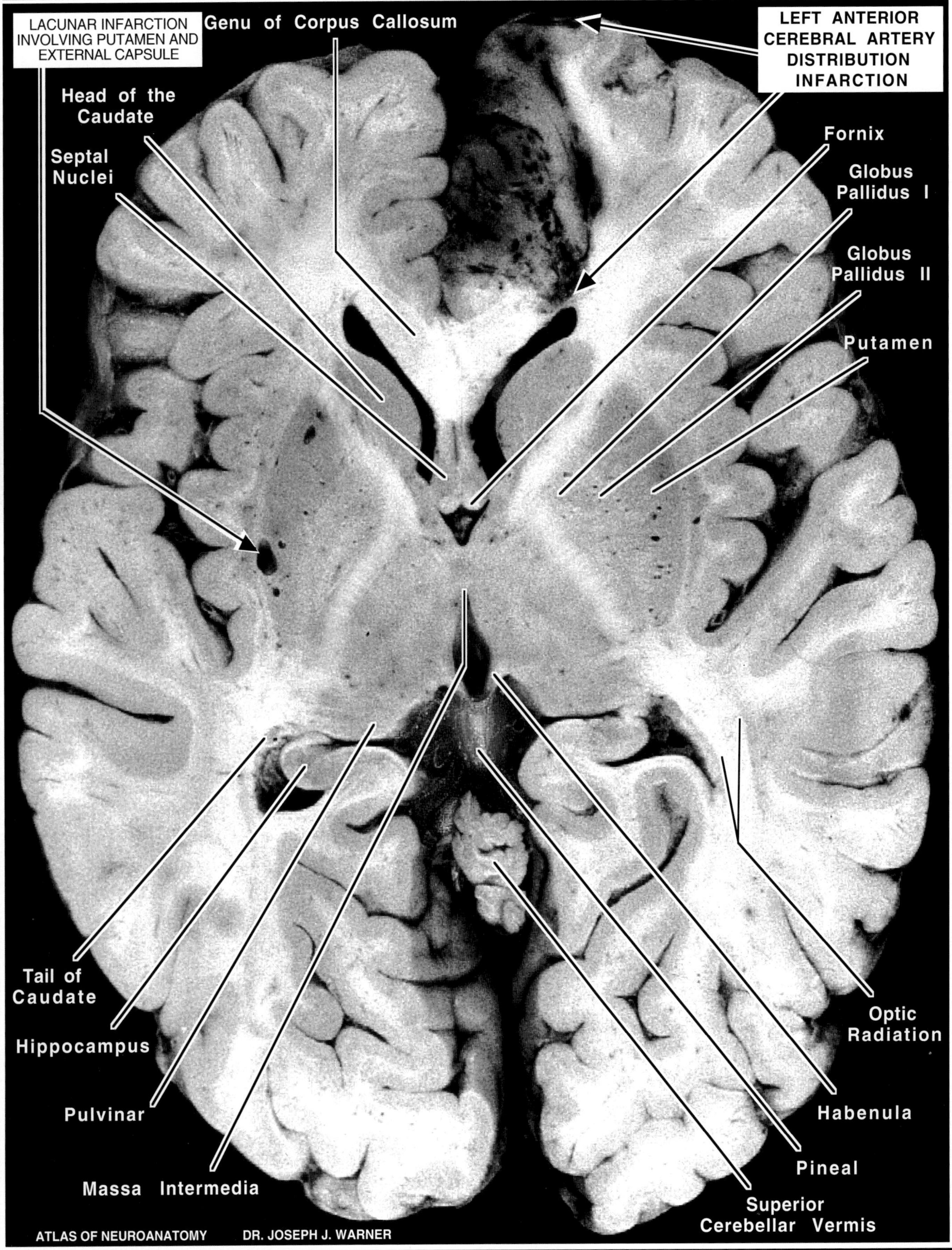

LACUNAR INFARCTION INVOLVING PUTAMEN AND EXTERNAL CAPSULE

Genu of Corpus Callosum

LEFT ANTERIOR CEREBRAL ARTERY DISTRIBUTION INFARCTION

Head of the Caudate

Septal Nuclei

Fornix

Globus Pallidus I

Globus Pallidus II

Putamen

Tail of Caudate

Hippocampus

Pulvinar

Massa Intermedia

Optic Radiation

Habenula

Pineal

Superior Cerebellar Vermis

ATLAS OF NEUROANATOMY DR. JOSEPH J. WARNER

COMPLEX PARTIAL STATUS EPILEPTICUS ASSOCIATED WITH A LEFT MIDDLE CEREBRAL ARTERY DISTRIBUTION INFARCTION (REMOTE): CASE PRESENTATION AND COMPUTERIZED TOMOGRAPHY

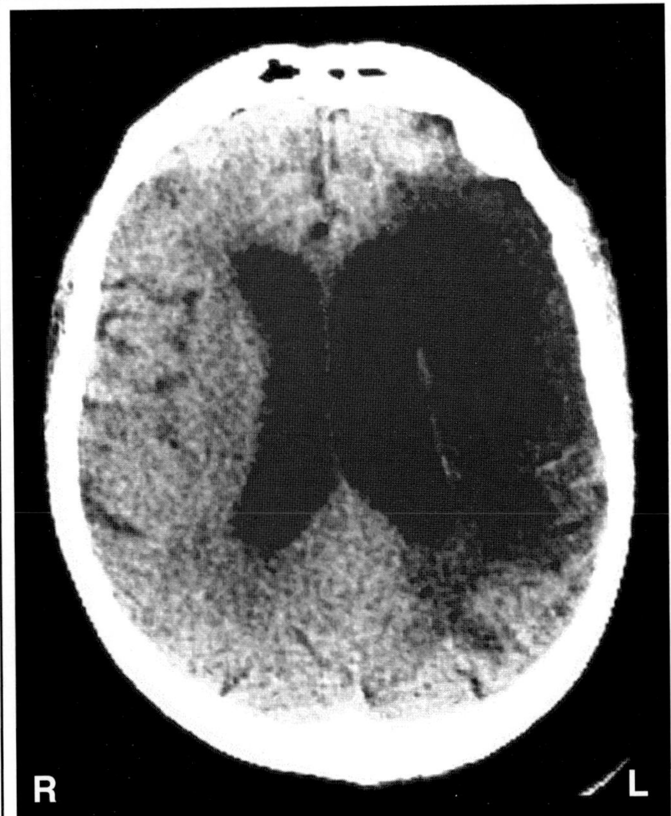

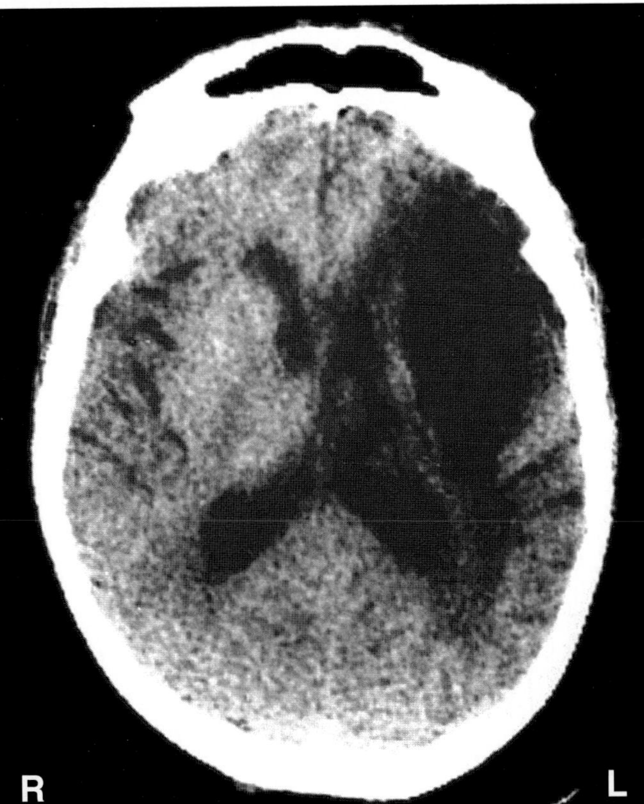

This 67-year-old right-handed male was brought to the hospital by family members who found him to be "confused" and lethargic. The patient had a previous history of a "stroke" two years earlier with a residual dense right hemiparesis and global aphasia. The patient had been able to acknowledge the presence of his family and appeared to appropriately recognize them prior to the recent change in his mental status. Although unable to converse, he had been able to communicate with gestures and by pointing. He had shown normal emotional responses to events in his environment. His previous medical history included coronary artery disease, hypertension, and a 40+ pack-year history of smoking. Neurologic findings included spontaneous movements of the left arm and leg, without any discernible movement on the right. A right upper motor neuron type facial paresis was present. The patient was minimally responsive to verbal and tactile stimuli, although his eyes were open and he appeared awake. He failed to follow visual targets, however demonstrated intermittent abrupt conjugate eye movements to the right followed by a left gaze preference.

Computerized tomography revealed a large area of decreased attenuation corresponding to the left middle cerebral artery distribution, with atrophy of the ipsilateral cerebral peduncle (see arrow).

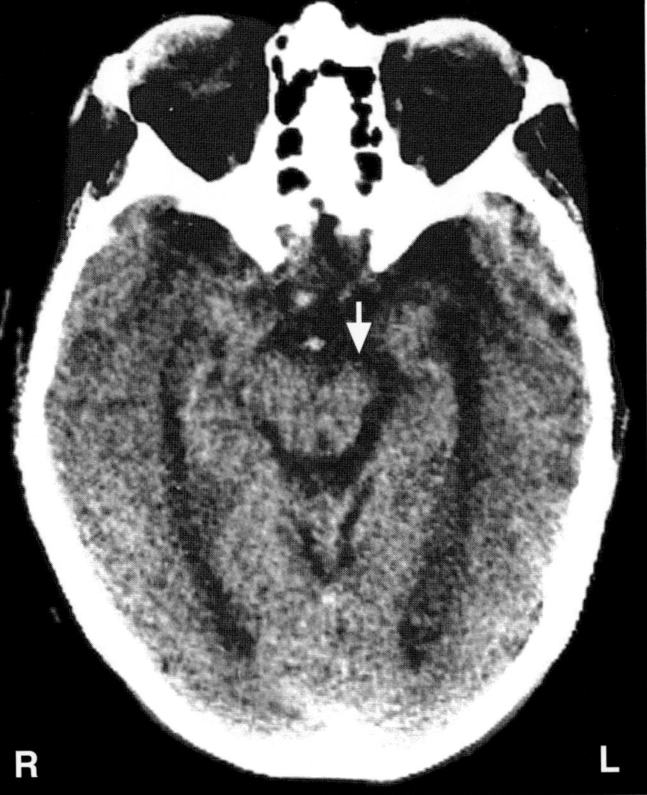

COMPUTERIZED TOMOGRAPHY (NON-CONTRAST)

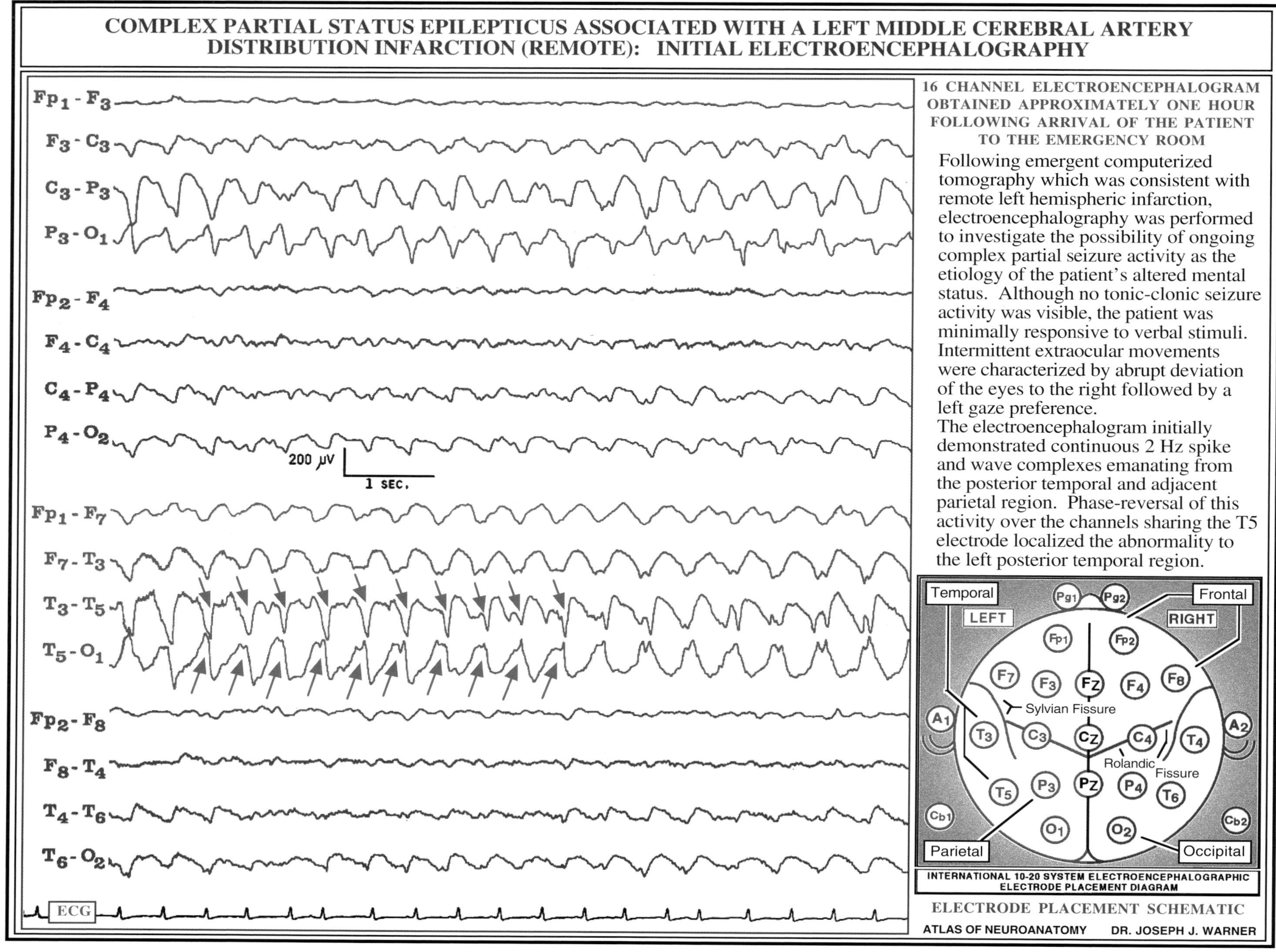
COMPLEX PARTIAL STATUS EPILEPTICUS ASSOCIATED WITH A LEFT MIDDLE CEREBRAL ARTERY DISTRIBUTION INFARCTION (REMOTE): INITIAL ELECTROENCEPHALOGRAPHY
Fp1 - F3
F3 - C3
C3 - P3
P3 - O1
Fp2 - F4
F4 - C4
C4 - P4
P4 - O2
200 µV
1 SEC.
Fp1 - F7
F7 - T3
T3 - T5
T5 - O1
Fp2 - F8
F8 - T4
T4 - T6
T6 - O2
ECG
16 CHANNEL ELECTROENCEPHALOGRAM OBTAINED APPROXIMATELY ONE HOUR FOLLOWING ARRIVAL OF THE PATIENT TO THE EMERGENCY ROOM
Following emergent computerized tomography which was consistent with remote left hemispheric infarction, electroencephalography was performed to investigate the possibility of ongoing complex partial seizure activity as the etiology of the patient's altered mental status. Although no tonic-clonic seizure activity was visible, the patient was minimally responsive to verbal stimuli. Intermittent extraocular movements were characterized by abrupt deviation of the eyes to the right followed by a left gaze preference.
The electroencephalogram initially demonstrated continuous 2 Hz spike and wave complexes emanating from the posterior temporal and adjacent parietal region. Phase-reversal of this activity over the channels sharing the T5 electrode localized the abnormality to the left posterior temporal region.
Temporal
Frontal
LEFT
RIGHT
Pg1
Pg2
Fp1
Fp2
F7
F3
FZ
F4
F8
Sylvian Fissure
A1
A2
T3
C3
CZ
C4
T4
Rolandic Fissure
T5
P3
PZ
P4
T6
Cb1
Cb2
O1
O2
Parietal
Occipital
INTERNATIONAL 10-20 SYSTEM ELECTROENCEPHALOGRAPHIC ELECTRODE PLACEMENT DIAGRAM
ELECTRODE PLACEMENT SCHEMATIC
ATLAS OF NEUROANATOMY
DR. JOSEPH J. WARNER

COMPLEX PARTIAL STATUS EPILEPTICUS ASSOCIATED WITH A LEFT MIDDLE CEREBRAL ARTERY DISTRIBUTION INFARCTION (REMOTE): ELECTROENCEPHALOGRAPHY AND CLINICAL COURSE

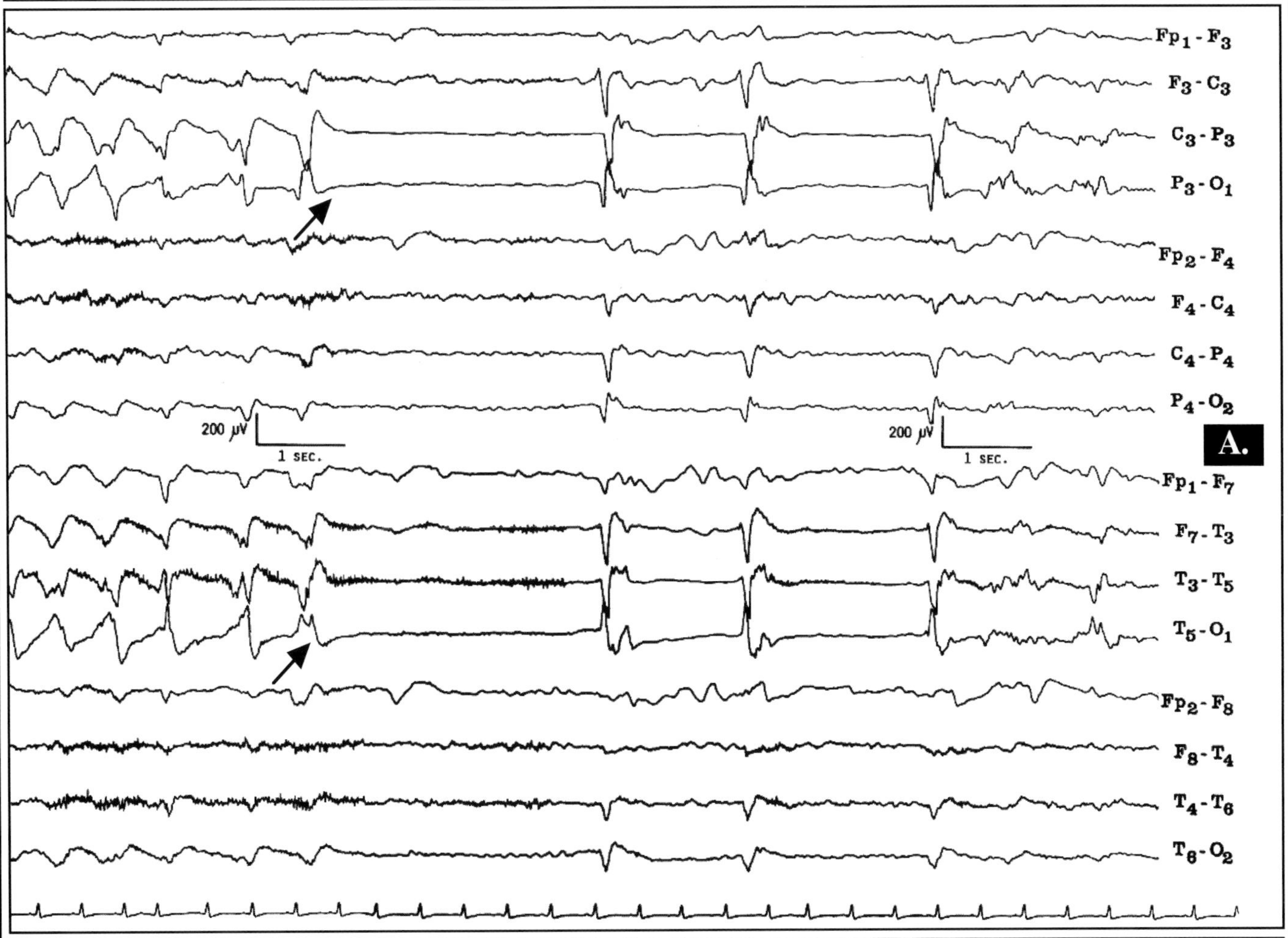

Fp1 - F3
F3 - C3
C3 - P3
P3 - O1
Fp2 - F4
F4 - C4
C4 - P4
P4 - O2
200 µV
1 SEC.
200 µV
1 SEC.
A.
Fp1 - F7
F7 - T3
T3 - T5
T5 - O1
Fp2 - F8
F8 - T4
T4 - T6
T6 - O2

The patient was treated with intravenous phenytoin and lorazepam to terminate the status epilepticus. The EEG (Panel A) demonstrates a sudden change in the pattern (arrows) from that of repetitive discharges to a suppression of activity with subsequent periodic discharges. This evolved into a pattern (Panel B) characterized by left hemispheric background slowing and focal epileptiform activity which shifted between the left posterior temporal and left parietal regions (arrows). The patient was intermittently responsive at this time, with evidence of a global aphasia and right hemiparesis.

Seizure activity recurred, despite continued anticonvulsant therapy. The electrocardiogram demonstrated supraventricular and ventricular arrhythmias with ST segment and T wave changes consistent with myocardial ischemia. Additional anticonvulsant intervention failed to control the recurrent refractory status epilepticus. The electroencephalographic pattern evolved into one of background suppression with periodic lateralized epileptiform discharges (Panel C).

Fp1 - F3
F3 - C3
C3 - P3
P3 - O1
Fp2 - F4
F4 - C4
C4 - P4
P4 - O2
B.
200 µV
1 SEC.
Fp1 - F7
F7 - T3
T3 - T5
T5 - O1
Fp2 - F8
F8 - T4
T4 - T6
T6 - O2

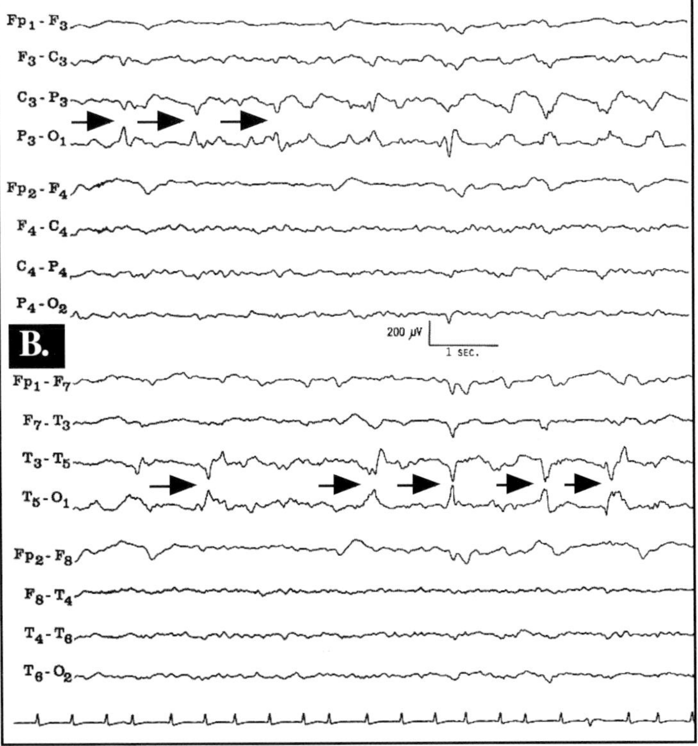

COMPLEX PARTIAL STATUS EPILEPTICUS ASSOCIATED WITH A LEFT MIDDLE CEREBRAL ARTERY DISTRIBUTION INFARCTION (REMOTE): FINAL EEG DEMONSTRATING PERIODIC LATERALIZED EPILEPTIFORM DISCHARGES

Fp1 - F3
F3 - C3
C3 - P3
P3 - O1
Fp2 - F4
F4 - C4
C4 - P4
P4 - O2
200 µV
1 SEC.
Fp1 - F7
F7 - T3
T3 - T5
T5 - O1
Fp2 - F8
F8 - T4
T4 - T6
T6 - O2
C.

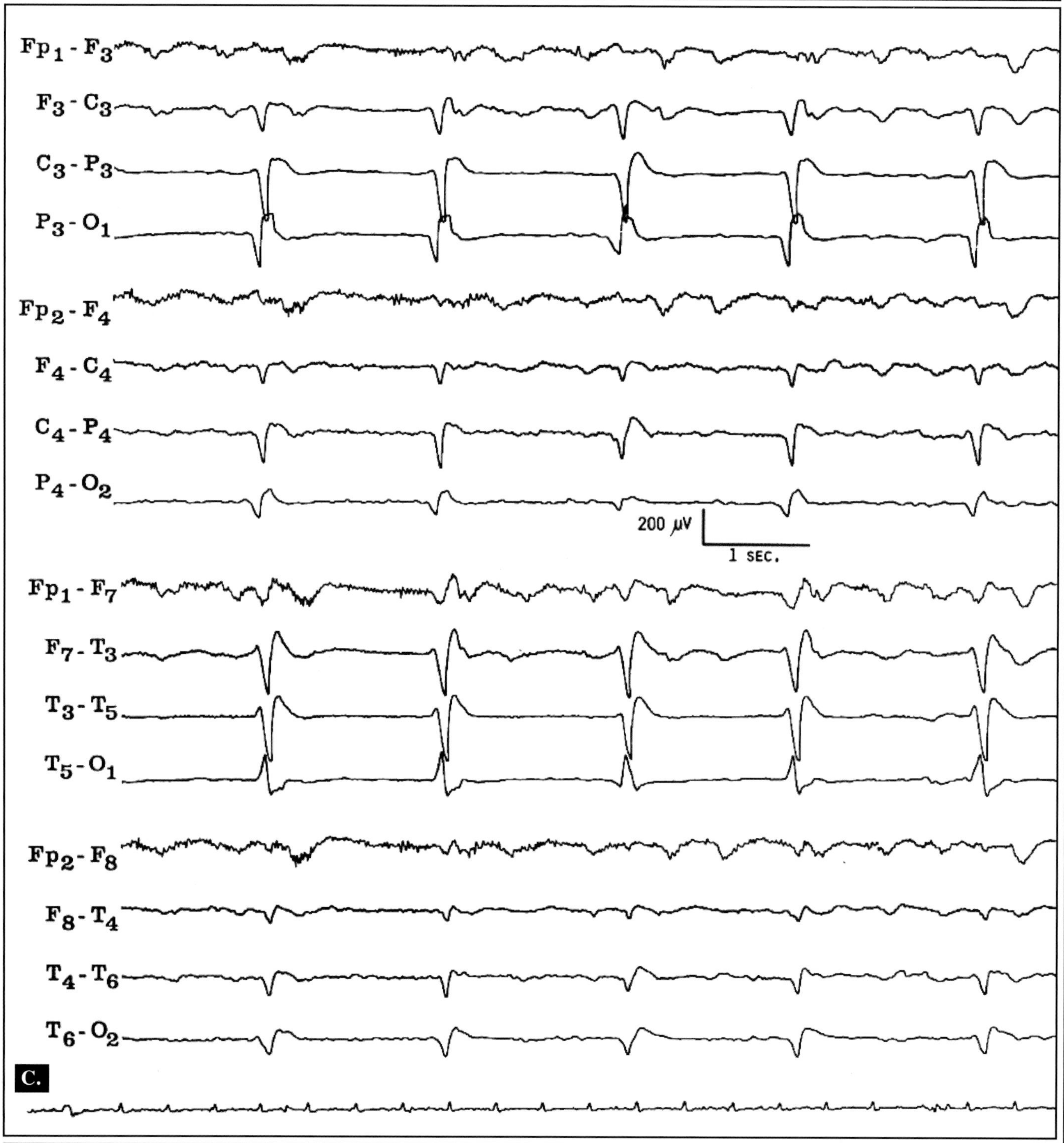

The patient developed refractory complex partial status epilepticus complicated by cardiac ischemia and arrhythmias. Electroencephalography (Panel C) demonstrated a pattern of periodic lateralized epileptiform discharges occurring every 1.75 to 2.0 seconds, with a suppression of normal background activity between discharges. Although of highest amplitude over the T5 (left posterior temporal) and P3 (left parietal) electrodes, this activity was transmitted to homologous areas of the right hemisphere as well. The patient sustained a cardiopulmonary arrest and was not resuscitated.

LEFT
RIGHT
Pg1
Pg2
Fp1
Fp2
F7
F3
Fz
F4
F8
A1
T3
C3
Cz
C4
T4
A2
T5
P3
Pz
P4
T6
Cb1
O1
O2
Cb2

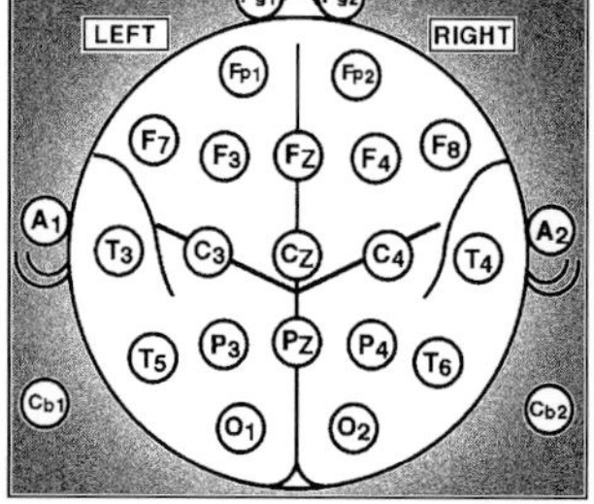

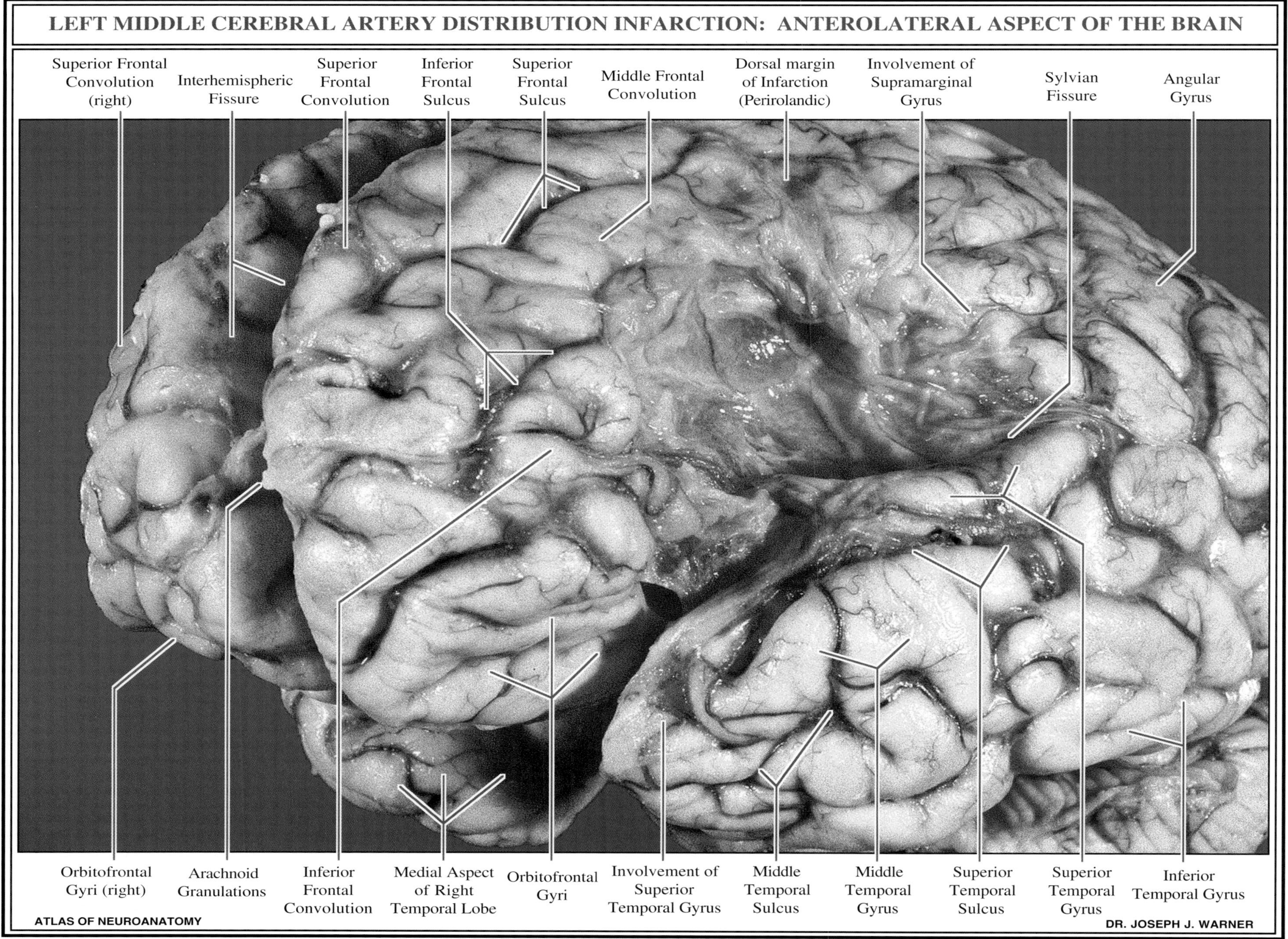
LEFT MIDDLE CEREBRAL ARTERY DISTRIBUTION INFARCTION: ANTEROLATERAL ASPECT OF THE BRAIN
Superior Frontal Convolution (right)
Interhemispheric Fissure
Superior Frontal Convolution
Inferior Frontal Sulcus
Superior Frontal Sulcus
Middle Frontal Convolution
Dorsal margin of Infarction (Perirolandic)
Involvement of Supramarginal Gyrus
Sylvian Fissure
Angular Gyrus
Orbitofrontal Gyri (right)
Arachnoid Granulations
Inferior Frontal Convolution
Medial Aspect of Right Temporal Lobe
Orbitofrontal Gyri
Involvement of Superior Temporal Gyrus
Middle Temporal Sulcus
Middle Temporal Gyrus
Superior Temporal Sulcus
Superior Temporal Gyrus
Inferior Temporal Gyrus
ATLAS OF NEUROANATOMY
DR. JOSEPH J. WARNER

COMPLEX PARTIAL STATUS EPILEPTICUS ASSOCIATED WITH A LEFT MIDDLE CEREBRAL ARTERY DISTRIBUTION INFARCTION (REMOTE): HORIZONTAL SECTION OF THE BRAIN, DORSAL TO VENTRAL PERSPECTIVE

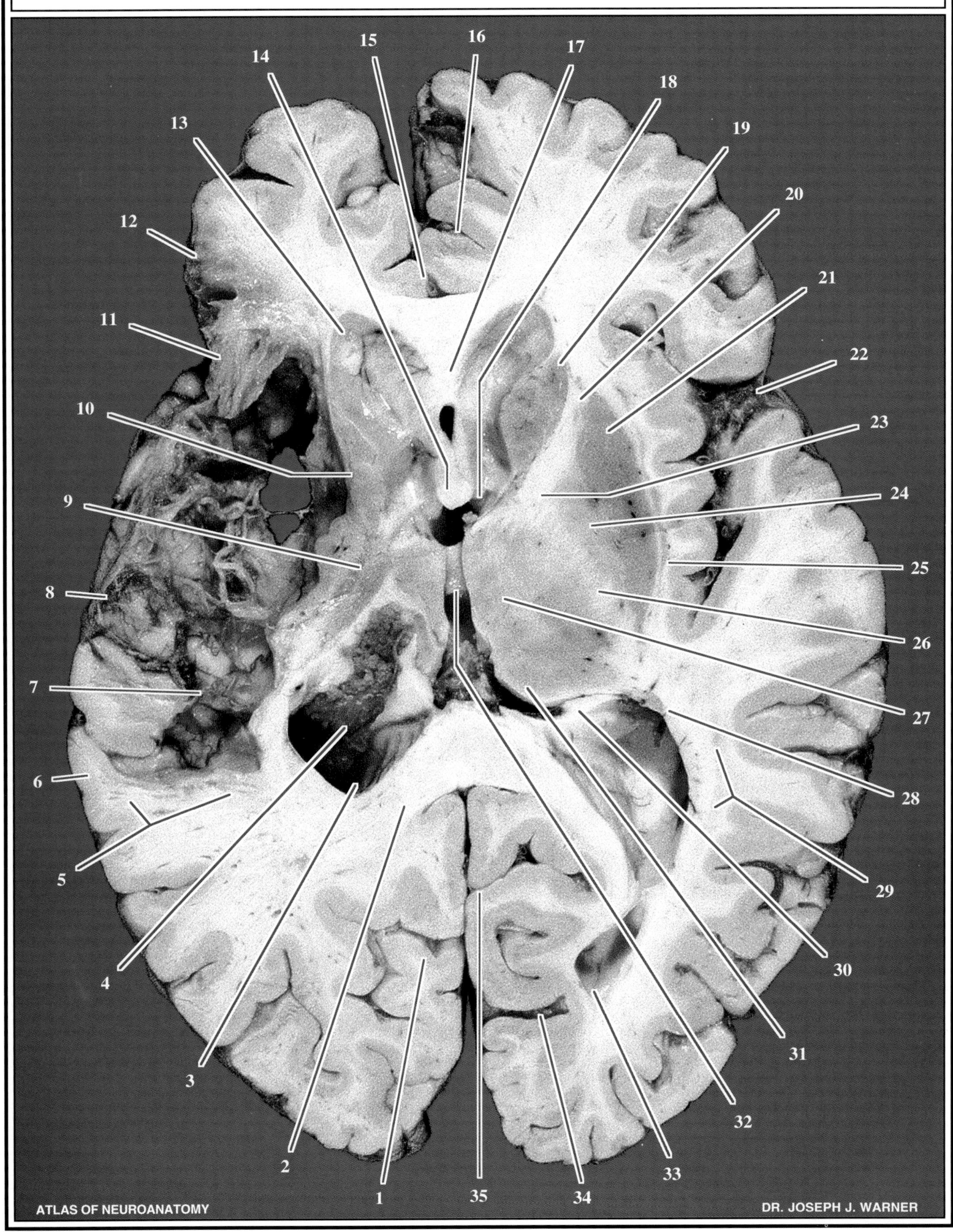

COMPLEX PARTIAL STATUS EPILEPTICUS ASSOCIATED WITH A LEFT MIDDLE CEREBRAL ARTERY DISTRIBUTION INFARCTION (REMOTE); HORIZONTAL SECTIONS OF THE BRAIN: (A) KEY TO STRUCTURES, (B) UNILATERAL DEGENERATION INVOLVING THE LEFT CEREBRAL PEDUNCLE

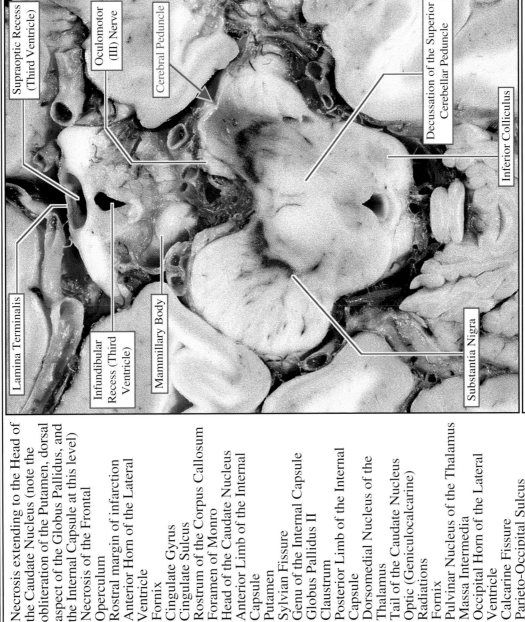

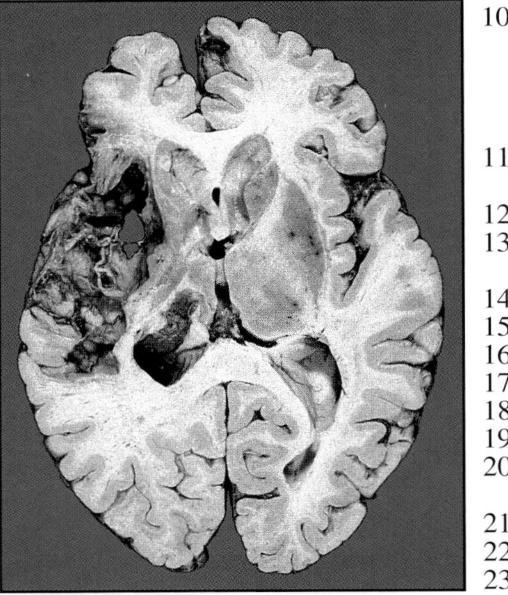

HORIZONTAL SECTION, LEVEL OF THE FORAMEN OF MONRO; DORSAL TO VENTRAL PERSPECTIVE: KEY TO NUMBERED STRUCTURES

1. Area 17 Striate Cortex
2. Splenium of the Corpus Callosum
3. Atrium of the Lateral Ventricle
4. Choroid Plexus
5. Caudal margin of infarction
6. Caudal Temporal Cortex (region approximating the focus of epileptiform activity on EEG)
7. Necrosis with cavitation of the Perisylvian region
8. Necrosis of the Superior Temporal Gyrus
9. Deep extension of lesion through the Internal Capsule into the Thalamus*
10. Necrosis extending to the Head of the Caudate Nucleus (note the obliteration of the Putamen, dorsal aspect of the Globus Pallidus, and the Internal Capsule at this level)
11. Necrosis of the Frontal Operculum
12. Rostral margin of infarction
13. Anterior Horn of the Lateral Ventricle
14. Fornix
15. Cingulate Gyrus
16. Cingulate Sulcus
17. Rostrum of the Corpus Callosum
18. Foramen of Monro
19. Head of the Caudate Nucleus
20. Anterior Limb of the Internal Capsule
21. Putamen
22. Sylvian Fissure
23. Genu of the Internal Capsule
24. Globus Pallidus II
25. Claustrum
26. Posterior Limb of the Internal Capsule
27. Dorsomedial Nucleus of the Thalamus
28. Tail of the Caudate Nucleus
29. Optic (Geniculocalcarine) Radiations
30. Fornix
31. Pulvinar Nucleus of the Thalamus
32. Massa Intermedia
33. Occipital Horn of the Lateral Ventricle
34. Calcarine Fissure
35. Parieto-Occipital Sulcus

*Sparing of the medial thalamus is attributable to the fact that the vascular supply to this region arises from the basilar bifurcation and the posterior cerebral arteries.

HORIZONTAL SECTION, LEVEL OF THE MESENCEPHALON (VENTRAL TO DORSAL VIEW): DEGENERATION OF THE CEREBRAL PEDUNCLE IPSILATERAL TO THE LEFT MIDDLE CEREBRAL ARTERY DISTRIBUTION INFARCTION

Anterograde corticospinal and corticobulbar tract degeneration affected the left cerebral peduncle, basis pontis, and medullary pyramid.

ACUTE RIGHT MIDDLE CEREBRAL ARTERY DISTRIBUTION INFARCTION WITH SEVERE MASS EFFECT AND TRANSTENTORIAL HERNIATION IN A CASE WITH PREVIOUS EMBOLIC INFARCTS

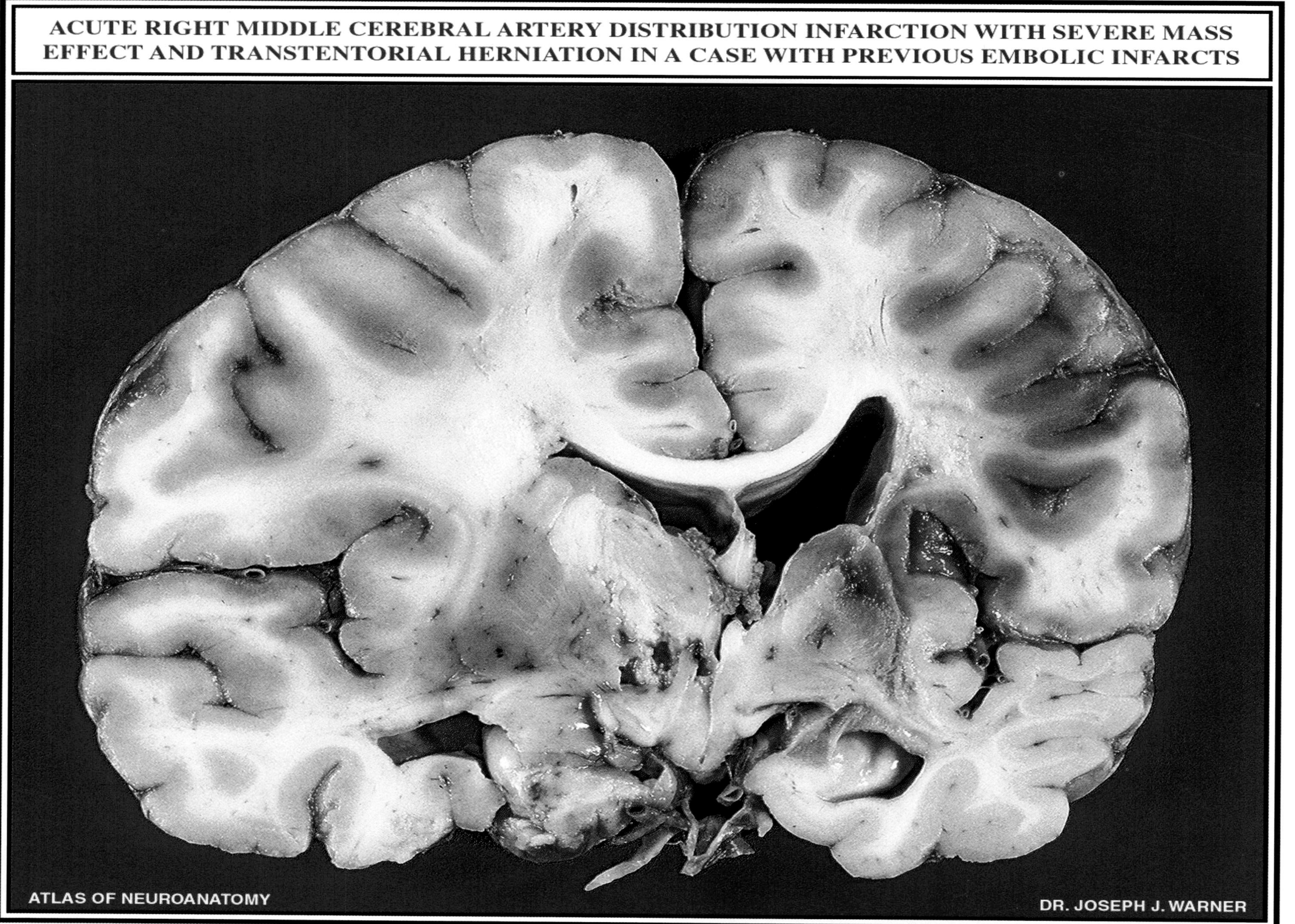

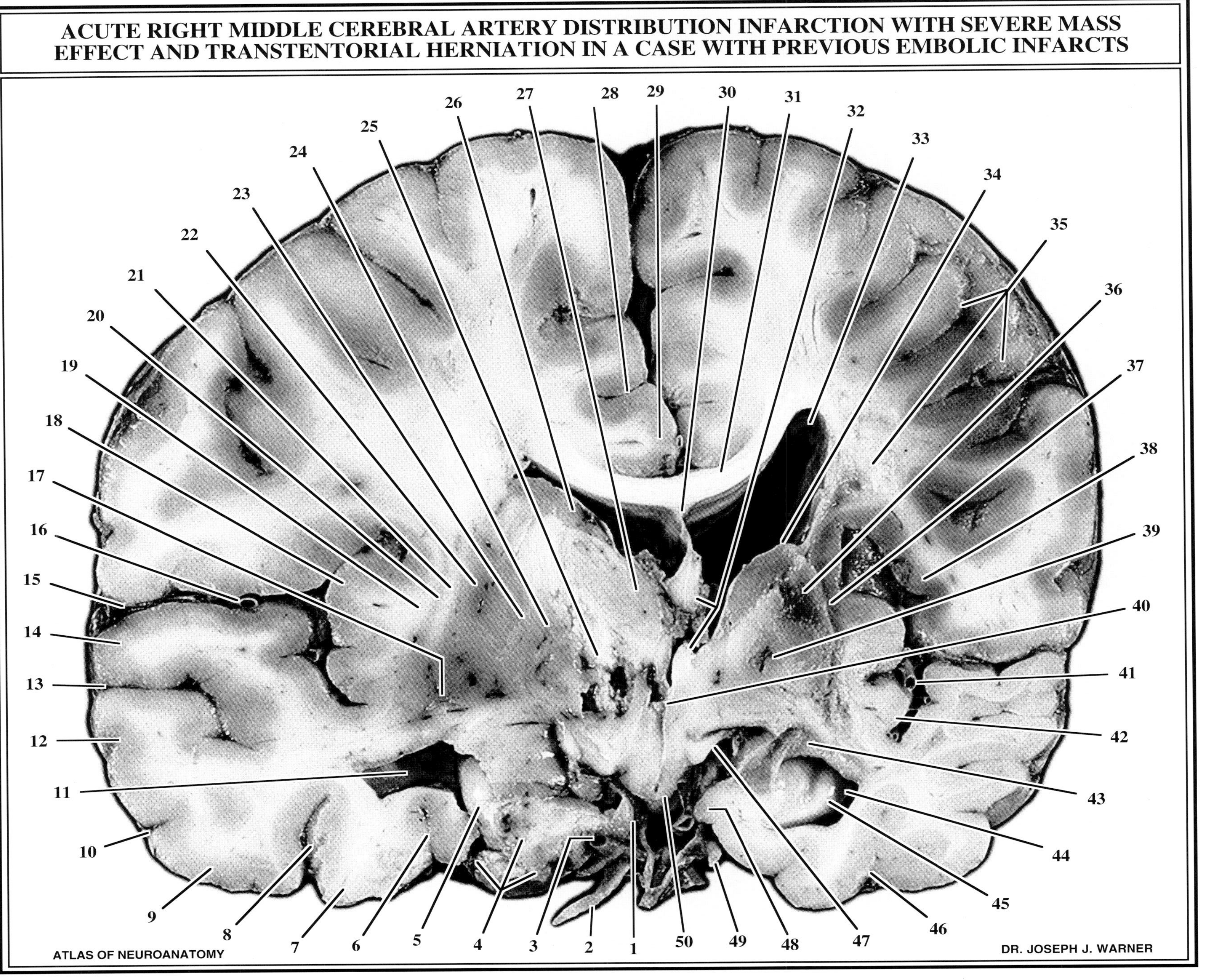
ACUTE RIGHT MIDDLE CEREBRAL ARTERY DISTRIBUTION INFARCTION WITH SEVERE MASS EFFECT AND TRANSTENTORIAL HERNIATION IN A CASE WITH PREVIOUS EMBOLIC INFARCTS
1
2
3
4
5
6
7
8
9
10
11
12
13
14
15
16
17
18
19
20
21
22
23
24
25
26
27
28
29
30
31
32
33
34
35
36
37
38
39
40
41
42
43
44
45
46
47
48
49
50
ATLAS OF NEUROANATOMY
DR. JOSEPH J. WARNER

ACUTE RIGHT MIDDLE CEREBRAL ARTERY DISTRIBUTION INFARCTION WITH SEVERE MASS EFFECT AND TRANSTENTORIAL HERNIATION IN A CASE WITH PREVIOUS EMBOLIC INFARCTS: CORONAL SECTION

KEY TO NUMBERED STRUCTURES

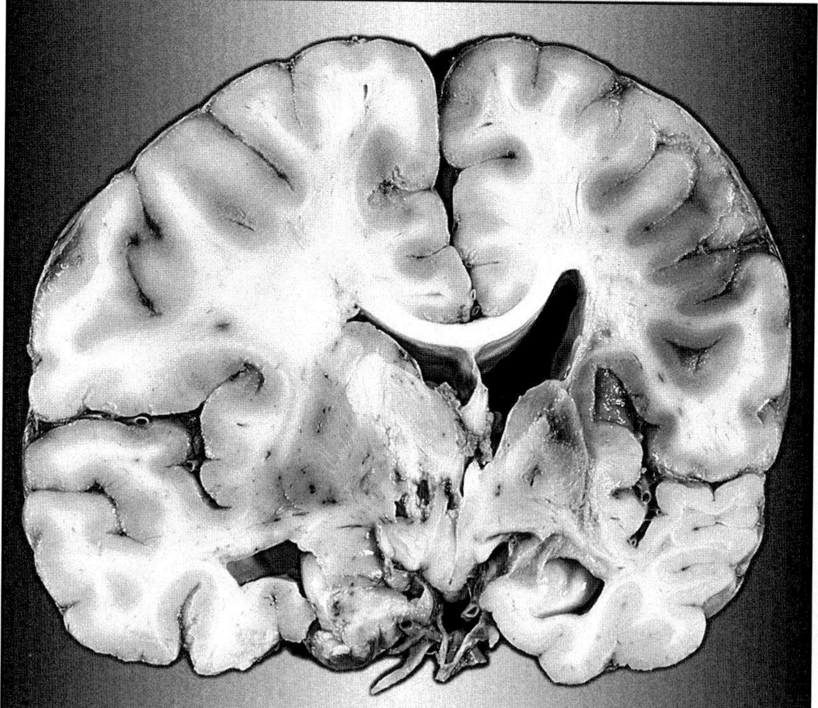

1. Uncus (necrotic and ventromedially displaced)
2. Oculomotor (III) Nerve
3. Posterior Communicating Artery
4. Hemorrhage, necrosis and edema involving the Parahippocampal Gyrus
5. Hippocampal Formation (medially displaced)
6. Collateral Sulcus
7. Fusiform Gyrus
8. Inferior Temporal Sulcus
9. Inferior Temporal Gyrus
10. Middle Temporal Sulcus
11. Temporal Horn of the Lateral Ventricle
12. Middle Temporal Gyrus
13. Superior Temporal Sulcus
14. Superior Temporal Gyrus
15. Sylvian Fissure
16. Middle Cerebral Artery
17. Necrosis of ventral Putamen
18. Insular Cortex
19. Extreme Capsule
20. Claustrum
21. External Capsule
22. Putamen
23. External Medullary Lamina
24. Globus Pallidus II
25. Genu of the Internal Capsule (necrotic)
26. Caudate Nucleus
27. Anterior Nuclear group of the Thalamus (rostromedially displaced secondary to edema)
28. Cingulate Sulcus
29. Cingulate Gyrus
30. Septum Pellucidum
31. Corpus Callosum
32. Fornix (passes through plane of section twice as postcommissural fibers recurve toward the mammillary bodies)
33. Body of the Lateral Ventricle
34. Caudate Nucleus
35. Zone of necrosis secondary to previous left middle cerebral artery embolus
36. Cavitation of the Putamen (previous infarction)
37. Necrosis of the subinsular region, including the Claustrum and the Extreme and External Capsules
38. Infarction of the Frontal Opercular region
39. Cavitation of the Globus Pallidus (previous infarction)
40. Third Ventricle (compressed and shifted)
41. Middle Cerebral Artery

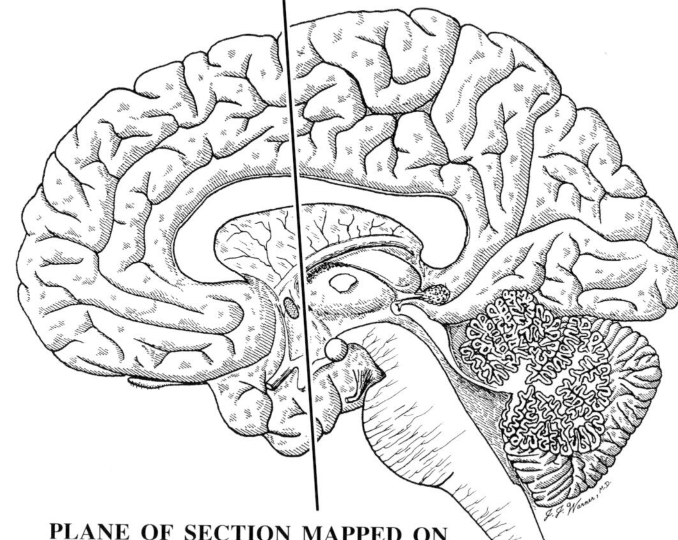

PLANE OF SECTION MAPPED ON A MIDLINE SAGITTAL DIAGRAM

42. Insular Cortex
43. Necrosis involving the region of the amygdala
44. Temporal Horn of the Lateral Ventricle
45. Hippocampal Formation
46. Inferior Temporal Sulcus
47. Optic Tract
48. Uncus
49. Oculomotor (III) Nerve
50. Hypothalamus

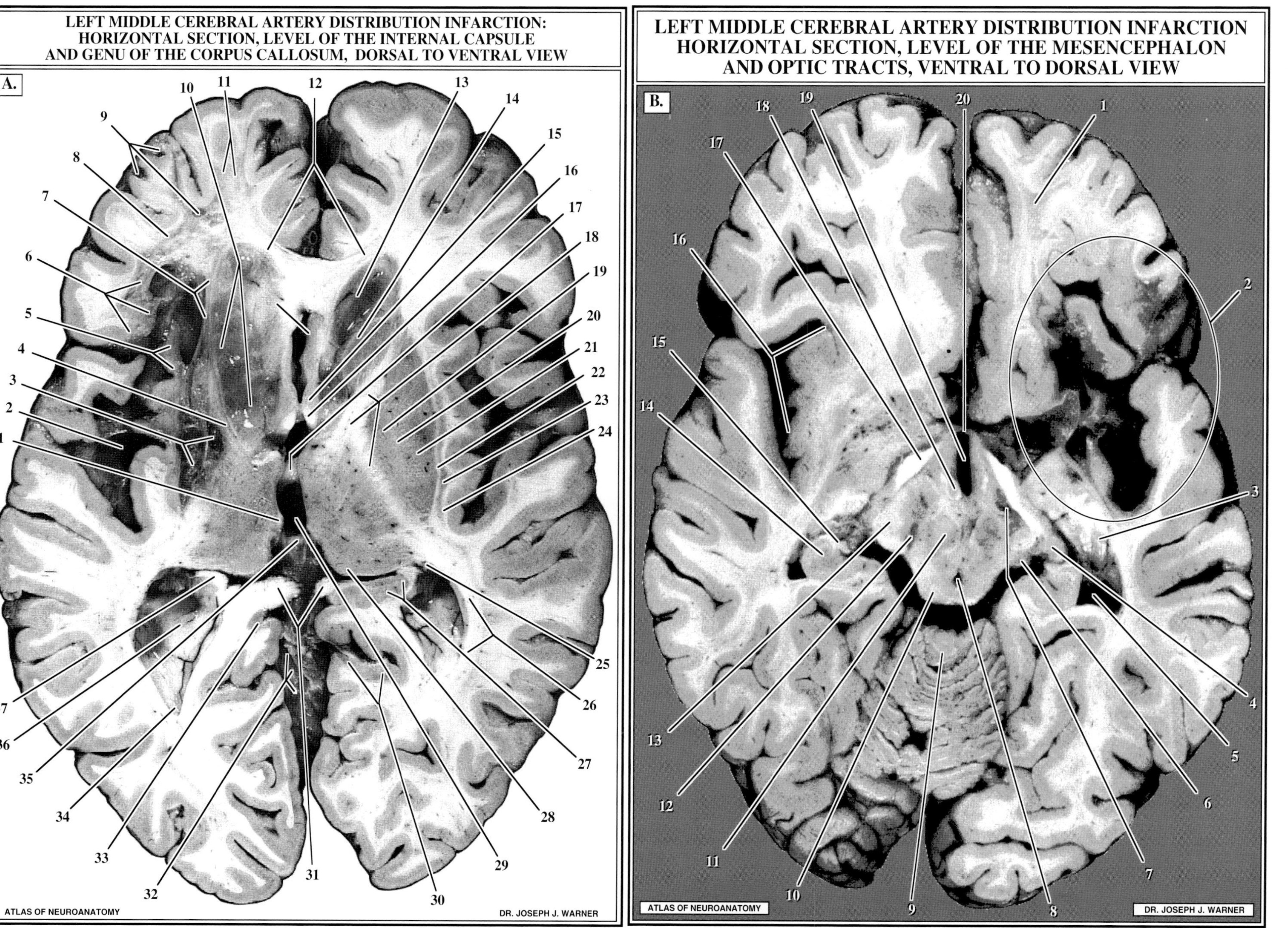

LEFT MIDDLE CEREBRAL ARTERY DISTRIBUTION INFARCTION: HORIZONTAL SECTION, LEVEL OF THE INTERNAL CAPSULE AND GENU OF THE CORPUS CALLOSUM, DORSAL TO VENTRAL VIEW

LEFT MIDDLE CEREBRAL ARTERY DISTRIBUTION INFARCTION HORIZONTAL SECTION, LEVEL OF THE MESENCEPHALON AND OPTIC TRACTS, VENTRAL TO DORSAL VIEW

LEFT MIDDLE CEREBRAL ARTERY DISTRIBUTION INFARCTION WITH IPSILATERAL DEGENERATION OF THE CEREBRAL PEDUNCLE: HORIZONTAL SECTION, LEVEL OF THE MESENCEPHALON AND OPTIC TRACTS

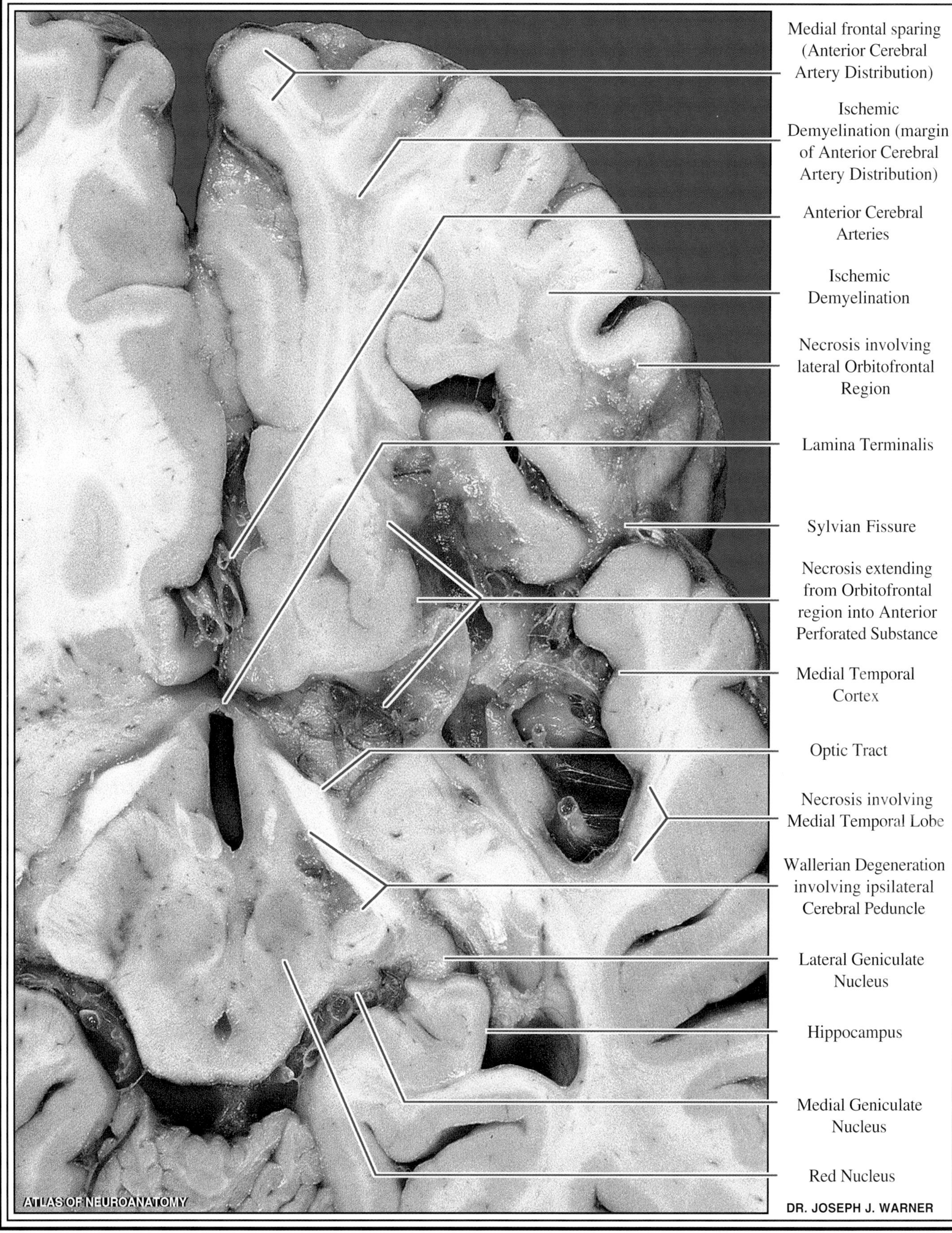

LEFT MIDDLE CEREBRAL ARTERY DISTRIBUTION INFARCTION: HORIZONTAL SECTION LEVELS MAPPED ON MIDLINE SAGITTAL DIAGRAM AND KEY TO NUMBERED STRUCTURES FOR EACH SECTION

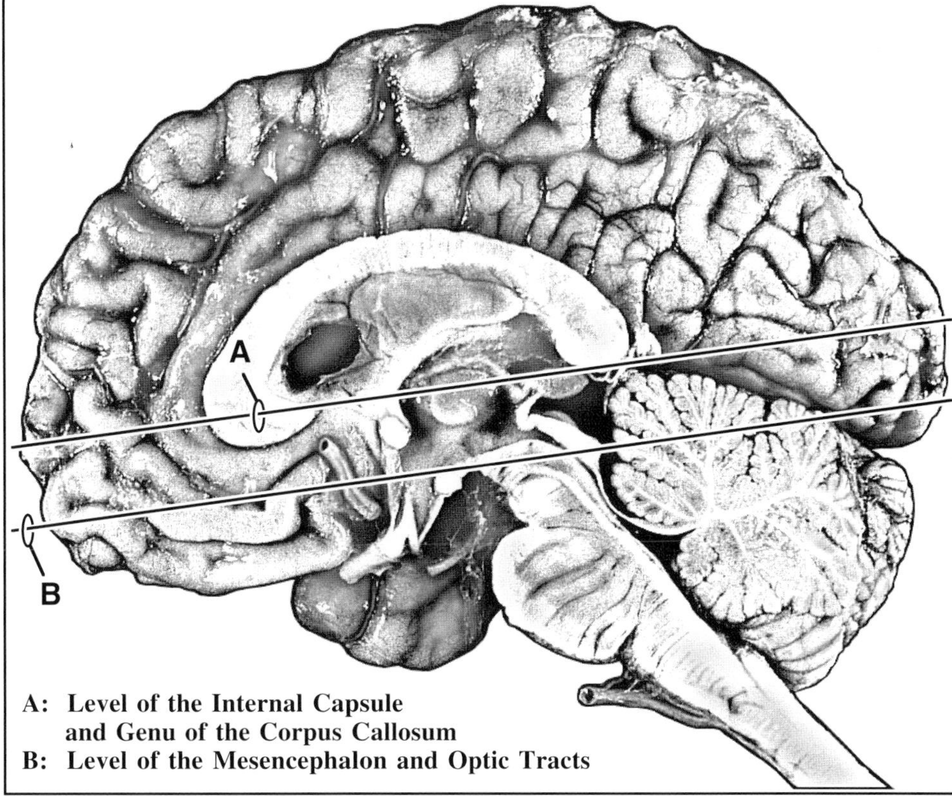

SECTION A: KEY

1. Stria Medullaris
2. Sylvian Fissure (enlarged)
3. Cavitation secondary to necrosis of Putamen and Globus Pallidus
4. Degeneration of Internal Capsule
5. Remnant of Insular Cortex
6. Infarction subjacent to Frontal Opercular region
7. Membrane of Glial tissue separating Anterior Horn of the Lateral Ventricle from cavitary area of Infarction
8. Ischemic White Matter degeneration
9. Ischemic necrosis on rostral margin of Middle Cerebral Artery Distribution
10. Anterior Horn of the Lateral Ventricle, enlarged due to atrophy of adjacent structures (including the Head of the Caudate Nucleus)
11. Ischemic Demyelination
12. Attenuation of Corpus Callosum (fiber degeneration due to adjacent infarction)
13. Anterior Horn of the Lateral Ventricle
14. Head of the Caudate Nucleus
15. Septal Nuclei
16. Fornix
17. Massa Intermedia
18. Internal Capsule (Anterior Limb, Genu, Posterior Limb)
19. Globus Pallidus II
20. External Medullary Lamina
21. Putamen
22. External Capsule
23. Claustrum
24. Extreme Capsule
25. Tail of the Caudate
26. Optic Radiations
27. Hippocampal Formation
28. Pulvinar
29. Third Ventricle
30. Striate Cortex (Area 17)
31. Splenium, Corpus Callosum
32. Superior Cerebellar Vermis
33. Retrosplenial Cortex
34. Occipital Horn of the Lateral Ventricle
35. Posterior Commissure
36. Atrium, Lateral Ventricle
37. Fornix

SECTION B: KEY TO NUMBERED STRUCTURES

1. Ischemic Demyelination
2. Major zone of Infarction in the distribution of the Left Middle Cerebral Artery
3. Tail of the Caudate Nucleus
4. Lateral Geniculate Nucleus
5. Atrium of the Lateral Ventricle
6. Medial Geniculate Nucleus
7. Wallerian degeneration involving the ipsilateral Cerebral Peduncle
8. Aqueduct of Sylvius
9. Cerebellar Vermis
10. Inferior Colliculus
11. Red Nucleus
12. Substantia Nigra
13. Cerebral Peduncle (intact)
14. Hippocampal Formation
15. Fornix
16. Insular Cortex
17. Optic Tract
18. Mammillary Body (superior aspect, refer to reference map)
19. Third Ventricle
20. Lamina Terminalis

CLINICAL HISTORY AND NEUROLOGIC FINDINGS

This patient presented with neurological deficits which included Broca's aphasia, characterized by nonfluent speech, inability to repeat, and relative sparing of comprehension (except for certain syntactical components of complex sentences). The patient was able to read and follow written commands, however he could not read aloud.

Additional findings included (1) a severe right hemiparesis, involving the face, arm, and leg; (2) mild to moderately diminished perception of light touch over the right face, arm, and to a lesser extent, the leg, with impaired proprioception and diminished perception of vibration involving the right arm and leg; and (3) initial conjugate right gaze paresis (with left gaze preference), which gradually resolved.

LEFT MIDDLE CEREBRAL ARTERY DISTRIBUTION INFARCTION, REMOTE: HORIZONTAL SECTION, LEVEL SUPERIOR TO THE CORPUS CALLOSUM, DORSAL TO VENTRAL VIEW

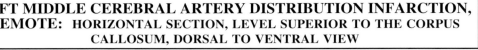

* DORSOLATERAL MARGIN OF INFARCTION

LEFT MIDDLE CEREBRAL ARTERY DISTRIBUTION INFARCTION (REMOTE): SECTIONS MAPPED ON A MIDLINE SAGITTAL DIAGRAM OF THE BRAIN

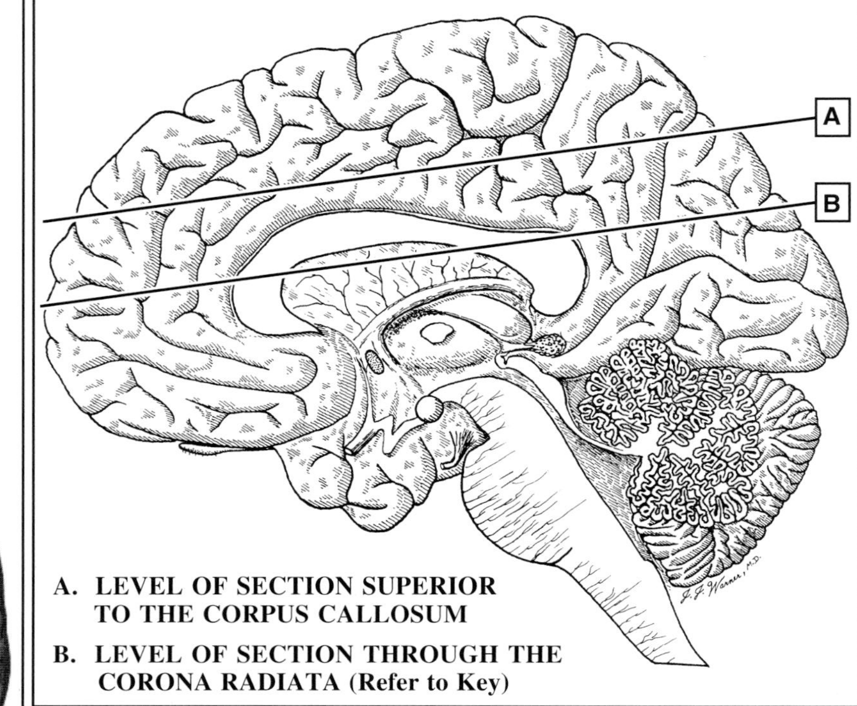

A. LEVEL OF SECTION SUPERIOR TO THE CORPUS CALLOSUM

B. LEVEL OF SECTION THROUGH THE CORONA RADIATA (Refer to Key)

SECTION B (Refer to Map), LEVEL OF THE CORONA RADIATA, DORSAL TO VENTRAL VIEW: KEY TO NUMBERED STRUCTURES

1. Infarction with cortical necrosis, subjacent white matter atrophy and gliosis
2. Anterior Cingulate Gyrus
3. Anterior Cerebral Arteries, callosomarginal branches
4. Corpus Callosum
5. Anterior Horn, Lateral Ventricle
6. Head of the Caudate Nucleus
7. Insular Cortex
8. Corona Radiata
9. Claustrum
10. Putamen
11. Sylvian Fissure
12. Choroid Plexus
13. Subacute Infarction, Middle and Posterior Cerebral Artery Watershed Distribution
14. Septum Pellucidum
15. Fornix
16. Caudate Nucleus

LEFT MIDDLE CEREBRAL ARTERY DISTRIBUTION INFARCTION, REMOTE:
HORIZONTAL SECTION, LEVEL OF THE CORONA RADIATA, DORSAL TO VENTRAL VIEW

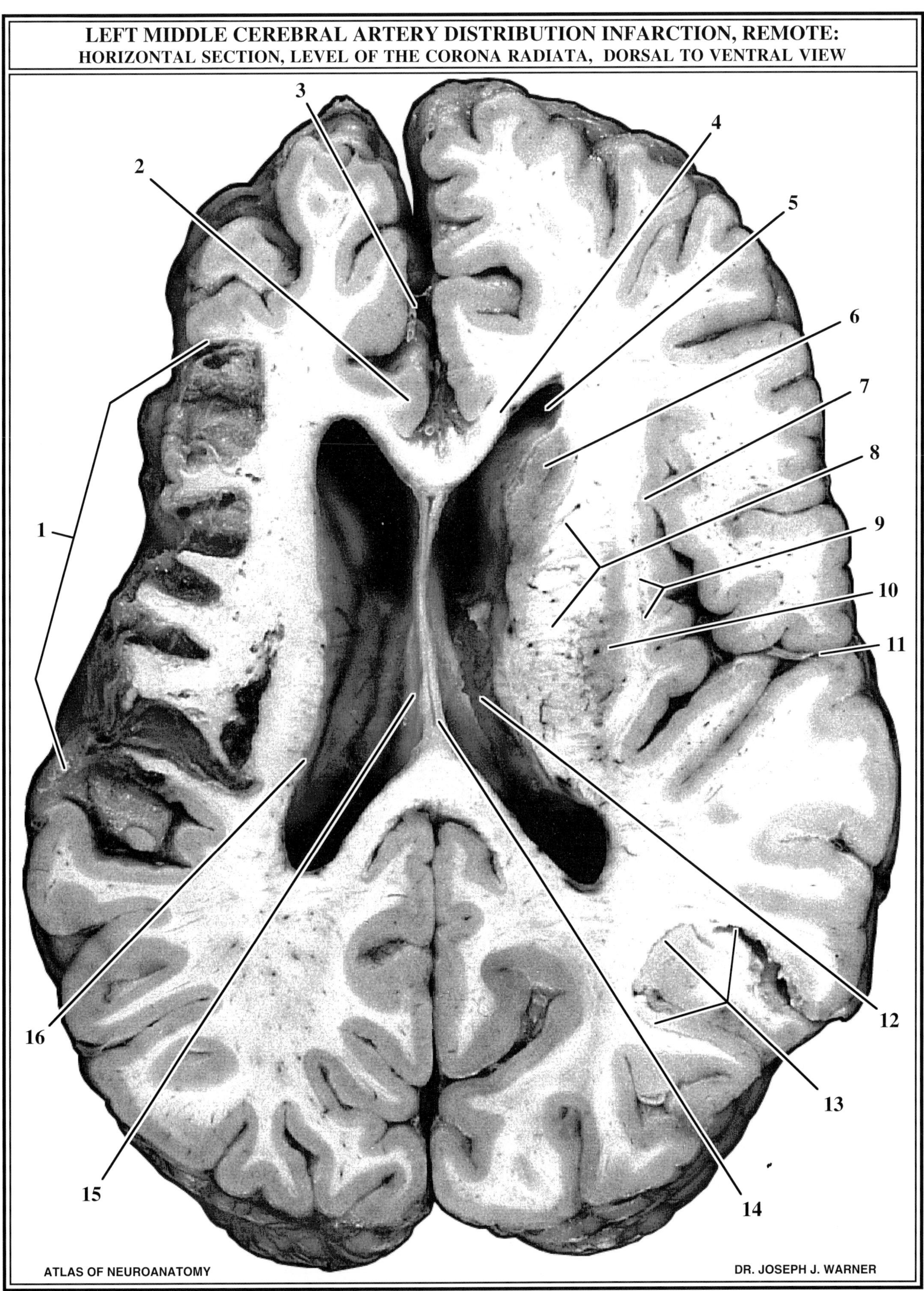

RIGHT MIDDLE CEREBRAL ARTERY DISTRIBUTION INFARCTION, REMOTE

A.

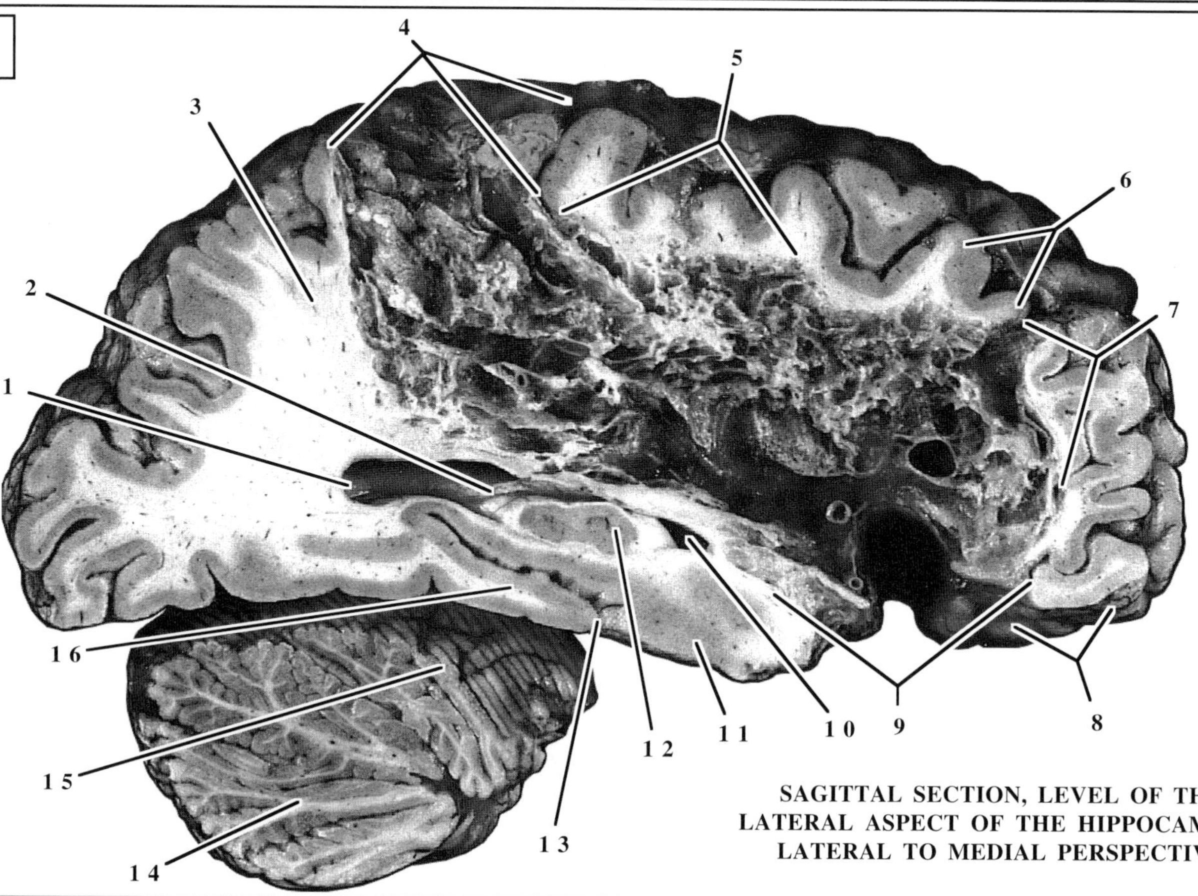

SAGITTAL SECTION, LEVEL OF THE LATERAL ASPECT OF THE HIPPOCAMPUS: LATERAL TO MEDIAL PERSPECTIVE

B.

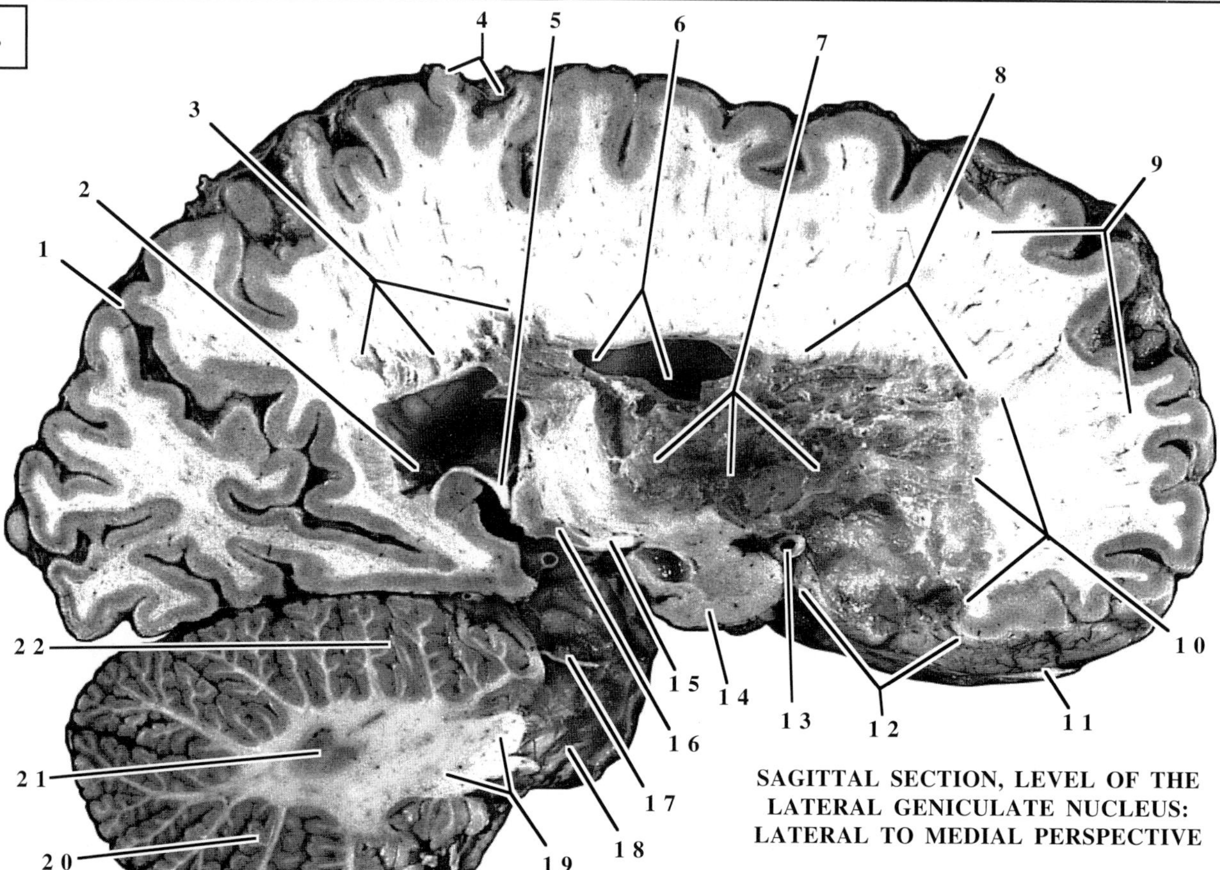

SAGITTAL SECTION, LEVEL OF THE LATERAL GENICULATE NUCLEUS: LATERAL TO MEDIAL PERSPECTIVE

RIGHT MIDDLE CEREBRAL ARTERY DISTRIBUTION INFARCTION

SAGITTAL SECTIONS MAPPED ON VENTRAL VIEW OF THE BRAIN AND KEY TO NUMBERED STRUCTURES

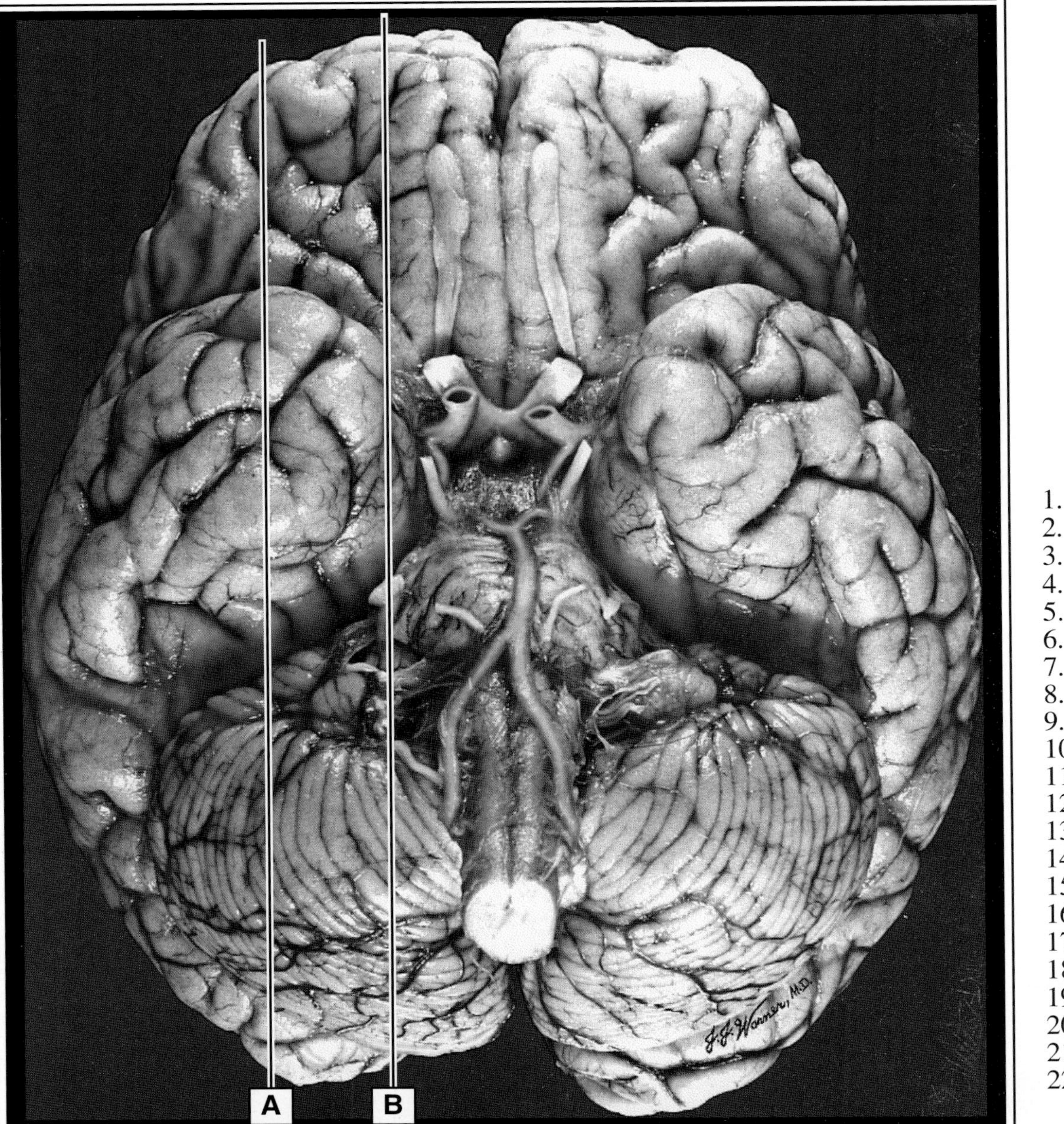

A: SAGITTAL SECTION, LEVEL OF THE LATERAL ASPECT OF THE HIPPOCAMPUS

1. Occipital Horn of the Lateral Ventricle
2. Choroid Plexus
3. White Matter, Parietal Lobe
4. Extension of infarction to Perirolandic Cortex
5. Dorsolateral margin of infarction
6. Middle Frontal Convolution
7. Rostral margin of Infarction
8. Orbitofrontal Gyri
9. Lateral frontal and superior temporal necrosis
10. Temporal Horn of the Lateral Ventricle
11. Parahippocampal Gyrus
12. Hippocampus
13. Collateral Sulcus
14. Posterior Lobe of the Cerebellum
15. Anterior Lobe of the Cerebellum
16. Fusiform Gyrus

B: SAGITTAL SECTION, LEVEL OF THE LATERAL GENICULATE NUCLEUS

1. Parieto-Occipital Sulcus
2. Atrium of Lateral Ventricle
3. Caudal extent of infarction
4. Cortical necrosis
5. Fornix
6. Body of Lateral Ventricle
7. Necrosis of Putamen, Globus Pallidus, Caudate
8. Superior margin of infarction in frontal lobe
9. White Matter subjacent to Superior Frontal Convolution
10. Rostral margin of infarction
11. Olfactory Bulb
12. Extension of infarction to Orbitofrontal Gyri
13. Middle Cerebral Artery
14. Medial Temporal Cortex, Uncus
15. Optic Tract
16. Lateral Geniculate Nucleus
17. Trochlear (IV) Nerve
18. Basis Pontis
19. Middle Cerebellar Peduncle
20. Posterior Lobe of the Cerebellum
21. Dentate Nucleus of the Cerebellum
22. Anterior Lobe of the Cerebellum

SUBACUTE INFARCTION INVOLVING THE LEFT MIDDLE CEREBRAL ARTERY DISTRIBUTION AND REMOTE RIGHT HEMISPHERIC INFARCTIONS WITH SECONDARY ASYMMETRIC CEREBRAL ATROPHY

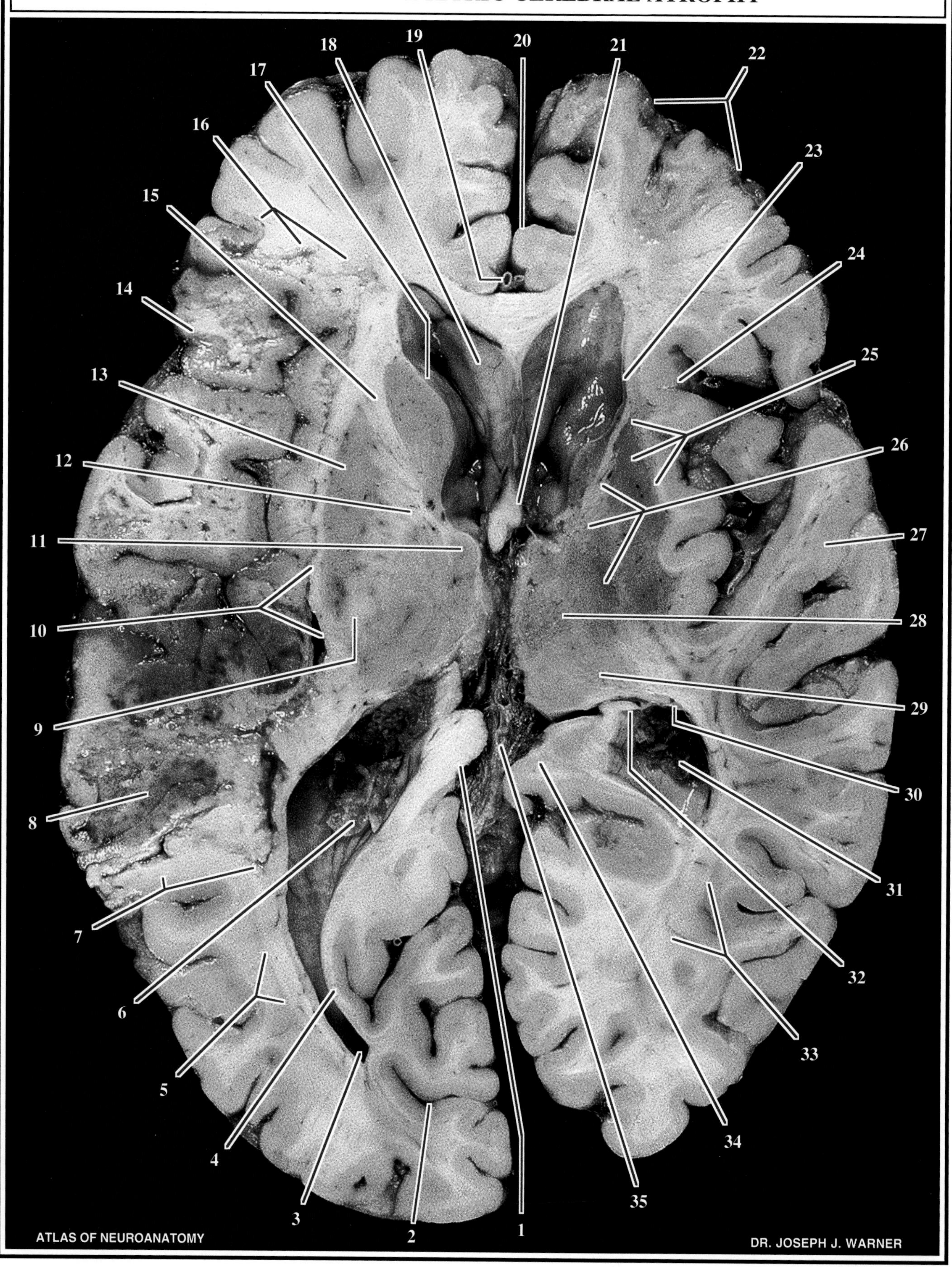

SUBACUTE INFARCTION INVOLVING THE LEFT MIDDLE CEREBRAL ARTERY DISTRIBUTION AND REMOTE RIGHT HEMISPHERIC INFARCTIONS WITH SECONDARY ASYMMETRIC CEREBRAL ATROPHY: (A) KEY TO STRUCTURES, (B) UNILATERAL DEGENERATION OF THE RIGHT MEDULLARY PYRAMID

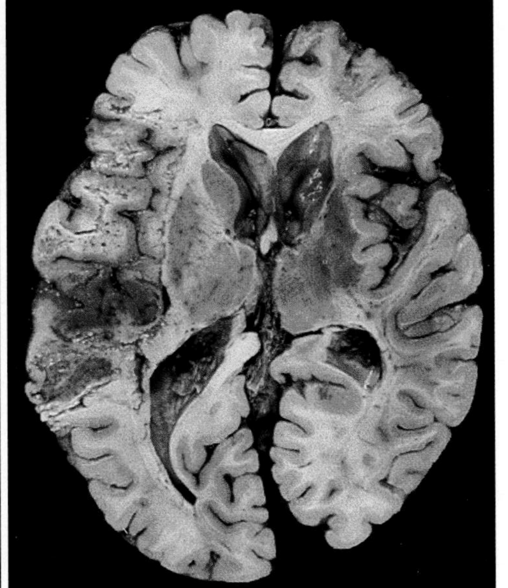

(A) HORIZONTAL SECTION, LEVEL OF THE ANTERIOR NUCLEUS OF THE THALAMUS; DORSAL TO VENTRAL PERSPECTIVE: KEY TO NUMBERED STRUCTURES

1. Splenium of the Corpus Callosum
2. Calcarine Fissure
3. Occipital Horn of the Lateral Ventricle
4. Calcar Avis
5. Optic (Geniculocalcarine) Radiations
6. Choroid Plexus
7. Caudal margin of necrosis
8. Hemorrhagic Necrosis of the Cortex
9. Posterior Limb of the Internal Capsule
10. Medial margin of necrosis
11. Anterior Nucleus of the Thalamus
12. Genu of the Internal Capsule
13. Putamen
14. Necrosis of the Frontal Operculum
15. Anterior Limb of the Internal Capsule
16. Rostral margin of necrosis
17. Head of the Caudate Nucleus
18. Rostrum of the Corpus Callosum ventral to the Anterior Horn of the Lateral Ventricle
19. Anterior Cerebral Arteries
20. Cingulate Gyrus
21. Fornix
22. Remote Infarction (note wedge-shaped extension toward the Ventricle)
23. Infarction and necrosis of the Head of the Caudate Nucleus (consistent with involvement of the distribution of the Recurrent Artery of Heubner)
24. Insular Cortex
25. Discoloration of the Putamen due to remote infarction
26. Degeneration of the Internal Capsule secondary to remote infarction
27. Heschl's Gyrus (frequently paired in the right hemisphere)
28. Necrosis within the Thalamus
29. Pulvinar Nucleus of the Thalamus
30. Tail of the Caudate Nucleus
31. Atrium of the Lateral Ventricle
32. Fornix
33. Optic (Geniculocalcarine) Radiations
34. Isthmus of the Gyrus Fornicatus
35. Great Vein of Galen (and Arachnoid)

In this case, remote infarctions of the right cerebral hemisphere were accompanied by anterograde degeneration of the ipsilateral corticospinal tracts, evidenced by unilateral atrophy of the right medullary pyramid. Discoloration and atrophy of the corticobulbar and corticospinal tracts could be traced through the cerebral peduncle and the basis pontis on the right. Insufficient time had elapsed after the left middle cerebral artery distribution infarction for the development of similar ipsilateral atrophy.

Posterior Inferior Cerebellar Artery
Fasciculus Gracilis
Fasciculus Cuneatus
Cerebellar Tonsil
Spinal Tract of the Trigeminal Nerve
Medial Lemniscus
Inferior Olivary Nucleus
Vagus (X) Nerve
Vertebral Artery
Left Medullary Pyramid
Degeneration of the right Medullary Pyramid

(B) HORIZONTAL SECTION THROUGH THE MEDULLA AND CEREBELLAR TONSILS DEMONSTRATING UNILATERAL DEGENERATION OF THE RIGHT MEDULLARY PYRAMID (VENTRAL TO DORSAL VIEW)

LEFT HEMISPATIAL NEGLECT ASSOCIATED WITH INFARCTION INVOLVING THE RIGHT MIDDLE CEREBRAL ARTERY AND PARTIAL ANTERIOR CEREBRAL ARTERY DISTRIBUTIONS: CASE PRESENTATION

This 42-year-old right-handed male reportedly fell at 1:00 a.m. (by his own account), at which time he noticed left-sided weakness. He initially remained at home, however was brought in to the hospital at 7:00 a.m. According to the family, the patient's speech was slurred. According to the Emergency Medical Services transport record, he was described as "awake" and "able to answer questions" as of approximately 6:30 a.m. The patient was examined at 10:00 a.m. He had become more lethargic during that time interval, however no loss of consciousness, posturing, or seizure activity was noted. *Nursing staff had noted that the patient reported movement of his left arm although it was observed to be motionless at the time.*

His history was remarkable for recent blunt trauma to the right anterolateral aspect of his neck during martial arts training. He also had a history of atherosclerotic coronary artery disease, with coronary artery bypass graft surgery at the age of 38. He had no history of previous stroke or transient neurologic symptomatology.

Examination at the time of initial neurologic consultation revealed the following findings. The patient was lethargic, but arousable to verbal stimuli. He was able to move the right upper and lower extremities, however could only move the left lower extremity on command. He followed midline commands without difficulty. He could direct his gaze to the left on command only briefly, with a baseline right gaze preference. The patient exhibited kinesthetic hallucinations during the examination, reporting movement of the fingers of his left hand while the limb was completely motionless. Left-sided extinction was elicited on double simultaneous auditory, visual, and tactile stimulation. Opticokinetic nystagmus testing revealed no leftward refixation saccades, whereas rightward saccades and pursuit to the left were intact. Visual fields were intact (except with double simultaneous stimulation). The optic fundi were characterized by blurred disc margins bilaterally, however no hemorrhages or microemboli were visualized. Extraocular movements were conjugate with a left gaze paresis. Moderate ptosis of the left eye was present with the pupils equal in size. A diminished response to pinprick sensation was discerned over the left side of the face. A left upper motor neuron type facial paresis was noted. Sensory testing revealed a subjective decrease in perception of all modalities over the left side of the body, with left tactile extinction as mentioned previously. A left hemiparesis was discerned on motor examination, with severe involvement of the face and upper extremity and relative sparing of the left lower extremity. No decorticate or decerebrate posturing was observed. Bilateral hyperreflexia and Babinski signs were present.

Emergent computerized tomography of the brain revealed a large area of decreased attenuation in the right hemisphere with midline shift evident within twelve hours of the onset of symptoms. No hemorrhagic component was seen.

The patient was re-examined two weeks later, after stabilization of his neurologic status. Neurobehavioural testing revealed the patient to be alert, cooperative, and somewhat jocular. The trimodal extinction persisted. Although the right gaze preference was less prominent, he did retain a tendency to orient to the right in response to verbal stimuli from his left. Elements of left hemispatial neglect were clearly demonstrable, including unilateral hemispatial neglect of drawing. Marked visuospatial dysfunction and constructional apraxia were noted. (Refer to test figures.) The left hemiparesis was slightly improved, with dense involvement of the face and distal upper extremity. He was able to move the left shoulder and leg, however weakness was discernible. The patient used his right arm to move the left and was unable to ambulate, using a wheelchair whenever out of bed.

The patient subsequently developed secondarily generalized tonic-clonic seizures, which were treated with phenytoin. Follow-up magnetic resonance imaging confirmed a large zone of infarction in the right middle cerebral artery distribution. In addition, evidence of infarction in the territory of proximal branches of the right anterior cerebral artery was discerned. (Refer to MRI figures.) These findings supported the likelihood of a lesion of the right internal carotid artery with possible distal arterial embolization. The history of right anterolateral cervical trauma suggested carotid dissection or contusion as a contributory cause.

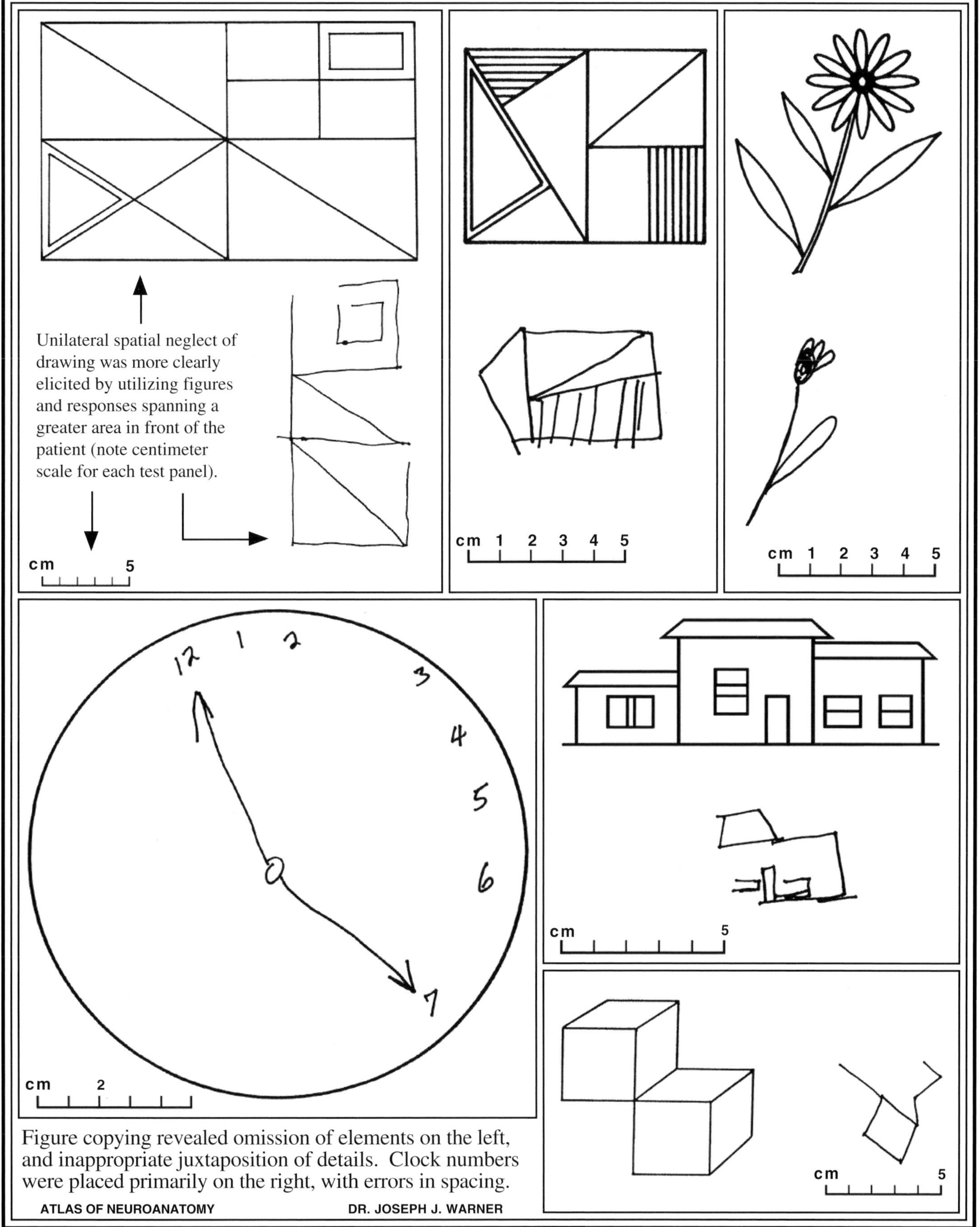
LEFT HEMISPATIAL NEGLECT ASSOCIATED WITH INFARCTION INVOLVING THE RIGHT MIDDLE CEREBRAL ARTERY AND PARTIAL ANTERIOR CEREBRAL ARTERY DISTRIBUTIONS: NEUROBEHAVIOURAL TESTING
Unilateral spatial neglect of drawing was more clearly elicited by utilizing figures and responses spanning a greater area in front of the patient (note centimeter scale for each test panel).
cm 5
cm 1 2 3 4 5
cm 1 2 3 4 5
12 1 2 3 4 5 6 7
cm 2
cm 5
cm 5
Figure copying revealed omission of elements on the left, and inappropriate juxtaposition of details. Clock numbers were placed primarily on the right, with errors in spacing.
ATLAS OF NEUROANATOMY
DR. JOSEPH J. WARNER

LEFT HEMISPATIAL NEGLECT ASSOCIATED WITH INFARCTION INVOLVING THE RIGHT MIDDLE CEREBRAL ARTERY AND PARTIAL ANTERIOR CEREBRAL ARTERY DISTRIBUTIONS: NEUROBEHAVIOURAL TESTING

A. MEDICAL RECORD — PROGRESS NOTES

Writing to dictation

"Hospital"

"I am here"

"I am here" (Trial 2)

"If I were here, she would go."

"No ifs, ands, or buts"

Elicited Sentences

"Describe the weather."

"Describe your work." (The patient was a correctional officer).

Note the patient's shift of the margin to his right.

Note perseveration "herere."

Note extreme rightward margin shift with continuation of sentences.

cm 1. 2. 3. 4. 5.

A. Testing the patient's writing, both to dictation and with spontaneous sentences, revealed a consistent tendency to utilize only the right side of the paper, despite repeated instructions to begin at the left margin. Furthermore, as the patient continued his sentences on new lines, the starting point shifted even more to his right.

B. For the letter circling task, the patient was requested to circle each and every "S" on the page. The distribution of the patient's responses, concentrated within the extreme right of the page, was characteristic of left hemispatial neglect. When asked to check his work, the patient failed to recognize any omissions.

T O X X O T X O T S
S O X S S T O S X T O X
S X X O T S O X S T T
T O X X S T O S X T O S
S O T S X T O S X O S
O O X S X S T T O X S
T X T S O S O T X X O T
O X O X T S X O T S X
S T X S S X O T S X S X
X O X T T S O S T O X T S T
T O X T S X S O O S X O
O O X S X T X T S S S O S
T T S X O S T O X S X X T
S S X T O O X S X O T X
X X X T O S T T S T O X
O S O O X X O X S T O S T
X X S S T O X O S X T O
S T T X T S O T X S O S
S X O O O X T S X T X
O O X T X O S X O T X O
X T T S O X S T O T S
O O S X T X T O S O X T X

cm

B.

LEFT HEMISPATIAL NEGLECT ASSOCIATED WITH INFARCTION INVOLVING THE RIGHT MIDDLE CEREBRAL ARTERY AND PARTIAL ANTERIOR CEREBRAL ARTERY DISTRIBUTIONS: MAGNETIC RESONANCE IMAGING

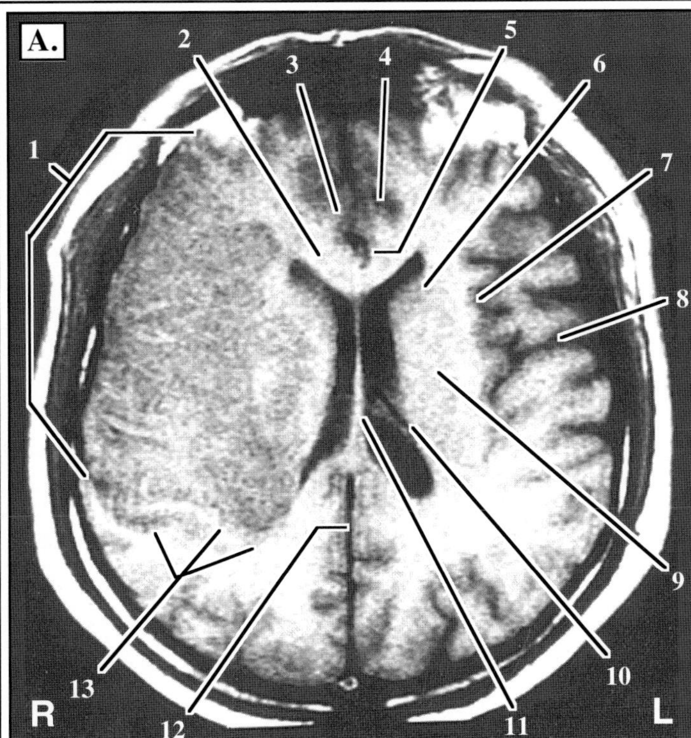

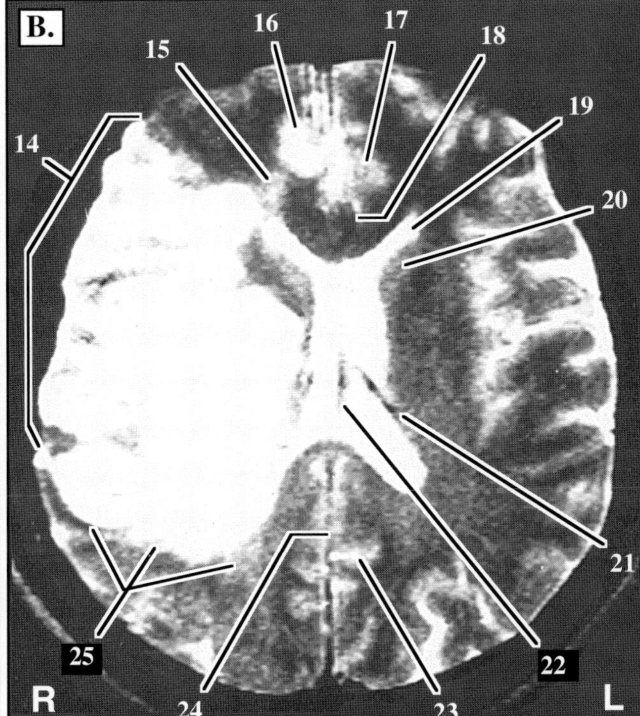

Magnetic resonance imaging after resolution of the mass effect associated with acute infarction demonstrates the distribution of the lesion. The majority of the middle cerebral arterial vascular distribution is involved, as shown on the T1 and T2 images. The rostral extent of the lesion includes the inferior and middle frontal convolutions as well as the caudal aspect of the orbitofrontal region. The entire perisylvian region has been involved (figures A-C), with medial extension to include the putamen, globus pallidus, genu and posterior limb of the internal capsule, and lateral aspect of the thalamus (figure C). The caudal margin of the lesion extends caudal to the Rolandic fissure, involving the parietal lobe. Sparing of the parasagittal aspect of the cerebral hemisphere indicates sparing of the majority of the anterior cerebral arterial distribution. However, signal change is seen within the medial prefrontal region consistent with infarction in the distribution of proximal branches of the anterior cerebral artery (figure B, #16, and figure C, #30). This pattern raises the possibility of a hemodynamically significant lesion involving the right internal carotid artery and/or artery to artery embolization from that vessel with infarction involving (1) the right middle cerebral artery territory and (2) limited areas within the vascular distribution of the right anterior cerebral artery. Note sparing of the vascular distribution of the posterior cerebral arteries and of vessels arising from the basilar bifurcation.

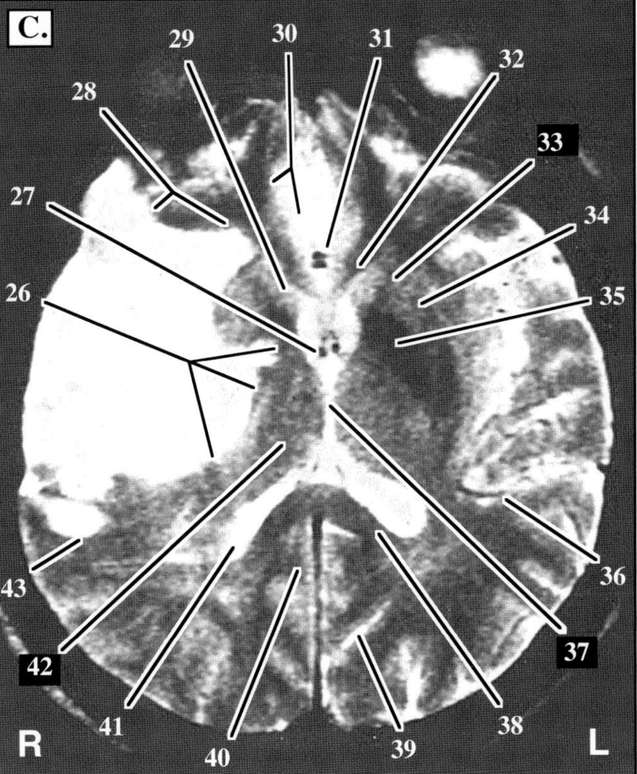

Magnetic resonance images in a plane approximately parallel to the Sylvian fissure: (A.) T1- and (B.) T2-weighted images immediately dorsal to the thalamus; (C.) T2 image, level passing through the splenium and ventral to the rostrum of the corpus callosum.

LEFT HEMISPATIAL NEGLECT ASSOCIATED WITH INFARCTION INVOLVING THE RIGHT MIDDLE CEREBRAL ARTERY AND PARTIAL ANTERIOR CEREBRAL ARTERY DISTRIBUTIONS: MAGNETIC RESONANCE IMAGING

KEY TO NUMBERED STRUCTURES

1. Zone of infarction within the territory of the right Middle Cerebral Artery
2. Corpus Callosum
3. Cingulate Gyrus
4. Cingulate Sulcus
5. Anterior Cerebral Arteries
6. Caudate Nucleus
7. Insular Cortex
8. Sylvian Fissure
9. Corona Radiata
10. Thalamostriate Vein
11. Septum Pellucidum
12. Falx Cerebri
13. Caudal margin of infarction
14. Zone of infarction
15. Infarction extending into lateral aspect of the Corpus Callosum
16. Infarction involving territory of proximal branch of the Anterior Cerebral Artery
17. Cingulate Sulcus
18. Anterior Cerebral Arteries
19. Lateral Ventricle
20. Caudate Nucleus
21. Thalamostriate Vein
22. Septum Pellucidum
23. Parieto-Occipital Sulcus
24. Falx Cerebri
25. Caudal margin of infarction
26. Medial Extension of Infarction (involving Putamen, Globus Pallidus, Genu and Posterior Limb of the Internal Capsule, and Lateral Thalamus)
27. Rostral aspect of the Internal Cerebral Veins (at the Venous Angle)
28. Rostral margin of infarction
29. Caudate Nucleus
30. Infarction involving territory of proximal branch of the Anterior Cerebral Artery
31. Anterior Cerebral Arteries
32. Rostrum of the Corpus Callosum
33. Anterior Limb of the Internal Capsule
34. Putamen
35. Globus Pallidus (note dark signal on T2 image)
36. Middle Cerebral Artery, branch within Sylvian Fissure
37. Third Ventricle
38. Splenium of the Corpus Callosum
39. Area 17 Striate Cortex
40. Cingulate Gyrus
41. Atrium of the Lateral Ventricle
42. Thalamus
43. Caudal margin of infarction extending into the Parietal Lobe

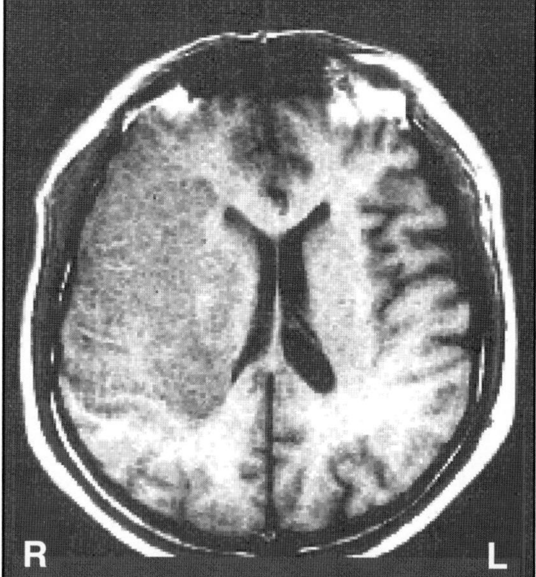

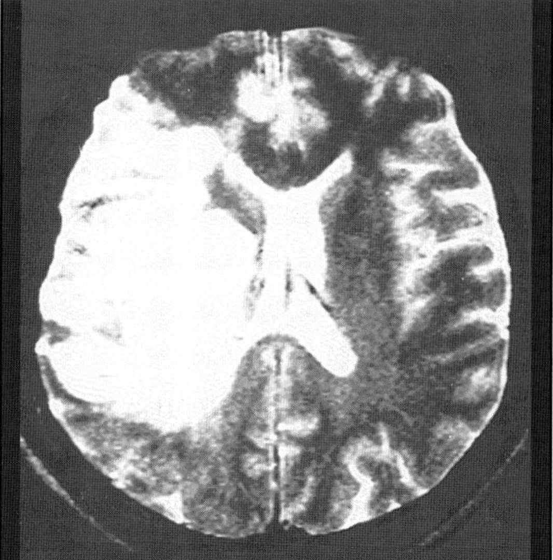

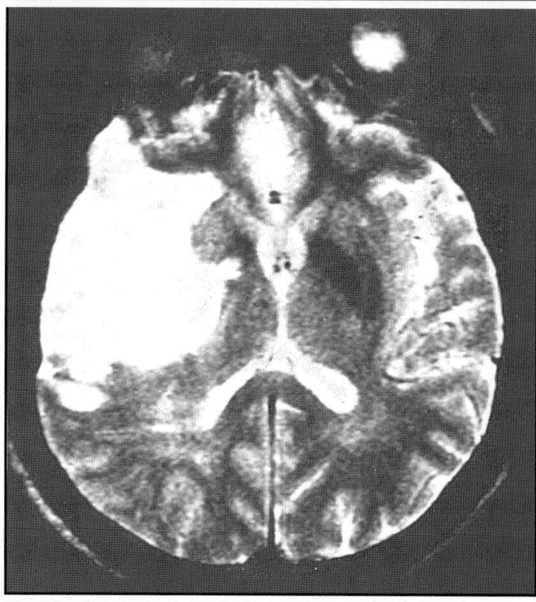

LEFT HEMISPATIAL NEGLECT ASSOCIATED WITH A RIGHT PARIETOTEMPORAL INTRACEREBRAL HEMORRHAGE: CASE PRESENTATION

This 55-year-old right-handed male was admitted to the hospital following the sudden onset of headache, followed by somnolence and loss of consciousness. Upon arrival to the emergency room, the patient was marginally responsive to verbal and tactile stimuli, and remained lethargic. Spontaneous movements of the extremities were decreased on the left, and his head and eyes were deviated to the right. Neurologic findings included (1) patient arousable, able to follow simple commands when stimulated, (2) increased head and eye deviation to the right whether stimulated from the left or right side, and (3) left hemiparesis with predominant involvement of the face and distal upper extremity. Computerized tomography revealed an area of increased attenuation in the right parietotemporal region with mass effect including contralateral shift of the midline and ipsilateral compression of the lateral ventricle.

Following stabilization, more detailed neurobehavioural testing was performed. The right gaze preference persisted, with the patient orienting to the right even when stimulated on his left side. Upon questioning by the examiner, the patient stated "There's nothing wrong with me... I want to go home." When shown his paretic left upper extremity, the patient replied "That isn't mine, that's your arm." Visual field testing revealed a dense left homonymous hemianopsia vs. left visual neglect. The patient localized left-sided tactile stimuli to homologous areas of the right side of his body (allesthesia). He demonstrated extinction of double simultaneous auditory and tactile stimulation on the left. Additional testing demonstrated unilateral spatial neglect of drawing, visuospatial dysfunction, and constructional apraxia. His affect was flat. In summary, the patient was unable to appropriately report, recognize, or respond to stimuli in the left side of space (left hemispatial neglect). Neurobehavioural findings included a denial of deficits with extrapersonalization of the left side of his body and anosognosia.

The patient was followed for approximately four years after the acute intracerebral hemorrhage. Re-examination was performed one month after the event. The previously detected allesthesia had resolved, however the left homonymous hemianopsia, left tactile and auditory extinction, and left hemiparesis persisted. His affect was markedly depressed. The patient appeared somnolent, yawning frequently during the interview and examination. He was significantly inattentive to serial task performance and demonstrated a tendency to perseverate during formal testing. Magnetic resonance imaging (performed following that visit) revealed changes consistent with the previous right parietotemporal intracerebral hemorrhage. (Refer to figures.)

Five months after the intracerebral hemorrhage, the patient presented with a history of neurobehavioural changes including dressing apraxia, intermittent confusion, inattention, social withdrawal, and depressed affect. The patient was reportedly emotionally labile, occasionally becoming inappropriately angry or aggressive with family members. His only complaint, when directly questioned, was that of "running into things on [his] left side." The patient was treated with Sertraline with an improvement of subjective complaints of fatigue, resolution of insomnia and excessive daytime somnolence, and an improvement in his affect. Antidepressant therapy was accompanied by an improvement in his level of attention and motivation to engage in activities with family and friends.

Ten months after the intracerebral hemorrhage, neurobehavioural testing was repeated and revealed persistent elements of hemispatial neglect, visuospatial planning deficits, and constructional apraxia. This pattern was observed with repeated testing over a span of four years. (Refer to figures.) Electroencephalography performed two years after the initial clinical presentation demonstrated diffuse right hemispheric slowing and suppression of normal background rhythms. These changes were consistent with the persistent effects of a structural lesion involving the right cerebral hemisphere. No evidence of epileptiform activity was discerned.

MAGNETIC RESONANCE IMAGING OF A PATIENT WITH LEFT HEMISPATIAL NEGLECT ASSOCIATED WITH A RIGHT PARIETOTEMPORAL INTRACEREBRAL HEMORRHAGE

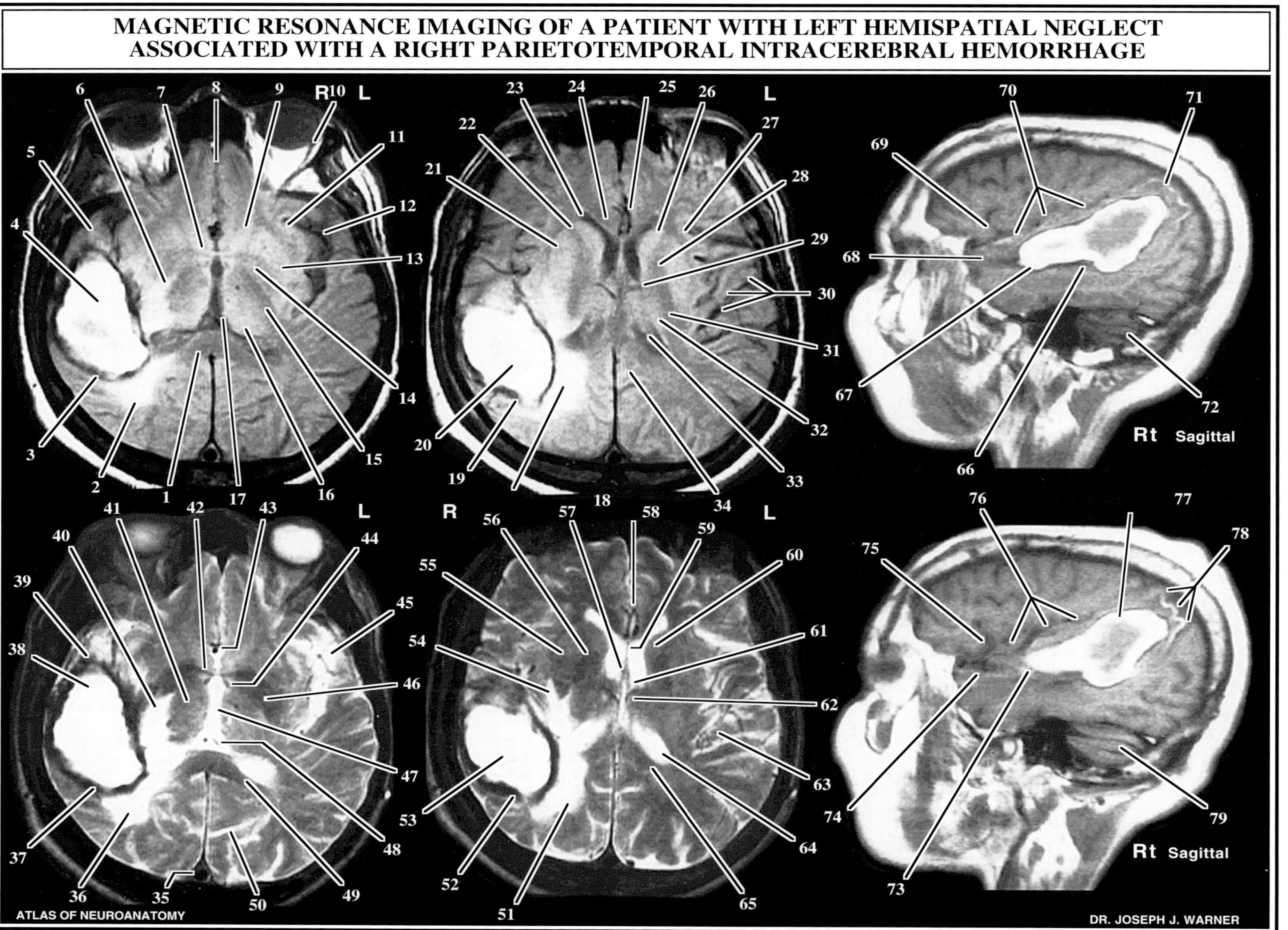

MAGNETIC RESONANCE IMAGING OF A PATIENT WITH LEFT HEMISPATIAL NEGLECT ASSOCIATED WITH A RIGHT PARIETOTEMPORAL INTRACEREBRAL HEMORRHAGE

KEY TO NUMBERED STRUCTURES

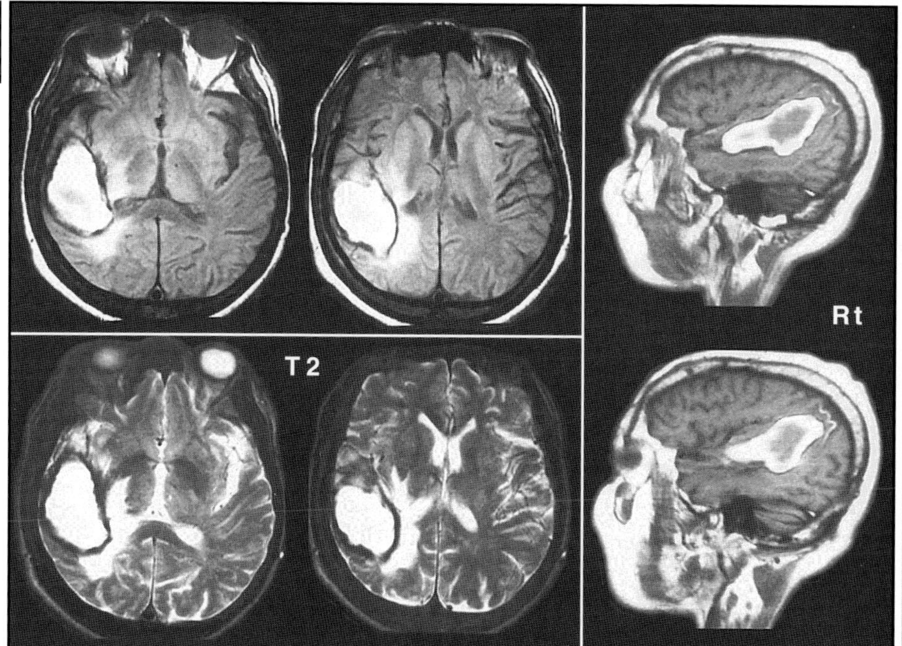

1. Splenium of the Corpus Callosum
2. Edema extending into the Parietal Lobe
3. Paramagnetic margin of hemorrhagic lesion
4. Parietotemporal intracerebral hemorrhage
5. Anterior aspect of the Temporal Lobe
6. Edema extending into the Internal Capsule
7. Anterior Commissure
8. Interhemispheric Fissure
9. Head of the Caudate Nucleus
10. Lateral Rectus Muscle
11. Insular Cortex
12. Sylvian Fissure
13. Putamen
14. Globus Pallidus
15. Posterior Limb of the Internal Capsule
16. Pulvinar Nucleus of the Thalamus
17. Habenula
18. Edema extending into the Parietal Lobe
19. Paramagnetic margin of hemorrhagic lesion
20. Parietotemporal intracerebral hemorrhage
21. Putamen
22. Anterior Limb of the Internal Capsule
23. Anterior Horn of the Lateral Ventricle
24. Genu of the Corpus Callosum
25. Anterior Cerebral Arteries
26. Head of the Caudate Nucleus
27. Insular Cortex
28. Genu of the Internal Capsule
29. Thalamostriate Vein adjacent to the Venous Angle
30. Heschl's Gyrus
31. Posterior Limb of the Internal Capsule
32. Thalamus
33. Choroid Plexus dorsal to the Thalamus
34. Posterior Cingulate Gyrus
35. Superior Sagittal Sinus
36. Edema extending into the Parietal Lobe
37. Paramagnetic margin of hemorrhagic lesion
38. Parietotemporal intracerebral hemorrhage
39. Rostral paramagnetic margin of lesion
40. Edema extending into the Globus Pallidus and Internal Capsule
41. Thalamus
42. Anterior Commissure
43. Anterior Cerebral Arteries
44. Postcommissural fibers of the Fornix
45. Sylvian Fissure
46. Globus Pallidus
47. Third Ventricle
48. Internal Cerebral Vein
49. Splenium of the Corpus Callosum
50. Area 17 Striate Cortex
51. Edema extending into the Parietal Lobe
52. Paramagnetic margin of hemorrhagic lesion
53. Parietotemporal intracerebral hemorrhage
54. Subinsular Edema
55. Putamen
56. Genu of the Internal Capsule
57. Septal Vein and Septal Nuclei
58. Anterior Cerebral Arteries
59. Septum Pellucidum
60. Head of the Caudate Nucleus
61. Foramen of Monro
62. Venous Angle
63. Planum Temporale
64. Lateral Ventricle
65. Corpus Callosum
66. Paramagnetic margin of hemorrhagic lesion
67. Rostral extension of hemorrhage into the Temporal Lobe
68. Superior Temporal Gyrus
69. Frontal Operculum
70. Sylvian Fissure (straightened)
71. Concentric signal suggesting recurrent marginal hemorrhage
72. Cerebellum
73. Extension of hemorrhage into the Temporal Lobe
74. Superior Temporal Gyrus
75. Frontal Operculum
76. Sylvian Fissure (straightened)
77. Parietotemporal intracerebral hemorrhage
78. Concentric signal suggesting recurrent marginal hemorrhage
79. Cerebellum

LEFT HEMISPATIAL NEGLECT ASSOCIATED WITH A RIGHT PARIETOTEMPORAL INTRACEREBRAL HEMORRHAGE: SEQUENTIAL NEUROBEHAVIOURAL TESTING

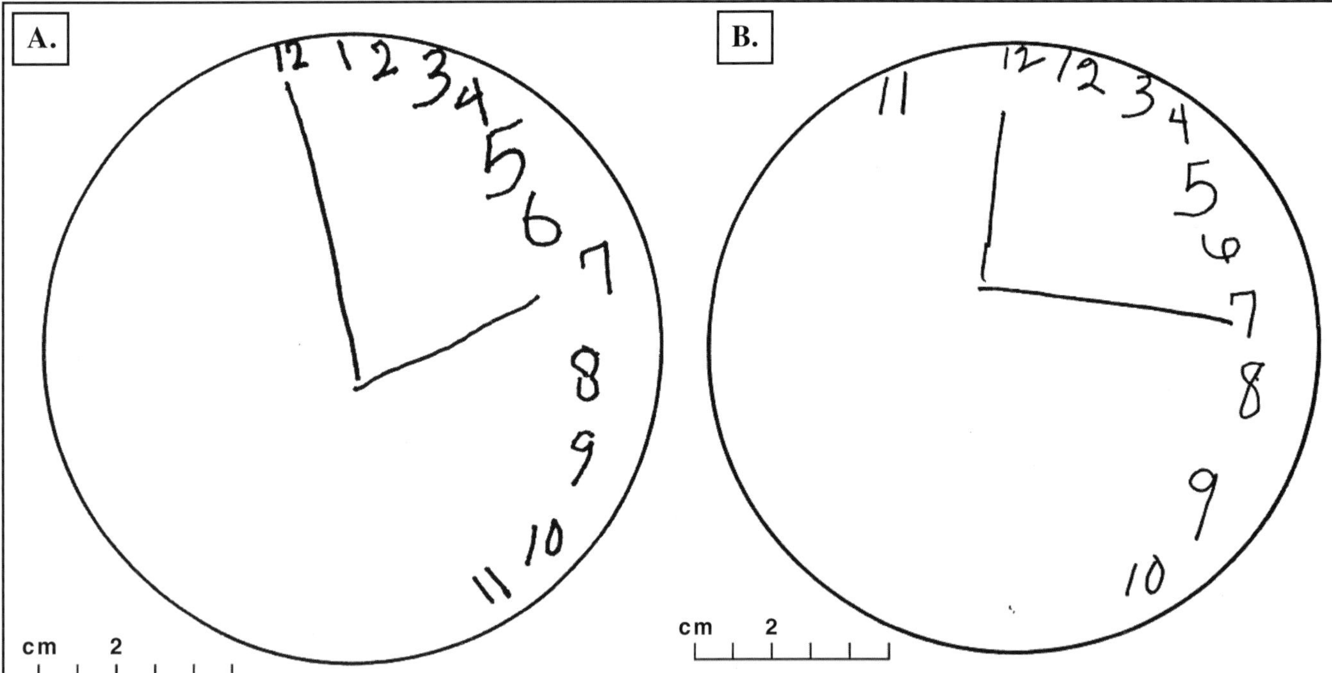

RESULTS OF THE CLOCK-FACE CONSTRUCTION TASK AT (A) 11 MONTHS AND (B) 24 MONTHS AFTER A RIGHT PARIETOTEMPORAL INTRACEREBRAL HEMORRHAGE

Placement of numbers in the right side of the circle in trial A with a failure to incorporate the left side of the circle into task execution is frequently observed in hemispatial neglect. In trial B, the patient placed the 11 appropriately after placing 12 through 10 in the right side of the circle. In neither trial A nor B did the patient recognize any abnormality of the clock when shown to him immediately after completion.

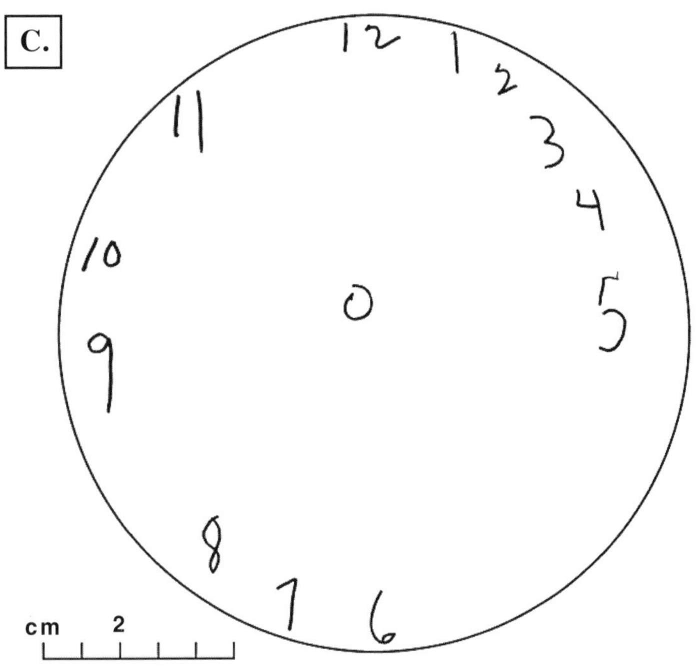

CLOCK-FACE CONSTRUCTION 43 MONTHS AFTER THE INTRACEREBRAL HEMORRHAGE

Note the errors in spacing with self-correction at the six and nine o'clock positions, indicative of a visuospatial planning deficit with relative sparing of spatial perception.

CLOCK-FACE CONSTRUCTION TASK

The patient is given a test sheet with a circle printed in the center and is subsequently instructed to place numbers on the sheet such as to create a clock face. Patients are reminded to distribute the numbers around the circle as they would be on an analog (non-digital) clock or watch. The patient is further instructed not to move the sheet along a left-right axis, nor to rotate the sheet during completion of the task. Once the patient starts, no further instruction nor prompting is given. Following completion, the patient is asked to assess the finished clock without more specific cues which might draw their attention to certain errors. In this way, the patient's perception of the completed clock is tested.

In this case, the patient failed to recognize any abnormality of his finished clock face when questioned in trials A and B. In trial C, the patient spontaneously recognized his error in spacing of the numbers, verbally stated that he had made the errors, and attempted to correct the spacing as he continued.

LEFT HEMISPATIAL NEGLECT ASSOCIATED WITH A RIGHT PARIETOTEMPORAL INTRACEREBRAL HEMORRHAGE: NEUROBEHAVIOURAL TESTING

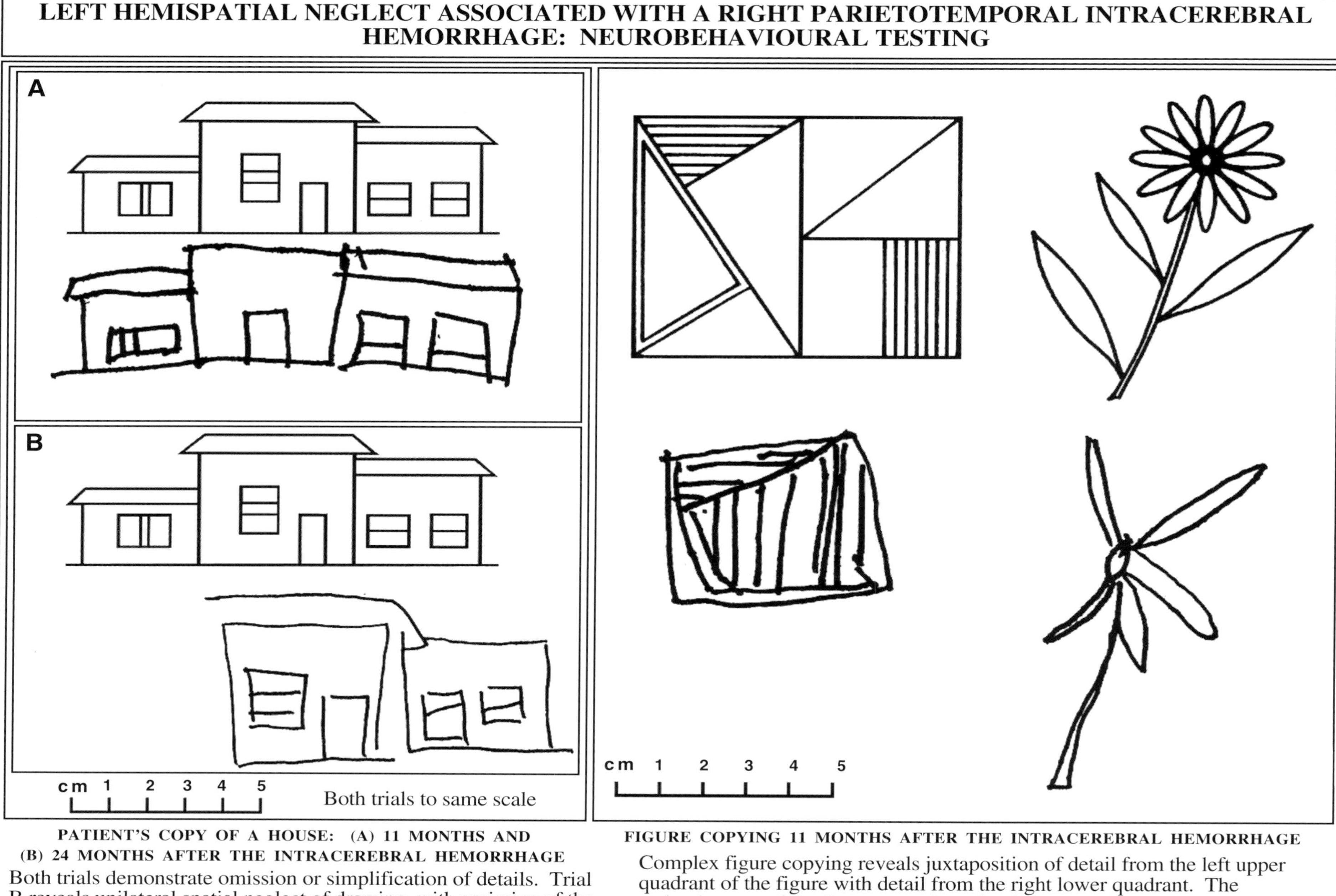

PATIENT'S COPY OF A HOUSE: (A) 11 MONTHS AND (B) 24 MONTHS AFTER THE INTRACEREBRAL HEMORRHAGE

Both trials demonstrate omission or simplification of details. Trial B reveals unilateral spatial neglect of drawing, with omission of the section of the building on the patient's left and failure to complete the left side of the roof over the center of the structure.

FIGURE COPYING 11 MONTHS AFTER THE INTRACEREBRAL HEMORRHAGE

Complex figure copying reveals juxtaposition of detail from the left upper quadrant of the figure with detail from the right lower quadrant. The patient's copy of the flower reveals omitted leaves and petals, especially from the left side of the original figure.

LEFT HEMISPATIAL NEGLECT ASSOCIATED WITH A RIGHT PARIETOTEMPORAL INTRACEREBRAL HEMORRHAGE: ELECTROENCEPHALOGRAM TWO YEARS AFTER INITIAL CLINICAL EVENT

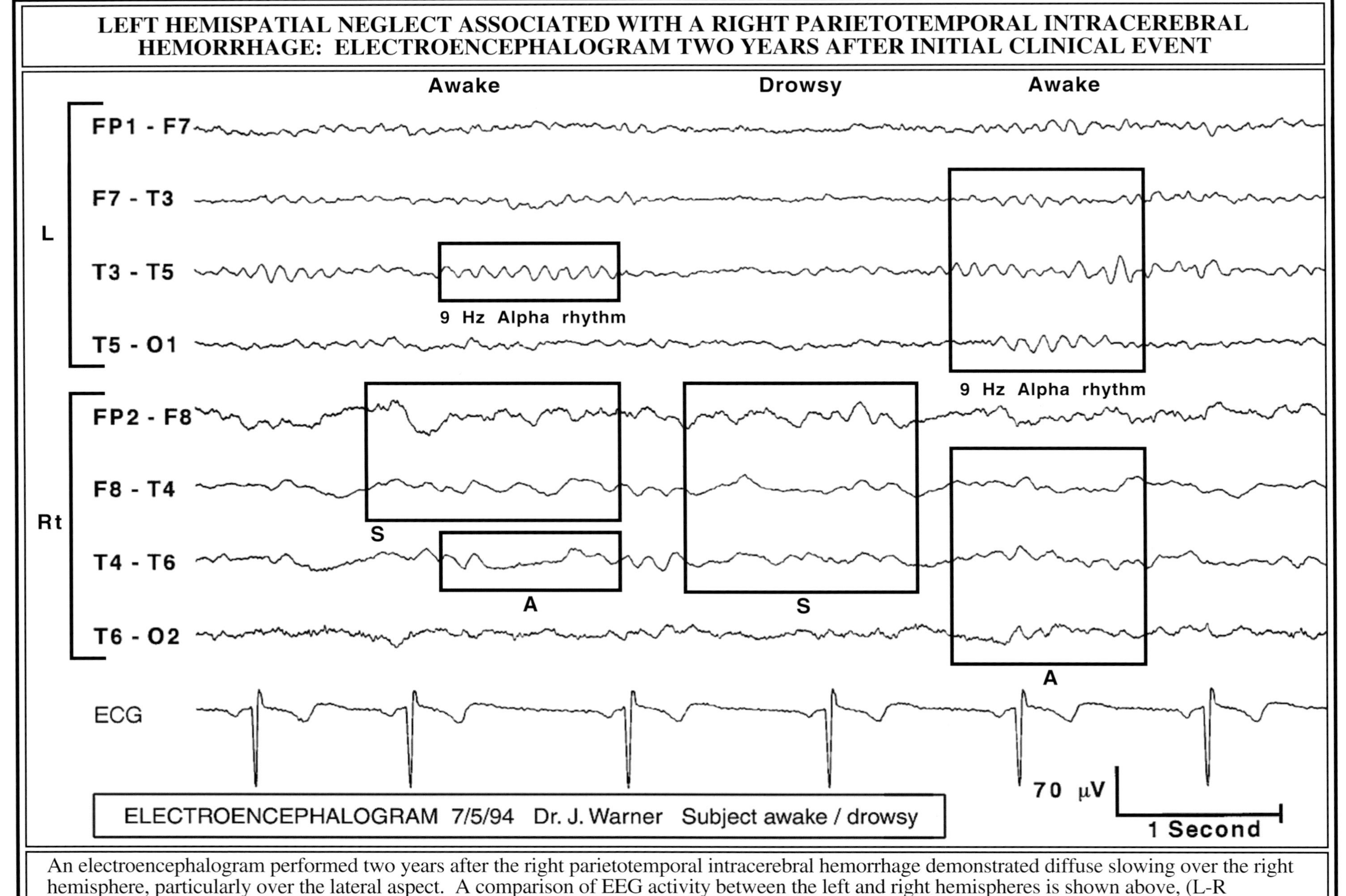

An electroencephalogram performed two years after the right parietotemporal intracerebral hemorrhage demonstrated diffuse slowing over the right hemisphere, particularly over the lateral aspect. A comparison of EEG activity between the left and right hemispheres is shown above, (L-R anteroposterior bipolar bitemporal montage). Electroencephalographic activity over the right cerebral hemisphere is characterized by changes including absence of alpha rhythm (A) and superimposed slow-wave activity in the theta and delta ranges (S), consistent with a structural lesion.

ATLAS OF NEUROANATOMY DR. JOSEPH J. WARNER

HEMORRHAGIC INFARCTION IN THE DISTRIBUTION OF THE RIGHT INTERNAL CAROTID ARTERY ASSOCIATED WITH BRACHIOCEPHALIC ARTERY OCCLUSION: CASE PRESENTATION AND COMPUTERIZED TOMOGRAPHY

This 62-year-old right-handed male presented with "cramping pain" and coldness of the right upper extremity. The symptoms were progressive over approximately one week. The patient had a prior history of hypertension and angina with coronary artery disease. There was an additional history of adenocarcinoma of the gastroesophageal junction with a resection via a left thoracotomy seven years prior to the current hospital admission. Thirteen years earlier, he had undergone a laryngectomy for carcinoma, with no recurrence.

The distal right upper extremity was cold to palpation. The patient developed marked cyanosis of the right hand, with no palpable radial or brachial pulse. The author was consulted when the patient developed intermittent weakness and numbness of the left arm. On examination, visual fields were full without extinction. Extraocular movements were normal, and there was no facial weakness. The patient had mild weakness of left shoulder abduction and left hip flexion, with normal strength of the distal extremities. Sensation was slightly diminished to all modalities over the proximal left upper and lower extremities and trunk. Reflexes were symmetrical. These finding were consistent with cerebral ischemia in a watershed distribution, leading to the presumptive diagnosis of innominate artery occlusion with right subclavian and carotid distribution ischemia. Vascular surgery was consulted. However, before further intervention could be undertaken, the patient developed a dense left hemiparesis with a right gaze preference. Computerized tomography revealed decreased attenuation in the anterior and middle cerebral artery distributions with hemorrhage into the caudate nucleus and putamen. There was also evidence of multiple cortical hemorrhages in the frontal, temporal, and parietal regions with subarachnoid extension and mass effect with contralateral midline shift.

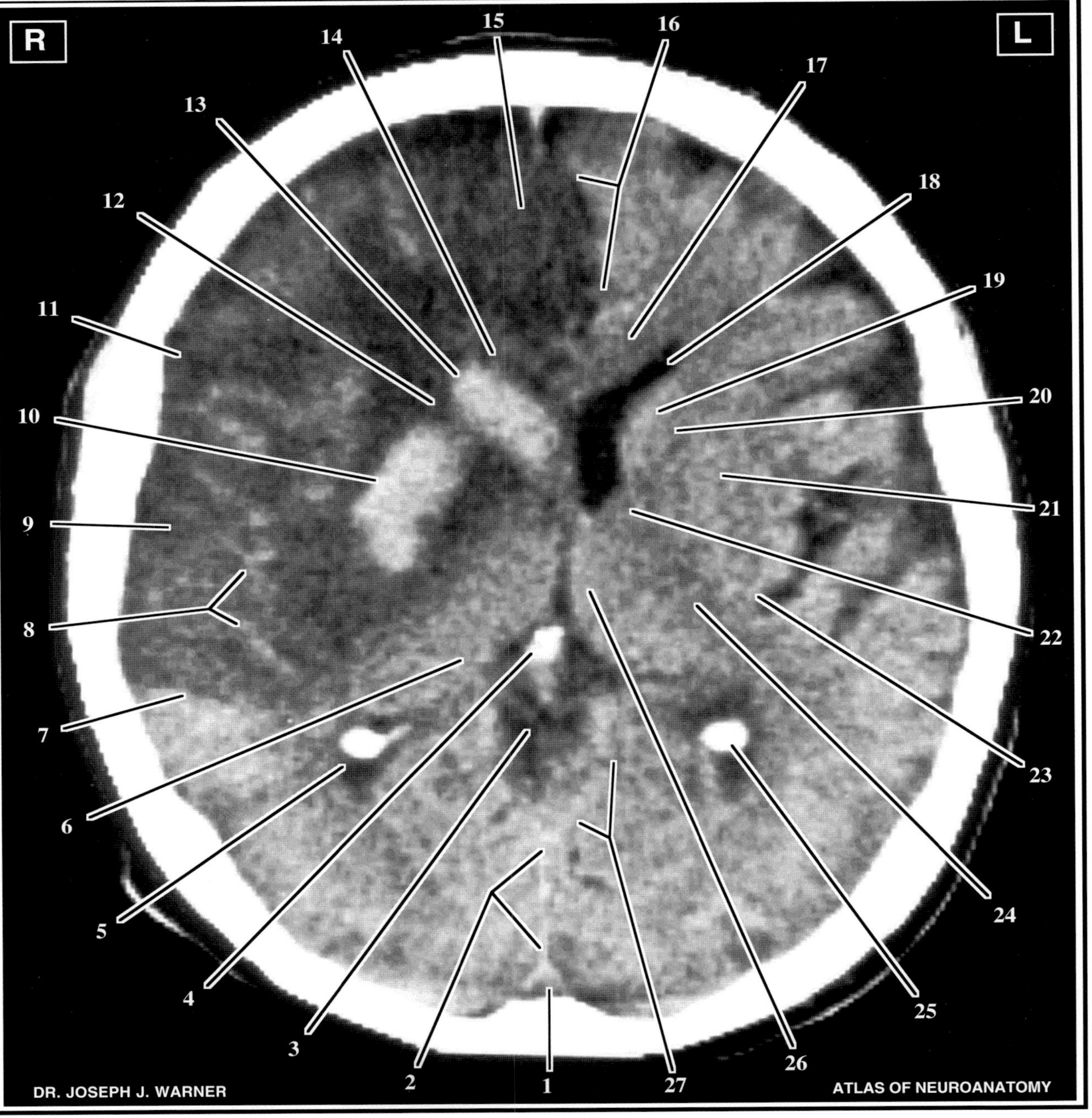

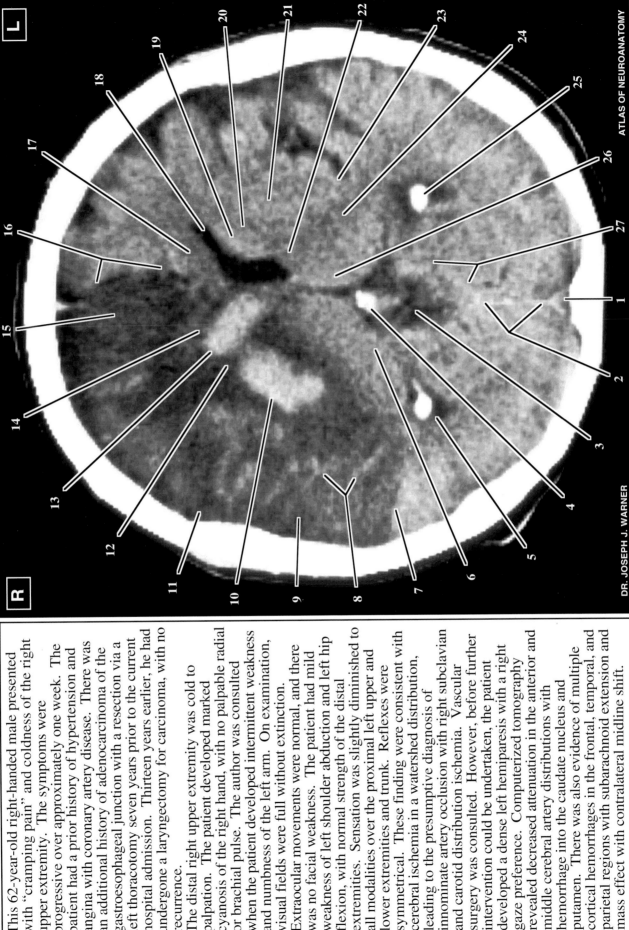

HEMORRHAGIC INFARCTION IN THE DISTRIBUTION OF THE RIGHT INTERNAL CAROTID ARTERY ASSOCIATED WITH BRACHIOCEPHALIC ARTERY OCCLUSION: KEY TO CT, CLINICAL COURSE, AND PATHOPHYSIOLOGY

KEY TO NUMBERED STRUCTURES

1. Superior Sagittal Sinus
2. Falx Cerebri
3. Quadrigeminal Cistern
4. Pineal Body
5. Atrium of the Lateral Ventricle
6. Pulvinar Nucleus of the Thalamus
7. Caudal margin of infarction and edema
8. Hemorrhage involving Insular Cortex and/or Subarachnoid Space
9. Decreased attenuation and sulcal effacement involving the Temporal Lobe
10. Hemorrhage into the Putamen
11. Decreased attenuation involving the Frontal Opercular region
12. Anterior Limb of the Internal Capsule
13. Hemorrhage into the Head of the Caudate Nucleus
14. Anterior Horn of the Lateral Ventricle (compressed)
15. Decreased attenuation with mass effect involving the medial aspect of the Frontal Pole
16. Shift of midline structures including the Anterior Cerebral Arteries
17. Corpus Callosum
18. Anterior Horn of the Lateral Ventricle
19. Head of the Caudate Nucleus
20. Anterior Limb of the Internal Capsule
21. Putamen
22. Genu of the Internal Capsule
23. Insular Cortex
24. Posterior Limb of the Internal Capsule
25. Choroid Plexus
26. Dorsomedial Nucleus of the Thalamus
27. Tentorial Incisura (dorsal aspect)

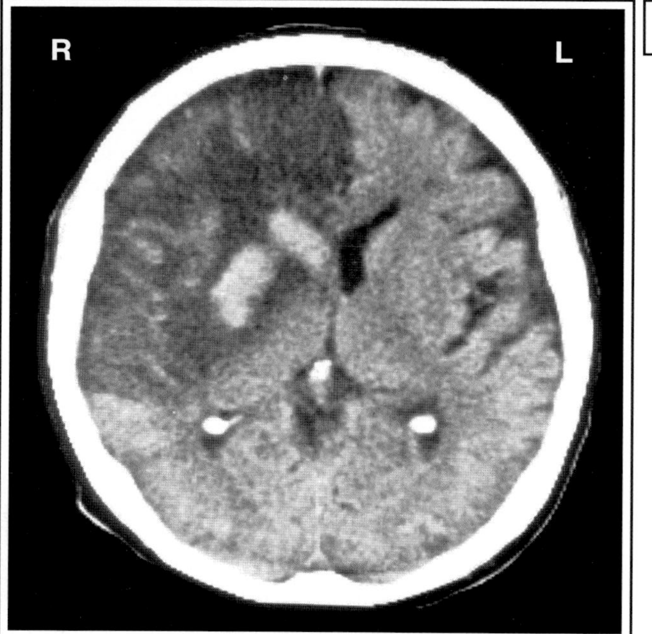

COMPUTERIZED TOMOGRAPHIC SECTION MAPPED ON A MIDLINE SAGITTAL DIAGRAM OF THE BRAIN

Cyanosis of the right hand progressed. The patient developed a severe metabolic acidosis, presumably related to the severe ischemia involving the right upper extremity. He became extremely lethargic, and subsequently developed left decerebrate posturing. The patient sustained a cardiopulmonary arrest and could not be resuscitated.

Neuropathologic examination was performed by the author. General pathologic findings at autopsy included severe aortic atherosclerosis. The heart was remarkable for coronary arterial atherosclerosis with slight biventricular hypertrophy. There was no significant valvular disease or chamber enlargement. No cardiac source of emboli was identified. The ostium of the brachiocephalic artery was severely stenotic, with a reduction in lumenal diameter to less than 3 mm. Neuropathologic findings included multiple atherosclerotic plaques involving the basilar and both vertebral arteries. The left supraclinoid portion of the internal carotid artery revealed moderate atherosclerosis. The right internal carotid artery was mildly atherosclerotic; however, thrombus was present within the supraclinoid segment of that vessel. Acute hemorrhagic infarction involving the anterior and middle cerebral arterial distributions with significant mass effect was confirmed. The pathophysiology of this case emphasizes the anatomy of the proximal aspect of the cerebrovascular system. The right common carotid artery arises from the brachiocephalic artery, in contrast to the left common carotid artery, which usually arises directly from the arch of the aorta. The right vertebral artery, arising distal to the common carotid, was not hemodynamically compromised, presumably due to collateral flow from the contralateral vertebral artery and/or retrograde flow along the basilar artery.

THE ARCH OF THE AORTA AND PROXIMAL CERVICOCRANIAL ARTERIES: ANATOMY AND THE HEMODYNAMIC EFFECTS OF SEVERE BRACHIOCEPHALIC ARTERY STENOSIS

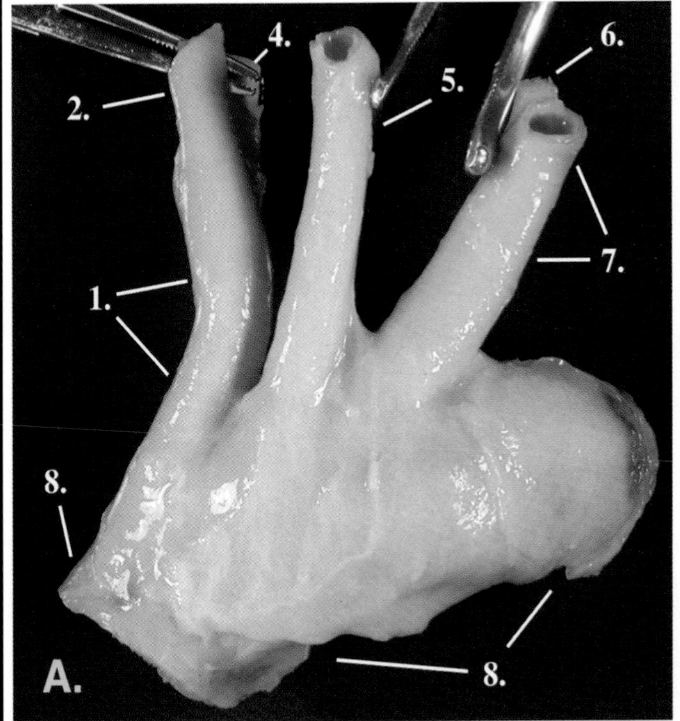

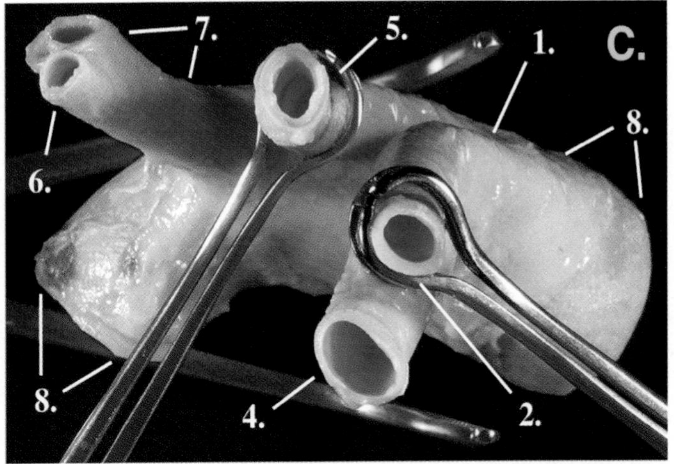

D. Diagrammatic representation of the aortic arch and cervicocranial arteries illustrating the finding of severe atherosclerotic stenosis of the brachiocephalic artery.

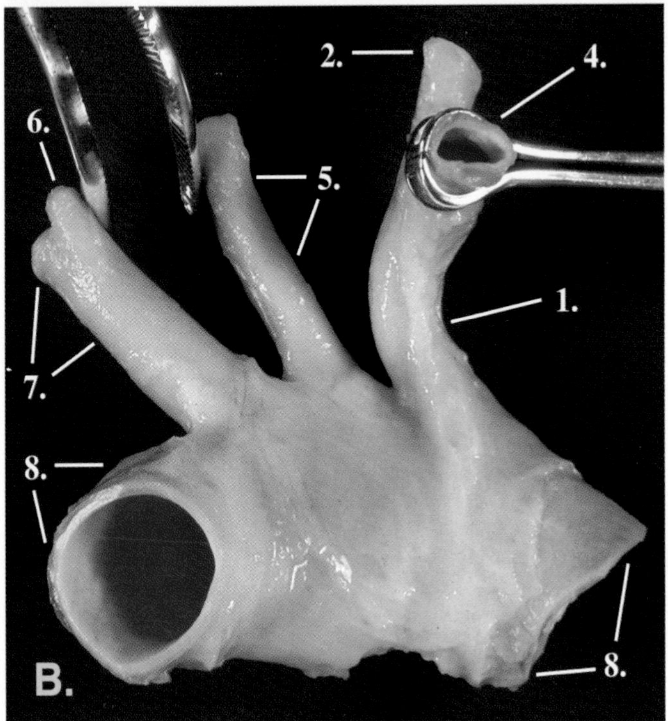

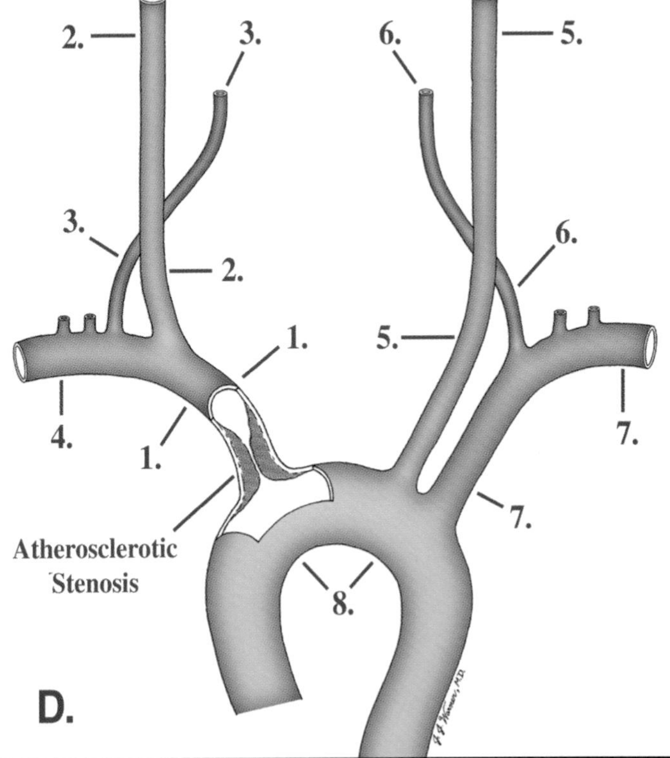

The Aortic Arch and Major Arteries
- A. Anterior (Ventral) Aspect
- B. Posterior (Dorsal) Aspect
- C. Superior (Rostral) Aspect

1. Brachiocephalic Artery
2. Right Common Carotid Artery
3. Right Vertebral Artery
4. Right Subclavian Artery
5. Left Common Carotid Artery
6. Left Vertebral Artery
7. Left Subclavian Artery
8. Arch of the Aorta

HEMORRHAGIC INFARCTION IN THE DISTRIBUTION OF THE RIGHT INTERNAL CAROTID ARTERY ASSOCIATED WITH BRACHIOCEPHALIC ARTERY OCCLUSION: HORIZONTAL SECTION OF THE BRAIN, LEVEL OF THE ANTERIOR NUCLEUS OF THE THALAMUS

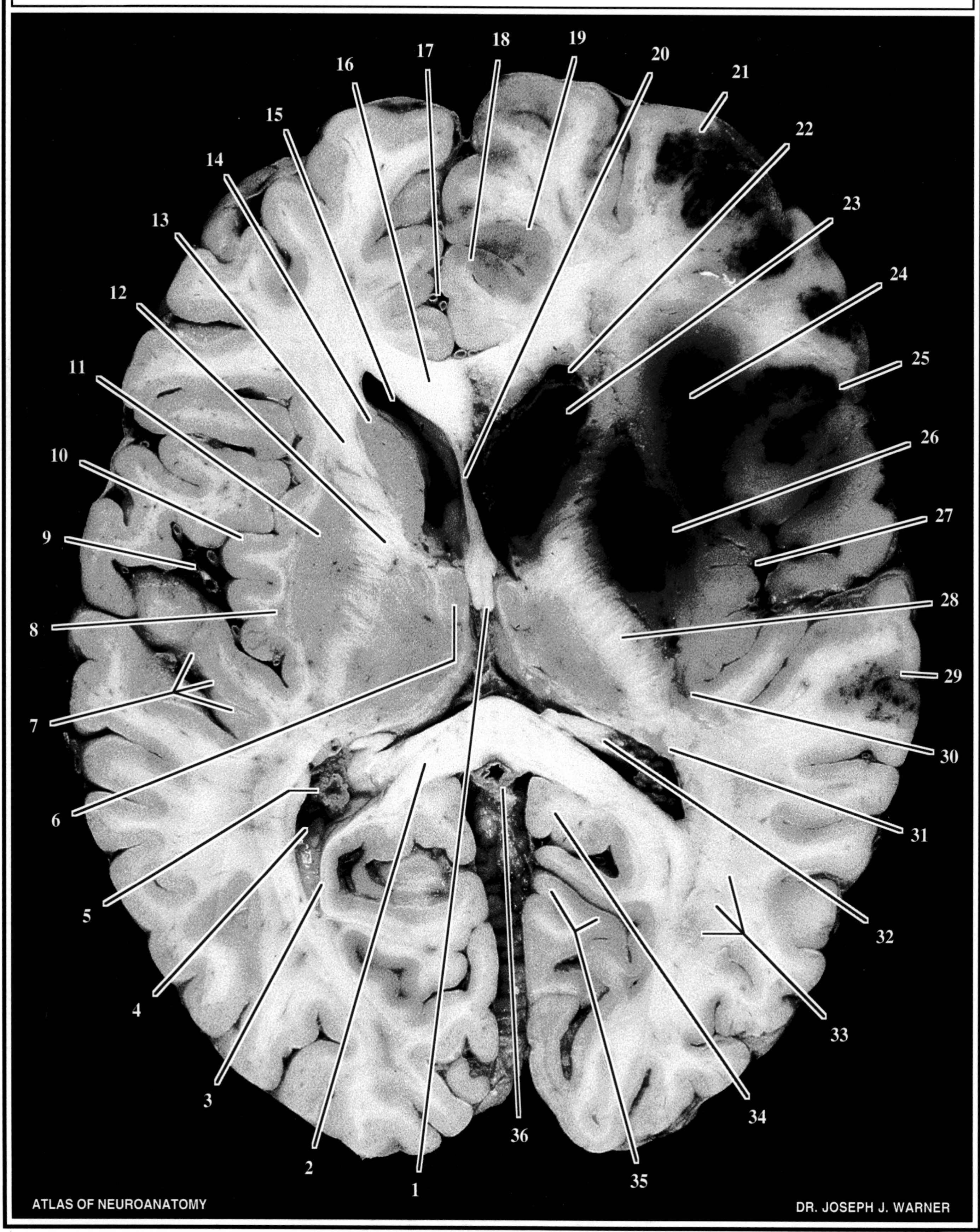

HEMORRHAGIC INFARCTION IN THE DISTRIBUTION OF THE RIGHT INTERNAL CAROTID ARTERY ASSOCIATED WITH BRACHIOCEPHALIC ARTERY OCCLUSION; HORIZONTAL SECTION OF THE BRAIN, LEVEL OF THE ANTERIOR NUCLEUS OF THE THALAMUS: KEY TO NUMBERED STRUCTURES AND CT CORRELATION

KEY TO NUMBERED STRUCTURES

1. Fornix
2. Splenium of the Corpus Callosum
3. Calcar Avis
4. Atrium of the Lateral Ventricle
5. Choroid Plexus
6. Anterior Nucleus of the Thalamus
7. Heschl's Gyrus
8. Claustrum
9. Middle Cerebral Artery, branch within the Sylvian Fissure
10. Insular Cortex
11. Putamen
12. Genu of the Internal Capsule
13. Anterior Limb of the Internal Capsule
14. Head of the Caudate Nucleus
15. Anterior Horn of the Lateral Ventricle
16. Genu of the Corpus Callosum
17. Anterior Cerebral Arteries
18. Leftward shift of the Cingulate Gyrus associated with ipsilateral mass effect
19. Zone of infarction and edema involving the region of the Cingulate Sulcus
20. Septum Pellucidum (shifted due to mass effect)
21. Hemorrhagic infarction of dorsolateral frontal cortex
22. Anterior Horn of the Lateral Ventricle (note compression due to ipsilateral mass effect)
23. Hemorrhage into the Head of the Caudate Nucleus*
24. Hemorrhagic infarction of Insula
25. Hemorrhagic infarction of Frontal Opercular region
26. Hemorrhage into the Putamen*
27. Necrosis of Perisylvian Cortex
28. Posterior Limb of the Internal Capsule
29. Hemorrhagic infarction of parietotemporal cortex
30. Caudal margin of necrotic change
31. Tail of the Caudate Nucleus
32. Fornix
33. Optic (Geniculocalcarine) Radiations
34. Isthmus of the Gyrus Fornicatus
35. Area 17 Striate Cortex
36. Great Vein of Galen at junction with the Inferior Sagittal Sinus

*Note dense hemorrhages into the Striatum, separated by the Anterior Limb of the Internal Capsule.

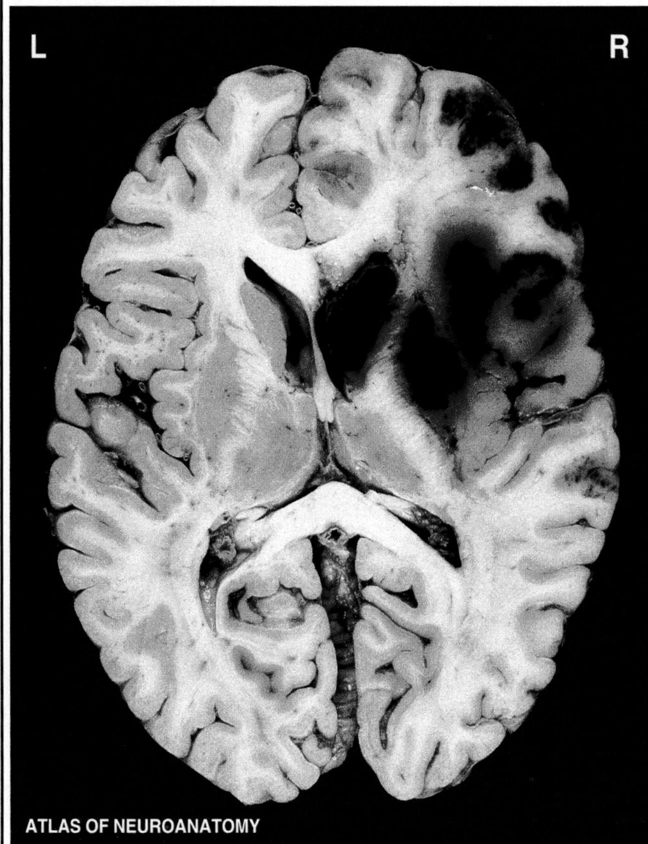

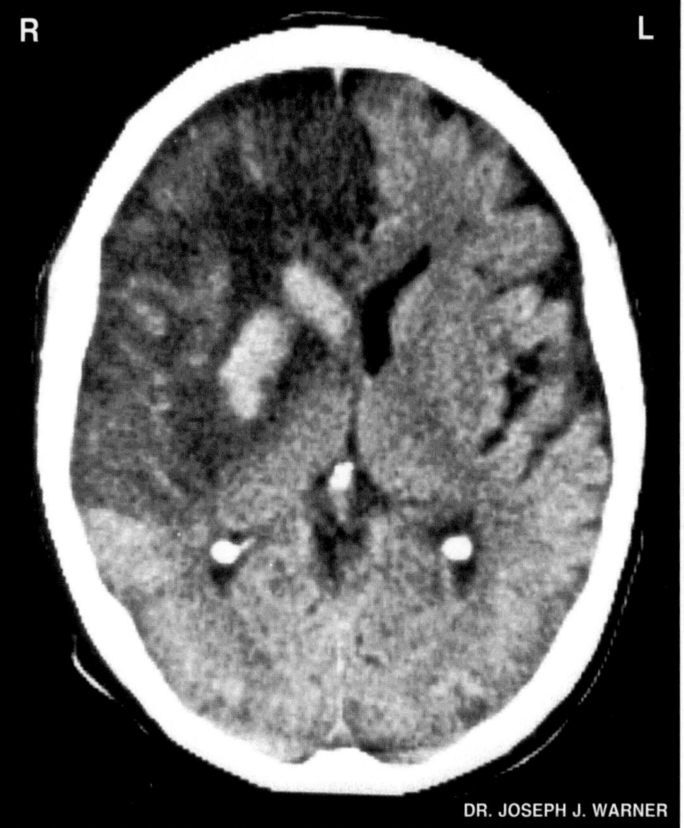

PONTINE INFARCTIONS ASSOCIATED WITH HYPERTENSION, VERTEBROBASILAR ARTERIOSCLEROSIS, AND SUPERIOR CEREBELLAR VERMAL DEGENERATION: MIDLINE SAGITTAL SECTION OF THE BRAIN

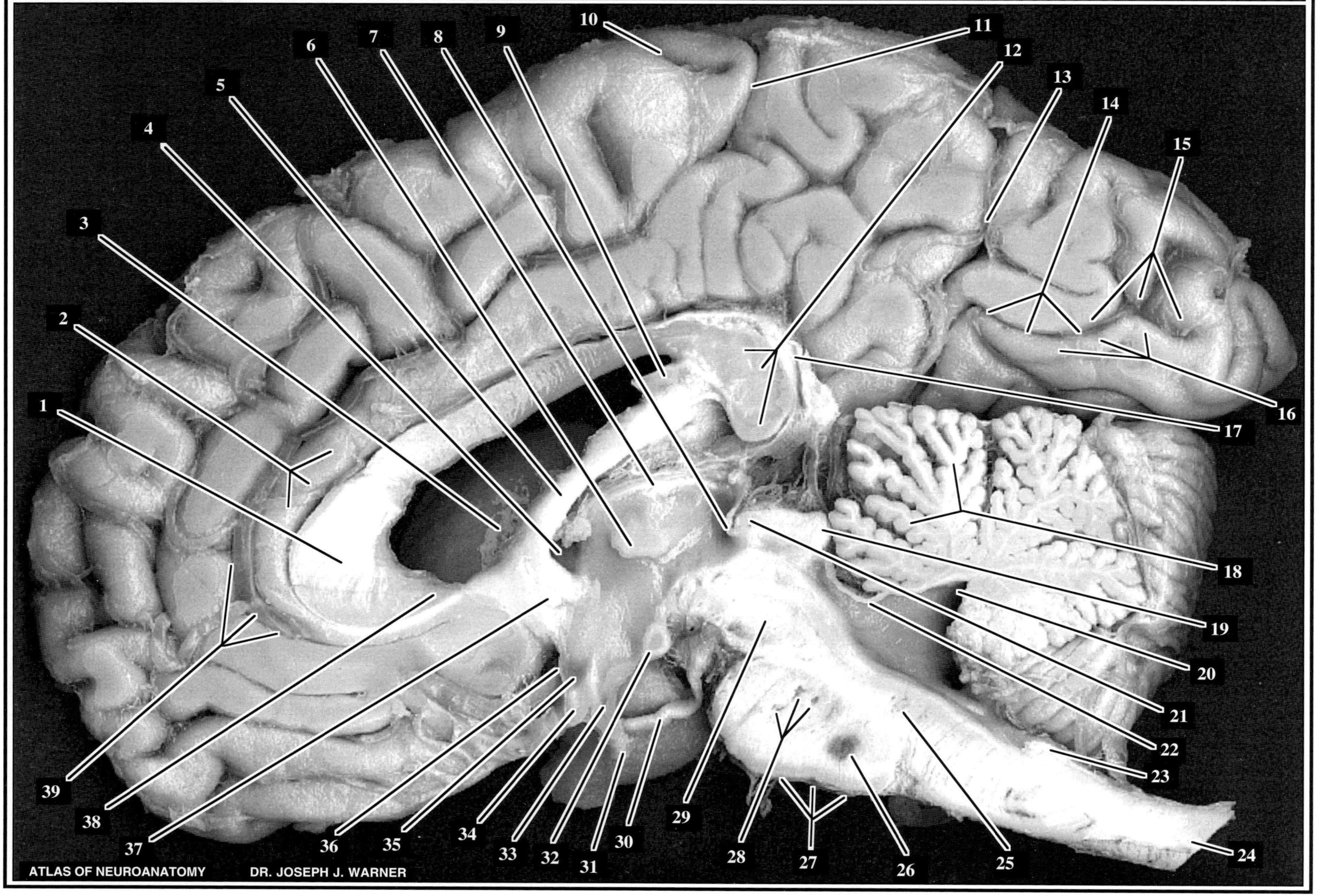

THALAMIC INFARCTION ASSOCIATED WITH HYPERTENSION AND VERTEBROBASILAR ARTERIOSCLEROSIS: SAGITTAL SECTION OF THE BRAIN

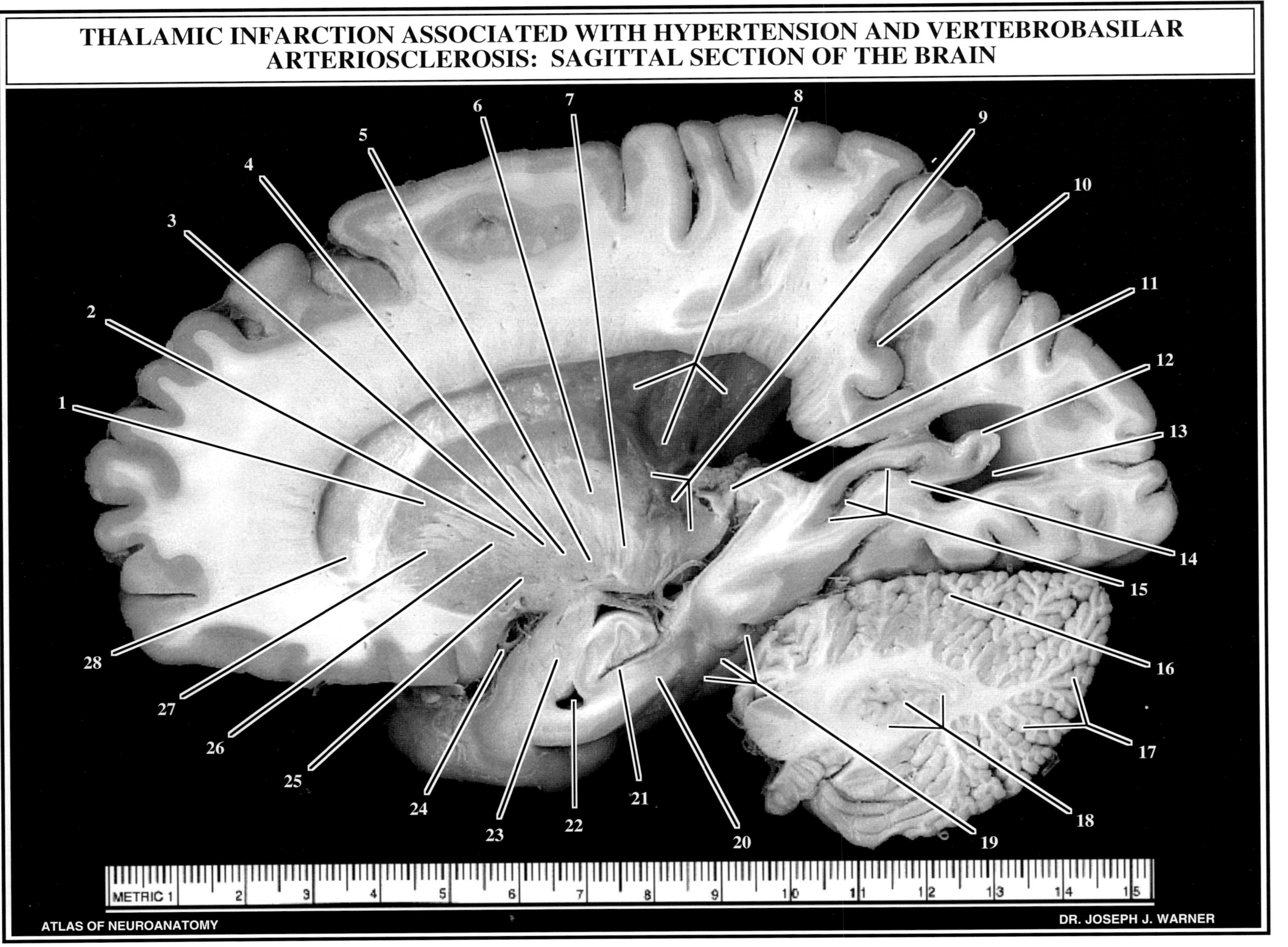

PONTINE AND RIGHT THALAMIC INFARCTIONS ASSOCIATED WITH HYPERTENSION AND VERTEBROBASILAR ARTERIOSCLEROSIS: SECTION MAPS AND KEY TO NUMBERED STRUCTURES

MIDLINE SAGITTAL SECTION (MAP A): KEY TO NUMBERED STRUCTURES

1. Genu of Corpus Callosum
2. Cingulate Gyrus
3. Head of the Caudate
4. Foramen of Monro
5. Fornix
6. Massa Intermedia
7. Stria Medullaris
8. Posterior Commissure
9. Septum Pellucidum
10. Central Sulcus (Rolandic Fissure)
11. Cingulate Sulcus, Pars Marginalis
12. Splenium of Corpus Callosum
13. Parieto-Occipital Sulcus
14. Calcarine Fissure

15, 16. Area 17 Striate Cortex

17. Inferior Sagittal Sinus
18. Superior Cerebellar Vermis (note selective atrophy)
19. Inferior Colliculus
20. Fourth Ventricle
21. Superior Colliculus
22. Anterior Medullary Velum
23. Fasciculus Gracilis
24. Rostral Cervical Spinal Cord
25. Infarction, Caudal Pontine Tegmentum
26. Hemorrhagic Infarction, Basis Pontis
27. Secondary atrophy, Basis Pontis
28. Multiple zones of necrosis from remote infarction
29. Decussation of the Superior Cerebellar Peduncle
30. Oculomotor (III) Nerve
31. Pituitary Stalk
32. Mammillary Body
33. Infundibular Recess of Third Ventricle
34. Optic Chiasm
35. Supraoptic Recess of the Third Ventricle
36. Lamina Terminalis
37. Anterior Commissure
38. Rostrum of Corpus Callosum
39. Anterior Cerebral Artery

SAGITTAL SECTION (MAP B): KEY TO NUMBERED STRUCTURES

1. Caudate Nucleus
2. External Medullary Lamina
3. Globus Pallidus II
4. Internal Medullary Lamina
5. Globus Pallidus I
6. Rostral Thalamus
7. Posterior Limb of Internal Capsule
8. Fiber degeneration, Corona Radiata*
9. Infarction of mid-caudal Thalamus
10. Parieto-Occipital Sulcus
11. Fornix
12. Calcar Avis
13. Occipital Horn of Lateral Ventricle
14. Area 17 Striate Cortex
15. Calcarine Fissure
16. Anterior Lobe of Cerebellum
17. Posterior Lobe of Cerebellum
18. Dentate Nucleus
19. Collateral Fissure
20. Parahippocampal Gyrus
21. Hippocampus
22. Temporal Horn of Lateral Ventricle
23. Amygdala
24. Middle Cerebral Artery
25. Anterior Commissure
26. Putamen
27. Anterior Limb of Internal Capsule
28. Anterior Horn of Lateral Ventricle

* secondary to thalamic infarction

MAP OF SAGITTAL SECTIONS REFERENCED TO A HORIZONTAL SECTION THROUGH THE LEVEL OF THE CENTROMEDIAN NUCLEUS OF THE THALAMUS

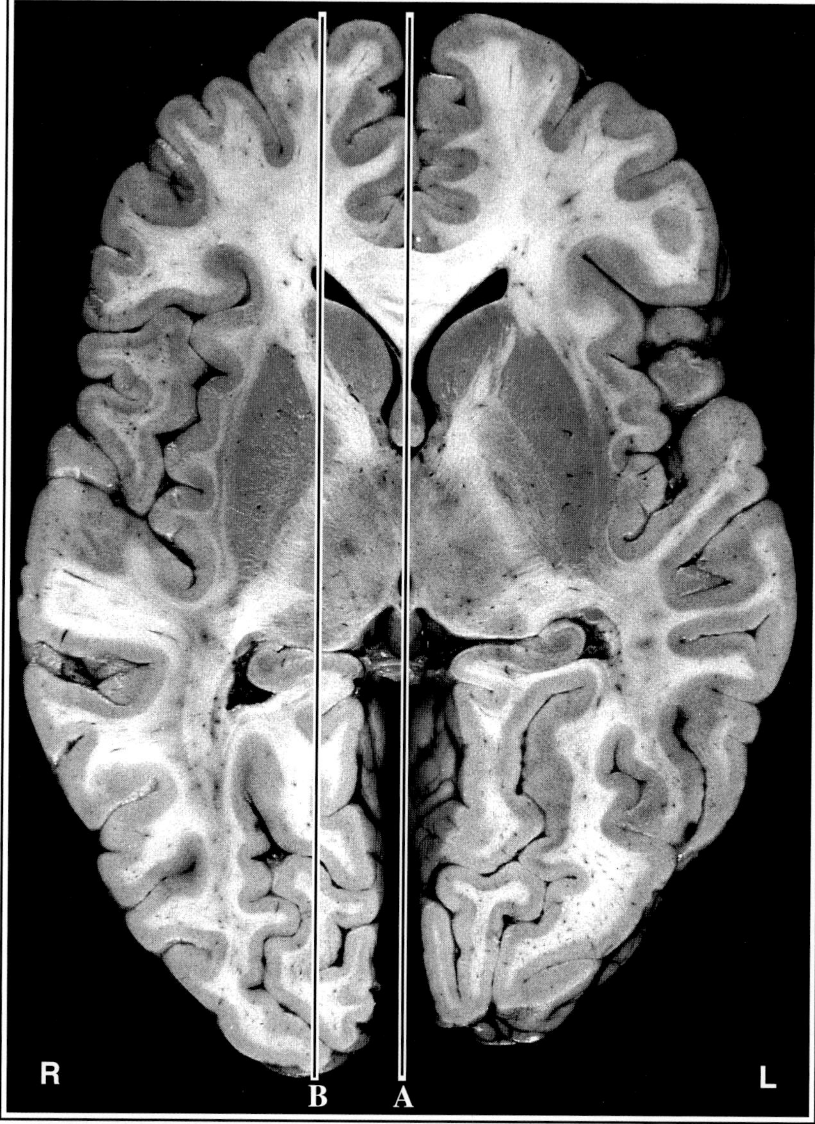

ROSTRAL BASILAR ARTERY OCCLUSION WITH BILATERAL POSTERIOR CEREBRAL ARTERY DISTRIBUTION INFARCTIONS: HORIZONTAL SECTION, LEVEL OF THE GENU OF THE CORPUS CALLOSUM AND GREAT VEIN OF GALEN

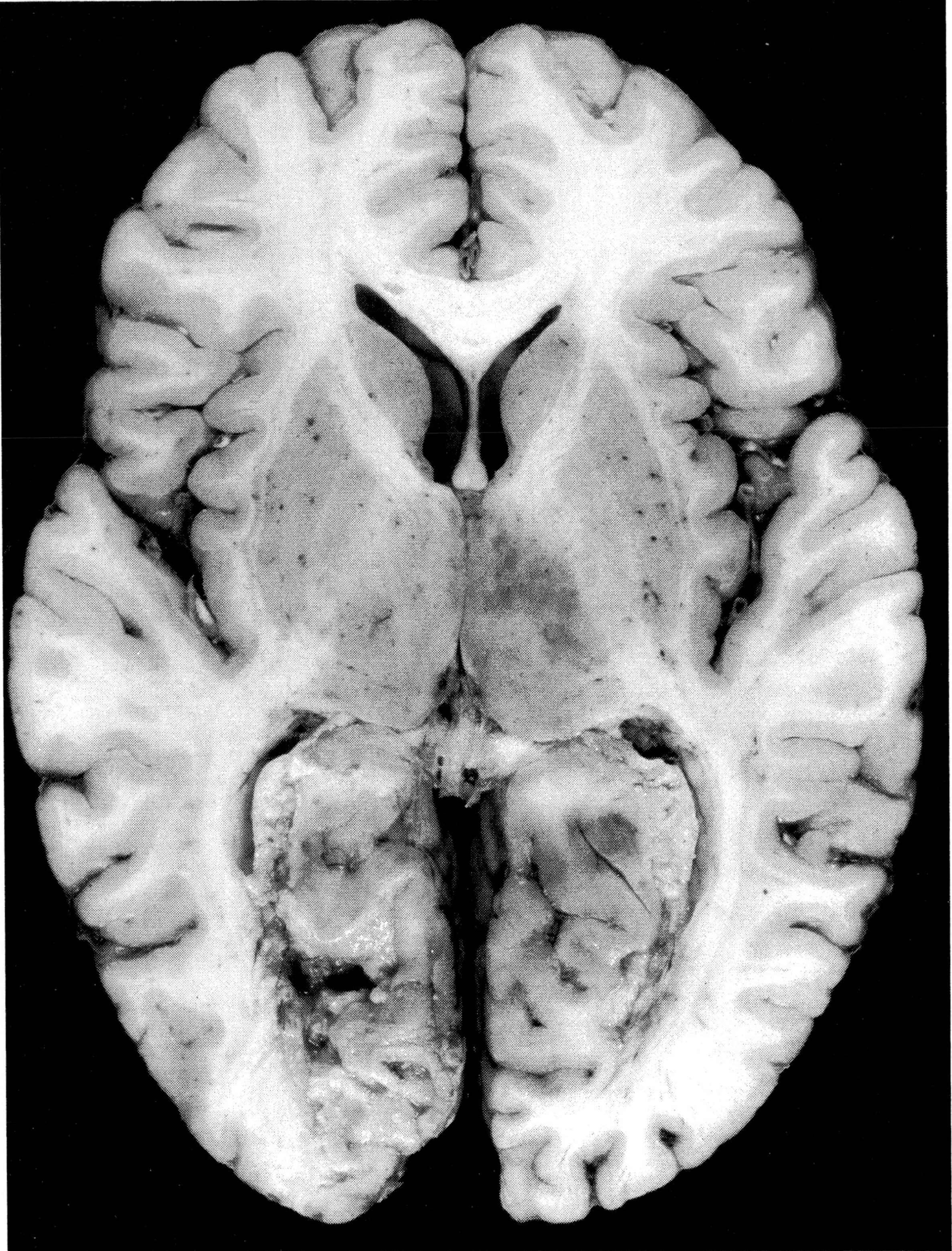

This section demonstrates bilateral necrosis of the medial occipital lobes extending to the splenium of the corpus callosum, and involving the optic radiations. Areas of discoloration (consistent with infarction) involve the left thalamus as well. The vascular supply to the thalamus includes thalamogeniculate (posterolateral), posterior choroidal, and posteromedial thalamoperforating arteries which arise rostral to the basilar bifurcation.

ROSTRAL BASILAR ARTERY OCCLUSION WITH INFARCTION INVOLVING THE ANTEROLATERAL MESENCEPHALON: SERIAL HISTOLOGIC SECTIONS PERPENDICULAR TO THE LONGITUDINAL AXIS OF THE BRAINSTEM, LEVEL OF THE MESENCEPHALIC - DIENCEPHALIC TRANSITION

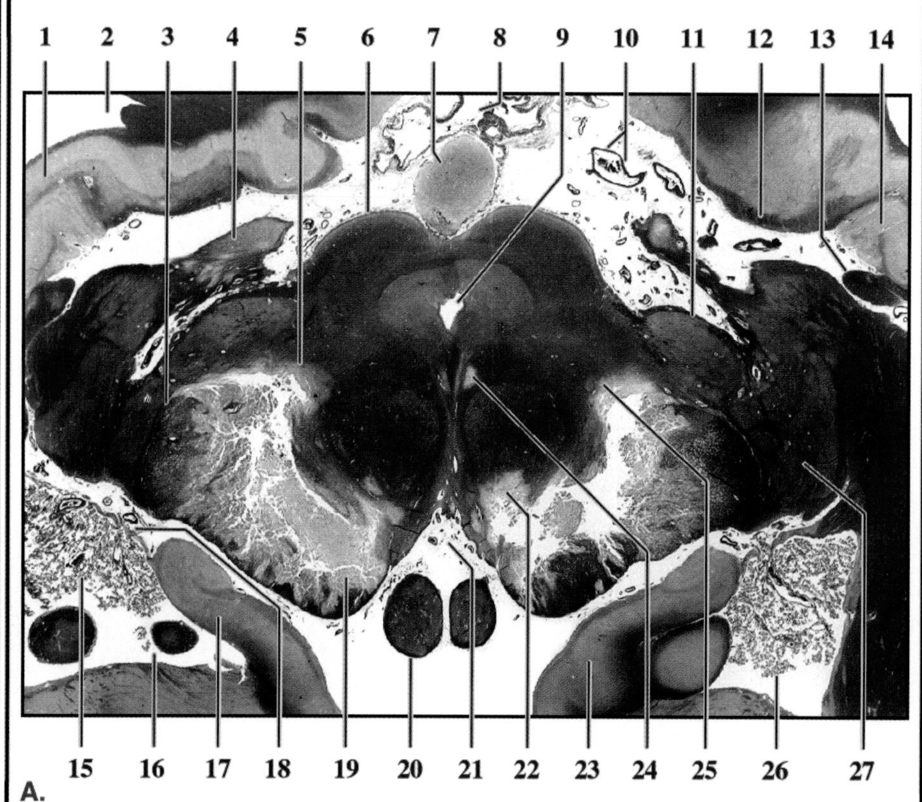

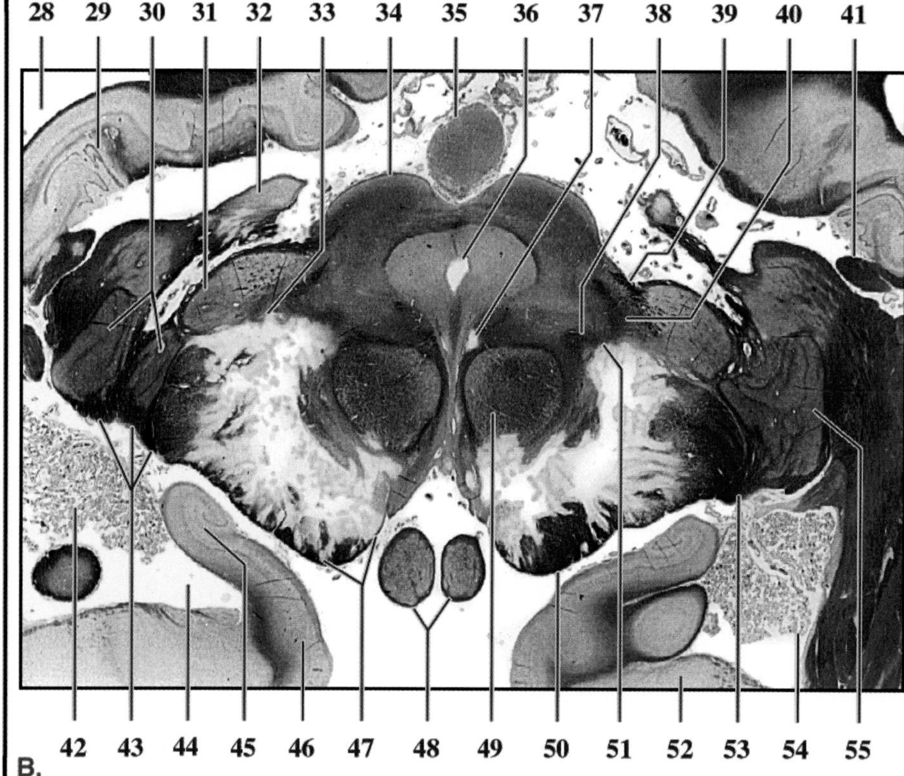

Sections 12 microns: (A) Phosphotungstic Acid Hematoxylin stain; (B) Kluver - Barrera Technique (LFB - Cresyl Violet)

KEY TO NUMBERED STRUCTURES

1. Hippocampus
2. Temporal Horn (Lateral Ventricle)
3. Dorsolateral margin of necrosis
4. Pulvinar Nucleus of the Thalamus
5. Lesion involving Medial Lemniscus
6. Superior Colliculus
7. Pineal Body
8. Great Vein of Galen
9. Aqueduct of Sylvius
10. Posterior Cerebral Artery
11. Medial Geniculate Nucleus
12. Superficial Medullary Stratum of the Subiculum
13. Fimbria of the Fornix
14. Hippocampus
15. Choroid Plexus
16. Temporal Horn (Lateral Ventricle)
17. Hippocampus
18. Tela Choroidea
19. Necrosis of the Cerebral Peduncle
20. Mammillary Body
21. Interpeduncular Fossa
22. Lesion involving Red Nucleus
23. Parahippocampal Gyrus
24. Degeneration involving the Oculomotor (III) Nuclear Complex
25. Lesion involving Medial Lemniscus
26. Choroid Plexus
27. Lateral Geniculate Nucleus
28. Temporal Horn, Lateral Ventricle
29. Dentate Gyrus of the Hippocampus
30. Lateral Geniculate Nucleus
31. Medial Geniculate Nucleus
32. Pulvinar Nucleus of the Thalamus
33. Dorsal margin of necrosis
34. Superior Colliculus
35. Pineal Body
36. Aqueduct of Sylvius
37. Degeneration involving Oculomotor (III) Nuclear Complex
38. Medial Lemniscus
39. Brachium of the Inferior Colliculus
40. Spinothalamic Tract
41. Fimbria of the Fornix
42. Choroid Plexus
43. Optic Tract
44. Temporal Horn (Lateral Ventricle)
45. Hippocampus
46. Parahippocampal Gyrus
47. Necrosis of Cerebral Peduncle
48. Mammillary Bodies
49. Red Nucleus
50. Cerebral Peduncle
51. Lesion involving Medial Lemniscus
52. Amygdala
53. Optic Tract
54. Choroid Plexus
55. Lateral Geniculate Nucleus

LEFT POSTERIOR CEREBRAL ARTERY DISTRIBUTION INFARCTION INVOLVING THE VENTROMEDIAL TEMPORAL LOBE (INCLUDING THE HIPPOCAMPUS) WITH IPSILATERAL DEGENERATION OF THE FORNIX: CORONAL T2-WEIGHTED MAGNETIC RESONANCE IMAGING

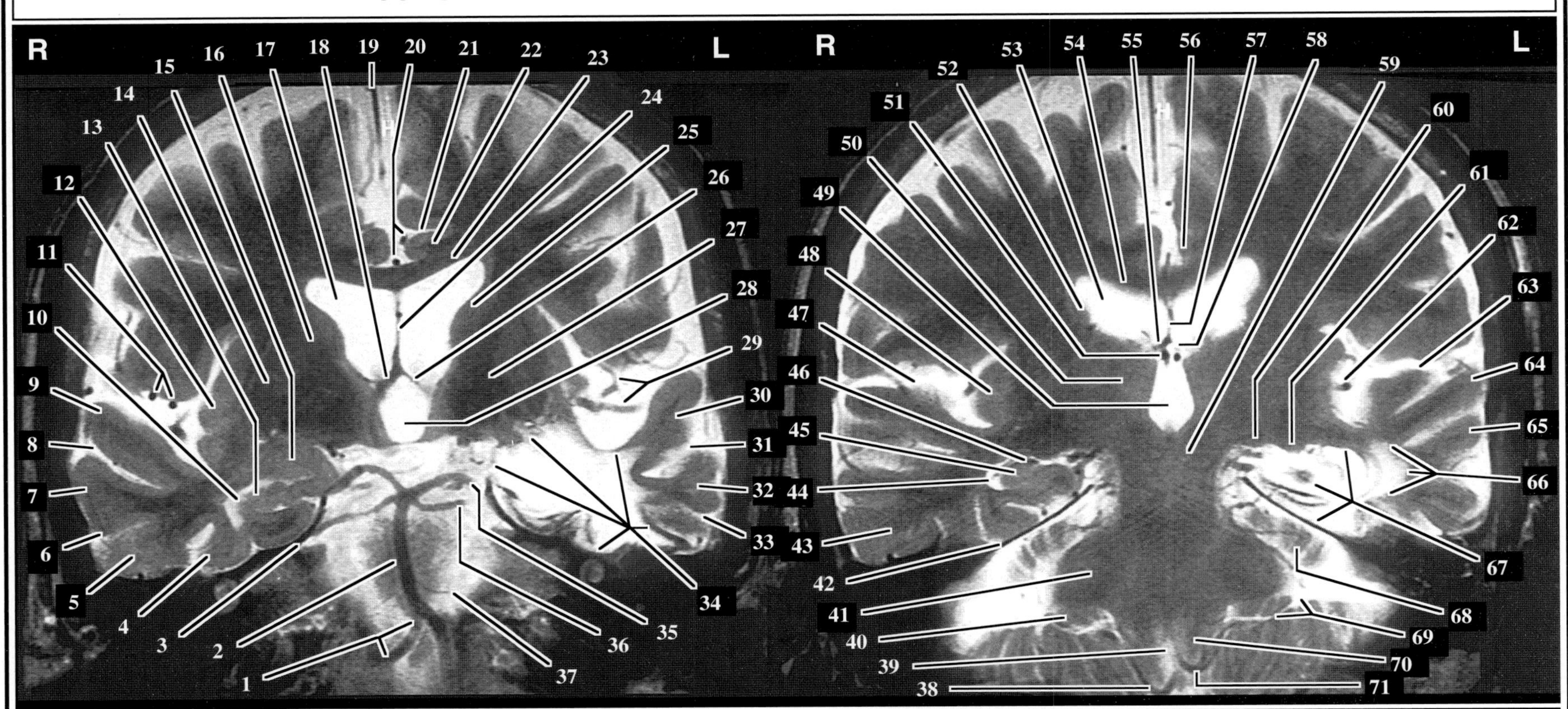

Both posterior cerebral arteries arise from the bifurcation of the basilar artery in 70% of individuals. The posterior communicating artery connects the internal carotid with the ipsilateral posterior cerebral artery. However, there is significant variability in this region of cerebrovascular anatomy. One or both posterior communicating arteries may be hypoplastic or absent. In many cases, one or both posterior communicating arteries may be of large caliber, with significant flow from the internal carotid to the posterior cerebral artery demonstrable during cerebral angiography In approximately 20% of cases, one posterior cerebral artery originates from the ipsilateral internal carotid artery, with the contralateral posterior cerebral artery arising from the basilar bifurcation. In the remainder of cases, both posterior cerebral arteries arise from the corresponding ipsilateral internal carotid artery. The posterior cerebral artery is divided into proximal and distal segments, with distinct territories of vascular distribution. Proximal segments include (A) the interpeduncular segment, (B) the crural or peduncular segment, (C) the ambient segment, and (D) the quadrigeminal segment. The distal segment gives rise to four main cortical branches: the anterior temporal, posterior temporal, parieto-occipital, and calcarine arteries. In this case, the infarction has spared the vascular distributions of the paramedian and thalamoperforating arteries (arising from the interpeduncular segment of the posterior cerebral artery and the termination of the basilar artery), and of the quadrigeminal arteries. The region of infarction corresponds to the distributions of the lateral posterior choroidal artery (arising from the crural or ambient segments) and distal cortical branches of the posterior cerebral artery. Note the degeneration of the fornix on the left, corresponding to ablation of the ipsilateral hippocampal formation.

LEFT POSTERIOR CEREBRAL ARTERY DISTRIBUTION INFARCTION INVOLVING THE VENTROMEDIAL TEMPORAL LOBE WITH IPSILATERAL DEGENERATION OF THE FORNIX, MAGNETIC RESONANCE IMAGING: KEY TO NUMBERED STRUCTURES

1. Vertebral Artery
2. Basilar Artery
3. Tentorium
4. Fusiform Gyrus
5. Inferior Temporal Gyrus
6. Middle Temporal Sulcus
7. Middle Temporal Gyrus
8. Superior Temporal Sulcus
9. Superior Temporal Gyrus
10. Temporal Horn of the Lateral Ventricle
11. Branches of the Middle Cerebral Artery
12. Insular Cortex
13. Hippocampal Formation
14. Putamen
15. Amygdala
16. Anterior Limb of the Internal Capsule
17. Body of the Lateral Ventricle
18. Fornix (adjacent to the Foramen of Monro)
19. Falx Cerebri
20. Anterior Cerebral Arteries
21. Cingulate Sulcus
22. Cingulate Gyrus
23. Corpus Callosum
24. Septum Pellucidum
25. Caudate Nucleus
26. Atrophy of the Fornix ipsilateral to the infarction
27. Globus Pallidus
28. Third Ventricle
29. Branches of the Middle Cerebral Artery
30. Superior Temporal Gyrus
31. Superior Temporal Sulcus
32. Middle Temporal Gyrus
33. Middle Temporal Sulcus
34. Infarction of the ventromedial Temporal Lobe (including the Amygdala and Hippocampus)
35. Posterior Cerebral Artery
36. Superior Cerebellar Artery
37. Anterior Inferior Cerebellar Artery
38. Posterior Inferior Cerebellar Artery
39. Fourth Ventricle
40. Flocculus
41. Middle Cerebellar Peduncle
42. Tentorium
43. Inferior Temporal Gyrus
44. Temporal Horn of the Lateral Ventricle
45. Hippocampus
46. Fimbria of the Fornix
47. Sylvian Fissure
48. Insular Cortex
49. Third Ventricle
50. Thalamus
51. Internal Cerebral Vein
52. Caudate Nucleus
53. Body of the Lateral Ventricle
54. Corpus Callosum
55. Fornix
56. Cingulate Gyrus
57. Septum Pellucidum
58. Atrophy of the Fornix ipsilateral to the infarction
59. Rostral Mesencephalic Tegmentum
60. Medial Geniculate Nucleus
61. Lateral Geniculate Nucleus
62. Middle Cerebral Artery
63. Sylvian Fissure dorsal to the Planum Temporale
64. Superior Temporal Gyrus
65. Middle Temporal Gyrus
66. Lateral margin of infarction in the Temporal Lobe
67. Zone of infarction involving the Ventromedial Temporal Lobe including the Hippocampus)
68. Anterior Lobe of the Cerebellum
69. Posterolateral Fissure of the Cerebellum
70. Superior Cerebellar Peduncle
71. Posterior Inferior Cerebellar Artery

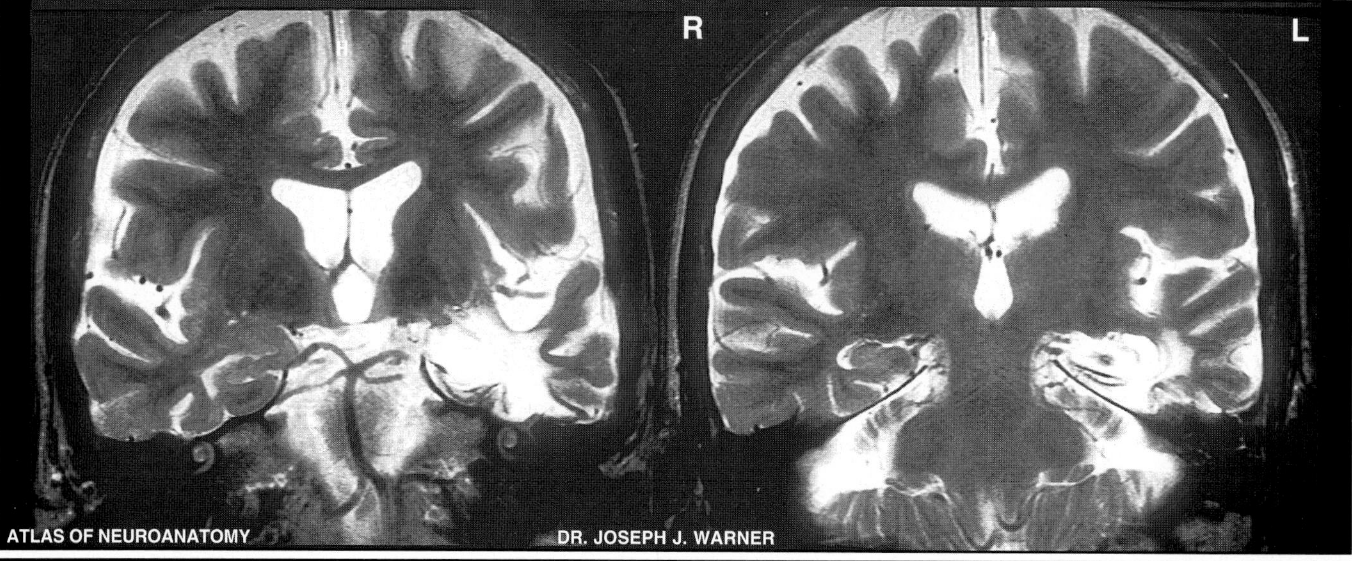

LEFT POSTERIOR CEREBRAL ARTERY DISTRIBUTION INFARCTION INVOLVING THE VENTROMEDIAL TEMPORAL LOBE (INCLUDING THE HIPPOCAMPUS) AND THE RETROSPLENIAL REGION: T2 WEIGHTED MAGNETIC RESONANCE IMAGING, PLANE PARALLEL TO THE SYLVIAN FISSURE

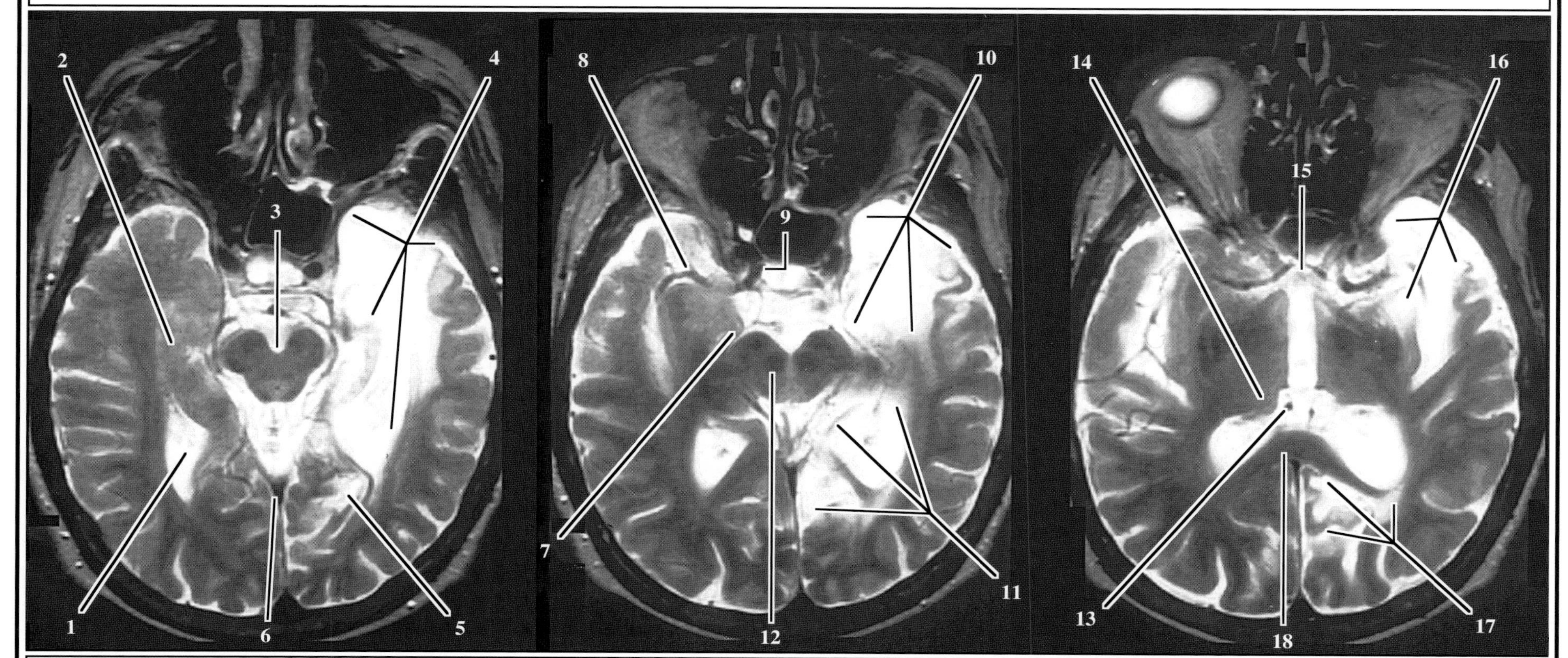

KEY TO NUMBERED STRUCTURES

1. Atrium of the Lateral Ventricle
2. Hippocampal Formation
3. Interpeduncular Fossa
4. Infarction involving the ventromedial aspect of the Temporal Lobe, including the Hippocampal formation
5. Zone of infarction involving the ventral and rostral aspect of the Occipital Lobe
6. Straight Sinus
7. Uncus
8. Middle Cerebral Artery
9. Internal Carotid Artery
10. Infarction involving the rostral and medial aspects of the Temporal Lobe, including the Uncus and remainder of the Parahippocampal Gyrus
11. Zone of infarction involving the rostral and medial aspect of the Occipital Lobe and adjacent Medial Temporal Region
12. Red Nucleus
13. Internal Cerebral Vein
14. Medial Pulvinar Nucleus of the Thalamus
15. Optic Chiasm
16. Infarction of rostral and medial regions of the Temporal Lobe
17. Extension of infarction affecting the medial Occipital Lobe, the Retrosplenial region, and lateral fibers of the Splenium of the Corpus Callosum
18. Splenium of the Corpus Callosum

Major structures of the mesencephalon, thalamus, and epithalamus are located within the central territory of the posterior cerebral artery (supplied by the proximal segment). The zone of infarction, in this case, has left these regions relatively spared.

OCULOMOTOR (III) NERVE PALSY WITH SPARING OF THE PARASYMPATHETIC COMPONENT

This 62-year-old male presented to the clinic with the acute onset of "double vision". The patient denied any accompanying neurologic symptomatology with the exception of paresthesiae in the distal lower extremities, which had been slowly progressive over a four year period. The patient's medical history was significant for insulin-dependent diabetes mellitus diagnosed at least five years earlier. The patient denied a history of hypertension or smoking. He had no prior history of stroke or transient neurologic symptoms.

Neurologic examination revealed marked ptosis of the right eyelid and deviation of the right eye laterally and slightly downward. Vertical misalignment of the ocular axes was exacerbated with upward gaze to the right, in midline, and to the left. Left lateral gaze revealed failure of adduction of the right eye, consistent with the patient's subjective complaint of increased diplopia when looking to the left. Convergence, elicited by fixation on a near target, was characterized by adduction of the left eye, however the right eye did not adduct. Both pupils were equally reactive to light and accommodation. Tangiential lighting of the pupils in a dark room did not reveal any discernible anisocoria. (Ptosis due to oculosympathetic paresis would be accompanied by ipsilateral miosis. The difference in pupillary diameter would be amplified in darkness because the contralateral pupil would dilate in response to increased sympathetic activity.)

The remainder of the cranial nerve examination revealed no deficit. Sensory examination revealed a bilateral gradient distal lower extremity decrease in pinprick, temperature, light touch, and vibratory sensation consistent with a peripheral neuropathy. Motor and cerebellar system examination was normal. Deep tendon reflexes were diminished at both ankles. Magnetic resonance imaging was normal.

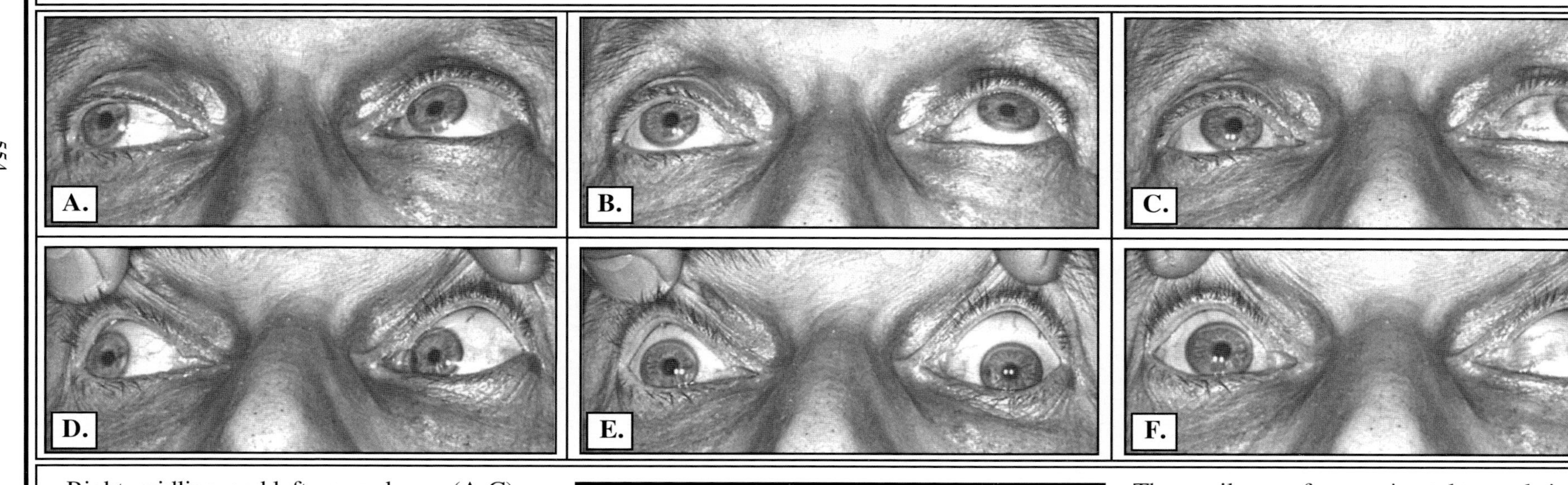

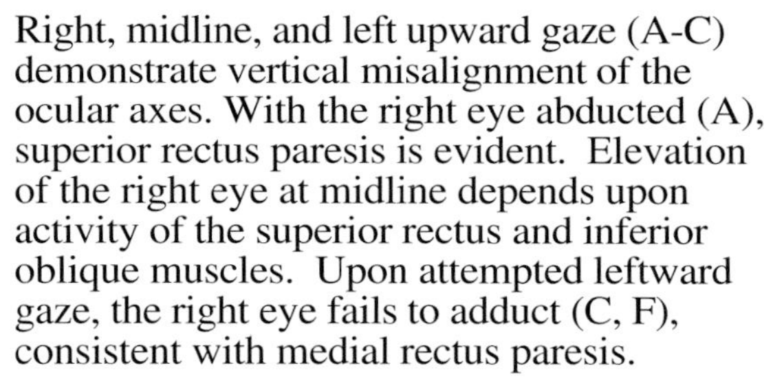

Right, midline, and left upward gaze (A-C) demonstrate vertical misalignment of the ocular axes. With the right eye abducted (A), superior rectus paresis is evident. Elevation of the right eye at midline depends upon activity of the superior rectus and inferior oblique muscles. Upon attempted leftward gaze, the right eye fails to adduct (C, F), consistent with medial rectus paresis.

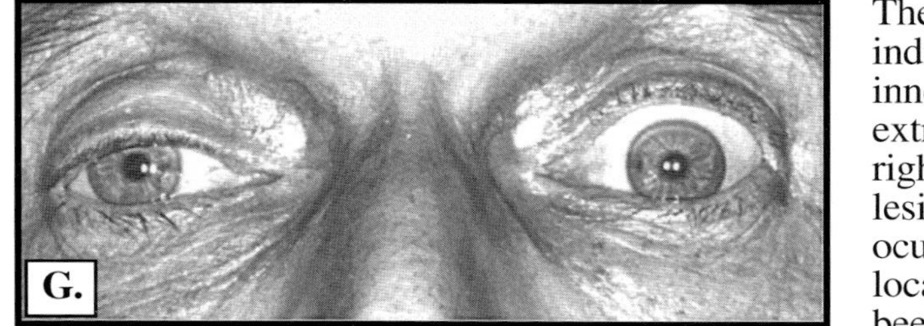

EYES DIRECTED AT EXAMINER

The pupils are of approximately equal size, indicating sparing of the parasympathetic innervation of right eye, despite weakness of extraocular movements (A-F) and ptosis of the right eyelid (G), consistent with an ischemic lesion involving the intrinsic fibers of the right oculomotor nerve. The parasympathetic fibers, located on the surface of the nerve, would have been involved with a compressive lesion.

LEFT ABDUCENS (VI) NERVE PALSY IN A PATIENT WITH DIABETES MELLITUS

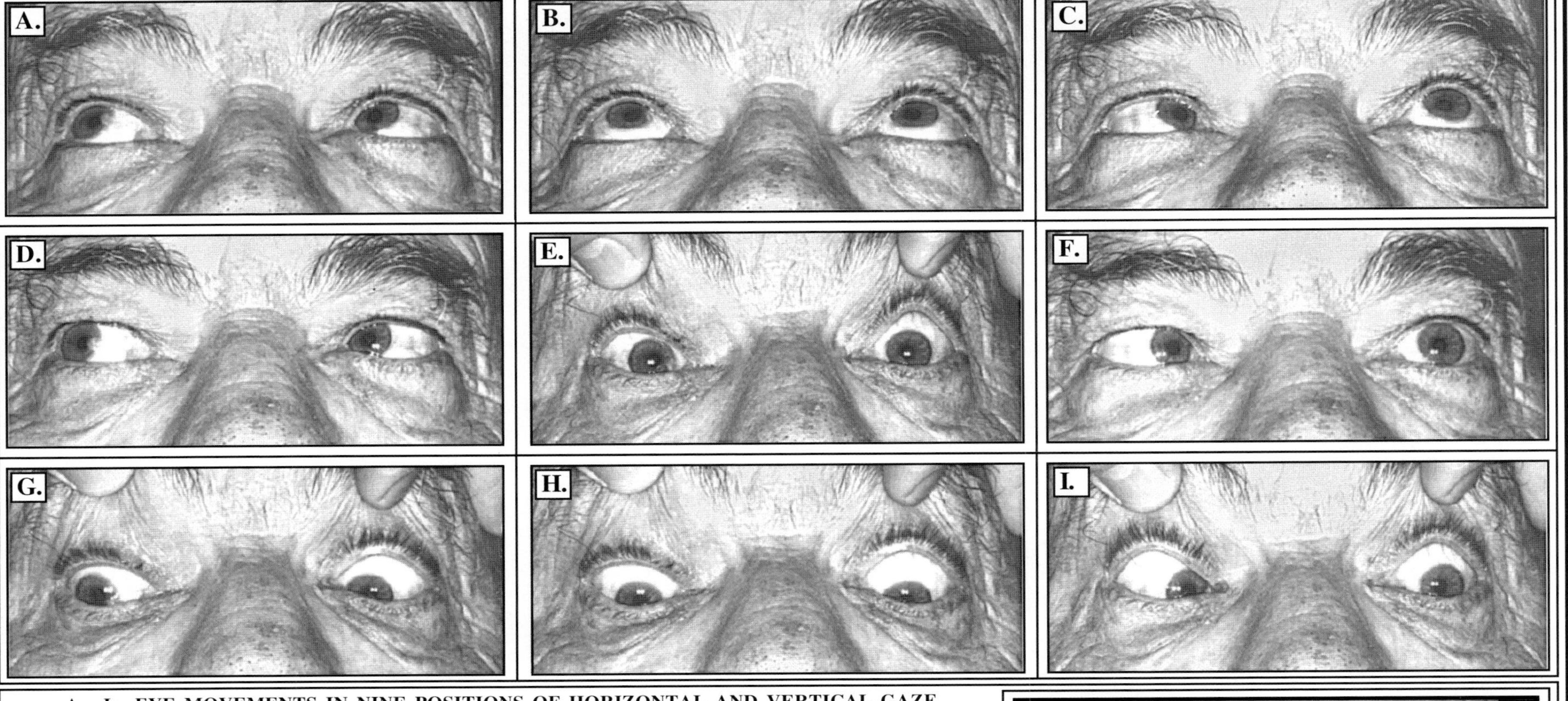

A - I: EYE MOVEMENTS IN NINE POSITIONS OF HORIZONTAL AND VERTICAL GAZE

This 70-year-old male presented with the complaint of an acute onset of double vision accompanied by a sensation of "pressure-like" pain in the left eye. The patient had a history of diabetes mellitus, first diagnosed approximately ten years earlier, which had been treated with oral hypoglycemic agents. One year prior to the current complaint, it was decided to place the patient on insulin due to marginal control. The patient had no prior history of stroke, syncope, seizures, or transient neurologic symptoms. His past medical history included chronic bronchitis and mild hypertension. Cranial nerve examination was consistent with an abducens (VI) nerve palsy on the left. (Refer to photography of eye movements, figures A-J). Leftward gaze (C, F, and I) was characterized by failure of abduction of the left eye and resulted in an exacerbation of the patient's diplopia On rightward gaze (A, D, and G), diplopia was minimal. The remainder of the neurologic examination was normal. Laboratory studies included normal vasculitis screen, CBC, and chemistry profile with a fasting glucose of 140. An intravenous edrophonium (Tensillon) test (performed to exclude the diagnosis of ocular myasthenia gravis) produced no change in the abducens paresis. Magnetic resonance imaging was remarkable only for mild cerebral atrophy, however no focal lesion was discerned.

J. EYES PHOTOGRAPHED WITH THE PATIENT'S GAZE DIRECTED AT A DISTANT VISUAL TARGET

In left lateral rectus paresis, unopposed activity of the left medial rectus muscle results in left eye adduction when the patient looks straight ahead.

MESENCEPHALIC INFARCTION WITH CONTRALATERAL HEMIPLEGIA

Magnetic Resonance Imaging revealed infarction involving the left cerebral peduncle. A transient left oculomotor nerve palsy observed in this case was likely due to ischemia and/or edema involving adjacent third nerve fascicles.

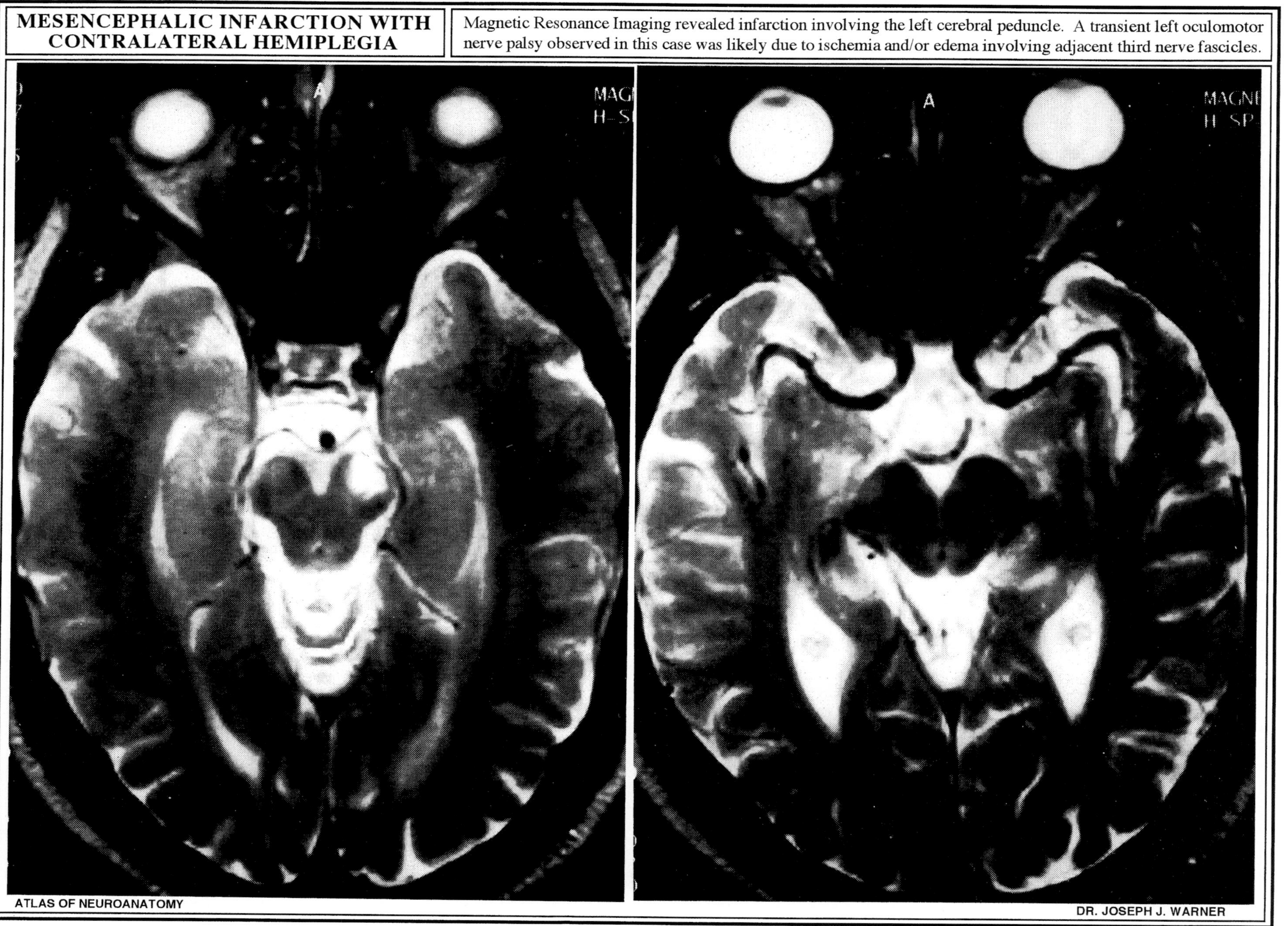

Case Presentation: History

A 58-year-old white male presented with the sudden onset of right facial numbness, nausea, vertigo, and a tendency to fall to the right. He subsequently noticed hoarseness of his voice and moderate difficulty swallowing. The patient had also complained of diminished sensation to temperature over the left side of his body, which he first noticed when he took a hot shower.

He denied loss of vision, diplopia, syncope, or weakness of his face, arms, or legs. He did acknowledge mild incoordination of the right arm and leg.

Neurologic Findings

- Right eye ptosis and meiosis (Horner's Syndrome)
- Rotatory nystagmus increased on leftward gaze
- Diminished pain and temperature sensation over the right side of the face, with sparing of light touch sensation
- Decreased sensation and response to gag reflex testing on the right
- Failure of right-sided palatal elevation with phonation
- Dysphonia (hoarseness) and dysphagia
- Mild right upper and lower extremity ataxia
- Tendency to veer to the right on gait testing
- Loss of pain and temperature sensation over the left side of the body

Diagnostic Investigation

Laboratory studies, chest x-ray, and electrocardiogram were normal.

Magnetic Resonance Imaging: Studies revealed increased T2 signal intensity involving the right lateral medulla. There was no evidence of flow through the right vertebral artery above the foramen magnum; and the posterior inferior artery flow void was not visualized on the right. No other intracranial abnormality was discerned. (Refer to figure.)

Clinical Course

Over the subsequent three months, the patient demonstrated gradual improvement in neurologic function, including resolution of the vertigo, ataxia, dysphonia, and dysphagia.

Between three and six months after the lateral medullary infarction, the patient experienced progressive right facial burning, with a sensation that he had "sniffed pepper into the right side of [his] nose." The diminished pain and temperature sensation persisted over the right side of his face and the left side of his body, although moderate recovery had occurred. The burning dysesthesiae were alleviated with oral carbamazepine therapy.

The patient was maintained on anticoagulation therapy, with no new or recurrent neurologic symptomatology. However, over the subsequent three years, he developed progressive symptoms related to obstructive pulmonary disease and cardiac ischemia secondary to coronary artery disease.

Analysis of Systems or Structures Involved, Based on Neurologic Findings

Case analysis begins with consideration of the history and symptomatology presented by the patient. The level of the neuraxis involved is established by signs and symptoms indicative of specific cranial nerve deficits. An initial review of neurologic findings indicates a level including the eighth, ninth, and tenth cranial nerves in the medulla. In addition to localization based on specific neurologic deficits, the rapid onset of symptoms suggests a vascular etiology. Thus, a lesion involving a particular vascular distribution becomes a major underlying factor in the analysis of this case. The selection of appropriate neurodiagnostic testing must be based upon a hypothesis with respect to the most likely lesion localization and pathogenesis. This process involves an integration of basic neuroanatomy, physiology, and systems organization with functional correlations. *(Refer to corresponding systems and neuroanatomic diagrams).*

1. Right oculosympathetic paresis: *ipsilateral (right) descending sympathetic fibers in the lateral medulla*
2. Nystagmus: *indicative of a lesion of the right vestibular nucleus or brainstem vestibular connections*
3. Right facial deficit of pain and temperature sensation: *right spinal tract and nucleus of the trigeminal system*
4. Deficits of pharyngeal and palatal sensation on the right: *nucleus and tractus solitarius, ninth (glossopharyngeal) and tenth (vagus) nerves, right medulla*
5. Right palatal paralysis, dysphonia, dysphagia: *nucleus ambiguus, ninth, tenth, and bulbar division of the eleventh (spinal accessory) nerves, right medulla*
6. Right upper and lower extremity ataxia, falling toward the right: *inferior cerebellar peduncle, cuneocerebellar and/or dorsal spinocerebellar tract, right lateral medulla*
7. Left hemibody (excluding face) deficit of pain and temperature sensation: *spinothalamic tract, right lateral medulla*

Localization to the right lateral medulla was confirmed by the magnetic resonance imaging studies. This lesion localization also correlates with the vascular distribution of the posterior inferior cerebellar artery. This cerebrovascular pathogenesis was further corroborated by the MRI, which demonstrated no evidence of flow through the vertebral artery nor the posterior inferior cerebellar artery on the side of the lesion. (Refer to MRI figure).

Lateral medullary infarction is also known by the eponym of Wallenburg's Syndrome. This lesion, classically associated with occlusive disease of the posterior inferior cerebellar artery (PICA), may also be observed with ipsilateral vertebral artery occlusion. Vertebral artery thrombosis or embolism may directly involve the orifice of the PICA. However, even if the PICA is not directly occluded, blood flow through this vessel may be compromised due to inadequate collateral flow following vertebral artery thromboembolism. (Refer to diagram of cerebrovasculature.) The pattern of collateral flow in the vertebrobasilar distribution is a major determinant of the degree of ischemic damage to the cerebellum in such cases. In this case, the infarction involved the majority of the lateral medulla, however cerebellar involvement was minimal (refer to MRI and pathology).

LATERAL MEDULLARY INFARCTION: T2 WEIGHTED MAGNETIC RESONANCE IMAGING (IMAGES INVERTED FOR COMPARISON TO CORRESPONDING ANATOMIC SECTIONS)

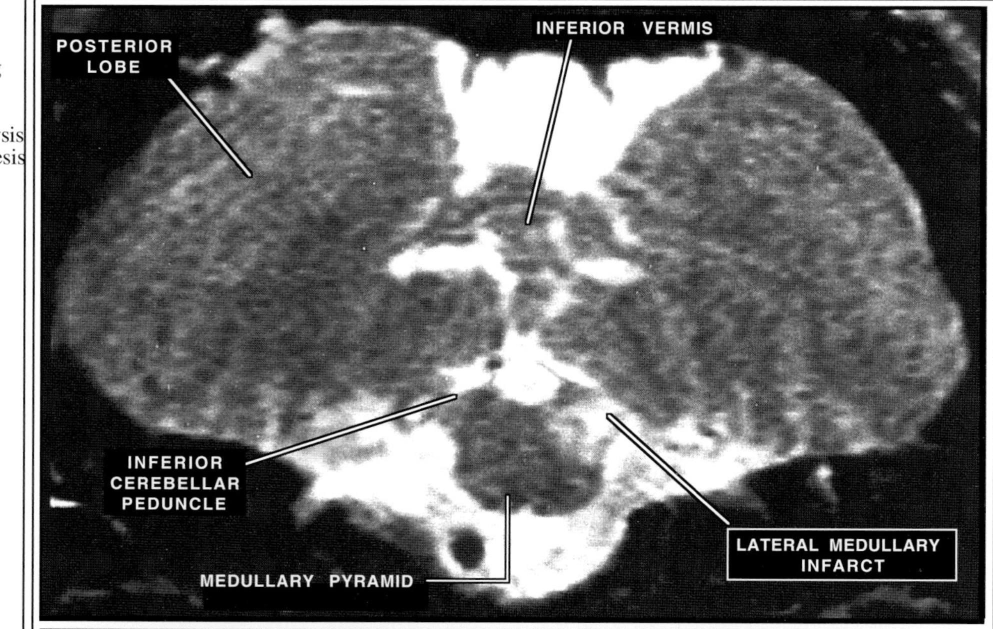

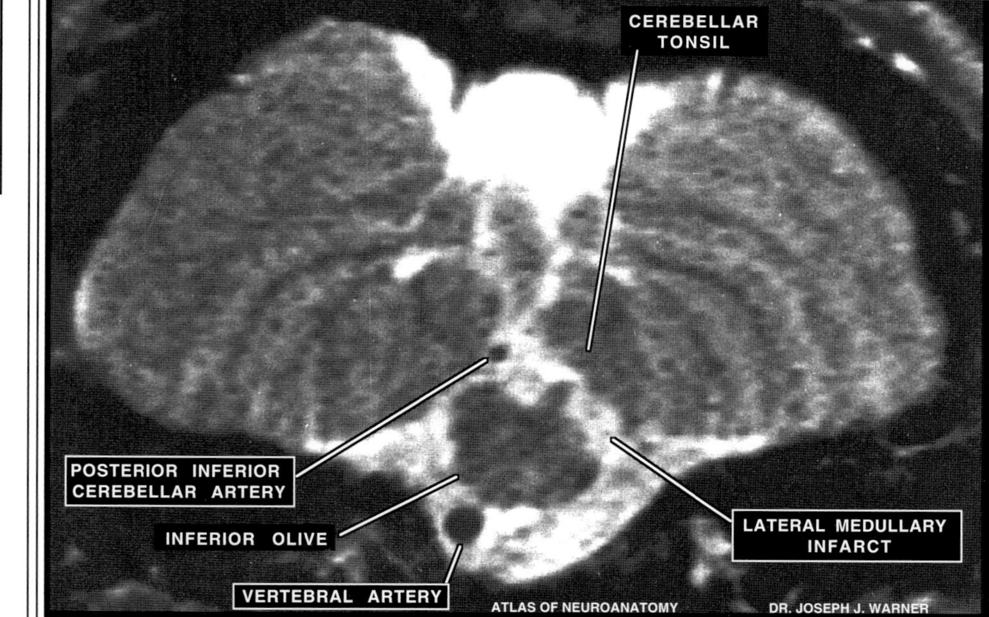

LATERAL MEDULLARY INFARCTION: VERTEBRAL ARTERY OCCLUSION AFFECTING THE VASCULAR DISTRIBUTION OF THE POSTERIOR INFERIOR CEREBELLAR ARTERY

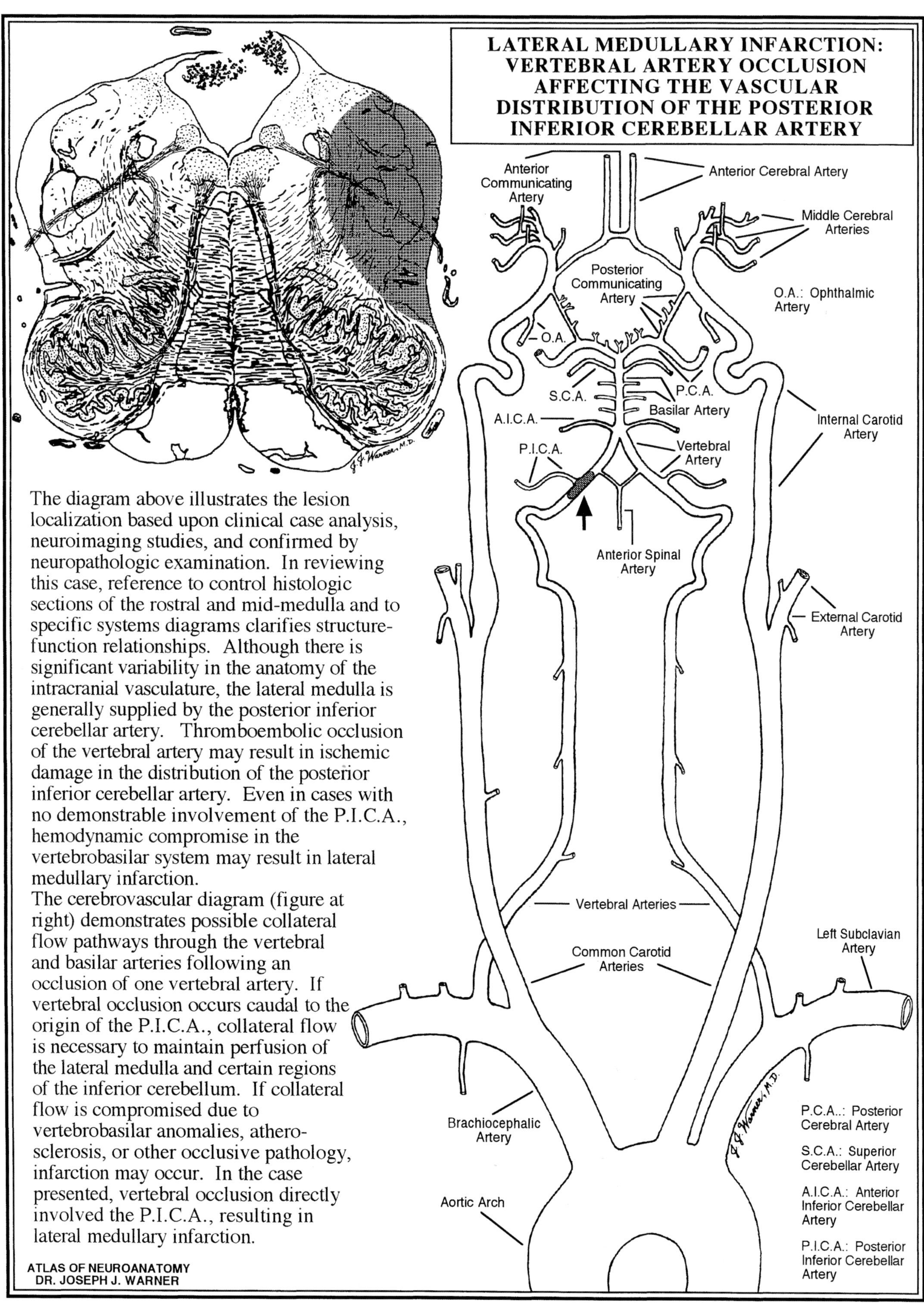

The diagram above illustrates the lesion localization based upon clinical case analysis, neuroimaging studies, and confirmed by neuropathologic examination. In reviewing this case, reference to control histologic sections of the rostral and mid-medulla and to specific systems diagrams clarifies structure-function relationships. Although there is significant variability in the anatomy of the intracranial vasculature, the lateral medulla is generally supplied by the posterior inferior cerebellar artery. Thromboembolic occlusion of the vertebral artery may result in ischemic damage in the distribution of the posterior inferior cerebellar artery. Even in cases with no demonstrable involvement of the P.I.C.A., hemodynamic compromise in the vertebrobasilar system may result in lateral medullary infarction.

The cerebrovascular diagram (figure at right) demonstrates possible collateral flow pathways through the vertebral and basilar arteries following an occlusion of one vertebral artery. If vertebral occlusion occurs caudal to the origin of the P.I.C.A., collateral flow is necessary to maintain perfusion of the lateral medulla and certain regions of the inferior cerebellum. If collateral flow is compromised due to vertebrobasilar anomalies, athero-sclerosis, or other occlusive pathology, infarction may occur. In the case presented, vertebral occlusion directly involved the P.I.C.A., resulting in lateral medullary infarction.

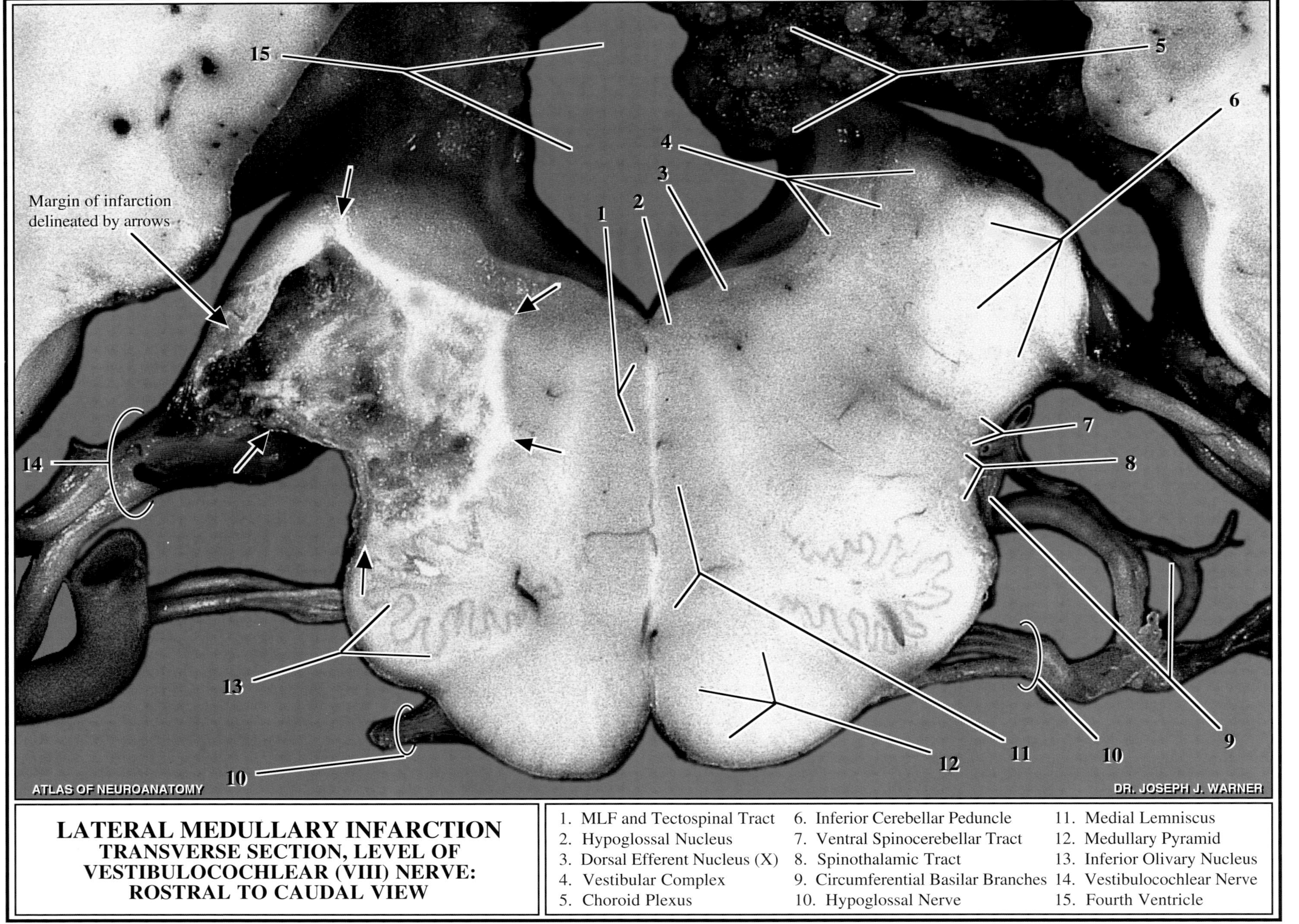

LATERAL MEDULLARY INFARCTION
TRANSVERSE SECTION, LEVEL OF VESTIBULOCOCHLEAR (VIII) NERVE: ROSTRAL TO CAUDAL VIEW

1. MLF and Tectospinal Tract
2. Hypoglossal Nucleus
3. Dorsal Efferent Nucleus (X)
4. Vestibular Complex
5. Choroid Plexus
6. Inferior Cerebellar Peduncle
7. Ventral Spinocerebellar Tract
8. Spinothalamic Tract
9. Circumferential Basilar Branches
10. Hypoglossal Nerve
11. Medial Lemniscus
12. Medullary Pyramid
13. Inferior Olivary Nucleus
14. Vestibulocochlear Nerve
15. Fourth Ventricle

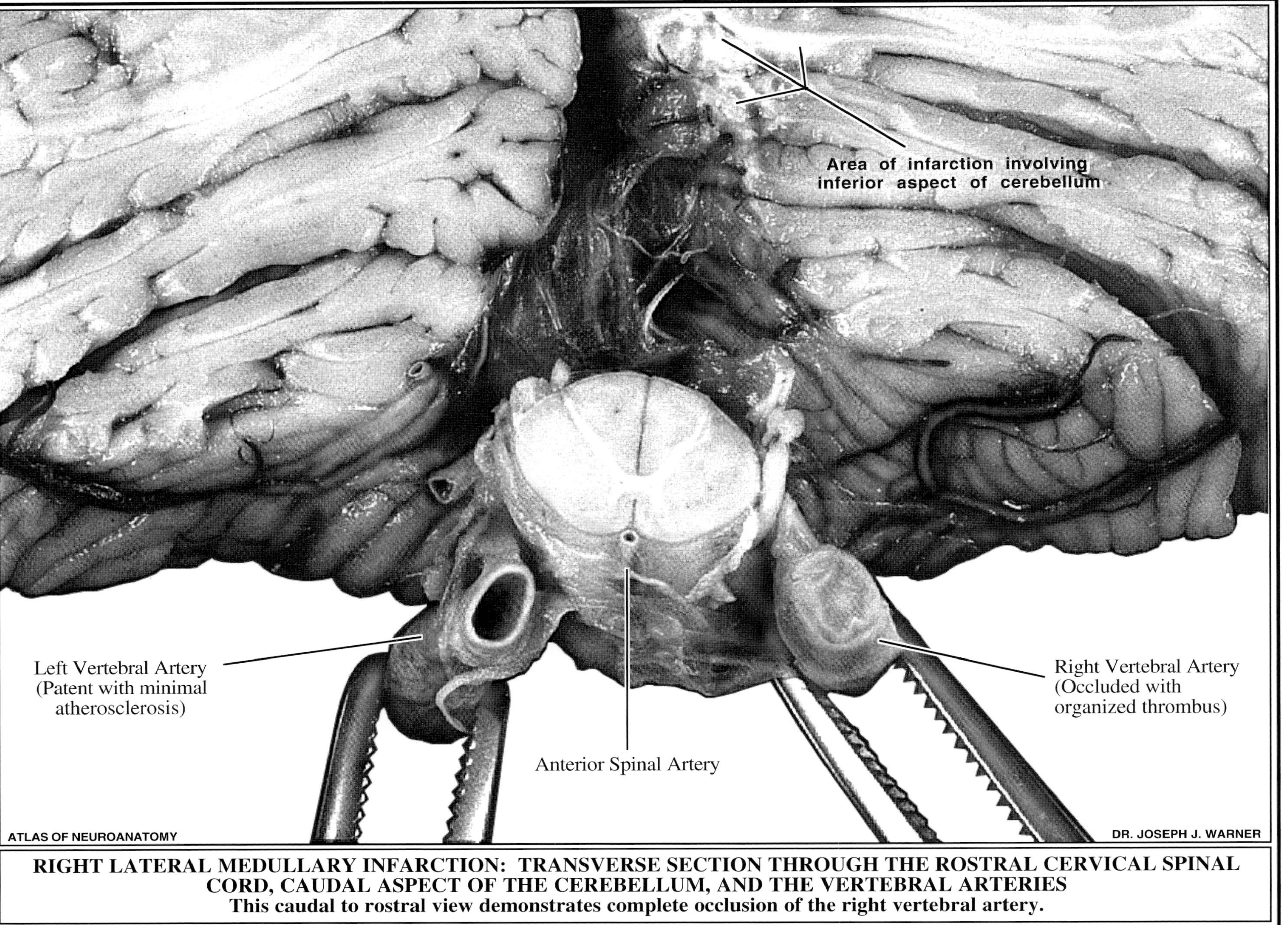

RIGHT LATERAL MEDULLARY INFARCTION: TRANSVERSE SECTION THROUGH THE ROSTRAL CERVICAL SPINAL CORD, CAUDAL ASPECT OF THE CEREBELLUM, AND THE VERTEBRAL ARTERIES
This caudal to rostral view demonstrates complete occlusion of the right vertebral artery.

DEGENERATIVE DISEASE OF THE CERVICAL SPINE WITH EXTRINSIC COMPRESSION OF THE SPINAL CORD: SAGITTAL SECTION

Mechanical stresses on the spine, (including trauma and axial forces exerted in the maintenance of posture) may produce degenerative joint disease, including facet sclerosis, osteophyte formation, and hypertrophy of the posterior longitudinal ligament and/or of the ligamentum flavum. Sudden mechanical forces applied to the intervertebral discs may result in herniation of the nucleus pulposis either centrally to affect the spinal canal or eccentrically to compromise the spinal roots as they course through the intervertebral foramena. Vertical herniation may occur into the vertebral bodies. Long-term degenerative disc disease may include disc dessication, loss of disc height, displacement of disc material, and reactive osteophyte formation of the adjacent vertebral bodies. Ligamentous hypertrophy frequently accompanies these changes. The pathophysiologic changes of cervical spondylosis may result in *radicular* compression, with segmental sensory symptoms, lower motor neuron deficits, and focal loss of deep tendon reflexes. If the *spinal cord* is compromised (either by direct compression or by vascular effects of extrinsic lesions), upper motor neuron findings may be detected below the level(s) of compression on neurologic examination. Due to the somatotopic lamination of long tracts in the spinal cord, early incontinence may occur, with involvement of sacral levels by extrinsic compressive lesions. Asymmetric compressive myelopathy may result in findings that suggest *Brown-Sequard Syndrome*, with *ipsilateral* loss of epicritic touch, proprioception, and vibratory sensation [dorsal columns]; *ipsilateral* upper motor neuron type weakness and hyperreflexia [corticospinal tract]; and *contralateral* loss of pain and temperature sensation below a level one to three segments caudal to the level of compression [spinothalamic tract].

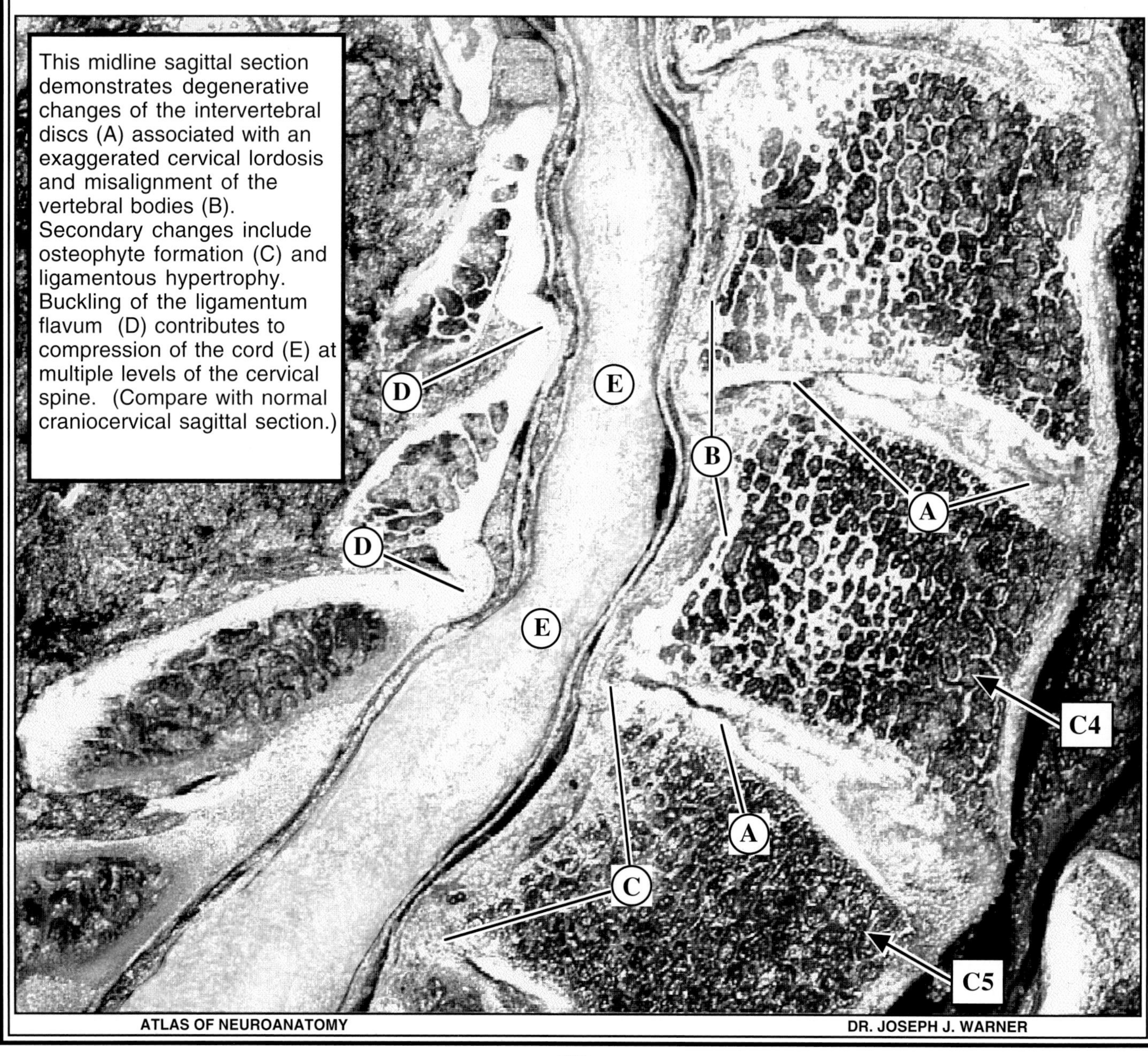

This midline sagittal section demonstrates degenerative changes of the intervertebral discs (A) associated with an exaggerated cervical lordosis and misalignment of the vertebral bodies (B). Secondary changes include osteophyte formation (C) and ligamentous hypertrophy. Buckling of the ligamentum flavum (D) contributes to compression of the cord (E) at multiple levels of the cervical spine. (Compare with normal craniocervical sagittal section.)

THORACOLUMBAR SPINAL CORD HEMORRHAGIC INFARCTION IN THE ANTERIOR SPINAL ARTERY DISTRIBUTION ASSOCIATED WITH DESCENDING AORTIC THROMBOEMBOLISM

This patient underwent surgery for an aneurysm of the descending aorta. Upon awakening from anesthesia, the patient complained of paralysis and altered sensation of the lower extremities. Neurologic examination revealed flaccid paralysis associated with impaired sensation to pain and temperature involving both lower extremities. Vibratory sensation and light touch were relatively spared.

The patient developed further complications from the surgery and sustained a cardiopulmonary arrest a few days post-operatively. Gross sections of the lumbosacral spinal cord at 8 mm intervals are shown (see figure at right). Bilateral softening of the anterolateral cord associated with grossly visible discoloration and hemorrhage in the gray matter was discernible.

LUMBAR SPINAL CORD: SERIAL ROSTRAL TO CAUDAL GROSS SECTIONS, 8 mm INTERVALS

1. Dorsal Root
2. Ventral Root
3. Anterior Spinal Artery
4. Arachnoid Membrane, thickened by acute inflammatory infiltrate
5. Ventral Median Fissure
6. Fasciculus Gracilis
7. Necrosis of Anterior Horn
8. Corticospinal Tract
9. Anterolateral Tracts
10. Hemorrhage into Anterior Horn
11. Dorsal Median Septum

The anterior spinal artery supplies the ventral and lateral structures of the spinal cord. The paired dorsal spinal arteries supply the dorsal aspect of the cord, including the dorsal columns. Infarction in the distribution of the anterior spinal artery therefore generally affects the ventromedial tracts, the anterolateral (including spinothalamic) tracts, the lateral corticospinal tracts, and a significant portion of the spinal gray, particularly susceptible to ischemia. Sparing of the dorsal columns is characteristic of this type of pathology. This correlates with the clinical findings of this case, in which only the dorsal column sensory modalities were spared.

The subsequent figure shows a 10X view of a transverse 15 micron trichrome myelin stained histological section of the caudal lumbar spinal cord. This section emphasizes the distribution of the anterior spinal artery, with pallor of myelin staining of affected white matter (including the lateral corticospinal, anterolateral, and ventromedial tracts), and necrosis with hemorrhage in the spinal gray. Note the relatively dark (normal) staining of the fasciculus gracilis.

LUMBAR SPINAL CORD, 15 μ, TRICHROME-STAINED SECTION: NUMERICAL KEY

1. Fasciculus Gracilis (note intact myelin staining)
2. Margin demarcating loss of normal myelin staining
3. Dorsal Root fibers
4. Dorsal Horn, including Substantia Gelatinosa
5. Perivascular Hemorrhages
6. Lateral Corticospinal Tract
7. Arachnoid thickened by inflammatory infiltrate
8. Hemorrhagic necrosis
9. Margin of necrosis with surrounding edema
10. Anterolateral Tracts
11. Ventral Horn
12. Ventral Root fibers
13. Ventral Median Fissure
14. Arachnoid inflammation

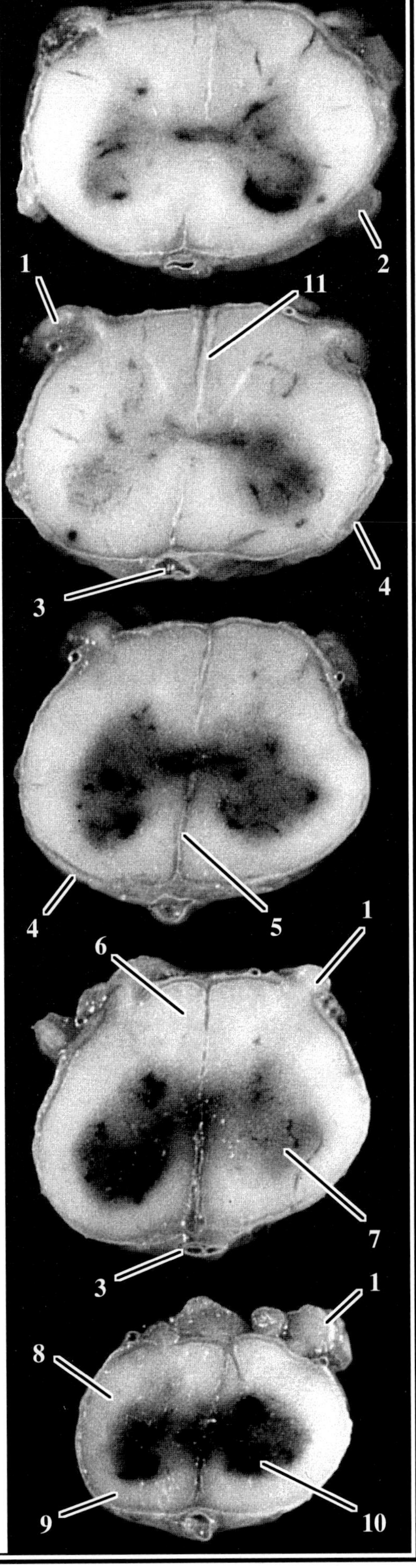

ANTERIOR SPINAL ARTERY DISTRIBUTION HEMORRHAGIC INFARCTION OF THE THORACOLUMBAR SPINAL CORD ASSOCIATED WITH DESCENDING AORTIC ANEURYSM: HISTOPATHOLOGY

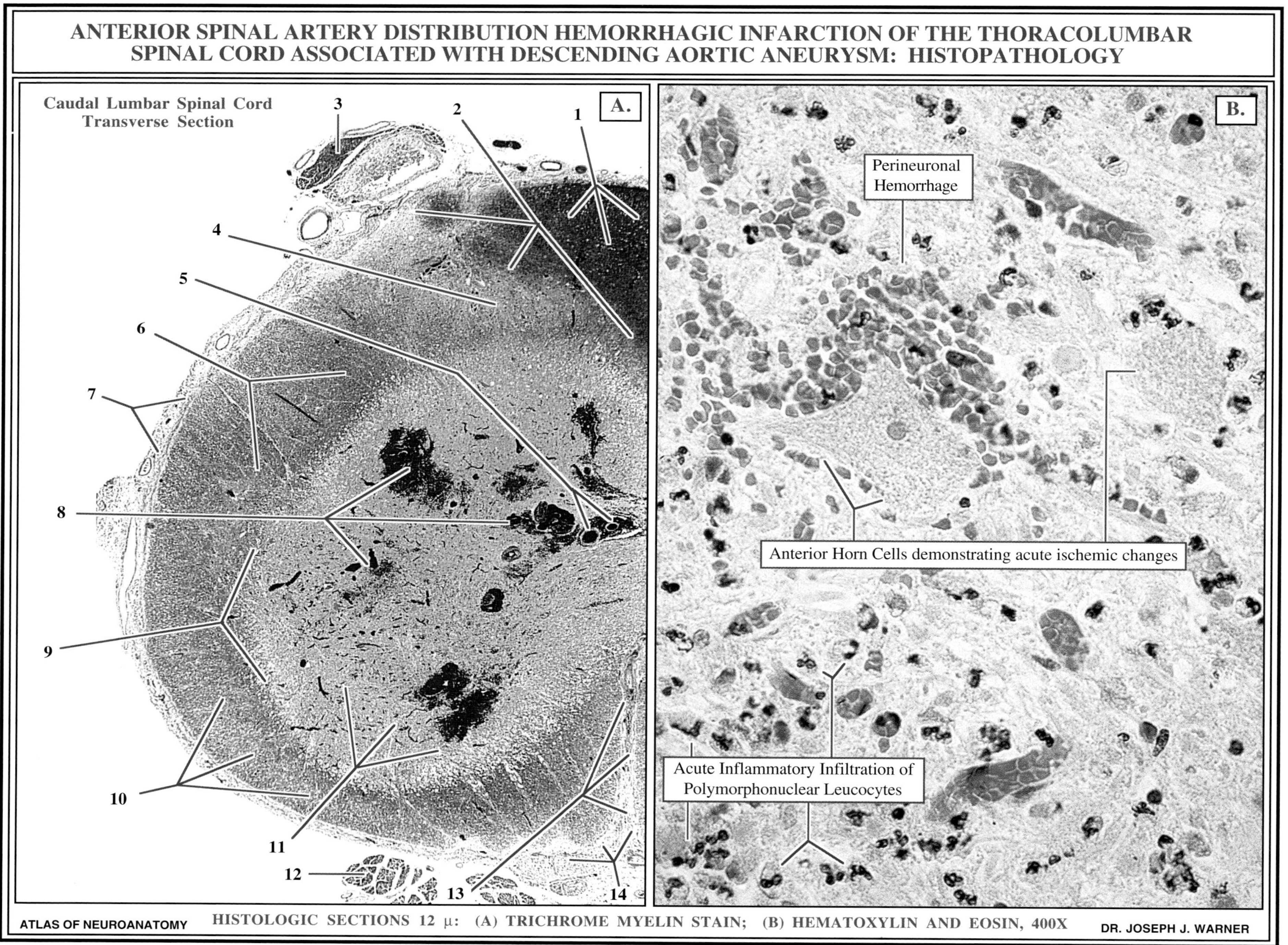

HISTOLOGIC SECTIONS 12 μ: (A) TRICHROME MYELIN STAIN; (B) HEMATOXYLIN AND EOSIN, 400X

DR. JOSEPH J. WARNER

HEAD TRAUMA WITH BASILAR SKULL FRACTURE, ACUTE EPIDURAL AND SUBDURAL HEMORRHAGES, AND CEREBRAL CONTUSIONS: DORSAL CRANIAL DISSECTION

A.

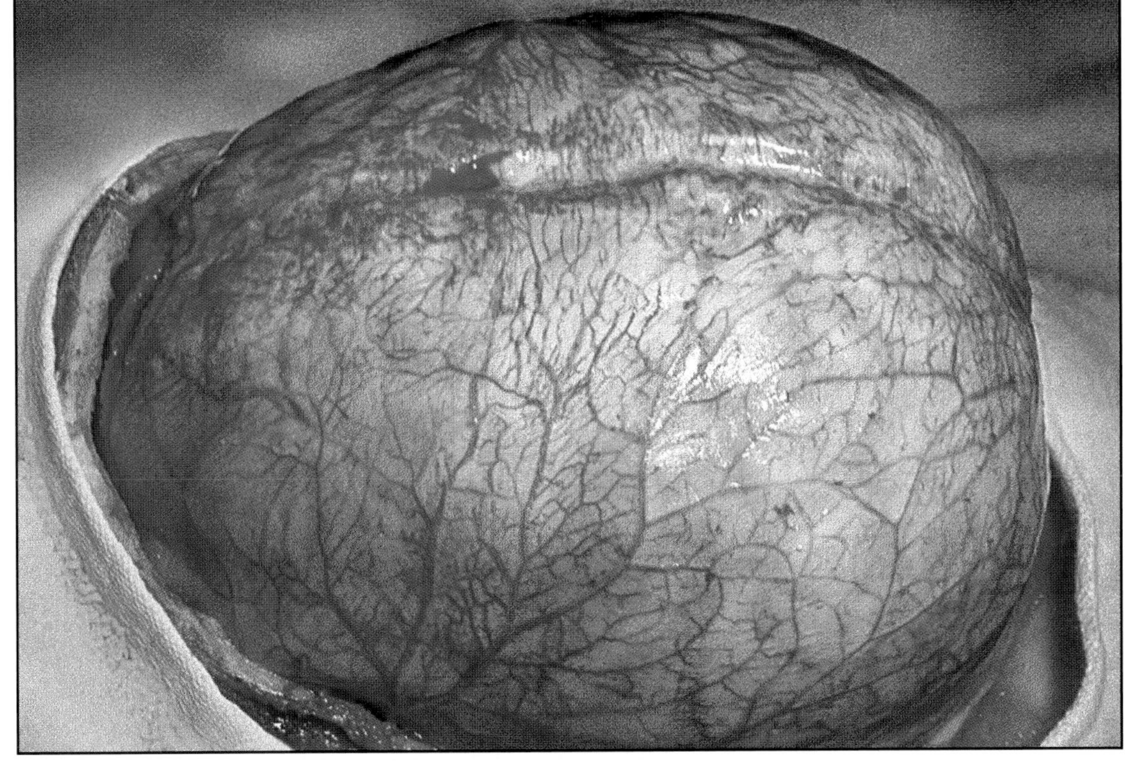

A. Dura intact, demonstrating frontal epidural hemorrhage with anterior branch laceration of the middle meningeal artery; B. Dura reflected, revealing acute diffuse subdural hemorrhage

B.

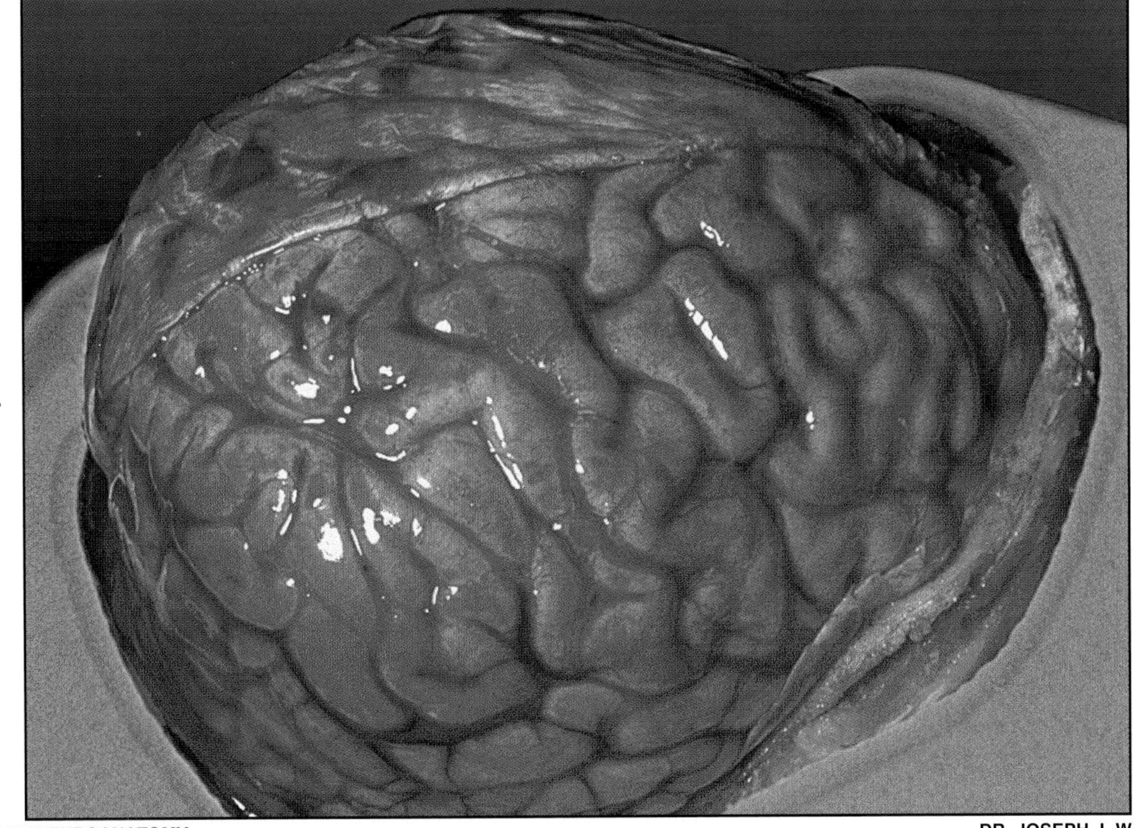

HEAD TRAUMA WITH BASILAR SKULL FRACTURE, ACUTE EPIDURAL AND SUBDURAL HEMORRHAGES, AND CEREBRAL CONTUSIONS

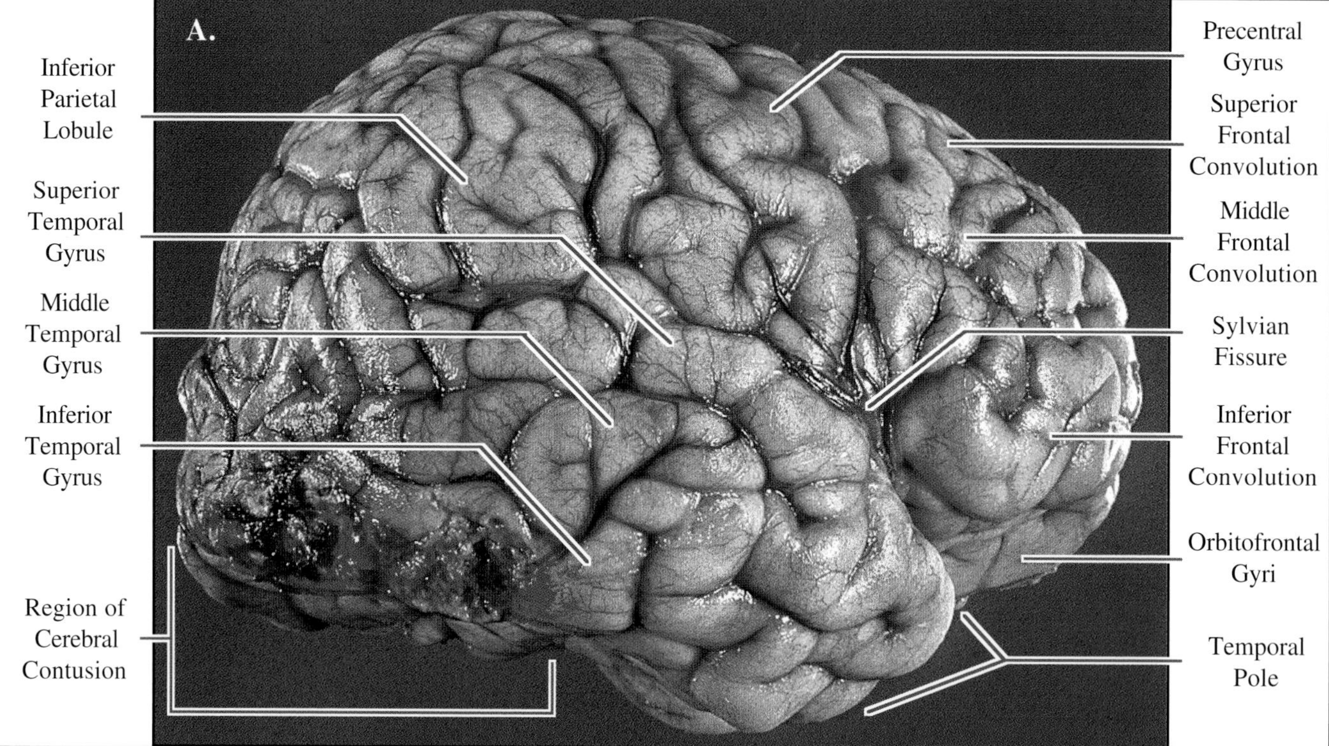

A. Lateral view of the right cerebral hemisphere
B. Ventral view of the brain, brainstem and cerebellum resected by intercollicular mesencephalic transection.

Areas of susceptibility to cerebral contusion include the temporal lobes and the orbitofrontal gyri. Parietal and occipital lobe contusions are far less common, unless related to skull fracture or to the coup-contrecoup phenomena. The latter mechanism involves the occurrence of maximal damage diametrically opposed to the point of impact with severe non-penetrating or blunt head trauma. In this case, the patient fell from a third-story window and sustained a left frontoparietal skull fracture with coronal suture separation and extension through the floor of the middle cranial fossa as a basilar skull fracture (1). Note the inferolateral occipital and temporal distribution of the cerebral contusion involving the right hemisphere (2).

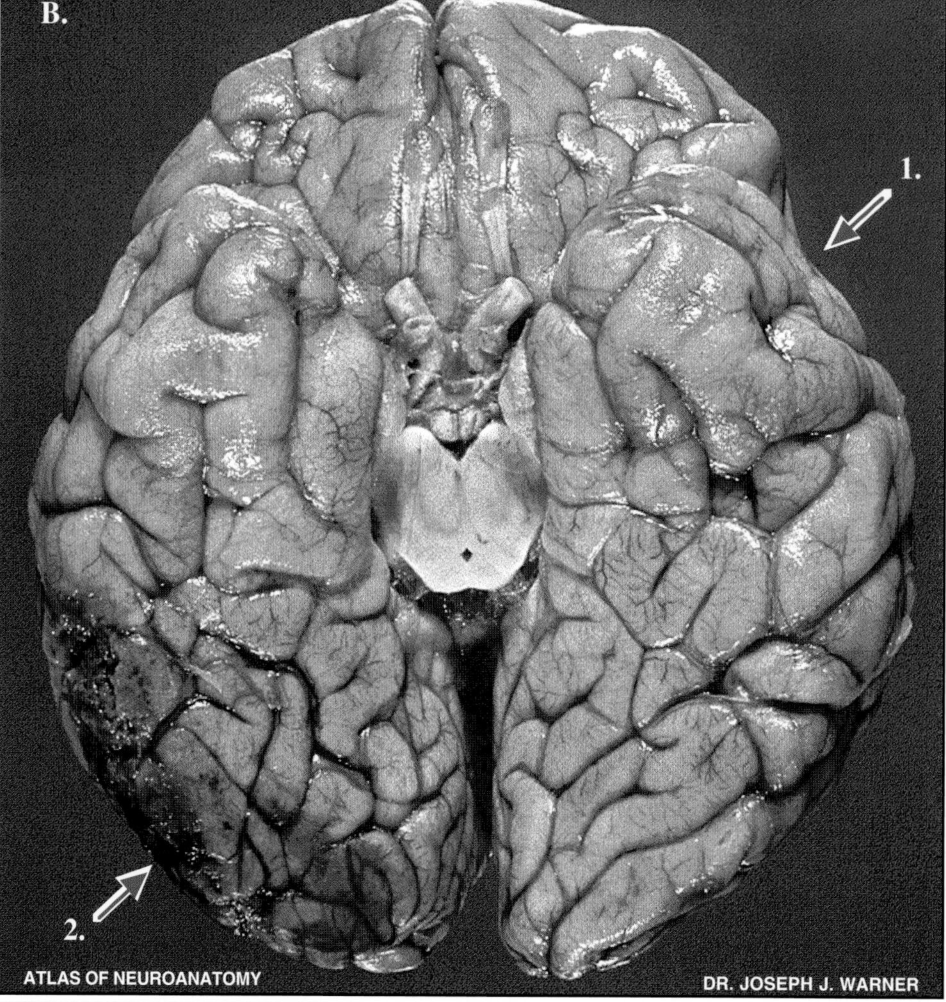

SUBDURAL HEMATOMA: COMPUTERIZED TOMOGRAPHIC SCANS OF THE SAME CASE IN THE SUBACUTE AND CHRONIC STAGES (SCANS SEPARATED BY A FIVE YEAR INTERVAL)

1. Head of the Caudate Nucleus
2. Anterior Horn of the Lateral Ventricle
3. Midline shift (mass effect)

Arrows: contrast-enhanced margin of subdural hematoma

4. Choroid Plexus
5. Falx Cerebri
6. Atrium of Lateral Ventricle
7. Thalamus
8. Septum Pellucidum
9. Head of the Caudate Nucleus
10. Anterior Horn of Lateral Ventricle
11. Corpus Callosum
12. Falx Cerebri
13. Atrophy ipsilateral to subdural fluid
14. Chronic Subdural Hygroma
15. Thalamus
16. Atrium of Lateral Ventricle
17. Falx Cerebri
18. Splenium of Corpus Callosum
19. Septum Pellucidum

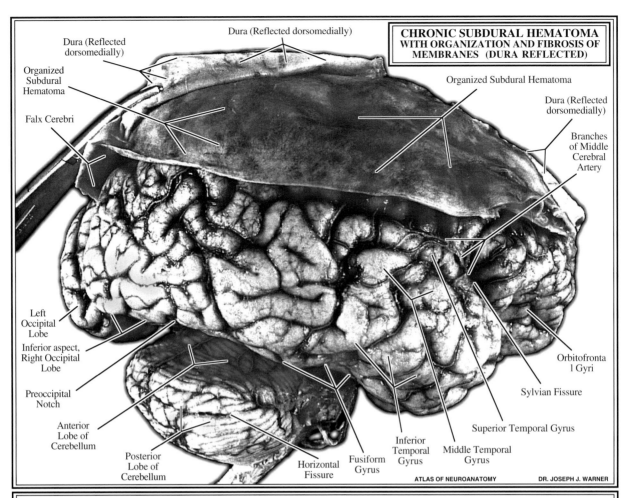

CHRONIC SUBDURAL HEMATOMA WITH ORGANIZATION AND FIBROSIS OF MEMBRANES (DURA REFLECTED)

Dura (Reflected dorsomedially)
Dura (Reflected dorsomedially)
Organized Subdural Hematoma
Falx Cerebri
Organized Subdural Hematoma
Dura (Reflected dorsomedially)
Branches of Middle Cerebral Artery
Left Occipital Lobe
Inferior aspect, Right Occipital Lobe
Preoccipital Notch
Anterior Lobe of Cerebellum
Posterior Lobe of Cerebellum
Horizontal Fissure
Fusiform Gyrus
Inferior Temporal Gyrus
Middle Temporal Gyrus
Superior Temporal Gyrus
Sylvian Fissure
Orbitofronta l Gyri

ATLAS OF NEUROANATOMY DR. JOSEPH J. WARNER

CHRONIC SUBDURAL HEMATOMA: ORGANIZED WITH CONNECTIVE TISSUE PROLIFERATION AND CALCIFICATION, T2 MAGNETIC RESONANCE IMAGING (FORTY YEARS AFTER CRANIOTOMY FOR EVACUATION OF ACUTE SUBDURAL HEMATOMA)

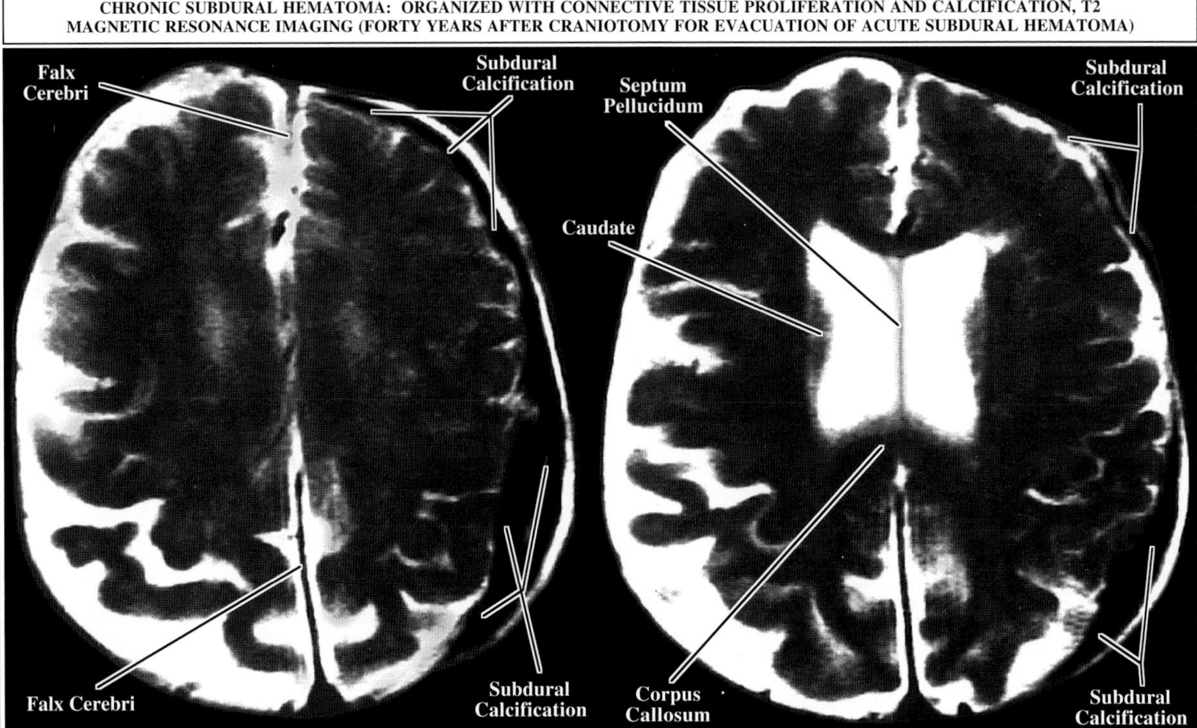

This 95-year-old male was admitted for evaluation of progressive confusion and short-term memory deficits. He had also developed urinary incontinence and a gait disorder. Otherwise, his affect and social interactions with family, friends, and staff were appropriate. The patient had a history of prior craniotomies for evacuation of acute bilateral subdural hematomas following head trauma. These procedures, confirmed by archival records, were performed forty years prior to the current evaluation.

Magnetic resonance imaging revealed significant cerebral atrophy, with prominent sulci and enlarged ventricles. A heavily calcified organized remote subdural hematoma was revealed (refer to figure of T2-weighted MRI images). Calcification was so dense as to be easily discernible on A-P and lateral skull x-rays. The crescent-shaped signal void contrasts with the high signal intensity of cerebrospinal fluid and intermediate signal intensities of the brain parenchyma.

ATLAS OF NEUROANATOMY DR. JOSEPH J. WARNER

CRANIOTOMY FOR ACUTE SUBDURAL HEMATOMA: SKULL X-RAY, LATERAL PROJECTION

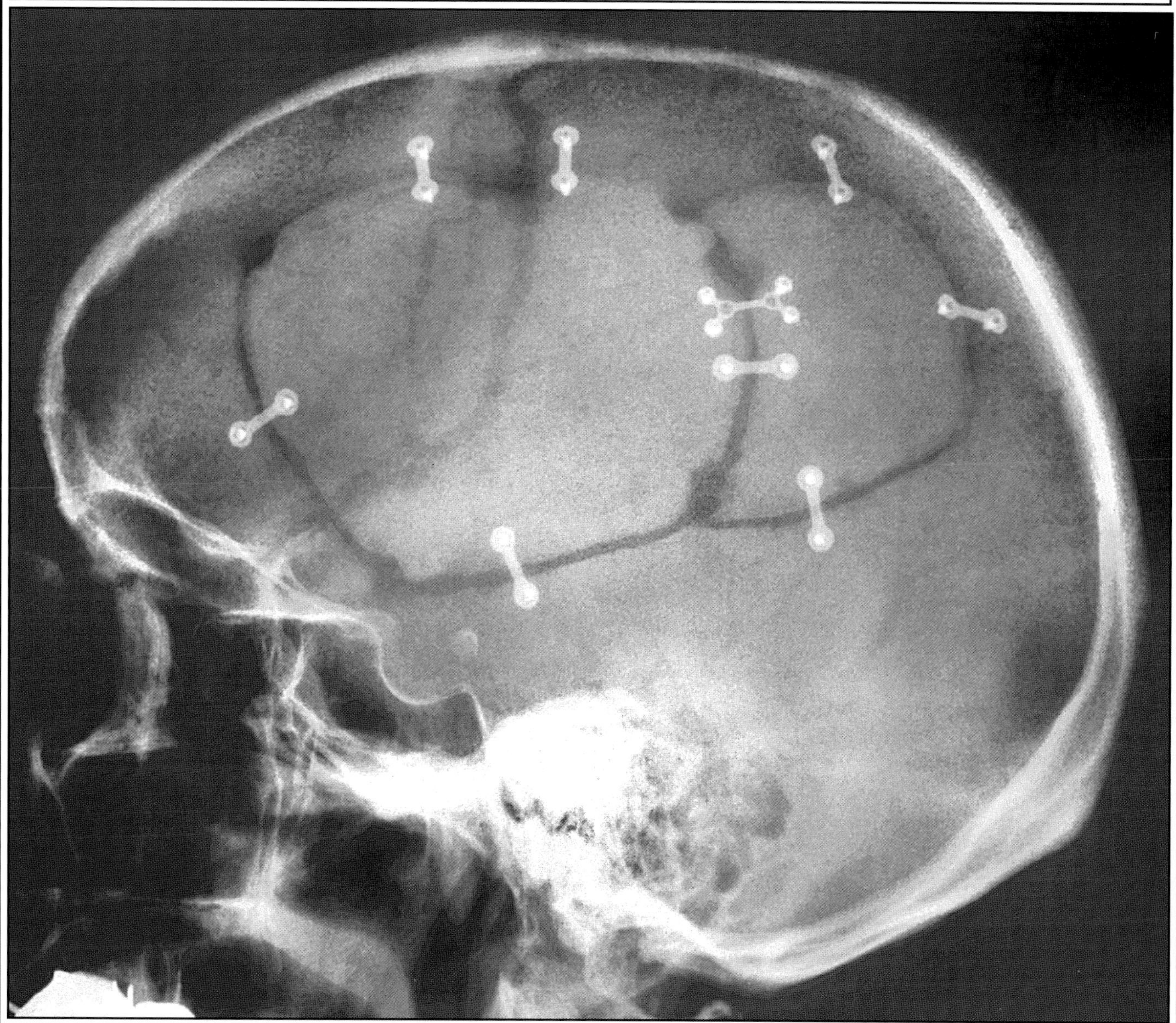

This 70-year-old right-handed female had presented with a gradually progressive gait disturbance associated with complaints of dysequilibrium. She had a previous history of cardiac catheterization via a left femoral arterial approach with subsequent femoral neuropathy attributed to hematoma formation at the site of arterial cannulation. Neurologic examination had revealed no focal deficits with the exception of pain over the region of the left quadriceps during motor testing. Prior magnetic resonance imaging revealed mild periventricular leukoencephalopathy consistent with ischemic demyelination, and cerebral atrophy. The patient sustained a fall, striking her head. She became unresponsive to verbal stimuli and was brought to the emergency room. Neurologic findings included a dilated and sluggishly reactive left pupil. Intermittent right decorticate posturing was observed as the patient's level of responsiveness deteriorated. Computerized tomography revealed a large, crescent-shaped area of increased attenuation over the left frontoparietal region consistent with an acute subdural hematoma. An extensive craniotomy was performed for evacuation of the hematoma as well as to identify and control sources of hemorrhage. The patient remained comatose for several days, then regained consciousness. Subsequent neurobehavioural testing revealed mild to moderate attentional and recent memory deficits. The patient developed a pain syndrome in the region of the craniotomy requiring subsequent occipital nerve blocks.

COLLOID CYST OF THE THIRD VENTRICLE

COMPUTERIZED TOMOGRAPHY WITH CONTRAST ENHANCEMENT

Colloid cyst of the third ventricle arises from ependymal cells located between the interventricular foramina of Monro and is generally attached to the roof of the ventricle. This benign tumor consists of a layer of epithelial cells surrounded by fibrous connective tissue and contains a gelatinous mixture of mucopolysaccharides. Although these cysts are congenital, they become symptomatic in adult life. The size, shape, and particularly the location of the colloid cyst produces intermittent "ball-valve" type obstruction of the foramina of Monro. Symptoms include severe bilateral frontal and occipital headaches, which may be positional. Episodes of impaired level of arousal, confusion, gait instability, incontinence, and lower extremity weakness may occur. Over time, the cyst may result in hydrocephalus involving the lateral ventricles, often associated with progressive clinical signs and symptoms. Treatment has traditionally consisted of resection of the colloid cyst. However, ventriculoperitoneal shunting has been successful; and in some cases, stereotaxic decompression of the cyst including endoscopy and microdissection.

Key to Numbered Structures

1. Colloid Cyst of the Third Ventricle
2. Anterior Horn of the Lateral Ventricle
3. Septum Pellucidum
4. Corpus Callosum
5. Head of the Caudate
6. Anterior Limb of the Internal Capsule
7. Putamen and Globus Pallidus II
8. Insula
9. Posterior Horn of Lateral Ventricle
10. Choroid Plexus in Atrium of Lateral Ventricle
11. Third Ventricle
12. Tentorial Incisura
13. Falx Cerebri
14. Great Vein of Galen
15. Thalamus
16. Genu of the Internal Capsule

COLLOID CYST OF THE THIRD VENTRICLE IN A 32-YEAR-OLD MALE WITH POSITIONAL HEADACHES, WHO DEVELOPED COMA APPROX. 8 - 12 HOURS AFTER LUMBAR PUNCTURE TO ASSESS POSSIBLE "MENINGITIS"

CLINICAL CASE PRESENTATION

This 32-year-old right-handed male presented to the emergency room of a local hospital complaining of severe positional headaches, progressive over at least two months prior to his evaluation. He sought medical attention when his headache became unusually intense. The patient did indicate that his headaches were exacerbated when he sat in a reclining chair, often relieved somewhat when he turned his head to the side. Upon presentation to the E.R., the physician performed a lumbar puncture to exclude the possibility of purulent meningitis or subarachnoid hemorrhage. The patient was given medications for pain and sent home. A magnetic resonance imaging study had been ordered; however, neither the colloid cyst nor the ventriculomegally had been appropriately reported. (Refer to preoperative M.R.I. photographs.)
That night, the patient reportedly went to bed. He developed "loud snoring"; subsequent sonorous, gasping respirations; and, according to a family member, could not be aroused. An emergency medical rescue unit was called. By the time of their arrival, the patient had irregular respirations, then sustained a period of respiratory arrest. Tracheostomy was performed and the patient was ventilated. He was subsequently airlifted to a tertiary care hospital. Neurosurgical consultation was obtained. Review of the M.R.I. confirmed the diagnosis of colloid cyst of the third ventricle. Subsequent neuroimaging studies demonstrated downward displacement of the cerebellar tonsils into the foramen magnum. Emergency ventriculostomy was performed, with an estimated intraventricular pressure of greater than 40 cm of CSF (>32 mm Hg, normal being 8 - 14 mm Hg). The opening pressure was thus estimated with the observation that cerebrospinal fluid "shot out" of the tube. The patient gradually stabilized, resumed a normal respiratory pattern, and sustained a gradual improvement in his level of arousal.

COLLOID CYST OF THE THIRD VENTRICLE IN A 32-YEAR-OLD MALE WITH A HISTORY OF SEVERE POSITIONAL HEADACHES AND COMA FOLLOWING LUMBAR PUNCTURE: PRE- AND POSTOPERATIVE M.R.I. STUDIES

CLINICAL COURSE AND TWO-YEAR FOLLOW-UP

Although the patient regained consciousness after ventriculostomy, his neurobehavioural status did not return to baseline. His wife stated that prior to the coma, "he was like a bulldog, memory for everything." After awakening, the patient was reported as "asking for his mother and father" (both deceased at the time). It was further stated that "he had no concept of what time was." Significant deficits in recent memory were noted. Following stabilization of the patient, a right frontal craniotomy was performed. Through this approach, the colloid cyst was resected, with clear identification of the fornix and surrounding structures.

Over the subsequent two years, the patient was followed. According to his wife, "when he first came home, he couldn't remember one minute to the next." His neurobehavioural deficits reportedly persisted. Euphoria alternated with rapid mood swings resulting in agitation, irritability, and intermittently aggressive behaviour. The patient was treated with phenytoin for probable complex partial seizures, with some moderation of these symptoms. Examination by the author revealed persistent recent memory and attentional deficits, along with a suggestion of mild euphoria. Repeat magnetic resonance imaging was obtained, which revealed a decrease in ventricular size and a well-defined tract in the right frontal lobe through which the colloid cyst was removed. Persistent attenuation of the corpus callosum was noted. However, midline structures adjacent to the foramen of Monro were clearly discernible, with no evidence of recurrence of the cyst. [Refer to figure below: (A) Preoperative sagittal T1-weighted M.R.I.; (B) Post-operative sagittal T1-weighted M.R.I.].

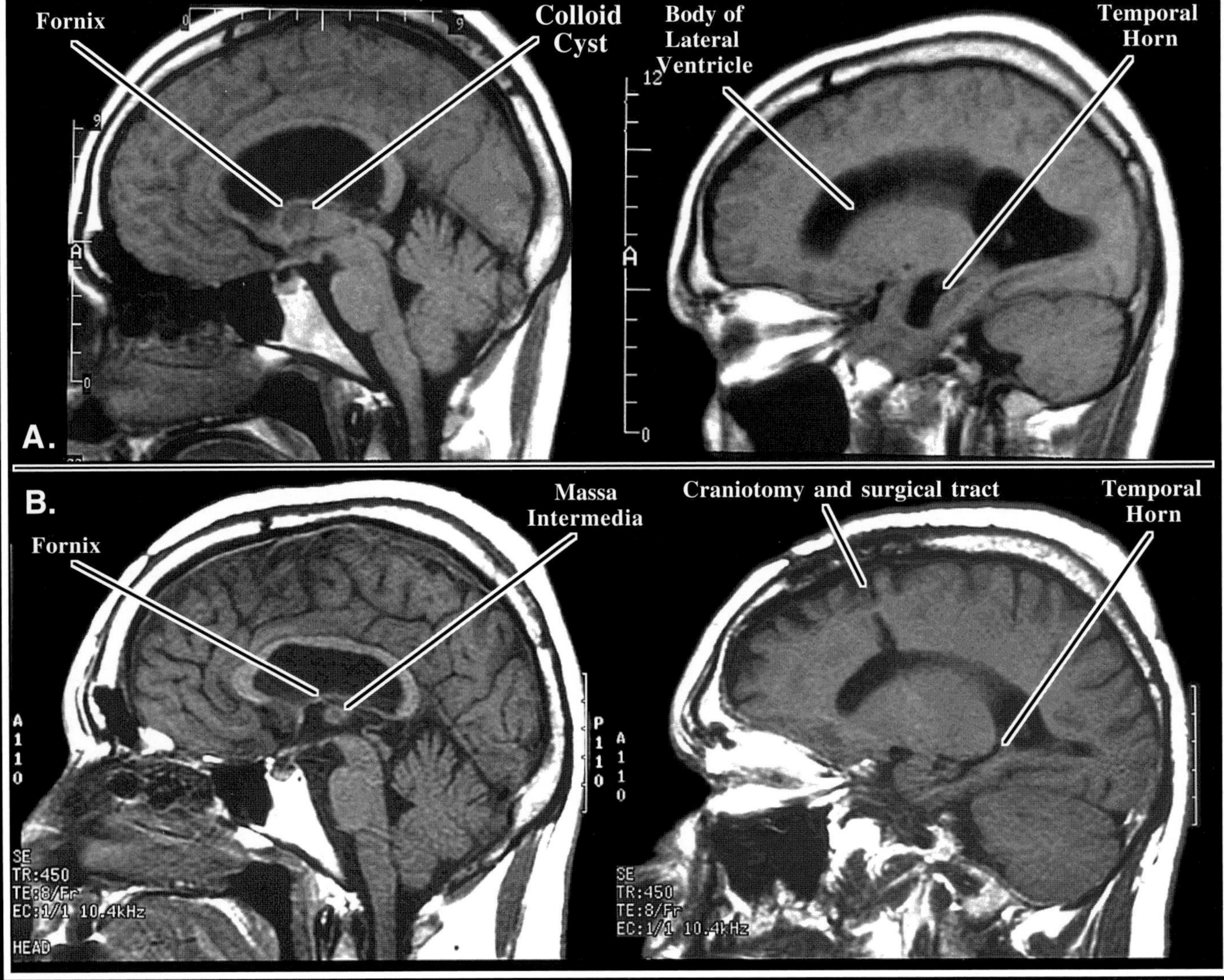

COLLOID CYST OF THE THIRD VENTRICLE, ADVANCED, WITH OBSTRUCTIVE HYDROCEPHALUS OF THE LATERAL VENTRICLES DUE TO OCCLUSION OF THE INTERVENTRICULAR FORAMINA OF MONRO

This case demonstrates marked hydrocephalus involving the lateral ventricles. The third ventricle, although deformed by the mass anteriorly and superiorly, was not enlarged. Neurologic findings included bilateral lower extremity spasticity, hyperreflexia, an ataxic gait, and postural instability.

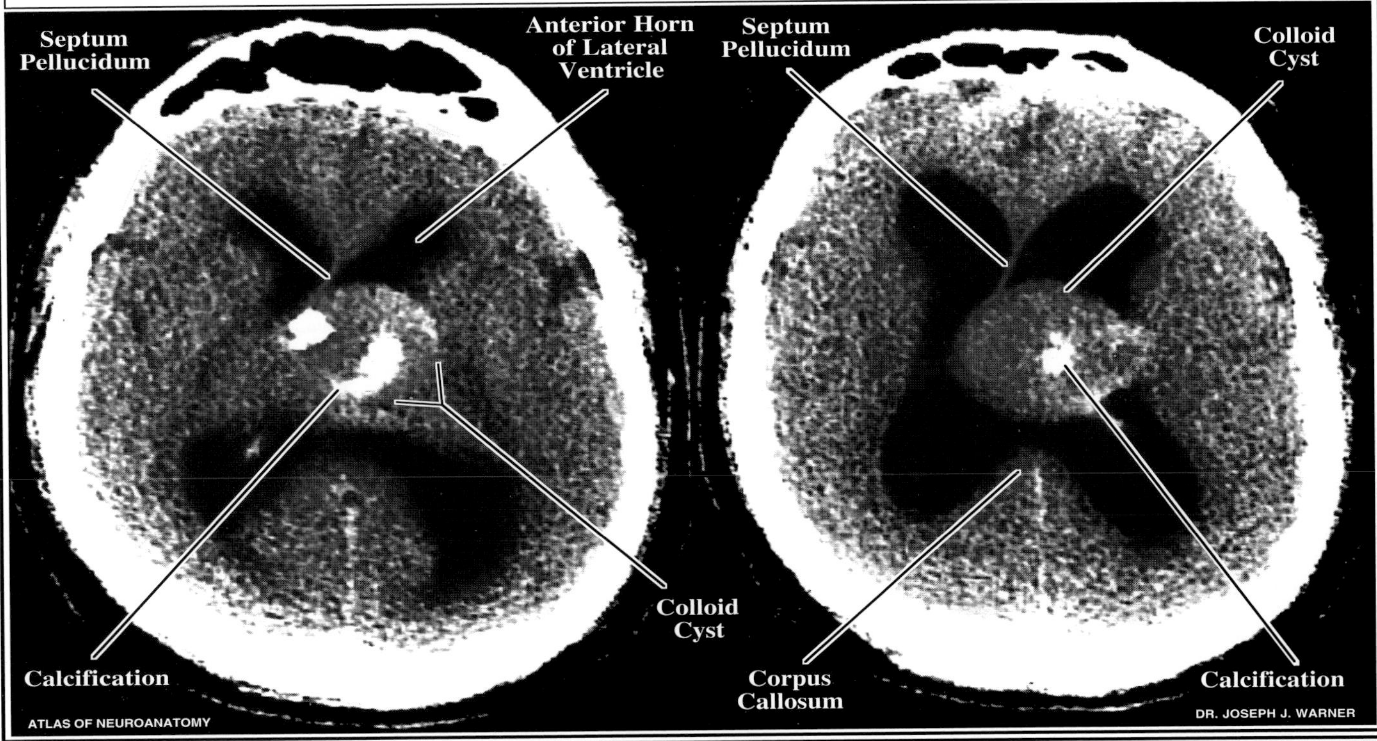

HYDROCEPHALUS DUE TO OBSTRUCTION OF THE FOURTH VENTRICLE AND AQUEDUCT OF SYLVIUS BY CARCINOMA OF THE LUNG METASTATIC TO THE CEREBELLUM

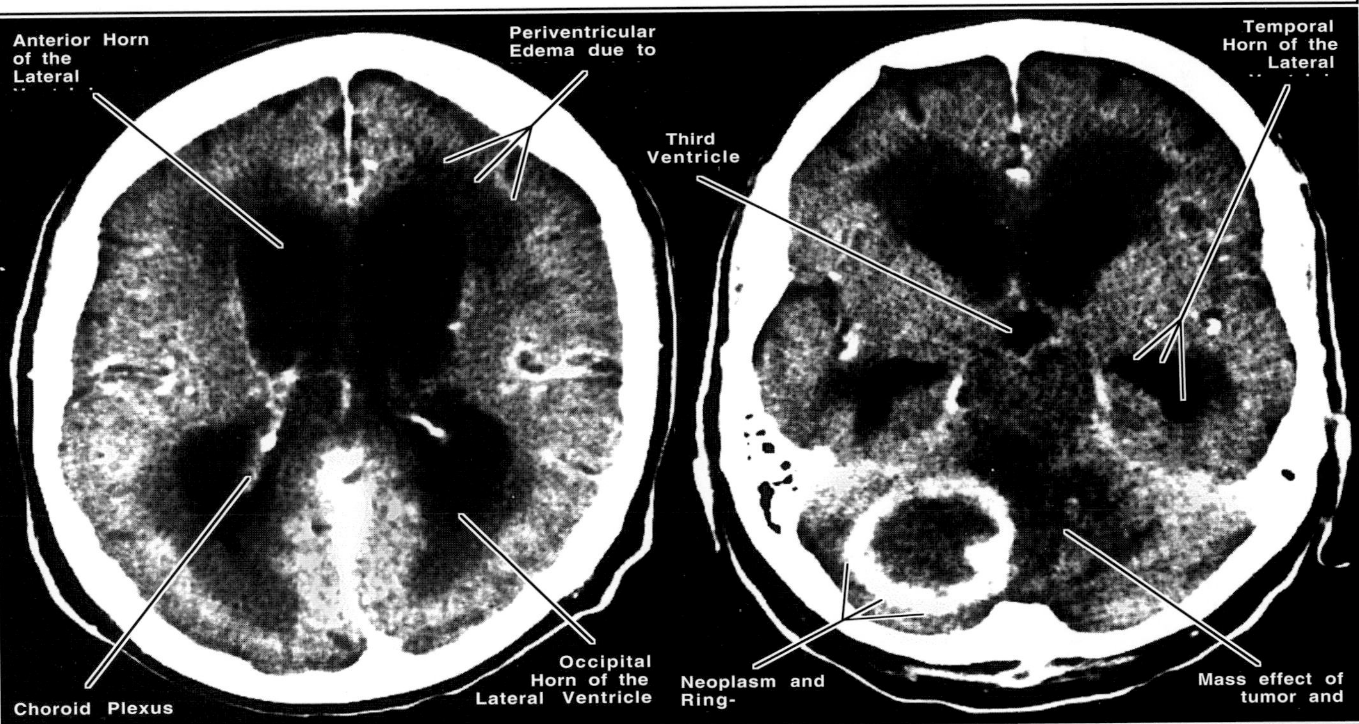

These contrast-enhanced computerized tomographic images demonstrate a classic form of obstructive (non-communicating) hydrocephalus. In this case, a tumor, metastatic from the lung, has exerted an expanding mass effect in the posterior fossa, compressing the fourth ventricle and aqueduct of Sylvius. The increase in intraventricular pressure due to the continued production of cerebrospinal fluid is associated with marked enlargement of the lateral and third ventricles, with periventricular edema. The tumor appears as an area of ring-enhancement following intravenous contrast administration, surrounded by edema extending across the midline.

ATLAS OF NEUROANATOMY DR. JOSEPH J. WARNER

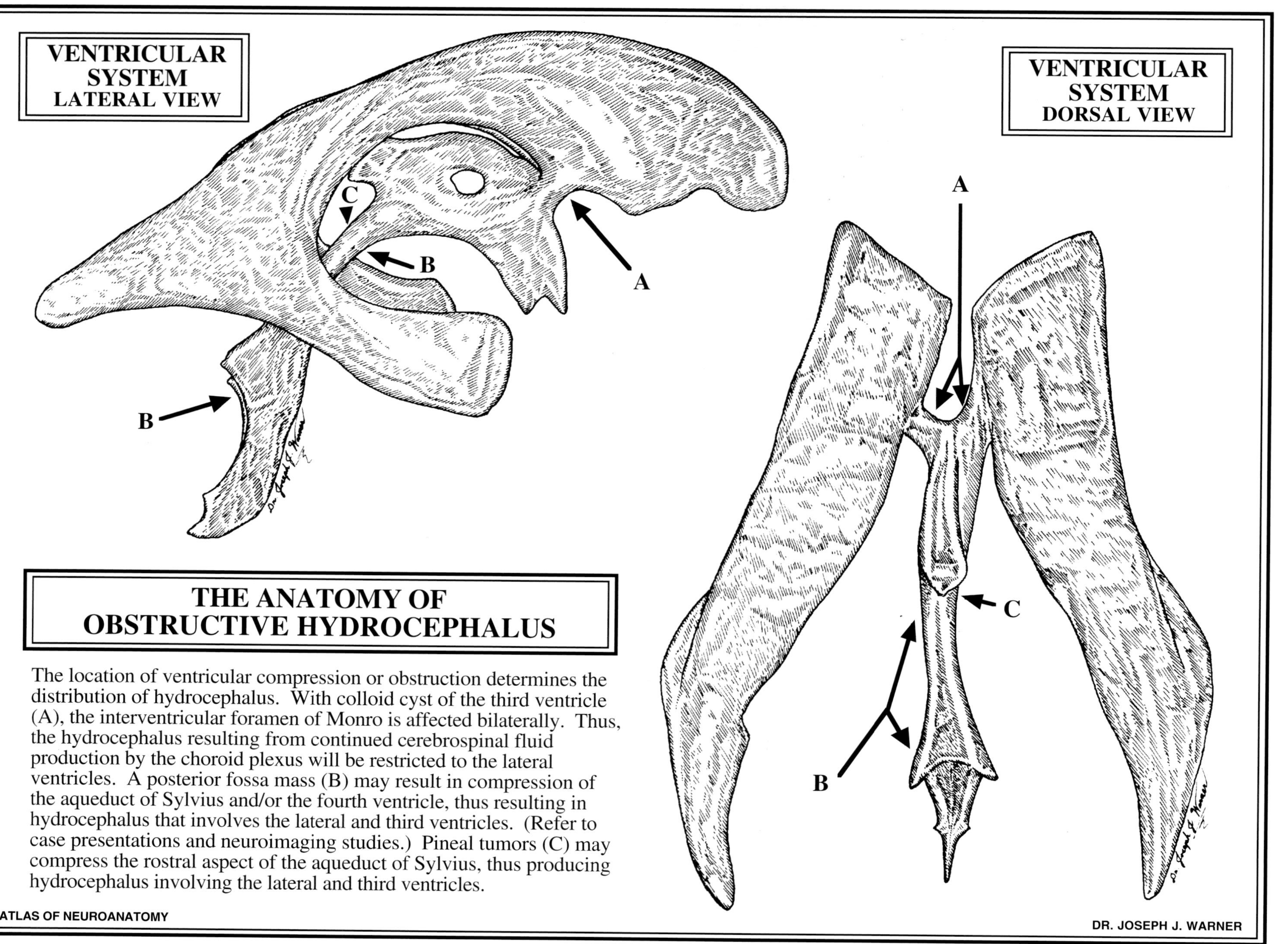

THE ANATOMY OF OBSTRUCTIVE HYDROCEPHALUS

The location of ventricular compression or obstruction determines the distribution of hydrocephalus. With colloid cyst of the third ventricle (A), the interventricular foramen of Monro is affected bilaterally. Thus, the hydrocephalus resulting from continued cerebrospinal fluid production by the choroid plexus will be restricted to the lateral ventricles. A posterior fossa mass (B) may result in compression of the aqueduct of Sylvius and/or the fourth ventricle, thus resulting in hydrocephalus that involves the lateral and third ventricles. (Refer to case presentations and neuroimaging studies.) Pineal tumors (C) may compress the rostral aspect of the aqueduct of Sylvius, thus producing hydrocephalus involving the lateral and third ventricles.

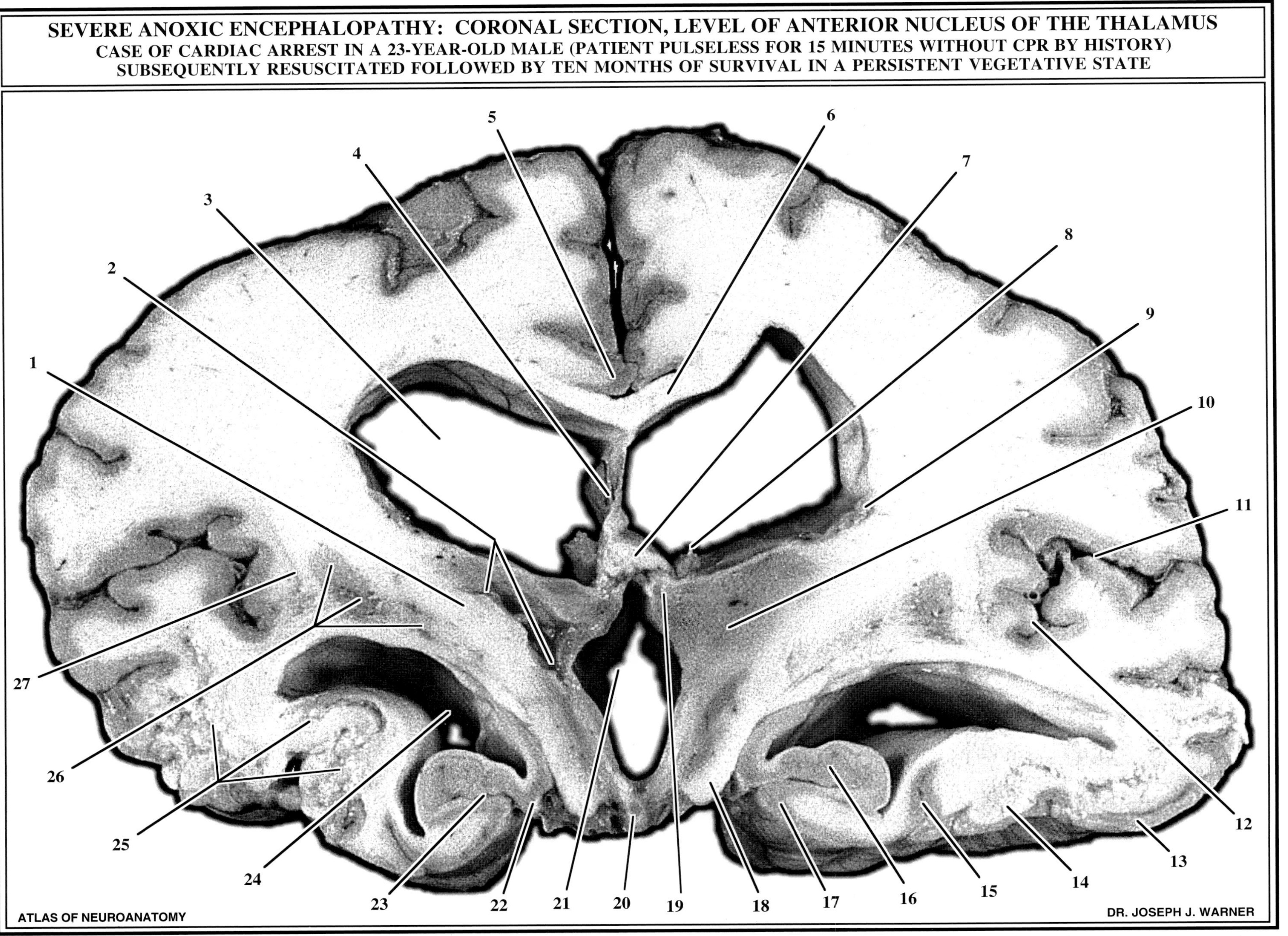
SEVERE ANOXIC ENCEPHALOPATHY: CORONAL SECTION, LEVEL OF ANTERIOR NUCLEUS OF THE THALAMUS
CASE OF CARDIAC ARREST IN A 23-YEAR-OLD MALE (PATIENT PULSELESS FOR 15 MINUTES WITHOUT CPR BY HISTORY)
SUBSEQUENTLY RESUSCITATED FOLLOWED BY TEN MONTHS OF SURVIVAL IN A PERSISTENT VEGETATIVE STATE
1
2
3
4
5
6
7
8
9
10
11
12
13
14
15
16
17
18
19
20
21
22
23
24
25
26
27
ATLAS OF NEUROANATOMY
DR. JOSEPH J. WARNER

SEVERE ANOXIC ENCEPHALOPATHY: CORONAL SECTION, LEVEL OF ANTERIOR NUCLEUS OF THE THALAMUS

SOLVENT BLUE 38 - CRESYL ECHT VIOLET STAIN, 15μ

(HISTOLOGICAL PREPARATION CORRESPONDING TO GROSS CORONAL SECTION IN PREVIOUS FIGURE)

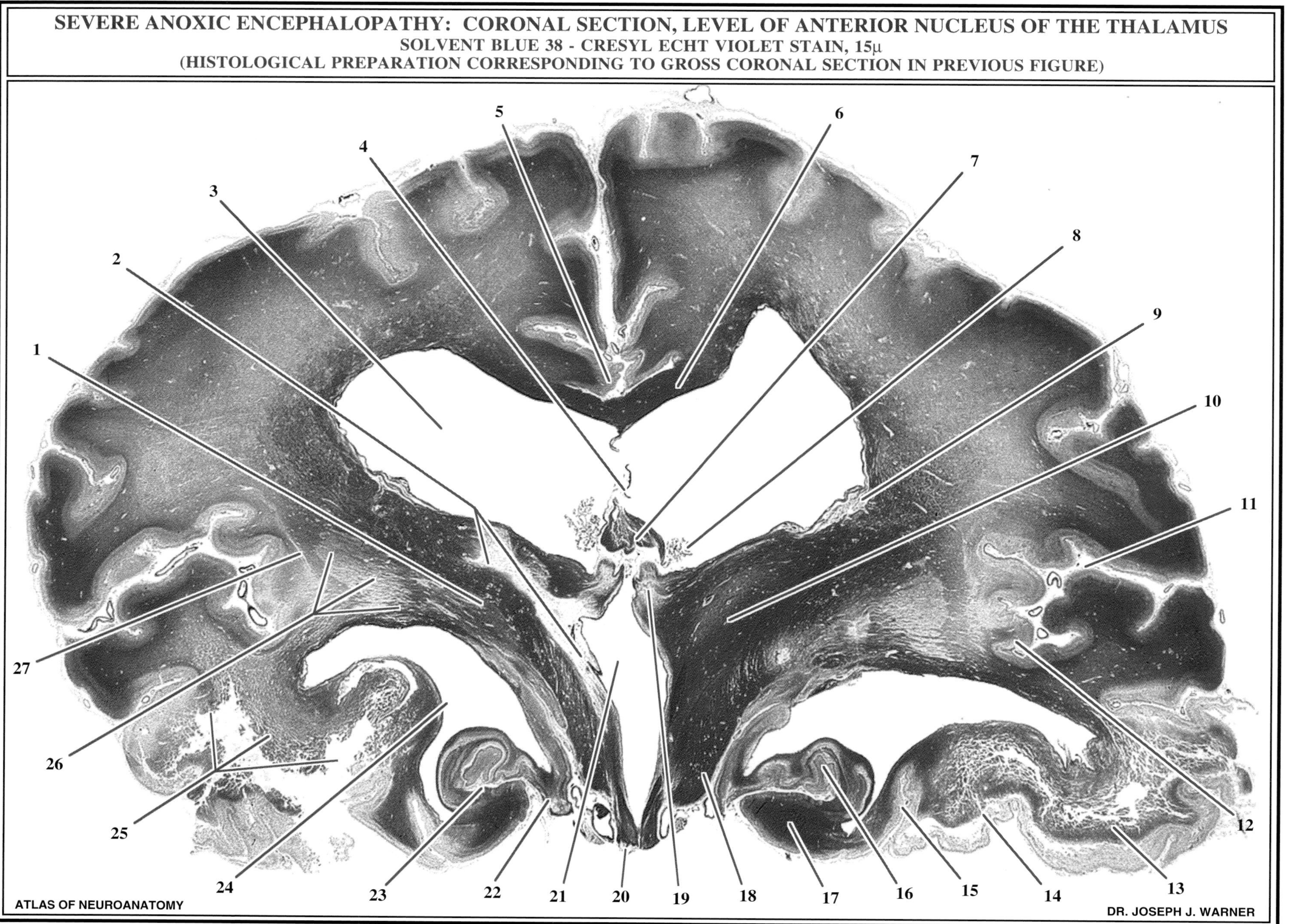

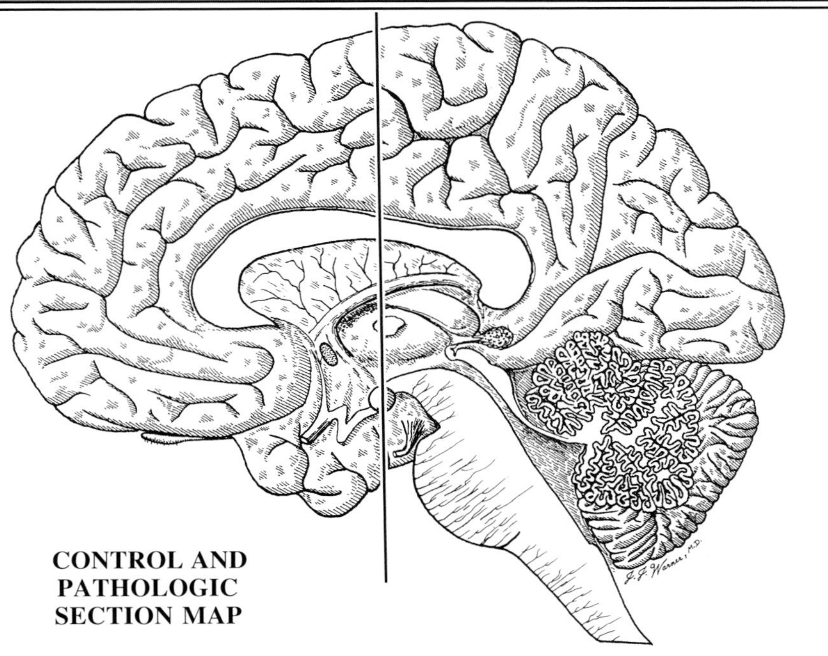

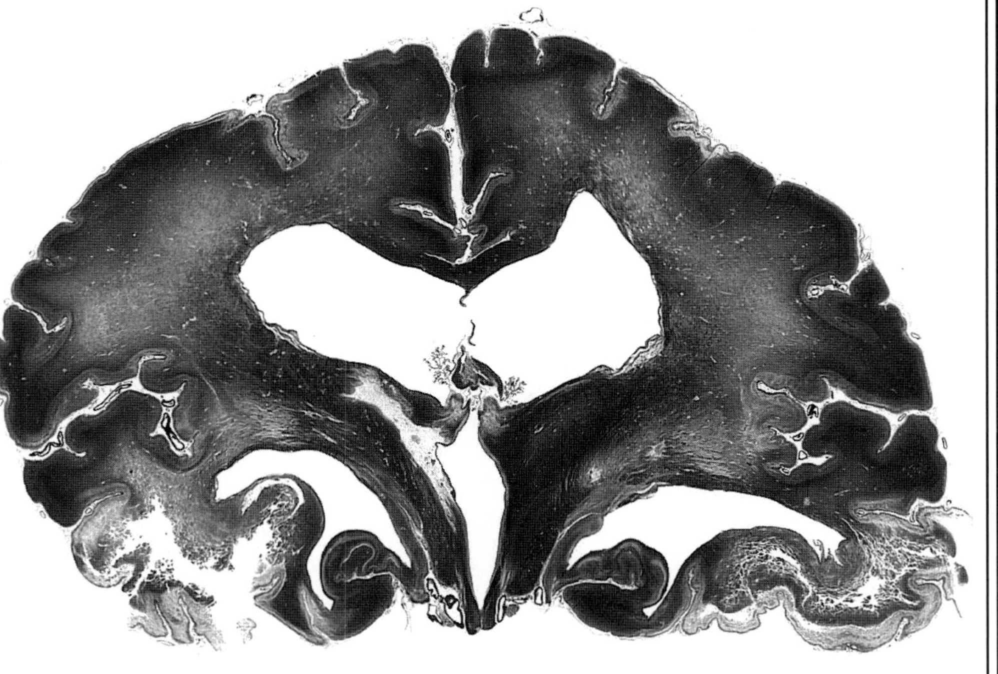

SEVERE ANOXIC ENCEPHALOPATHY: CORONAL SECTION, LEVEL OF ANTERIOR NUCLEUS OF THE THALAMUS

SECTION MAP AND COMPARISON WITH CONTROL SECTION

CONTROL AND PATHOLOGIC SECTION MAP

KEY TO NUMBERED STRUCTURES FOR GROSS AND CORRELATED HISTOLOGICAL SECTIONS

1. Internal Capsule
2. Cavitation of Thalamus
3. Body of Lateral Ventricle
4. Septum Pellucidum
5. Cingulate Gyrus
6. Corpus Callosum
7. Fornix
8. Choroid Plexus
9. Caudate Nucleus
10. Ventroanterior, Ventrolateral Nucleus of the Thalamus
11. Sylvian Fissure
12. Insular Cortex
13. Inferior Temporal Gyrus
14. Fusiform Gyrus
15. Collateral Sulcus
16. Hippocampus
17. Parahippocampal Gyrus
18. Cerebral Peduncle
19. Anterior Nucleus of the Thalamus
20. Mammillary Body
21. Third Ventricle
22. Uncus
23. Hippocampal Fissure
24. Temporal Horn of Lateral Ventricle
25. Necrotic Temporal White Matter
26. Putamen and Globus Pallidus (degenerated)
27. Claustrum

ATLAS OF NEUROANATOMY DR. JOSEPH J. WARNER

MEDULLA, HORIZONTAL (OBLIQUE TRANSVERSE) SECTION , 15 μ KLUVER-BARRERA TECHNIQUE: CASE OF SEVERE ANOXIC ENCEPHALOPATHY INCLUDING BILATERAL CEREBRAL CORTICAL NECROSIS

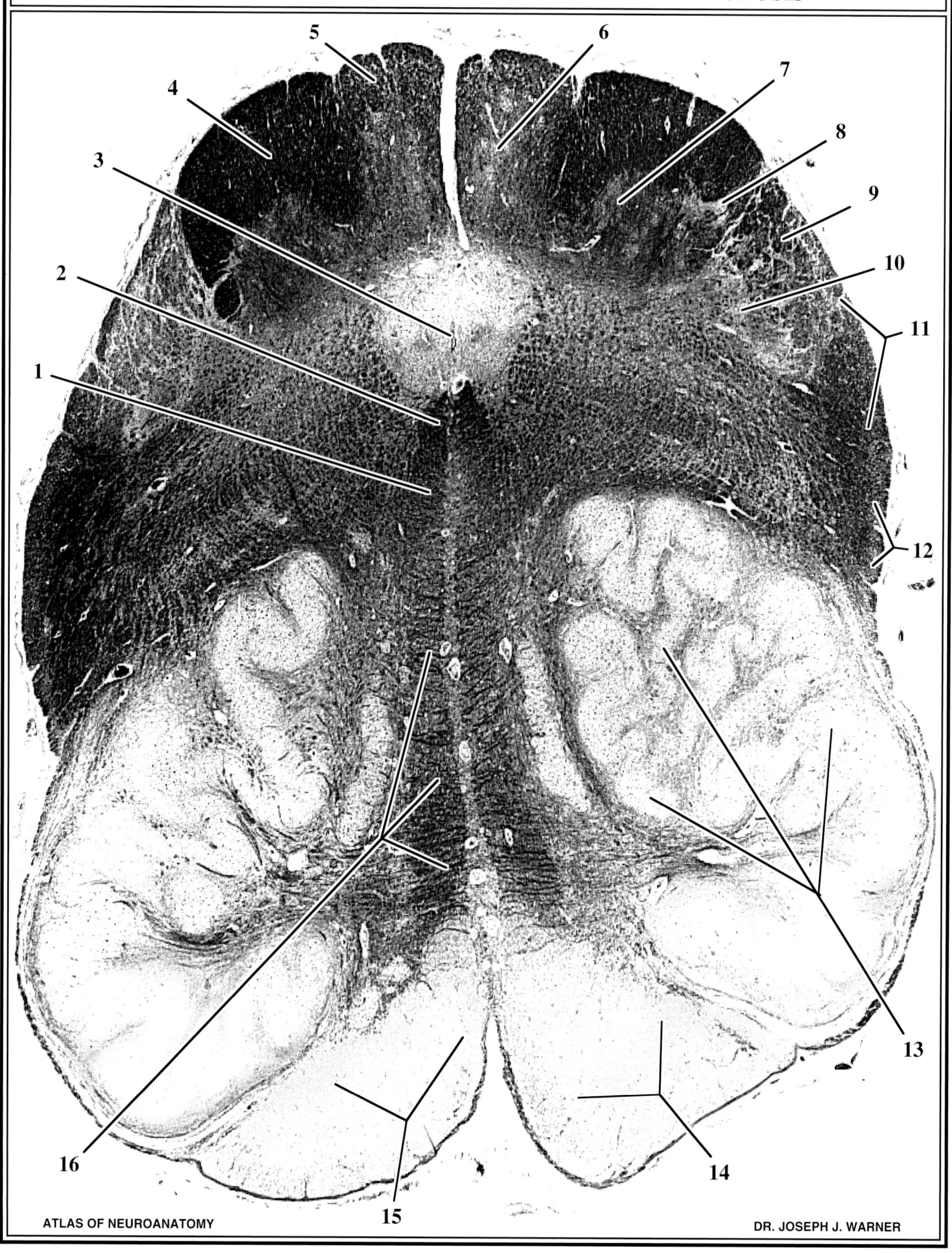

ATLAS OF NEUROANATOMY

DR. JOSEPH J. WARNER

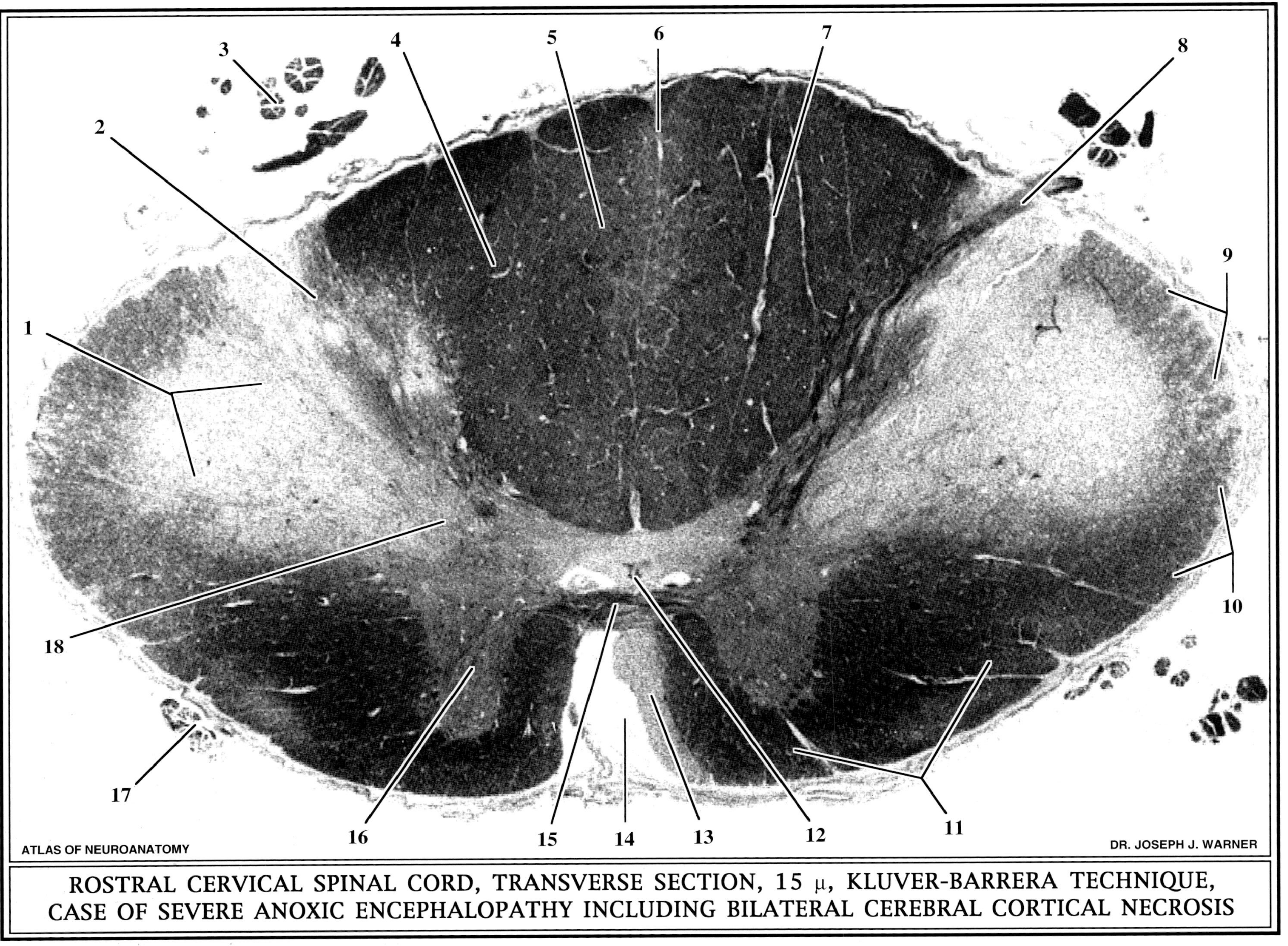

ROSTRAL CERVICAL SPINAL CORD, TRANSVERSE SECTION, 15 μ, KLUVER-BARRERA TECHNIQUE, CASE OF SEVERE ANOXIC ENCEPHALOPATHY INCLUDING BILATERAL CEREBRAL CORTICAL NECROSIS

SEVERE ANOXIC ENCEPHALOPATHY WITH NECROSIS OF THE CEREBRAL CORTEX, THALAMUS, BASAL GANGLIA, AND CEREBELLAR CORTEX

MEDULLA, HORIZONTAL (OBLIQUE TRANSVERSE) SECTION, 15 μ, KLUVER-BARRERA TECHNIQUE

KEY TO NUMBERED STRUCTURES

1. Tectospinal Tract
2. Medial Longitudinal Fasciculus
3. Central Canal
4. Fasciculus Cuneatus
5. Fasciculus Gracilis
6. Nucleus Gracilis
7. Nucleus Cuneatus
8. Accessory Cuneate Nucleus
9. Spinal Tract of the Trigeminal Nerve
10. Spinal Nucleus of the Trigeminal Nerve
11. Dorsal and Ventral Spinocerebellar Tracts
12. Spinothalamic Tract
13. Inferior Olivary Nucleus

14, 15. Medullary Pyramids*

16. Medial Lemniscus

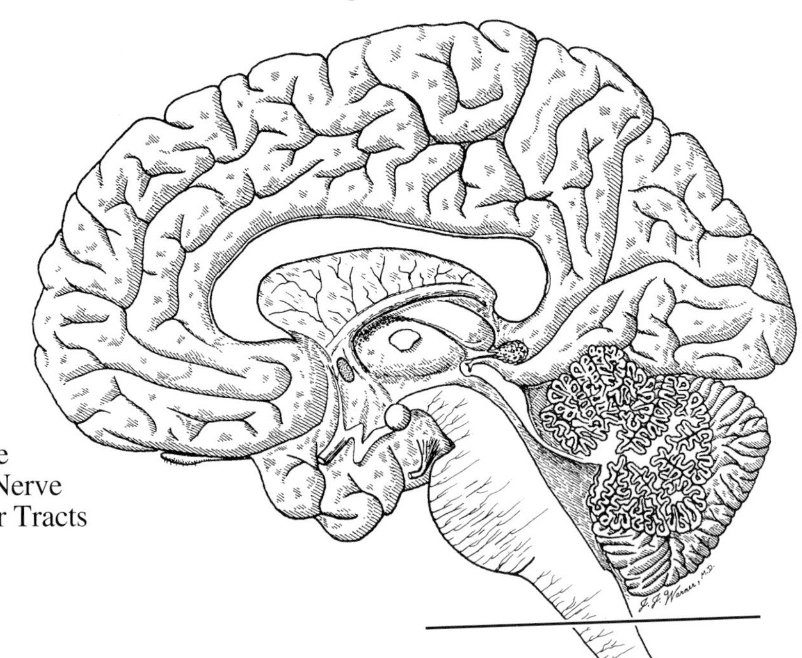

ROSTRAL CERVICAL SPINAL CORD, TRANSVERSE SECTION, 15 μ, KLUVER-BARRERA TECHNIQUE

KEY TO NUMBERED STRUCTURES

1. Lateral Corticospinal Tract*
2. Dorsal Root Entry Zone
3. Dorsal Root Fascicles
4. Fasciculus Cuneatus
5. Fasciculus Gracilis
6. Dorsal Median Septum
7. Dorsal Intermediate Septum
8. Dorsal Root
9. Dorsal Spinocerebellar Tract
10. Ventral Spinocerebellar Tract
11. Anterolateral (including Spinothalamic) Tracts
12. Central Canal
13. Ventromedial Tracts (including Ventral Corticospinal Tract)*
14. Ventral Median Fissure
15. Ventral White Commissure
16. Ventral (Anterior) Horn
17. Ventral Root
18. Intermediate Spinal Gray

*The Kluver-Barrera technique combines a myelin stain (Solvent Blue 38) with a Nissl stain. Thus, the loss or degeneration of myelinated fibers will appear as an area of significant pallor in histological sections (in contrast to normal staining of white matter structures).

The neuropathological findings of this case are clearly illustrative of the course of descending tracts originating in the cerebral hemispheres, which were severely affected by a fifteen-minute period of cardiopulmonary arrest (witnessed by family who were unable to initiate cardiopulmonary resuscitation). This patient, a 22-year-old male, was subsequently resuscitated and survived in a persistent vegetative state for nine additional months. During this time, the anterograde degeneration of descending tracts developed fully following ablation of their cell bodies of origin in the cerebral hemispheres. Therefore, the corticospinal tracts are delineated as regions of demyelination and fiber degeneration that may be traced from the brainstem through the spinal cord. The medullary pyramids clearly demonstrate these changes, as do the lateral and uncrossed (ipsilateral) corticospinal tracts in the cervical cord section as presented. This change is in clear contrast to the ascending tracts and tracts originating from more caudal brainstem structures.

CEREBRAL ANOXIA: EFFECTS ON HIPPOCAMPAL PYRAMIDAL CELLS

A

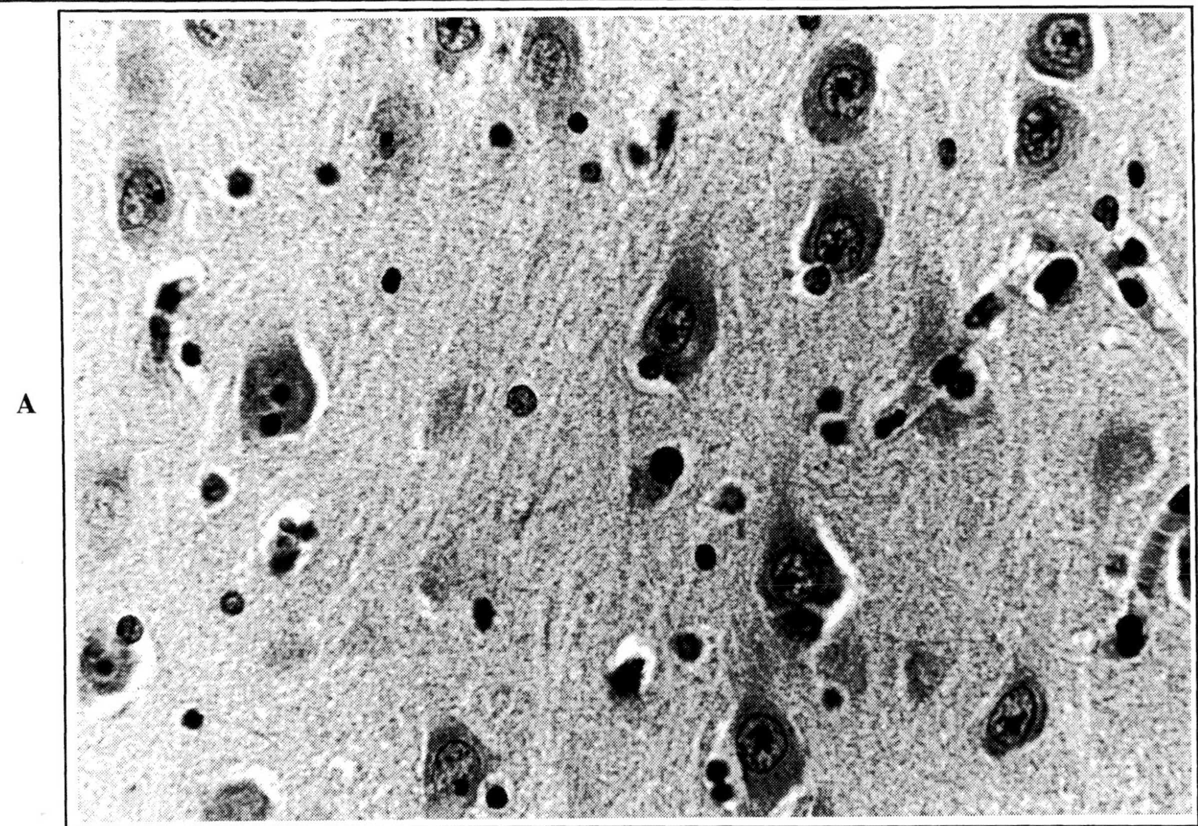

A. Pyramidal cells in CA3 of the hippocampus of a normal patient. (H & E, 400X)

B

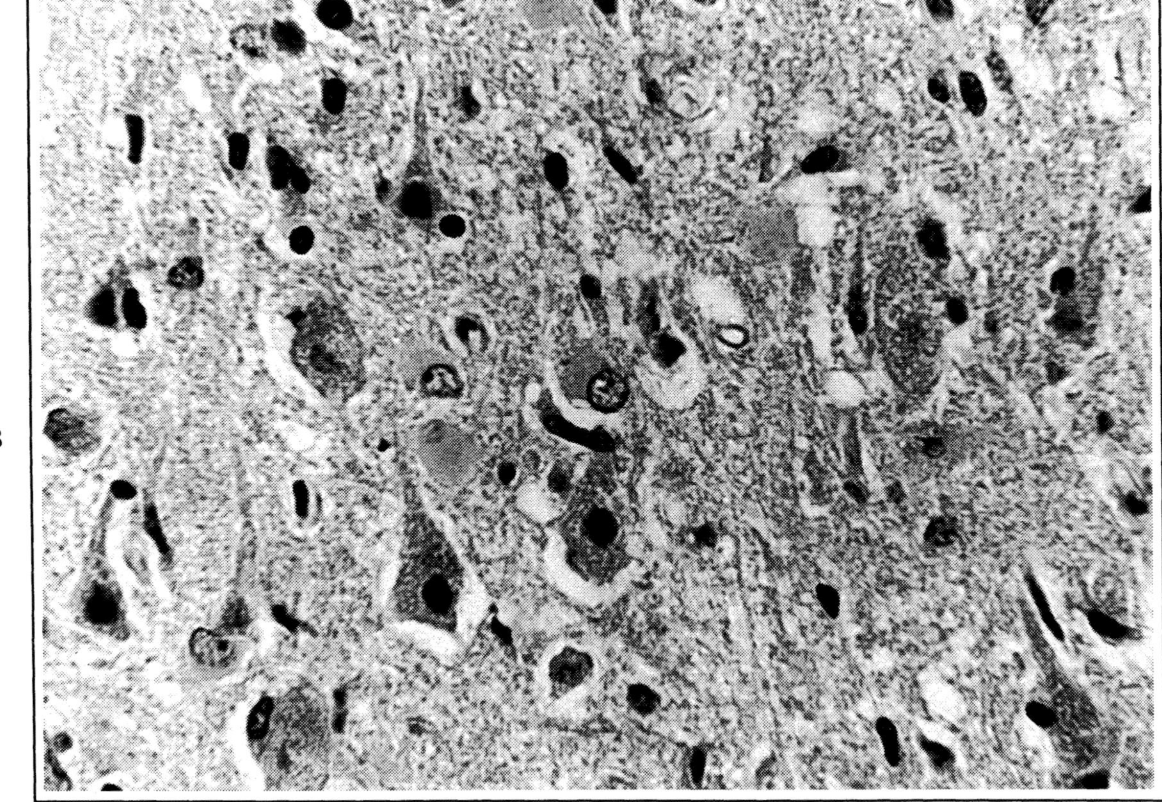

B. Hippocampal pyramidal cells (CA3) of a patient resuscitated from a cardiac arrest. Nuclei are hyperchromatic and pyknotic, and the cytoplasm is eosinophilic and granular in appearance.

MAGNETIC RESONANCE IMAGING IN A PATIENT WITH CHRONIC PROGRESSIVE MULTIPLE SCLEROSIS

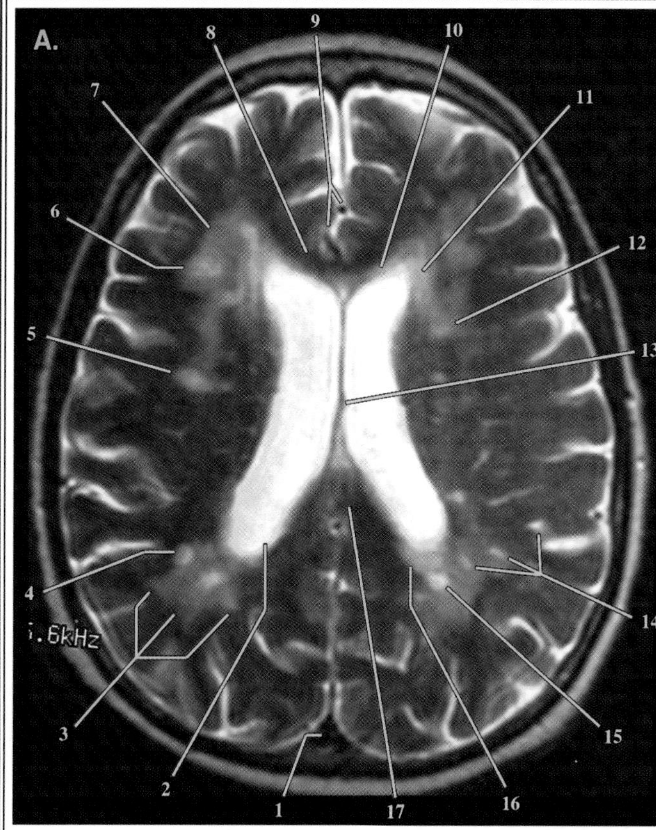

A. T2-Weighted Magnetic Resonance Image: Horizontal Plane

B. Fluid Attenuated Inversion Recovery Image: Coronal Plane

KEY TO NUMBERED STRUCTURES

1. Superior Sagittal Sinus
2. Body of the Lateral Ventricle
3. Diffuse Demyelination
4. Focal Demyelinating Lesion
5. Focus of Demyelination in the Corona Radiata
6. Confluence of Focal Lesions
7. Diffuse Demyelination
8. Corpus Callosum
9. Anterior Cerebral Arteries
10. Demyelination Extending into Corpus Callosum
11. Periventricular Demyelination
12. Focal and Diffuse Demyelination involving the Corona Radiata
13. Septum Pellucidum
14. Focal Demyelinating Lesions
15. Focal and Diffuse Demyelination
16. Periventricular Demyelination
17. Forceps Major of the Corpus Callosum
18. Interhemispheric Fissure
19. Cavum Septum Pellucidum
20. Foci of Demyelination Ventral and Rostral to the Caudate Nucleus
21. Sylvian Fissure
22. Periventricular Demyelination
23. Extension of Demyelination into the Inferior Frontal Convolution
24. Diffuse Demyelination
25. Focal Demyelination in the Superior and Middle Frontal Convolutions
26. Cingulate Sulcus
27. Cingulate Gyrus
28. Intense signal of Periventricular Demyelination
29. Diffuse Demyelination
30. Inferior Frontal Convolution
31. Head of the Caudate Nucleus
32. Temporal Pole
33. Anterior Horn of the Lateral Ventricle
34. Subcallosal Gyrus

HISTOPATHOLOGY OF MULTIPLE SCLEROSIS: FOCAL AND CONFLUENT DEMYELINATING LESIONS

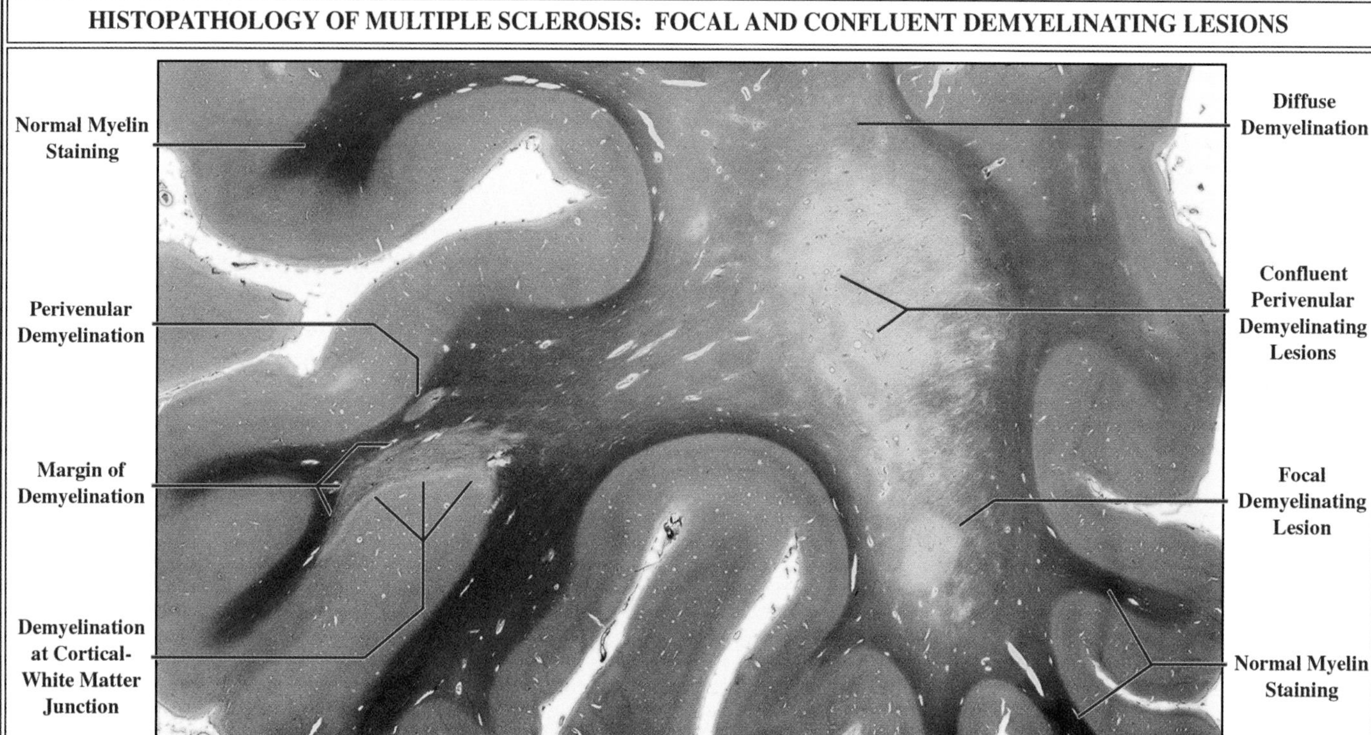

Histologic Section 12 μ, LFB-PAS Technique

MULTIPLE SCLEROSIS, ADVANCED, WITH SEVERE CEREBRAL ATROPHY: COMPLETE CORONAL SECTION, LEVEL OF THE ANTERIOR NUCLEUS OF THE THALAMUS; 15 μ, SOLVENT BLUE 38 - PERIODIC ACID - SCHIFF REACTION

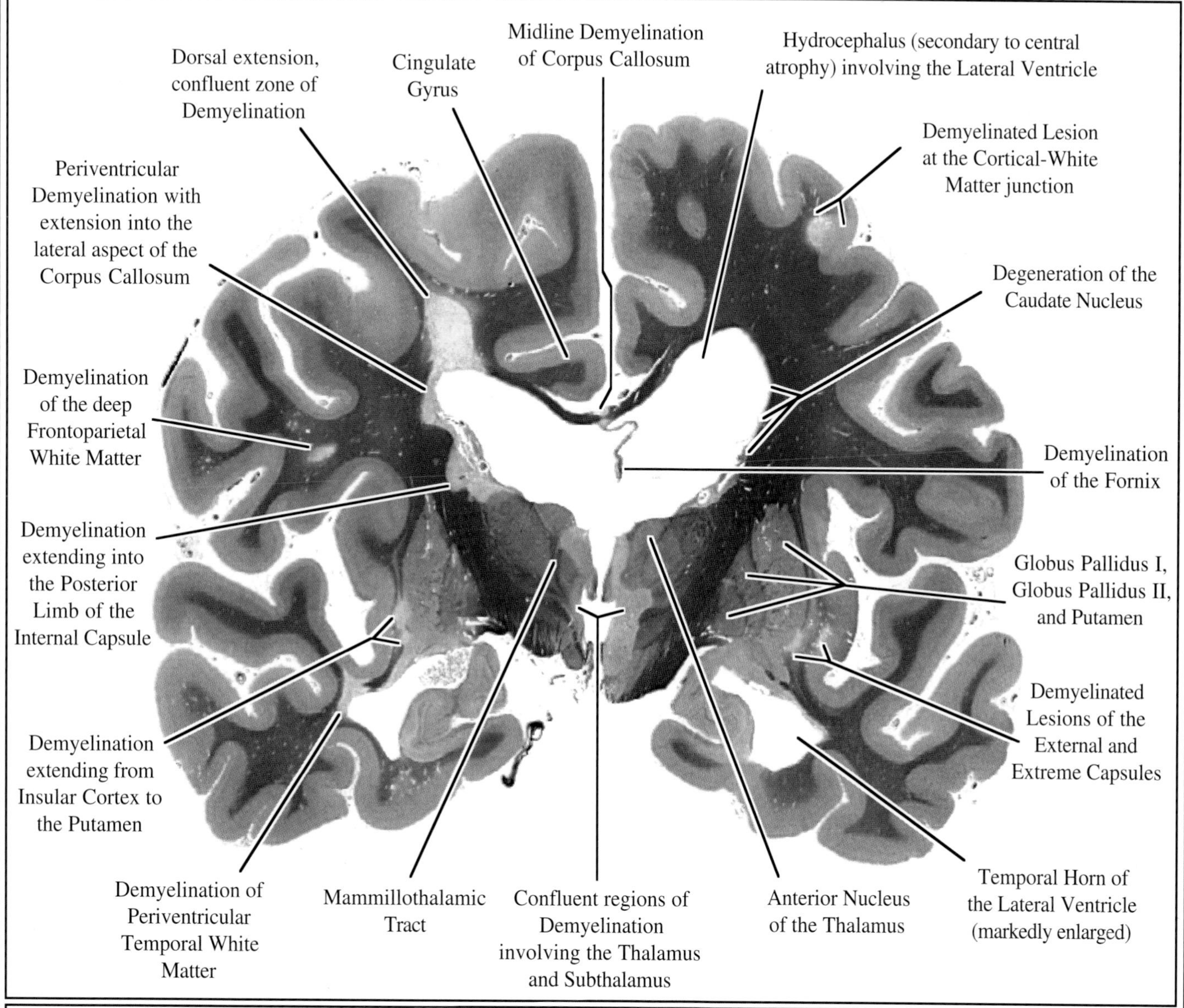

DEMYELINATING DISEASES: MULTIPLE SCLEROSIS

Multiple sclerosis (M.S.) is one of a group of disorders of the nervous system classified as the demyelinating diseases. The various entities within this classification share certain pathophysiologic criteria including destruction of the myelin sheaths surrounding nerve fibers, *relative* sparing of neurons and axon cylinders, perivascular inflammation, and multifocal perivenous lesions (which may subsequently become confluent). The lesions of M.S. have a predilection for certain regions of the central nervous system which often result in specific signs and symptoms considered as characteristic of the disease. Depending on the distribution of the lesions, symptoms may include somatosensory, motor, visual, cranial nerve, and cognitive or other behavioural abnormalities. Certain findings, such as bilateral internuclear ophthalmoplegia (due to involvement of both medial longitudinal fasciculi), are highly suggestive of the diagnosis of M.S. Separation of the lesions (and clinical manifestations) over space and time is an important diagnostic criterion. Therefore, a relapsing-remitting course and neurologic findings which suggest more than one lesion localization are diagnostic. Variations of the progression of the disease are recognized, including a chronic progressive type, and (less frequently) an acute, fulminant form which may result in coma and death over a period of weeks without intervening remission.

MULTIPLE SCLEROSIS: PERIVENULAR DEMYELINATING LESION OF THE FRONTAL WHITE MATTER

(SECTION 15 μ, SOLVENT BLUE 38 - PERIODIC ACID - SCHIFF REACTION, 40X)

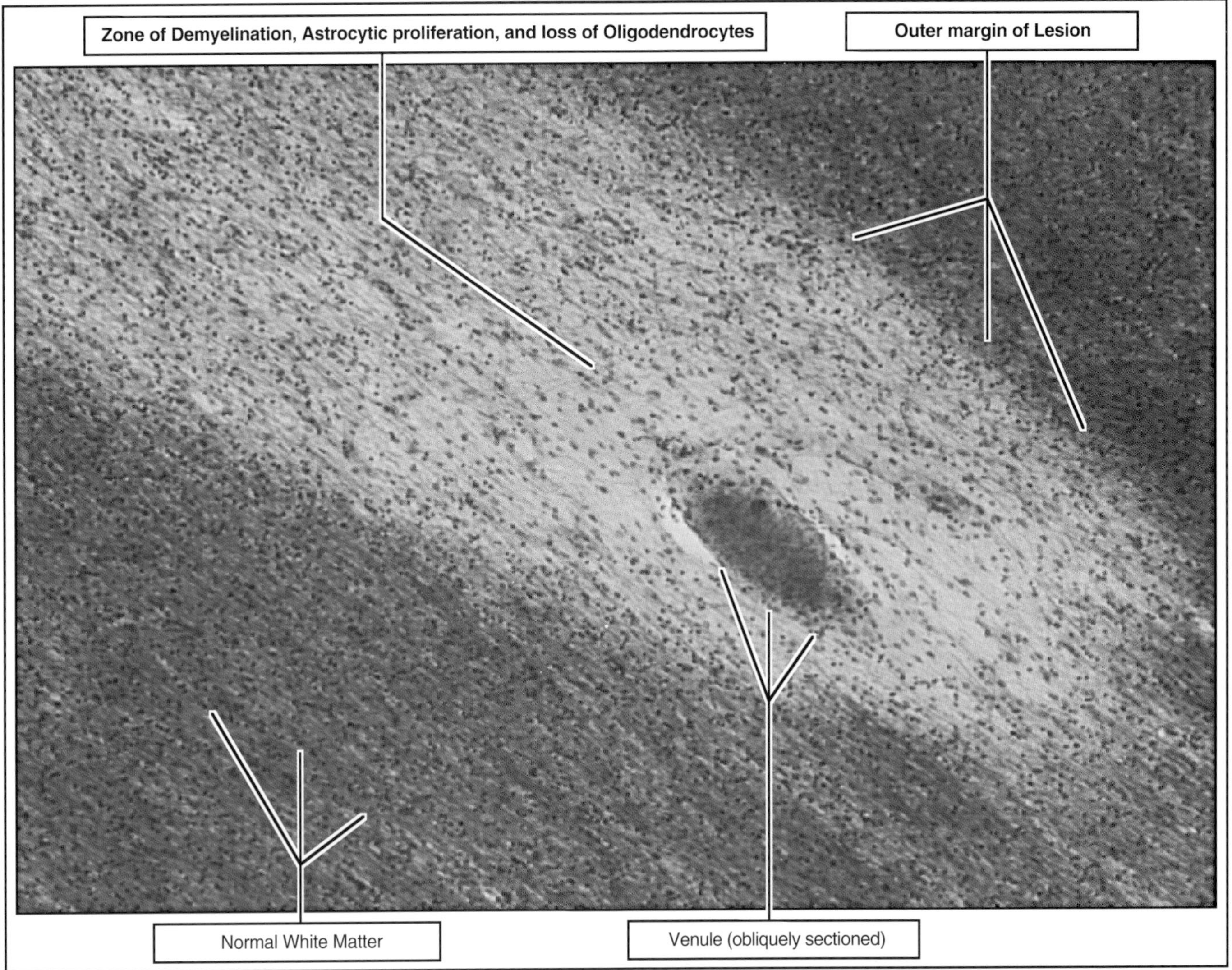

THE PATHOGENESIS OF MULTIPLE SCLEROSIS

The pathogenesis of multiple sclerosis is associated with an autoimmune process directed toward myelin. Antibodies to oligodendrocytes have been identified in a significant proportion of patients with multiple sclerosis. Autoimmunization of T lymphocytes against myelin basic protein has been invoked in the pathogenesis of certain post-infectious cases. Elevated cerebrospinal fluid IgG levels and oligoclonal banding have been associated with M.S. For many years, these findings have been utilized as diagnostic indicators for M.S., although their specificity has been argued. Antecedent viral infections, trauma, vaccinations, or other events which might stimulate immune mechanisms have been invoked as precipitating factors. Most therapeutic modalities have been directed toward the suppression or modification of the immune process, although interpretation of the results is complicated by the relapsing-remitting course and the variability of progression of M.S. between patients.

There is a well-established familial tendency toward the development of M.S. Studies have shown that approximately 15 to 20% of patients with M.S. have an affected relative, with the highest risk occurring in siblings. Ebers et al. demonstrated a 33% concordance rate in 27 pairs of monozygotic twins, as compared to 2.3% in 43 pairs of dizygotic twins. Further studies, which showed an increased frequency of certain histocompatibility antigens with M.S. (as compared to control subjects), gave additional support to the hypothesis that hereditary factors are involved in certain groups of M.S cases. (Conclusions with respect to genetic heritability must assess the possible role of shared environmental factors.)

MULTIPLE SCLEROSIS: ACUTE DEMYELINATING LESION DEMONSTRATING PERIVASCULAR INFLAMMATORY INFILTRATION AND ASTROCYTIC REACTION SECTION 12 μ, HEMATOXYLIN AND EOSIN STAIN, 100X

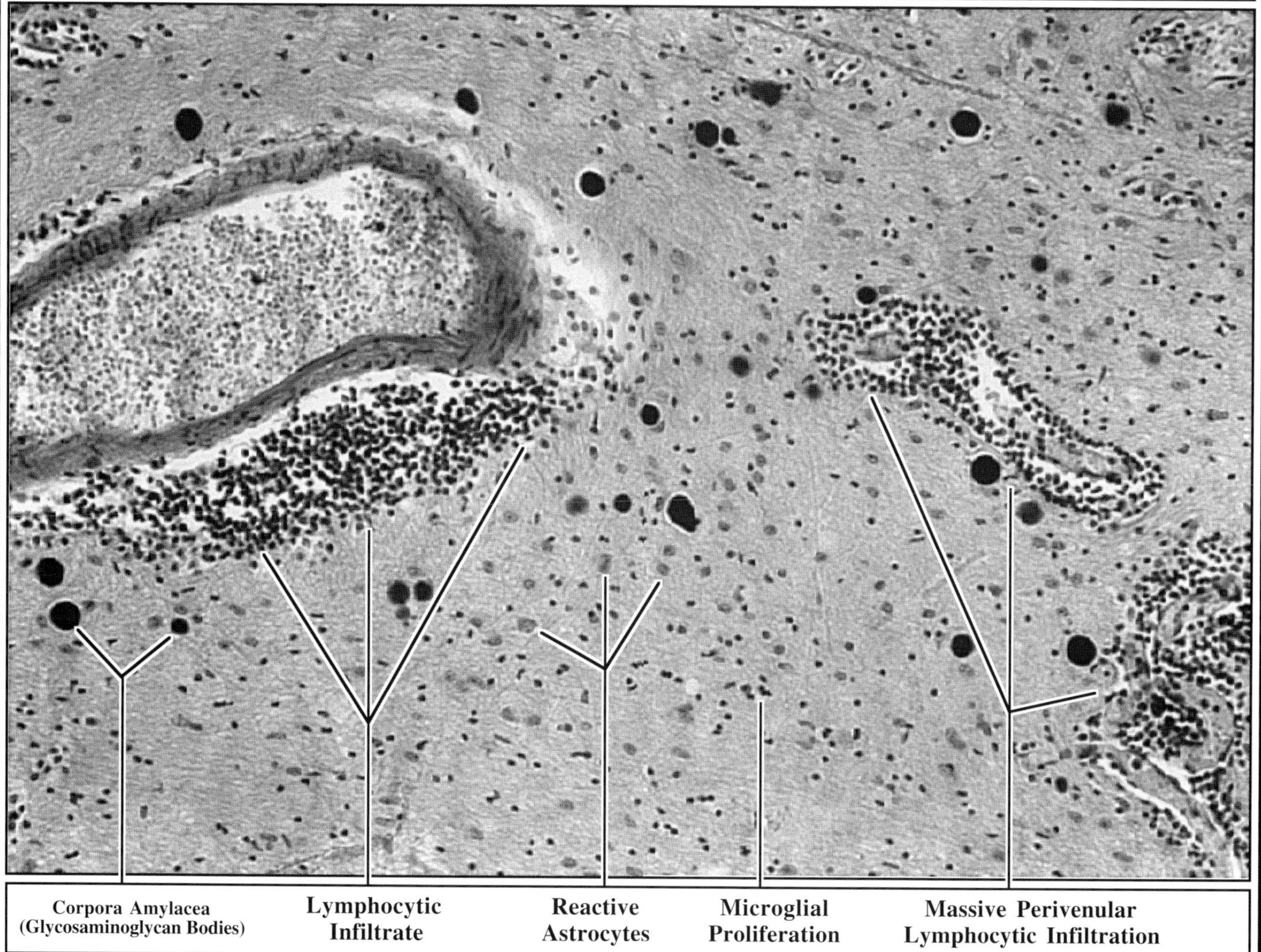

Corpora Amylacea (Glycosaminoglycan Bodies) | Lymphocytic Infiltrate | Reactive Astrocytes | Microglial Proliferation | Massive Perivenular Lymphocytic Infiltration

ETIOLOGY AND HISTOPATHOLOGY OF MULTIPLE SCLEROSIS

An interesting epidemiologic factor in M.S. involves the influence of geographic origin. With a prevalence of 1 per 100,000 in equatorial regions, 6 to 14 per 100,000 in the southern United States and southern Europe, and 30 to 80 per 100,000 in Canada, northern Europe, and the northern United States, a latitudinal gradient is clearly observed. A less well-defined latitudinal gradient has been demonstrated in the southern hemisphere. The precipitating factors of M.S. are complex and raise questions regarding the pathogenesis of this disease. The possibility of more than one disease entity producing the clinical manifestations of M.S. has been an active area of investigation. However, most of the clinical and basic science research into the mechanisms of M.S. and related demyelinating diseases supports an autoimmune pathogenesis.

The pathologic findings of M.S. are also consistent with an autoimmune etiology. Histologic findings depend upon the age of the demyelinating lesion. Acute or recent lesions demonstrate areas of myelin loss that range from perivascular (venous) foci to larger regions formed by the confluence of multiple foci. Axons are relatively spared in areas of early demyelination. Initially, there is a variable degeneration of oligodendroglia. Perivascular infiltrates of mononuclear cells and lymphocytes characterize acute lesions. At subsequent stages, reactive astrocytic proliferation continues, and transformation of microglia is associated with macrophage accumulation. Lesions in later stages (chronic or long-term) are characterized by astrocytosis, fibrous gliosis, diminished cellularity, and variable sparing of axonal processes. Lesions associated with a massive inflammatory response and edema often demonstrate axonal disruption and secondary degenerative changes. A predilection for periventricular white matter may be related to the presence of subependymal veins lining the ventricles (especially adjacent to the lateral ventricles).

BINSWANGER'S DISEASE: CLINICOPATHOLOGIC CORRELATIONS OF SUBCORTICAL ISCHEMIC DEMYELINATION

Binswanger's disease has classically been defined by the presence of subcortical arteriolar sclerosis, ischemic periventricular leukoencephalopathy, and a "frontal-subcortical" type dementia. The clinical course is often characterized by progressive dementia, accompanied by a stepwise decline in neurologic function, suggestive of the occurrence of small cerebral infarcts or subcortical lacunes. The subtle and often transient symptomatology of these infarcts might be either unrecognized or misdiagnosed as transient ischemic attacks or reversible ischemic neurologic deficits. However, this clinical course appears to correlate with the pathology of Binswanger's disease, which includes not only the finding of subcortical arteriolar sclerosis, but of leukomalacia in the white matter adjacent to the lateral ventricles. This diffuse change may be accompanied by microinfarctions or focal areas of ischemic change with patchy necrosis.

The pathologic finding of myelin loss in periventricular white matter has been termed ischemic demyelination. This term is also used by neuroradiologists to describe certain periventricular white matter changes observed on computerized tomography and magnetic resonance imaging. However, ischemic demyelination remains a pathologic diagnosis. With the refinements in magnetic resonance imaging and its increasing use in neurodiagnostic evaluations, the detection of white matter changes has become more prevalent. The specificity of these changes as well as their clinical and pathologic significance remains to be determined. The term leukoaraiosis has been used to describe the radiologic findings of decreased attenuation of periventricular white matter on CT and increased signal intensity on T2-weighted magnetic resonance imaging with sparing of subcortical white matter. This term has also been associated with specific white matter changes characteristic of Binswanger's disease.

NEUROBEHAVIOURAL TESTING IN A PATIENT WITH BINSWANGER'S DISEASE

Neurobehavioural testing revealed a tendency for perseveration (refer to the patient's copy of the house and attempted cube drawing). Many perseverative responses were affixed to the original (stimulus) figures, demonstrating the "stimulus-bound" phenomenon with an inability to generate independent components of the drawing.

This finding was accompanied by elements of perseveration throughout the examination, including verbal tasks and sensory, motor, and cerebellar testing (requiring the patient to respond to questions and/or commands).

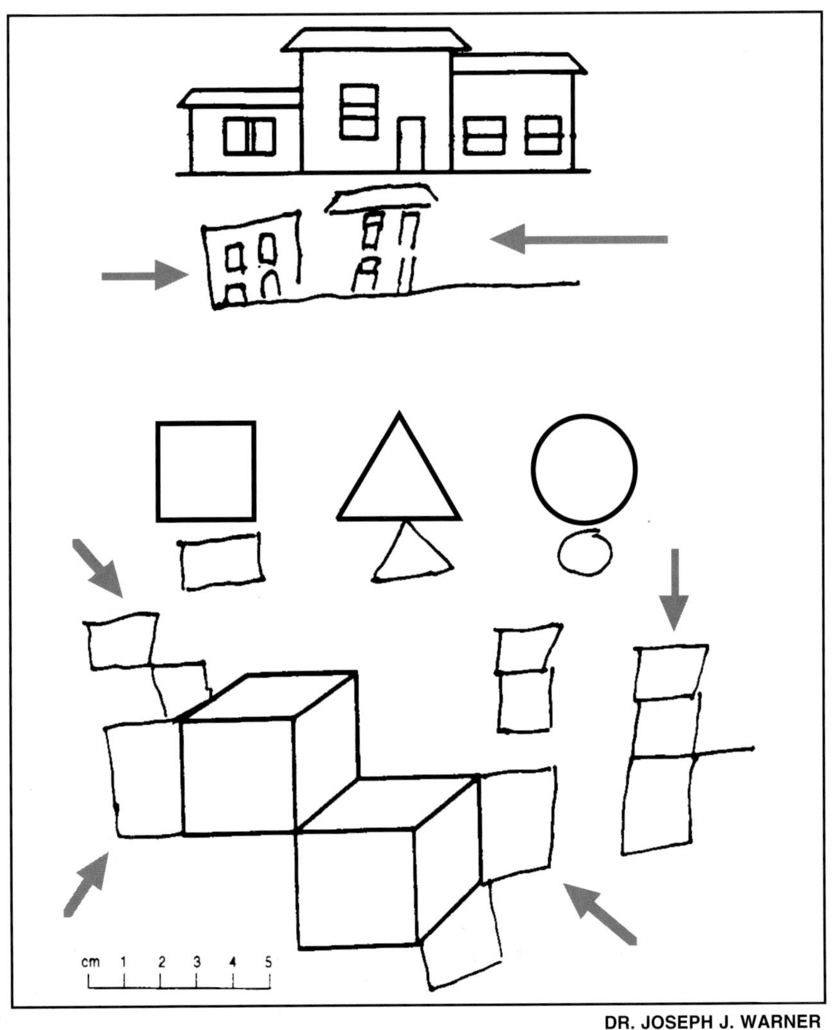

BINSWANGER'S DISEASE: CLINICOPATHOLOGIC CORRELATIONS

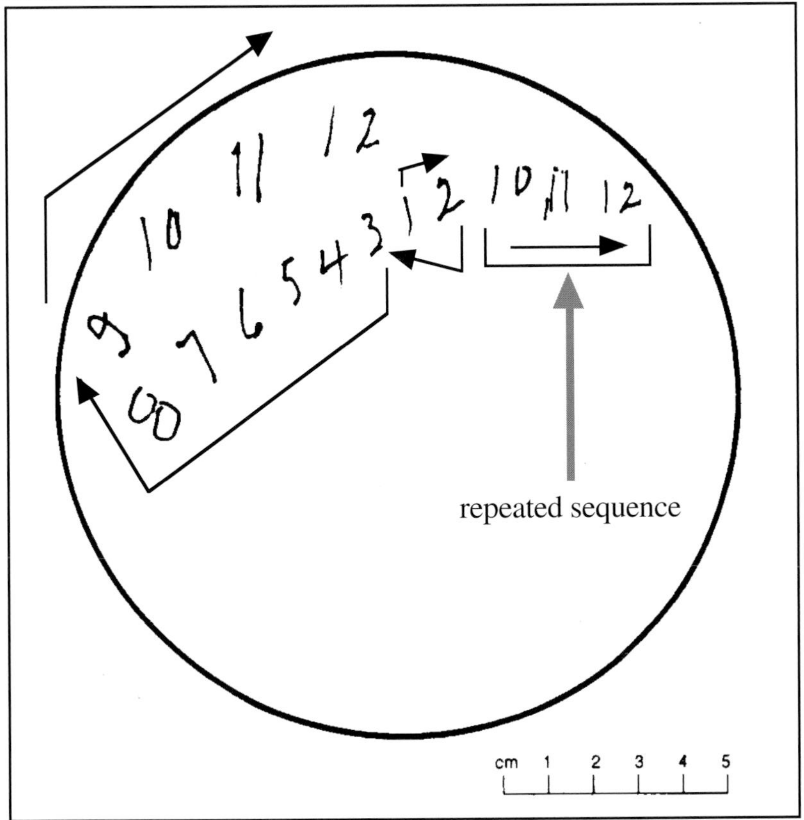

NEUROBEHAVIOURAL TESTING IN A PATIENT WITH BINSWANGER'S DISEASE (Continued)

In this task, the patient was requested to construct a clock face within the circle provided. The patient's response is shown, which is characterized by severe visuospatial disorganization. Perseveration was evident as the patient repeated the sequence "10 - 11 - 12" (refer to figure). The arrows indicate the order in which the patient placed the numbers in the clock face.

PATHOGENESIS

On pathologic examination, the brain may appear externally normal. However, cerebral atrophy is a frequent finding. On cut section, the white matter is characterized by a softened consistency, often with focal zones of necrosis or cavitation consistent with microinfarction. Central atrophy accompanied by ventricular enlargement is commonly observed. The initial white matter change may consist of a pallor in myelin staining with a decrease in the number of oligodendrocytes with varying degrees of astrocytic proliferation. Fiber loss is observed in advanced cases, attributable either to severe demyelination or to diffuse subcortical ischemia. It has been proposed on this basis that Binswanger's disease represents a "disconnection dementia" with secondary cortical atrophy. The primary pathogenetic factor is thought to be related to a transarteriolar diffusion barrier rather than arterial occlusive disease.

Figure copying (refer to figure below) again demonstrated a tendency for the patient to "attach" her responses to the stimulus figure. The patient tended to "dissect" the flower, copying individual details without synthesizing an independent figure. Constructional apraxia is evident.

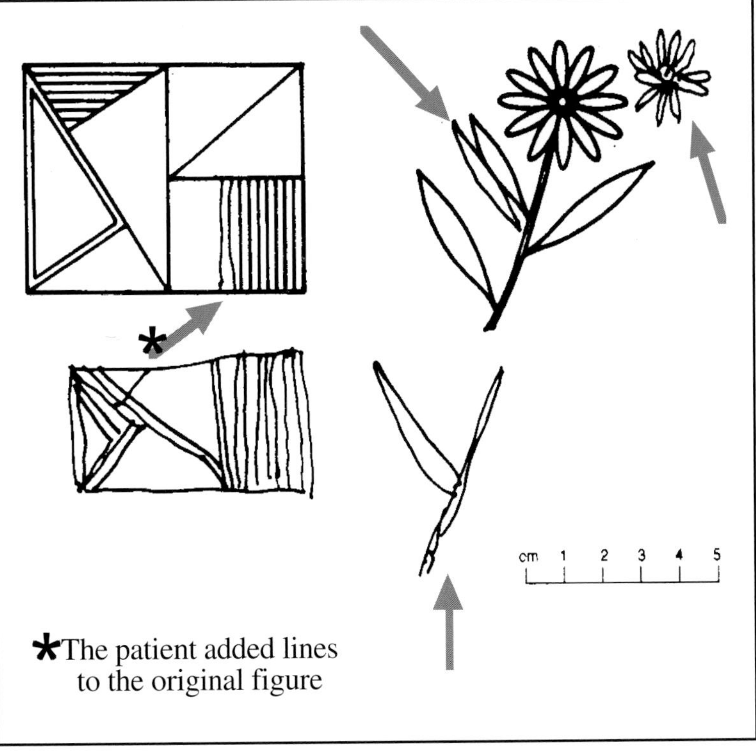

*The patient added lines to the original figure

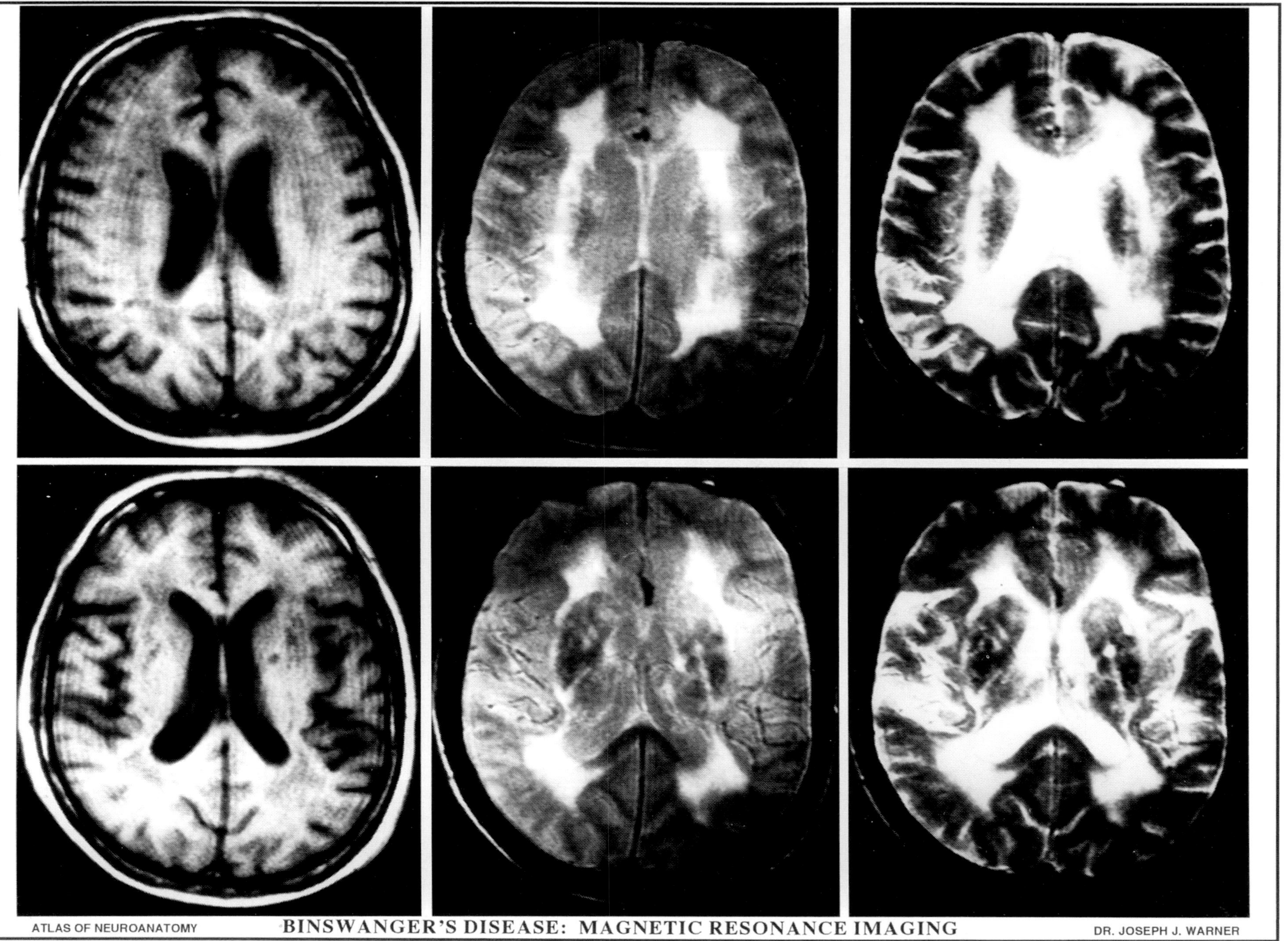

BINSWANGER'S DISEASE: MAGNETIC RESONANCE IMAGING

SUBCORTICAL ARTERIOLAR SCLEROSIS IN A CASE OF BINSWANGER'S DISEASE (ROSTRAL CENTRUM SEMIOVALE)

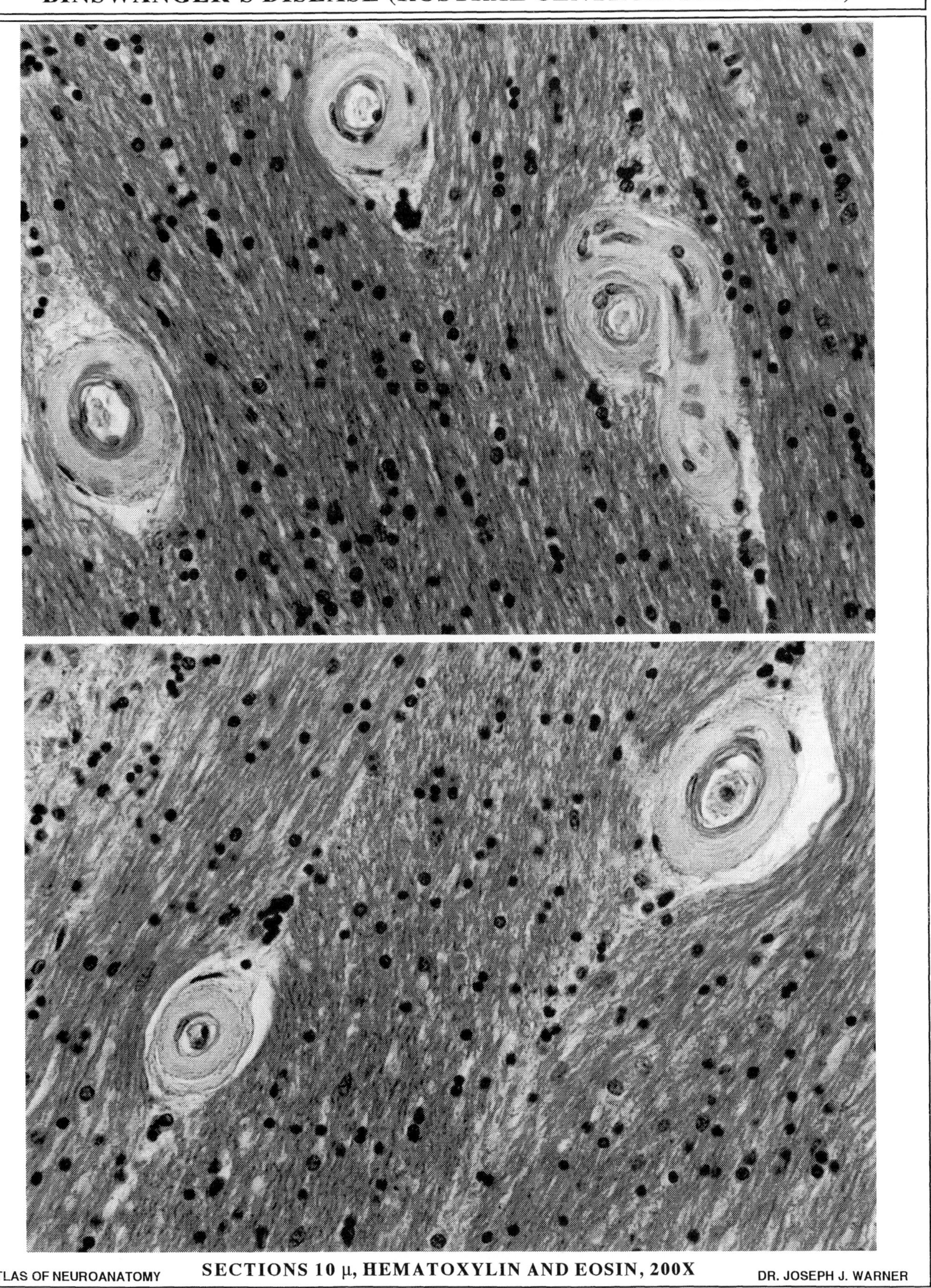

SECTIONS 10 μ, HEMATOXYLIN AND EOSIN, 200X

ALZHEIMER'S DISEASE: CORONAL SECTION OF THE BRAIN AT THE LEVEL OF THE MAMMILLARY BODIES AND THE ANTERIOR NUCLEUS OF THE THALAMUS

A

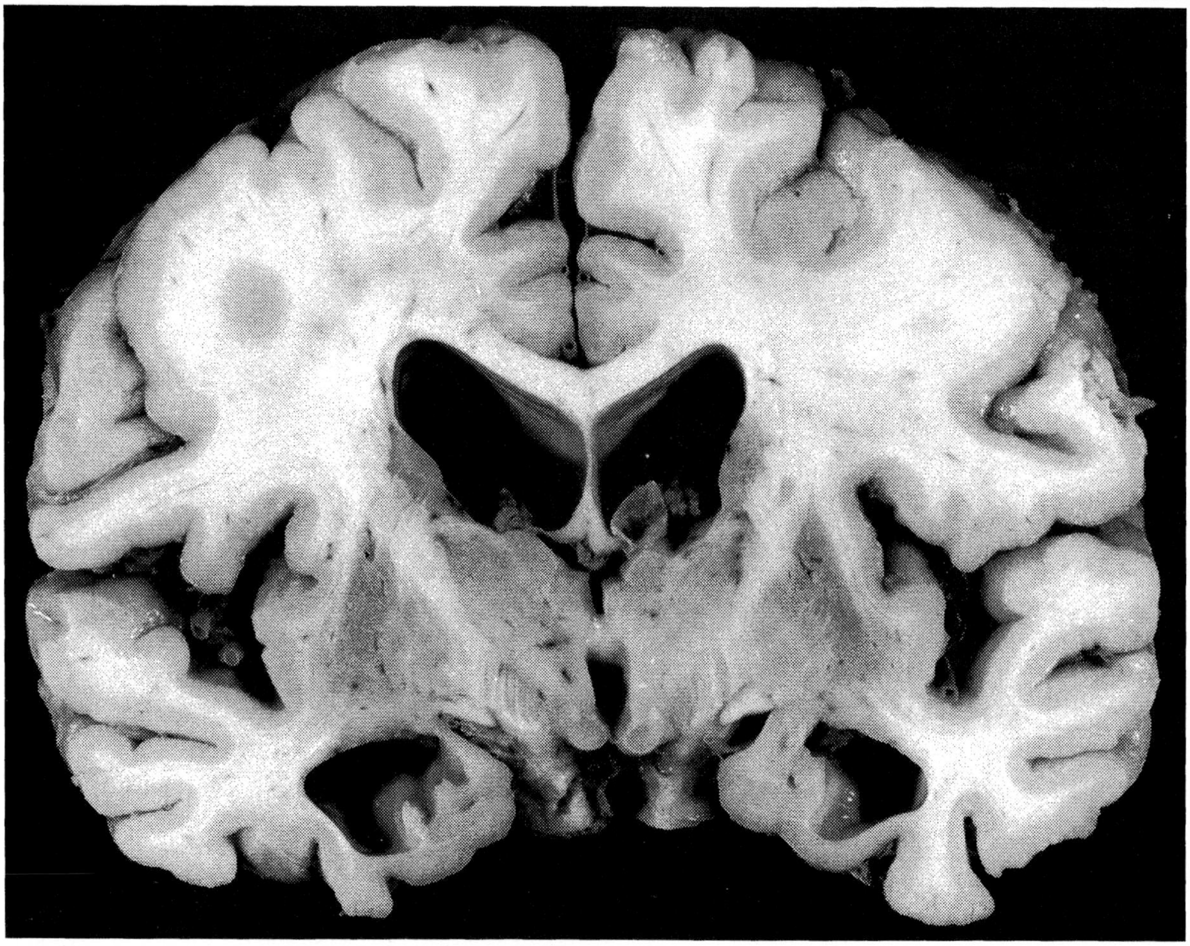

Coronal section, case of Alzheimer's Disease (A)
Coronal section from a control subject (B)
(Refer to section map [C] on the sagittal diagram).

This gross coronal section of the brain (A) from a patient with Alzheimer's disease demonstrates moderate atrophy of the cortex, thalamus and basal ganglia, with widening of the Sylvian fissure and ventricular enlargement. There is severe degeneration of the hippocampal formation. A control section (B) at the same level and orientation (C) is included for comparison.

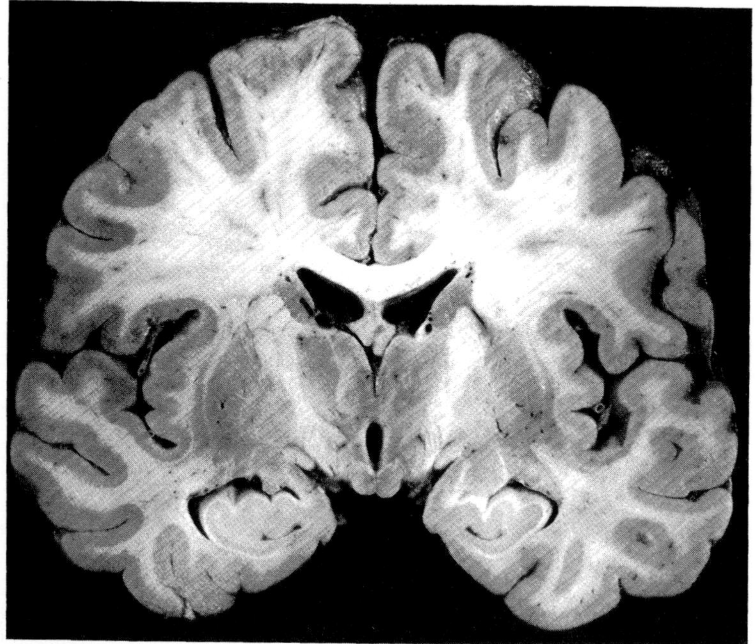

B

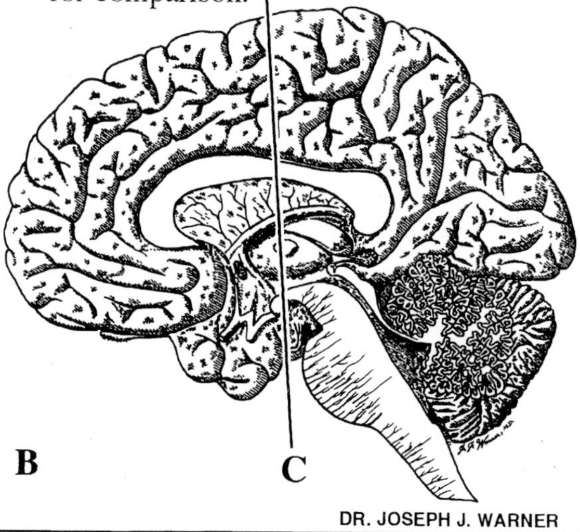

C

GROSS CORONAL SECTIONS: (A) NORMAL BRAIN; (B) ALZHEIMER'S DISEASE

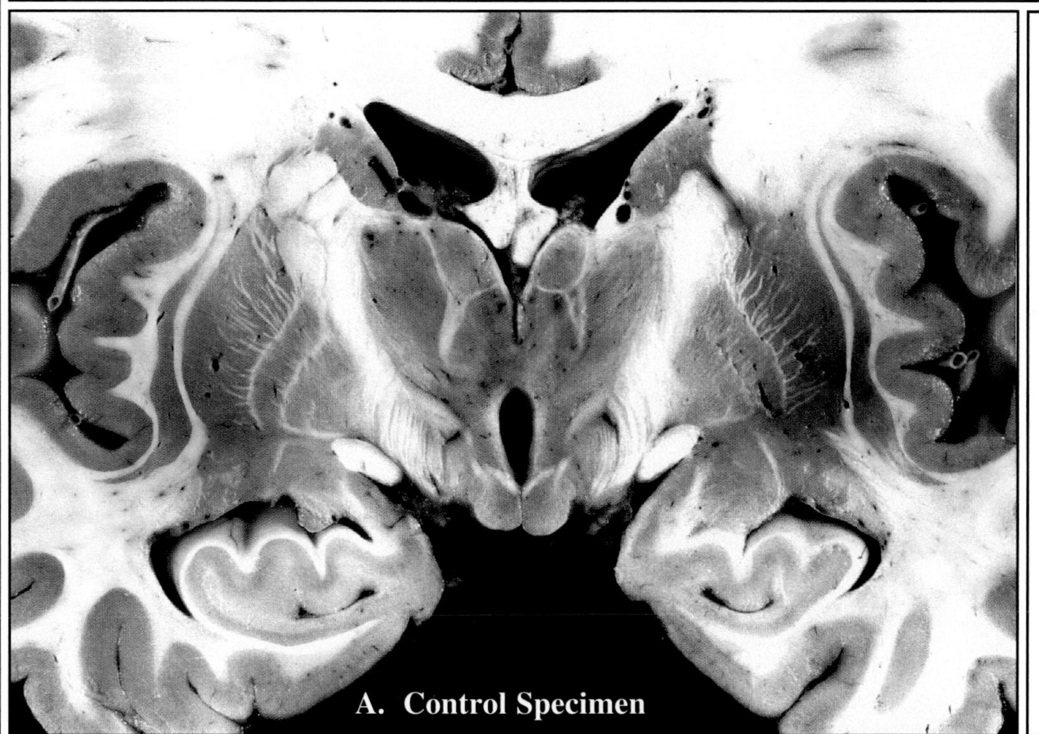

A. Control Specimen

CORONAL SECTIONS: LEVEL OF THE ANTERIOR NUCLEUS OF THE THALAMUS AND THE MAMMILLARY BODIES

Severe atrophy of the hippocampus is clearly shown on section B. Cerebral atrophy is evident, with widening of the Sylvian fissure, loss of normal gyral morphology in the insula, and ventriculomegaly. Corresponding Kluver-Barrera stained sections from these gross specimens are presented on the following page.

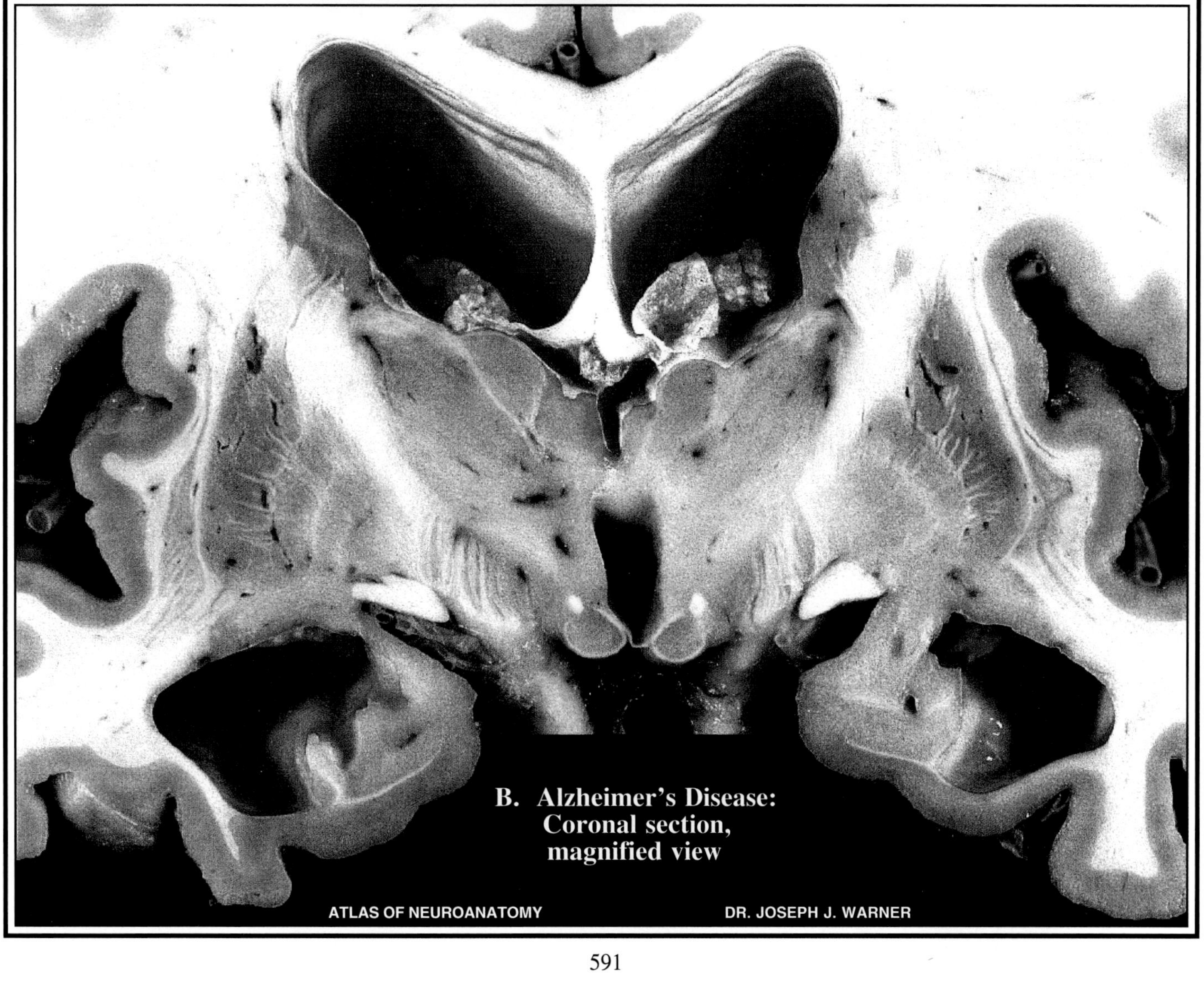

B. Alzheimer's Disease: Coronal section, magnified view

CORONAL HISTOLOGIC SECTIONS THROUGH THE ANTERIOR NUCLEUS OF THE THALAMUS: A DIRECT COMPARISON BETWEEN A NORMAL SUBJECT AND A CASE OF ALZHEIMER'S DISEASE

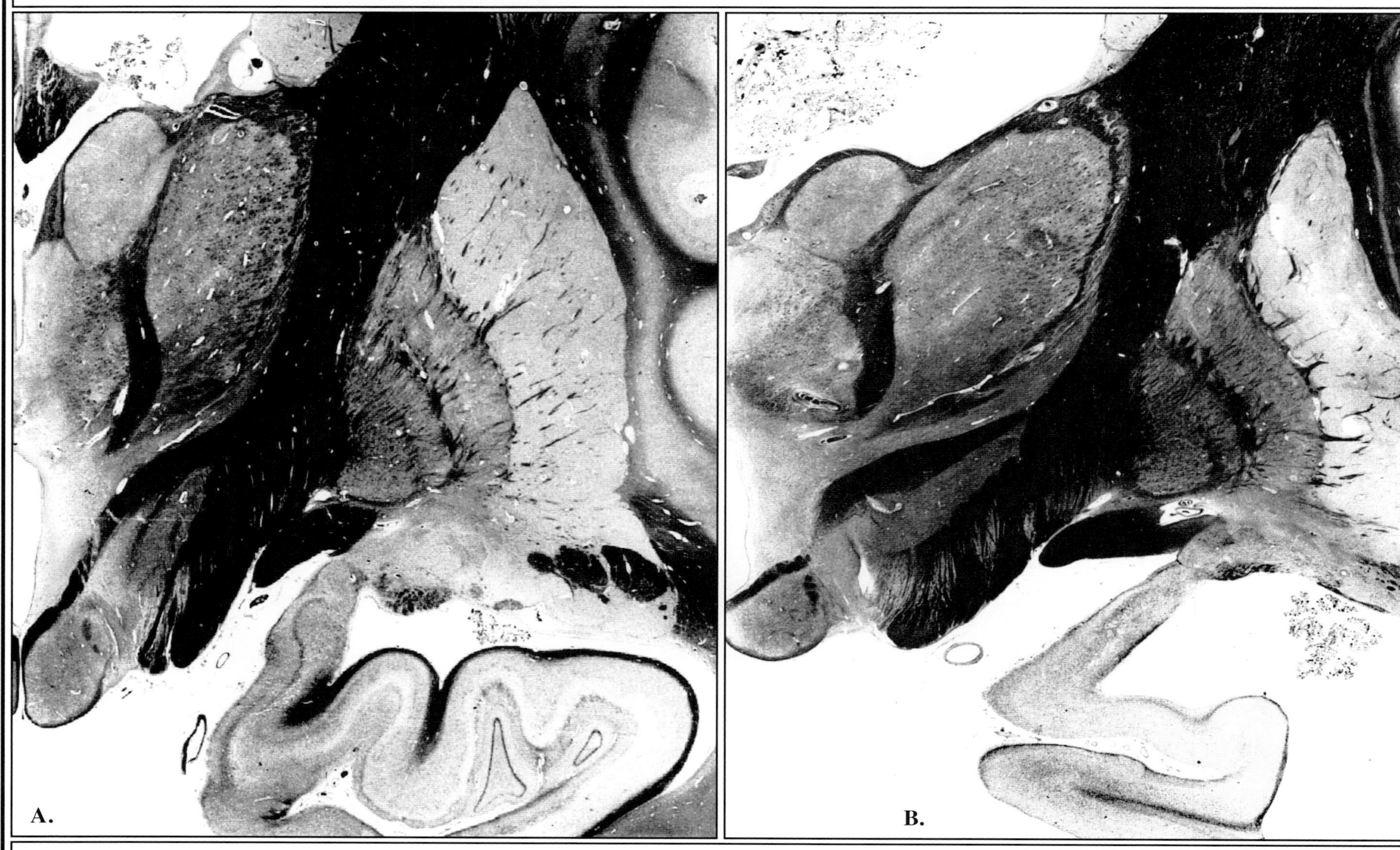

A direct comparison of a section from a case of Alzheimer's disease (B) and a normal brain (A) reveals several major abnormalities. The hippocampus, fornix, and parahippocampal gyrus are severely atrophic in the Alzheimer's case. Cerebral atrophy is accompanied by significant enlargement of the lateral ventricle. The putamen and caudate nucleus demonstrate areas of pallor and atrophy as well.

A and B: Coronal Sections, 15 μ, Kluver-Barrera Technique

HISTOPATHOLOGY OF ALZHEIMER'S DISEASE: NEURITIC PLAQUES

A

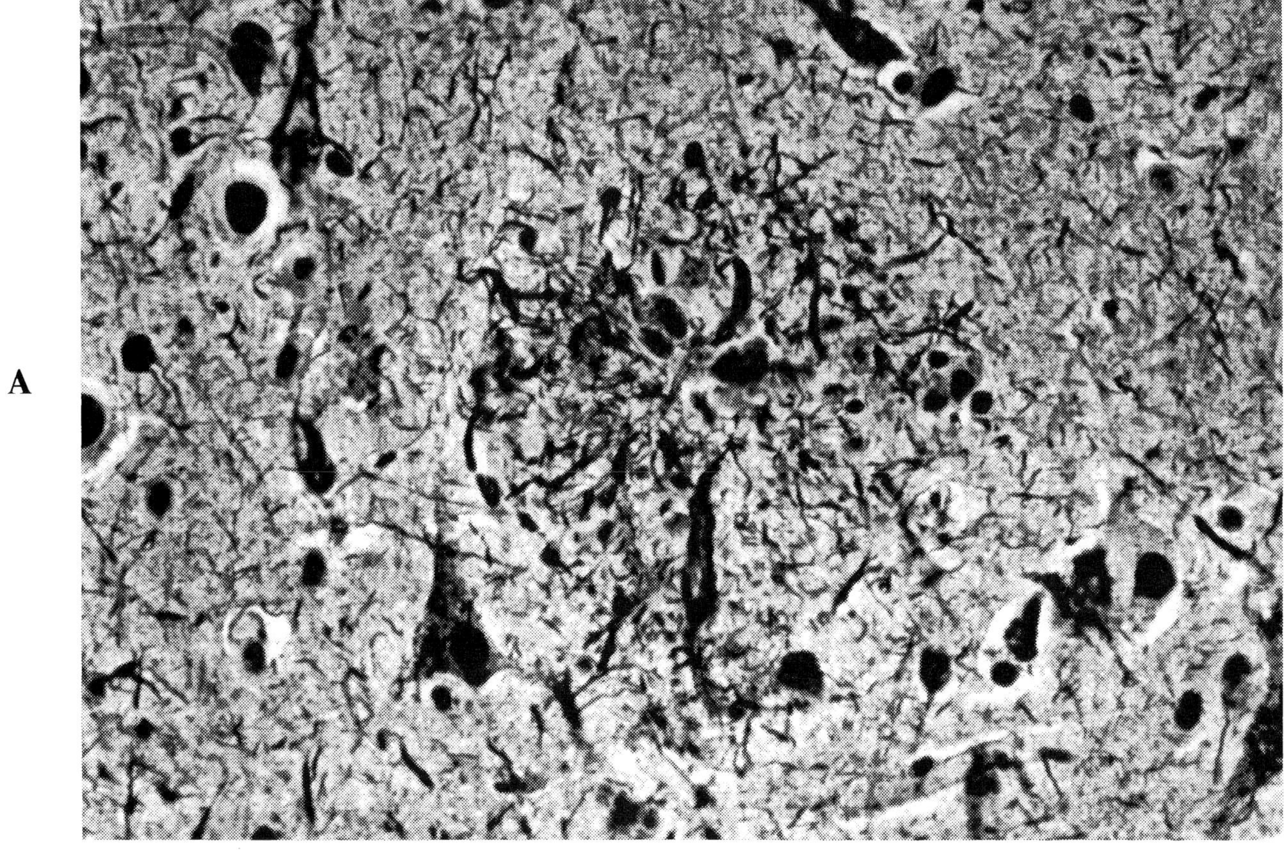

(A) Neuritic (Senile) Plaque, temporal neocortex, 12 μ section, Bodian silver stain, 400X

(B) Two neuritic plaques are demonstrated in this Bielschowsky silver-stained 12 μ section of frontal cortex, 400X. The plaque to the right has a well-defined amyloid core.

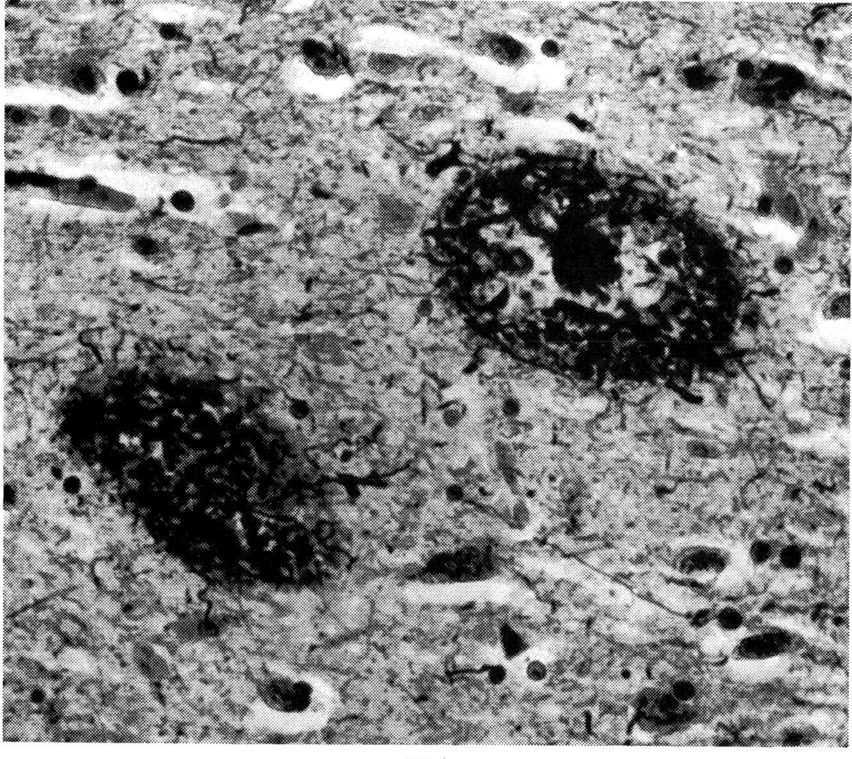

B

In 1907, Alzheimer reported the case of a 51-year-old female with a five year history of progressive dementia. He described miliary lesions in the brain characterized as clumping and distortion of fibrils in neuronal cytoplasm in Bielschowsky silver-impregnated sections. Miliary lesions were first described in senile brains in 1892 by Blocq and Marinesco. Such lesions were named "senile plaques" by Simchowicz in 1910.

Neuritic (senile) plaques consist of material associated with degenerated nerve terminals, including abnormal mitochondria, lysosomes, and dysmorphic or fragmented neurofibrils (components of dystrophic neurites). Plaques may be diffuse or may contain a well-defined amyloid core. Beta-amyloid protein deposition is associated with these degenerative lesions.

HISTOPATHOLOGY OF ALZHEIMER'S DISEASE: NEUROFIBRILLARY TANGLES AND GRANULOVACUOLAR DEGENERATION

Characteristic pathologic changes of Alzheimer's disease include the presence of neuritic plaques, neurofibrillary tangles, granulovacuolar degeneration, neuronal loss, and astrocytic proliferation. Neurofibrillary tangles are argyrophilic fibrillary deposits within neuronal cytoplasm (refer to figures A and C), shown by electron microscopy to consist of paired helical filaments. Granulovacuolar degeneration (refer to figures B and C) is characterized by the presence of intraneuronal vacuolar structures containing eosinophilic inclusions.

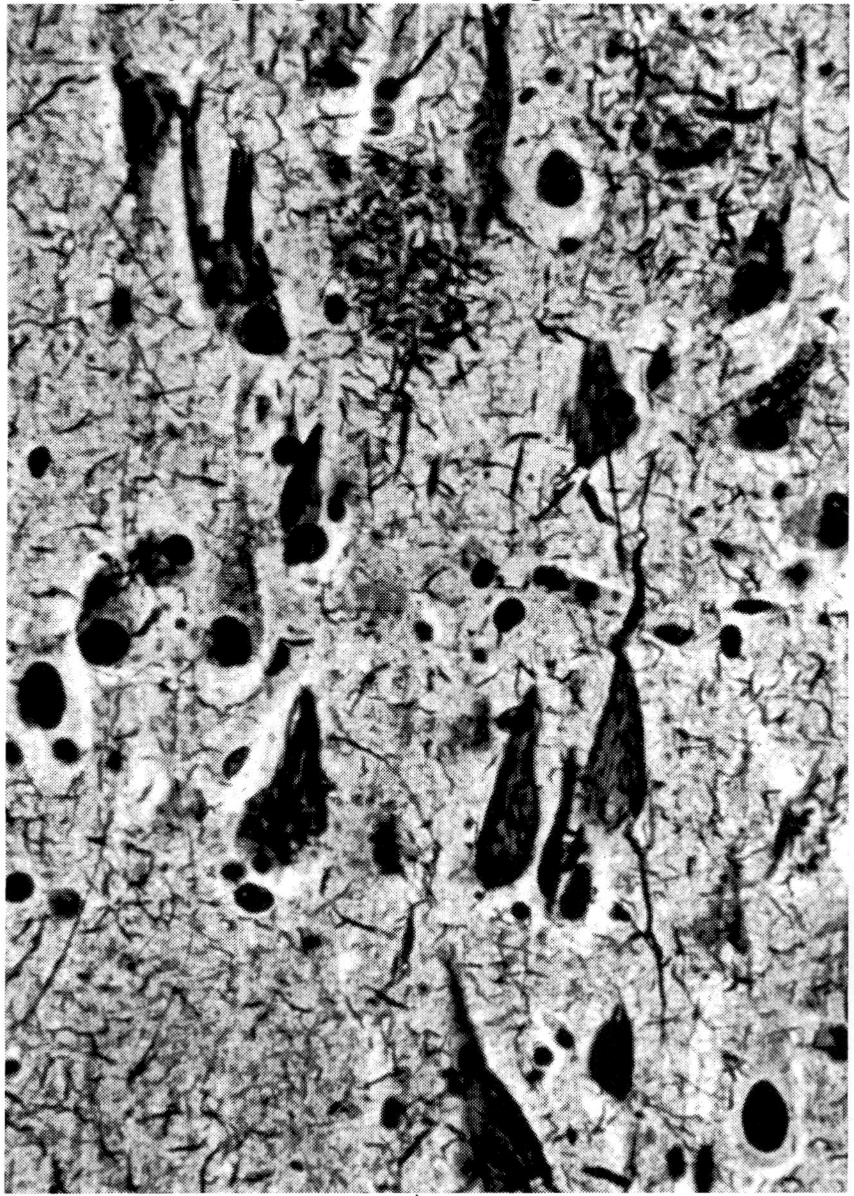

A. Neurofibrillary tangles within temporal cortical neurons, Bodian silver stain, 12 μ, 400X

B, C. Temporal cortex, Hematoxylin and Eosin, 12 μ, 400X

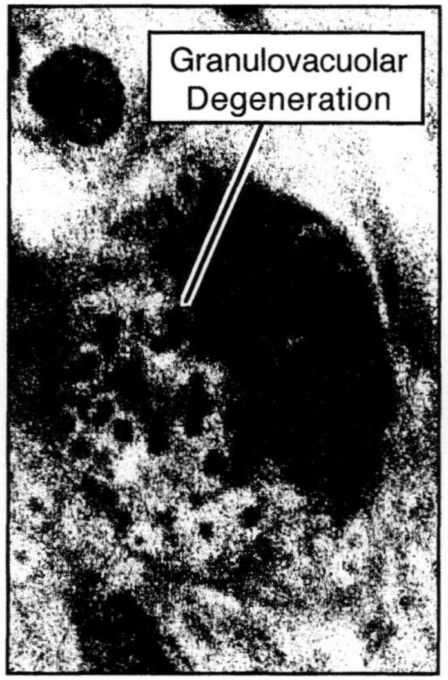

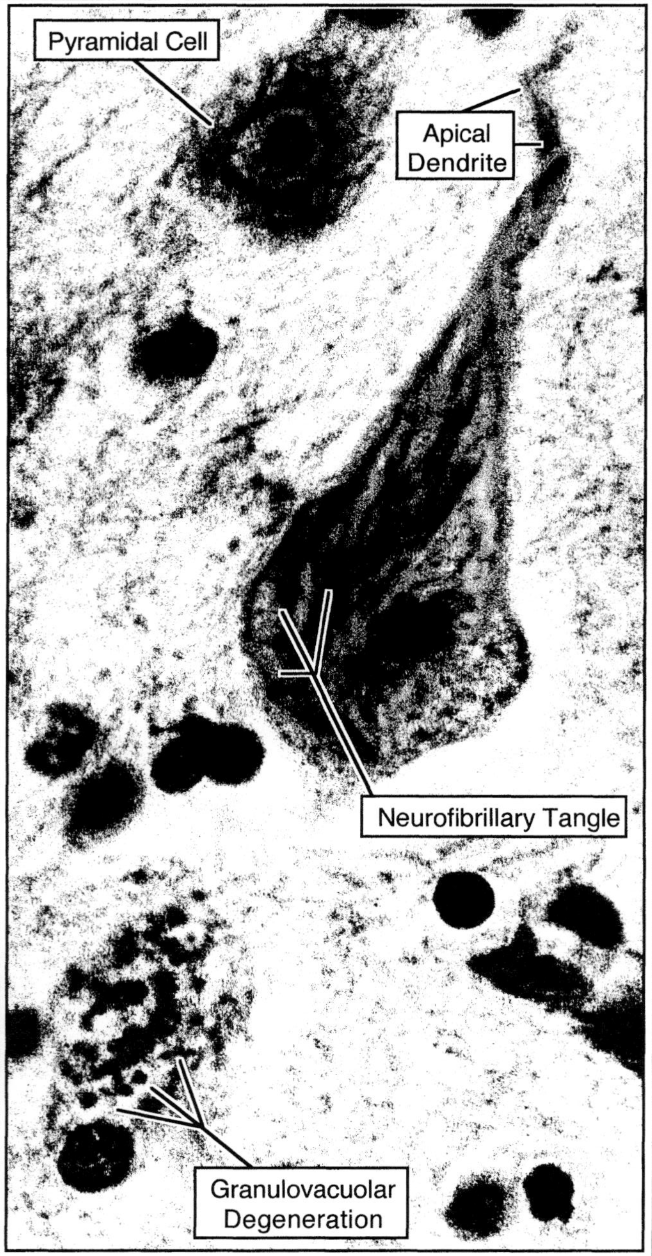

Granulovacuolar Degeneration

Pyramidal Cell

Apical Dendrite

Neurofibrillary Tangle

Granulovacuolar Degeneration

A

B

C

ALZHEIMER'S DISEASE: FRONTAL CORTEX, BIELSCHOWSKY SILVER STAIN 12 μ SECTION, 40X MAGNIFICATION

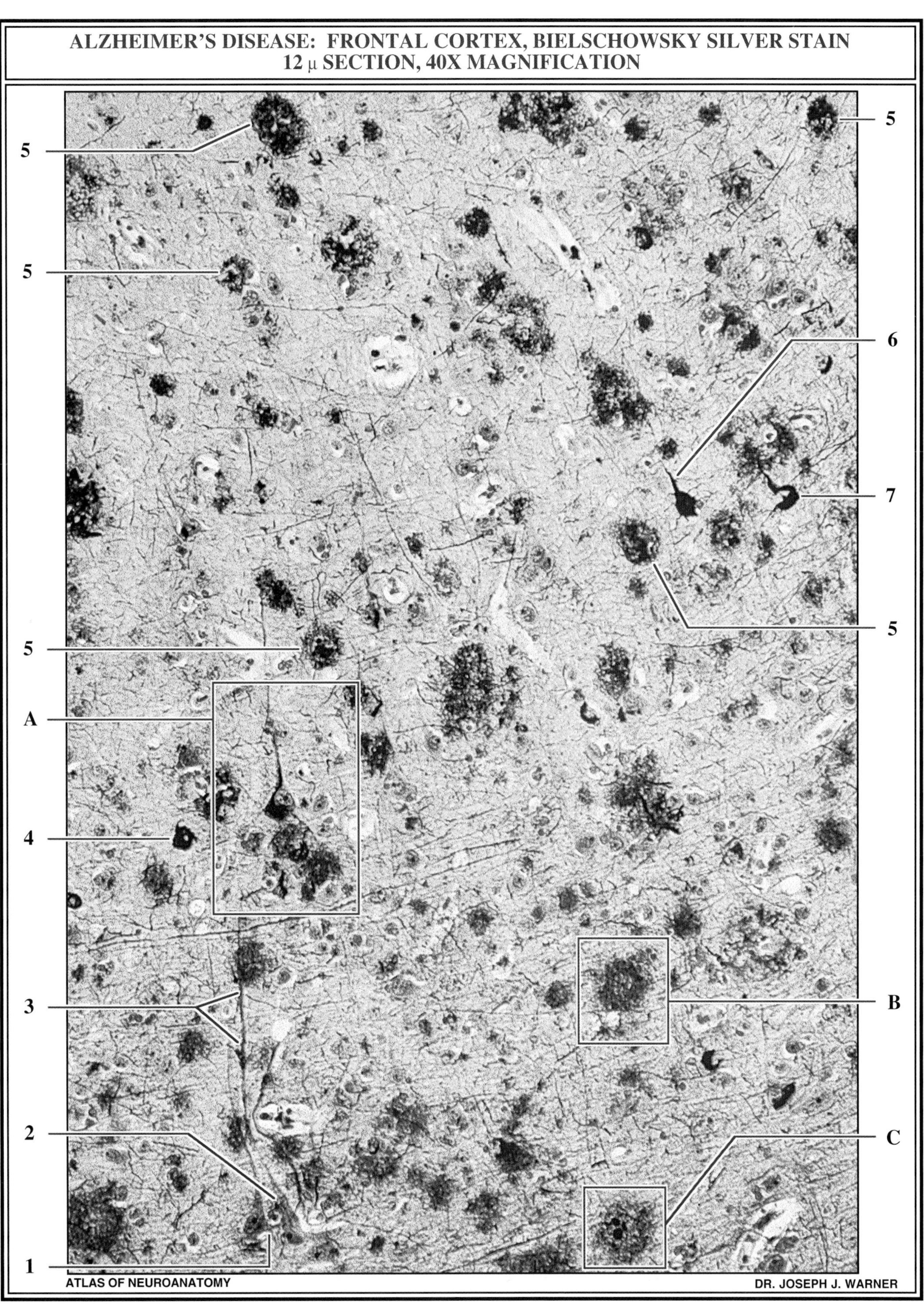

HISTOPATHOLOGIC CHANGES OF ALZHEIMER'S DISEASE: FRONTAL CORTEX, BIELSCHOWSKY SILVER STAIN

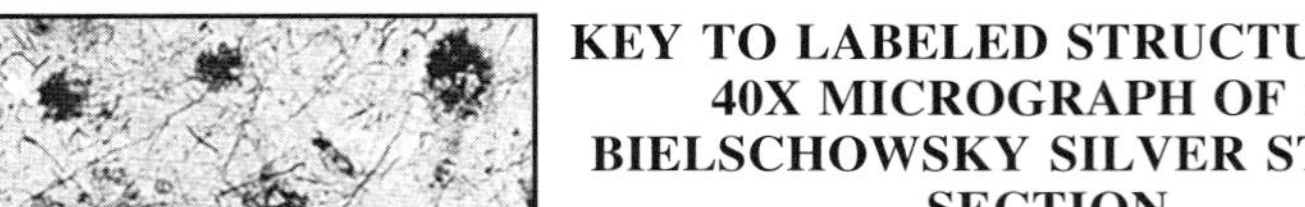

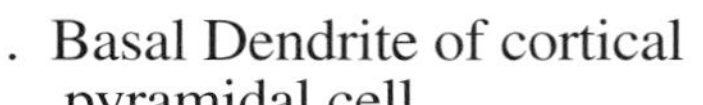

Frontal Cortex, 12 μ Section, Bielschowsky Silver stain, 40X

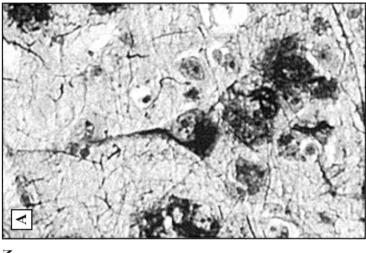

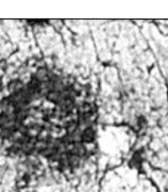

KEY TO LABELED STRUCTURES ON 40X MICROGRAPH OF 12μ BIELSCHOWSKY SILVER STAINED SECTION

1. Basal Dendrite of cortical pyramidal cell
2. Pyramidal cell body
3. Apical Dendrite of cortical pyramidal cell
4. Dense neurofibrillary tangle in degenerating pyramidal cell
5. Neuritic (Senile) Plaques
6. Apical Dendrite of pyramidal cell occupied by neurofibrillary tangle
7. Pyramidal cell body with neurofibrillary tangle

A. Neurofibrillary Tangle within a cortical pyramidal cell

B, C. Neuritic plaques, each with a well-defined amyloid core

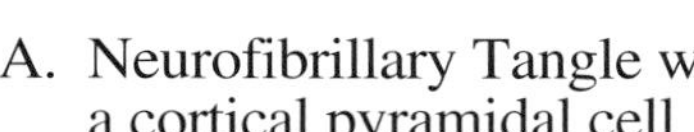

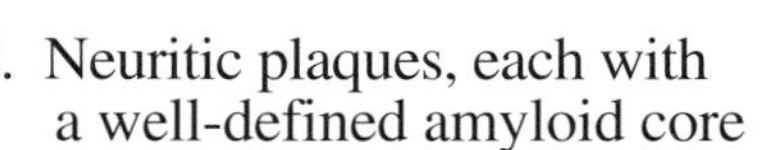

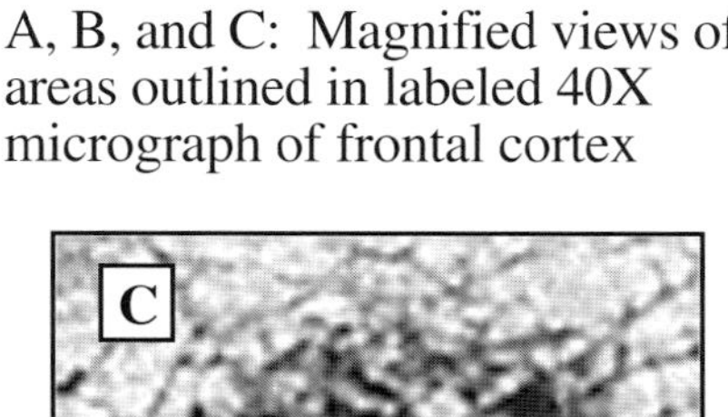

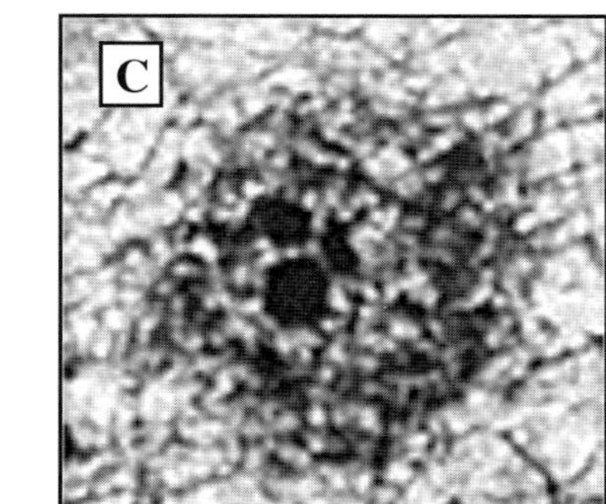

A, B, and C: Magnified views of areas outlined in labeled 40X micrograph of frontal cortex

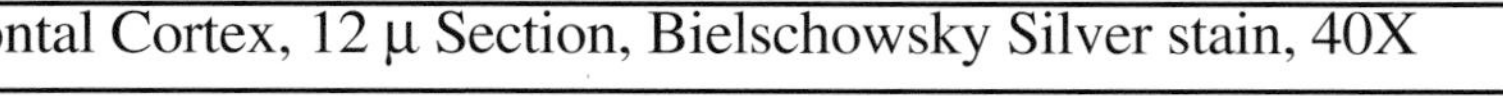

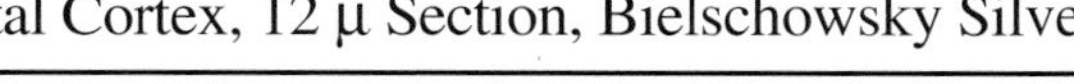

THE HIPPOCAMPAL PYRAMIDAL CELL LAYER: COMPARATIVE HISTOLOGY OF A NORMAL SUBJECT AND A CASE OF ALZHEIMER'S DISEASE

A

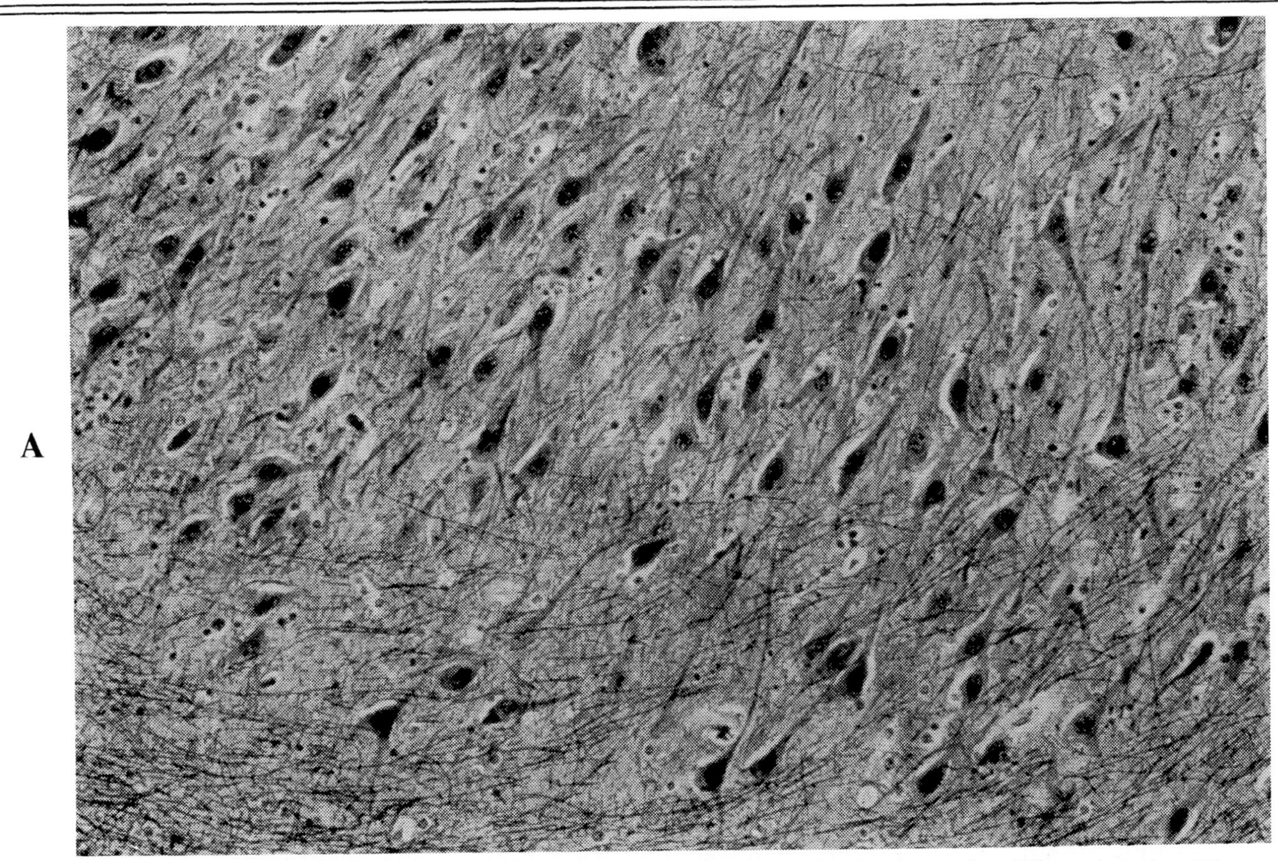

Hippocampal Formation, Pyramidal Cell Layer: Bielschowsky Silver stain, 12 μ section, 100X; from a Control subject (A) and case of Alzheimer's Disease (B)

B

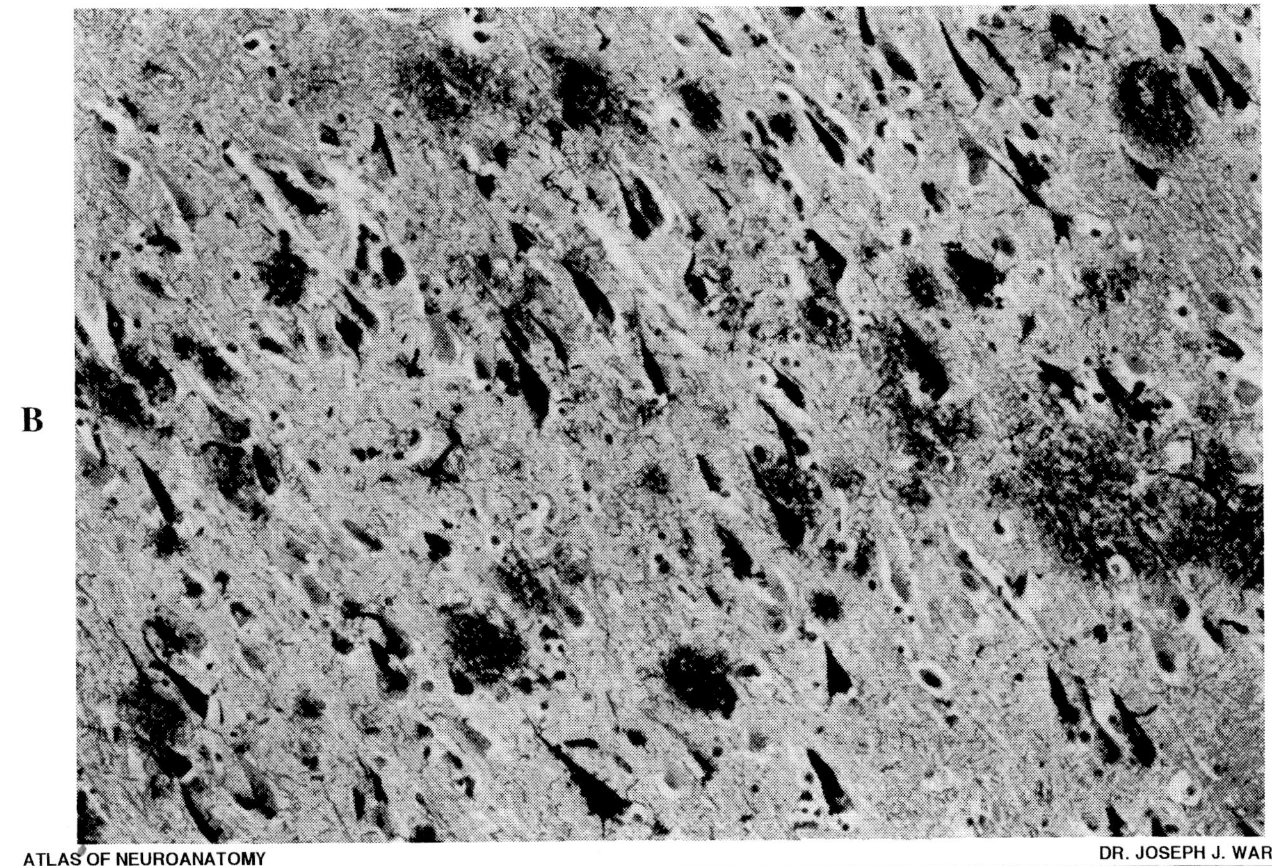

ALZHEIMER'S DISEASE: BIELSCHOWSKY SILVER STAINED SECTIONS OF THE HIPPOCAMPUS AND TEMPORAL NEOCORTEX

A.

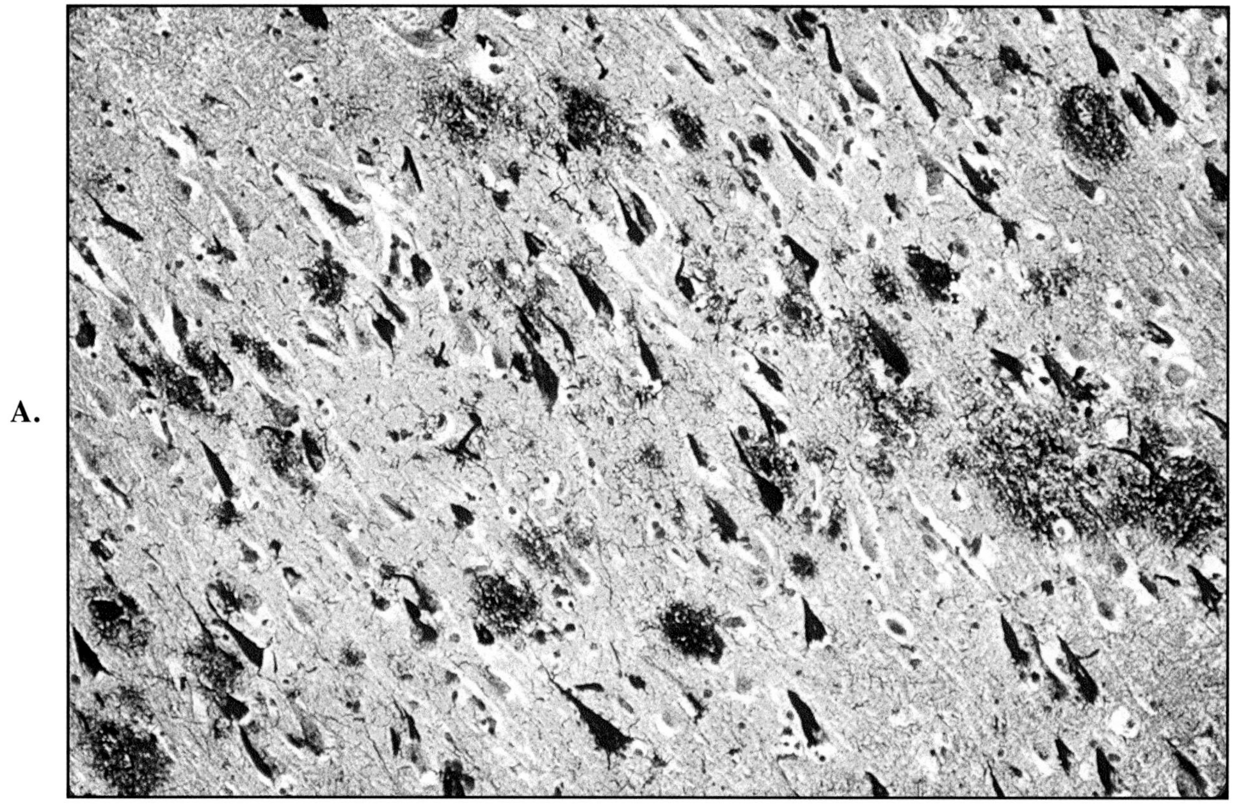

A. Hippocampal formation: argyrophilic neurofibrillary tangles occupy the majority of the pyramidal cells, with interspersed neuritic plaques; 100X
B. Temporal neocortex: neuritic (senile) plaque with a well-defined core; 400X

B.

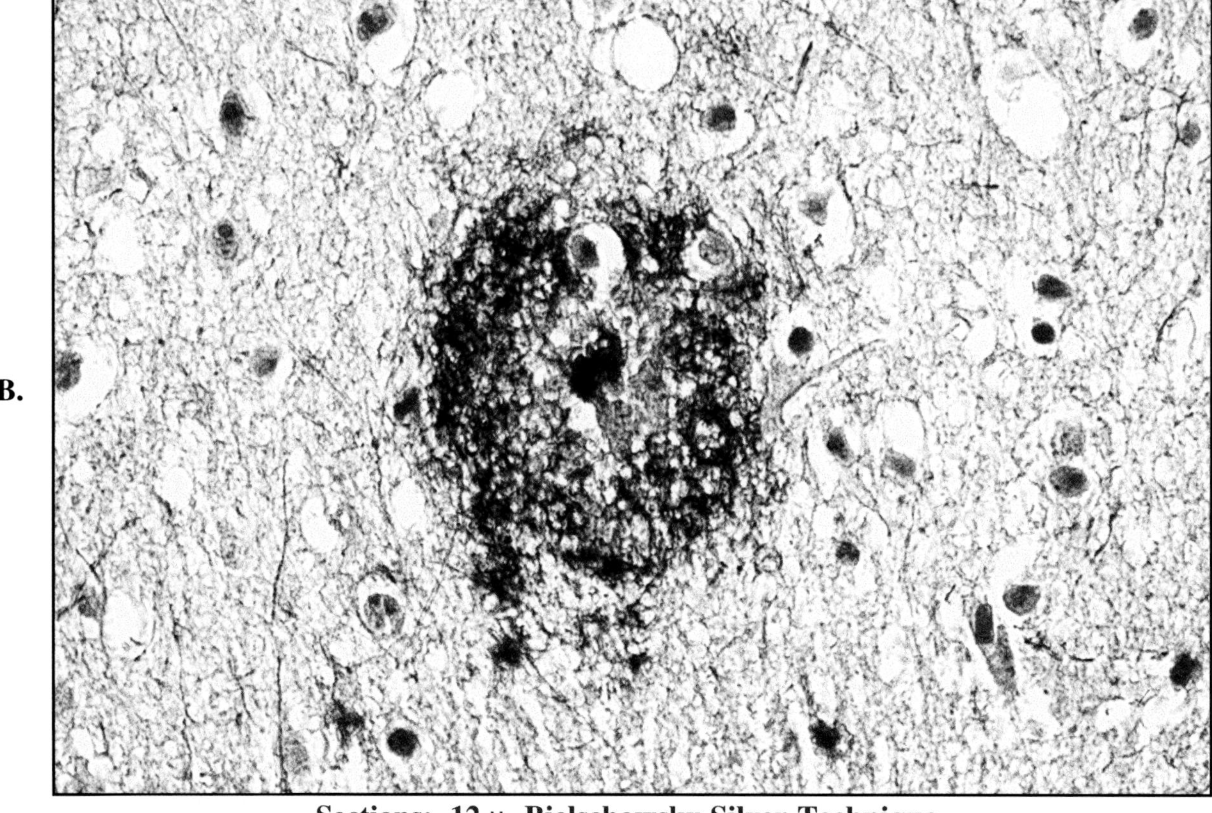

Sections: 12 μ, Bielschowsky Silver Technique

Dear mother: Friday nite Jan 9th

Just a line to tell you I am fine! I am fine.. Just a line to tell you I am fine. I am fine Just to tell you I am fine, There's a word to tell you I am fine there's a note to tell you I am fine, I am fine to tell you that I am fine. Just a note to tell you I am fine, There's a note to tell you I am fine.

Just a note to tell you I am fine. Just a note to tell you I am fine.

There's a note to tell you I am fine. There's a note to tell you I am fine. There's a note to tell you I am fine. There's a note to tell you I am fine. There's a note to tell you I am fine. There's a note to tell you I am fine. There's a note to tell you I am fine.

Letter written by the patient to his deceased mother (page 1)

CASE PRESENTATION

Clinical History

This 55-year-old male presented with a history of "personality changes" including irritability, agitation, and inappropriate social behaviour. The patient became increasingly aggressive, and had begun to demonstrate "bad judgment" in his role as an assistant business manager. Family complained that he had "poor memory" with a marked tendency to repeat sentences and phrases in conversation and when asked questions.

Neurobehavioural Findings

Neurobehavioural testing revealed a marked tendency for perseveration (continuation of a response to a stimulus that is no longer appropriate). This was elicited throughout multiple verbal and nonverbal testing modalities, as well as during the elemental neurologic examination. The family brought a letter written by the patient to his deceased mother. The two-page letter demonstrated severe verbal perseveration (refer to figure).

Clinical Course

As the illness progressed, he developed a marked gait disturbance, with postural instability and gait apraxia. Repeat neurological examination revealed frontal release signs including a visual suck reflex, as well as snout and root reflex responses.

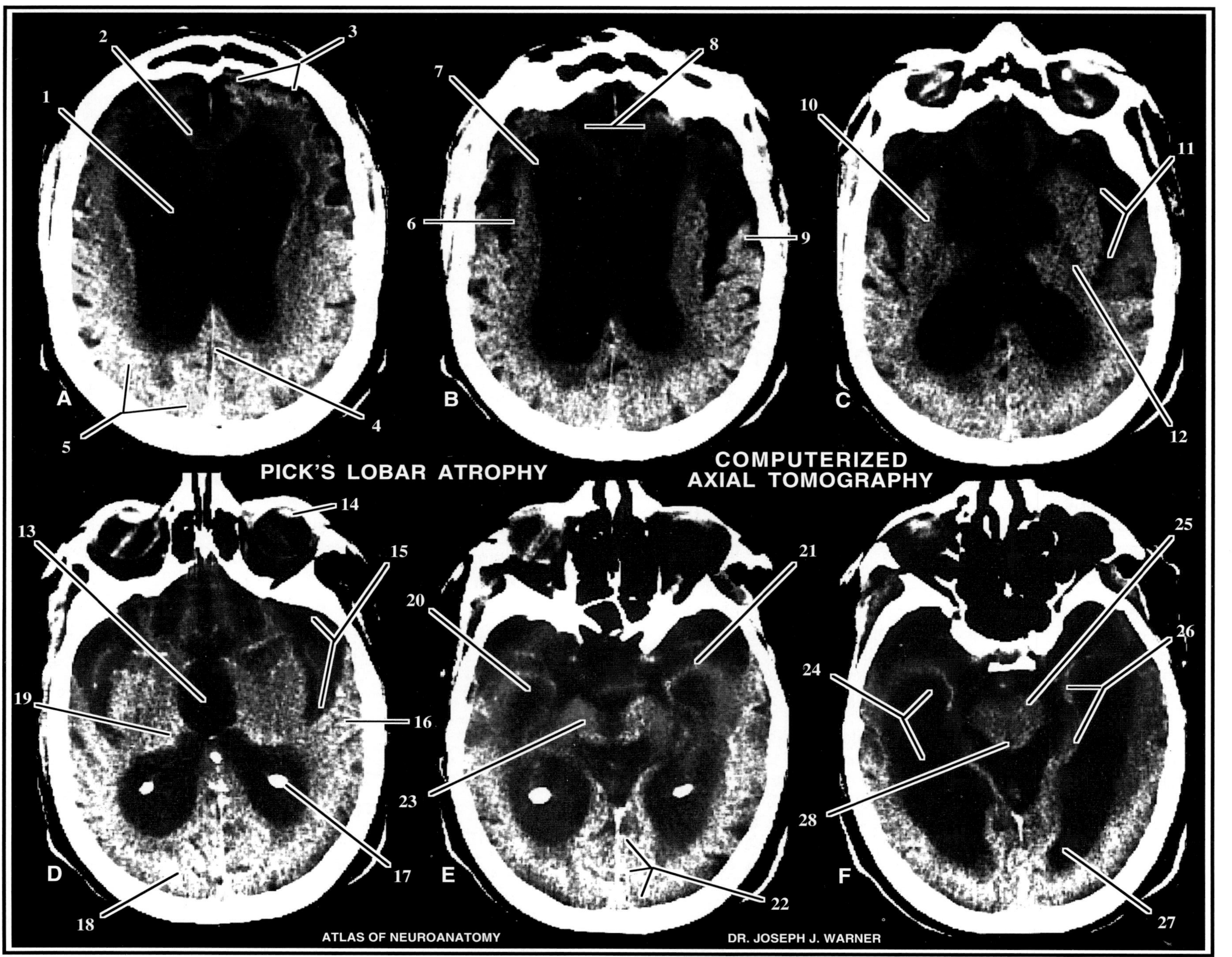
PICK'S LOBAR ATROPHY
COMPUTERIZED AXIAL TOMOGRAPHY
A
B
C
D
E
F
1
2
3
4
5
6
7
8
9
10
11
12
13
14
15
16
17
18
19
20
21
22
23
24
25
26
27
28
ATLAS OF NEUROANATOMY
DR. JOSEPH J. WARNER

All laboratory studies were normal, with the exception of electroencephalographic evidence of bilateral frontal and temporal theta and delta slow wave activity. Computerized tomography demonstrated marked atrophy involving the frontotemporal regions bilaterally, with central atrophy and ventriculomegaly. A clinical diagnosis of Pick's lobar atrophy was made on the basis of neurobehavioural findings including evidence of severe frontal lobe dysfunction, the progressive course, and the demonstration of disproportionate frontal and temporal atrophy on neuroimaging studies.

Subsequent computerized tomographic scanning revealed severe frontotemporal atrophy, and hydrocephalus "ex vacuo" associated with basal ganglia and thalamic degeneration. The parieto-occipital regions, although demonstrating mild atrophy, were relatively spared. (Refer to figure depicting representative images from this case and explanatory key to numbered structures.)

CASE: PICK'S LOBAR ATROPHY
KEY TO COMPUTERIZED TOMOGRAPHIC FINDINGS

1. Body of Lateral Ventricle
2. Corpus Callosum (attenuated and radiolucent)
3. Severe Frontal Cortical Atrophy
4. Falx Cerebri
5. Parieto-Occipital region (note the relative sparing in contrast to severe frontal atrophy)
6. Insula (cortical atrophy evident)
7. Anterior Horn of Lateral Ventricle (note severe ventriculomegaly with loss of the caudate density)
8. Widening of the rostral (frontal) aspect of the Interhemispheric Fissure
9. Temporal Lobe Neocortex
10. Atrophic remnant of Putamen, Anterior Limb of Internal Capsule, and Caudate Nucleus
11. Sylvian Fissure (widened)
12. Posterior Limb of Internal Capsule
13. Third Ventricle (severely enlarged)
14. Lens (rostral orbit)
15. Sylvian Fissure (widened)
16. Posterior Temporal region
17. Choroid Plexus in Atrium of Lateral Ventricle
18. Superior aspect, Occipital Lobe
19. Thalamus
20. Temporal Horn of Lateral Ventricle
21. Temporal Pole (atrophic)
22. Medial Occipital Lobe (note relative sparing)
23. Mesencephalic-Diencephalic Junction
24. Severe ventriculomegaly involving the Temporal Horn
25. Cerebral Peduncle, Caudal Mesencephalon
26. Hippocampus and Parahippocampal Gyrus
27. Occipital Pole, Lateral Ventricle
28. Aqueduct of Sylvius (normal)

Sections A through F are arranged in a dorsal to ventral sequence. Section orientation in these images approximates the plane parallel to the lateral aspect of the Sylvian fissures rather than the anatomically horizontal plane. This section orientation is optimal for visualization of structures of the temporal lobe, including a longitudinal view of the hippocampus and temporal (inferior) horn of the lateral ventricle. (Refer to diagram at right.)

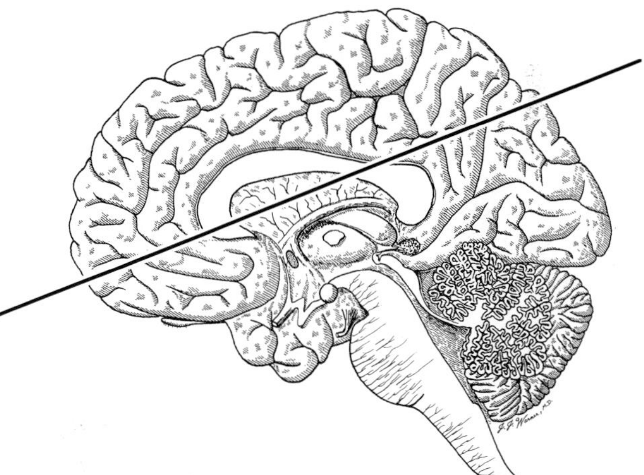

Pathologic Examination

Severe atrophy involved the frontal and temporal lobes to a disproportionately severe degree in comparison to other brain regions. The posterior aspect of the superior temporal gyrus and parieto-occipital regions were relatively spared. The insular cortex was grossly atrophic inferiorly, however only minimally affected superiorly. Severe central atrophy, with thalamic and basal ganglia degeneration, was accompanied by marked enlargement of the third ventricle. Together with the lobar atrophy, degeneration of deep gray matter structures was accompanied by significant ventriculomegaly. The aqueduct of Sylvius and fourth ventricle were not significantly enlarged. Histologic study revealed intense gliosis, neuronal loss, and Pick bodies. Few neuritic plaques or neurofibrillary tangles were discerned. No inflammatory changes of the meninges were evident, and the microvasculature appeared normal. The gross and histological findings confirmed the diagnosis of Pick's lobar atrophy.

PICK'S LOBAR ATROPHY: VENTRAL ASPECT OF THE BRAIN

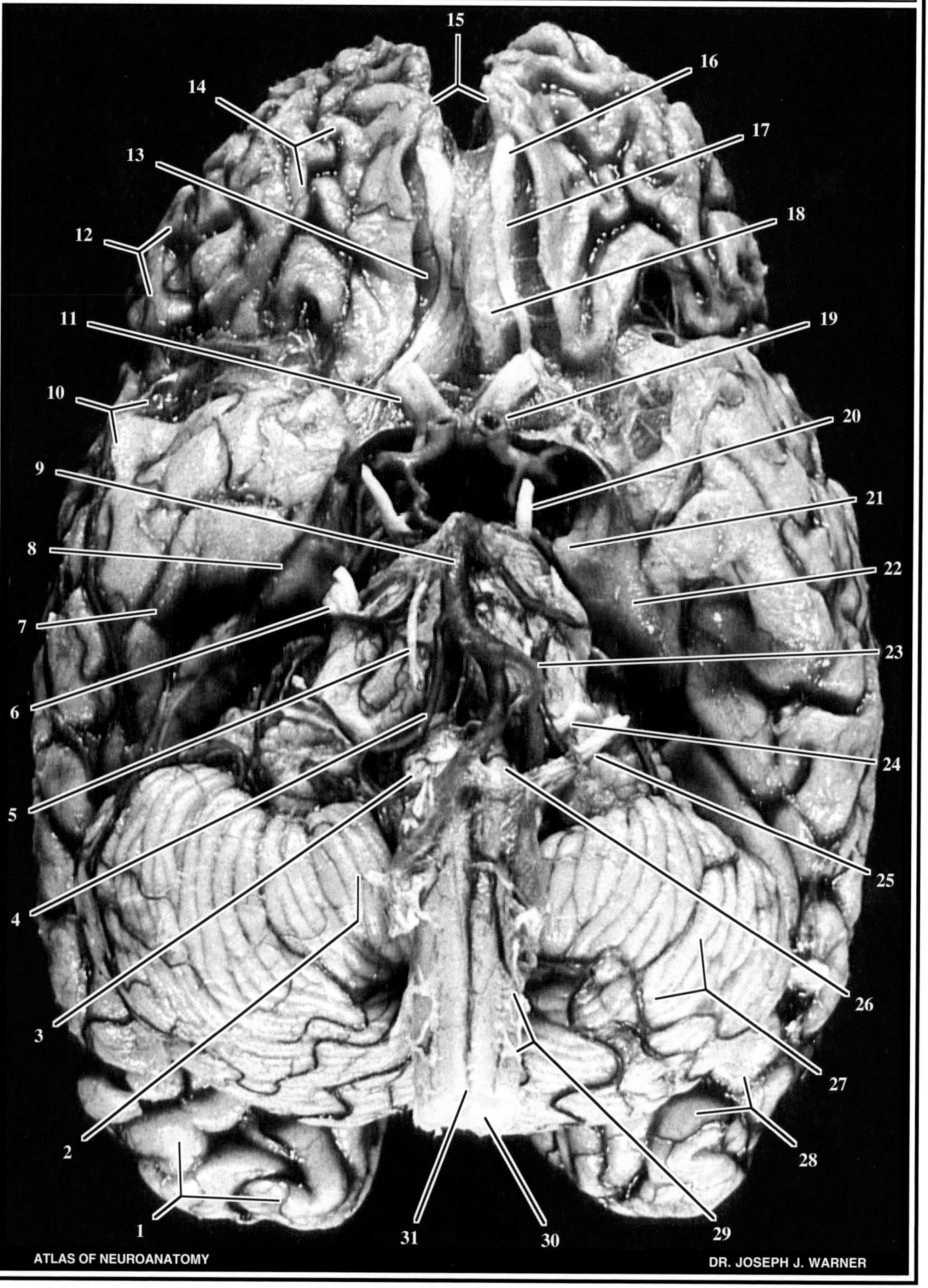

15
14
16
13
17
12
18
11
19
10
20
9
21
8
22
7
6
23
5
24
25
4
26
3
27
2
28
1
31
30
29

PICK'S LOBAR ATROPHY: VENTRAL ASPECT OF THE BRAIN, KEY TO NUMBERED STRUCTURES

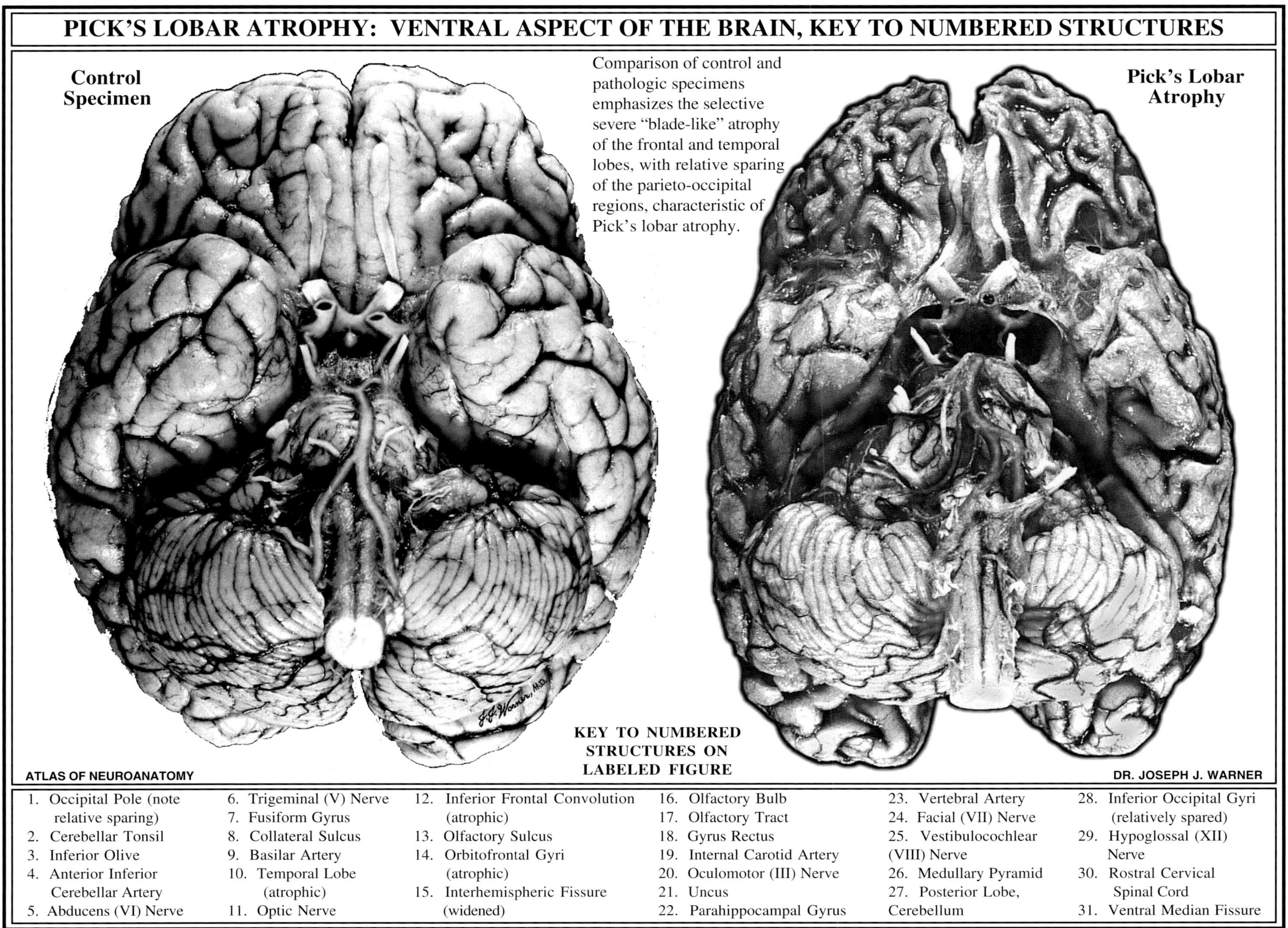

Comparison of control and pathologic specimens emphasizes the selective severe "blade-like" atrophy of the frontal and temporal lobes, with relative sparing of the parieto-occipital regions, characteristic of Pick's lobar atrophy.

KEY TO NUMBERED STRUCTURES ON LABELED FIGURE

1. Occipital Pole (note relative sparing)
2. Cerebellar Tonsil
3. Inferior Olive
4. Anterior Inferior Cerebellar Artery
5. Abducens (VI) Nerve
6. Trigeminal (V) Nerve
7. Fusiform Gyrus
8. Collateral Sulcus
9. Basilar Artery
10. Temporal Lobe (atrophic)
11. Optic Nerve
12. Inferior Frontal Convolution (atrophic)
13. Olfactory Sulcus
14. Orbitofrontal Gyri (atrophic)
15. Interhemispheric Fissure (widened)
16. Olfactory Bulb
17. Olfactory Tract
18. Gyrus Rectus
19. Internal Carotid Artery
20. Oculomotor (III) Nerve
21. Uncus
22. Parahippocampal Gyrus
23. Vertebral Artery
24. Facial (VII) Nerve
25. Vestibulocochlear (VIII) Nerve
26. Medullary Pyramid
27. Posterior Lobe, Cerebellum
28. Inferior Occipital Gyri (relatively spared)
29. Hypoglossal (XII) Nerve
30. Rostral Cervical Spinal Cord
31. Ventral Median Fissure

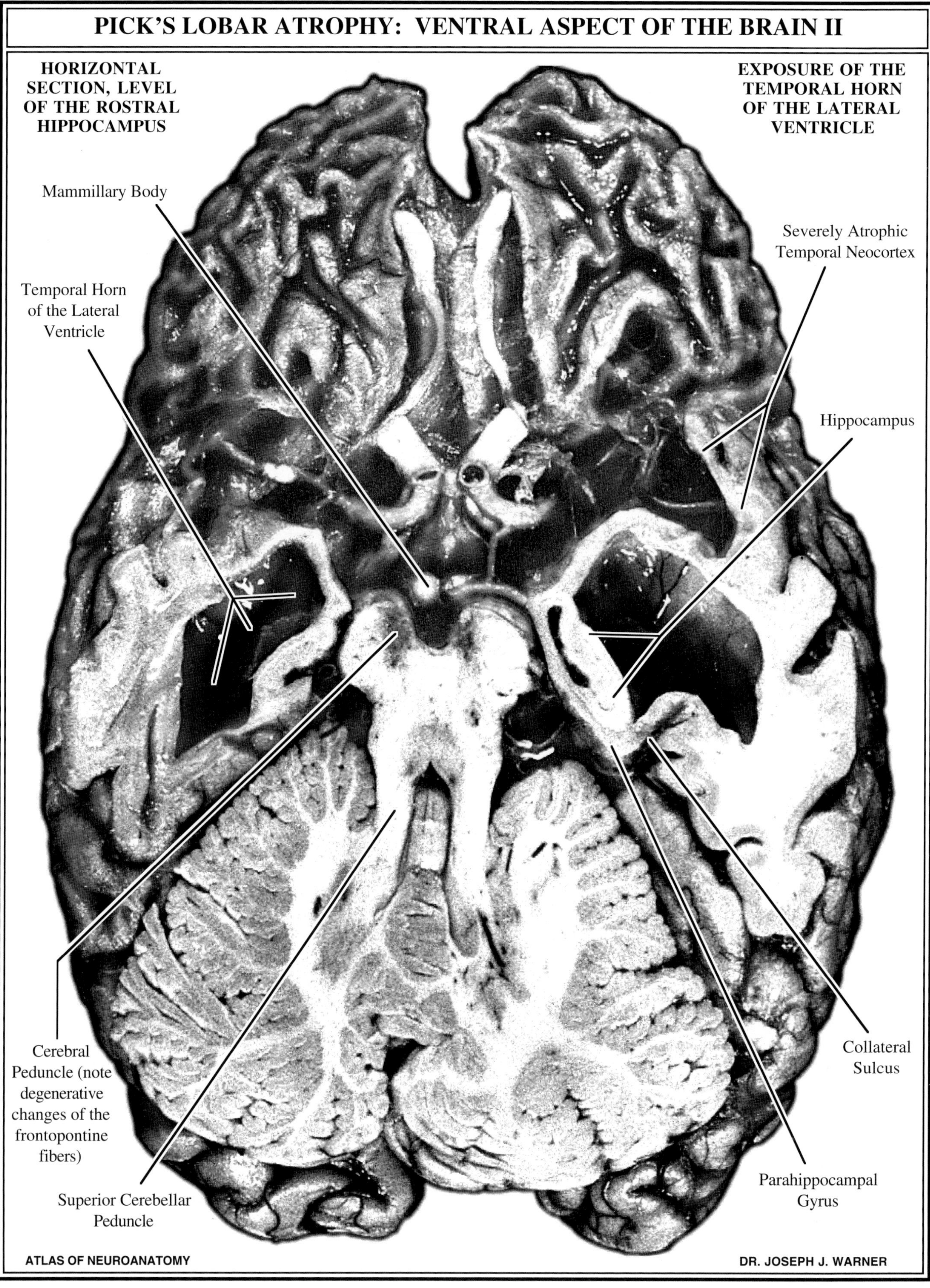
PICK'S LOBAR ATROPHY: VENTRAL ASPECT OF THE BRAIN II
HORIZONTAL SECTION, LEVEL OF THE ROSTRAL HIPPOCAMPUS
EXPOSURE OF THE TEMPORAL HORN OF THE LATERAL VENTRICLE
Mammillary Body
Severely Atrophic Temporal Neocortex
Temporal Horn of the Lateral Ventricle
Hippocampus
Cerebral Peduncle (note degenerative changes of the frontopontine fibers)
Collateral Sulcus
Parahippocampal Gyrus
Superior Cerebellar Peduncle
ATLAS OF NEUROANATOMY
DR. JOSEPH J. WARNER

CONTROL STUDY: HORIZONTAL SECTION OF THE BRAIN, LEVEL OF THE ROSTRAL HIPPOCAMPUS AND THE SUPERIOR CEREBELLAR PEDUNCLES

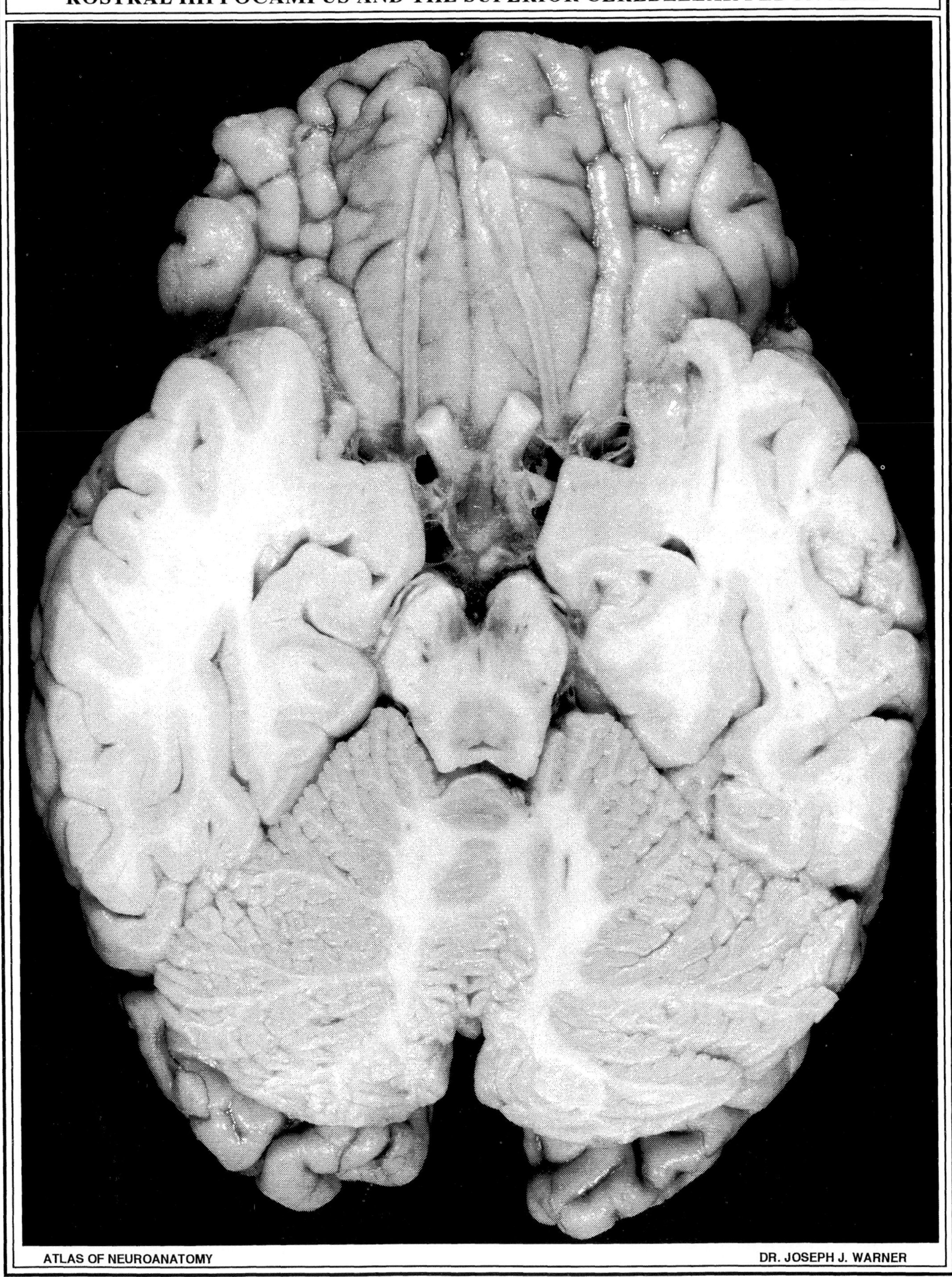

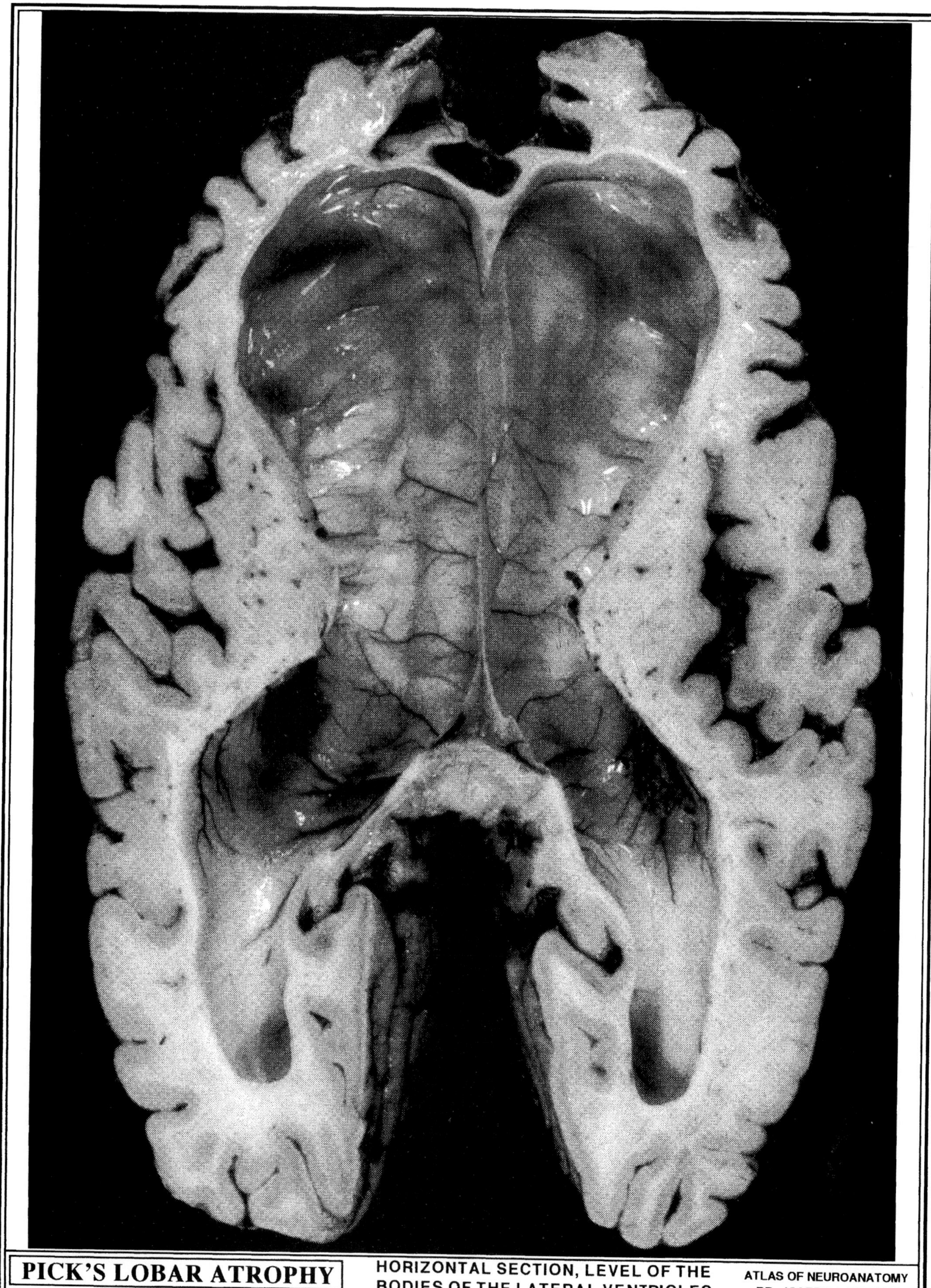

PICK'S LOBAR ATROPHY

HORIZONTAL SECTION, LEVEL OF THE BODIES OF THE LATERAL VENTRICLES

ATLAS OF NEUROANATOMY
DR. JOSEPH J. WARNER

PICK'S LOBAR ATROPHY: MAGNETIC RESONANCE IMAGING

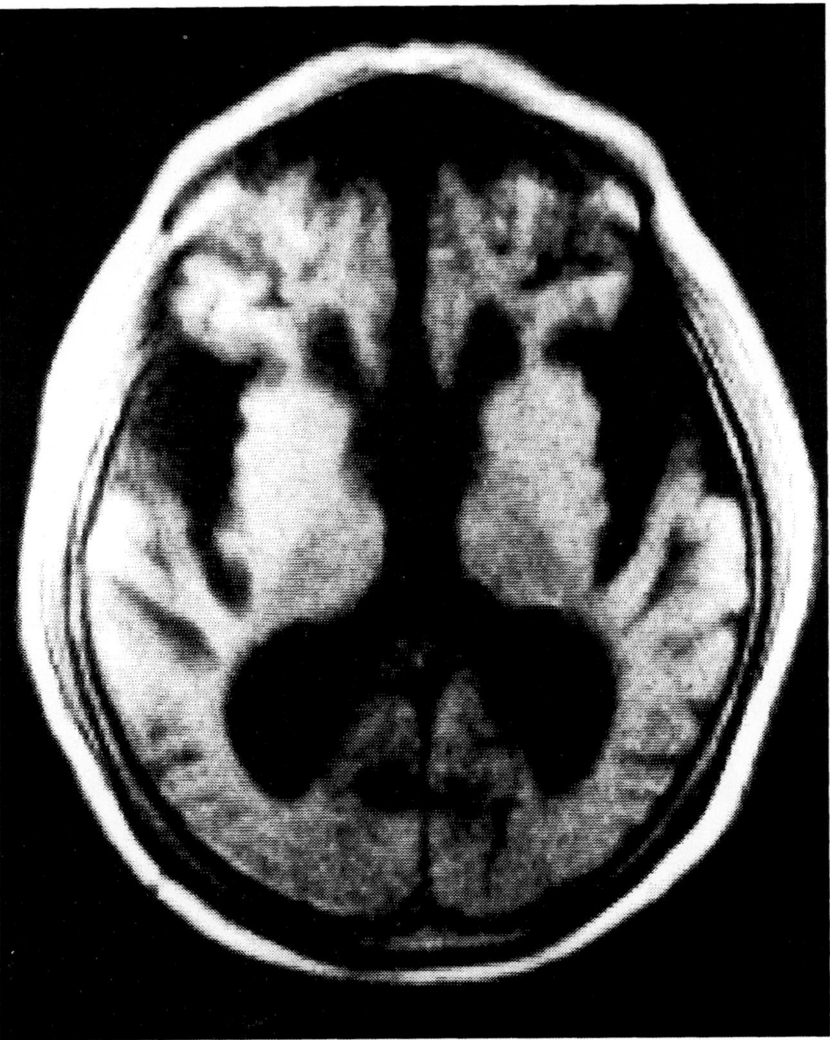

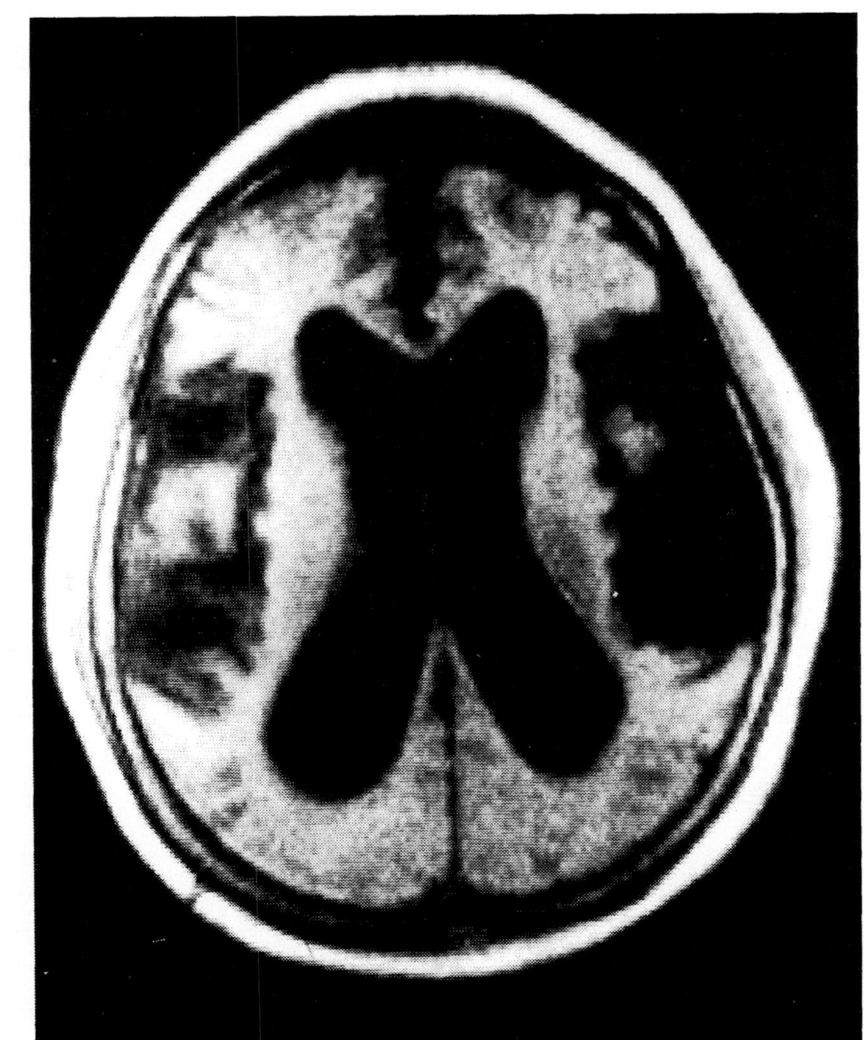

In this case of Pick's Lobar Atrophy, magnetic resonance imaging (T1 weighted, horizontal plane) demonstrates significant atrophy involving the frontal and temporal lobes. This is accompanied by significant widening of the Interhemispheric and Sylvian Fissures. In contrast to the previous case, the caudate nucleus, although reduced in size, remains discernible lateral to the anterior horn of the lateral ventricles. The thalamus is moderately involved. Relative sparing of the occipital regions is a characteristic finding in this degenerative disease.

DR. JOSEPH J. WARNER

HERPES SIMPLEX ENCEPHALITIS: MAGNETIC RESONANCE IMAGING SEVEN YEARS FOLLOWING THE ACUTE ONSET OF NEUROBEHAVIOURAL CHANGES, SEIZURES, AND COMA

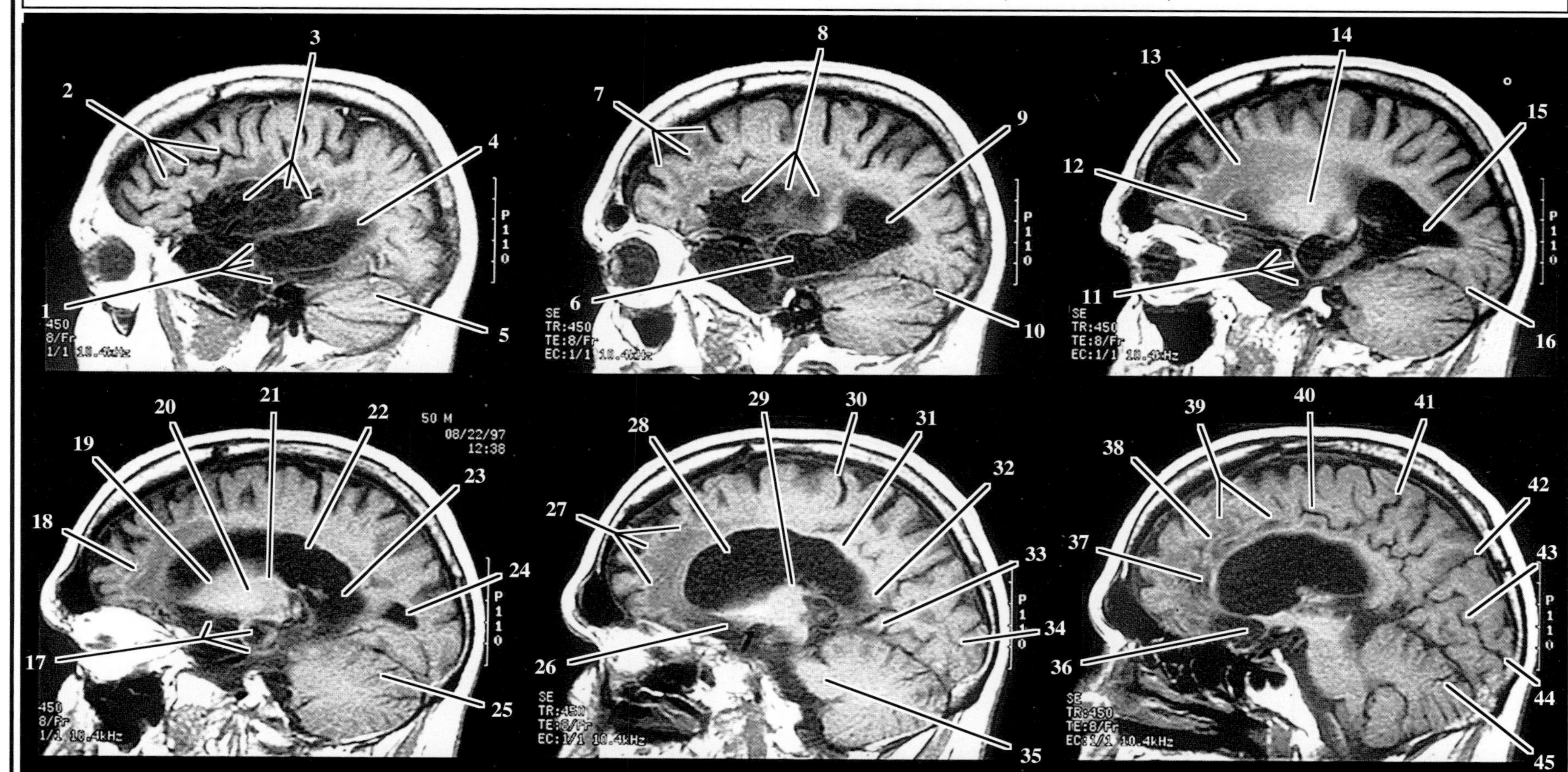

This right-handed male presented at the age of 43 years with the rapid onset of personality changes, including irritability, agitation, and emotional lability. He subsequently developed partial seizures characterized by "staring into space" during which he was unresponsive to verbal stimuli. These episodes were followed by paroxysmal loss of consciousness and secondarily generalized tonic-clonic seizures. The patient was febrile on hospital admission. His clinical course included progressive lethargy with intermittent tonic-clonic seizure activity. He became comatose within approximately 3 to 4 days of the initial behavioural changes. The patient was treated with acyclovir and anticonvulsants, however remained comatose for several days. The patient's level of arousal gradually improved despite baseline fluctuations. Repeated neurologic assessment revealed global aphasia. The patient was followed on a long-term basis. Major deficits included a global aphasia which evolved into a nonfluent aphasia with approximately 50 to 75 percent comprehension of simple commands. Repetition was severely impaired, with superimposed dysarthria. Recurrent seizure activity was observed despite anticonvulsant treatment, which included phenytoin and sodium valproate. These seizures were characterized by repetitive hand and buccolingual movements (automatisms) during which he was unresponsive to verbal stimuli. Through questioning with yes-no responses, the patient was apparently amnestic for these episodes.

HERPES SIMPLEX ENCEPHALITIS: MAGNETIC RESONANCE IMAGING SEVEN YEARS FOLLOWING THE ACUTE ONSET OF NEUROBEHAVIOURAL CHANGES, SEIZURES, AND COMA

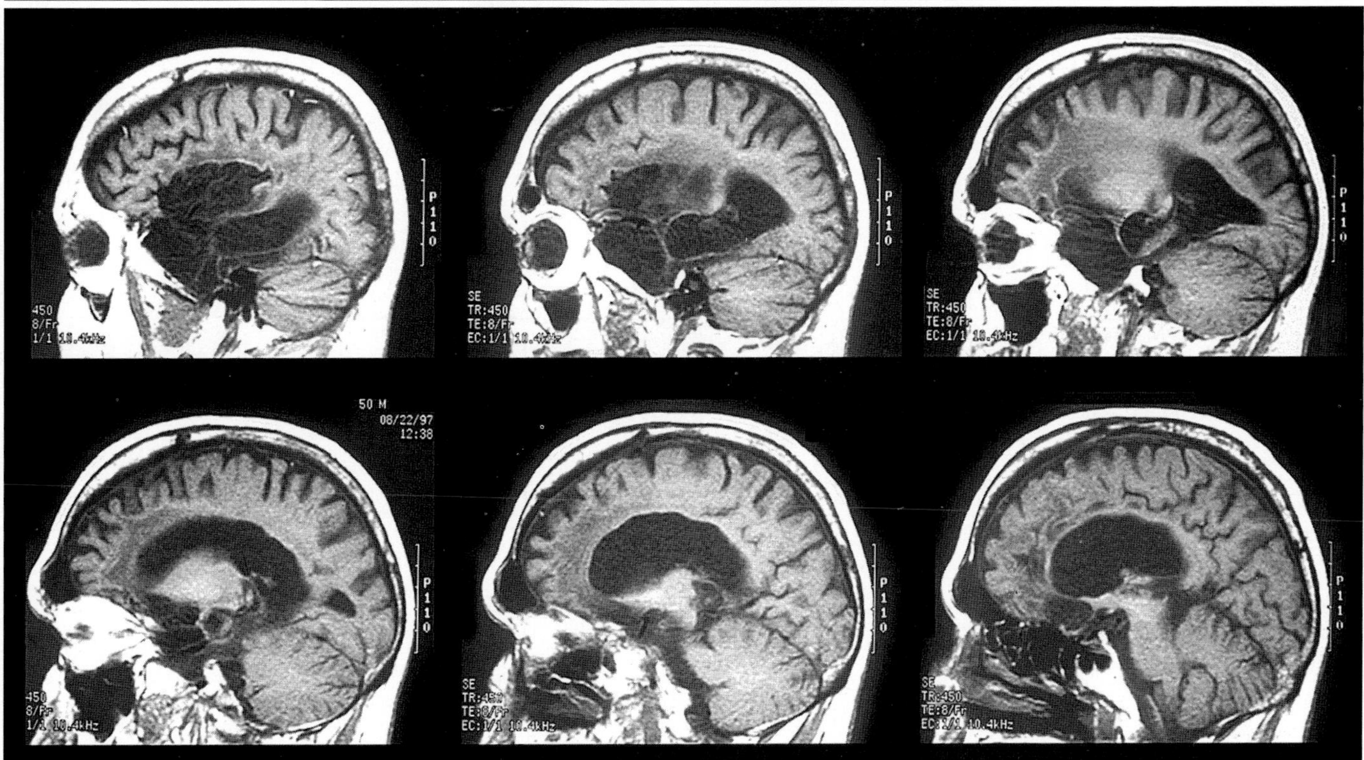

KEY TO NUMBERED STRUCTURES

1. Severe encephalomalacia involving the Temporal Pole
2. Inferior Frontal Sulcus
3. Insular and Frontoparietal Opercular encephalomalacia
4. Atrium of the Lateral Ventricle
5. Cerebellum
6. Temporal Horn of the Lateral Ventricle (markedly dilated secondary to severe atrophy)
7. Middle Frontal Convolution
8. Insular encephalomalacia
9. Atrium of the Lateral Ventricle
10. Tentorium
11. Anterior and Medial Temporal encephalomalacia
12. Deep Insular encephalomalacia
13. Secondary changes in Prefrontal White Matter
14. Lateral aspect of the Putamen
15. Atrium of the Lateral Ventricle
16. Tentorium
17. Severe encephalomalacia of the Medial Temporal and Basal Forebrain regions
18. Prefrontal atrophy and White Matter changes
19. Head of the Caudate Nucleus
20. Genu of the Internal Capsule
21. Thalamus
22. Body of the Lateral Ventricle
23. Atrium of the Lateral Ventricle
24. Occipital Horn of the Lateral Ventricle
25. Primary Fissure of the Cerebellum
26. Severe encephalomalacia of the Basal Forebrain region
27. Secondary changes in the Prefrontal White Matter
28. Body of the Lateral Ventricle
29. Medial Thalamus
30. Rolandic Fissure
31. Corpus Callosum (attenuated)
32. Splenial fibers of the Corpus Callosum and Isthmus of the Gyrus Fornicatus
33. Lingular Gyrus
34. Area 17 Striate Cortex
35. Middle Cerebellar Peduncle
36 Severe encephalomalacia of the Paraterminal and Subcallosal Gyri
37. Encephalomalacia of the anterior Cingulate Gyrus
38. Cingulate Sulcus
39. Encephalomalacia of the Cingulate Gyrus
40. Cingulate Sulcus
41. Pars Marginalis of the Cingulate Sulcus
42. Parieto-Occipital Sulcus
43. Area 17 Striate Cortex
44. Calcarine Fissure
45. Primary Fissure of the Cerebellum

CLINICAL CORRELATIONS: THE LIMBIC SYSTEM

Herpes simplex encephalitis is among the most severe of the various forms of acute encephalitis, and it is the most common. Approximately 2000 cases occur annually, representing about 10 percent of all cases of encephalitis in the United States. Fatality ranges from 30 to 70 percent of cases. Most patients who survive are left with severe neurological deficits. The onset of the disease is associated with neurobehavioural signs and symptoms that suggest inferomedial frontal and temporal lobe involvement. The neurological manifestations may include anosmia, olfactory or gustatory hallucinations, emotional disinhibition, personality changes, inappropriate or "bizarre" behaviour, and psychosis.

As the clinical course continues, patients may develop seizures, confusion and severe inattention, and progressive deterioration in level of arousal evolving from stupor to coma. Memory deficits are generally evident in the convalescent stage of the infection, which may include anterograde amnesia with variable sparing memory for events occurring prior to onset of the disease. The neuroanatomic distribution of this necrotizing encephalitis is quite characteristic, thus enabling clinicians to make the diagnosis with a high degree of accuracy. Computerized tomography and magnetic resonance imaging studies demonstrate acute inflammatory changes and edema affecting the inferior frontal and temporal regions, not characteristic of trauma, neoplastic or cerebrovascular disease. Transtentorial herniation is a major complication due to intense edema of the frontotemporal regions.

HERPES SIMPLEX ENCEPHALITIS: CORONAL SECTION
LEVEL OF THE NUCLEUS ACCUMBENS, CAUDAL TO ROSTRAL PERSPECTIVE

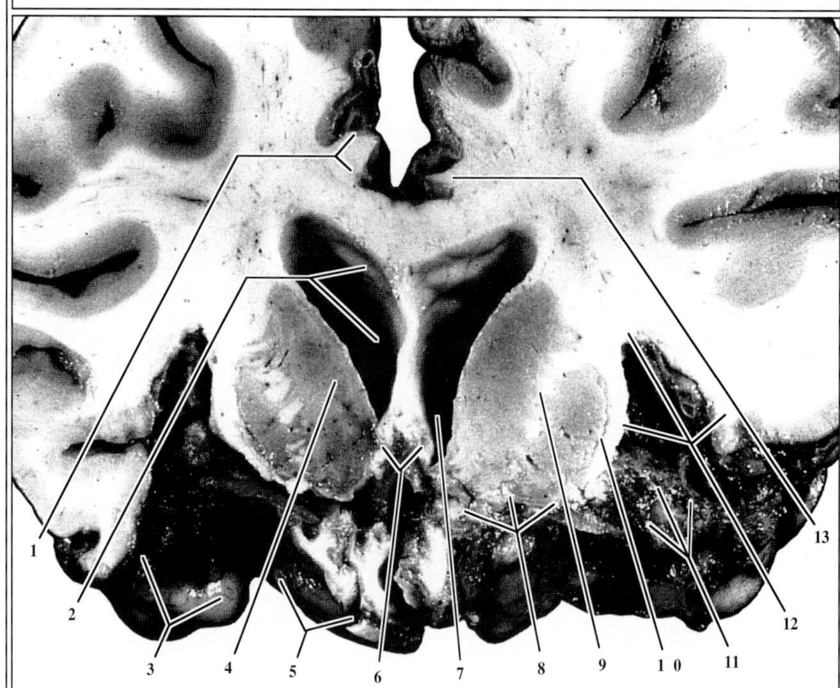

In the case shown, the patient survived the acute phase of the illness. However, residua included severe anterograde amnesia, anosmia and altered taste sensation, temporal lobe seizures, and significant behavioural changes from his previous baseline. The patient remained in a long-term care facility, however sustained an intercurrent infection with complications and expired. Pathologic examination was performed.

HERPES SIMPLEX ENCEPHALITIS

CORONAL SECTION
LEVEL OF THE SUBTHALAMIC NUCLEUS
15μ SECTION, H & E STAIN

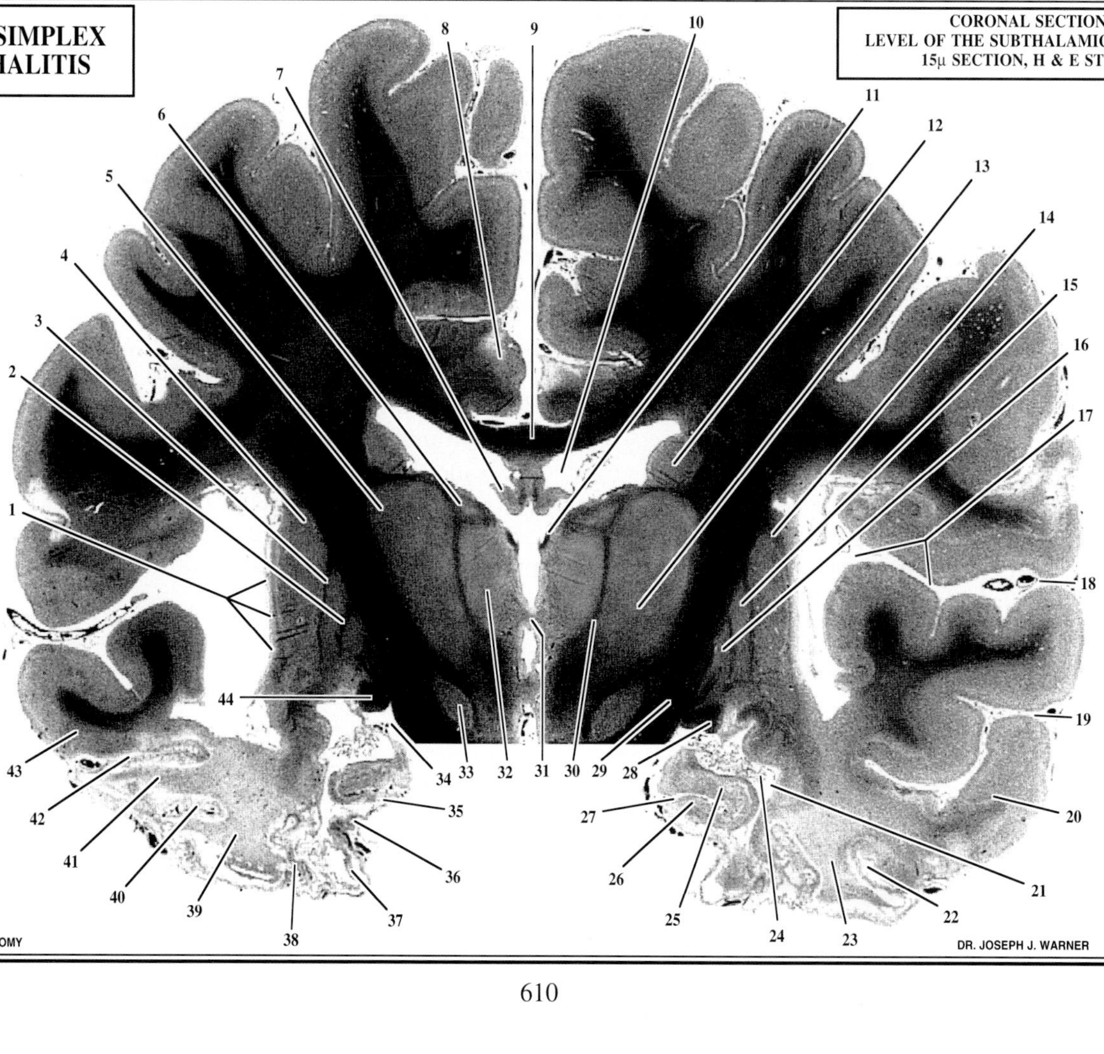

DR. JOSEPH J. WARNER

HERPES SIMPLEX ENCEPHALITIS: MAP OF CORONAL SECTIONS AND EXPLANATORY KEY TO NUMBERED STRUCTURES

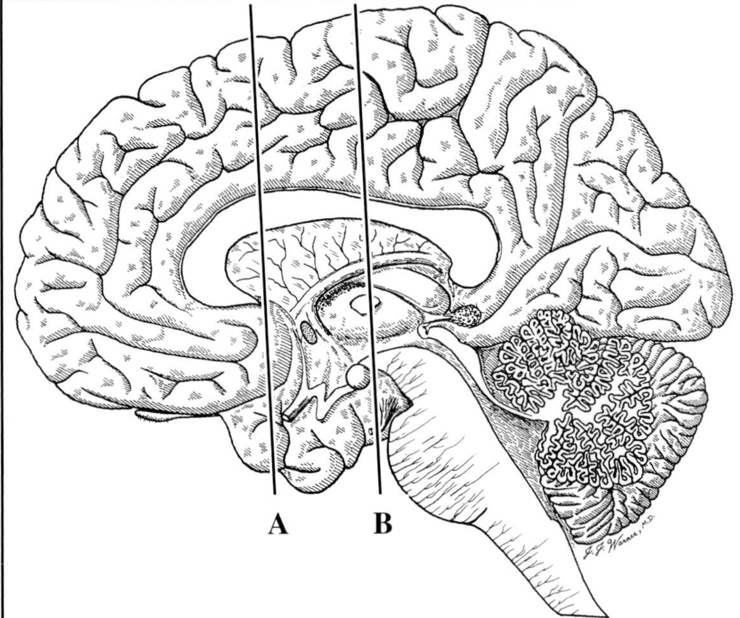

A. CORONAL SECTION: LEVEL OF THE NUCLEUS ACCUMBENS

1. Cingulate Gyrus, cortical necrosis
2. Body and Genu of Corpus Callosum
3. Intact Frontal Gyri rostral to the major regions of necrosis
4. Head of the Caudate Nucleus
5. Orbitofrontal Gyri
6. Necrosis of Septal area
7. Anterior Horn of the Lateral Ventricle
8. Necrosis of the Nucleus Accumbens
9. Anterior Limb of the Internal Capsule
10. Lateral margin of the Putamen (necrotic)
11. Necrotic rostral Temporal Pole
12. Necrosis of rostral extent of the Insula and inferior Frontal Opercular Region
13. Degenerative changes of the Cingulum

B. CORONAL SECTION. LEVEL OF THE SUBTHALAMIC NUCLEUS

1. Insular Cortex*
2. Internal Medullary Lamina
3. External Medullary Lamina
4. Putamen
5. Lateral Posterior Nucleus of the Thalamus
6. Lateral Dorsal Nucleus of the Thalamus
7. Fornix*
8. Cingulate Gyrus*
9. Corpus Callosum
10. Body of Lateral Ventricle
11. Stria Medullaris
12. Caudate Nucleus
13. Ventroanterior, Ventrolateral Nucleus of the Thalamus
14. External Capsule
15. Globus Pallidus II
16. Globus Pallidus I
17. Sylvian Fissure
18. Branch of Middle Cerebral Artery
19. Superior Temporal Sulcus
20. Middle Temporal Gyrus*
21. Temporal Horn of the Lateral Ventricle
22. Middle Temporal Sulcus* (altered from its normal anatomic position due to severe temporal lobe necrosis and atrophy)
23. Inferior Temporal Gyrus*
24. Choroid Plexus
25. Hippocampal Formation*
26. Subiculum*
27. Hippocampal Fissure*
28. Termination of Optic Tract in Lateral Geniculate Nucleus
29. Cerebral Peduncle
30. Internal Medullary Lamina of the Thalamus
31. Massa Intermedia
32. Dorsomedial Nucleus of the Thalamus
33. Subthalamic Nucleus
34. Choroidal Fissure
35. Parahippocampal Gyrus*
36. Collateral Sulcus*
37. Fusiform Gyrus*
38. Inferior Temporal Sulcus*
39. Inferior Temporal Gyrus*
40. Middle Temporal Sulcus*
41. Middle Temporal Gyrus*
42. Superior Temporal Sulcus*
43. Superior Temporal Gyrus*
44. Caudal aspect of Optic Tract

* *Demonstrating necrosis or related degenerative changes*

NORMAL VS. PATHOLOGIC NEUROANATOMY AND FUNCTIONAL CORRELATIONS

The pathologic changes demonstrated in this and other cases should be studied by direct comparison with control sections at corresponding levels. The contrast between the normal and pathologic neuroanatomy serves to emphasize important structural relationships and a more meaningful correlation with the clinical signs and symptoms associated with the disease process. This direct comparative study not only serves to clarify pathologic changes and clinical correlations, but also reinforces the conceptualization of normal neuroanatomic relationships, systems organization, and functional considerations.

NEUROANATOMY AND PATHOPHYSIOLOGY

The characteristic findings of Herpes simplex encephalitis are exemplified by the neuropathologic findings in this case. The inferior frontal and temporal lobe lesions are evident along with areas of necrosis involving portions of the cingulate gyrus, bilateral insular cortex, septal nuclei, nucleus accumbens, and other basal forebrain structures. The temporal lobes are almost entirely obliterated (including both hippocampi), with the exception of the superior temporal gyri. Rostral orbitofrontal cortex is relatively spared, however tissue destruction becomes quite significant adjacent to olfactory receptive areas. The involvement of limbic system structures correlates well with many of the neurobehavioural changes associated with Herpes simplex encephalitis.

The rather consistent neuroanatomic distribution of pathology associated with this disease raises interesting questions with respect to an apparent predilection of the virus for these specific regions vs. selective vulnerability. Two routes of viral entry have been proposed, which may account for the pattern of involvement seen in these cases. It is known that Herpes simplex virus, although clinically latent, is harbored in the trigeminal ganglion. Under certain physiologic conditions, the virus may travel distally in trigeminal nerve fibers that innervate the leptomeninges of the anterior and middle cranial fossae, thus affecting the frontal and temporal lobes. Another explanation involves distal migration of the virus along trigeminal fibers, thus infecting the nasal mucosa. The olfactory epithelium thus serves as a neural "bridge," allowing the virus to follow the afferent olfactory pathways into the inferior frontal and medial temporal areas. Sparing of the olfactory bulbs in up to 40% of cases examined pathologically suggests the former pathway.

HERPES SIMPLEX ENCEPHALITIS: VENTRAL VIEW OF THE BRAIN

This specimen demonstrates necrotic changes and atrophy secondary to the acute necrotizing encephalitis of Herpes simplex virus, with a predilection for the ventromedial frontal and temporal lobes and associated limbic structures.

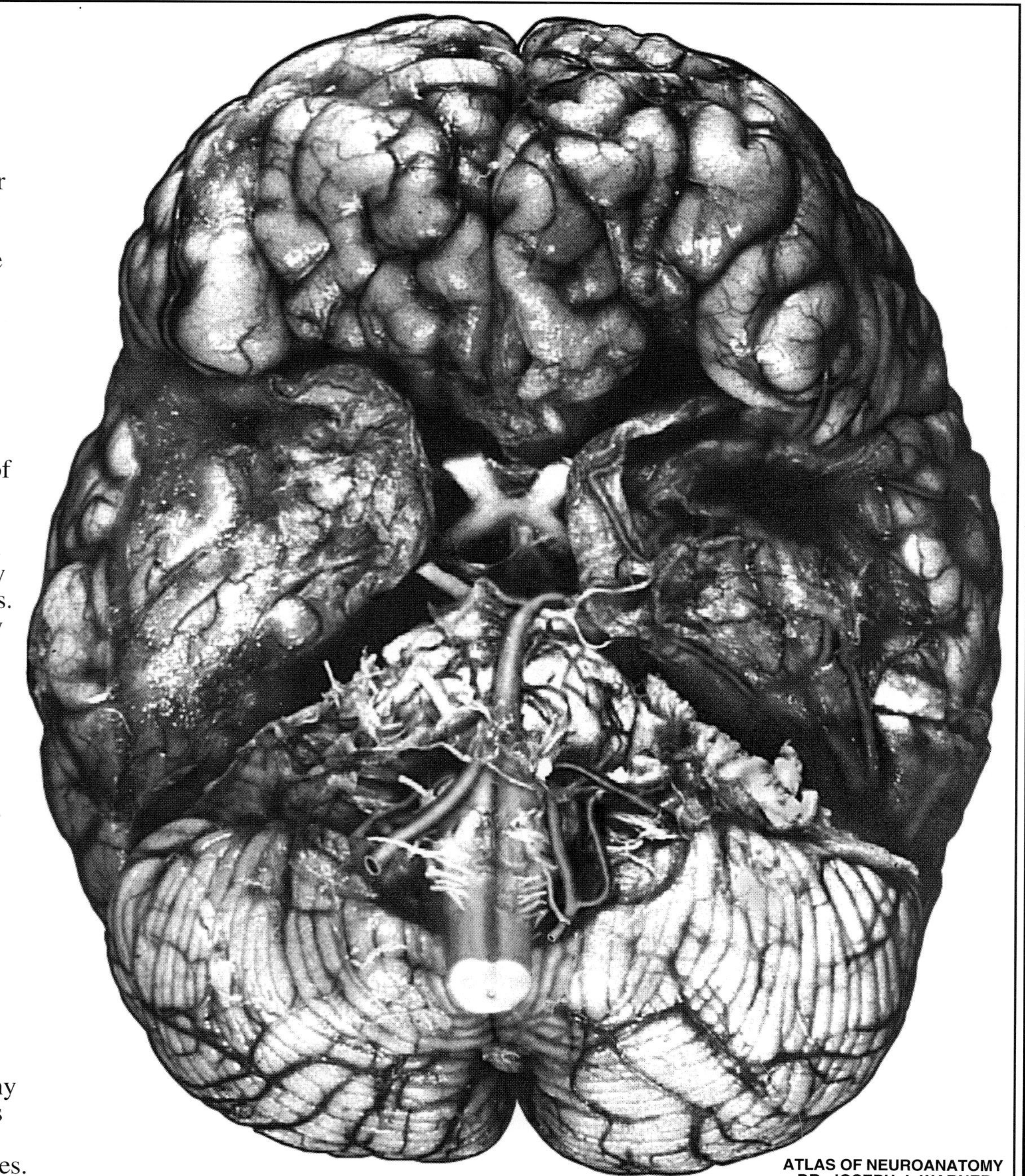

STRIATONIGRAL DEGENERATION: COMPLETE CORONAL SECTION, LEVEL OF THE MAMMILLARY BODIES

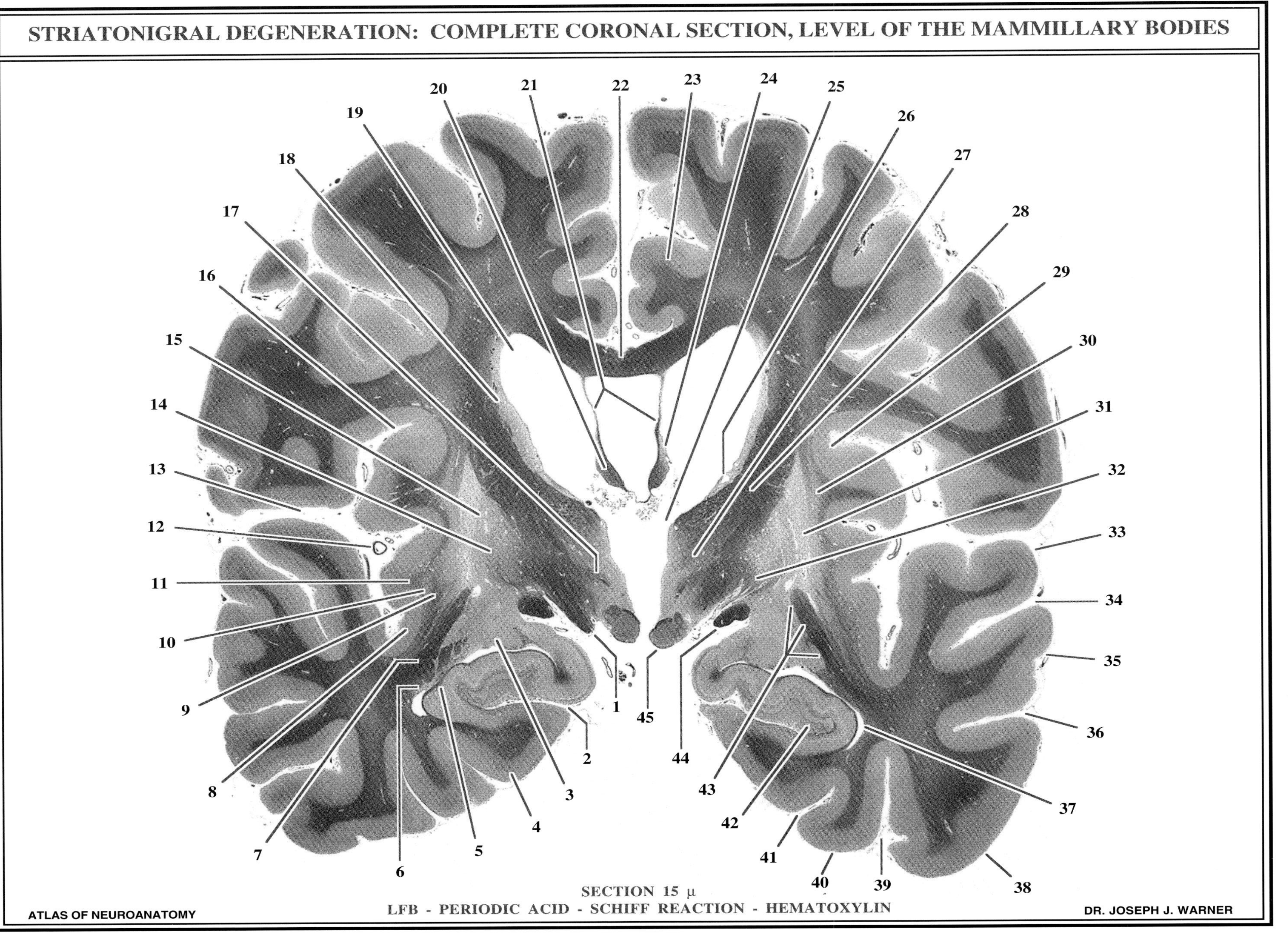

SECTION 15 μ
LFB - PERIODIC ACID - SCHIFF REACTION - HEMATOXYLIN

DR. JOSEPH J. WARNER

STRIATONIGRAL DEGENERATION: COMPLETE CORONAL SECTION OF THE BRAIN, LEVEL OF THE MAMMILLARY BODIES; 15μ, LFB - PAS - HEMATOXYLIN TECHNIQUE

SECTION MAP ON MIDLINE SAGITTAL DIAGRAM

KEY TO NUMBERED STRUCTURES

1. Cerebral Peduncle
2. Hippocampal Fissure
3. Amygdala
4. Parahippocampal Gyrus
5. Alveus
6. Tail of the Caudate Nucleus
7. Lateral Fibers of the Anterior Commissure
8. Insular Cortex
9. External Capsule
10. Claustrum
11. Extreme Capsule
12. Middle Cerebral Artery
13. Sylvian Fissure
14. Internal Medullary Lamina
15. External Medullary Lamina
16. Circular Sulcus
17. Lenticular Fasciculus, rostral aspect of the Fields of Forel
18. Head of the Caudate Nucleus (severely atrophic)
19. Lateral Ventricle
20. Fornix
21. Cavum Septum Pellucidum
22. Corpus Callosum
23. Cingulate Gyrus
24. Septal Nuclei
25. Foramen of Monro
26. Thalamostriate Vein
27. Anterior Nuclear Group of the Thalamus
28. Genu of the Internal Capsule
29. Insular Cortex
30. Claustrum
31. Putamen (severely atrophic)
32. Globus Pallidus I
33. Superior Temporal Gyrus
34. Superior Temporal Sulcus
35. Middle Temporal Gyrus
36. Middle Temporal Sulcus
37. Temporal Horn of the Lateral Ventricle
38. Inferior Temporal Gyrus
39. Inferior Temporal Sulcus
40. Fusiform Gyrus
41. Collateral Sulcus
42. Hippocampal Formation
43. Anterior Commissure
44. Optic Tract
45. Mammillary Body

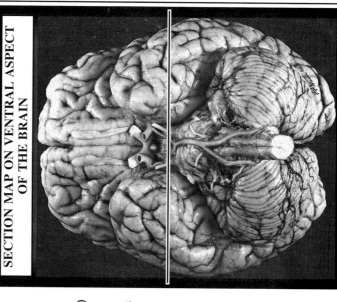

SECTION MAP ON VENTRAL ASPECT OF THE BRAIN

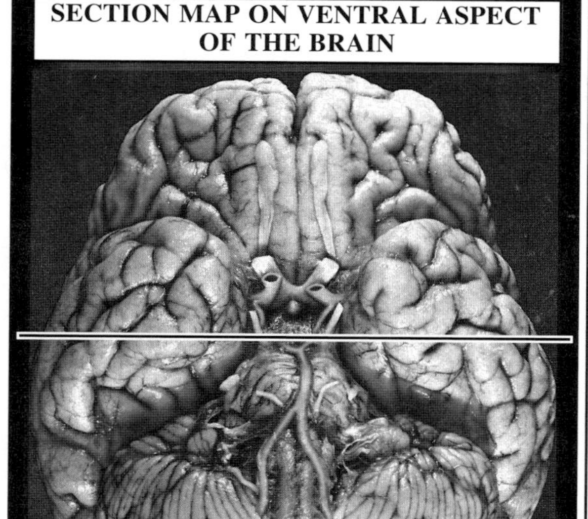

HUNTINGTON'S CHOREA: COMPUTERIZED TOMOGRAPHY

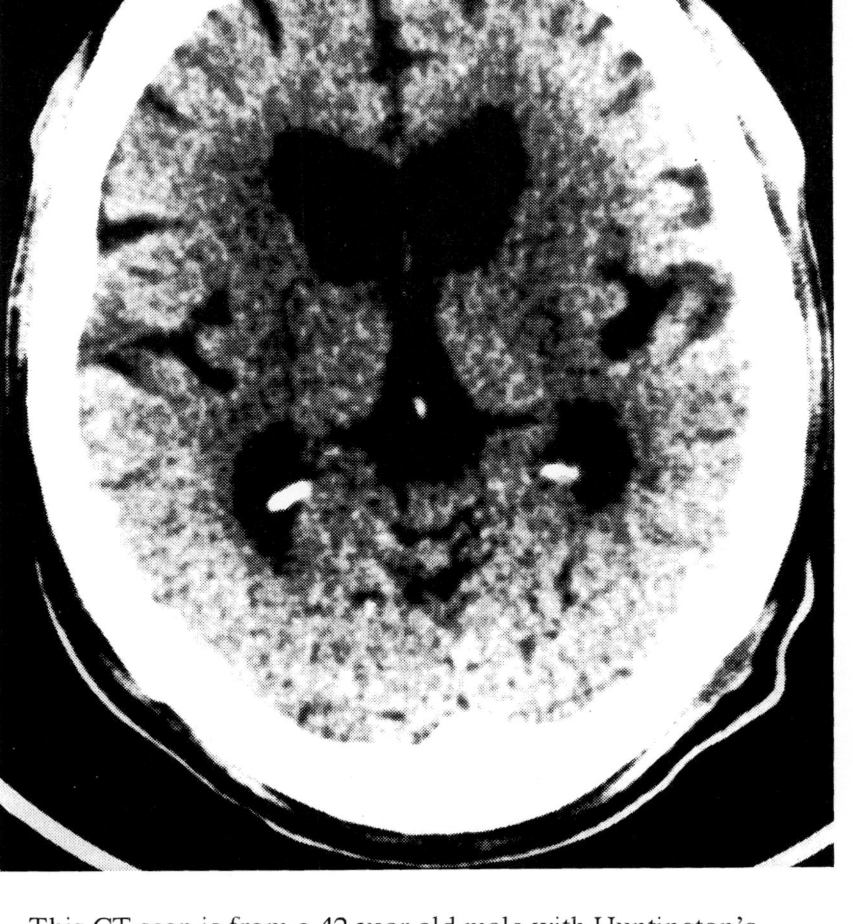

This CT scan is from a 42-year-old male with Huntington's Chorea. The scan demonstrates moderate cortical atrophy with characteristic loss of the contour of the head of the caudate nucleus along the anterior horns of the lateral ventricles. Ventricular enlargement is secondary to atrophic changes.

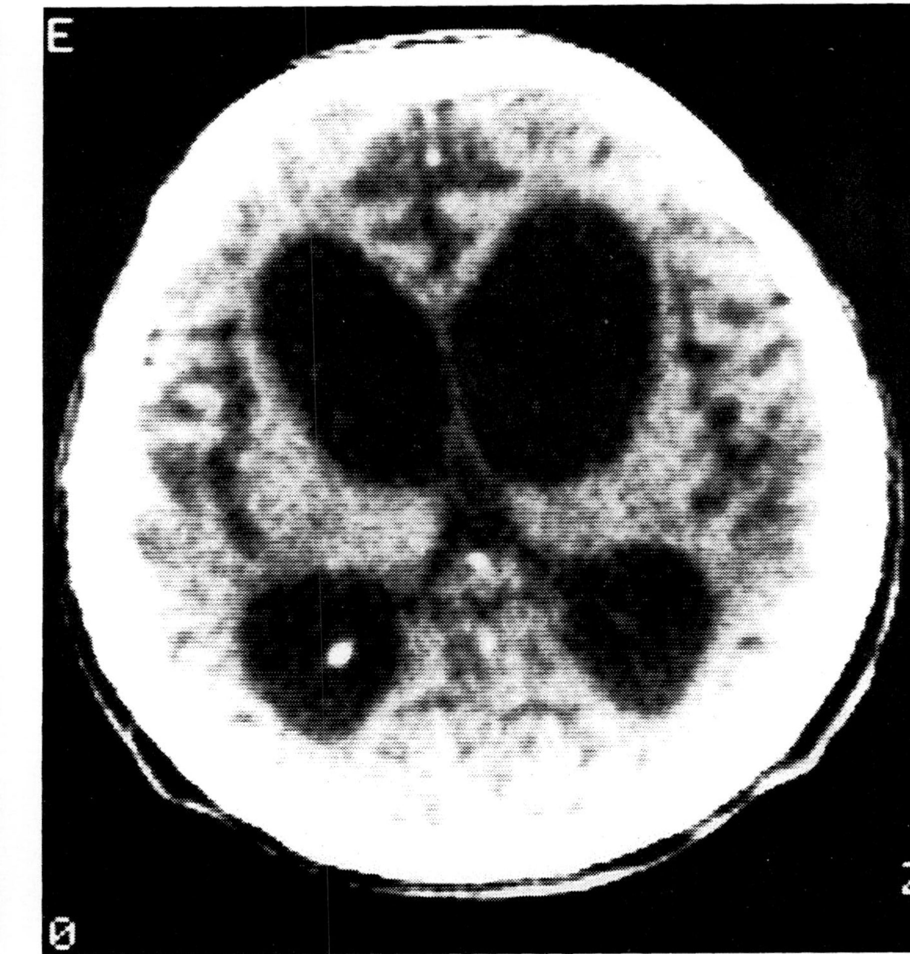

This scan is from one of two affected male siblings with advanced Huntington's Chorea. The CT demonstrates severe central atrophy with secondary ventricular enlargement. The anterior horns of the lateral ventricles demonstrate no discernible contour of the head of the caudate nucleus. The striatum and thalamus were characterized by significant atrophy as well. Note the relative disparity between the severity of the central vs. cortical atrophy.

PINEAL CYST PRESENTING WITH PARALYSIS OF UPWARD GAZE AND GAIT ATAXIA

CLINICAL CASE PRESENTATION

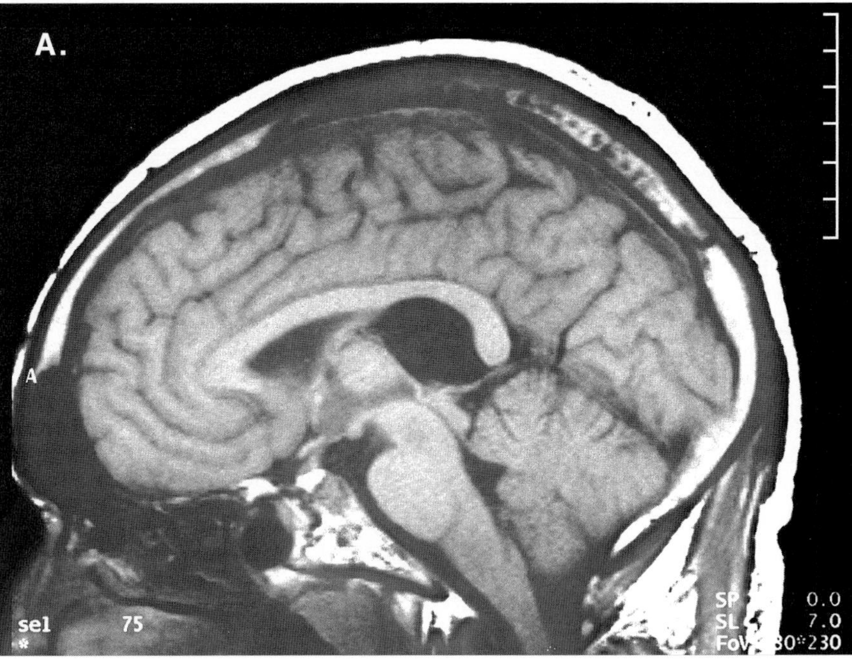

This 70-year-old right-handed male presented with progressive gait instability and limitation of upward gaze. The patient had noted "trouble with coordination" particularly when walking, with a tendency to "lose [his] equilibrium." An astute observer, this patient responded to a question about his vision with the following detailed account. He stated that he was an avid bird watcher and enjoyed this pastime in the woods surrounding his home. He indicated that he would go out every day, and "look up into the trees at the birds." The patient stated, "I had more trouble over the past couple of years because I couldn't look up without bending my whole neck back."

On further analysis, the patient explained that he could not move his eyes fully, and that head and neck movement was necessary to look up. Neurological examination revealed a normal mental status, with appropriate affect and attention to tasks. Cranial nerve testing demonstrated a vertical (upward) gaze paresis with little motility superior to the horizontal meridian. Horizontal and downward vertical eye movements were full and conjugate without nystagmus. Pupils were equal at 3 mm diameter and reactive to light. Accommodation was somewhat limited. Other findings included minimal bilateral upper extremity dysmetria with mild intention/terminal tremor, and a broad-based, ataxic gait. Bilateral lower extremity hyperreflexia was present without Babinski signs.

Magnetic resonance imaging was performed (see figure A) which demonstrated a 2 by 3 cm cyst dorsal to the corpora quadrigemina and the posterior commissure. The cyst was associated with a ventral displacement of the posterior commissure and caudal aspect of the stria medullaris, with a dorsal shift of the caudal third of the corpus callosum. The Aqueduct of Sylvius was stenotic adjacent to the posterior commissure. There was no significant hydrocephalus involving the lateral ventricles.

PATHOPHYSIOLOGY

Mass lesions of the pineal include tumors with histologic characteristics of the pineal gland, such as pineocytomas and pineoblastomas. Other neoplasms of the pineal include germinomas or atypical teratomas and tumors of glial origin. Pineal cysts may be found as incidental findings at autopsy, with single or multiloculated fluid-filled cavities ranging in size from 1 or 2 millimeters in diameter to larger cysts that exert a discernible mass effect on surrounding neural structures. Such lesions may become clinically evident, presenting with signs of increased intracranial pressure related to the development of hydrocephalus. Characteristic localizing findings may include elements of Parinaud syndrome. Cranial nerve examination may reveal paralysis of upward gaze, impaired pupillary light reflexes, and loss of convergent eye movements. Compromise of the dorsal mesencephalic tegmentum, including attenuation and/or compression of the posterior commissure, may result in extraocular motility and pupillary reflex deficits. Activation of extraocular muscles which elevate the eyes involves dorsal projections from each interstitial nucleus of Cajal, which pass through the posterior commissure and terminate on the contralateral superior rectus and inferior oblique subnuclei of the oculomotor nuclear complex. A lesion affecting this pathway would thereby result in a selective upgaze paralysis of both eyes. Progressive compression of the aqueduct of Sylvius may produce subacute obstructive hydrocephalus. In mass lesions of the pineal, ataxia of the limbs may be related to mesencephalic compression affecting the superior cerebellar peduncles or their decussation. Alternatively, hydrocephalus may result in motor dysfunction (including spasticity) particularly evident in the lower extremities.

PINEAL CYST PRESENTING WITH PARALYSIS OF UPWARD GAZE AND GAIT ATAXIA: MAGNETIC RESONANCE IMAGING (SAGITTAL PLANE)

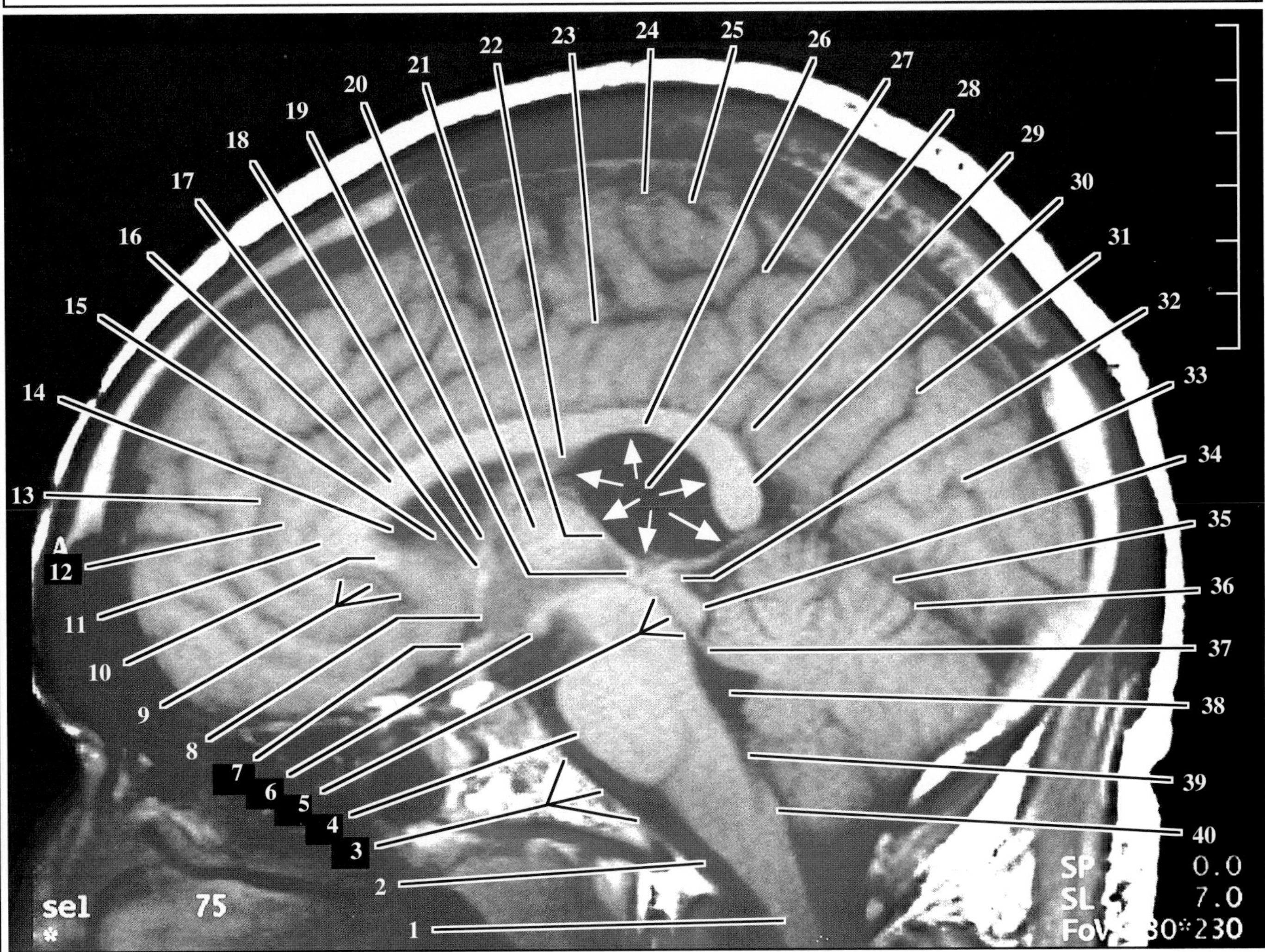

KEY TO NUMBERED STRUCTURES

1. Rostral Cervical Spinal Cord
2. Foramen Magnum
3. Clivus
4. Basis Pontis
5. Aqueduct of Sylvius
6. Mammillary Body
7. Optic Chiasm
8. Supraoptic Recess of the Third Ventricle
9. Anterior Cerebral Arteries
10. Rostrum of the Corpus Callosum
11. Genu of the Corpus Callosum
12. Cingulate Gyrus
13. Cingulate Sulcus
14. Anterior Horn of the Lateral Ventricle
15. Head of the Caudate Nucleus
16. Body of the Corpus Callosum
17. Anterior Commissure
18. Foramen of Monro
19. Posterior Commissure (displaced ventral to the Pineal Cyst)
20. Medial Thalamus (rostrally displaced)
21. Stria Medullaris (note distortion with rostral and ventral displacement by the Pineal Cyst)
22. Fornix
23. Cingulate Sulcus
24. Precentral Gyrus
25. Central Sulcus (Rolandic Fissure)
26. Dorsal distortion of the Body of the Corpus Callosum
27. Pars Marginalis (extension of the Cingulate Sulcus)
28. Pineal Cyst (arrows indicate cyst wall with displacement of adjacent structures)
29. Cingulate Gyrus
30. Splenium of the Corpus Callosum
31. Parieto-Occipital Sulcus
32. Superior Colliculus
33. Calcarine Fissure
34. Inferior Colliculus
35. Tentorium
36. Primary Fissure of the Cerebellum
37. Anterior (Superior) Medullary Velum
38. Fourth Ventricle
39. Foramen of Magendie
40. Gracile Tubercle

LEFT PERISYLVIAN MENINGIOMA IN A PATIENT WITH EPISODIC WERNICKE'S APHASIA

Computerized Tomography with Intravenous Contrast

R Transaxial L

L Coronal R

This 53-year-old right-handed female presented for the evaluation of a frequent episodic speech disturbance. Her primary care physician considered a diagnosis of transient ischemic attacks. Further evaluation revealed that each episode consisted of the sudden onset of speech arrest followed by 10 to 15 minutes during which (1) she was unable to comprehend verbal or written commands, and (2) repetition and spontaneous speech was characterized by numerous phonemic paraphasic errors. Electroencephalography revealed frequent left temporal epileptiform discharges. Computerized tomography demonstrated a large, dural - based contrast enhancing mass in region of the left Sylvian Fissure. Prior to surgical intervention, anticonvulsant therapy (phenytoin) was initiated, with no recurrent symptomatology.

FRONTAL MENINGIOMA IN A PATIENT WITH PROGRESSIVE NEUROBEHAVIOURAL CHANGES

CASE PRESENTATION

This 20-year-old right-handed male was brought in by his parents for an evaluation of gradually progressive behavioural changes. The parents became concerned over recent, distinctly uncharacteristic behaviour. He was described as becoming irritable, easily agitated, and "short-fused." He had frequent disagreements with family members and friends. The family became extremely concerned when he was arrested for "shoplifting" because such was in marked contrast to his previously "normal behaviour." The patient acknowledged difficulty in "concentrating on his college classes." He also developed episodes of "staring off into space" during which he did not respond to people around him. He seemed "confused" after each episode, which lasted "a couple of minutes." The patient had a previous history of good academic performance in school. He had been well-liked by his classmates and teachers and participated in various extracurricular school activities. He had no record of behavioural problems or learning disability. There was no history of illicit drug use.

When the examiner (the author) first observed the patient, a striking prominence of the patient's forehead was noted. In order to avoid affronting the patient or family, they were asked whether they had noticed any changes in his overall appearance. The father became mildly irritated and replied that neither he nor his wife had noticed anything unusual. However, he elaborated that "when relatives would come to visit for the holidays, they would ask if [the patient] had bumped his head or something." The parents, however, gave his physical appearance no significance. Further investigation of this history, however, revealed evidence that a slight, but gradually progressive change in his head configuration was first noticed by his relatives at least seven or eight years earlier.

Neurological examination was normal. The patient was alert, cooperative, and his affect was appropriate. Cortical function testing revealed no significant abnormality. Tests were performed by the patient in a meticulous manner. (Refer to test panels.)

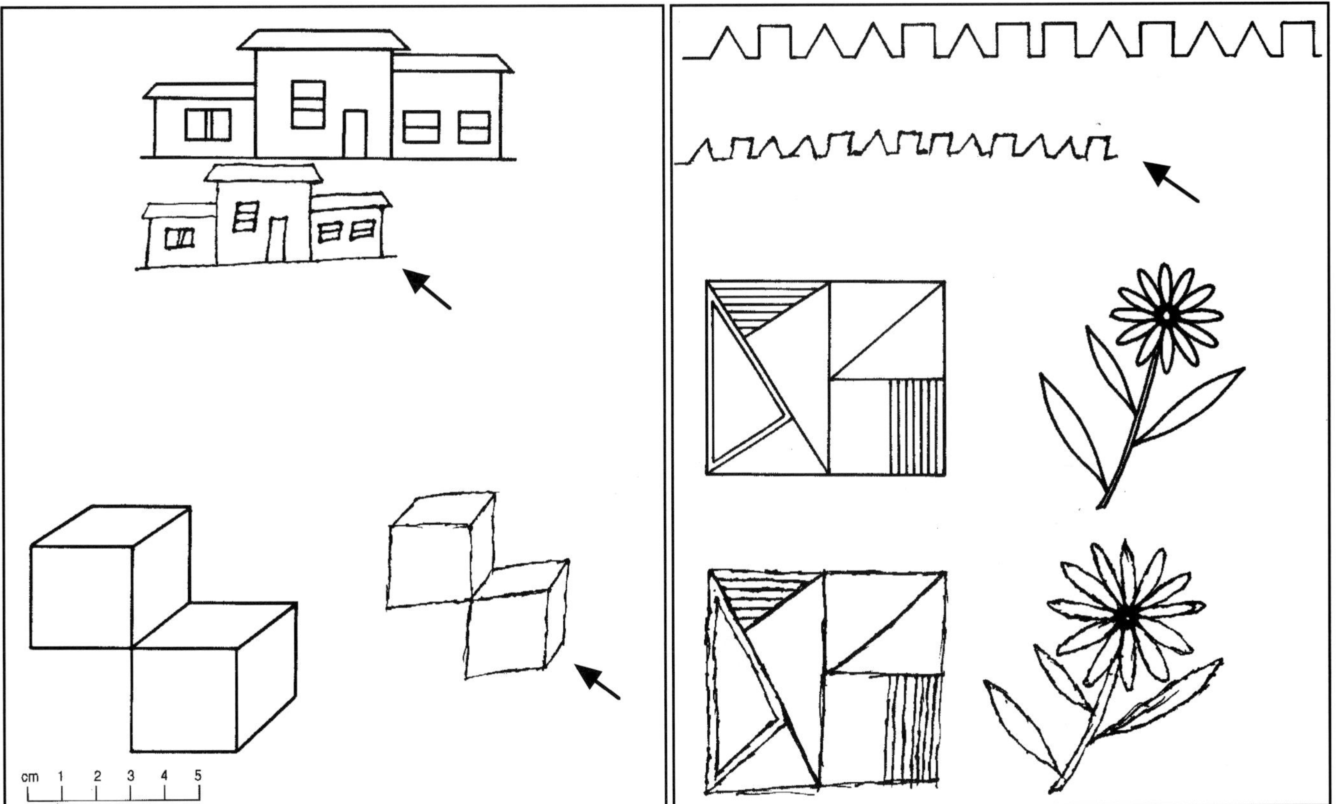

Patient was able to copy figures using multiple sketch strokes of the pen. Although his responses are smaller than the stimulus figures on some tests (refer to arrows), this was not a consistent finding. Completion time was not significantly prolonged, and instructions did not need to be reinforced or repeated.

FRONTAL MENINGIOMA IN A PATIENT WITH PROGRESSIVE NEUROBEHAVIOURAL CHANGES

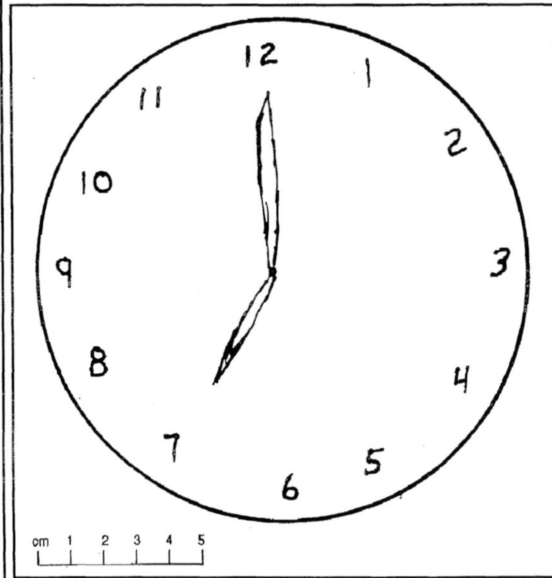

Clock drawing revealed an equivocal spatial planning deficit (note relative spaces between 4, 5, 6, and 7). The remainder of the testing was unremarkable.

An electroencephalogram revealed bilateral frontotemporal paroxysmal sharp wave discharge activity and amplitude suppression over the rostral head regions. These findings, in the context of the history of episodic alterations of responsiveness, were suggestive of complex partial seizure activity arising from the frontal and anterior temporal regions.

Computerized tomography demonstrated a large, dural-based frontal mass lesion with anteroposterior mass effect and associated edema which was relatively mild considering the magnitude of the lesion. Hyperostosis frontalis and frontal bossing were clearly evident rostral to the lesion.

A heterogeneous pattern of increased X-ray attenuation prior to contrast administration was suggestive of regions of calcification within the mass. Marked contrast enhancement was observed, with enlarged vessels associated with the mass lesion. These findings were consistent with a large meningioma. (Refer to figure).

The patient was treated with anticonvulsants and the meningioma was resected in a four stage procedure. On follow-up, the patient was doing well, residing with family. There was no recurrence of seizure activity. He had been left with mild attentional and recent memory deficits, however these improved over the next several months.

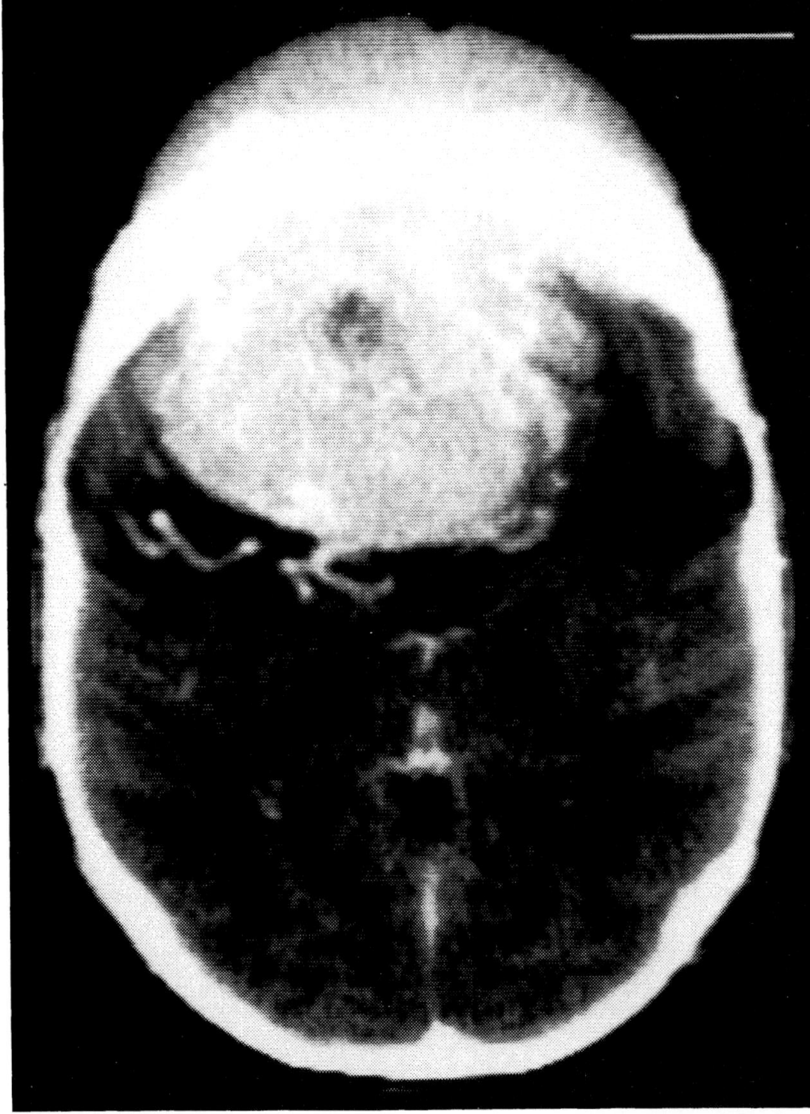

FRONTAL MENINGIOMA: COMPUTERIZED TOMOGRAPHY WITH INTRAVENOUS CONTRAST

PATHOLOGIC CHARACTERISTICS OF MENINGIOMAS

Although meningiomas are considered as tumors arising from the meninges, the specific cell types of origin remain to be elucidated. It has been proposed that the histogenesis may involve arachnoid cap cells or fibroblastic elements of the meningeal layers. The multipotentiality of function of arachnoid cells may account for the marked variability in the histologic appearance of these tumors. Electron microscopic studies have not demonstrated fundamental differences between meningothelial and fibroblastic subtypes of meningiomas. The determination of which of the meningeal layers gives rise to these tumors is not readily apparent; therefore, the classification of meningiomas is based upon histologic characteristics rather than specific cellular or tissue sources.

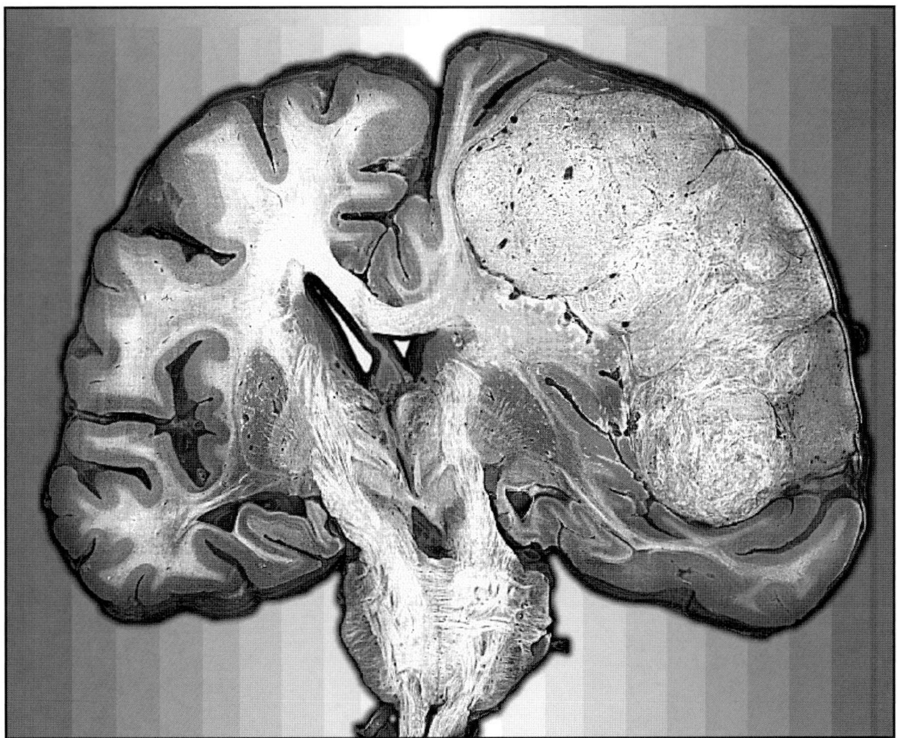

DURAL-BASED MENINGIOMA ARISING OVER THE CEREBRAL CONVEXITY

Dural-based meningiomas arise in various anatomic regions. Of those arising over the cerebral convexities, approximately 50% involve the sagittal sinus. The remainder of the dural-based group, lateral sites are common, including the Sylvian fissure. Other well-known locations include the olfactory groove, sphenoid ridges, and the parasellar region. The anterior half of the cranial vault is involved with a far greater frequency than the posterior half.

Meningiomas may arise from the tela choroidea or the choroid plexus. These intraventricular masses, although not dural-based, are often not histologically distinguishable from the surface lesions. The incidence of hyperostosis in association with meningiomas has been estimated at between 4 and 5 percent (Cushing and Eisenhardt, 1938). This figure has been supported by subsequent clinical and neuropathologic studies. The mechanism for the stimulation of bone formation remains unclear and may occur in the absence of any demonstrable infiltration of bony structures with tumor cells. Of interest is the fact that many histologic types of meningiomas may produce bony spicules. New bone formation as well as calcifications (including Psammoma bodies) may result in radio-opacity of the tumor.

HISTOLOGIC TYPES OF MENINGIOMAS

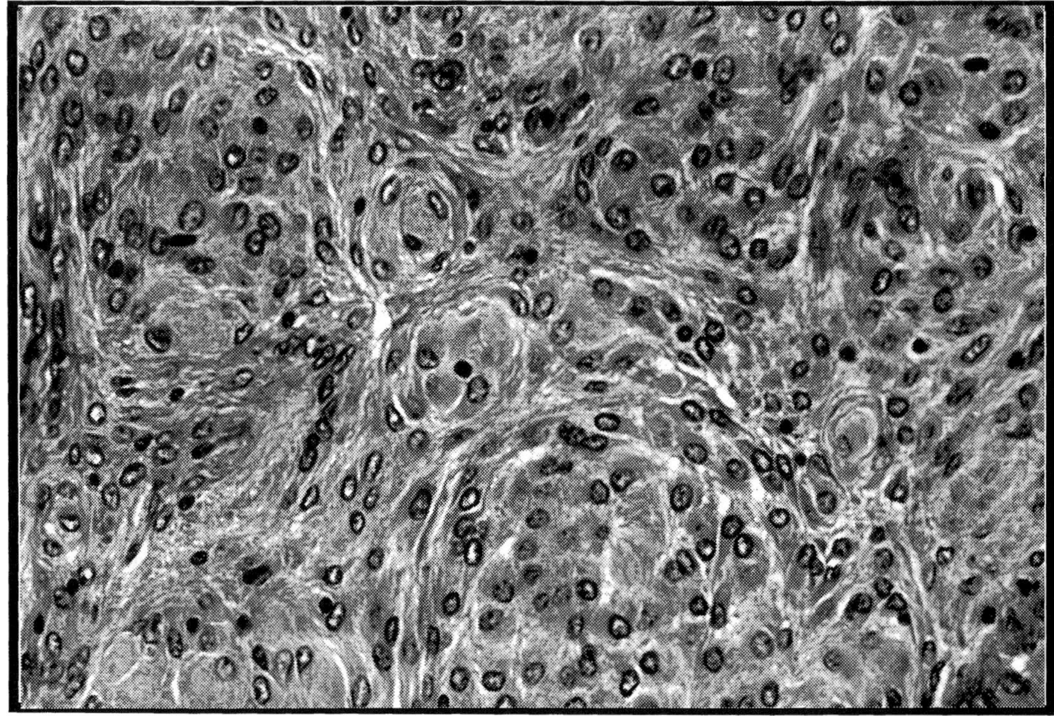

1. Meningotheliomatous or Syncytial Type (Hematoxylin and Eosin, 200X)

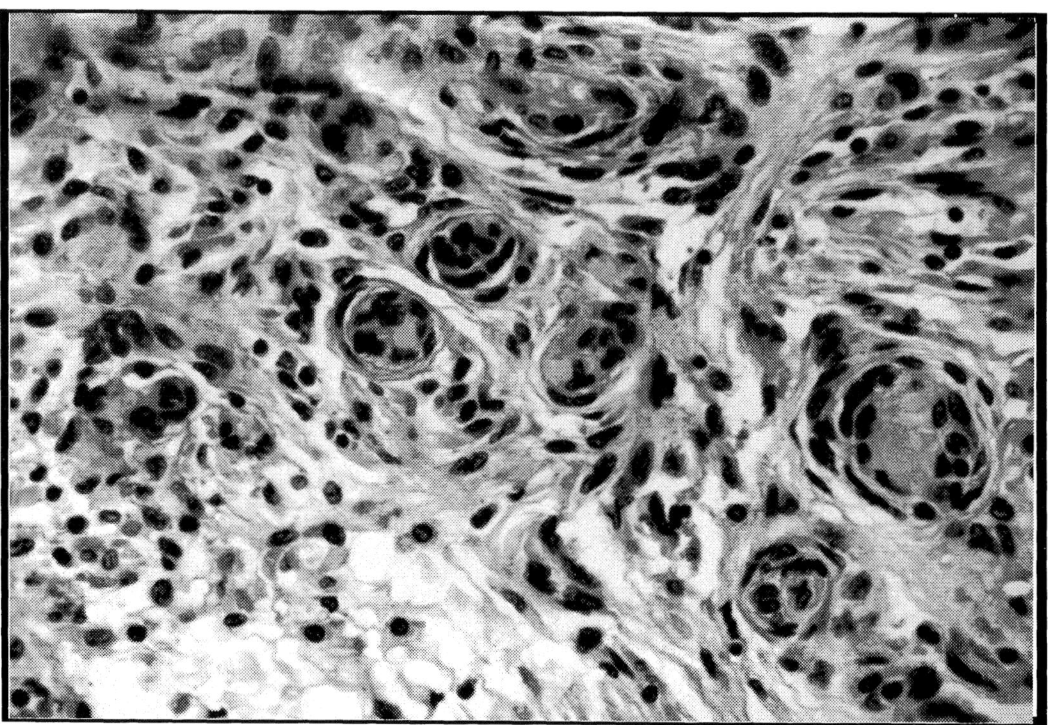

2. Transitional Type demonstrating whorl formations (Hematoxylin and Eosin, 200X)

HISTOLOGIC TYPES OF MENINGIOMAS

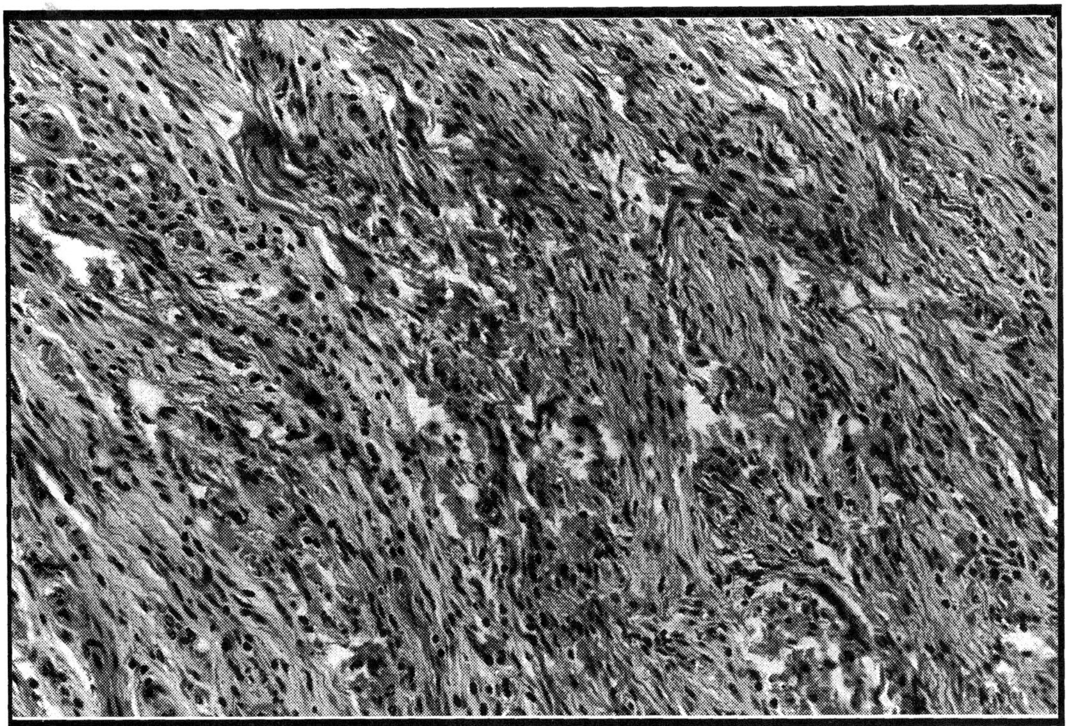

3. Fibroblastic or Fibrous Type (Hematoxylin and Eosin, 100X)

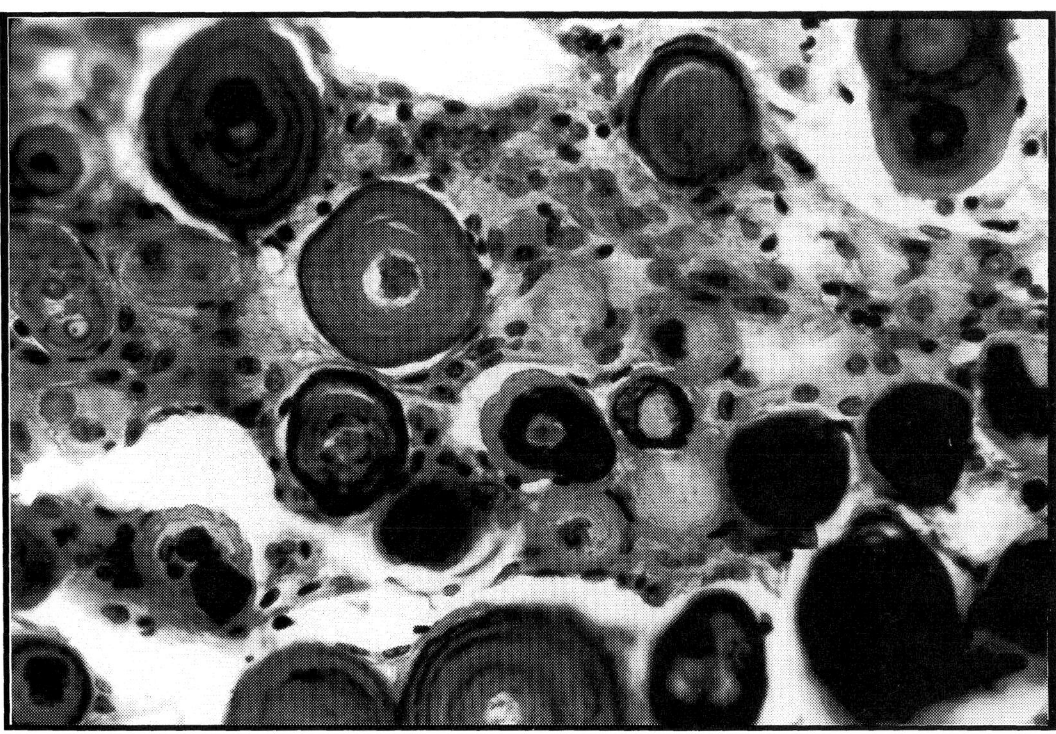

4. Psammomatous Type with typical concentrically calcified Psammoma bodies (Hematoxylin and Eosin, 200X)

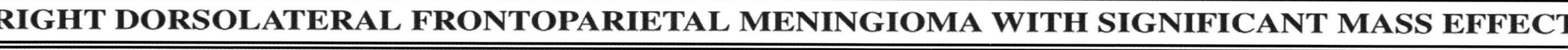

RIGHT DORSOLATERAL FRONTOPARIETAL MENINGIOMA WITH SIGNIFICANT MASS EFFECT

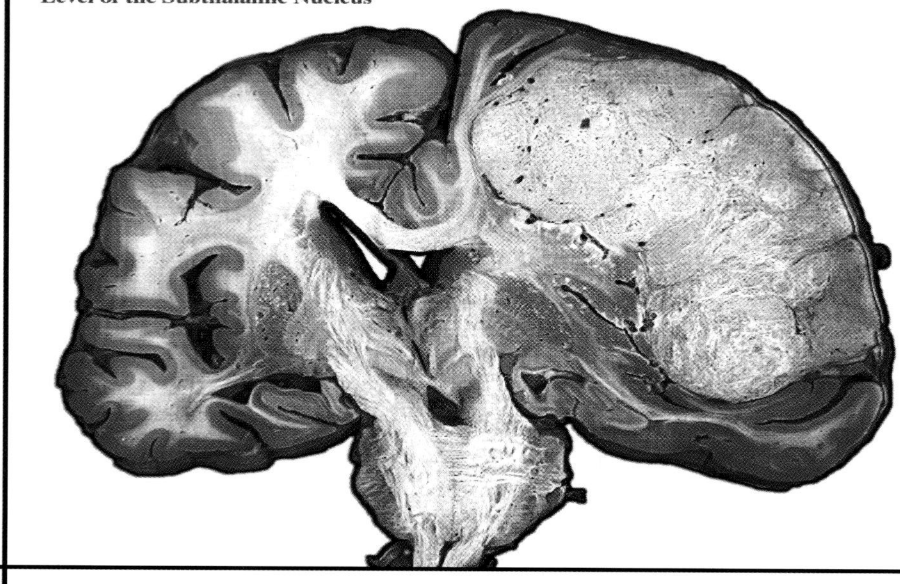

Level of the Anterior Commissure

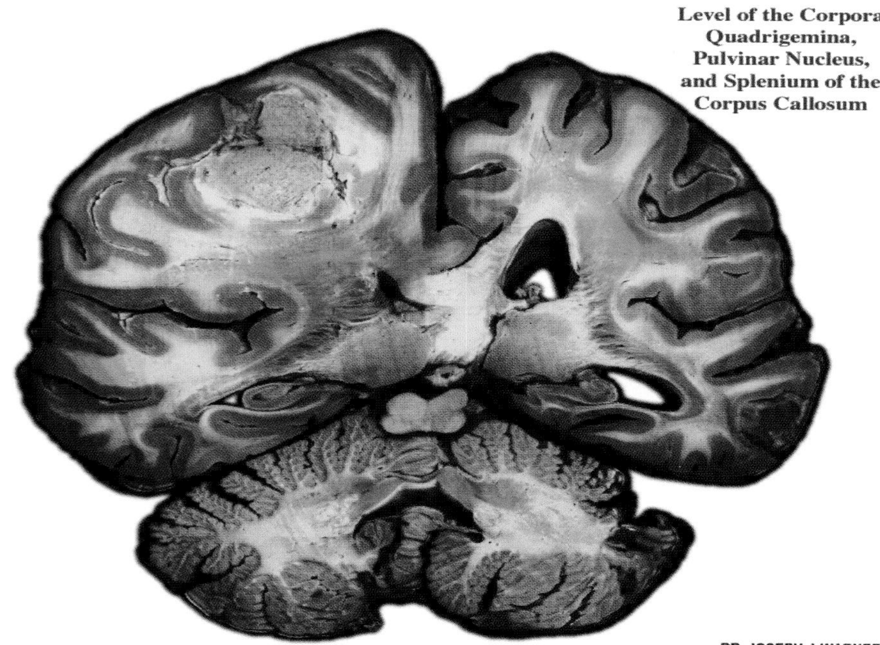

Level of the Subthalamic Nucleus

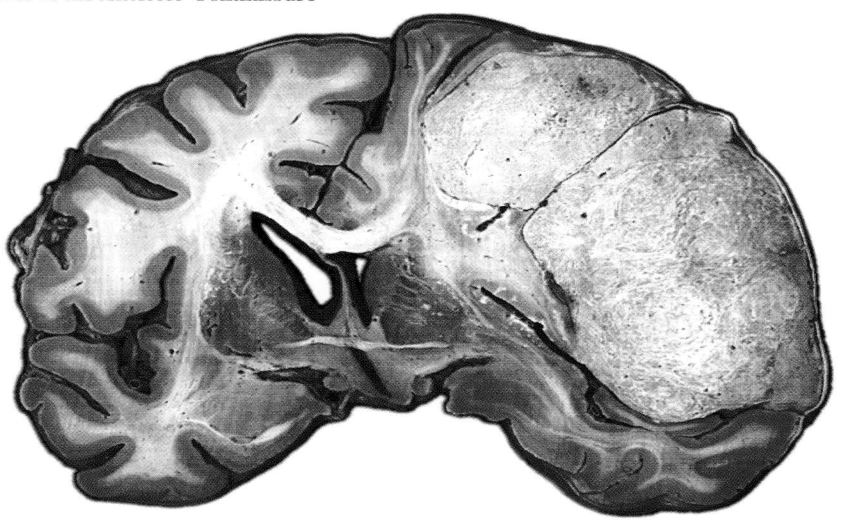

Level of the Centromedian Nucleus and Decussation of the Superior Cerebellar Peduncles

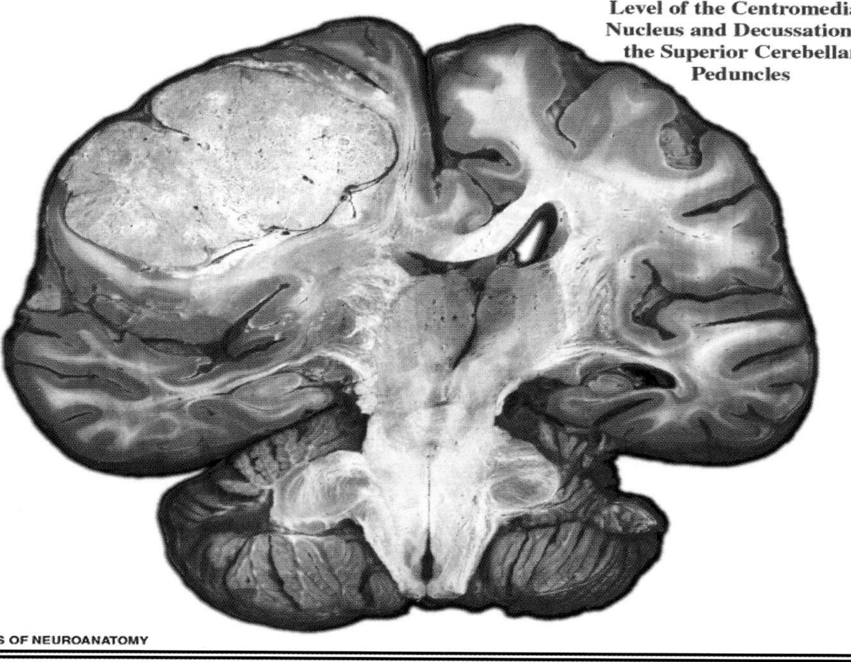

Level of the Corpora Quadrigemina, Pulvinar Nucleus, and Splenium of the Corpus Callosum

SECTIONS APPROXIMATELY PARALLEL TO THE LONGITUDINAL AXIS OF THE BRAINSTEM: CUPRIC ACETATE - ACETIC ACID - FORMALIN PROTOCOL (WARNER)

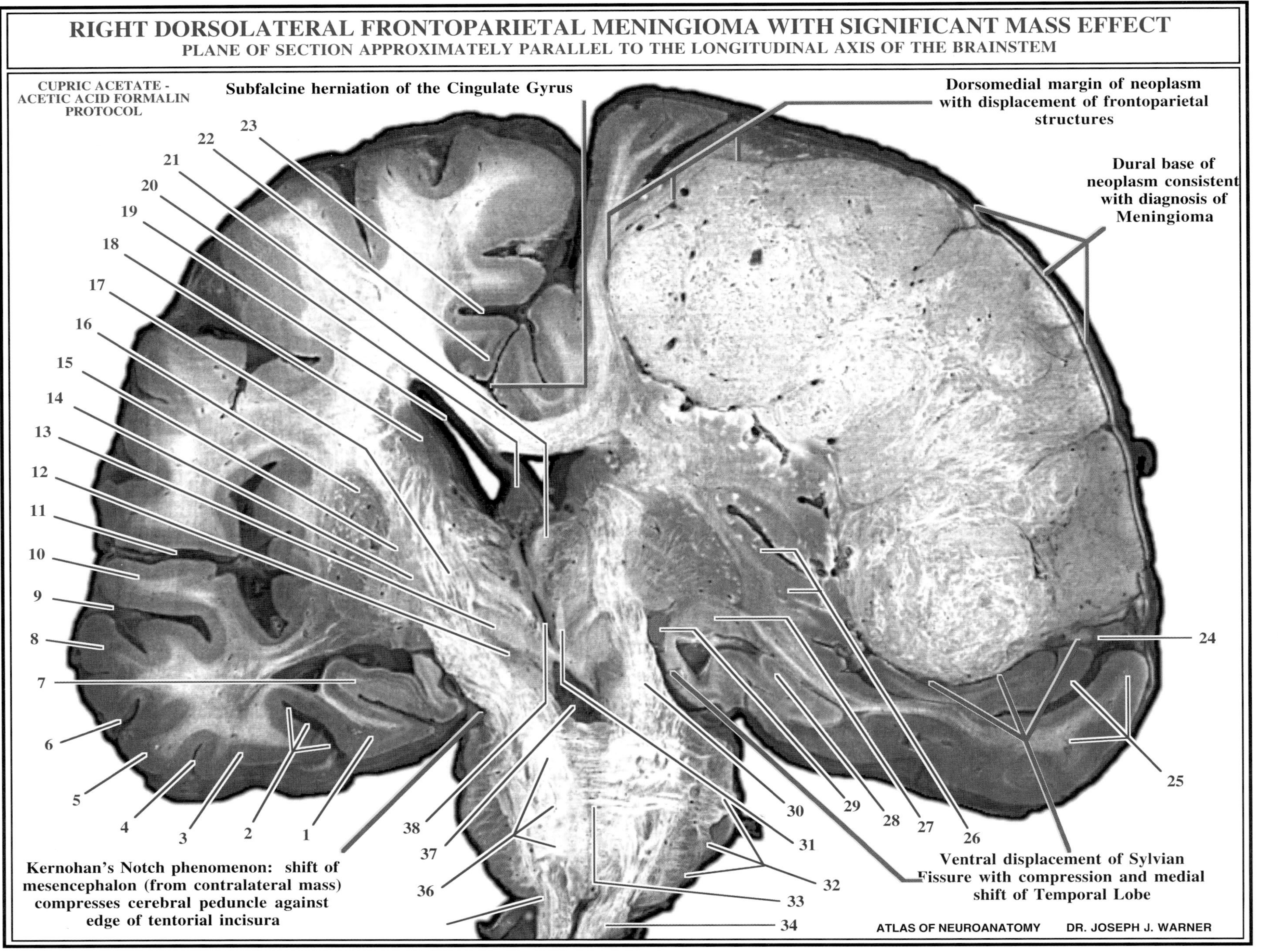
RIGHT DORSOLATERAL FRONTOPARIETAL MENINGIOMA WITH SIGNIFICANT MASS EFFECT
PLANE OF SECTION APPROXIMATELY PARALLEL TO THE LONGITUDINAL AXIS OF THE BRAINSTEM
CUPRIC ACETATE - ACETIC ACID FORMALIN PROTOCOL
Subfalcine herniation of the Cingulate Gyrus
Dorsomedial margin of neoplasm with displacement of frontoparietal structures
Dural base of neoplasm consistent with diagnosis of Meningioma
Ventral displacement of Sylvian Fissure with compression and medial shift of Temporal Lobe
Kernohan's Notch phenomenon: shift of mesencephalon (from contralateral mass) compresses cerebral peduncle against edge of tentorial incisura
1
2
3
4
5
6
7
8
9
10
11
12
13
14
15
16
17
18
19
20
21
22
23
24
25
26
27
28
29
30
31
32
33
34
36
37
38
ATLAS OF NEUROANATOMY
DR. JOSEPH J. WARNER

RIGHT DORSOLATERAL FRONTOPARIETAL MENINGIOMA WITH SIGNIFICANT MASS EFFECT, PLANE OF SECTION APPROXIMATELY PARALLEL TO THE LONGITUDINAL AXIS OF THE BRAINSTEM: SECTION ORIENTATION AND KEY TO NUMBERED STRUCTURES

KEY TO NUMBERED STRUCTURES

1. Parahippocampal Gyrus
2. Collateral Sulcus
3. Fusiform Gyrus
4. Inferior Temporal Sulcus
5. Inferior Temporal Gyrus
6. Middle Temporal Sulcus
7. Hippocampus
8. Middle Temporal Gyrus
9. Superior Temporal Sulcus
10. Superior Temporal Gyrus
11. Sylvian Fissure
12. Substantia Nigra
13. Subthalamic Nucleus
14. Globus Pallidus I
15. Globus Pallidus II
16. Putamen
17. Posterior Limb, Internal Capsule
18. Caudate Nucleus
19. Body of the Lateral Ventricle
20. Fornix
21. Anterior Nucleus, Thalamus
22. Cingulate Cortex
23. Cingulate Sulcus
24. Sylvian Fissure
25. Superior and Middle Temporal Gyri
26. Insular Cortex
27. Amygdala
28. Hippocampus
29. Optic Tract
30. Cerebral Peduncle
31. Mammillothalamic Tract
32. Middle Cerebellar Peduncle (Ventral Aspect)
33. Transverse Pontocerebellar Fibers
34. Medullary Pyramid
35. Pontomedullary Sulcus
36. Corticospinal, Corticobulbar Tracts
37. Interpeduncular Fossa
38. Third Ventricle

Note: The long term Cupric Acetate-Acetic Acid-Formalin post-fixation with Image Spectral Histogram Extension (Warner) results in blue staining of white matter tracts oriented either obliquely or transverse to the plane of section and enhances structural differentiation. The tumor does not demonstrate such staining.

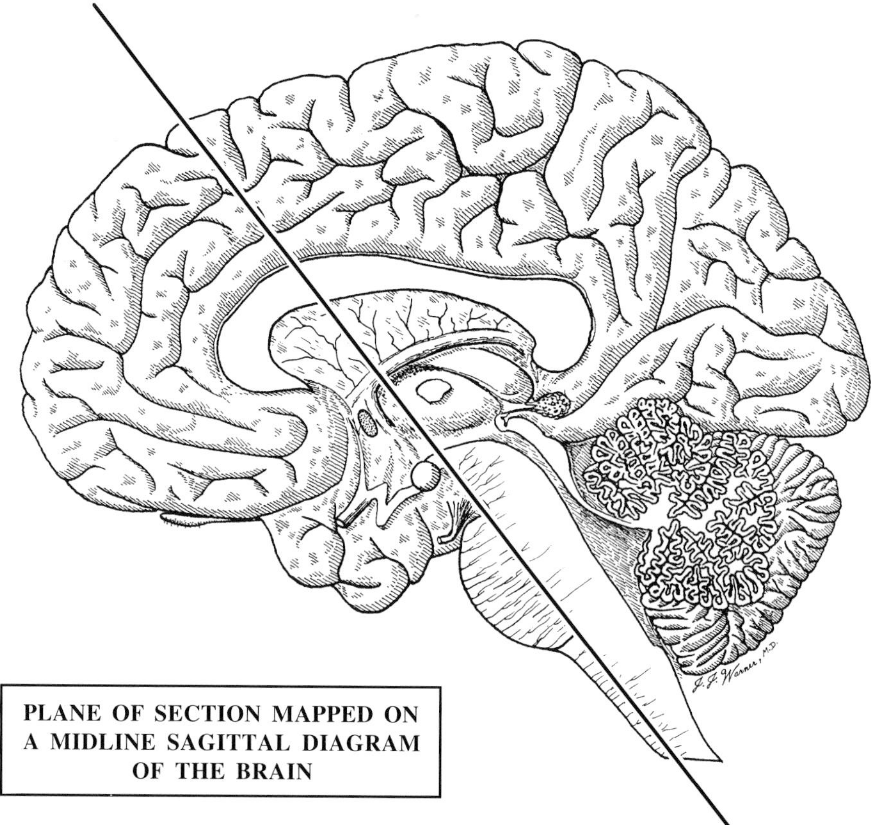

PLANE OF SECTION MAPPED ON A MIDLINE SAGITTAL DIAGRAM OF THE BRAIN

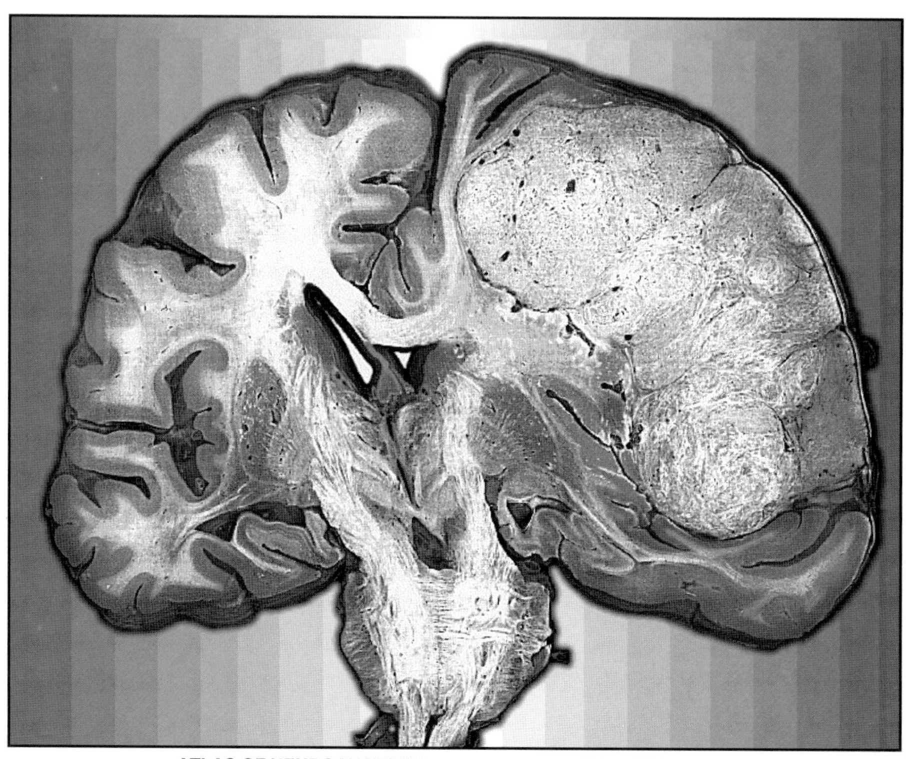

CASE PRESENTATION

This 32-year-old male presented with a history of gradually progressive weakness of the right face, arm, and leg, with an intermittent "tingling" sensation of the right side of his body, which evolved into a feeling of numbness. The patient developed speech difficulties, characterized by family members as "slurring" of his words, and also "coming out with the wrong words." They commented that he seemed to have some trouble understanding others when they spoke to him. The patient complained of early morning headaches. He later sustained seizures, beginning in the right arm, then spreading to involve the right side of the face and leg, followed by generalized tonic-clonic activity.

Neurologic findings included global aphasia, right hemiparesis involving the face, arm, and leg, and diminished perception of various sensory modalities over the right side of the body (including the face). Impaired opticokinetic nystagmus (saccades and pursuit) was discerned when the test strip was passed from the patient's right to his left.

Computerized tomography with intravenous contrast was performed (see figure). The scan revealed a large ring-enhancing lesion with a radiolucent center involving the left cerebral hemisphere, and evidence of edema extending throughout the frontoparietal white matter. Significant mass effect was present, with a left to right midline shift and compression of the ipsilateral lateral ventricle.

A diagnosis of glioblastoma multiforme was made. The patient was given intravenous dexamethasone, phenytoin, and administered 5000 r of cranial radiation therapy in divided doses. Despite therapeutic intervention, the patient deteriorated. A left gaze preference was observed. He became progressively somnolent, then comatose. His left pupil dilated, followed by right-sided decorticate posturing. Subsequently, no movements of either side could be elicited. The patient developed decerebrate posturing and sustained a cardiopulmonary arrest six months after the diagnosis was made. He was not resuscitated.

GLIOBLASTOMA MULTIFORME INVOLVING THE LEFT CEREBRAL HEMISPHERE: HORIZONTAL SECTION, LEVEL OF THE ANTERIOR NUCLEUS OF THE THALAMUS, 15μ, H & E STAINED

The brain was sectioned in the horizontal plane in order to approximate the orientation of the computerized tomographic images of the case. (Refer to figure of CT.) Neuropathologic examination confirmed the diagnosis of glioblastoma multiforme. Areas of contrast enhancement on the CT scan correlated with hypercellularity on the margins of the neoplasm. The shift of midline structures is well demonstrated on the CT and histologic sections.

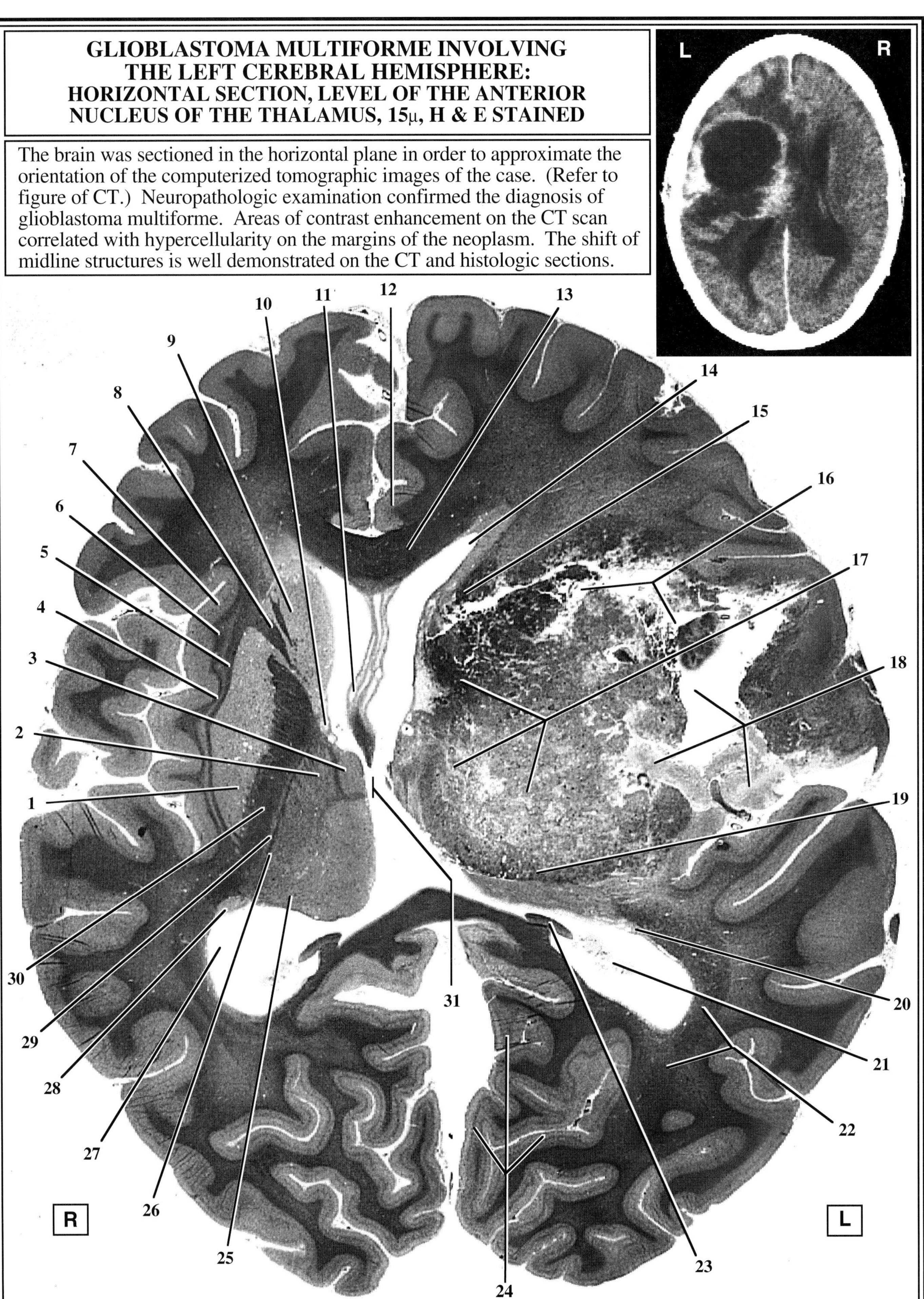

GLIOBLASTOMA MULTIFORME INVOLVING THE LEFT CEREBRAL HEMISPHERE: COMPUTERIZED TOMOGRAPHY AND HISTOPATHOLOGIC SECTION CORRELATION SECTION MAPS AND KEY TO NUMBERED STRUCTURES

CT SCAN (SECTION MAP A): KEY TO NUMBERED STRUCTURES

1. Contrast enhancement in area of neoplastic proliferation
2. Central tumor necrosis
3. Rostral margin of tumor
4. Vasogenic edema, Frontal Lobe
5. Corpus Callosum
6. Body of Lateral Ventricle
7. Septum Pellucidum
8. Choroid Plexus
9. Atrium of Lateral Ventricle
10. Falx Cerebri
11. Striate Cortex (Area 17)
12. Occipital Horn of Lateral Ventricle
13. Vasogenic edema
14. Contrast enhancement of tumor dorsal to Thalamus

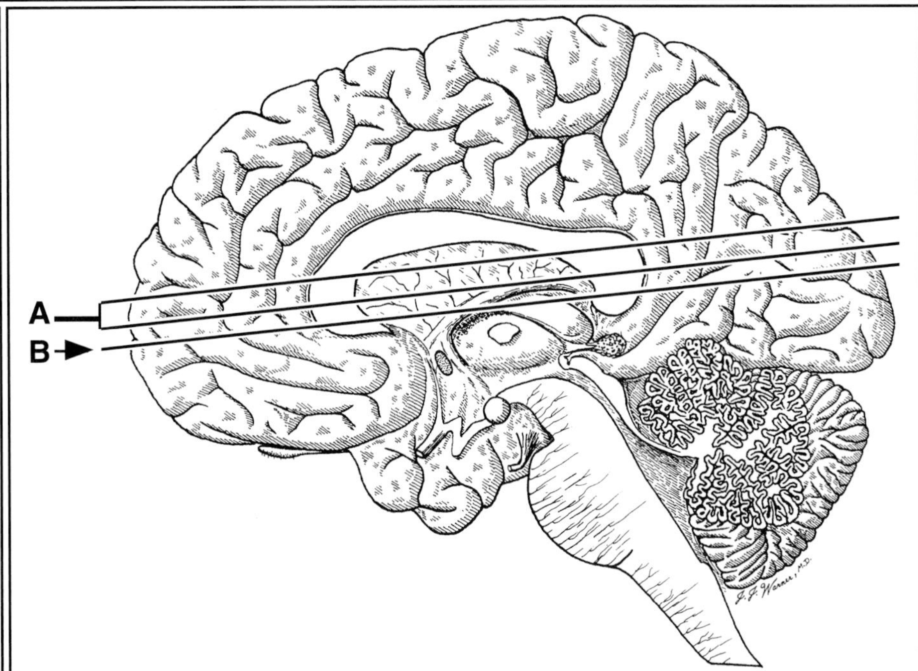

HORIZONTAL SECTION, LEVEL OF THE ANTERIOR NUCLEUS OF THE THALAMUS (SECTION MAP B): 15μ, H & E STAIN; KEY TO NUMBERED STRUCTURES

1. Putamen
2. Ventroanterior Nucleus of the Thalamus
3. Anterior Nucleus of the Thalamus
4. Claustrum
5. External Capsule
6. Extreme Capsule
7. Insular Cortex
8. Anterior Limb of Internal Capsule
9. Head of the Caudate Nucleus
10. Thalamostriate Vein
11. Septal Vein within Septum Pellucidum
12. Cingulate Gyrus
13. Corpus Callosum
14. Anterior Horn of the Lateral Ventricle
15. Neoplastic invasion of the Caudate
16. Tumor necrosis with cavitation
17. Tumor invasion/replacement of Internal Capsule, Putamen, and Globus Pallidus
18. Necrosis in region of Insula, Sylvian Fissure
19. Tumor margin advancing through Thalamus
20. Tail of the Caudate Nucleus
21. Choroid Plexus
22. Optic Radiations
23. Fornix
24. Striate Cortex (Area 17)
25. Pulvinar
26. External Medullary Lamina of the Thalamus
27. Atrium of the Lateral Ventricle
28. Tail of the Caudate Nucleus
29. Reticular Nucleus of the Thalamus
30. Posterior Limb of the Internal Capsule
31. Midline shift (left to right, mass effect)

Glioblastoma multiforme comprises 20% of all intracranial tumors according to the combined series of Zulch, Cushing, and Olivecrona (a total of 15,000 cases). Of all tumors of glial cell origin, glioblastoma multiforme accounts for 55%, and for 90% of gliomas of the cerebral hemispheres in adults. The peak incidence of this tumor is in mid-adulthood, and (according to Zulch and Rubinstein) is twice as frequent in males as in females. Glioblastoma is generally thought to arise from anaplasia of mature astrocytes. The histologic findings include hypercellularity, pseudopalisading of cells and zones of necrosis, tumor giant cells, frequent mitotic figures, cellular pleomorphism and hyperchromaticity. Associated findings include endothelial proliferation of small vessels, vascular thrombosis, and hemorrhage. Cells of the glioblastoma may break free and move through the cerebrospinal fluid, seeding other regions of the central nervous system. Such dissemination and growth of cells may give rise to meningeal gliomatosis or foci of malignant cells on spinal roots. Extraneural metastasis is rare. Clinical symptomatology is initially nonspecific, and the tumor may reach a remarkably large size with extensive involvement of the brain before specific localizing signs or symptoms are evident. Survival is less than 20% one year after the onset of symptoms, and 10% after two years. Treatment includes cranial radiation, chemotherapeutic protocols, and in certain cases, surgical tumor resection. Such interventions have met with limited clinical success.

GLIOBLASTOMA MULTIFORME: HISTOPATHOLOGY

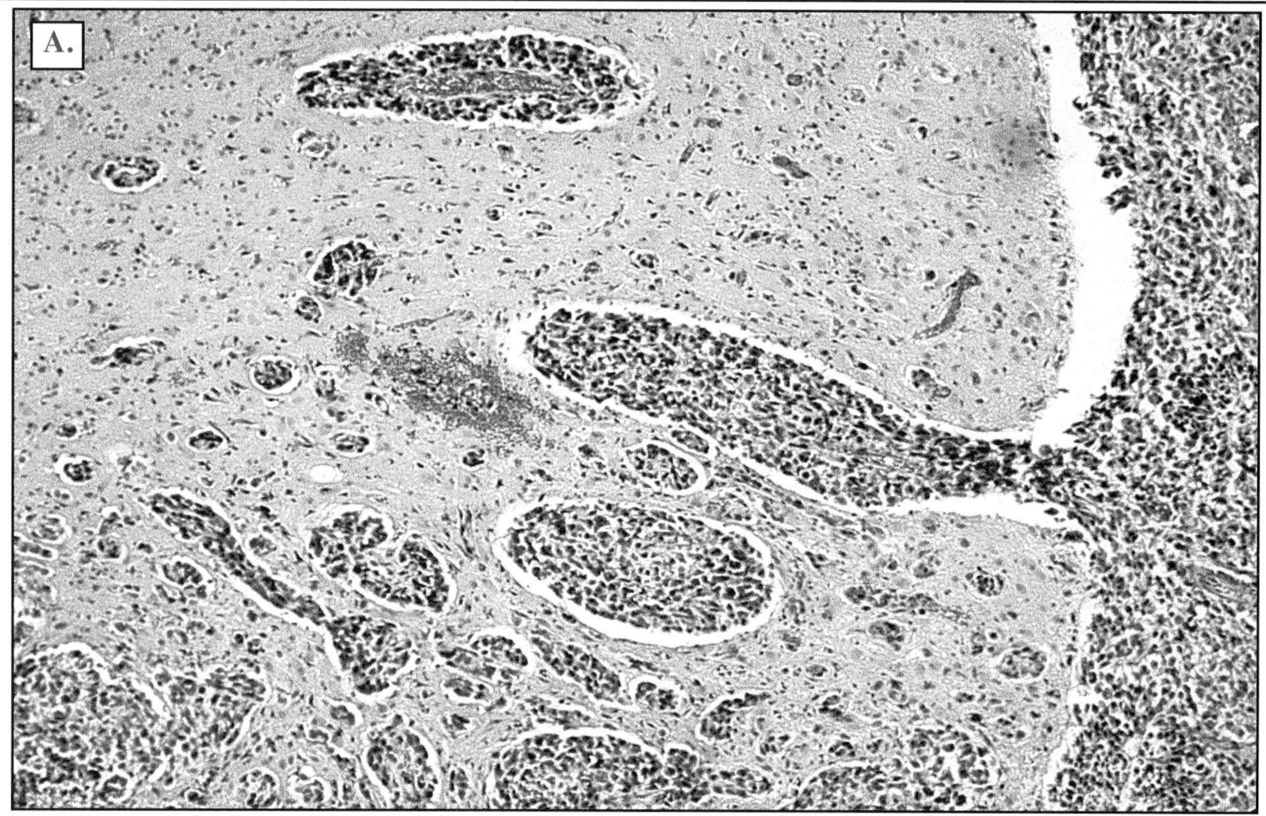

A. Subarachnoid tumor proliferation with cortical invasion through Virchow-Robin Spaces (100X).
B. Cellular pleomorphism with pseudopalisading and necrosis within the glioblastoma (40X).

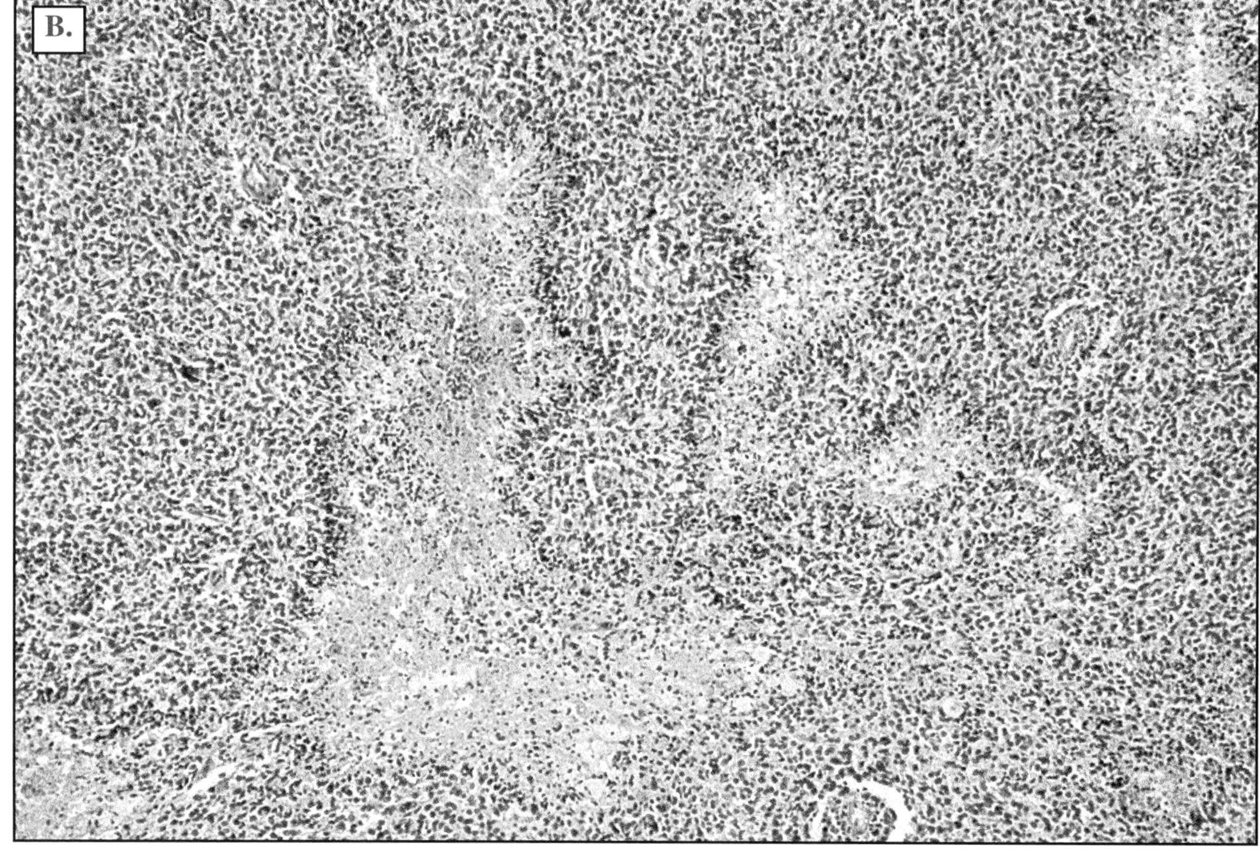

HISTOLOGIC SECTIONS 10 μ, HEMATOXYLIN AND EOSIN STAIN

GLIOBLASTOMA MULTIFORME: HYPERCELLULARITY ASSOCIATED WITH NEOVASCULARIZATION

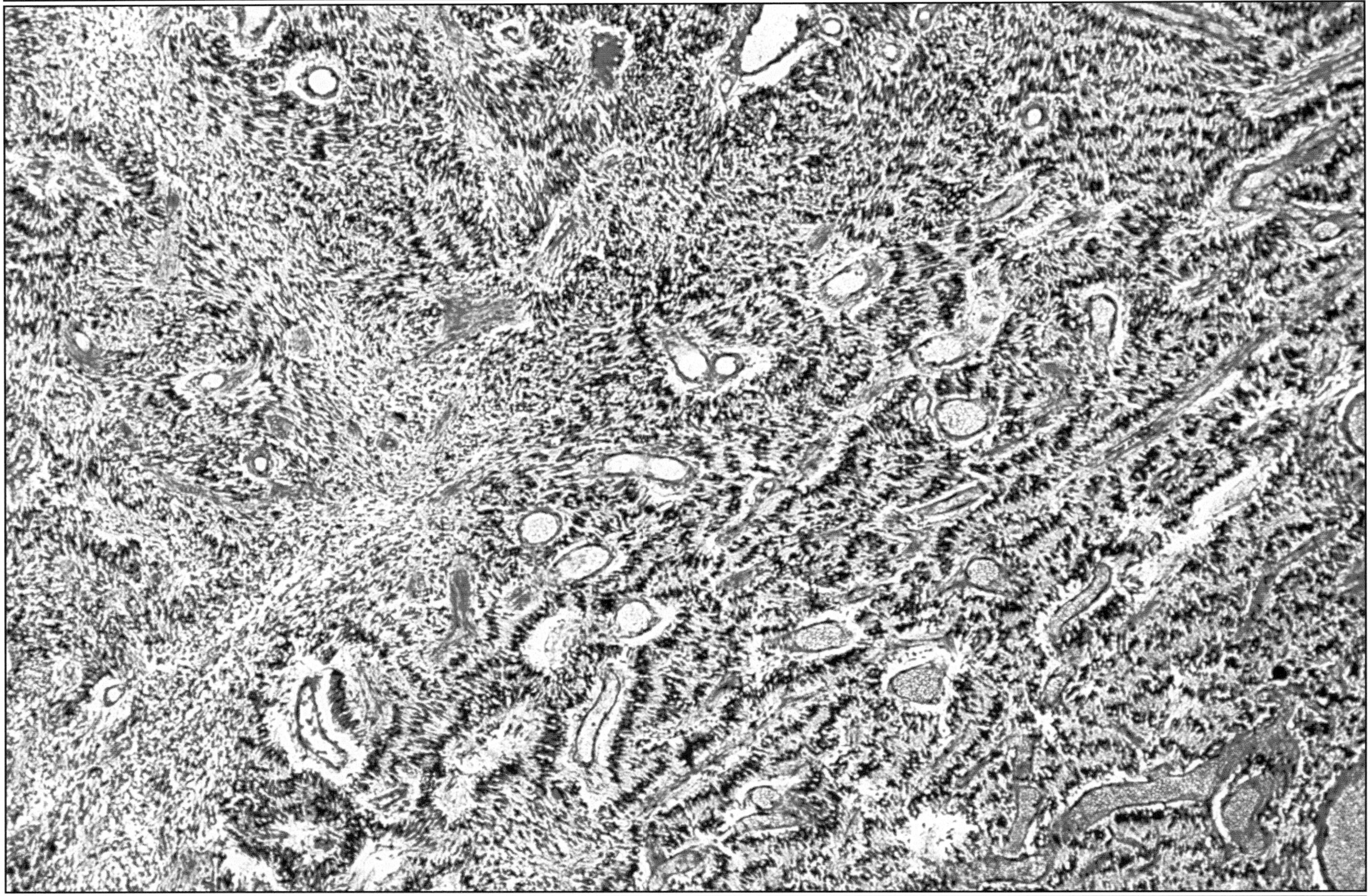

HISTOLOGIC SECTION: 10 μ, PHOSPHOTUNGSTIC ACID HEMATOXYLIN, 40X

DR. JOSEPH J. WARNER

GLIOBLASTOMA MULTIFORME: HISTOPATHOLOGIC CHARACTERISTICS

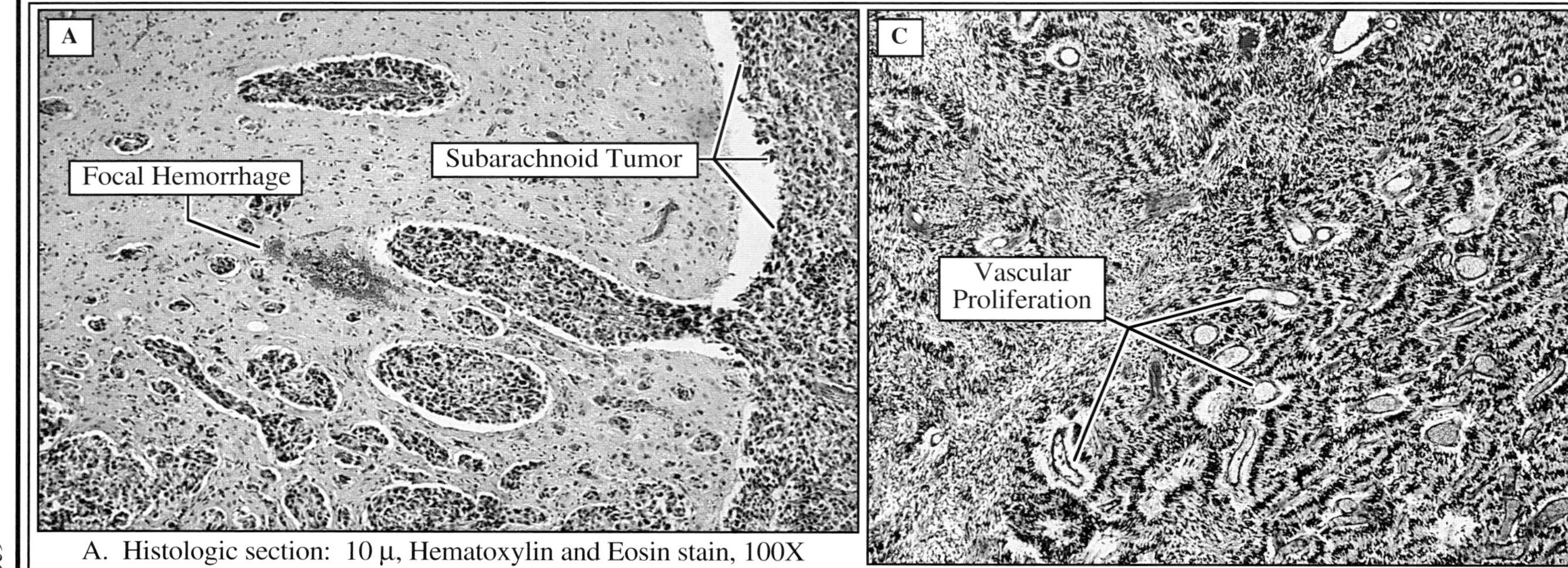

A. Histologic section: 10 µ, Hematoxylin and Eosin stain, 100X

B. Histologic section: 10 µ, Hematoxylin and Eosin stain, 50X

C. Histologic section: 10 µ, Phosphotungstic Acid Hematoxylin, 40X

A. *Subarachnoid tumor proliferation with cortical invasion via the Virchow-Robin spaces.*

This photomicrograph illustrates one of the mechanisms of tumor dissemination that involves growth into the subarachnoid space with invasion of the parenchyma not contiguous with the site of origination of the primary neoplasm. A focal hemorrhage is also demonstrated.

B. *Cellular pleomorphism with pseudopalisading and necrosis within the glioblastoma.*

A diagnostic feature of glioblastoma, foci of necrosis surrounded by pseudopalisading cells are frequently detected in biopsy as well as pathologic examination.

C. *Hypercellularity with palisading of cells associated with neovascularization.*

Formations involving neovascular growth and specific arrangements of tumor cells are among the histopathologic characteristics of glioblastoma. Glomeruloid formation, pseudoglandular cellular patterns, epithelioid metaplasia, and multinucleated giant cells may be encountered within the same region of the tumor.

GLIOBLASTOMA MULTIFORME: HISTOPATHOLOGY

A.

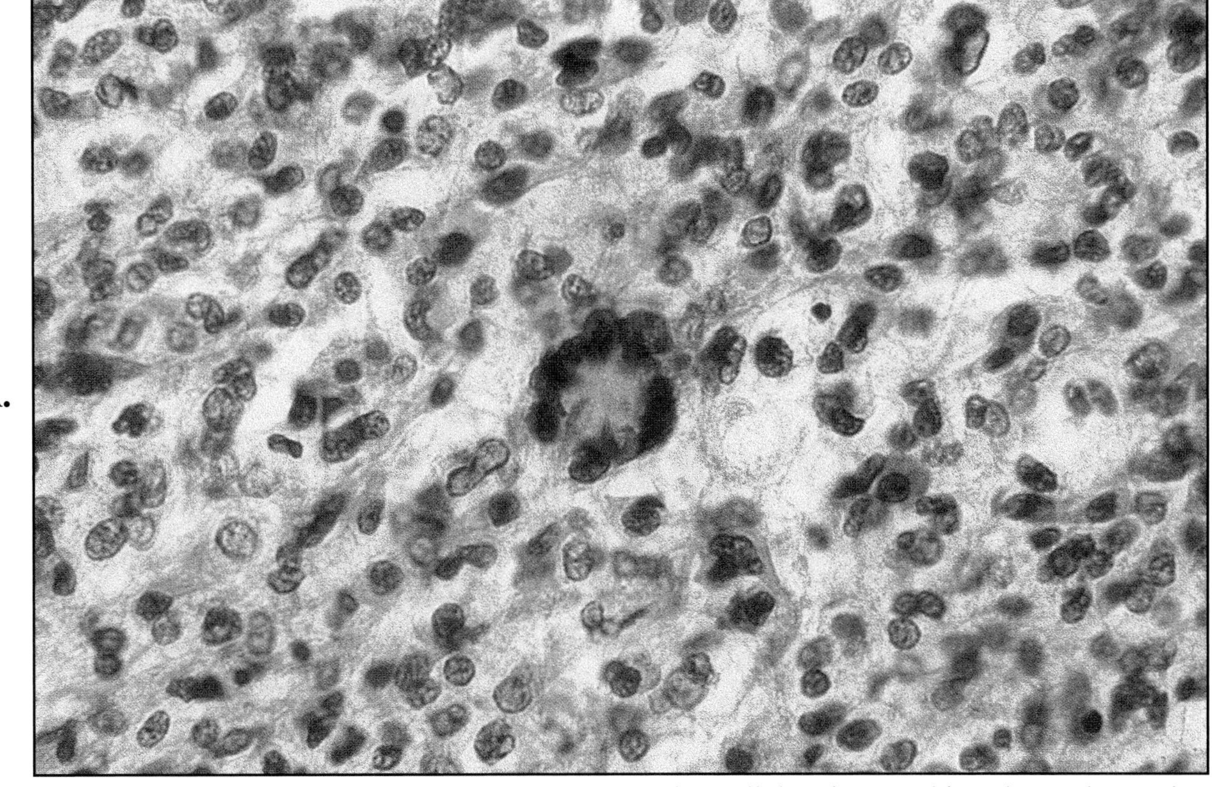

A. Glioblastoma multiforme: 10µ section demonstrating cellular pleomorphism, hyperchromatic nuclei, and a multinucleated tumor giant cell; hematoxylin and eosin, 400X original magnification

B.

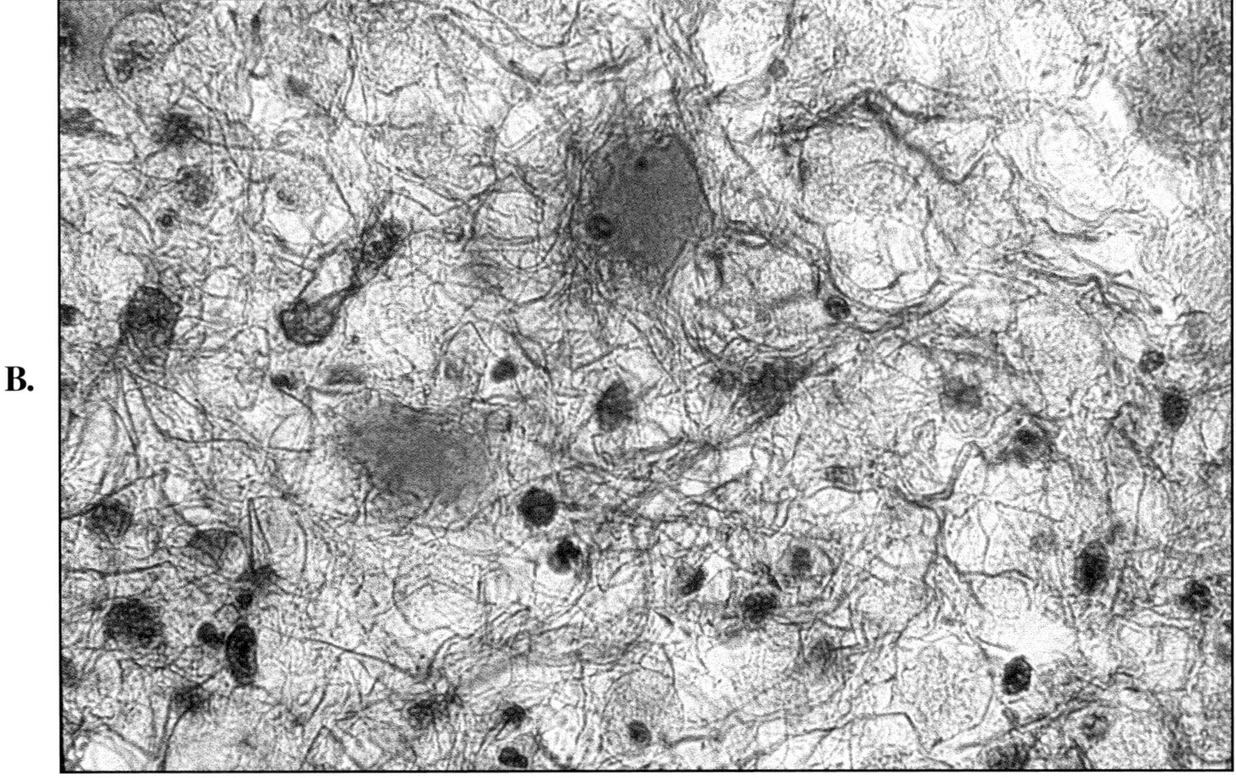

B. Reactive astrocytes in an area of chronic edema adjacent to tumor margin, demonstrating cytoplasmic changes, eccentric nuclear displacement, and abundant glial processes; 10µ section, phosphotungstic acid hematoxylin technique, 400X original magnification

GLIOBLASTOMA MULTIFORME: ASSOCIATED HISTOPATHOLOGY

A.

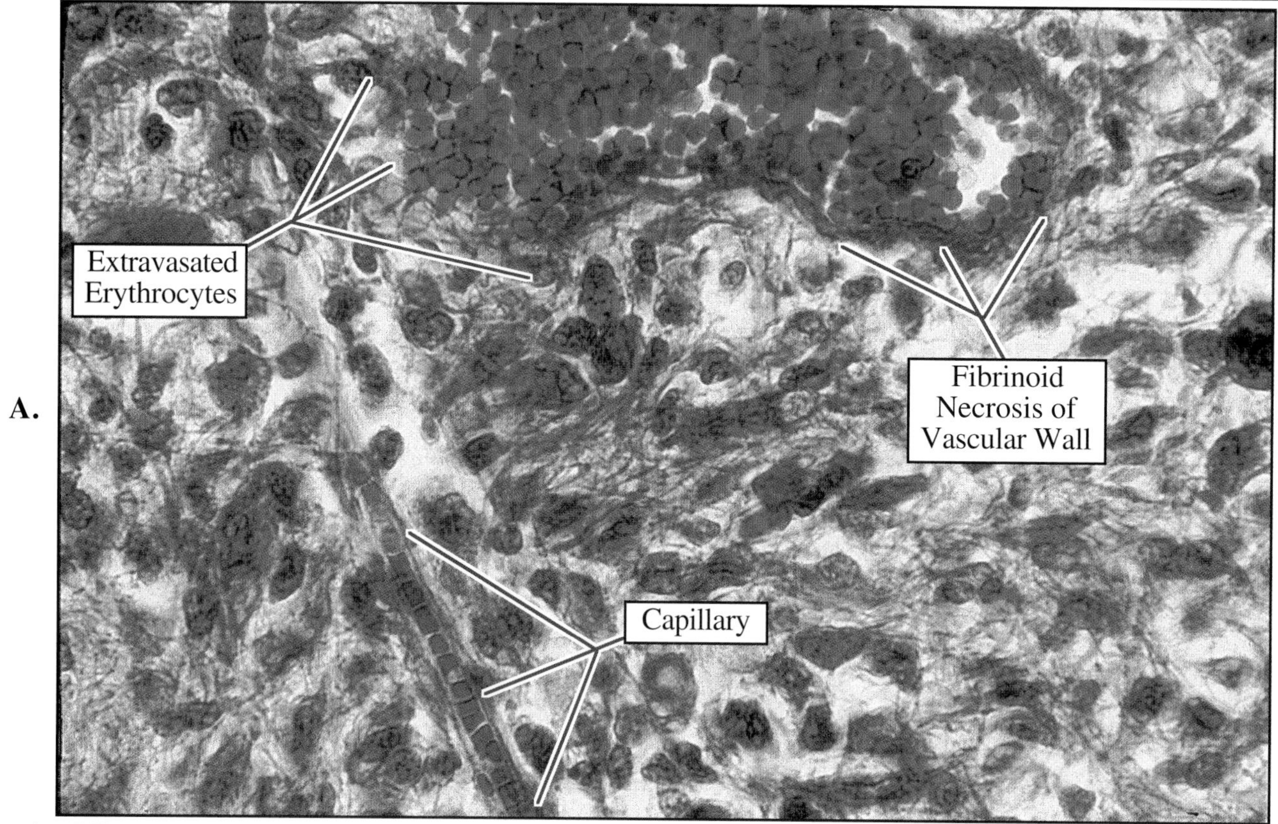

A. Microscopic hemorrhage in highly vascular region of neoplasm; 400X magnification
B. Necrotic margin of tumor, demonstrating numerous macrophages (M) with eccentric nuclei (N), hypervascularity, and an absence of neoplastic cells; 400X magnification

B.

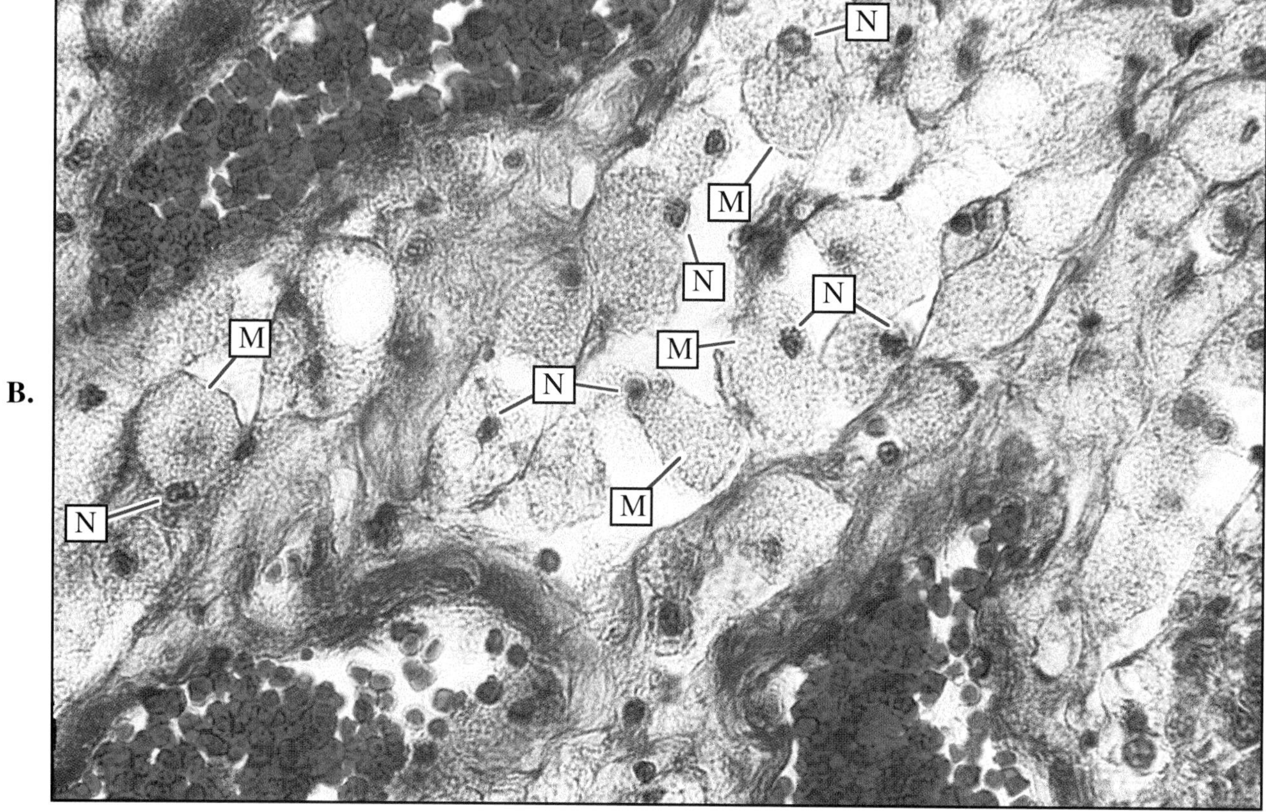

HISTOLOGIC SECTIONS 12μ, TRICHROME STAIN

GLIOBLASTOMA MULTIFORME PRESENTING WITH COMPLEX PARTIAL SEIZURE ACTIVITY

This 58-year-old right-handed white male was admitted to the hospital with a history of a "blackout" during which he was involved in a motor vehicle accident. The recent history was significant for left supraorbital headaches, which the patient had attributed to previous surgery for retinal detachment in the left eye. Approximately two weeks prior to admission, the patient was working in his home when he complained of a metallic taste in his mouth associated with an unpleasant olfactory sensation of "burning tires." He complained of "not feeling right" and indicated that he needed to sit down because he felt "like he was going to pass out." The patient had furthermore described "a feeling that he had never felt before." According to observations by the family, the patient also had a recent history of rapid mood changes, episodic depression, and "fatigue." According to co-workers, there were noticeable changes in his behavior three to five months prior to admission. These changes included abrupt temperament, outbursts of anger, and occasional agitation associated with forgetfulness.

One day prior to admission, the patient was driving his vehicle and experienced a "strange taste in [his] mouth." Approximately 30 seconds later, he reportedly "blacked out." The patient was amnestic for subsequent events. According to available evidence, the patient drove off the road, down an embankment, and struck a road sign. He continued to maneuver the vehicle, crossing the median of a divided highway. The patient subsequently drove the vehicle for several miles on a damaged wheel rim. He took the vehicle in to have the wheel repaired. At this point, the patient apparently regained his ability to remember ongoing events. He recalled having the repair work done and being questioned regarding the circumstances of the vehicular damage. He indicated that he told the repair personnel, "I don't want to talk about it" and experienced frustration at being unable to remember the accident. Following the repair work, he drove to his home. Upon arriving at his home, the patient continued his planned activities for the day as if this incident had never occurred. Later that evening, his wife called him, at which time he informed her that he had experienced a "blackout," and that his vehicle was damaged.

The patient did not seek medical attention until the following day. He was complaining of severe pain above his left eye and sought evaluation by his ophthalmologist. Examination revealed papilledema. Further diagnostic investigation included computerized tomography, which demonstrated a large ring-enhancing mass lesion in the left temporal lobe with associated edema and compression of the ipsilateral cerebral peduncle. Neurosurgical consultation was obtained. The patient was initiated on dexamethasone and phenytoin for a presumptive diagnosis of seizure activity associated with a mass lesion. Magnetic resonance imaging was performed which demonstrated a four by five centimeter mass in the left temporal lobe and extensive edema involving white matter of the temporal, frontal, and parietal lobes. Associated findings included subfalcine herniation of the cingulate gyrus, contralateral midline shift, ipsilateral compression of the lateral ventricle, and sulcal effacement extending to the vertex of the left hemisphere.

Three days after admission, a left craniotomy was performed. A resection, estimated at approximately 80% of the tumor volume, was followed by implantation of a chemotherapy wafer, Frozen section and permanent histologic section studies confirmed the diagnosis of glioblastoma multiforme.

Neurobehavioural testing was obtained in the early afternoon of the eleventh post-operative day. Findings included a deficit in the Thurstone controlled word fluency test (six "s" responses in one minute), mild dysgraphia with occasional spelling errors, and one error on serial subtractions (from one hundred by sevens). Comprehension, repetition, object and color naming, and spontaneous speech were normal. However, an analysis of spontaneous speech performed within one hour of awakening in the morning revealed infrequent phonemic paraphasic errors. No evidence of dyscalculia, allochiria, agnosia, or apraxia was discernible. Letter circling test was normal, however, a geometric shape selection task revealed numerous omissions, especially in the right superior quadrant, No significant constructional apraxia or visuospatial dysfunction was evident. Clock drawing did reveal a mild deficit in visuospatial planning.

DR. JOSEPH J. WARNER

GLIOBLASTOMA MULTIFORME OF THE LEFT TEMPORAL LOBE: MAGNETIC RESONANCE IMAGING

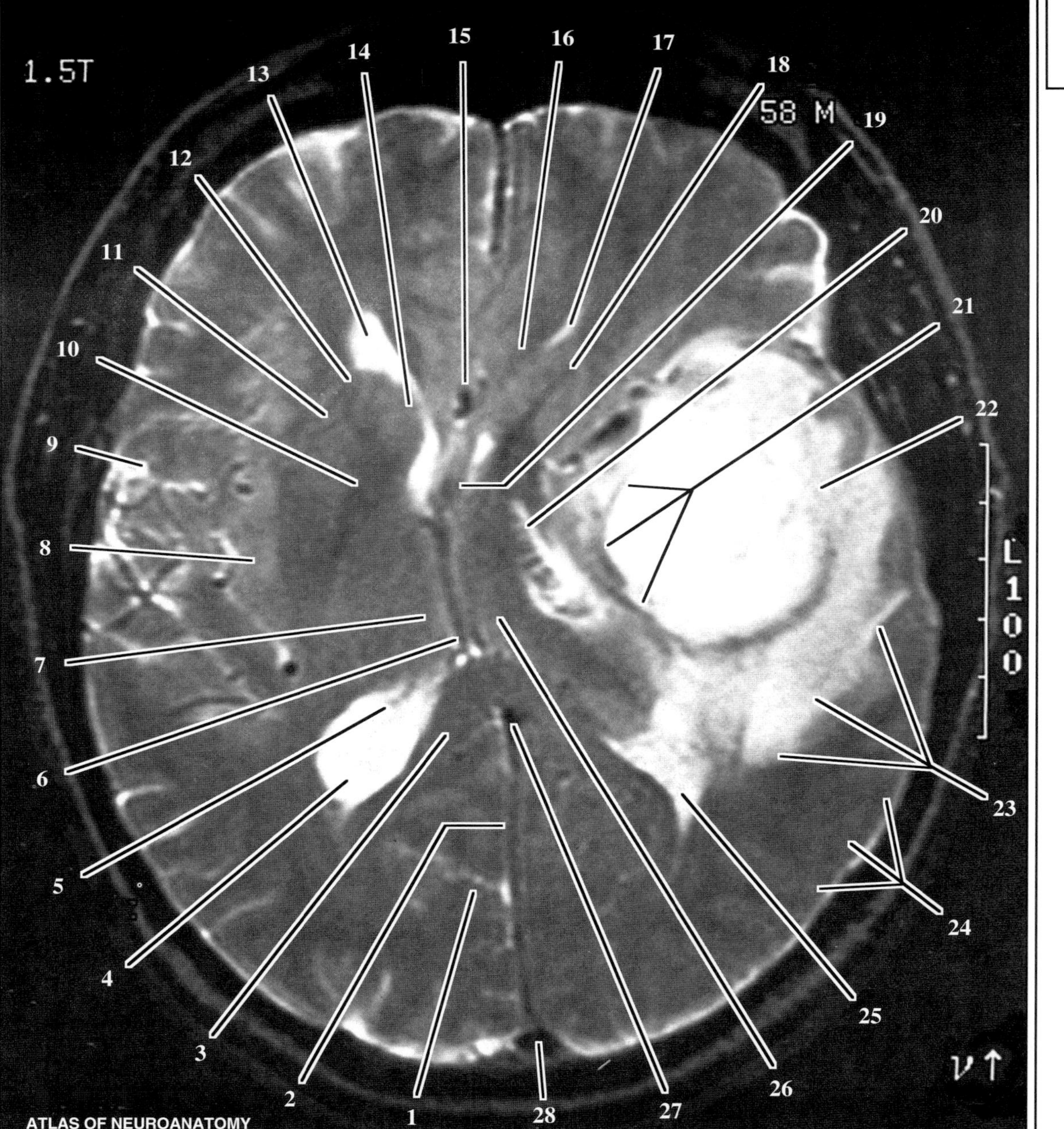

T2-weighted Magnetic Resonance Imaging (horizontal plane): KEY TO NUMBERED STRUCTURES

1. Area 17 Striate Cortex
2. Falx Cerebri
3. Splenium of the Corpus Callosum
4. Atrium of the Lateral Ventricle
5. Choroid Plexus
6. Internal Cerebral Vein
7. Thalamus
8. Insular Cortex
9. Sylvian Fissure
10. Globus Pallidus (dark signal on T2)
11. Putamen
12. Anterior Limb of the Internal Capsule
13. Anterior Horn of the Lateral Ventricle
14. Head of the Caudate Nucleus
15. Anterior Cerebral Artery
16. Rostrum of the Corpus Callosum
17. Anterior Horn of the Lateral Ventricle (note compression and contralateral shift due to mass effect)
18. Anterior Limb of the Internal Capsule
19. Fornix (and Septal Nuclei) contralaterally shifted by mass effect
20. Vasogenic edema invading the Posterior Limb of the Internal Capsule
21. Margin of Glioblastoma medial to region of necrosis and cavitation
22. Tumor and edema extending into Superior Temporal Gyrus
23. Vasogenic edema extending into the inferior parietal region
24. Effacement of the Sulcal pattern
25. Atrium of the Lateral Ventricle
26. Thalamus
27. Inferior Sagittal Sinus
28. Superior Sagittal Sinus

DR. JOSEPH J. WARNER

GLIOBLASTOMA MULTIFORME OF THE LEFT TEMPORAL LOBE: MAGNETIC RESONANCE IMAGING

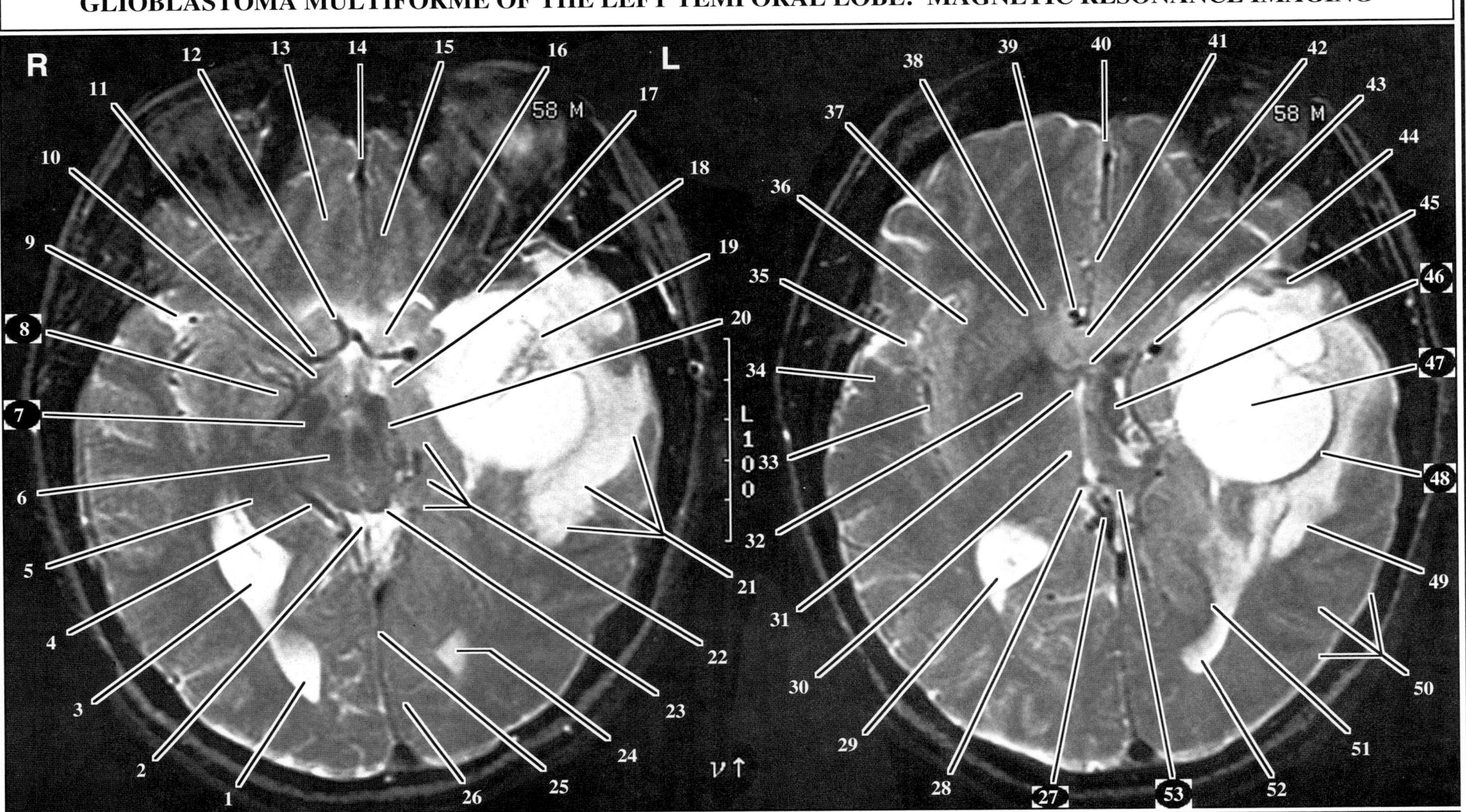

This T2-weighted magnetic resonance imaging study in the horizontal plane demonstrates a large mass located in the left temporal lobe, with rostral and medial shift of the insula. The temporal lobe is significantly enlarged, with compression of the mesencephalon by the medial and ventral shift of the uncus. The morphology of the mesencephalon includes a shearing effect, especially of its ventral aspect, with marked compression of the cerebral peduncle ipsilateral to the mass. Increased T2 signal is visible in the left cerebral peduncle as well. The contralateral cerebral peduncle is shifted toward the edge of the tentorial incisura, and each red nucleus is compressed with anteroposterior elongation. The medial displacement of the uncus and remainder of the parahippocampal gyrus has shifted the course of the ipsilateral optic tract. Vasogenic edema is visible adjacent to the glioblastoma, extending from the temporal lobe in a caudal and dorsal direction. The tumor demonstrates multicentric areas of necrosis with well-defined margins. Edema is not clearly distinguished from areas of tumor proliferation in the T2 study.

GLIOBLASTOMA MULTIFORME OF THE LEFT TEMPORAL LOBE: T2 WEIGHTED MAGNETIC RESONANCE IMAGING

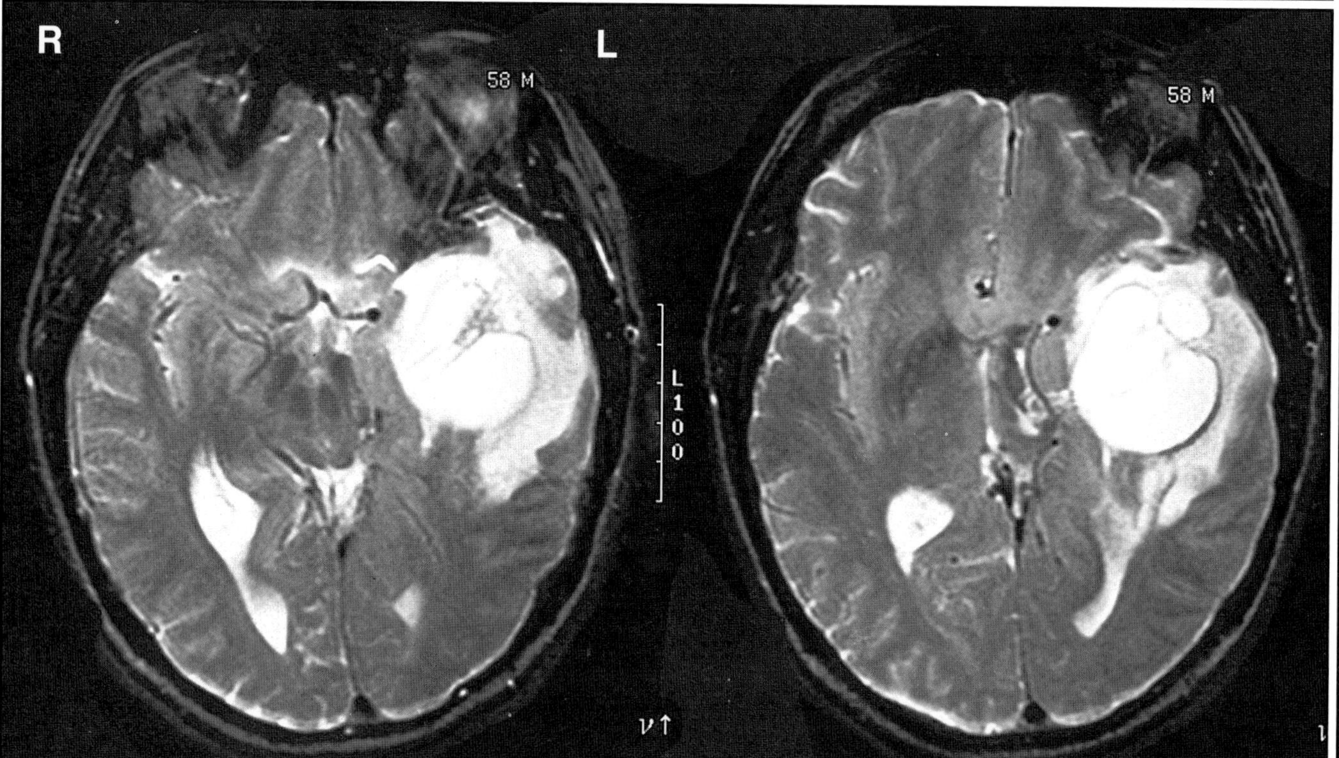

KEY TO NUMBERED STRUCTURES

1. Occipital Horn of the Lateral Ventricle
2. Quadrigeminal Cistern
3. Atrium of the Lateral Ventricle
4. Posterior Cerebral Artery
5. Hippocampal Formation
6. Red Nucleus
7. Cerebral Peduncle
8. Uncus
9. Sylvian Fissure
10. Optic Tract
11. Proximal segment, Anterior Cerebral Artery
12. Anterior Cerebral Artery (distal to the Anterior Communicating Artery)
13. Olfactory Sulcus
14. Falx Cerebri (attachment at Crista Galli)
15. Gyrus Rectus
16. Anterior Perforated Substance
17. Rostral aspect of the Temporal Lobe
18. Uncus (medially displaced)
19. Glioblastoma Multiforme, central region
20. Cerebral Peduncle (note heterogeneous T2 signal ipsilateral to the temporal lobe mass)
21. Posterolateral margin of edema and tumor
22. Parahippocampal Gyrus (medially displaced)
23. Superior Colliculus
24. Occipital Horn of the Lateral Ventricle
25. Falx Cerebri
26. Area 17 Striate Cortex
27. Confluence of the Internal Cerebral Veins
28. Habenula
29. Atrium of the Lateral Ventricle
30. Dorsomedial Nucleus of the Thalamus
31. Fornix
32. Globus Pallidus I
33. Middle Cerebral Artery, insular course
34. Temporal Neocortex
35. Sylvian Fissure
36. Insular Cortex
37. Anterior Limb of the Internal Capsule
38. Ventral aspect of the Caudate Nucleus
39. Anterior Cerebral Artery
40. Falx Cerebri
41. Shift of Interhemispheric Fissure
42. Subfalcine Herniation of the Cingulate Gyrus
43. Anterior Commissure
44. Middle Cerebral Artery
45. Sylvian Fissure (displaced due to mass effect)
46. Internal Capsule (medially shifted)
47. Central necrosis within Glioblastoma
48. Margin of "cystic" change (often corresponds to region of hypercellularity and/or vascular proliferation on histologic study)
49. Margin of tumor and/or associated edema
50. Effacement of sulcal morphology
51. Calcar Avis
52. Occipital Horn of the Lateral Ventricle

GLIOBLASTOMA MULTIFORME OF THE LEFT TEMPORAL LOBE: MAGNETIC RESONANCE IMAGING

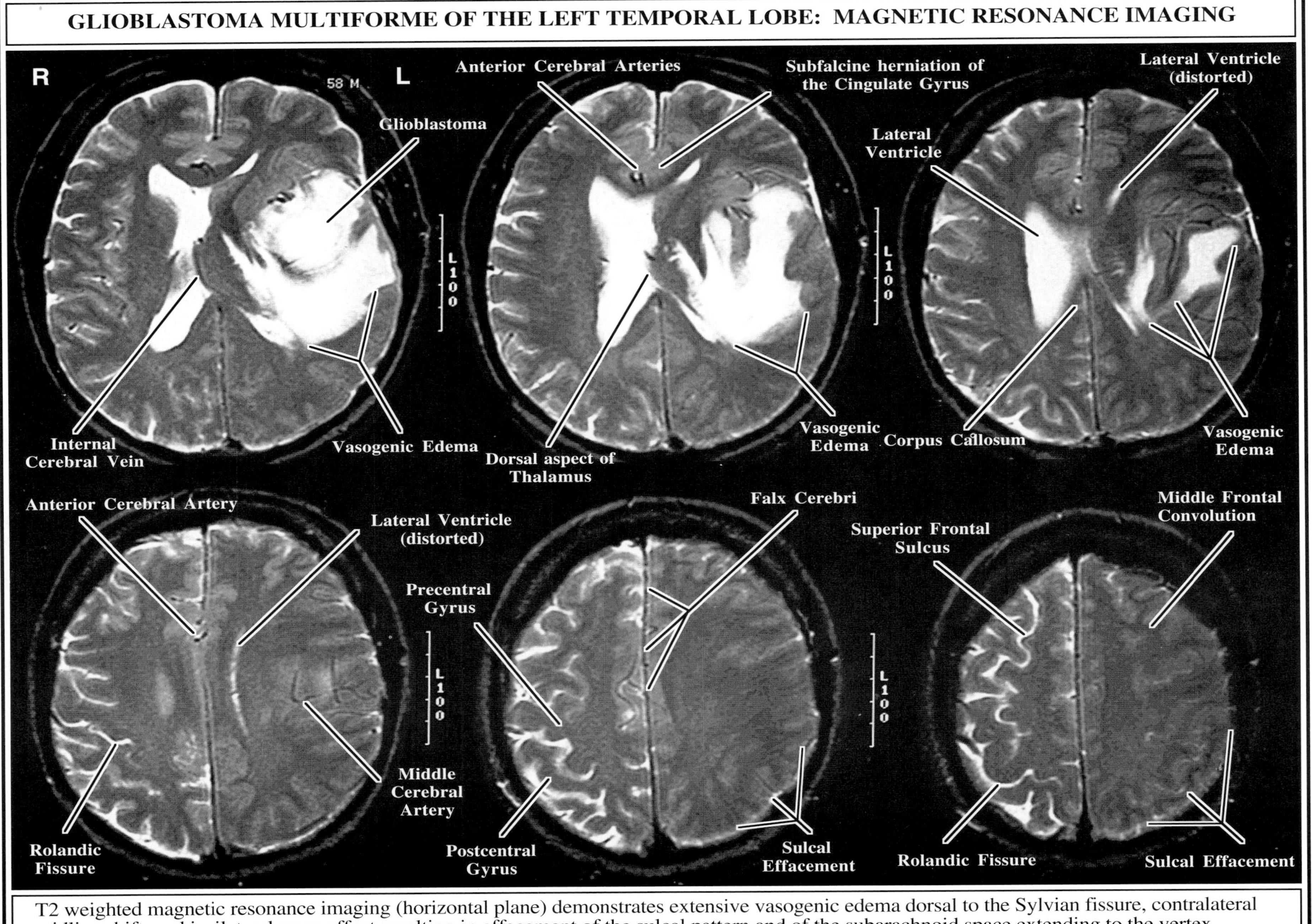

T2 weighted magnetic resonance imaging (horizontal plane) demonstrates extensive vasogenic edema dorsal to the Sylvian fissure, contralateral midline shift, and ipsilateral mass effect resulting in effacement of the sulcal pattern and of the subarachnoid space extending to the vertex.

 DR. JOSEPH J. WARNER

GLIOBLASTOMA MULTIFORME OF THE LEFT TEMPORAL LOBE: GADOLINIUM - ENHANCED MAGNETIC RESONANCE IMAGING

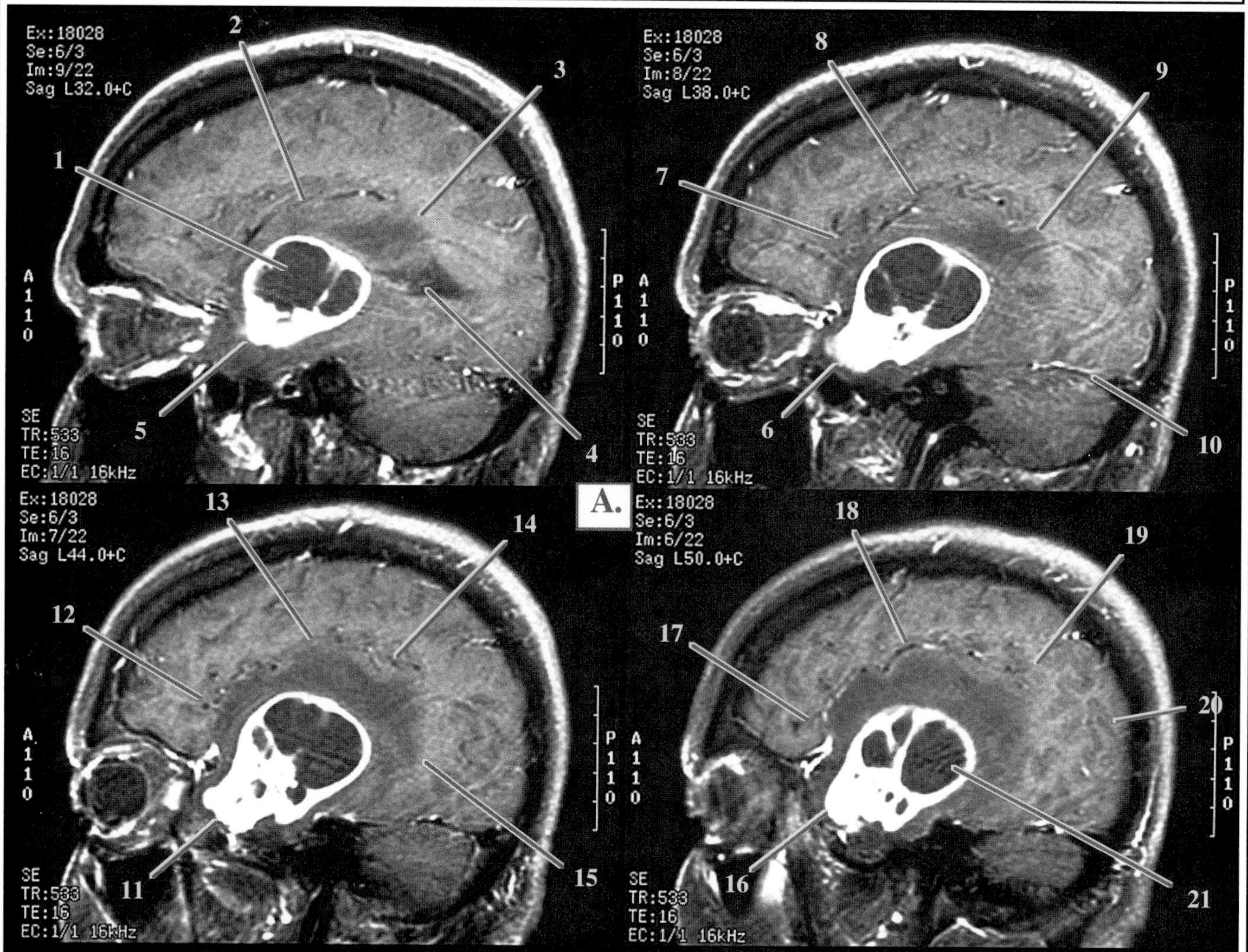

A.

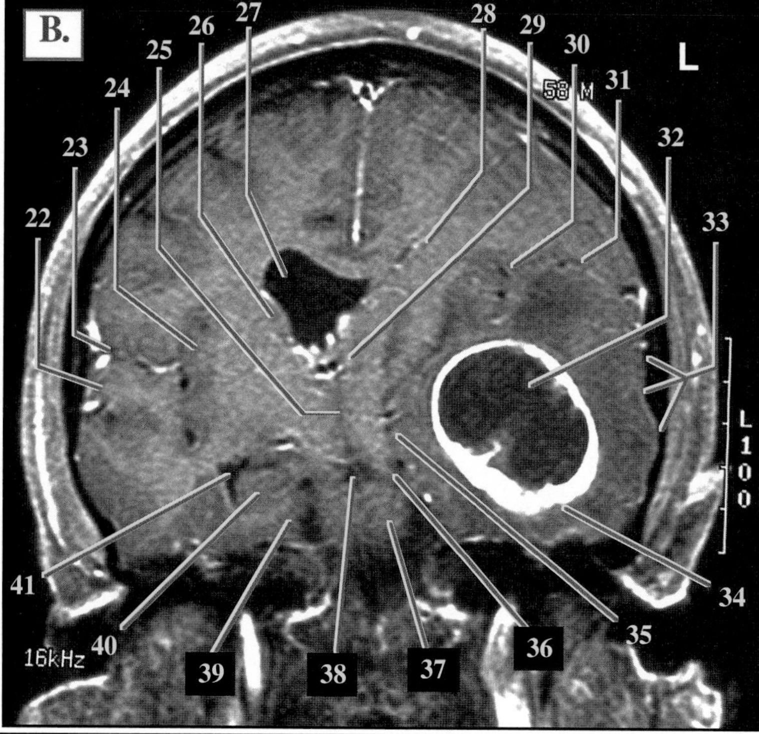

GADOLINIUM-ENHANCED MAGNETIC RESONANCE IMAGING

A. Imaging in the sagittal plane demonstrates ring-enhancement of the mass with central signal characteristics suggestive of necrosis and/or cavitation. The mass is accompanied by severe dorsal displacement of the Sylvian fissure and distortion of the morphology of the entire temporal lobe. Heschl's gyrus and the planum temporale are effaced and displaced by mass effect within the temporal lobe. The left lateral ventricle is compressed with only the atrium and occipital horn discernible caudally.

B. Coronal section demonstrates the ring-enhancing mass and edema. Dorsal shift of the Sylvian fissure and contralateral midline shift are quite pronounced. The anterior horn of the right lateral ventricle is somewhat enlarged, raising a question of obstruction near the foramen of Monro.

GLIOBLASTOMA MULTIFORME OF THE LEFT TEMPORAL LOBE: GADOLINIUM - ENHANCED MAGNETIC RESONANCE IMAGING

KEY TO NUMBERED STRUCTURES FOR THE SAGITTAL AND CORONAL PLANES

1. Signal attenuation consistent with central necrosis
2. Dorsal displacement of Sylvian Fissure
3. Margin of edema extending into parietal lobe
4. Atrium of the Lateral Ventricle
5. Rostral margin of Gadolinium enhancement
6. Gadolinium enhancement in Temporal Pole
7. Insular Cortex
8. Dorsal displacement of Sylvian Fissure
9. Caudal margin of edema
10. Tentorium Cerebelli
11. Gadolinium enhancement in Temporal Pole
12. Rostral region of the Insula
13. Dorsal displacement of the Sylvian Fissure
14. Planum Temporale
15. Edema involving the Parietotemporal Region
16. Gadolinium enhancement in Temporal Pole
17. Frontal Opercular Region
18. Dorsal displacement of the Sylvian Fissure
19. Caudal aspect of the Planum Temporale
20. Gyral effacement involving the Parietal Lobe
21. Signal attenuation consistent with central necrosis
22. Superior Temporal Gyrus
23. Sylvian Fissure
24. Insular Cortex
25. Third Ventricle (compressed and shifted)
26. Caudate Nucleus
27. Body of the Lateral Ventricle
28. Compression of the Lateral Ventricle ipsilateral to the mass lesion
29. Internal Cerebral Veins
30. Middle Cerebral Arterial branch within the Sylvian Fissure
31. Dorsal displacement of the Sylvian Fissure
32. Signal attenuation consistent with central necrosis
33. Effacement of gyral pattern of the Temporal Lobe
34. Inferolateral margin of Gadolinium enhancement
35. Medial margin of edema and displacement of the Insular Cortex
36. Cerebral Peduncle
37. Basis Pontis
38. Interpeduncular Fossa
39. Parahippocampal Gyrus
40. Hippocampus
41. Temporal Horn of the Lateral Ventricle

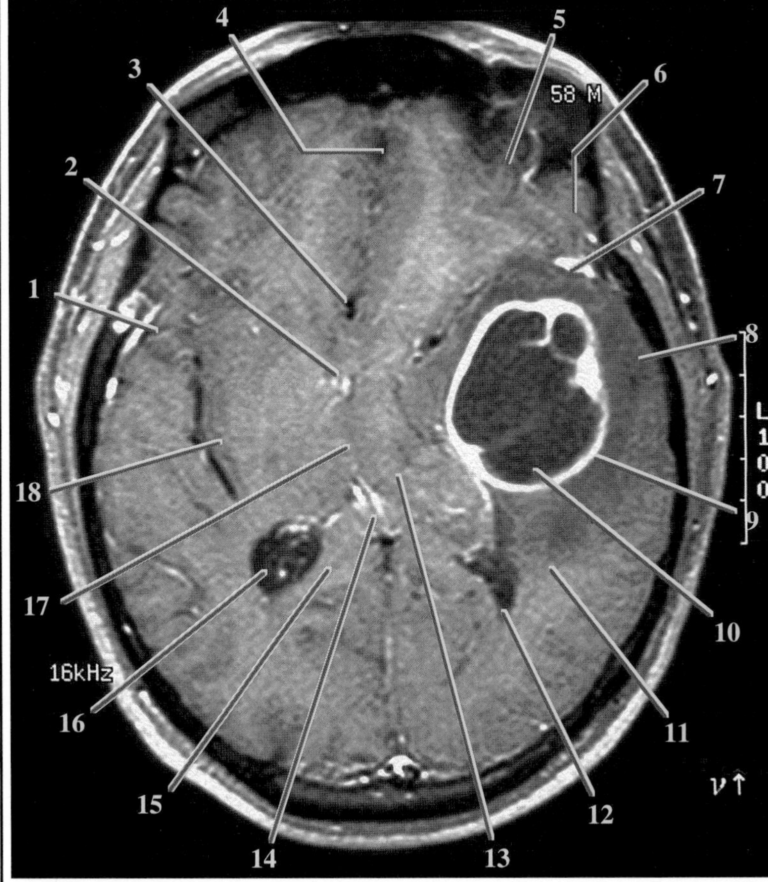

GADOLINIUM-ENHANCED IMAGE IN THE HORIZONTAL PLANE

1. Sylvian Fissure
2. Internal Cerebral Veins adjacent to the Venous Angle
3. Anterior Cerebral Arteries
4. Interhemispheric Fissure
5. Orbitofrontal Gyri
6. Frontal Opercular Region
7. Sylvian Fissure
8. Effacement of gyral morphology of the Temporal Lobe
9. Margin of Gadolinium enhancement
10. Signal attenuation consistent with central necrosis
11. Caudal margin of edema
12. Atrium of the Lateral Ventricle
13. Thalamus
14. Internal Cerebral Veins adjacent to the Great Vein of Galen
15. Lateral fibers, Splenium of the Corpus Callosum
16. Atrium of the Lateral Ventricle
17. Third Ventricle (compressed)
18. Insular Cortex

GLIOBLASTOMA MULTIFORME OF THE LEFT TEMPORAL LOBE: POST-OPERATIVE MAGNETIC RESONANCE IMAGING (HORIZONTAL PLANE)

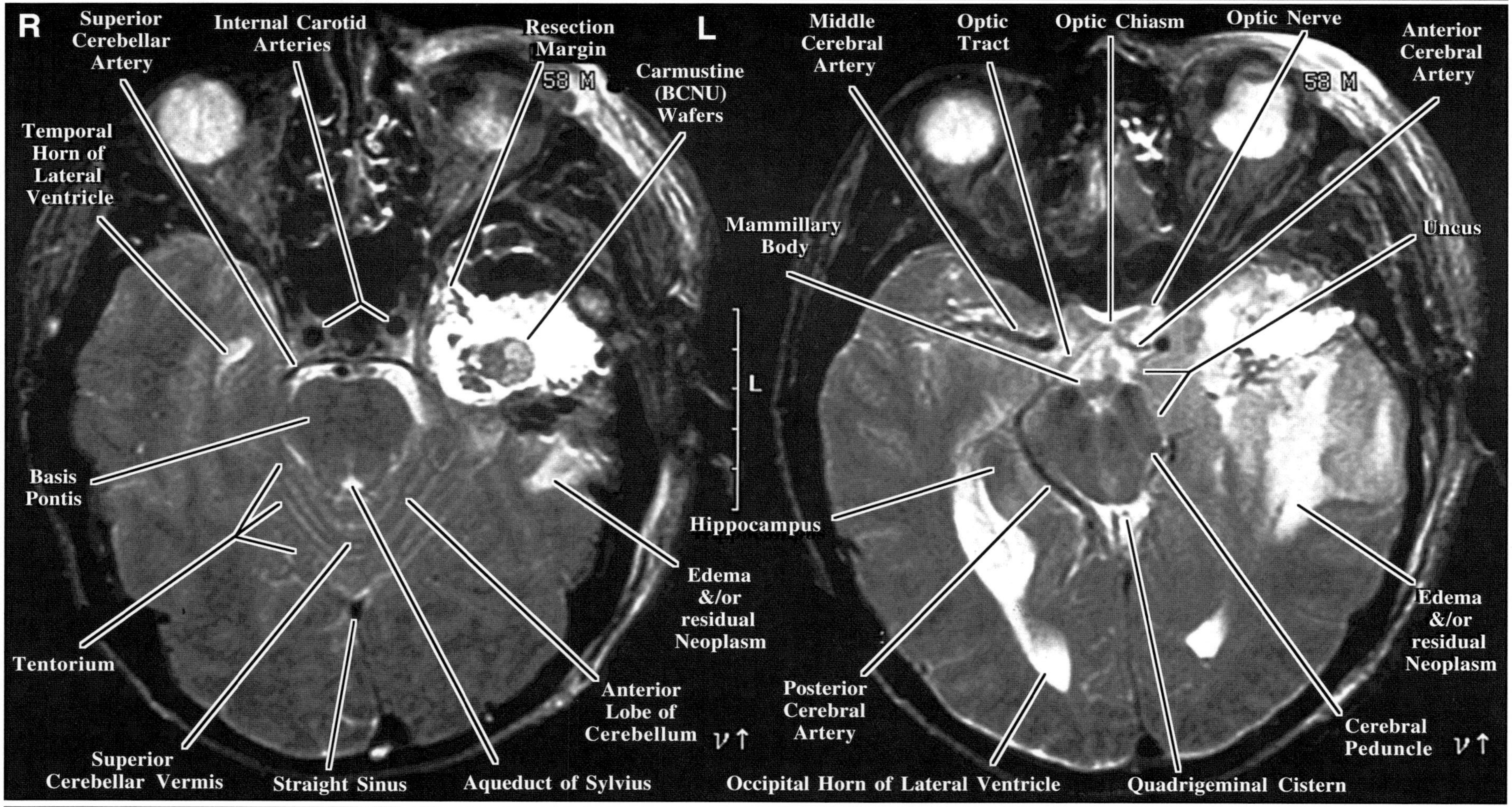

The patient underwent a left craniotomy with subtotal resection of the tumor. Frozen sections as well as permanent histologic sections confirmed the diagnosis of glioblastoma multiforme. At the time of the craniotomy, eight Gliadel(TM) wafers, each containing 7.7 mg of carmustine [1,3-bis(2-chloroethyl)-1-nitrosourea, BCNU] in a polifeprosan 20 copolymer matrix, were implanted in the cavity left by tumor resection. This post-operative T2-weighted magnetic resonance study was performed five days after the initial preoperative neuroimaging. Although the resected tumor volume was estimated at 80% during surgery, a significant persistent mass effect is demonstrated, with midline shift, mesencephalic compression, and sulcal effacement. The implanted wafers are discernible in these images, within the region of resection in the middle cranial fossa. (Extracranial edema is shown adjacent to the craniotomy site, especially involving the periorbital region.)

*BCNU exerts its oncolytic effect through alkylation of DNA and RNA, with the subsequent formation of DNA cross-links.

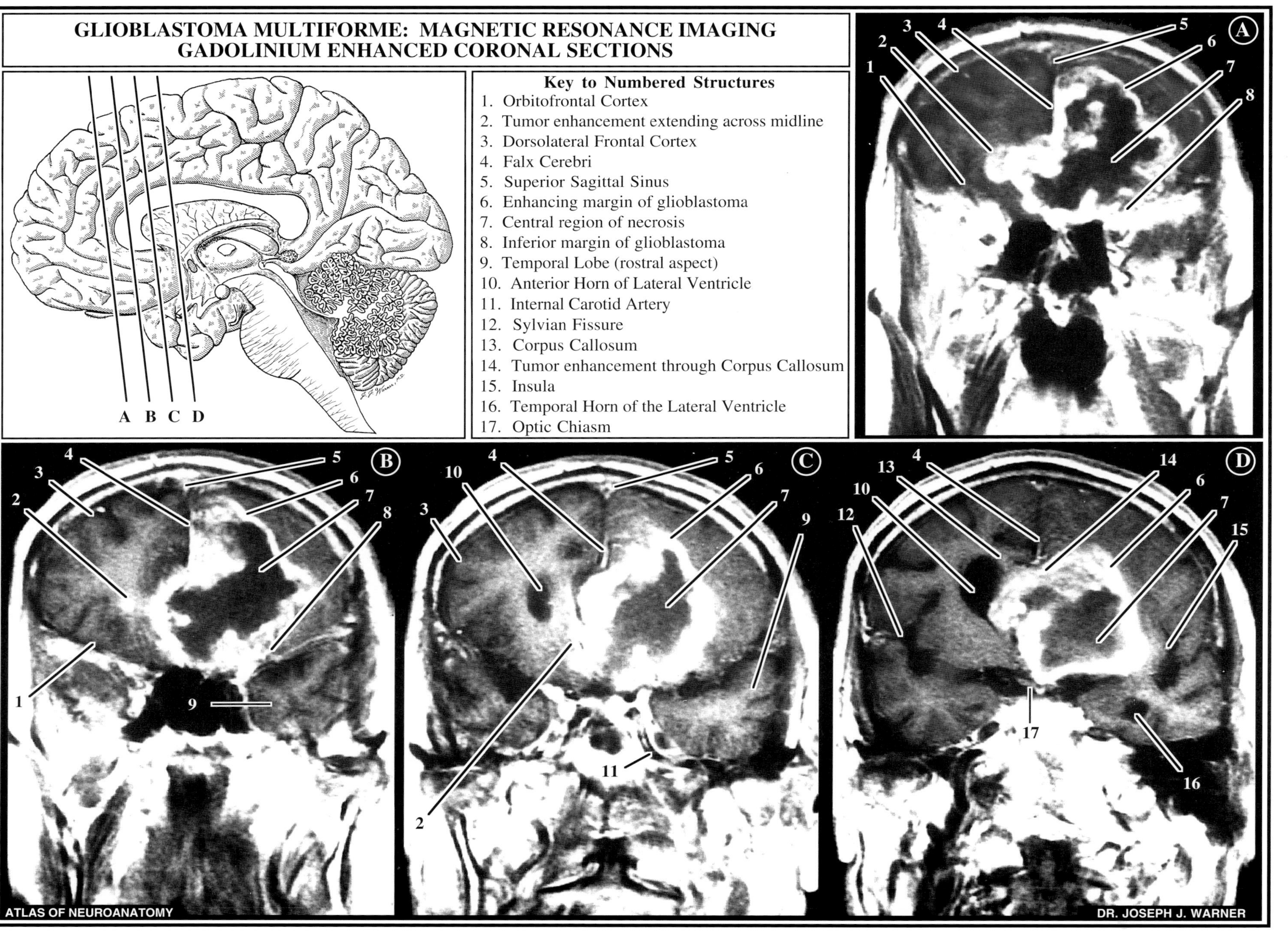
GLIOBLASTOMA MULTIFORME: MAGNETIC RESONANCE IMAGING
GADOLINIUM ENHANCED CORONAL SECTIONS
A B C D
Key to Numbered Structures
1. Orbitofrontal Cortex
2. Tumor enhancement extending across midline
3. Dorsolateral Frontal Cortex
4. Falx Cerebri
5. Superior Sagittal Sinus
6. Enhancing margin of glioblastoma
7. Central region of necrosis
8. Inferior margin of glioblastoma
9. Temporal Lobe (rostral aspect)
10. Anterior Horn of Lateral Ventricle
11. Internal Carotid Artery
12. Sylvian Fissure
13. Corpus Callosum
14. Tumor enhancement through Corpus Callosum
15. Insula
16. Temporal Horn of the Lateral Ventricle
17. Optic Chiasm
A
B
C
D
ATLAS OF NEUROANATOMY
DR. JOSEPH J. WARNER

GLIOBLASTOMA MULTIFORME: GADOLINIUM-ENHANCED MAGNETIC RESONANCE IMAGING AND CORRESPONDING PATHOLOGY

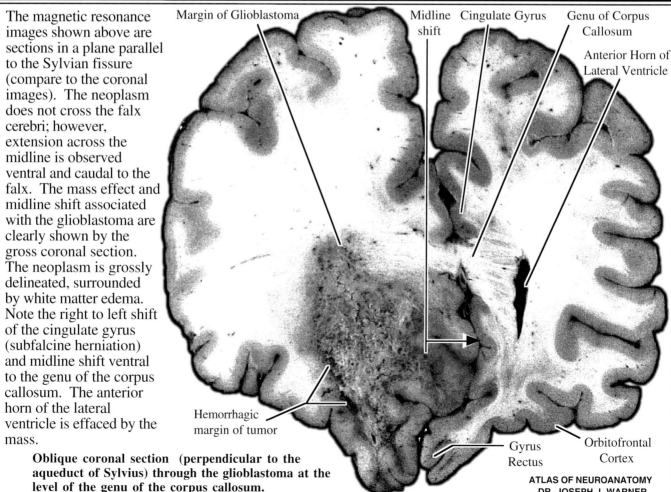

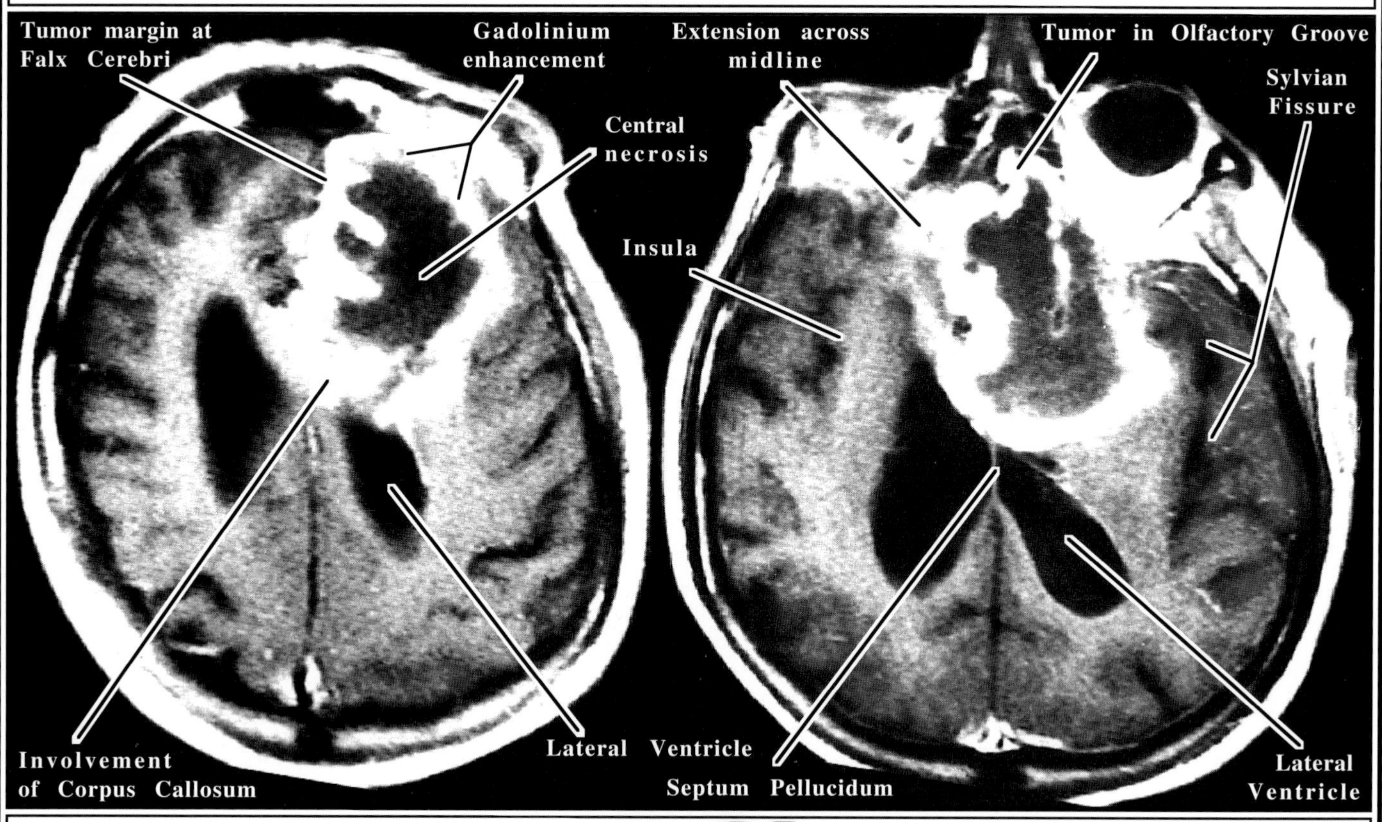

The magnetic resonance images shown above are sections in a plane parallel to the Sylvian fissure (compare to the coronal images). The neoplasm does not cross the falx cerebri; however, extension across the midline is observed ventral and caudal to the falx. The mass effect and midline shift associated with the glioblastoma are clearly shown by the gross coronal section. The neoplasm is grossly delineated, surrounded by white matter edema. Note the right to left shift of the cingulate gyrus (subfalcine herniation) and midline shift ventral to the genu of the corpus callosum. The anterior horn of the lateral ventricle is effaced by the mass.

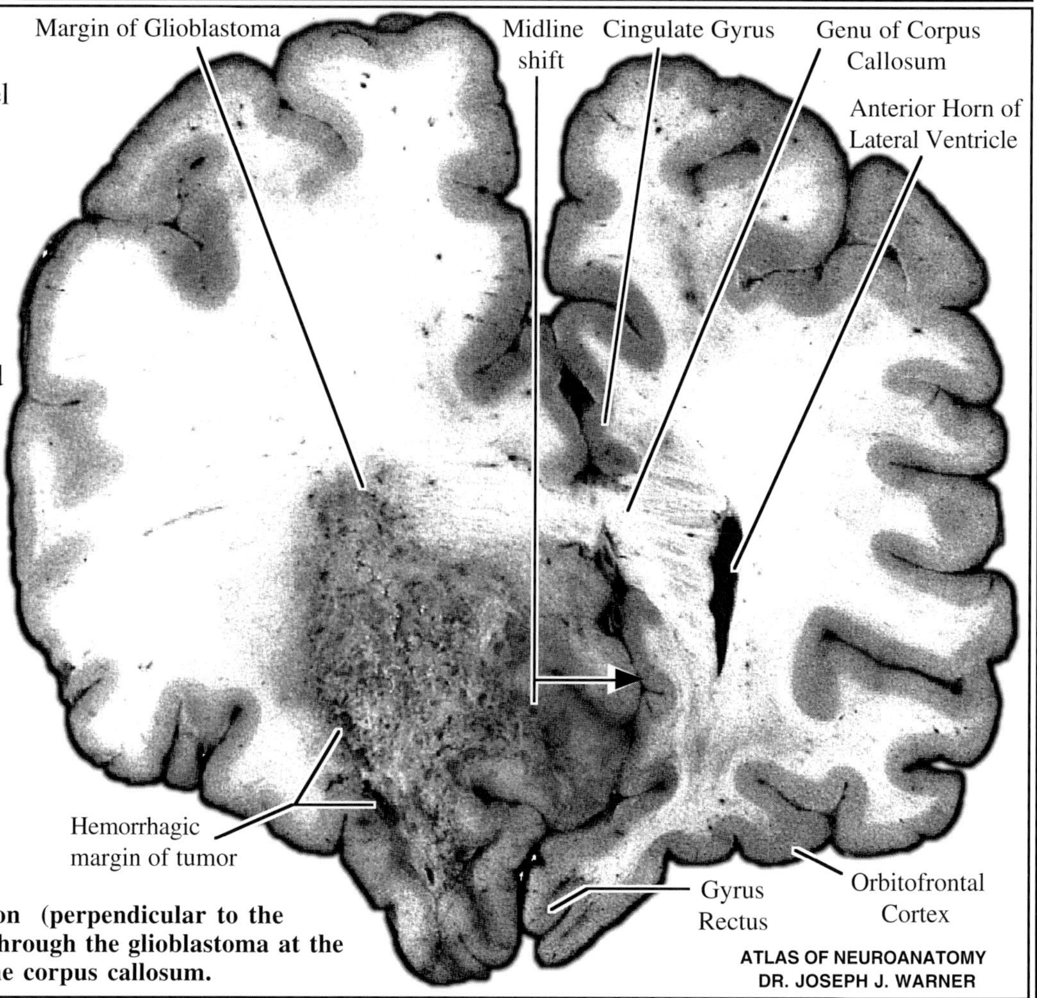

Oblique coronal section (perpendicular to the aqueduct of Sylvius) through the glioblastoma at the level of the genu of the corpus callosum.

ATLAS OF NEUROANATOMY
DR. JOSEPH J. WARNER

GLIOBLASTOMA OF THE LEFT CEREBRAL HEMISPHERE WITH EXTENSION INTO THE SEPTUM PELLUCIDUM AND CONTRALATERAL FRONTAL LOBE

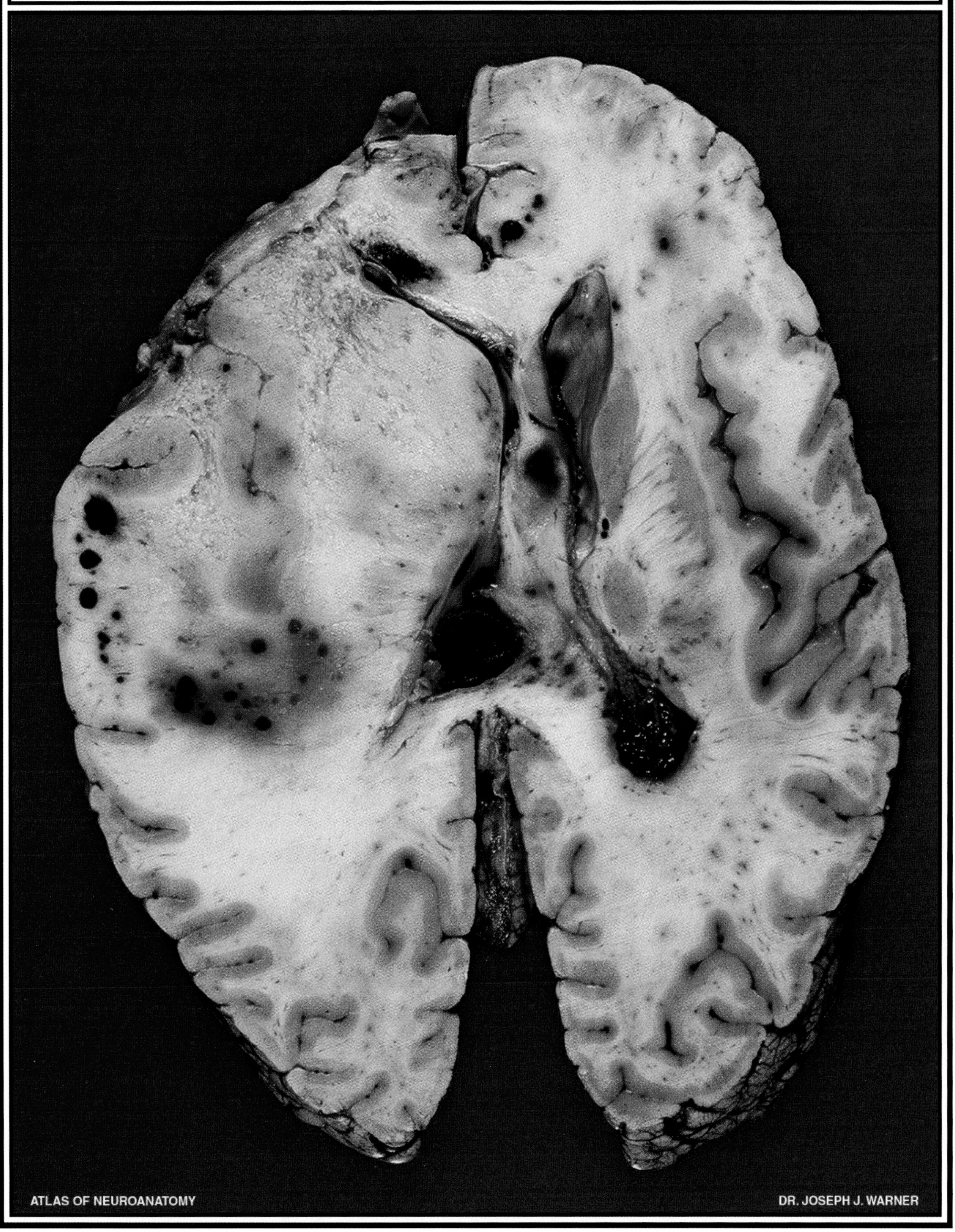

GLIOBLASTOMA MULTIFORME OF THE LEFT CEREBRAL HEMISPHERE WITH EXTENSION INTO THE SEPTUM PELLUCIDUM, FORNIX, AND THE CONTRALATERAL FRONTAL LOBE

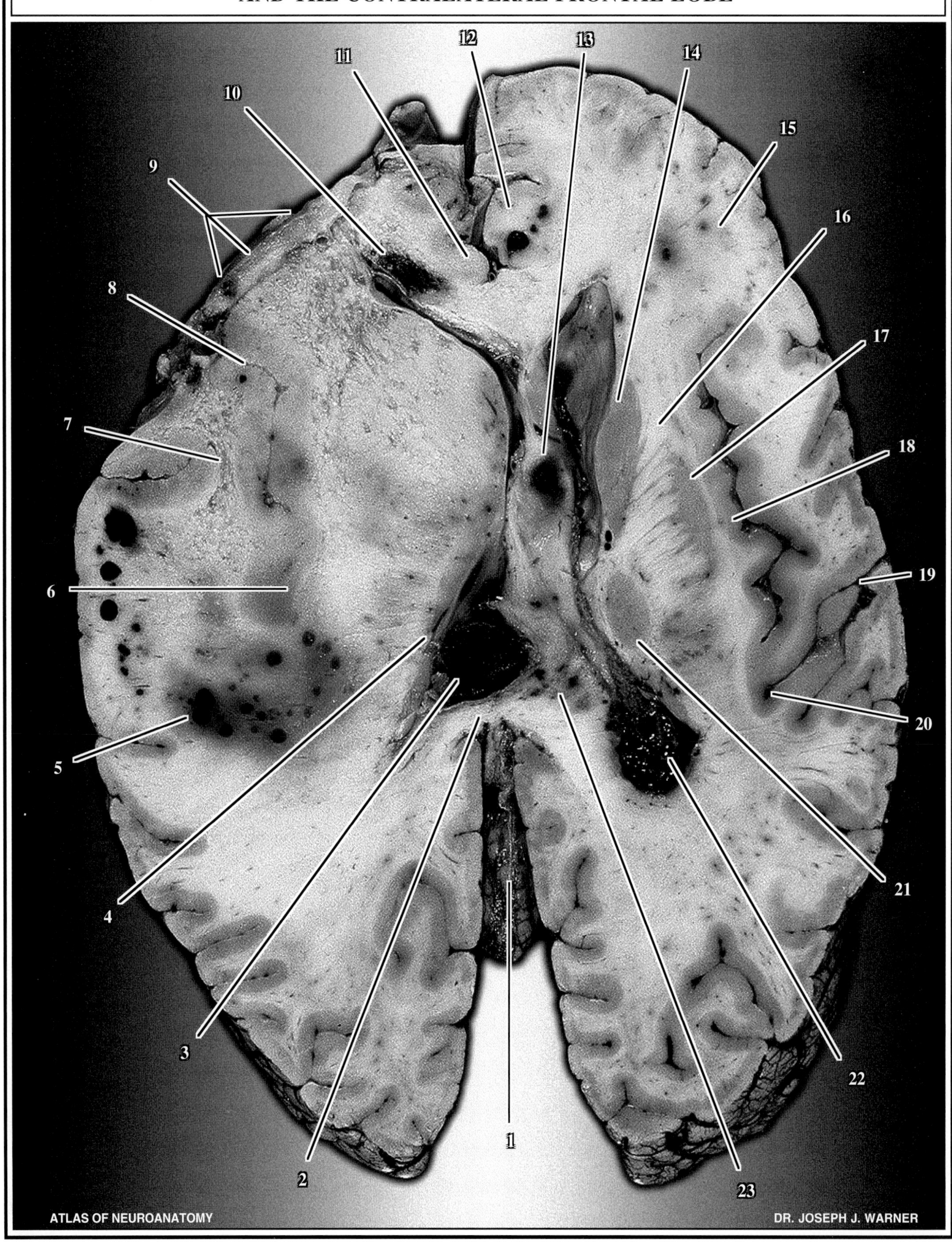

GLIOBLASTOMA MULTIFORME OF THE LEFT CEREBRAL HEMISPHERE WITH EXTENSION INTO THE SEPTUM PELLUCIDUM, FORNIX, AND THE CONTRALATERAL FRONTAL LOBE: (A) KEY TO GROSS HORIZONTAL SECTION; (B) PHOSPHOTUNGSTIC ACID HEMATOXYLIN-STAINED 15 μ SECTION

GROSS HORIZONTAL SECTION (A): KEY TO NUMBERED STRUCTURES

1. Superior Cerebellar Vermis
2. Corpus Callosum
3. Hemorrhage into Lateral Ventricle
4. Caudate Nucleus
5. Hemorrhages into tumor margin
6. Insula (invaded by tumor)
7. Necrosis of subcortical white matter
8. Sylvian Fissure (displaced)
9. Dural thickening (post-craniotomy) with tumor invasion
10. Hemorrhage and tumor involving Corpus Callosum
11. Subfalcine Herniation of the Cingulate Gyrus
12. Tumor invasion of contralateral Cingulate Gyrus
13. Hemorrhage into tumor invading Fornix
14. Caudate Nucleus
15. Tumor extension into dorsolateral Frontal Lobe
16. Anterior Limb of the Internal Capsule / Corona Radiata
17. Putamen
18. Insular Cortex
19. Sylvian Fissure
20. Subarachnoid Hemorrhage
21. Dorsal aspect of the Thalamus
22. Hemorrhage into Lateral Ventricle
23. Tumor with multifocal hemorrhages in the Septum Pellucidum and Corpus Callosum

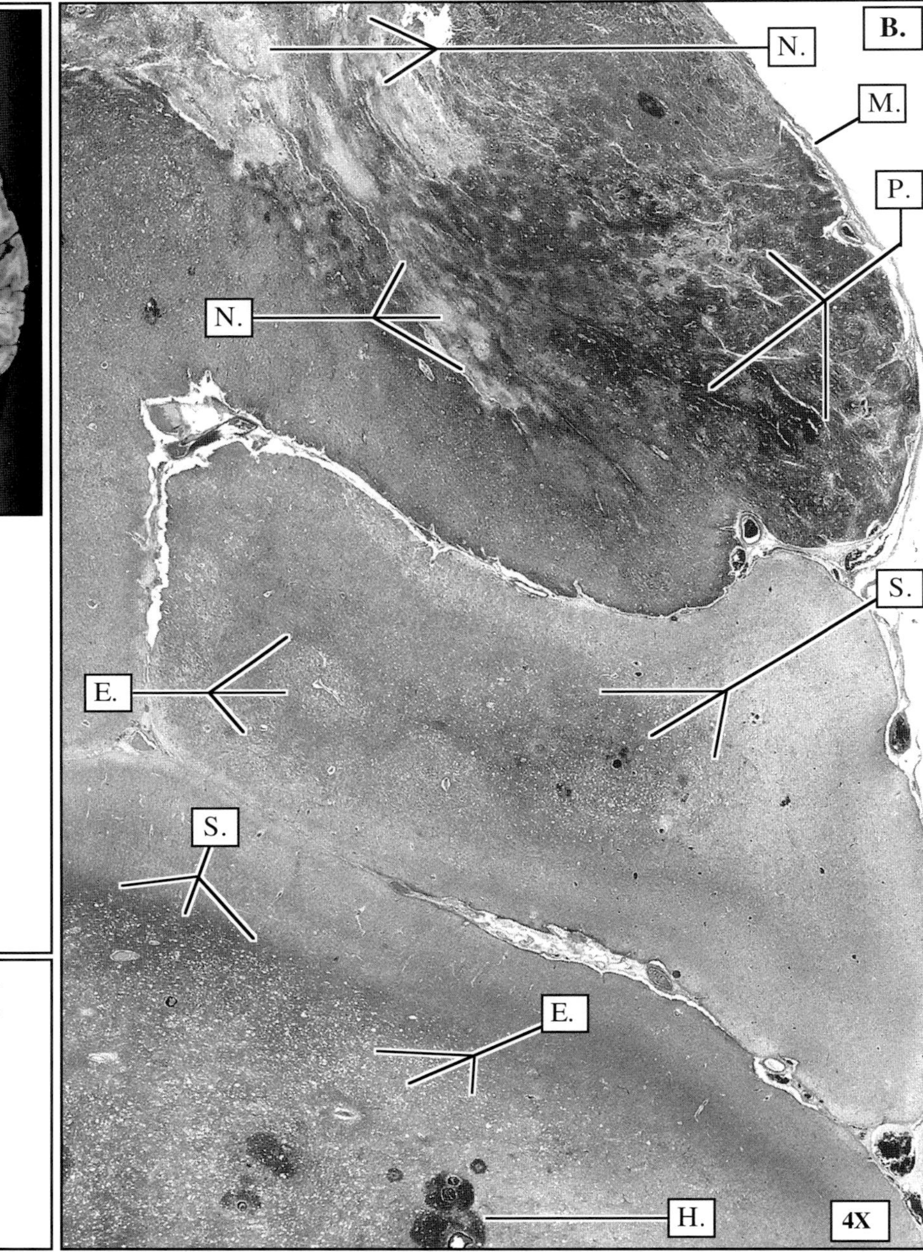

LEFT DORSOLATERAL FRONTAL LOBE (B), HORIZONTAL SECTION: PHOSPHOTUNGSTIC ACID HEMATOXYLIN, 15 μ

M. Arachnoid Membrane
P. Region of hypercellularity and active tumor proliferation
S. Extension of tumor into subcortical white matter
E. Regions of chronic edema and gliosis adjacent to tumor
H. Multiple hemorrhages associated with tumor
N. Necrosis within areas of active tumor proliferation

LEFT CEREBRAL HEMISPHERIC MASS (GLIOBLASTOMA MULTIFORME) WITH TRANSTENTORIAL UNCAL HERNIATION: HORIZONTAL SECTION

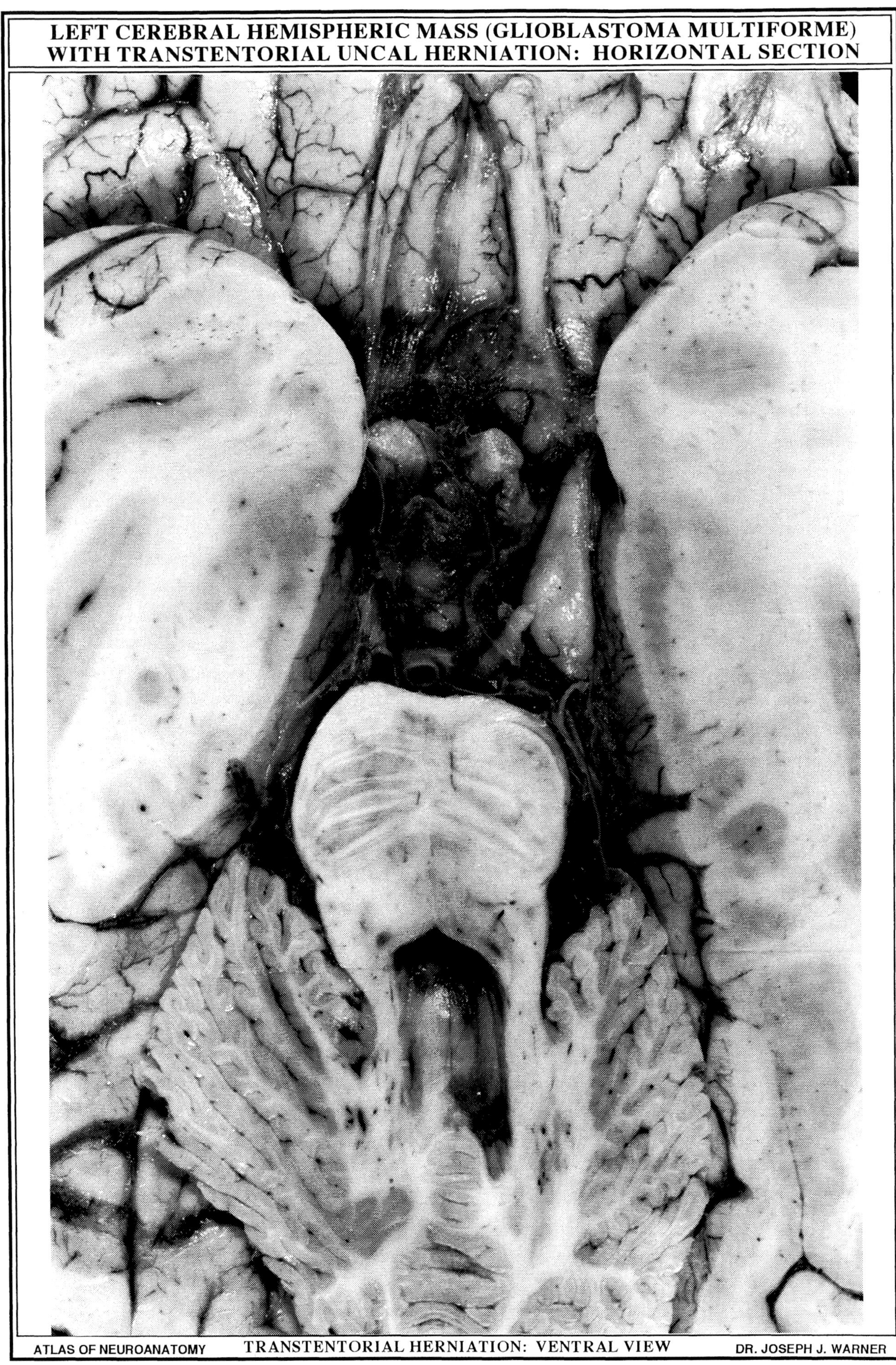

TRANSTENTORIAL HERNIATION: VENTRAL VIEW

BILATERAL VERTEBRAL ARTERIOGRAPHY (POST-MORTEM) IN A CASE OF GLIOBLASTOMA MULTIFORME: LATERAL PROJECTION

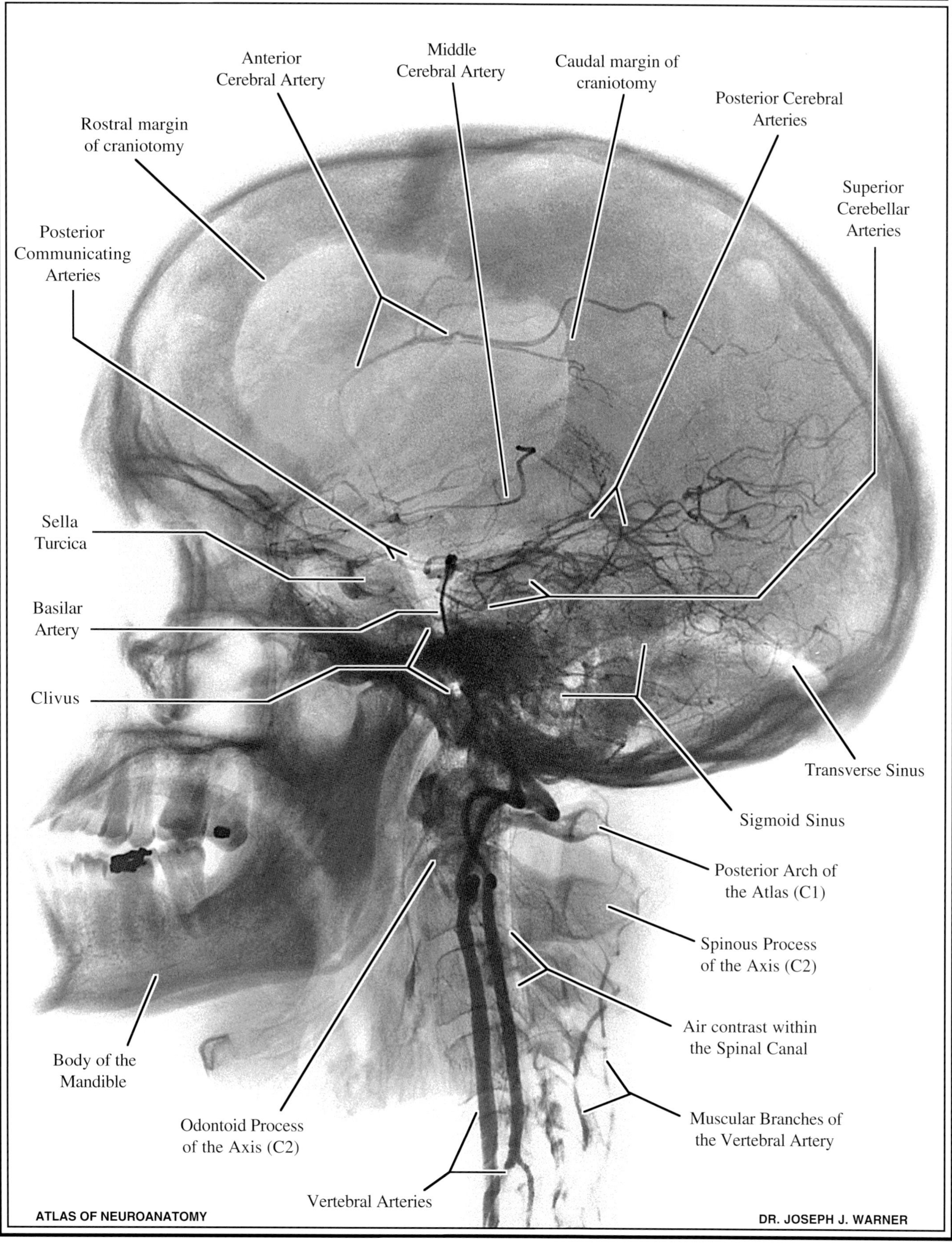

BILATERAL CAROTID AND VERTEBRAL ARTERIOGRAPHY (POST-MORTEM) IN A CASE OF GLIOBLASTOMA MULTIFORME: LATERAL PROJECTION

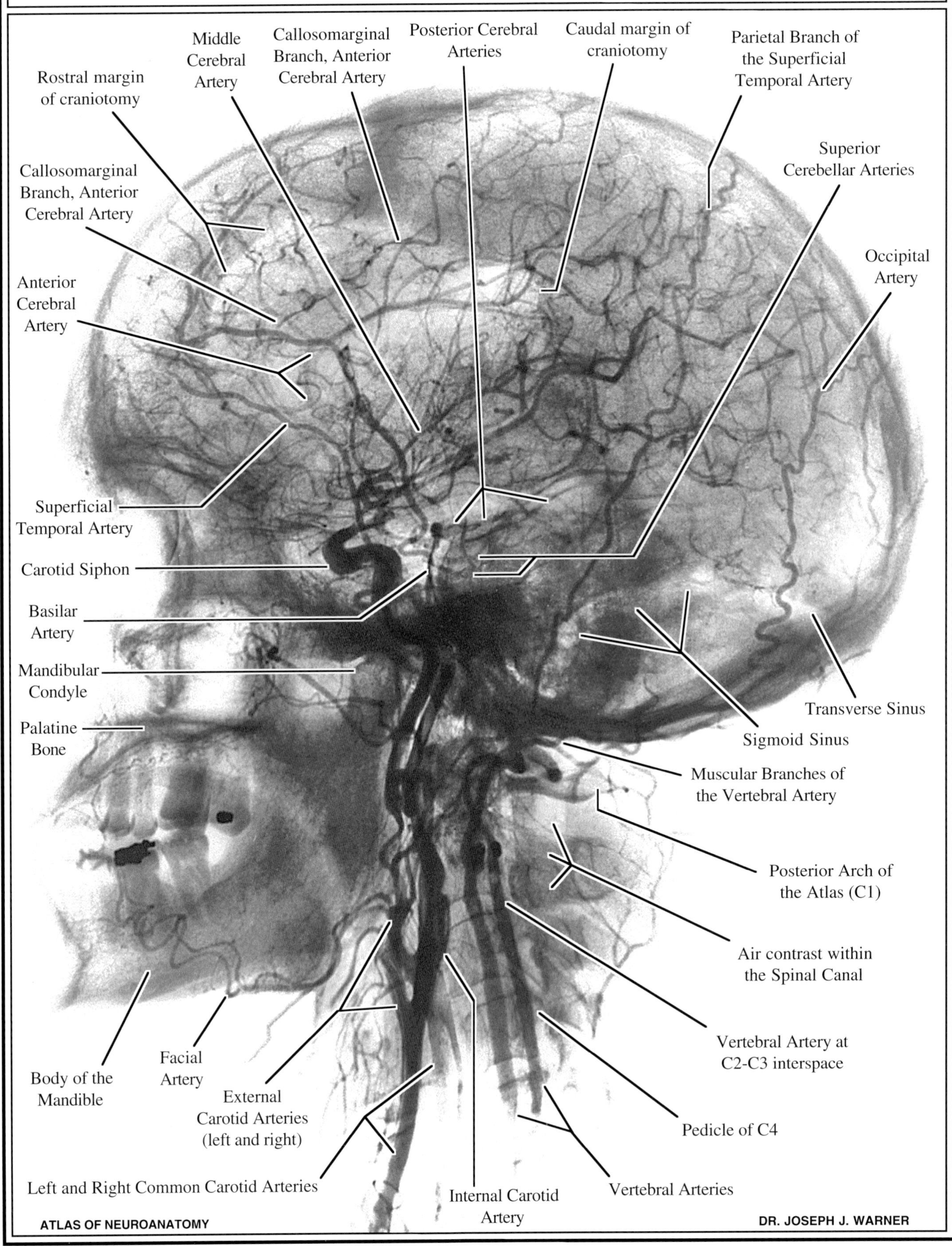

VENTRICULOGRAPHY VIA CERVICAL SPINAL INJECTION (POST-MORTEM) IN A CASE OF GLIOBLASTOMA MULTIFORME: LATERAL PROJECTION

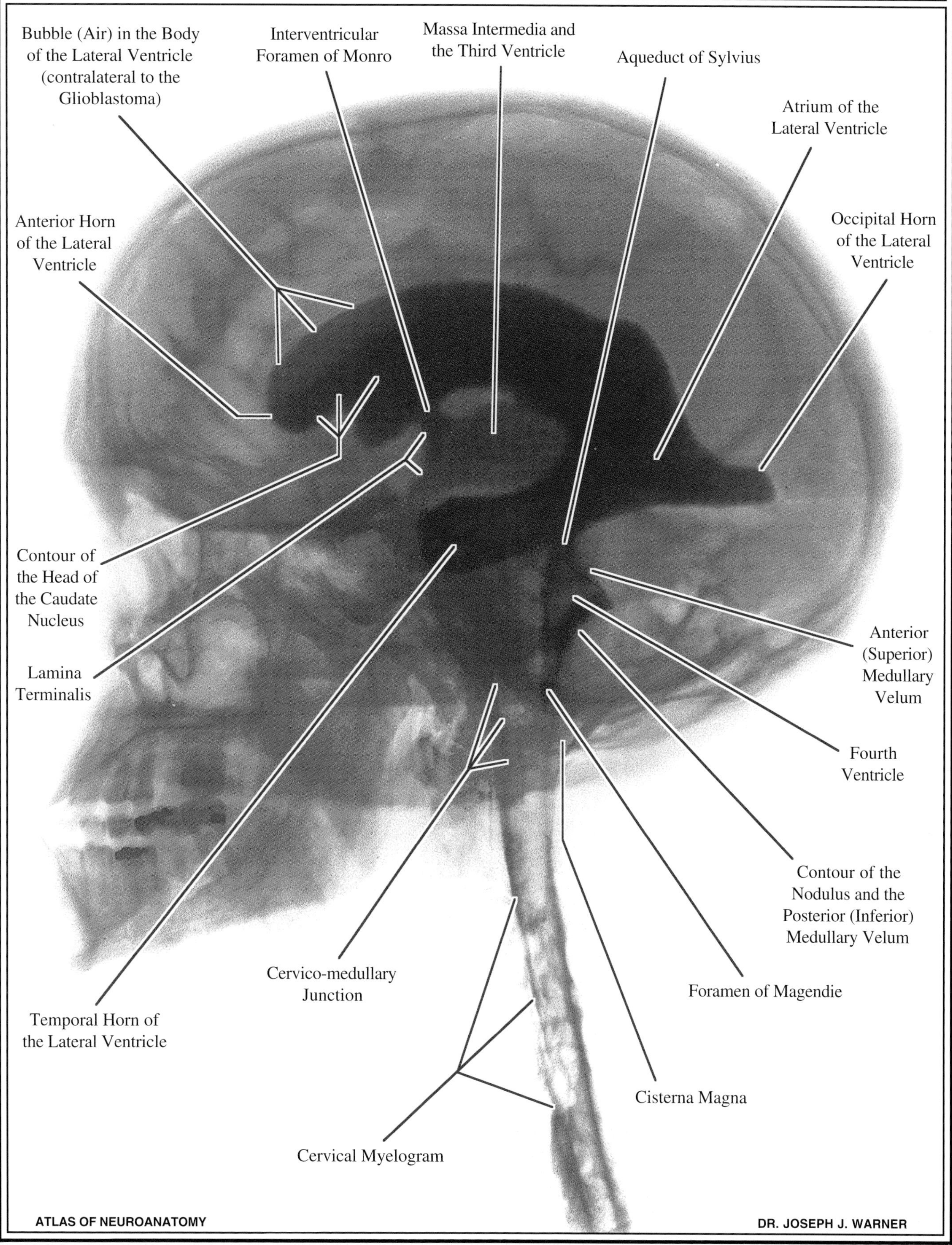

VENTRICULOGRAPHY VIA CERVICAL SPINAL INJECTION (POST-MORTEM) IN A CASE OF GLIOBLASTOMA MULTIFORME: CAUDAL TO ROSTRAL PROJECTION

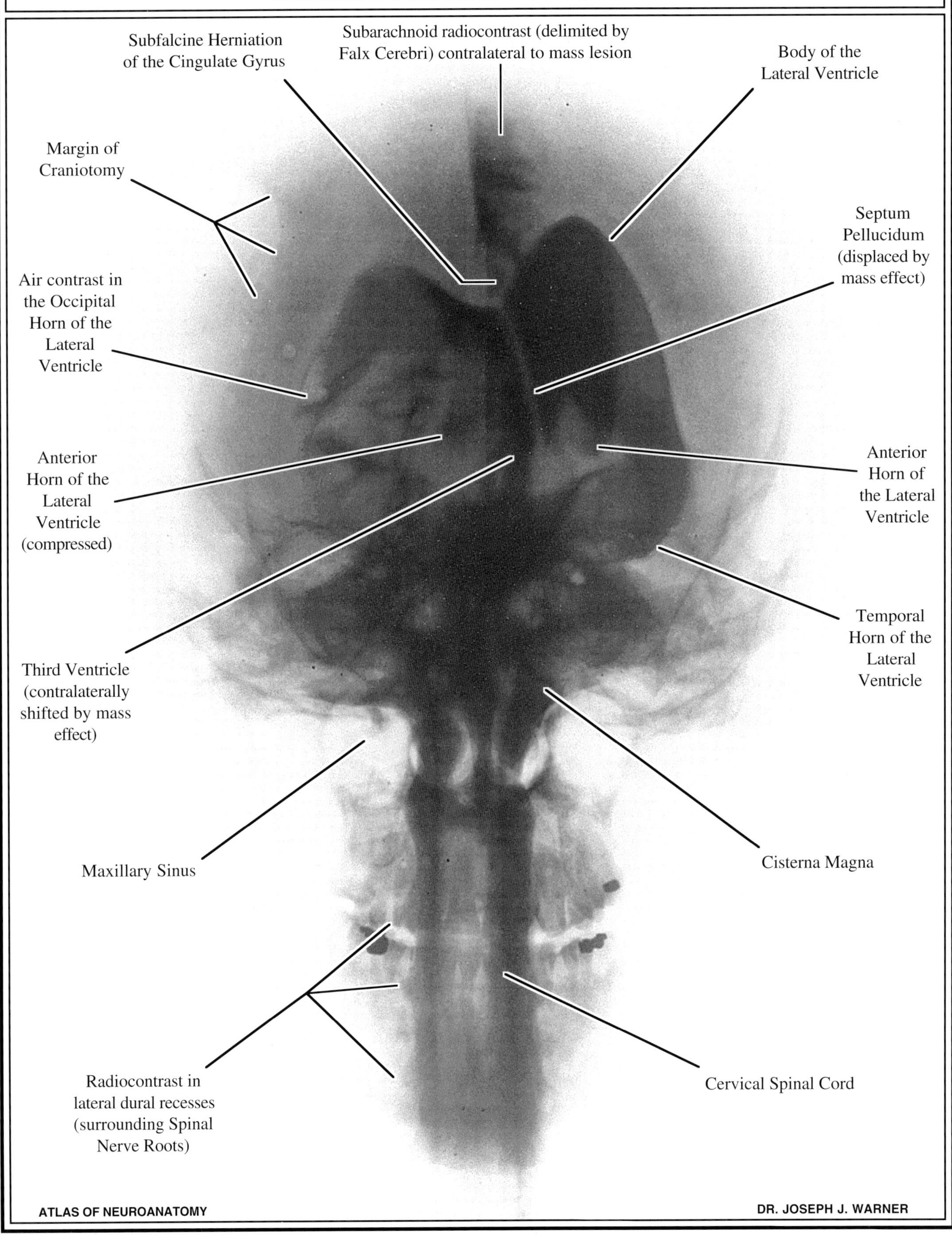

RADIOCONTRAST VENTRICULOGRAPHY (ROSTRAL TO CAUDAL PROJECTION) AND MAGNETIC RESONANCE IMAGING (CORONAL PLANE) IN A CASE OF GLIOBLASTOMA MULTIFORME: STRUCTURAL CORRELATIONS

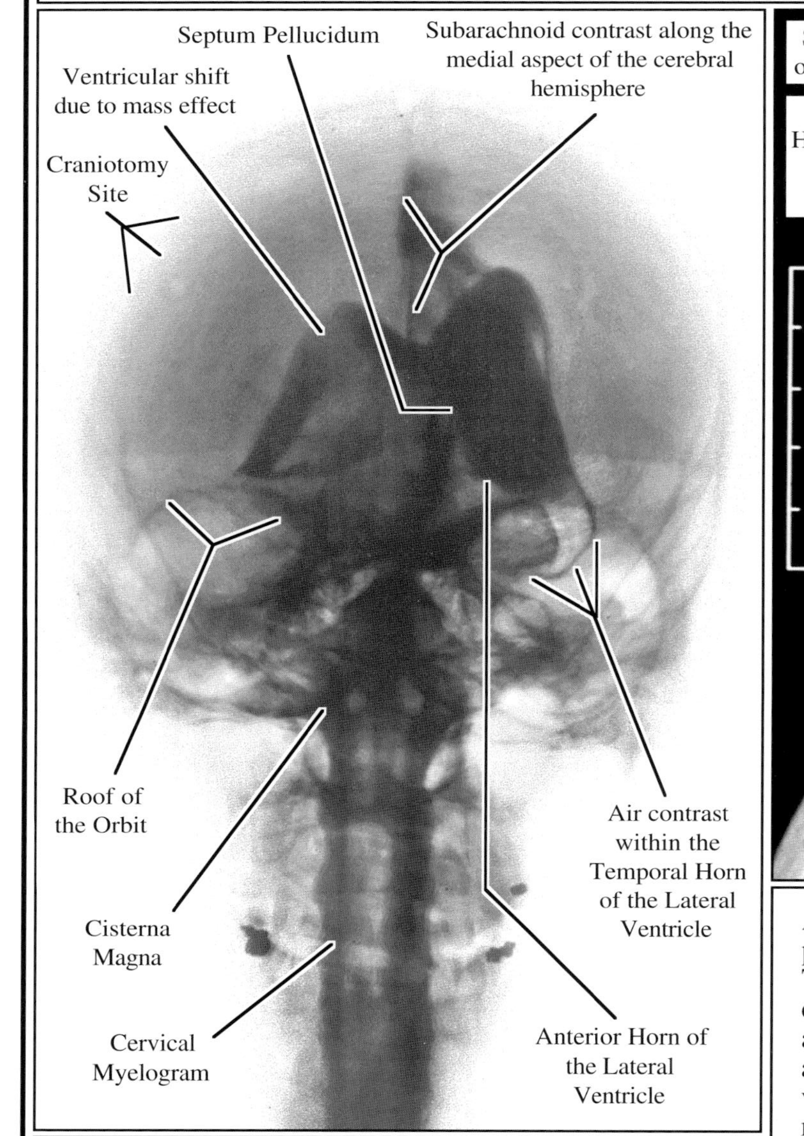

Contralateral to the mass, air contrast appears in the temporal horn. The ependymal and subependymal tissue has been stained by iodinated radiocontrast.

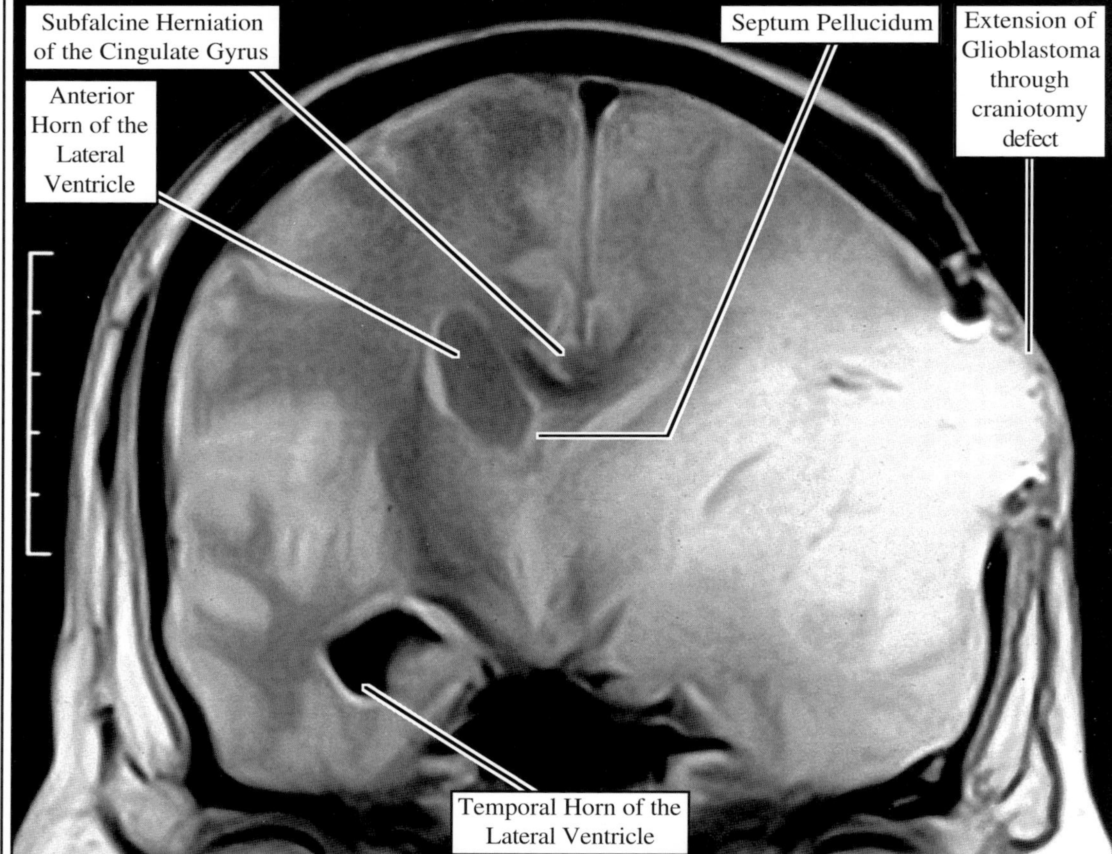

A comparison of the ventriculogram and the magnetic resonance image in the coronal plane clearly demonstrates the effect of the mass lesion on the ventricular system. The temporal horn of the lateral ventricle is not visualized ipsilateral to the mass. Air contrast within the contralateral temporal horn appears as a signal void on the fluid-attenuated inversion recovery MRI section. The bodies of the lateral ventricles are not as clearly contrasted on MRI, as they contain an aqueous solution. The radiocontrast ventriculogram provides a three-dimensional projection that demonstrates the complex morphologic effects of the mass lesion on the ventricular system. Correlative examination of these images emphasizes the spatial relationships between the ventricular system and surrounding structures for the study of (1) normal neuroanatomy and (2) morphologic alterations in neuropathologic states.

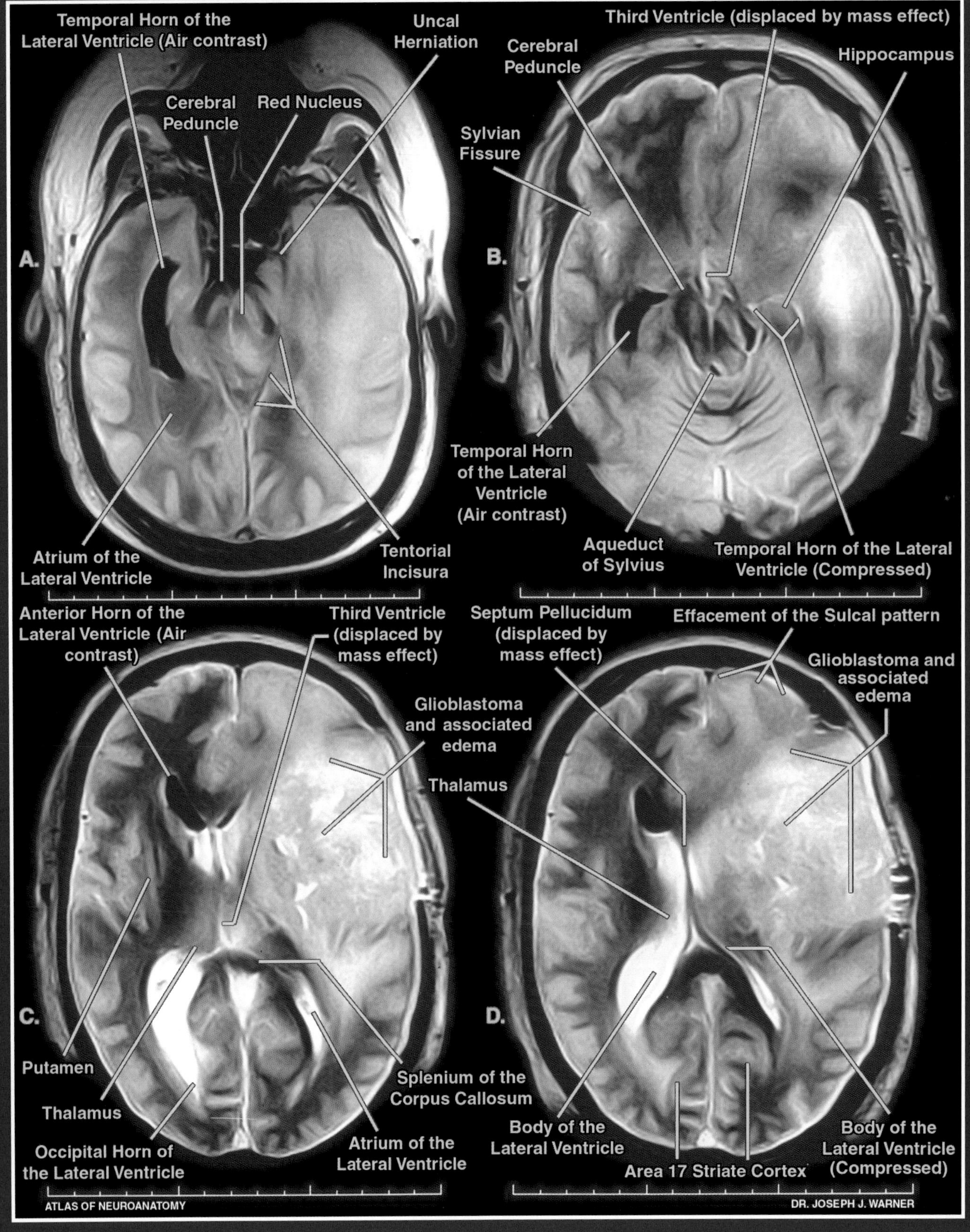
MAGNETIC RESONANCE IMAGING (POST-MORTEM) IN A CASE OF GLIOBLASTOMA MULTIFORME: SECTIONS ORIENTED (A) PARALLEL TO THE SYLVIAN FISSURE AND (B,C,D) IN THE HORIZONTAL PLANE FOR CORRELATION WITH VENTRICULOGRAPHY AND ANGIOGRAPHY
A.
Temporal Horn of the Lateral Ventricle (Air contrast)
Uncal Herniation
Cerebral Peduncle
Red Nucleus
Atrium of the Lateral Ventricle
Tentorial Incisura
B.
Third Ventricle (displaced by mass effect)
Cerebral Peduncle
Hippocampus
Sylvian Fissure
Temporal Horn of the Lateral Ventricle (Air contrast)
Aqueduct of Sylvius
Temporal Horn of the Lateral Ventricle (Compressed)
C.
Anterior Horn of the Lateral Ventricle (Air contrast)
Third Ventricle (displaced by mass effect)
Glioblastoma and associated edema
Thalamus
Putamen
Thalamus
Occipital Horn of the Lateral Ventricle
Splenium of the Corpus Callosum
Atrium of the Lateral Ventricle
D.
Septum Pellucidum (displaced by mass effect)
Effacement of the Sulcal pattern
Glioblastoma and associated edema
Body of the Lateral Ventricle
Area 17 Striate Cortex
Body of the Lateral Ventricle (Compressed)
ATLAS OF NEUROANATOMY
DR. JOSEPH J. WARNER

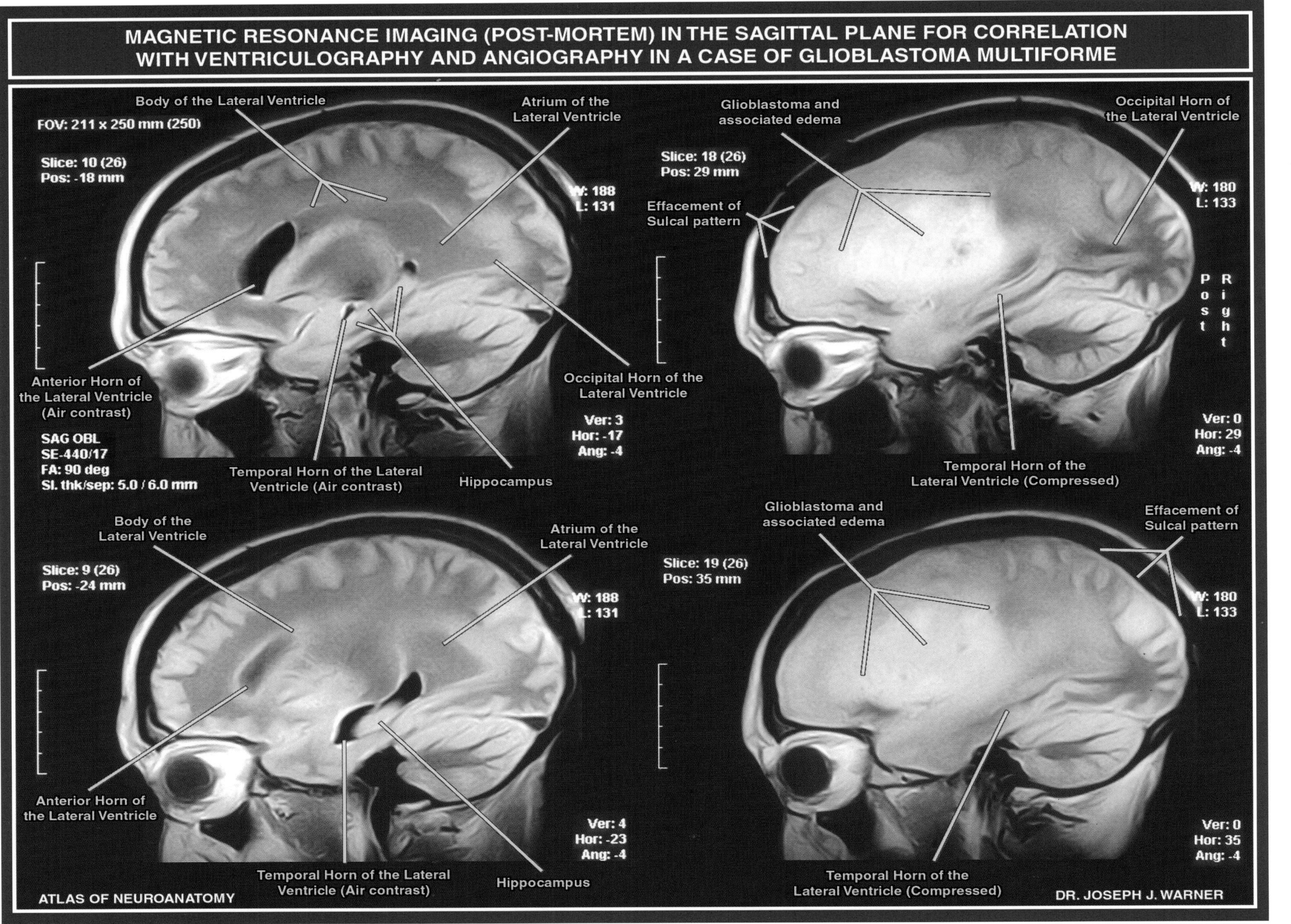
MAGNETIC RESONANCE IMAGING (POST-MORTEM) IN THE SAGITTAL PLANE FOR CORRELATION WITH VENTRICULOGRAPHY AND ANGIOGRAPHY IN A CASE OF GLIOBLASTOMA MULTIFORME
Body of the Lateral Ventricle
FOV: 211 x 250 mm (250)
Slice: 10 (26)
Pos: -18 mm
Atrium of the Lateral Ventricle
W: 188
L: 131
Anterior Horn of the Lateral Ventricle (Air contrast)
Occipital Horn of the Lateral Ventricle
Ver: 3
Hor: -17
Ang: -4
SAG OBL
SE-440/17
FA: 90 deg
Sl. thk/sep: 5.0 / 6.0 mm
Temporal Horn of the Lateral Ventricle (Air contrast)
Hippocampus
Glioblastoma and associated edema
Occipital Horn of the Lateral Ventricle
Slice: 18 (26)
Pos: 29 mm
Effacement of Sulcal pattern
W: 180
L: 133
P o s t
R i g h t
Ver: 0
Hor: 29
Ang: -4
Temporal Horn of the Lateral Ventricle (Compressed)
Body of the Lateral Ventricle
Atrium of the Lateral Ventricle
Slice: 9 (26)
Pos: -24 mm
W: 188
L: 131
Anterior Horn of the Lateral Ventricle
Ver: 4
Hor: -23
Ang: -4
Temporal Horn of the Lateral Ventricle (Air contrast)
Hippocampus
Glioblastoma and associated edema
Effacement of Sulcal pattern
Slice: 19 (26)
Pos: 35 mm
W: 180
L: 133
Ver: 0
Hor: 35
Ang: -4
Temporal Horn of the Lateral Ventricle (Compressed)
ATLAS OF NEUROANATOMY
DR. JOSEPH J. WARNER

Case Presentation: History

A 62-year-old white male presented with a one-week history of numbness of the right hand which progressed over three days to involve the entire right forearm. He also noticed a concomitant sensation of numbness of the left perioral and intraoral region. This subsequently spread to the entire left side of the face and left periauricular region.

A prominent symptom noticed by the patient was an inability to look to his left. He gave a history of first noticing this problem when he "couldn't look to the left when pulling [his car] out into the road from a driveway." The patient denied any actual visual disturbance, such as diplopia, visual field loss, etc. He did give a vague history of "light strokes" approximately two years earlier associated with transient unilateral weakness and no discernible residua.

Neurologic Findings

- Left conjugate gaze paresis
- Impaired leftward saccades and pursuit evoked by opticokinetic nystagmus testing
- Decreased sensation to all modalities over the left side of the face
- Diminished direct and consensual reflex responses to left corneal stimulation
- Mild weakness of the lower 2/3 of the face on the right
- Dysesthesiae evoked by pinprick sensory testing of the right upper extremity
- Bilateral upper extremity ataxia, with dysmetria and dysdiadochokinesis

Analysis of Systems or Structures Involved Based on Neurologic Findings

Level of the neuraxis involved is established by a prominent deficit of conjugate gaze in conjunction with alternating sensory findings compatible with pontine dysfunction. A review of the neurologic findings indicates involvement that includes the level of the trigeminal nerve of the left.

- Left conjugate gaze paresis: This finding indicates a unilateral lesion involving either the frontal eye fields or the paramedian pontine reticular formation (PPRF). Lesions involving the frontal eye fields would result in an impairment of saccades and volitional refixation to the contralateral side. PPRF involvement would be accompanied by an ipsilateral conjugate gaze paresis. *In this case, a left conjugate gaze paresis is attributable to an ipsilateral PPRF lesion* because the localization of other findings (including laterality) indicates a pontine level rather than a cerebral lesion.

- Impaired leftward saccades and pursuit eye movements: Projections of the frontal eye fields include the contralateral PPRF. The parietal pursuit center is a primarily ipsilateral projection system. *A PPRF lesion would therefore affect ipsilateral saccades and pursuit eye movements.* The findings in this case clearly indicate a left PPRF lesion.

Analysis of Systems or Structures Involved Based on Neurologic Findings

- Decreased sensation to all modalities over the left side of the face: *Left trigeminal nerve and/or fascicles traversing the left middle cerebellar peduncle and lateral pons.* If the right trigeminothalamic or thalamocortical system were involved, the corneal reflex would be intact.

- Diminished direct and consensual reflex response to left corneal stimulation: *Left trigeminal nerve or fascicles entering the lateral pons*

- Mild weakness of the lower 2/3 of the face on the right; (Right upper motor neuron type facial paresis): *Left corticobulbar fibers rostral to the level of the seventh cranial nerve*

- Right upper extremity dysesthesiae to sensory testing: (often associated with impaired lemniscal modalities and intact spinothalamic function) may indicate involvement of the *left medial lemniscus*. Considering the somatotopic organization within the medial lemniscus, the upper extremity findings would indicate that *the medial aspect of this tract is specifically involved*, sparing the lower extremity representation (lateral fibers) at the pontine level.

- Bilateral upper extremity ataxia: distal movements of the upper extremities involve the neocerebellar system, including pontocerebellar projections (middle cerebellar peduncles), as well as dentatorubrothalamic projections through the superior cerebellar peduncles. Findings in this case may indicate *involvement of the middle cerebellar peduncles or superior cerebellar peduncles adjacent to their decussation.*

Diagnostic Investigation

Chest X-ray revealed a 2.2 x 1.2 cm left upper lobe density, increased in size in comparison with previous radiographs, consistent with a diagnosis of possible neoplasm.

Cranial computerized tomography with and without intravenous radiocontrast injection demonstrated a contrast-enhancing lesion, 1 cm in diameter, located in the left pontine tegmentum with mass effect on adjacent structures.

Magnetic Resonance Imaging, gadolinium contrast: A spheroidal lesion, 1 cm in diameter, was demonstrated in the left pontine tegmentum, with mass effect distorting the fourth ventricle and basis pontis. This was associated with vasogenic edema involving the middle cerebellar peduncles, more pronounced on the left, including the level of the trigeminal nerve.

Clinical Course

After 2400 rads of whole brain radiation, clinical deterioration ensued with Magnetic Resonance Imaging evidence of rapid tumor enlargement and adjacent edema. Neurologic improvement followed 3000 rads of whole brain radiation and dexamethasone therapy. Clinical status declined, with aspiration pneumonitis and subsequent cardiopulmonary arrest (10 weeks after initial neurologic diagnosis).

Pathologic Examination

- Autopsy confirmed an adenocarcinoma of the lung, left upper lobe, metastatic.

- A solitary metastasis, approximately 1.2 cm in diameter, occupied the left pontine tegmentum, with associated edema and mass effect, peripheral hemorrhage and adjacent gliosis. (The neuroanatomic localization and structural involvement correlated with the case analysis as outlined above.)

CARCINOMA OF THE LUNG METASTATIC TO THE PONS: MAGNETIC RESONANCE IMAGING

GADOLINIUM-ENHANCED, HORIZONTAL SECTIONS AT THE LEVEL OF ROSTRAL AND MID-PONS

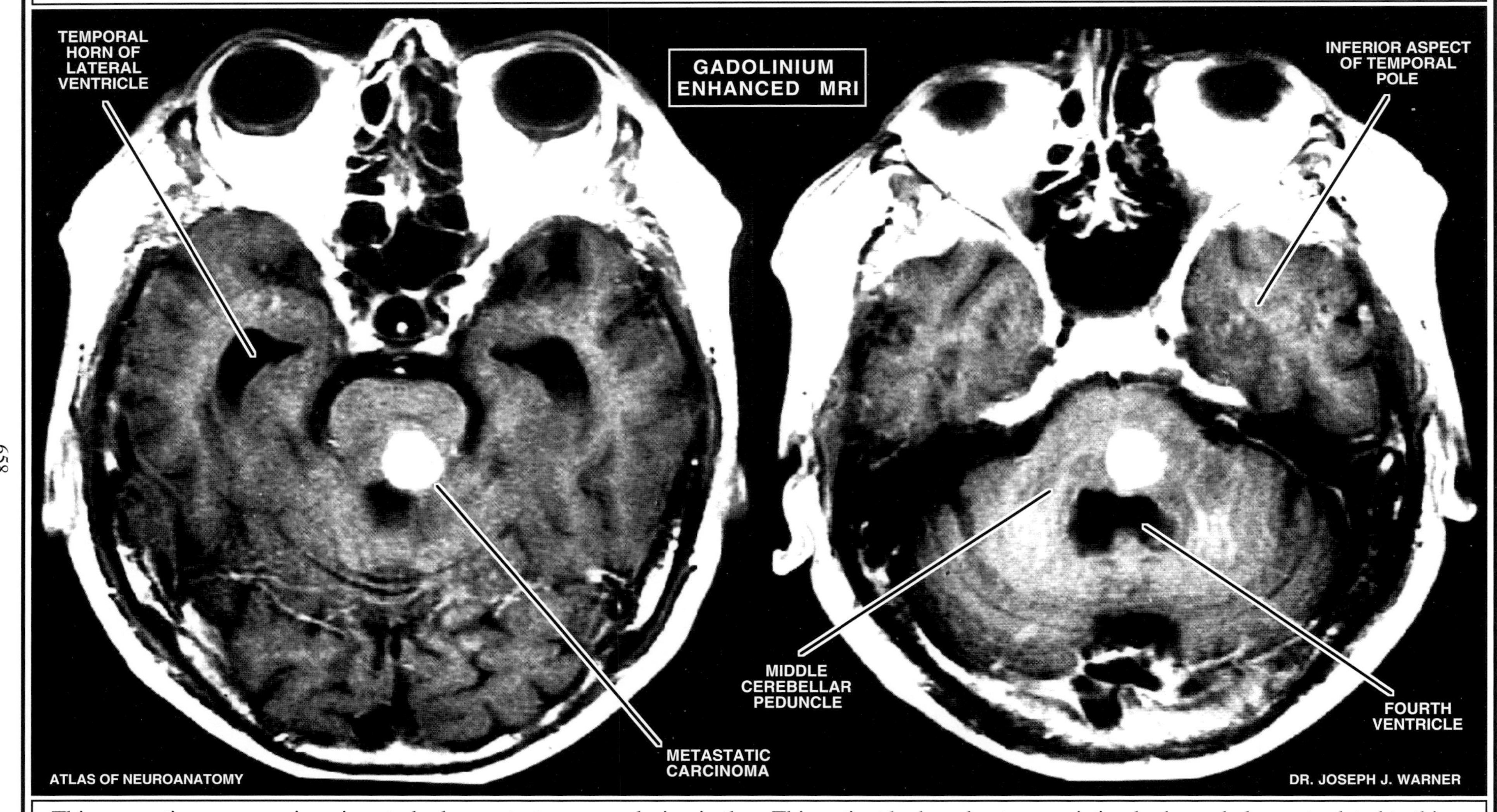

This magnetic resonance imaging study demonstrates a mass lesion in the pontine tegmentum, involving the rostral and mid-pontine levels. A moderate degree of deformation of the contour of the fourth ventricle is discernible. As is frequently the case with neoplastic lesions (in contrast to sudden events such as infarction or hemorrhage), specific signs and symptoms appear insidiously, such that by the time the patient presents for diagnostic investigation, the mass has already attained significant size.

This patient had moderate preexisting hydrocephalus, not related to this metastatic lesion nor to a previous infarction (refer to history). Enlargement of the temporal horn of the lateral ventricles and of the fourth ventricle suggests a more caudal obstruction of cerebrospinal fluid outflow. The localization of the lesion correlates with the clinical signs and symptoms as presented in the case analysis, including the ipsilateral gaze paresis, contralateral gaze preference, sensory and cerebellar signs.

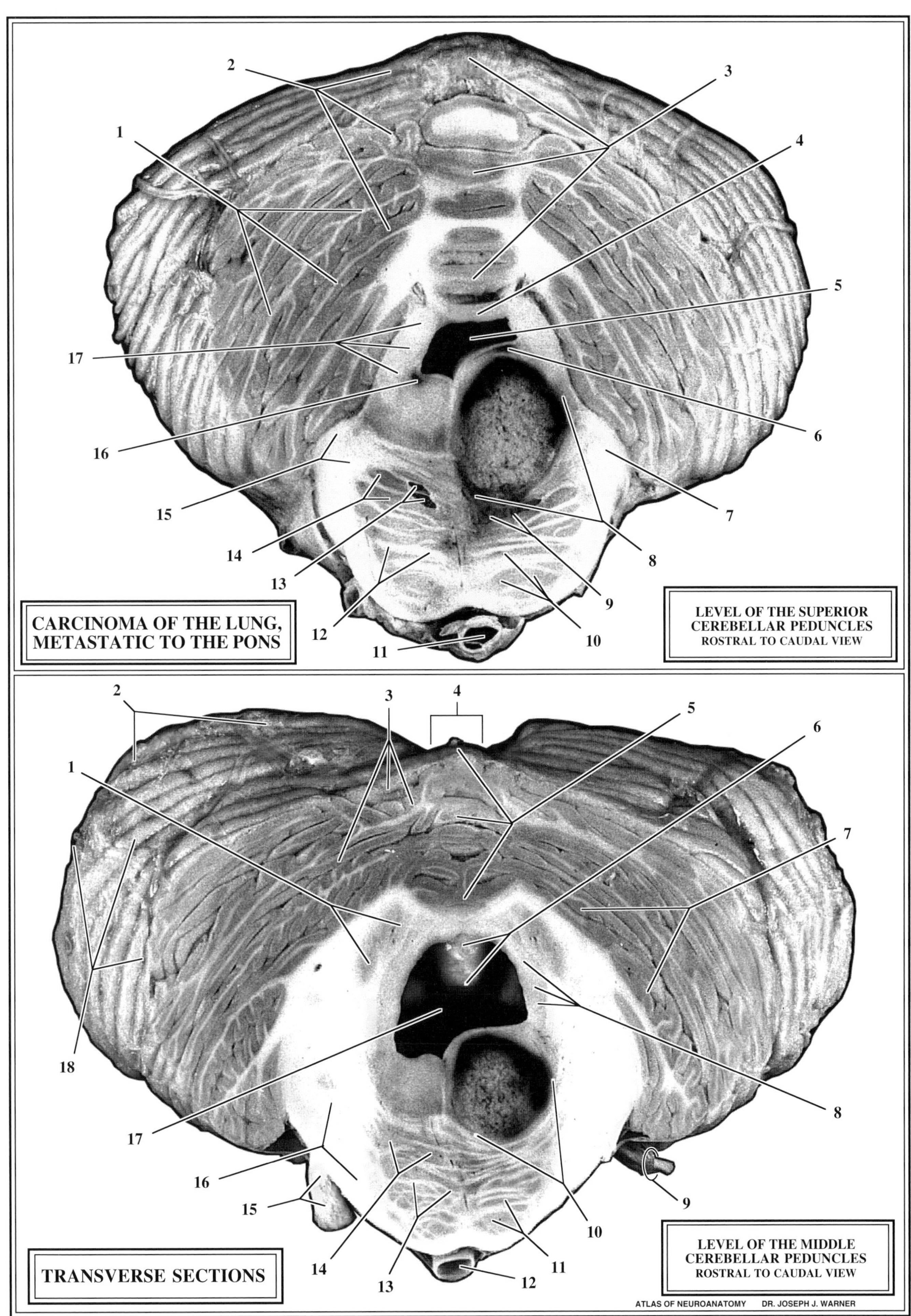

CARCINOMA OF THE LUNG, METASTATIC TO THE PONS
LEVEL OF THE SUPERIOR CEREBELLAR PEDUNCLES
ROSTRAL TO CAUDAL VIEW
1
2
3
4
5
6
7
8
9
10
11
12
13
14
15
16
17
TRANSVERSE SECTIONS
LEVEL OF THE MIDDLE CEREBELLAR PEDUNCLES
ROSTRAL TO CAUDAL VIEW
1
2
3
4
5
6
7
8
9
10
11
12
13
14
15
16
17
18
ATLAS OF NEUROANATOMY DR. JOSEPH J. WARNER

CARCINOMA OF THE LUNG METASTATIC TO THE PONS: MAP OF SECTION ORIENTATIONS AND KEY TO STRUCTURES

REFERENCED TO PARASAGITTAL SECTION, 15μ, KLUVER-BARRERA TECHNIQUE

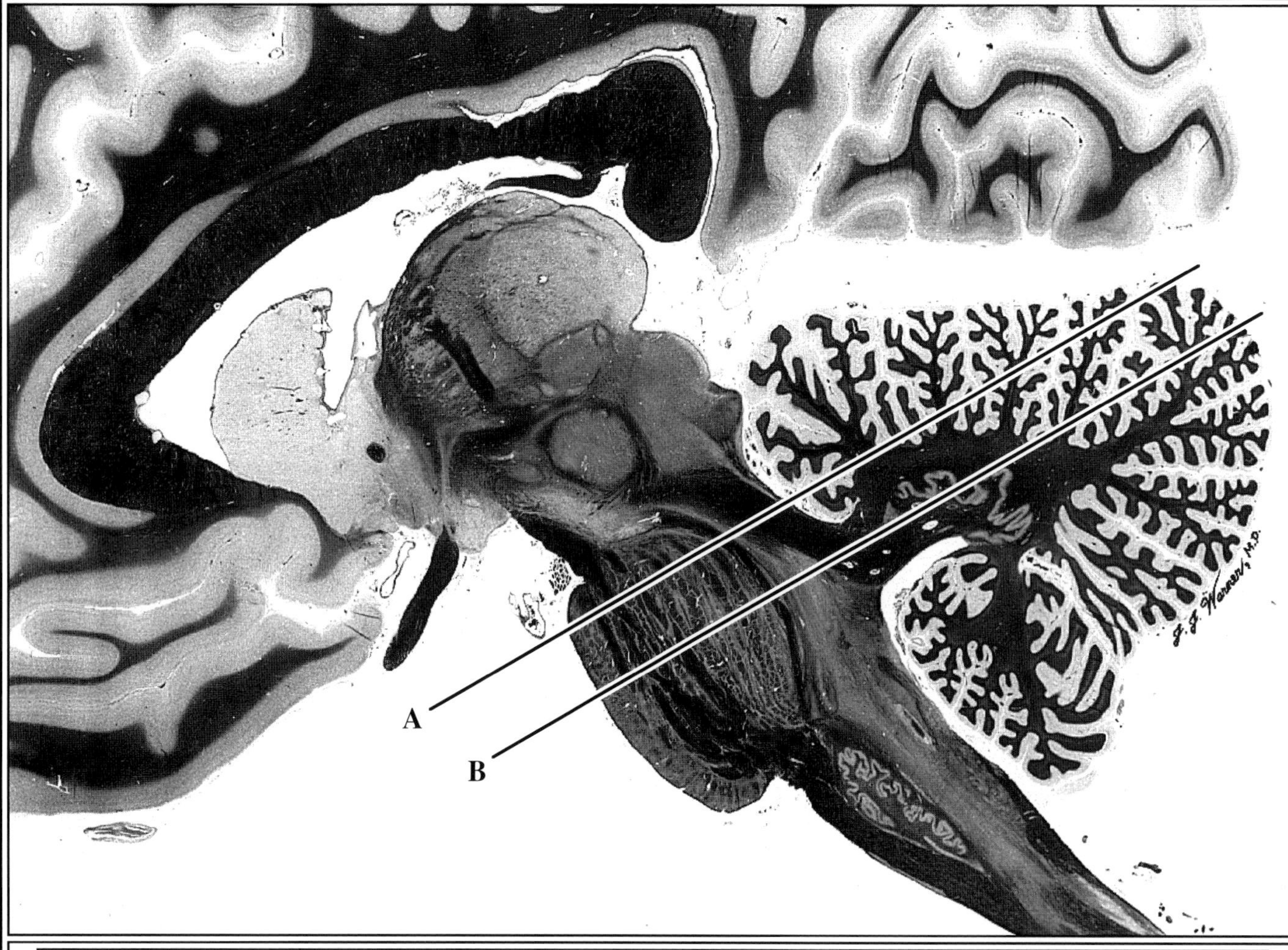

KEY TO NUMBERED STRUCTURES FOR EACH LEVEL (REFER TO ORIENTATION MAPS)

A. CARCINOMA OF THE LUNG, METASTATIC TO THE PONTINE TEGMENTUM: SECTION OF THE PONS AND CEREBELLUM, LEVEL OF THE SUPERIOR CEREBELLAR PEDUNCLES

1. Anterior Lobe of the Cerebellum
2. Intermediate Zone
3. Cerebellar Vermis
4. Superior (Anterior) Medullary Velum
5. Fourth Ventricle
6. Locus Coeruleus, deformed by mass effect of the tumor
7. Middle Cerebellar Peduncle (rostral aspect)
8. Metastatic Carcinoma of the Lung with peripheral hemorrhage
9. Lacunar Infarct (remote)
10. Corticobulbar, Corticospinal Tracts
11. Basilar Artery
12. Transverse Pontocerebellar Fibers
13. Lacunar Infarct (remote)
14. Pontine Nuclei (Gray)
15. Middle Cerebellar Peduncle (rostral aspect)
16. Locus Coeruleus
17. Superior Cerebellar Peduncle

B. CARCINOMA OF THE LUNG, METASTATIC TO THE PONTINE TEGMENTUM: SECTION OF THE PONS AND CEREBELLUM, LEVEL OF THE MIDDLE CEREBELLAR PEDUNCLES

1. Dentate Nucleus, Cerebellum
2. Superior Semilunar Lobule
3. Intermediate Zone, Cerebellum
4. Posterior Incisura
5. Cerebellar Vermis
6. Nodulus
7. Anterior Lobe of the Cerebellum
8. Superior Cerebellar Peduncle (caudal aspect)
9. Facial (VII) Nerve
10. Metastatic Carcinoma of the Lung with peripheral hemorrhage
11. Corticobulbar, Corticospinal Tracts
12. Basilar Artery
13. Transverse Pontocerebellar Fibers
14. Pontine Nuclei (Gray)
15. Trigeminal (V) Nerve
16. Middle Cerebellar Peduncle
17. Fourth Ventricle
18. Posterior Lobe of the Cerebellum

CHARACTERISTICS OF METASTATIC CARCINOMA INVOLVING THE CENTRAL NERVOUS SYSTEM

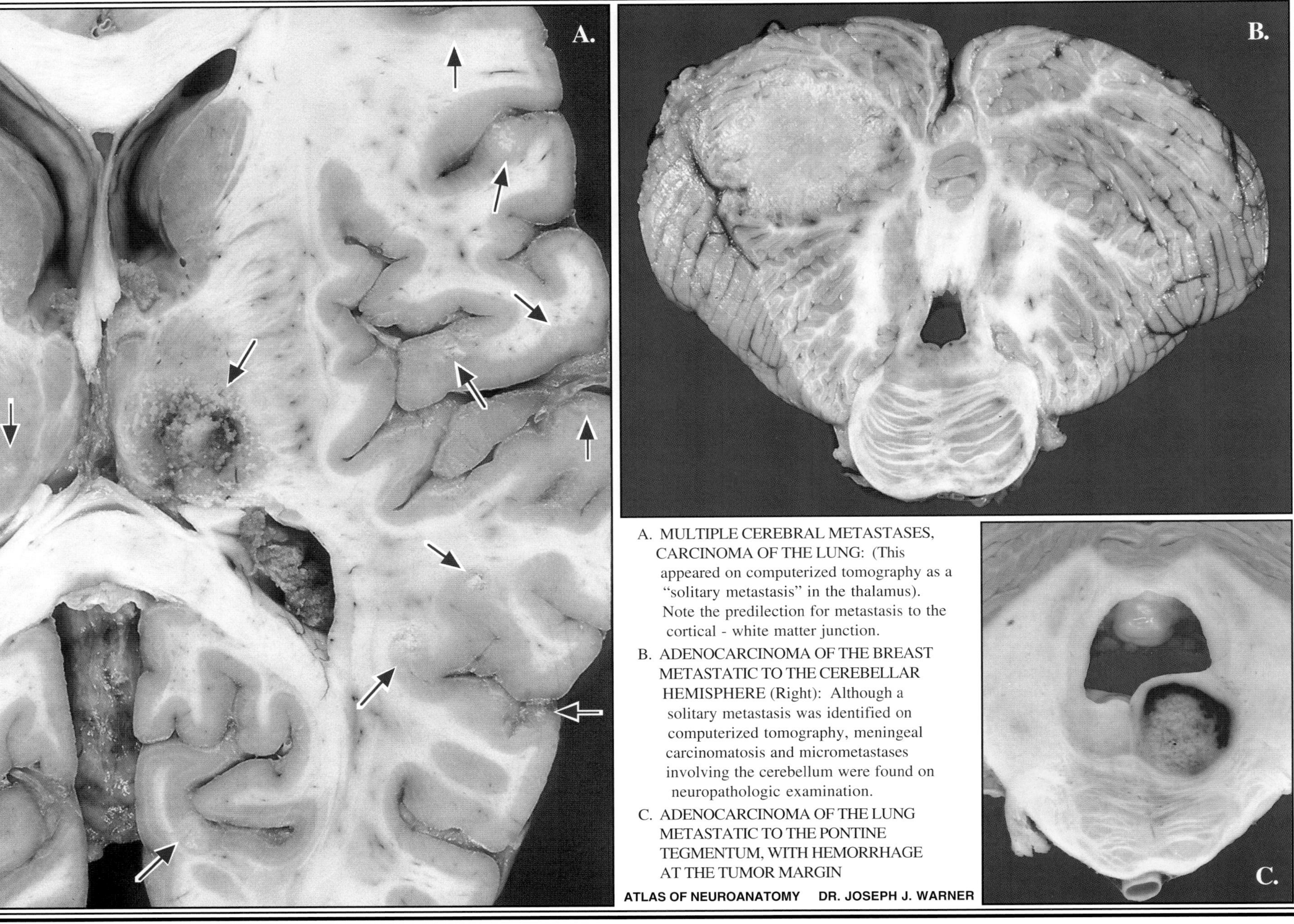

A. MULTIPLE CEREBRAL METASTASES, CARCINOMA OF THE LUNG: (This appeared on computerized tomography as a "solitary metastasis" in the thalamus). Note the predilection for metastasis to the cortical - white matter junction.

B. ADENOCARCINOMA OF THE BREAST METASTATIC TO THE CEREBELLAR HEMISPHERE (Right): Although a solitary metastasis was identified on computerized tomography, meningeal carcinomatosis and micrometastases involving the cerebellum were found on neuropathologic examination.

C. ADENOCARCINOMA OF THE LUNG METASTATIC TO THE PONTINE TEGMENTUM, WITH HEMORRHAGE AT THE TUMOR MARGIN

ACUTE BACTERIAL ENDOCARDITIS: MULTIPLE SEPTIC EMBOLI TO THE BRAIN WITH VASCULAR NECROSIS, PARENCHYMAL AND SUBARACHNOID HEMORRHAGE, AND MICROABSCESS FORMATION

CASE PRESENTATION

This 41-year-old female was admitted to the hospital with a history of fever, altered mental status, and left hemiparesis. Six days prior to admission, the patient developed a fever of 103 degrees F. Symptoms included chills, diffuse pain, marked fatigue, and a severe headache associated with photophobia. The severity of the headache and fever fluctuated, with transient improvement. One day prior to admission, she developed mild left hand weakness and presented to an outside hospital for evaluation. Physical examination at that time demonstrated hepatomegally and icterus, with slight weakness of the left hand. She was, however, reportedly alert and oriented at that time. A complete blood count revealed 15,000 white cells per mm^3, with 55% polymorphonuclear leukocytes. The patient was diagnosed as having a viral syndrome, and she was started on aspirin. That night, she became confused and lethargic. She could name objects and answer simple questions. Examination revealed a new left hemiparesis associated with a left Babinski sign. New petechiae were noted as well. She developed tachypnea. Repeat laboratory studies showed a white blood count of 20,000 and a platelet count of 10,000 per mm^3. The patient was transferred from the outside hospital due to her deteriorating clinical status.

Her past medical history was unremarkable with the exception of anxiety and depression. Medications found in her medicine cabinet by family members included Tofranil, Mellaril, Vistaril, Benadryl, and Darvocet. She had also been receiving "allergy shots." The patient was a nurse, who had been well and working up to the time of her illness. She was in the midst of divorce proceedings, and there was a prior history of ethanol abuse.

Upon admission, her blood pressure was 95/60, with a pulse of 120 per minute, shallow respirations at 35 per minute, and a temperature of 104.6 degrees F. Examination revealed the patient to be obtunded, moving only to noxious stimuli. General physical findings included marked icterus, diaphoresis, and diffuse petechial hemorrhages over the skin. There was slight meningismus detected upon attempted passive neck movement. There was no palpable lymphadenopathy. Auscultation of the chest revealed bibasilar rales and coarse rhonchi. Cardiovascular findings included normal cardiac sounds except for a new systolic murmur and non-palpable systolic point of maximum impulse. Marked hepatomegaly was noted, without detectable splenomegaly. Neurologic findings included markedly impaired level of arousal, with the patient unresponsive to verbal or tactile stimulation. There was occasional spontaneous eye opening. Weakness of the lower 2/3 of the face was noted on the left. Oculocephalic maneuvers produced conjugate eye movements. A left hemiparesis was noted upon attempts to elicit movement. Deep tendon reflexes were 2+ in the right upper extremity, 3+ in the left upper extremity, 3+ quadriceps and 4+ at the ankles bilaterally, with bilateral sustained clonus and Babinski signs. Laboratory findings included mildly elevated transaminase levels, total bilirubin of 4.2, LDH of 600, and alkaline phosphatase of 259. The white count was 24,500 per mm^3, with 89% polymorphonuclear leukocytes. Platelet count was 11,000 per mm^3. Arterial blood gases on room air revealed a pH of 7.47, pO_2 of 64, and a pCO_2 of 25.

Electrocardiogram demonstrated no ischemic changes. A chest X-ray revealed left-sided interstitial infiltrates. Urinalysis demonstrated many red blood cells and coarse granular casts.

Computerized tomography of the brain demonstrated a large right parietal intracerebral hemorrhage with rupture into the ventricular system. A smaller left frontal hemorrhage was noted, as was effacement of the sulcal pattern consistent with bilateral cerebral edema. Blood was detectable in the right lateral ventricle suggestive of rupture of the right parietal hemorrhage into the ventricular system. Blood cultures were drawn, which subsequently grew *Staphylococcus aureus* on samples from four separate sites. The patient was treated with platelet and fresh frozen plasma transfusions. Later on the day of admission, the patient sustained a generalized tonic-clonic seizure, followed by prolonged periods of apnea. The patient was intubated. She became deeply comatose, unresponsive to noxious stimuli, and developed spontaneous sustained hyperventilation. Two hours after the seizure, the patient was significantly hypotensive and was started on intravenous Dopamine. Thirty minutes later, she developed intermittent ventricular tachycardia, supraventricular tachycardia, and nodal rhythms. A repeat electrocardiogram revealed new changes including left anterior hemiblock, right bundle branch block, and ST changes consistent with acute anterior myocardial infarction. The patient sustained a cardiac arrest three hours later, and resuscitative efforts were unsuccessful. Pathologic examination was performed. Findings were consistent with acute bacterial endocarditis, with septic embolization of the systemic circulation.

ACUTE BACTERIAL ENDOCARDITIS: MULTIPLE SEPTIC EMBOLI WITH INTRACEREBRAL AND SUBARACHNOID HEMORRHAGE

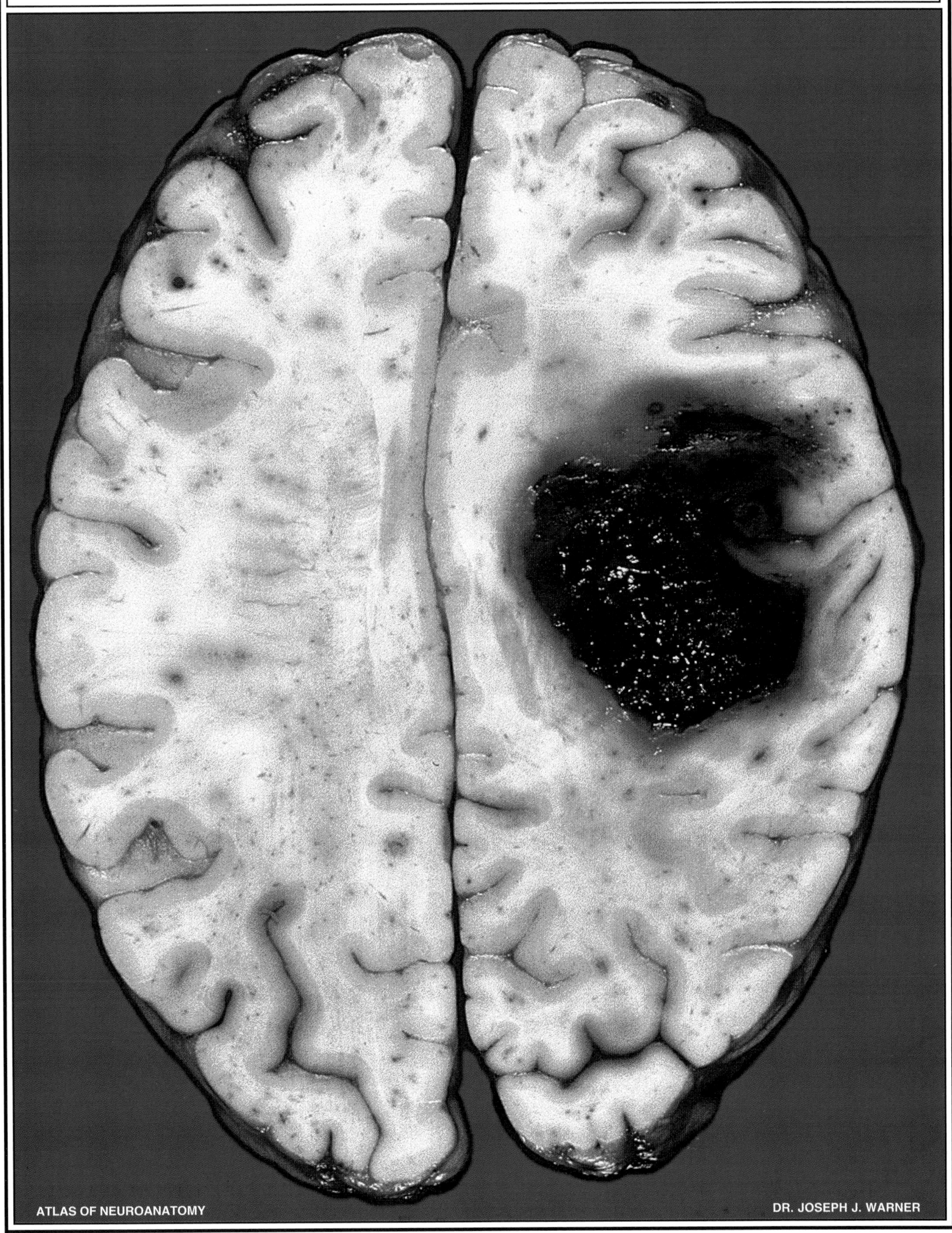

ACUTE BACTERIAL ENDOCARDITIS: MULTIPLE SEPTIC EMBOLI WITH INTRACEREBRAL AND SUBARACHNOID HEMORRHAGE

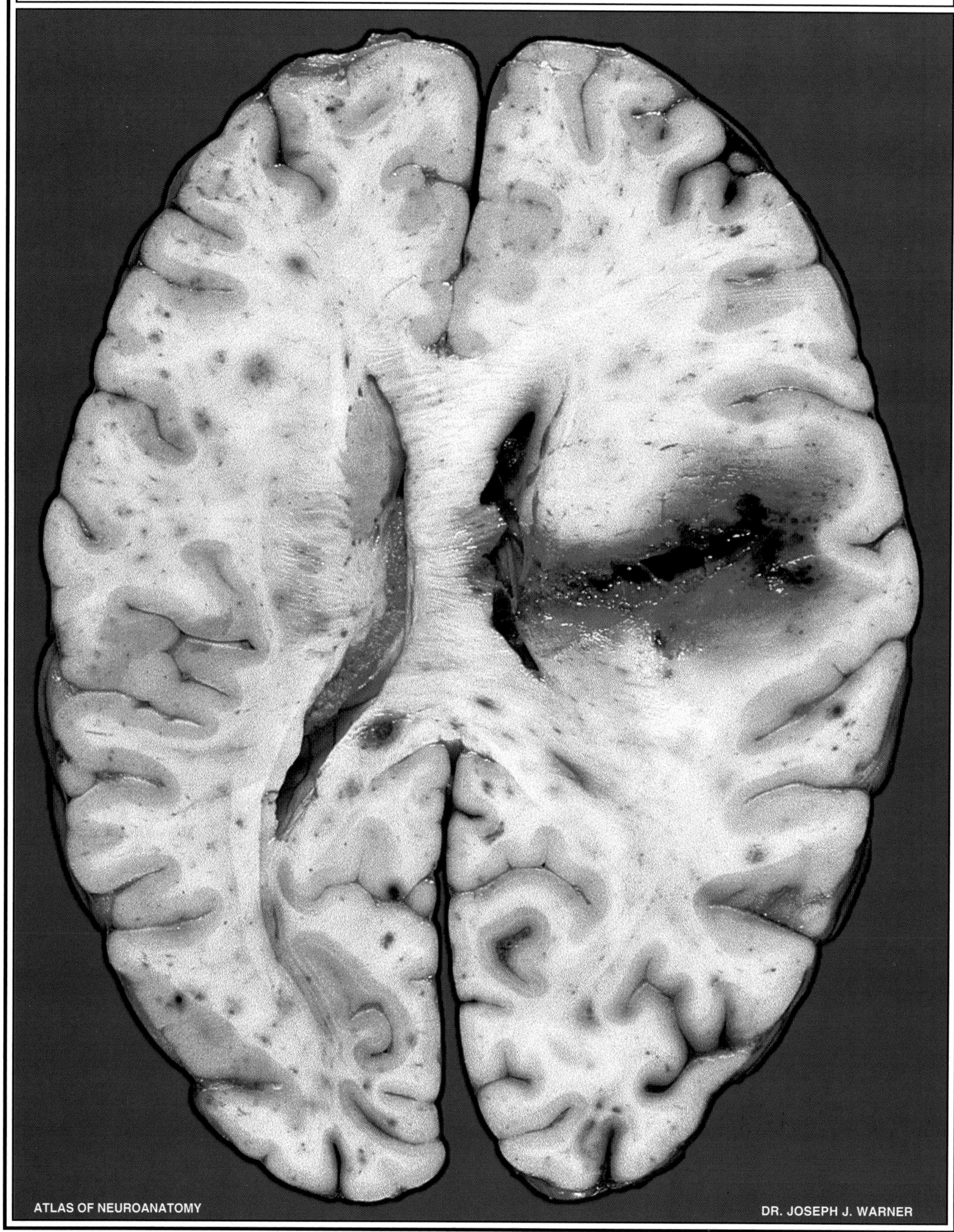

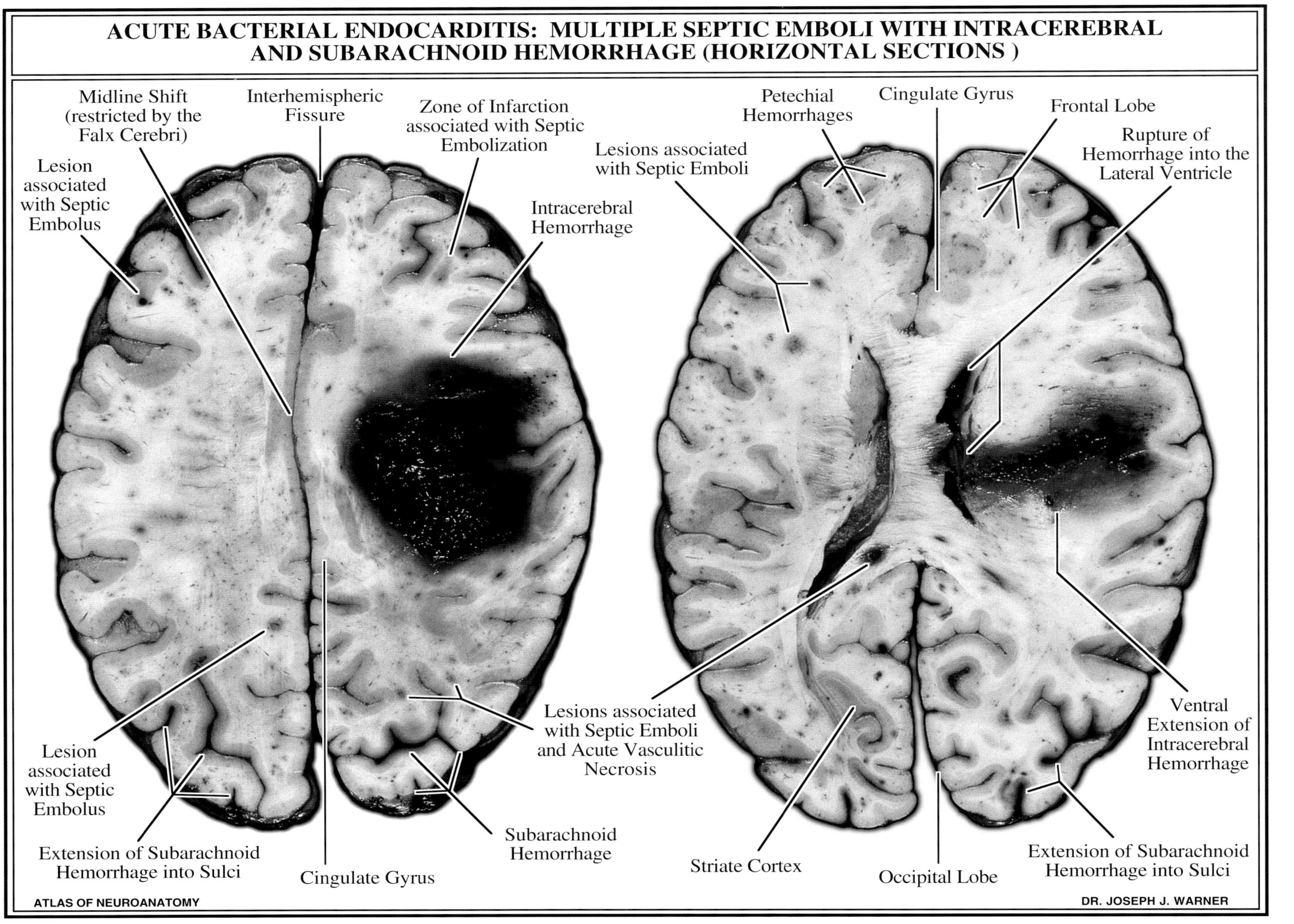
ACUTE BACTERIAL ENDOCARDITIS: MULTIPLE SEPTIC EMBOLI WITH INTRACEREBRAL AND SUBARACHNOID HEMORRHAGE (HORIZONTAL SECTIONS)
Midline Shift (restricted by the Falx Cerebri)
Interhemispheric Fissure
Zone of Infarction associated with Septic Embolization
Lesion associated with Septic Embolus
Intracerebral Hemorrhage
Lesion associated with Septic Embolus
Extension of Subarachnoid Hemorrhage into Sulci
Cingulate Gyrus
Subarachnoid Hemorrhage
Lesions associated with Septic Emboli and Acute Vasculitic Necrosis
Petechial Hemorrhages
Cingulate Gyrus
Frontal Lobe
Lesions associated with Septic Emboli
Rupture of Hemorrhage into the Lateral Ventricle
Ventral Extension of Intracerebral Hemorrhage
Striate Cortex
Occipital Lobe
Extension of Subarachnoid Hemorrhage into Sulci
ATLAS OF NEUROANATOMY
DR. JOSEPH J. WARNER

ACUTE BACTERIAL ENDOCARDITIS WITH SEPTIC EMBOLI TO THE BRAIN: VASCULAR NECROSIS, CEREBRAL ISCHEMIA, AND MICROABSCESS FORMATION

FRONTAL CORTEX, HEMATOXYLIN AND EOSIN, 100X

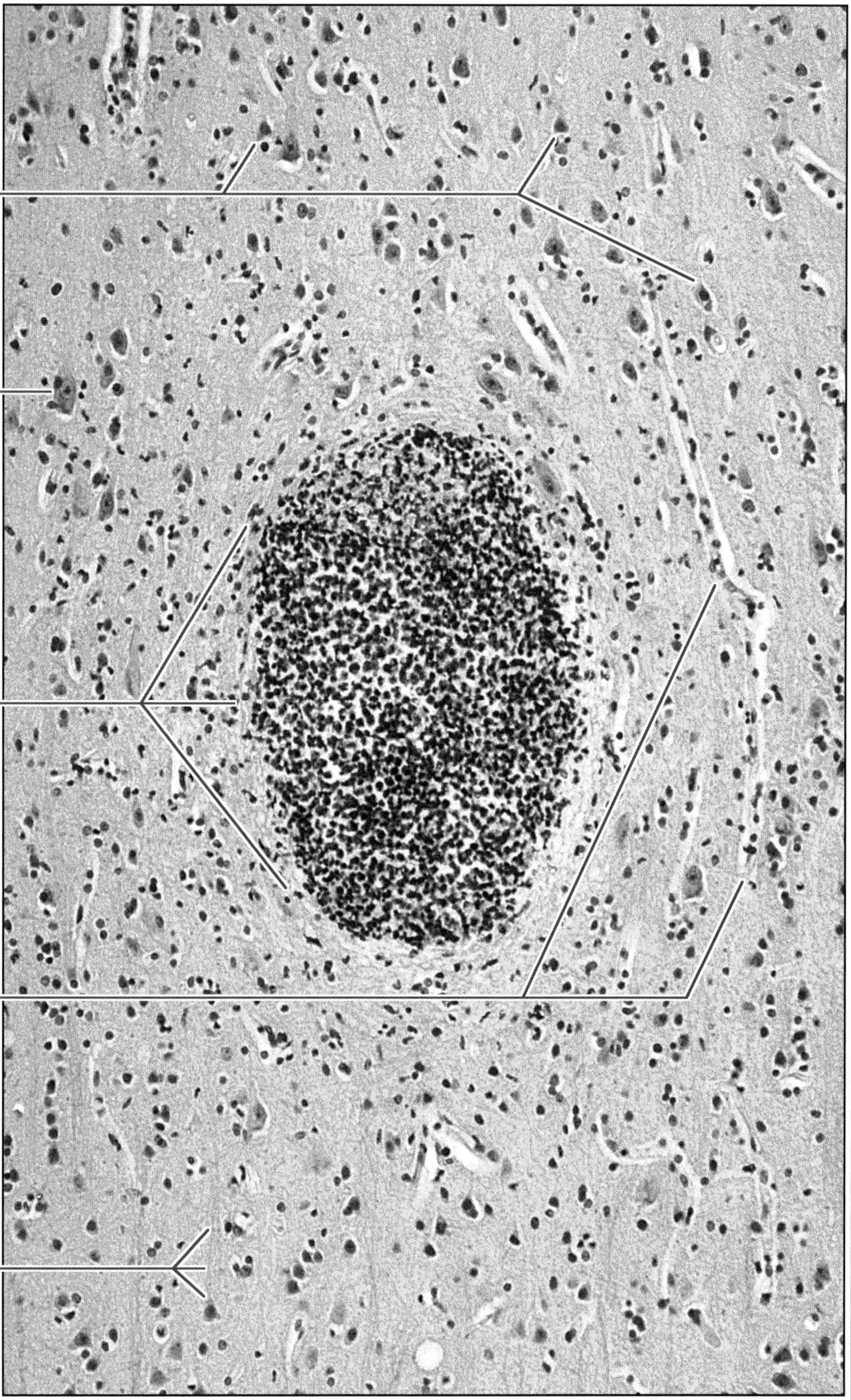

Pyramidal cells demonstrating ischemic changes, including pyknotic nuclei and eosinophilic cytoplasm

Large pyramidal cell with cytoplasmic eosinophilia (the nucleus and nucleolus remain discernible)

Cerebral cortical microabscess with acute inflammatory infiltrate of polymorphonuclear leukocytes

In this case, similar lesions were found in association with (1) septic emboli containing Gram positive cocci and (2) necrotizing vasculitis involving small arteries and arterioles.

Capillary

Apical dendrite of small cortical pyramidal cell

HISTOLOGIC SECTION: 10 μ

ACUTE BACTERIAL ENDOCARDITIS: MULTIPLE SEPTIC EMBOLI TO THE BRAIN WITH VASCULAR NECROSIS, PARENCHYMAL AND SUBARACHNOID HEMORRHAGE, AND MICROABSCESS FORMATION

A.

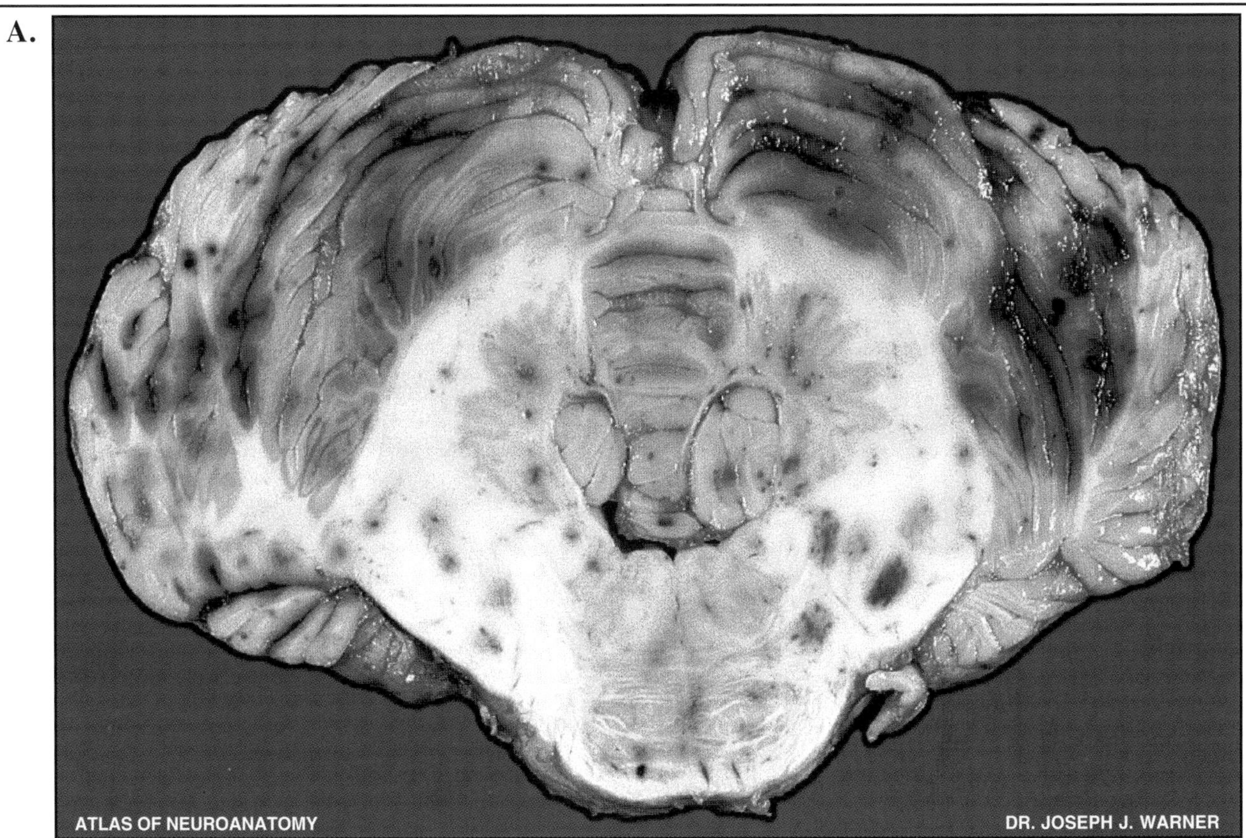

A. Pons and Cerebellum: transverse section demonstrating multiple hemorrhagic lesions

B.

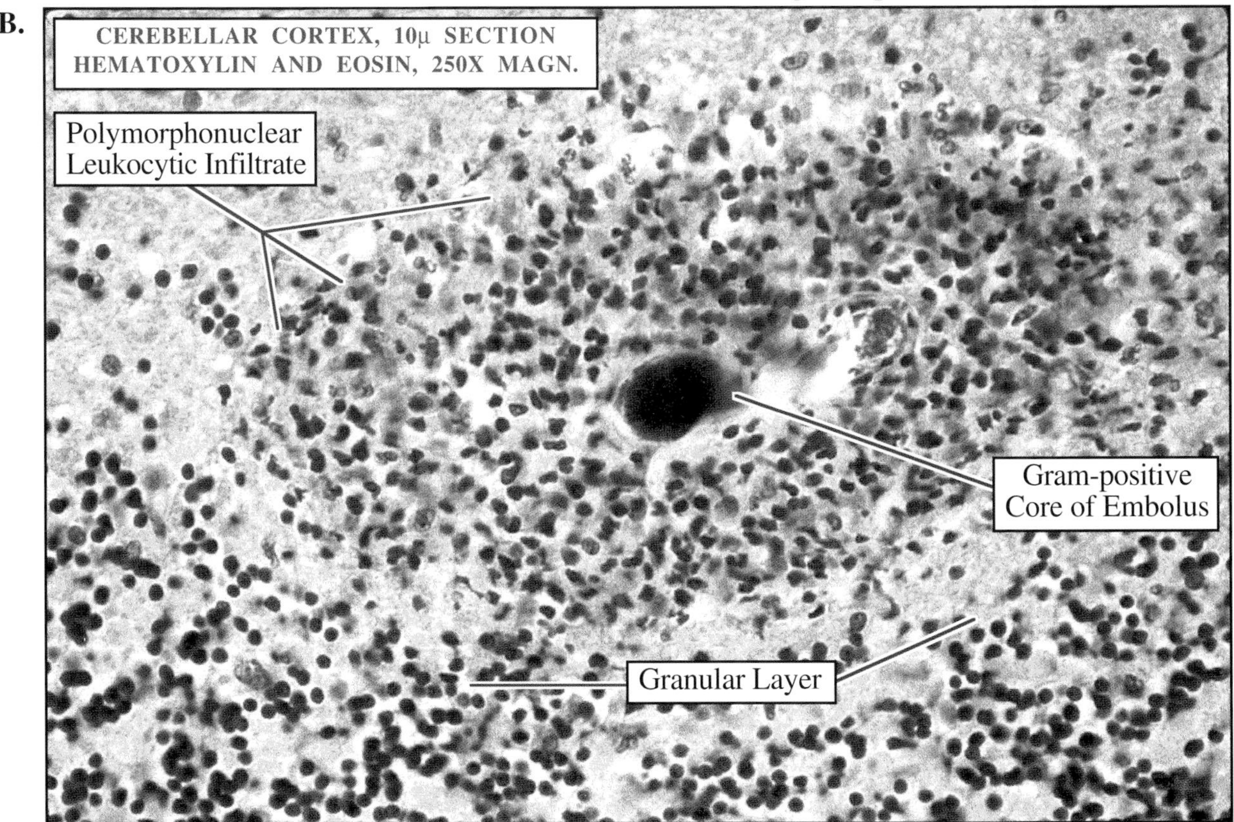

B. Septic Embolus containing gram-positive cocci, surrounded by polymorphonuclear leukocytes.

ACUTE BACTERIAL ENDOCARDITIS: MULTIPLE SEPTIC EMBOLI TO THE BRAIN WITH VASCULAR NECROSIS, HEMORRHAGE, AND MICROABSCESS FORMATION

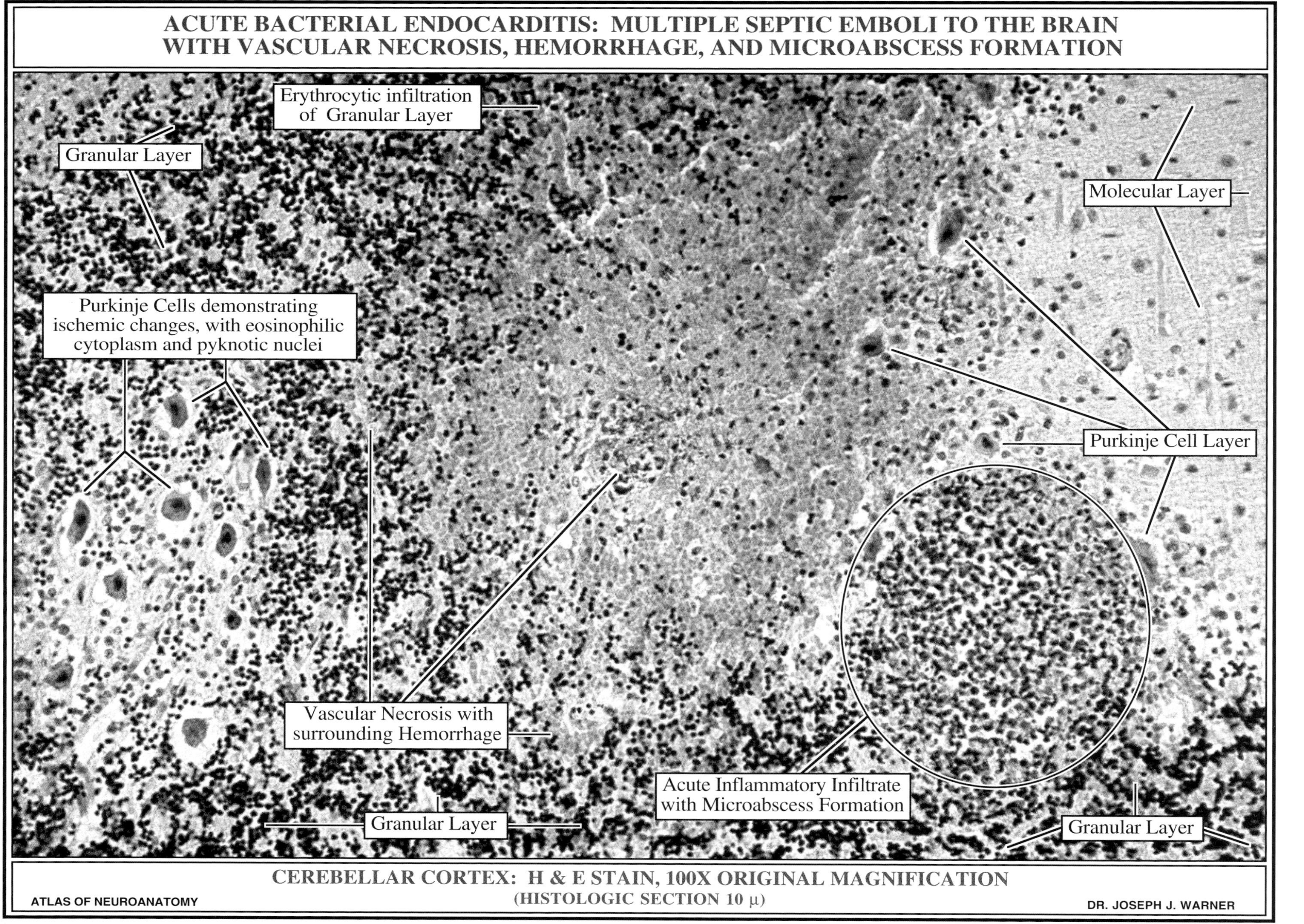

CEREBELLAR CORTEX: H & E STAIN, 100X ORIGINAL MAGNIFICATION
(HISTOLOGIC SECTION 10 μ)

AGENESIS OF THE CORPUS CALLOSUM (WITH ABSENT CINGULATE GYRUS): MIDLINE SAGITTAL SECTION

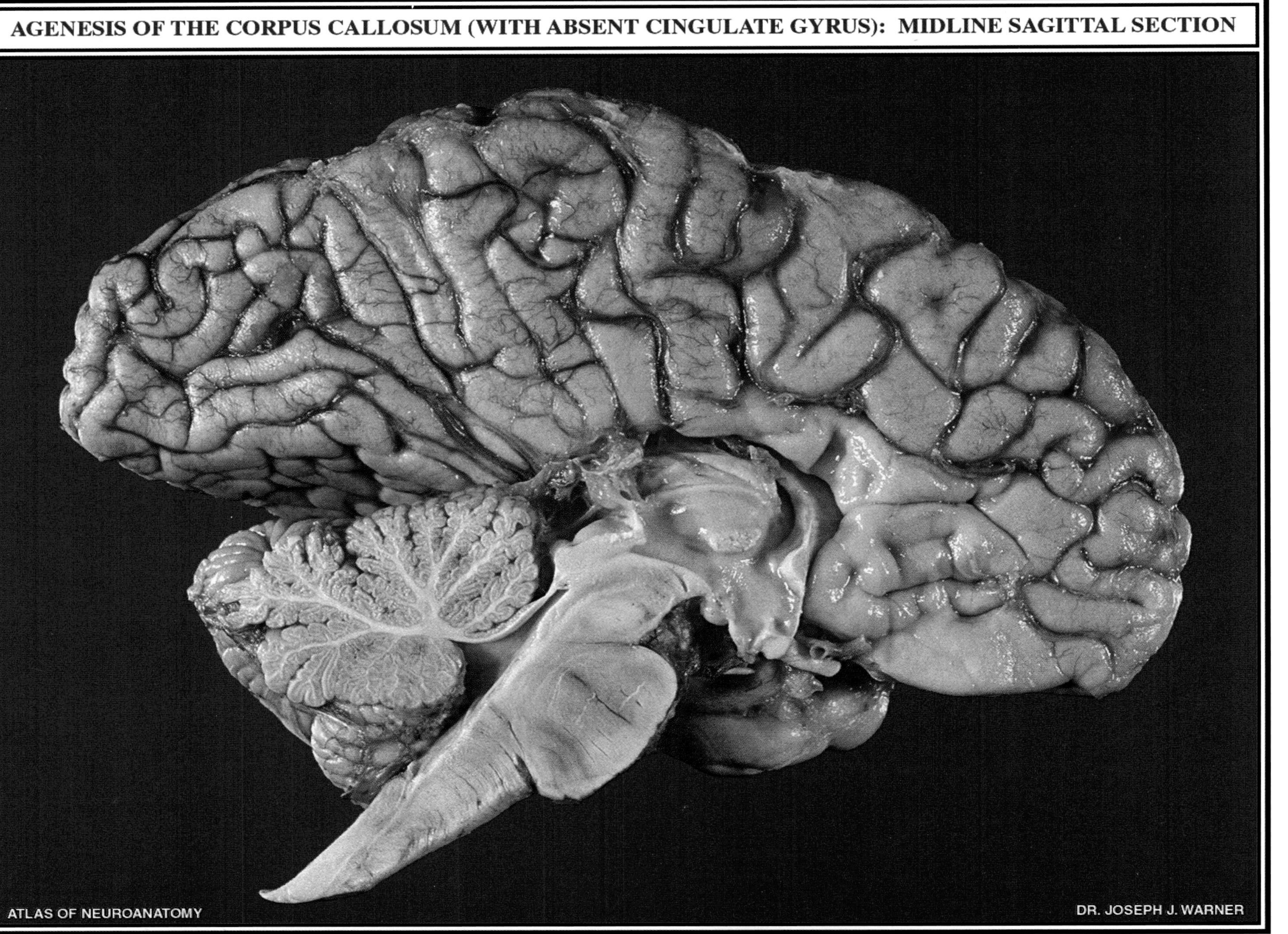

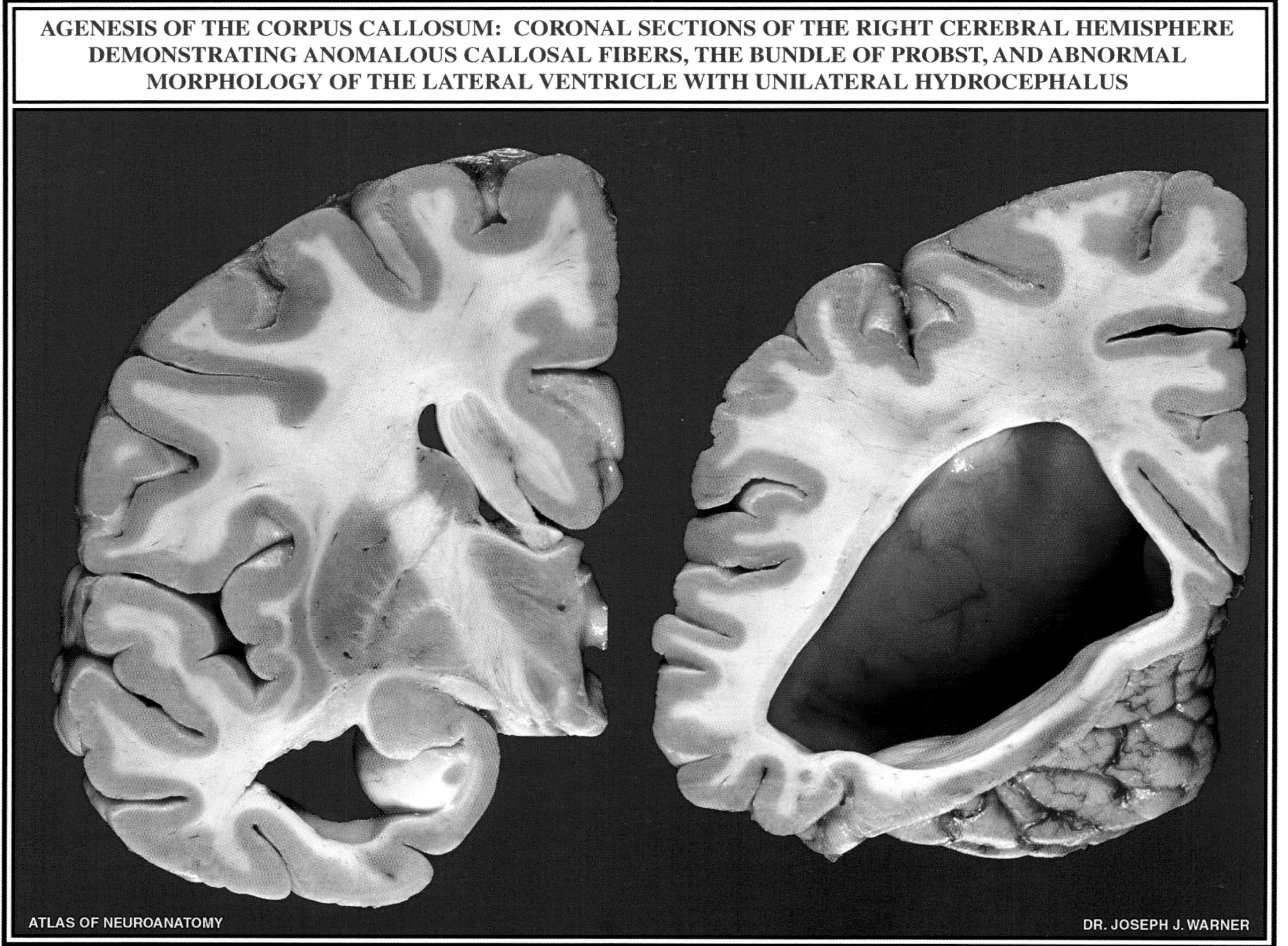

AGENESIS OF THE CORPUS CALLOSUM: CORONAL SECTIONS OF THE RIGHT CEREBRAL HEMISPHERE DEMONSTRATING ANOMALOUS CALLOSAL FIBERS, THE BUNDLE OF PROBST, AND ABNORMAL MORPHOLOGY OF THE LATERAL VENTRICLE WITH UNILATERAL HYDROCEPHALUS

AGENESIS OF THE CORPUS CALLOSUM: CORONAL SECTIONS OF THE RIGHT CEREBRAL HEMISPHERE DEMONSTRATING ANOMALOUS CALLOSAL FIBERS, THE BUNDLE OF PROBST, AND ABNORMAL MORPHOLOGY OF THE LATERAL VENTRICLE WITH UNILATERAL HYDROCEPHALUS

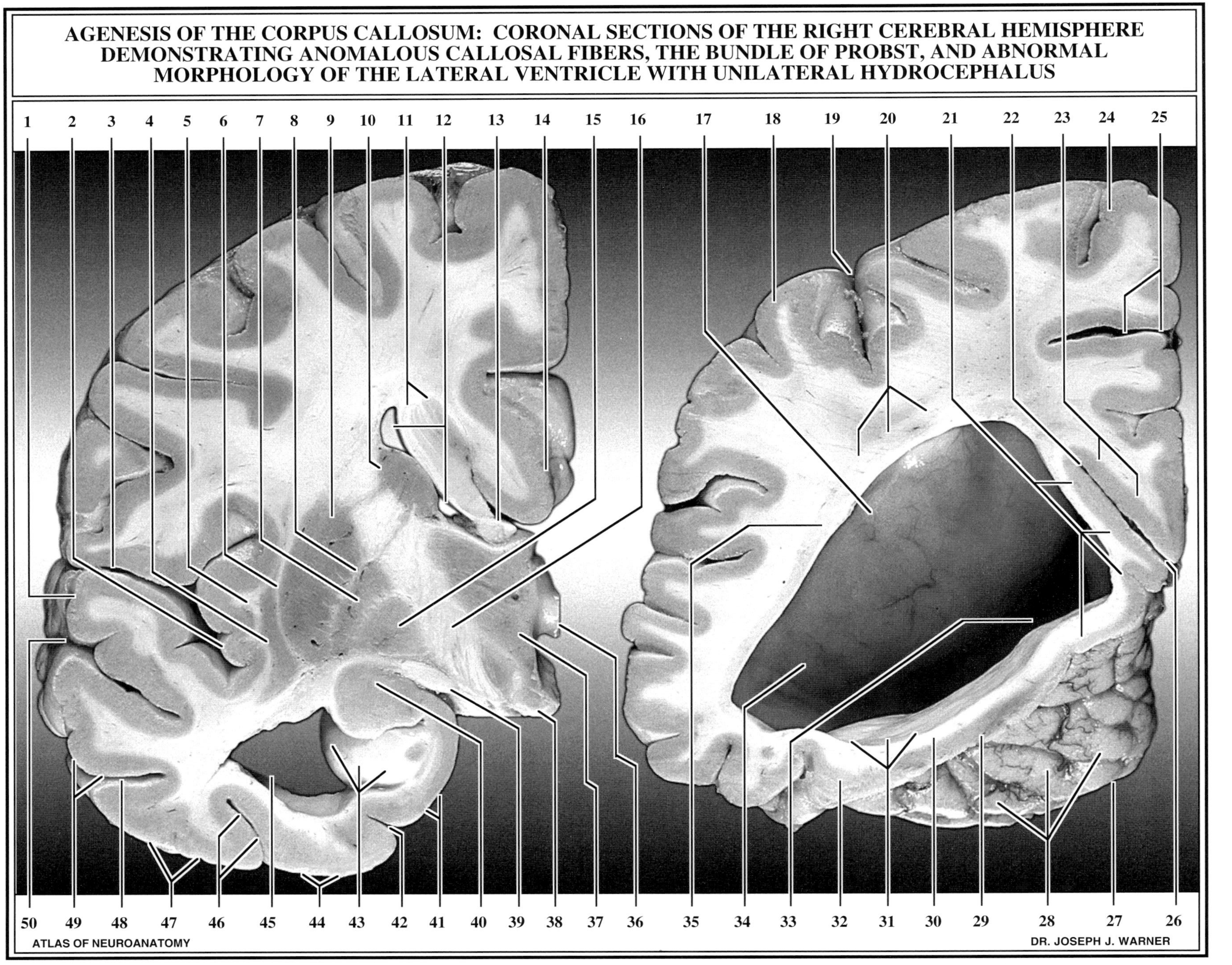

AGENESIS OF THE CORPUS CALLOSUM: CORONAL SECTIONS OF THE RIGHT CEREBRAL HEMISPHERE DEMONSTRATING ANOMALOUS CALLOSAL FIBERS, THE BUNDLE OF PROBST, AND ABNORMAL MORPHOLOGY OF THE LATERAL VENTRICLE WITH UNILATERAL HYDROCEPHALUS

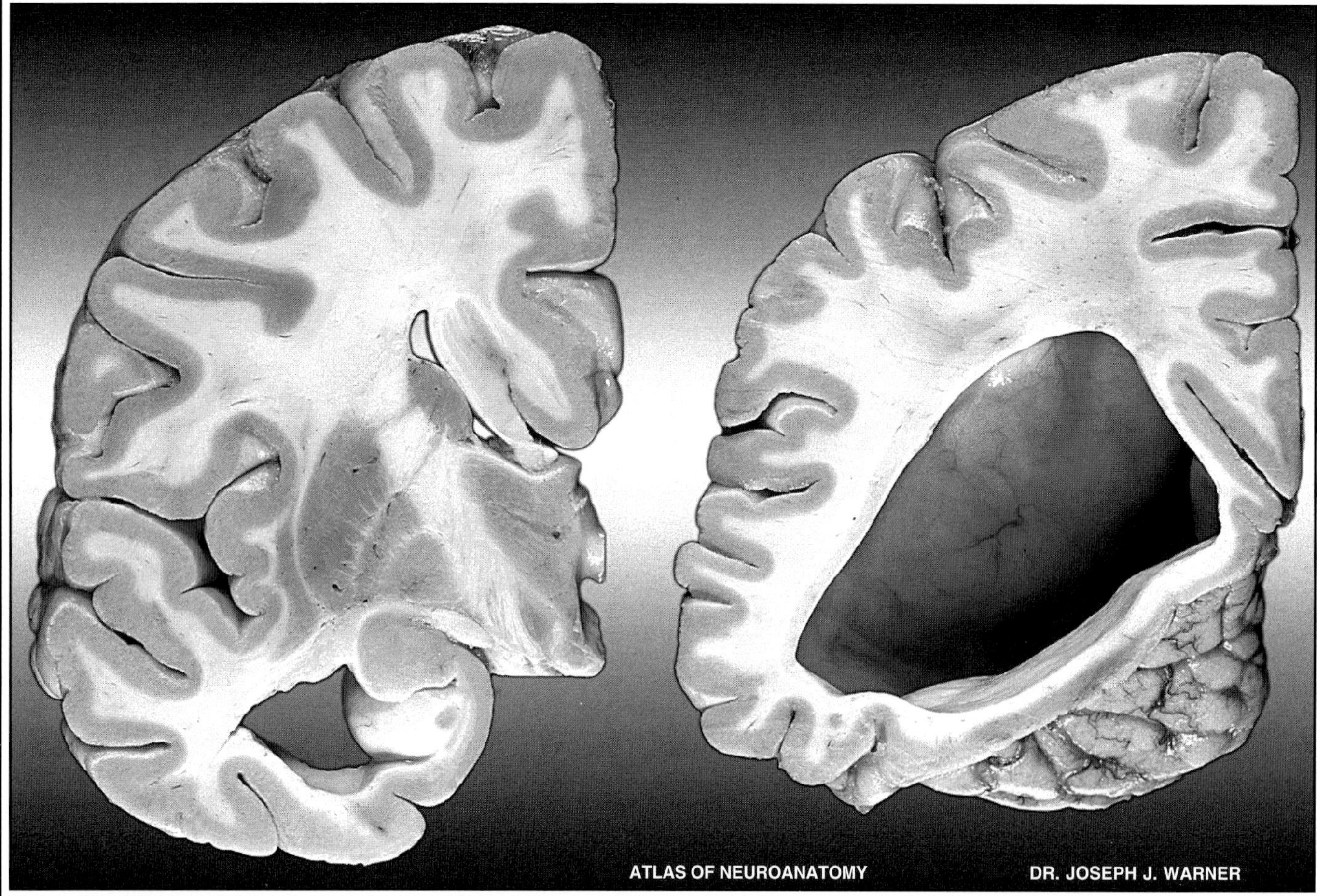

1. Superior Temporal Gyrus
2. Insular Cortex
3. Sylvian Fissure
4. Claustrum
5. Extreme Capsule
6. External Capsule
7. Globus Pallidus II
8. External Medullary Lamina
9. Putamen
10. Caudate Nucleus
11. Aberrant Callosal Fibers
12. Body of the Lateral Ventricle*
13. Bundle of Probst* and fibers of the Fornix
14. Radially oriented sulcus (Cingulate Gyrus not defined)
15. Globus Pallidus I
16. Posterior Limb of the Internal Capsule
17. Dorsolateral wall of the Occipital Horn of the Lateral Ventricle (thin mantle of cortex and white matter)
18. Inferior Parietal Lobule (caudal extent)
19. Interparietal Sulcus (caudal aspect)
20. Optic Radiations
21. Area 17 Striate Cortex
22. Calcarine Fissure
23. Area 17 Striate Cortex
24. Superior Parietal Lobule (caudal)
25. Parieto-Occipital Sulcus
26. Calcarine Fissure
27. Occipital Pole
28. Tentorial surface, Occipital Lobe
29. Inferior Occipitotemporal Cortex
30. Inferior Occipitotemporal White Matter
31. Floor of the Atrium of the Lateral Ventricle
32. Fusiform Gyrus
33. Occipital Horn of the Lateral Ventricle
34. Atrium of the Lateral Ventricle
35. Optic Radiations
36. Massa Intermedia
37. Thalamus
38. Mammillary Body
39. Optic Tract
40. Amygdala
41. Parahippocampal Gyrus
42. Collateral Sulcus
43. Hippocampal formation
44. Fusiform Gyrus
45. Temporal Horn of the Lateral Ventricle
46. Inferior Temporal Sulcus
47. Inferior Temporal Gyrus
48. Middle Temporal Sulcus
49. Middle Temporal Gyrus
50. Superior Temporal Sulcus

Fibers in the region of the corpus callosum course rostrocaudally as the Bundle of Probst. The steep angle of the roof of the lateral ventricle ("bat-wing configuration) is a characteristic radiologic feature of agenesis of the corpus callosum.

INDEX

V

W